D. K. C. Cooper · E. Kemp · J. L. Platt · D. J. G. White (Eds.)

Xenotransplantation

Springer

Berlin
Heidelberg
New York
Barcelona
Budapest
Hong Kong
London
Milan
Paris
Santa Clara
Singapore
Tokyo

D. K. C. Cooper · E. Kemp
J. L. Platt · D. J. G. White (Eds.)

Xenotransplantation

The Transplantation of Organs and Tissues Between Species

Second Edition
With 191 Figures, 12 in Color and 49 Tables

Springer

David K.C. Cooper, M.A., M.D., Ph.D., M.S., F.R.C.S.
Transplantation Biology Research Center,
Massachusetts General Hospital, Harvard Medical School,
Boston 02129, USA

Ejvind Kemp, M.D.
Department of Nephrology, Odense University Hospital,
5000 Odense, Denmark

Jeffrey L. Platt, M.D.
Departments of Surgery, Pediatrics and Immunology,
Duke University Medical Center, Durham, NC 27710, USA

David J.G. White, M.A., Ph.D., M.R.C.Path
Department of Surgery, University of Cambridge,
Cambridge CB22QQ, United Kingdom

ISBN-13: 978-3-642-64460-3 e-ISBN-13: 978-3-642-60572-7
DOI: 10.1007/978-3-642-60572-7

Library of Congress Cataloging-in-Publication Data
Xenotransplantation : the transplantation of organs and tissues between species / D. K. C. Cooper ... [et al.], (eds.). – – 2nd ed. p. cm. Includes bibliographical references and index.
1. Xenografts. 2. Transplantation of organs, tissues, etc. 3. Transplantation immunology. I. Cooper, D. K. C. (David K. C.), 1939– .
[DNLM: 1. Transplantation, Heterologous, WO 660 X52 1997] QR188.8.X46 1997 617.9'5– –dc21 DNLM/DLC for Library of Congress

Production: PRO EDIT GmbH, D-69126 Heidelberg
Cover design: design & production GmbH, D-69121 Heidelberg
Typesetting: Hermann Hagedorn GmbH, D-68519 Viernheim

SPIN: 10482034 27/3136-5 4 3 2 1 0 - Printed on acid-free paper

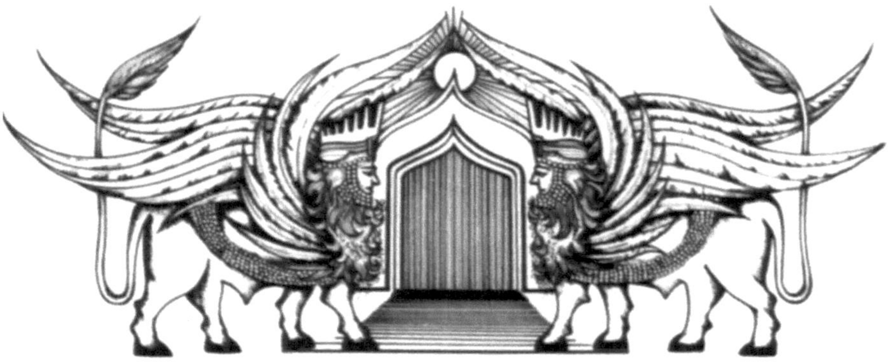

Frontispiece

The cover of this book depicts a Lamassu, one of the "fabulous" beasts of mythology. Like many similar creatures, it provides a highly successful example of xenotransplantation, having a human head set on an animal's body – sometimes that of a lion, but more often that of a bull – with wings that are believed to represent spiritual elevation. Its elegantly bearded head wears a headdress shaped like a crown, denoting the divine character of this "Great Winged Bull of Babylon." Lamassu were considered to be kindly figures, specifically acting as guardian divinities of cities.

Foreword

This is a time of excitement and progress in the field of xenotransplantation. The work described in this book traces the development of the science of cross-species transplantation, summarizes the current state of our knowledge, and focuses on approaches directed toward future clinical application.

The important question is not *whether* xenotransplantation will succeed, but rather *how* and *under what* circumstances xenografts will provide predictable enough results to warrant clinical application. The fact that the best results to date in clinical xenografting were achieved over three decades ago should not be a matter of discouragement, but rather a stimulus to apply new approaches to this area of work.

The shortage of human organs for transplantation is cited frequently as the driving force behind the increased interest in xenotransplantation. This shortage is an undeniable fact, but there are additional potential advantages of xenotransplantation, such as the ability to schedule replacement surgery on an elective basis and the modification of animals, organs, and tissues to improve acceptability in the human host.

The advances in the basic science of xenotransplantation outlined in this book give hope that the immunologic barriers to xenotransplantation will be overcome and that transplanted organs and tissues will succeed consistently in humans. However, if our experience with human allografts provides an analogy, we may anticipate that clinical progress in xenografts will be plagued by failures and rewarded by successes, often without a complete understanding of the mechanisms involved.

It is essential that clinical research in xenotransplantation be confined to carefully defined circumstances in which established treatments are not available and the risks, to the patients and others, are as clearly understood as possible. We may be assured that xenografts will be scrutinized by the scientific community and the public, and we must be certain that our efforts are perceived as appropriate exploration of new approaches to human illnesses.

The work described in this book gives reason for cautious optimism that we are approaching a new era in the replacement of organs, tissues, and cells in the treatment of human disease.

May, 1996

Keith Reemtsma
New York, USA

Preface

D.K.C. Cooper

Successful clinical xenotransplantation, together with immunological tolerance, has been one of the "holy grails" of transplant surgeons for most of the present century. Men of vision, such as Nobel laureate Alexis Carrel, saw its potential as early as 1907. Carrel was remarkably astute in his observations [1]:

> The organs of the anthropoid apes are perhaps able to tolerate human plasma. But nothing precise is known in that respect. Besides, anthropoid apes are very expensive, and difficult to handle. Their use would probably be impracticable. The ideal method would be to transplant on man organs of animals easy to secure and operate on, such as hogs, for instance. But it would in all probability be necessary to immunize organs of the hog against the human serum. The future of transplantation of organs for therapeutic purposes depends on the feasibility of hetero (xeno)transplantation.

This paragraph, written in the first decade of this century, could just have easily been written – with one or two refinements – within the past 5 years. Although we are not actually planning to "immunize" hog organs against human serum, Carrel's concept is not greatly different from the genetic engineering of donor pigs.

Since 1907, bursts of experimental and/or clinical activity have taken place at intervals, frequently accompanied by predictions that xenotransplantation would become a clinical option "within the foreseeable future." In the Introduction to the first edition of this volume, we drew attention to just such a prediction by no less an authority than Sir Peter Medawar, another Nobel laureate, who made the following remarks in 1969 [2]:

> A new solution is therefore called for: the use of heterografts – that is to say, of grafts transplanted from lower animals into man. Of the use of heterografts I can say only this: that in the laboratory we are achieving greater success with grafts *between* species today than we achieved with grafts *within* species 15 years ago. We shall solve the problem by using heterografts one day if we try hard enough, and maybe in less than 15 years.

His optimistic prediction – like so many – has unfortunately not been fulfilled, thus confirming the wisdom of the following pronouncement (which Keith Reemtsma attributes to a leading American politician): "Predictions are risky, especially about the future!"

No wonder that those with a more cynical outlook have said that "the future of transplantation is xenotransplantation, and always will be!"

Nevertheless, since the first edition of this volume was published in 1991, we do appear to have made some real progress in our understanding of the immunobiology of xenotransplantation and in developing potential therapeutic strategies that might overcome the considerable hurdles that face us. We therefore have reason for cautious optimism. However, as we have learned from past experience, progress in research is never as fast as we would wish; disappointments and setbacks will almost certainly confront us during the next few years. The ever-perceptive Sir Roy Calne perhaps accurately summarized our present position recently with his own prediction: "Clinical xenotransplantation is just around the corner, but it may be a very long corner!"

If we are successful, however, the rewards will be immense, and we shall have contributed to one of the greatest medical advances of the modern era. Unfortunately, until that time, there will always be those who question the need for xenotransplantation, and its feasibility and ethics. To those we can reply in the words of one of George Bernard Shaw's characters who, in the play *Back to Methuselah*, said,

"You see things: and you say 'why?'
Always 'why?'
But I dream things that never were:
And I say 'why not?'"

References

1. Carrel, A. The surgery of blood vessels, etc. Johns Hopkins Hosp. Bull. 18, 18, 1907
2. Medawar P. Quoted by Reemtsma, K. Heterotransplantation. Transplant. Proc. 1, 251, 1969

Acknowledgments. The editors owe a great debt of gratitude to Crystal Taylor, of CompOne Services Ltd., Oklahoma City, who has typed or retyped almost the entire manuscript and has done so with great efficiency and accuracy. Without her contribution, this work would have taken much longer to prepare.

The illustration used on the cover of this volume was drawn by Jenny Kukielski of Earls Colne in the United Kingdom, who also contributed that used on the cover of the first edition. We wish to express our appreciation to our many coauthors, who have generously contributed their knowledge, experience and time in making this volume available.

May 1996

David K.C. Cooper
Ejvind Kemp
Jeffrey Platt
David J.G. White

Contents

Contributing Authors

Abouna, G.M., M.D., M.S., F.R.C.S., F.R.C.S(C)
Professor and Chairman, Department of Surgery, and Dean, College of Medicine and Medical Sciences, Arabian Gulf University, Bahrain. Professor of Surgery, Hahnemann University, Philadelphia, Pennsylvania, USA

Andersson, A., M.D., Ph.D.
Professor of Diabetes Research, Department of Medical Cell Biology, Uppsala University, Uppsala, Sweden

Andreani, P., M.D.
Research Fellow, Institute of Experimental and Transplantation Surgery, University of Milan, Milan, Italy

Auchincloss, H. Jr., M.D.
Associate Professor of Surgery, Harvard Medical School, Massachusetts General Hospital, Boston, Massachusetts, USA

Aurell, M., M.D., Ph.D.
Professor, Institute of Internal Medicine, Department of Nephrology, Sahlgrenska University Hospital, University of Goteborg, Goteborg, Sweden

Aziz, S., M.D.
Associate Professor, Division of Cardiothoracic Surgery, Department of Surgery, University of Washington Medical Center, Seattle, Washington, USA

Bach, F.H., M.D.
Lewis Thomas Professor, AWD
Director, Sandoz Center for Immunobiology, New England Deaconess Hospital, Harvard Medical School, Boston, Massachusetts, USA

Bartlett, R.R., Ph.D.
Director, Immunopharmacology Laboratory, Hoechst AG, Wiesbaden, Germany

Bazin, H., D.V.M., Ph.D.
Professor and Head, Experimental Immunology Unit, Faculty of Medicine, University of Louvain, Brussels, Belgium

Besse, T., M.D.
Assistant, Experimental Surgery Unit, Faculty of Medicine, University of Louvain, Brussels, Belgium

Bjorck, S., M.D., Ph.D.
Assistant Professor, Institute of Internal Medicine, Department of Nephrology, Sahlgrenska University Hospital, University of Goteborg, Goteborg, Sweden

Brazelton, T.R., B.A.
Stanford Medical Scholar Recipient, Laboratory for Transplantation Immunology, Department of Cardiothoracic Surgery, Stanford University Medical Center, Stanford, California, USA

Breimer, M.E., M.D., Ph.D.
Assistant Professor, Institute of Surgical Sciences, Department of General Surgery, Sahlgrenska University Hospital, University of Goteborg, Goteborg, Sweden

Cairns, T.D.H., M.A., M.B., M.R.C.P.
Consultant Physician, Renal and Transplant Unit, St. Mary's Hospital, London, UK

Cardoso, J., M.D.
Surgeon, CRI INSERM, Laboratory for Surgical Research, Faculty of Medicine, Groupe Hospitalier Cochin, Paris, France

Carobbi, A., M.D.
Instructor in Surgery, University of Pisa, Pisa, Italy

Chapman, L.E., M.D., M.S.P.H.
Epidemiology Section Chief, Retrovirus Disease Branch, Division of AIDS, STD, and TB Laboratory Research, National Center for Infectious Diseases, Centers for Disease Control and Prevention, Atlanta, Georgia, USA

Cheung, A., M.D.
Cardiothoracic Surgery Fellow, Laboratory for Transplantation Immunology, Department of Cardiothoracic Surgery, Stanford University Medical Center, Stanford, California, USA

Chick, W.L., M.D.
President and Scientific Director, BioHybrid Technologies Inc., Shrewsbury, Massachusetts, USA

Cohney, S., M.B., B.S., F.R.A.C.P., M.R.C.P.
Postgraduate Research Student, Molecular Immunogenetics Laboratory, Austin Research Institute, Austin and Repatriation Medical Centre, University of Melbourne, Heidelberg, Melbourne, Victoria, Australia

Contreras, J., M.D.
Fellow in Transplantation, Department of Surgery, University of Alabama School of Medicine, Birmingham, Alabama, USA

Cooper, D.K.C., M.A., M.D., Ph.D., M.S., F.R.C.S.
Immunologist (Surgery), Transplantation Biology Research Center, Massachusetts General Hospital, Harvard Medical School, Boston, Massachusetts, USA, and Associate Member, Scientific Staff, Oklahoma Medical Research Foundation, Oklahoma City, Oklahoma, USA

Cormont, F., B.Sc.
Scientist and Research Associate, Experimental Immunology Unit, Faculty of Medicine, University of Louvain, Brussels, Belgium

Cozzi, E., M.D.
Clinical Research Associate, Department of Surgery, University of Cambridge, Cambridge, UK

Cramer, D.V., D.V.M., Ph.D.
Director, Transplantation Biology, St. Vincent Medical Center, Los Angeles, California, USA

Cummings, R.D., Ph.D.
Professor, Department of Biochemistry and Molecular Biology, University of Oklahoma Health Sciences Center, Oklahoma City, Oklahoma, USA

d'Apice, A.J.F., M.D., F.R.A.C.P., F.R.C.P.A.
Director, Immunology Research Centre, Department of Clinical Immunology, St. Vincent's Hospital, University of Melbourne, Fitzroy, Melbourne, Victoria, Australia

Dalmasso, A.P., M.D.
Professor, Department of Laboratory Medicine and Pathology, Veterans Affairs Medical Center and University of Minnesota Medical School, Minneapolis, Minnesota, USA

Demetris, A.J., M.D.
Associate Professor of Pathology and Director of Transplant Pathology, Pittsburgh Transplantation Institute, University of Pittsburgh Medical Center, Pittsburgh, Pennsylvania, USA

Dinsmore, J.H., Ph.D.
Director, Cell Transplantation Research, Diacrin Inc., Charlestown, Boston, Massachusetts, USA

Donato, M.F., M.D.
Assistant Director, Institute of Internal Medicine, Ospedale Maggiore-IRCCS, Milan, Italy

Doyle, H.R., M.D.
Assistant Professor of Surgery, University of Pittsburgh, and Staff Physician, Transplant Division, Veterans Administration Medical Center, Pittsburgh, Pennsylvania, USA

Fassati, L.R., M.D.
Associate Professor, Institute of Experimental and Transplantation Surgery, University of Milan, and Director, Liver Transplantation Center, Ospedale Maggiore-IRCCS, Milan, Italy

Faustman, D., M.D., Ph.D.
Director, Immunobiology Laboratory, Massachusetts General Hospital, Harvard Medical School, Boston, Massachusetts, USA

Ferran, C., M.D.
Research Fellow, Sandoz Center for Immunobiology, New England Deaconess Hospital, Harvard Medical School, Boston, Massachusetts, USA

Fishman, J.A., M.D.
Associate Physician and Assistant Professor of Medicine, Infectious Disease Unit, and Clinical Director, Transplantation Infectious Disease Unit, Massachusetts General Hospital, Harvard Medical School, Boston, Massachusetts, USA

Fodor, W., Ph.D.
Director of Xenotransplantation, Alexion Pharmaceuticals Inc., New Haven, Connecticut, USA

Frank, M.M., Ph.D.
Professor and Chairman, Department of Pediatrics, Duke University Medical School, Durham, North Carolina, USA

Fung, J.J., M.D.
Associate Professor of Surgery and Chief, Division of Transplant Surgery, Pittsburgh Transplantation Institute, University of Pittsburgh Medical Center, Pittsburgh, Pennsylvania, USA

Galili, U., Ph.D.
Professor, Department of Microbiology and Immunology, Medical College of Pennsylvania and Hahnemann University, Philadelphia, Pennsylvania, USA

Galmarini, D., M.D.
Research Fellow, Liver Transplantation Center, Ospedale Maggiore-IRCCS, Milan, Italy

Gammie, J.S., M.D.
Research Fellow, Division of Cellular Therapeutics, University of Pittsburgh, Pittsburgh, Pennsylvania, USA

Gatti, S., M.D., Ph.D.
Assistant Director, Liver Transplantation Center, Ospedale Maggiore-IRCCS, Milan, Italy

Gautreau, C., M.D.
Biologist, CRI INSERM, Blood Transfusion Institute, Hopital Cochin, Paris, France

George, J., Ph.D.
Assistant Professor, Department of Cardiothoracic Surgery, University of Alabama School of Medicine, Birmingham, Alabama, USA

Gianello, P., M.D., Ph.D.
Professor and Associate Head, Experimental Surgery Unit, Faculty of Medicine, University of Louvain, Brussels, Belgium

Goldberg, L.C., M.D., M.R.C.P.
Research Fellow, Renal and Transplant Unit, St. Mary's Hospital, London, UK

Goodman, D.J., M.D.
Research Fellow, Sandoz Center for Immunobiology, New England Deaconess Hospital, Harvard Medical School, Boston, Massachusetts, USA. Currently, Research Fellow, Immunology Research Centre, Department of Clinical Immunology, St. Vincent's Hospital, University of Melbourne, Fitzroy, Melbourne, Victoria, Australia

Gridelli, B., M.D.
Assistant Professor, Institute of Experimental and Transplantation Surgery, University of Milan, and Associate Director, Liver Transplantation Center, Ospedale Maggiore-IRCCS, Milan, Italy

Groth, C.G., M.D., Ph.D.
Professor of Transplantation Surgery, Department of Transplantation Surgery, Karolinska Institute at Huddinge Hospital, Huddinge, Sweden

Haisch, C., M.D.
Associate Professor, Department of Surgery, East Carolina University School of Medicine, Greenville, North Carolina, USA

Hammer, C., Dr.med.,Dr.med.vet.
Professor, Institute of Surgical Research, Klinikum Grosshadern, Ludwig-Maximilians-University of Munich, Munich, Germany

Hancock, W.W., M.B.B.S., Ph.D., F.R.C.P.A.
Associate Professor of Pathology, Harvard Medical School, and Department of Pathology, Sandoz Center for Immunobiology, New England Deaconess Hospital, Boston, Massachusetts, USA

Havaux, X., B.Sc.
Scientist and Research Associate, Experimental Immunology Unit, Faculty of Medicine, University of Louvain, Brussels, Belgium

Heiser, A., Dr.rer.nat.
Post-doctoral Research Scientist, Department of Immunology, Christian-Albrecht University of Kiel, Kiel, Germany

Hellerstrom, C., M.D., Ph.D.
Professor of Medical Cell Biology, Department of Medical Cell Biology, Uppsala University, Uppsala, Sweden

Holzknecht, Z.E., B.Sc.
Research Scientist, Department of Surgery, Duke University Medical Center, Durham, North Carolina, USA

Houssin, D., M.D.
Professor of Surgery, Laboratory for Surgical Research, Faculty of Medicine, Groupe Hospitalier Cochin, Paris, France

Hunt, B.J., M.R.C.P., M.R.C.Path.
Consultant and Honorary Senior Lecturer in Haematology, Guy's and St. Thomas' Trust, London, and Honorary Senior Lecturer in Cardiothoracic Surgery at the National Heart and Lung Institute, London, UK

Ildstad, S.T., M.D.
Director, Division of Cellular Therapeutics, University of Pittsburgh, Pittsburgh, Pennsylvania, USA

Inverardi, L., M.D.
Research Associate Professor of Medicine, Cell Transplantation Center, Diabetes Research Institute, University of Miami School of Medicine, Miami, Florida, USA

Itescu, S., M.D., F.R.A.C.P.
Director, Transplantation Immunology, Department of Surgery, Columbia-Presbyterian Medical Center, and Assistant Professor of Experimental Surgery and Pediatrics, Columbia University College of Physicians and Surgeons, New York, New York, USA

Jurd, K.M., B.Sc.(Hons), Ph.D.
Clinical Scientist, Department of Haematology, Guy's and St. Thomas' Trust, London, UK

Kemp, E., M.D.
Professor and Head, Department of Nephrology, Odense University Hospital, Odense, Denmark

Kobayashi, T., M.D.
Surgeon, Department of Surgery II, Nagoya University School of Medicine, Nagoya, Japan. Formerly, Clinical and Research Fellow, Oklahoma Transplantation Institute, Baptist Medical Center, Oklahoma City, Oklahoma, USA

Koren, E., M.D., Ph.D.
Senior Scientist, Genentech Inc., South San Francisco, California, USA. Formerly, Associate Member, Oklahoma Medical Research Foundation, Oklahoma City, Oklahoma, USA

Korsgren, O., M.D., Ph.D.
Assistant Professor of Medical Cell Biology, Department of Clinical Immunology and Transfusion Medicine, Uppsala University Hospital, Uppsala, Sweden

Kosanke, S.D., D.V.M., Ph.D.
Associate Professor, Department of Pathology, and Assistant Director, Division of Animal Resources, Oklahoma University Health Sciences Center, Oklahoma City, Oklahoma, USA

Langford, G.A., Ph.D.
Research Associate, Department of Surgery, University of Cambridge, Cambridge, UK

Lanza, R.P., M.D.
Director, Transplantation Biology, BioHybrid Technologies Inc., Shrewsbury, Massachusetts, USA

Larkin, E.W., M.D.
Associate Professor, Department of Pathology and Laboratory Medicine, East Carolina University School of Medicine, Greenville, North Carolina, USA

Larsen, S., M.D.
Professor and Head, Institute of Pathology, Herlev Hospital, University of Copenhagen, Herlev, Denmark

Latinne, D., M.D.
Associate Professor and Associate Head, Experimental Immunology Unit, Faculty of Medicine, University of Louvain, Brussels, Belgium

Lee, J., M.Sc.
Clinical Scientist, Renal and Transplant Unit, St. Mary's Hospital, London, UK

Leventhal, J.R., M.D.
Resident, Department of Surgery, University of Minnesota, Minneapolis, Minnesota, USA. Currently, Transplant Fellow, Division of Organ Transplantation, Department of Surgery, Northwestern University Medical School, Chicago, Illinois, USA

Li, S.F., M.D.
Research Fellow, Oklahoma Transplantation Institute, Baptist Medical Center, Oklahoma City, Oklahoma, USA

Lin, S.S., M.D.
Research Fellow, Departments of Surgery and Immunology, Duke University Medical Center, Durham, North Carolina, USA

Logan, J.S., Ph.D.
Vice-President of Research and Development, Nextran, Princeton, New Jersey, USA

Luo, Y., M.D., Ph.D.
Research Fellow, Oklahoma Transplantation Institute, Baptist Medical Center, Oklahoma City, Oklahoma, USA

Marchman, W., M.D.
Resident, Department of Surgery, East Carolina University School of Medicine, Greenville, North Carolina, USA

Marino, I.R., M.D.
Associate Professor of Surgery, Pittsburgh Transplantation Institute, University of Pittsburgh, and Associate Director, Transplant Division, Veterans Administration Medical Center, Pittsburgh, Pennsylvania, USA. Professore a contratto Università di Milano ed Università di Perugia, Italy. Director, European Medical Division, University of Pittsburgh Medical Center, Pittsburgh, Pennsylvania, USA

Marsh, H. Jr., Ph.D.
Senior Director of Immunobiology, T Cell Sciences Inc., Needham, Massachusetts, USA

Matis, L.A., M.D.
Vice-President, Research-Immunology, Alexion Pharmaceuticals Inc., New Haven, Connecticut, USA

McKenzie, I.F.C., M.D., Ph.D., F.R.A.C.P., F.R.C.P.A.
Professor and Director, Austin Research Institute, Austin and Repatriation Medical Centre, University of Melbourne, Heidelberg, Melbourne, Victoria, Australia

Michler, R.E., M.D.
Director, Cardiac Transplant Service, Columbia-Presbyterian Medical Center, Associate Professor of Surgery and Director, Cardiac Transplantation Research Laboratory, Department of Surgery, Columbia University College of Physicians and Surgeons, New York, New York, USA

Mieles, L., M.D.
Liver Transplant Surgeon, Children's Hospital, University of Pittsburgh, Pittsburgh, Pennsylvania, USA. Formerly, Chief, Abdominal Organ Transplantation Program, Oklahoma Transplantation Institute, Baptist Medical Center, Oklahoma City, Oklahoma, USA

Millan, M.T., M.D.
Research Fellow, Sandoz Center for Immunobiology, New England Deaconess Hosiptal, Harvard Medical School, Boston, Massachusetts, USA

Milotic, F., M.D.
Research Fellow, Oklahoma Medical Research Foundation, Oklahoma City, Oklahoma, USA. Currently, Staff Physician, Emergency Services, Rijeka Hospital, Rijeka, Croatia

Minanov, O.P., M.D.
Postdoctoral Research Fellow, Department of Surgery, Columbia University College of Physicians and Surgeons, New York, New York, USA

Möller, E., M.D., Ph.D.
Professor and Chairman, Department of Clinical Immunology, Karolinska Institute at Huddinge Hospital, Huddinge, Sweden

Morris, R.E., M.D.
Director of Transplantation Immunology and Research Professor, Department of Cardiothoracic Surgery, Stanford University Medical Center, Stanford, California, USA

Moses, R.D., M.D.
Assistant Professor of Surgery, Tufts University School of Medicine, St. Elizabeth's Medical Center, Boston, Massachusetts, USA

Murase, N., M.D.
Associate Professor of Surgery, Pittsburgh Transplantation Institute, University of Pittsburgh Medical Center, Pittsburgh, Pennsylvania, USA

Myburgh, J.A., M.B., Ch.M., F.R.C.S.
Professor Emeritus and Honorary Research Professorial Fellow, Department of Surgery, University of Witwatersrand, Parktown, Johannesburg, Transvaal, South Africa

Neethling, F.A., M.Med.Sci.
Postdoctoral Research Fellow, Transplantation Biology Research Center, Massachusetts General Hospital, Harvard Medical School, Boston, Massachusetts, USA. Formerly, Research Fellow, Oklahoma Transplantation Institute, Baptist Medical Center, Oklahoma City, Oklahoma, USA

Nisol, F.
Technician, Experimental Immunology Unit, Faculty of Medicine, University of Louvain, Brussels, Belgium

Norin, A.J., B.S., Ph.D.
Professor, Departments of Medicine and Anatomy and Cell Biology, and Director of the Transplantation Immunology and Immunogenetics Laboratory, SUNY Health Science Center at Brooklyn, Brooklyn, New York, USA

Nour, B., M.D.
Chief, Pediatric Liver Transplant Surgery, and Adult Liver Transplant Surgeon, Oklahoma Transplantation Institute, Baptist Medical Center, Oklahoma City, Oklahoma, USA

Oriol, R., M.D.
Medical Scientist, National Institute for Health and Medical Research (CRNS), INSERM, U178, Villejuif, France

Osman, N., Ph.D.
Research Fellow, Molecular Immunogenetics Laboratory, Austin Research Institute, Austin and Repatriation Medical Centre, University of Melbourne, Heidelberg, Melbourne, Victoria, Australia

Pardi, R., M.D.
Assistant Professor of Medicine, University of Milan School of Medicine, and Head, Human Immunology Unit, Scientific Institute San Raffaele-DIBIT, Milan, Italy

Parker, W.R., Ph.D.
Assistant Research Professor, Department of Surgery, Duke University Medical Center, Durham, North Carolona, USA

Pearse, M.J., B.Sc(Hons)., Ph.D.
Senior Scientist, Immunology Research Centre, Department of Clinical Immunology, St. Vincent's Hospital, University of Melbourne, Fitzroy, Melbourne, Victoria, Australia

Persing, D.H., M.D., Ph.D.
Director, Molecular Microbiology Laboratory, Divisions of Experimental Pathology and Clinical Microbiology, Department of Laboratory Medicine and Pathology, Mayo Clinic, Rochester, Minnesota, USA

Pierson, R.N. III, M.D.
Assistant Professor of Surgery, and Director, Heart and Lung Transplantation, Department of Cardiac and Thoracic Surgery, School of Medicine, Vanderbilt University, Nashville, Tennessee, USA

Pino-Chavez, G., M.D.
Research Fellow, Imutran Laboratories, and Department of Pathology, Papworth Hospital, Papworth Everard, Cambridge, UK

Pittman, K., B.S.
Research Technician, Department of Surgery, East Carolina University School of Medicine, Greenville, North Carolina, USA

Platt, J.L., M.D.
Joseph W. and Dorothy W. Beard Professor, Departments of Surgery, Pediatrics and Immunology, Duke University Medical Center, Durham, North Carolina, USA

Rao, A.S., M.D., D.Phil.
Associate Professor of Surgery and Pathology, and Director, Cellular Transplantation Laboratory, Pittsburgh Transplantation Institute, University of Pittsburgh Medical Center, Pittsburgh, Pennsylvania, USA

Rollins, S.A., Ph.D.
Director of Complement Biology, Alexion Pharmaceuticals Inc., New Haven, Connecticut, USA

Rose, A.G., M.D., F.R.C.Path.
Director, Jesse E. Edwards Registry of Cardiovascular Disease, St. Paul Heart and Lung Center, St. Paul, Minnesota, USA

Rose, M.L., Ph.D.
Reader in Transplant Immunology, Heart Science Centre, Harefield Hospital, Harefield, Middlesex, UK

Ryan, U.S., Ph.D.
President, Chief Operating Officer and Chief Scientific Officer, T Cell Sciences Inc., Needham, Massachusetts, USA

Rydberg, L., M.D., Ph.D.
Assistant Professor, Institute of Laboratory Medicine, Department of Clinical Chemistry and Transfusion Medicine, Sahlgrenska University Hospital, University of Goteborg, Goteborg, Sweden

Saadi, S., M.D., Ph.D.
Assistant Research Professor, Department of Surgery, Duke University Medical Center, Durham, North Carolina, USA

Sachs, D.H., M.D.
Paul S. Russell/Warner-Lambert Professor of Surgery (Immunology), and Director, Transplantation Biology Research Center, Massachusetts General Hospital, Harvard Medical School, Boston, Massachusetts, USA

Samuelsson, B.E., M.D., Ph.D.
Professor, Institute of Laboratory Medicine, Department of Clinical Chemistry and Transfusion Medicine, Sahlgrenska University Hospital, University of Goteborg, Goteborg, Sweden

Sandrin, M.S., Ph.D.
Principal Research Fellow and Head, Molecular Immunogenetics Laboratory, Austin Research Institute, Austin and Repatriation Medical Centre, University of Melbourne, Heidelberg, Melbourne, Victoria, Australia

Satake, M., M.D.
Research Fellow, Department of Clinical Immunology, Karolinska Institute at Huddinge Hospital, Huddinge, Sweden

Shah, A.S., M.D.
Postdoctoral Research Fellow, Department of Surgery, Columbia University College of Physicians and Surgeons, New York, New York, USA

Smit, J.A., D.Phil.
Principal Immunologist, Department of Surgery, University of Witwatersrand, Parktown, Johannesburg, Transvaal, South Africa

Soares, M., M.D.
Research Fellow, Experimental Immunology Unit, Faculty of Medicine, University of Louvain, Brussels, Belgium. Currently, Postdoctoral Fellow and Research Associate, Sandoz Center for Immunobiology, New England Deaconess Hospital, Harvard Medical School, Boston, Massachusetts, USA

Squinto, S.P., Ph.D.
Vice-President, Research-Molecular Sciences, Alexion Pharmaceuticals Inc., New Haven, Connecticut, USA

Stark, J.H., Ph.D.
Research Officer, Department of Surgery, University of Witwatersrand, Johannesburg, Transvaal, South Africa

Starklint, H., M.D.
Consultant, Institute of Pathology, Viejle Hospital, Viejle, Denmark

Starzl, T.E., M.D., Ph.D.
Distinguished Professor of Surgery and Director, Pittsburgh Transplantation Institute, University of Pittsburgh, and Director, Transplant Division, Veterans Administration Medical Center, Pittsburgh, Pennsylvania, USA

Suzuki, K., M.D.
Visiting Scientist, Division of Cardiothoracic Surgery, Department of Surgery, University of Washington Medical Center, Seattle, Washington, USA

Svalander, C.T., M.D., Ph.D.
Assistant Professor, Institute of Laboratory Medicine, Department of Pathology, Sahlgrenska University Hospital, University of Goteborg, Goteborg, Sweden

Sykes, M., M.D.
Associate Professor of Surgery (Immunology), Harvard Medical School, and Senior Investigator, Transplantation Biology Research Center, Massachusetts General Hospital, Boston, Massachusetts, USA

Tange, M.J., M.B., B.S., F.R.A.C.P.
Research Fellow, Immunology Research Centre, Department of Clinical Immunology, St. Vincent's Hospital, University of Melbourne, Fitzroy, Melbourne, Victoria, Australia

Taniguchi, S., M.D.
Surgeon, Division of Thoracic and Cardiovascular Surgery, Department of Surgery III, Nara Medical College, Nara, Japan. Formerly, Clinical and Research Fellow, Oklahoma Transplantation Institute, Baptist Medical Center, Oklahoma City, Oklahoma, USA

Taube, D.H., M.A., M.B., F.R.C.P.
Consultant Physician, Renal and Transplant Unit, St. Mary's Hospital, London, UK

Thomas, F.T., M.D.
Professor, Department of Surgery, University of Alabama School of Medicine, Birmingham, Alabama, USA

Thomas, J.M., M.D.
Professor and Director, Histocompatibility Laboratory, Department of Surgery, University of Alabama School of Medicine, Birmingham, Alabama, USA

Thorning, D., M.D.
Associate Professor of Pathology, University of Washington Medical Center, and Chief of Anatomic Pathology and Diagnostic Electron-microscopy, Veterans Affairs Puget Sound Health Care System, Seattle, Washington, USA

Tibell, A., M.D.
Staff Surgeon, Department of Transplantation Surgery, Karolinska Institute at Huddinge Hospital, Huddinge, Sweden

Ulrichs, K., Dr.rer.nat.
Professor, Experimental Transplantation Immunology Unit, Department of Surgery, Julius-Maximilian University of Wurzburg, Wurzburg, Germany

Valdivia, L.A., M.D., Ph.D.
Assistant Professor of Surgery, Pittsburgh Transplantation Institute, University of Pittsburgh Medical Center, Pittsburgh, Pennsylvania, USA

Wallwork, J., M.A., B.Sc., M.B., Ch.B., F.R.C.S(Ed).
Consultant Cardiothoracic Surgeon, and Director, Transplant Service, Papworth Hospital, Papworth Everard, Cambridge, UK

Wennberg, L., M.D.
Resident, Department of Transplantation Surgery, Karolinska Institute at Huddinge Hospital, Huddinge, Sweden

White, D.J.G., M.A., Ph.D., M.R.C.Path.
Immunologist and Lecturer, Department of Surgery, University of Cambridge, and Director of Research and Development, Imutran Laboratories, Cambridge, UK

Yannoutsos, N., Ph.D.
Research Associate, Department of Cell Biology, Erasmus University, Rotterdam, The Netherlands

I Introduction

1 Introduction

J.L. Platt, E. Kemp, and D.K.C. Cooper

Since the first edition of this book was published in 1991, the field of xenotransplantation has enjoyed a striking and gratifying rate of progress. This reflects in part the high level of enthusiasm among those in the field of transplantation for the idea that xenotransplantation may finally be approaching clinical application. This progress also reflects a change in the approach to inquiry in this field. The empirical approach, testing therapeutic agents singly or in combination for effects on graft survival, has been supplanted by attention to research design, focusing on the immunologic and other biological hurdles to xenotransplantation. Although this rapidly evolving field has not yet progressed to clinical reality, it would surprise none of us if this goal was soon achieved.

One important change is in our overall understanding of the mechanisms of hyperacute rejection and in the experimental models that reflect these mechanisms. It is now apparent that some of the classical models in xenotransplantation, such as the guinea pig-to-rat organ transplant and the pig-to-dog organ transplant, do not fully represent the immunological mechanisms which give rise to hyperacute rejection in primate recipients. The rejection of organs from pigs or other lower mammals by primates is now known to be initiated by the binding of xenoreactive antibodies to those organs, which leads to complement activation and an ensuing series of pathophysiologic events. In contrast, rejection in guinea pig-to-rat and pig-to-dog models may occur independently of antibody binding. Furthermore, the antibodies comprising the xenoreactive antibody repertoire in these lower animals differ substantially from the xenoreactive antibodies in humans.

While it might have been presumed that the antibody–antigen interactions that give rise to hyperacute rejection reflect many specificities in the xenograft donor, research in recent years has taught us the surprising lesson that practically all of the xenoreactive antibodies of importance in primates, including humans, are directed against Galα1–3Gal, a carbohydrate expressed on the vascular endothelium of New World monkeys and lower mammals but not by humans, apes and Old World monkeys. Not only is there one major epitope, but it now appears that the xenoreactive antibodies which recognize that epitope are more homogeneous than previously imagined. While much of the early work on these antibodies focused on IgG, it is now clear that the isotype which fixes complement and which is likely responsible for initiating hyperacute rejection consists largely of IgM.

Another area of striking progress has been in our understanding of how the complement system becomes involved in xenograft rejection. Some years ago it was hypothesized that a xenograft might be especially sensitive to complement because of the relative incompatibility of the complement regulatory proteins (such as decay accelerating factor and CD59) intrinsic to the xenograft with the complement system of the recipient. This idea has now been tested and proven correct. Thus the occurrence of hyperacute xenograft rejection in primate recipients depends on two factors: (1) the interaction of antibody with Galα1-3Gal, leading to activation of the complement cascade and (2) the heightened susceptibility of a xenograft to complement-mediated injury.

A further area of progress has been in our understanding of the cellular and molecular events which, triggered by the host's complement system or immune and inflammatory cells, cause injury to the xenograft. The pathological picture of xenograft rejection would appear to result from changes in the functioning of vascular endothelial cells in the graft, which include changes in the barrier, coagulant, and inflammatory properties of the endothelium.

It was once thought widely that hyperacute rejection is the major barrier to xenotransplantation. This view is rapidly being reconsidered as investigators have recently recognized that another type of rejection, variously termed "acute vascular xenograft rejection" or "delayed xenograft rejection," which arises in discordant xenografts when hyperacute rejection is averted, causes a second daunting hurdle. This type of rejection appears to be distinct from hyperacute rejection, not only in its time of onset but also in its pathogenesis. Whether it represents mainly an immunologic insult or an incompatibility of the graft to the host is not yet clear, nor is it clear whether this hurdle will be overcome in a clinically acceptable manner. However, some encouraging results have surfaced, suggesting that interfering with antibody-antigen interactions may overcome this problem also.

Until recently, the cellular immune response to a xenotransplant could only be estimated on the basis of in vitro studies, which have proved notoriously fickle in the prediction of alloimmune responses. However, the recent use of mutant mice with defined immune defects has clarified some aspects of the cellular immune response which might be relevant to xenotransplantation. Furthermore, a better understanding of the molecular events associated with T cell activation has allowed more critical inquiry into the likely mechanisms by which human T cells would become engaged and activated upon exposure to xenogeneic grafts or antigen presenting cells exposed to antigens from such grafts. In contrast to a previous theory held by some in this field, new evidence suggests that the cellular immune response may be as powerful, or even more powerful, than the cellular immune response to allotransplantation. In addition, the potential role of natural killer (NK) cells has emerged as an important area of study. That the cellular immune response to a xenotransplant may prove to be the major limiting factor to clinical application remains a possibility.

Some advances have emerged in part from advances in therapeutics. The use of specific inhibitors of the antibody-antigen interaction and of complement activation, and the application of transgenic techniques to this field have yielded many gains. Anti-αGal antibody can now be depleted from the plasma by the use of extracorporeal immunoadsorption using immunoaffinity columns of αGal oligosaccharides, a technique which significantly delays humoral xenograft rejection.

The concept of infusing specific oligosaccharides to "neutralize" or inhibit these antibodies in the circulation has been introduced. Complement depletion or inhibition by such agents as purified cobra venom factor or soluble complement receptor 1 similarly overcome hyperacute rejection, although not delayed vascular rejection.

The development of transgenic pigs expressing human complement regulatory proteins has made it possible not only to test the contribution of these proteins to the immunological hurdle to xenotransplantation, but has also provided a potent tool for interfering with complement-mediated injury while leaving host defenses intact. Similarly, the concepts of (a) preventing the synthesis of Galα1–3Gal by knockout techniques of genetic engineering or (b) competitively inhibiting its synthesis by the introduction of another glycosyltransferase, e.g., α1,2-fucosyltransferase, have been advanced, and there already exist genetically engineered animals in which the expression of Galα1–3Gal has been notably diminished by these approaches. Increasing interest in the cellular immune response to a xenotransplant has led to increasing interest in the development of approaches that may bring about immunological tolerance.

With the increasing awareness that clinical application of these therapeutic advances is drawing closer, awareness of the nonimmunologic problems facing us has been heightened. Concerns have been raised regarding the risks of transferring serious infection from donor animal to human host; to differentiate this type of disease transfer from the usual zoonosis, the terms "xenozoonosis" or "xenosis" have been suggested. Initial studies have been carried out to determine and minimize these risks, but more sophisticated research in this area is clearly required. Other concerns, such as the possibility of inducing malignant change from the transfer of endogenous retroviruses, may emerge as longer-term survival of xenografts is achieved. Likewise, comparative studies of human and donor species morphology and physiology may become a central issue, particularly with regard to donor organ function in the human metabolic environment.

Discussions regarding the "ethics" of xenotransplantation have been progressing for many years, but many of the questions raised relate to uncertainties in regard to the risks of infection, etc. This discussion will become greatly simplified as our knowledge of these matters expands.

What can we expect as the coming years unfold? A few groups have indicated that they are poised to carry out clinical xenotransplants using nonhuman primates as organ donors, though there is a growing feeling that these species will not resolve the problem of donor supply and that this is not the direction in which we should proceed. Tissue grafts from primates and lower species, such as the pig, for the treatment of various human diseases are also anticipated. Indeed, the application of xenogeneic cells and tissues for purposes other than organ replacement appears to be gaining ground, with exciting dimensions. Some protocols have already been approved by regulatory agencies, and early studies have been undertaken.

The overwhelming challenge, however, is the application of xenotransplantation as an approach to permanent organ replacement. While this may seem a distant prospect, the use of animal organs as "bridging" transplants may accelerate progress towards this end. Not only do xenogeneic cells, tissue, and organs offer the opportunity of an unlimited supply, they also offer the opportunity for genetic engineering. Indeed, it can be envisioned that xenotransplantation may become a far broader field than allotransplantation ever was.

We are surely participating in one of the great medical adventures of the modern era, which has the potential to revolutionize the treatment, not only of end-stage organ disease, but also of an increasing variety of other disease processes. Hopefully, before the time comes for the third edition of this volume to be prepared, we shall have seen the results of our research efforts successfully translated to the clinical arena.

II Immunobiology of Xenograft Rejection

2 Hyperacute Xenograft Rejection

J.L. Platt

Introduction

An organ from a donor of one species transplanted into a recipient of another species is subject to hyperacute xenograft rejection. Some combinations of donor and recipient species give rise almost invariably to hyperacute xenograft rejection; these combinations have been called "discordant" [1]. Some combinations of donor and recipient species are less apt to give rise to hyperacute xenograft rejection; these combinations have been called "concordant." Since in a given species combination, hyperacute xenograft rejection occurs nearly always or not at all, hyperacute xenograft rejection has been widely believed to have a genetic basis and to be a reflection of phylogenetic distance between the donor and the recipient [2–4]. During the past several years, the molecular basis for hyperacute xenograft rejection has been elucidated, at least in part, and thus it has become possible to define the mechanisms of susceptibility to rejection without resorting to the imprecision of a phylogenetic classification. The sections that follow will summarize the mechanisms contributing to the susceptibility to hyperacute xenograft rejection and how these mechanisms contribute to the devastating pathological changes characteristic of that lesion.

Mechanisms of Susceptibility to Hyperacute Xenograft Rejection

The development of hyperacute rejection depends absolutely on the activation of complement. In every experimental model studied thus far, activation of complement is detected when hyperacute rejection is observed and if activation of complement is inhibited, hyperacute rejection does not occur. Thus, in considering the immunology of hyperacute rejection, the mechanism(s) by which the complement system become activated is a central issue.

On a theoretical basis, there are three mechanisms which might account for the activation of complement in a xenograft and thus to the initiation of hyperacute xenograft rejection (Fig. 1).

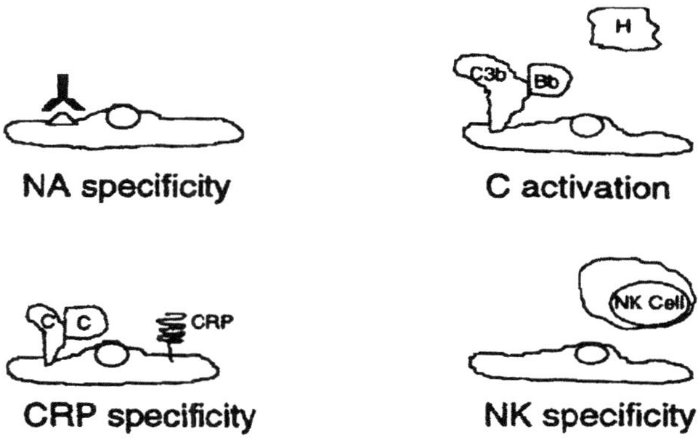

Fig. 1. Mechanisms of initiation of hyperacute xenograft rejection. Activation of complement (*C*) is a critical step in the development of hyperacute acute rejection. Complement motivation may be initiated by the binding of xenoreactive antibodies (*XA*) (*upper left*) or by the spontaneous formation of C3bBb complexes due in part to failure of factor H to control complex formation on heterologous surfaces (*upper right*) and/or by direct activation on donor cells. Complement activation is likely amplied because complement regulatory proteins (*CRP*) in the donor organ fail to control the reactions adequately. In addition, tissue injury might be mediated by natural killer (*NK*) cells

Activation of the Classical Complement Pathway

The classic concept has been that the rejection of a xenogeneic organ is initiated by xenoreactive antibodies which, binding the corresponding antigens in the organ transplant, activate complement. This mechanism clearly predominates in pig-to-primate xenografts. The essential role of xenoreactive antibodies in initiating hyperacute rejection in pig-to-primate organ xenografts is suggested by the following observations:

1. Tissue samples from organs undergoing hyperacute rejection invariably contain immunoglobulin of the recipient codeposited with components of the classical complement pathway along the endothelial lining of blood vessels but only focal deposits of alternative pathway components [5–7].
2. Depletion of xenoreactive antibodies from a xenograft recipient prolongs graft survival, even when the complement system of the recipient remains intact [7–9].
3. Transplantation of a porcine organ into a newborn baboon which lacks xenoreactive antibodies but which has an intact complement system does not result in hyperacute rejection [10].

Among the recent advances in understanding the pathogenesis of hyperacute xenograft rejection is the discovery that human xenoreactive antibodies recognize predominantly Galα1–3Gal [11], a sugar first described by Eckhardt [12]. The phylogenetic expression of this sugar and of natural IgG antibodies specific for it were elucidated by Galili [13]. Galα1–3Gal is synthesized by lower mammals and New World monkeys, which express a functional α1,3-galactosyltransferase gene, but not by humans, apes and Old World monkeys, which have instead two pseudogenes [14, 15]. The enzyme α1,3-galactosyltransferase adds galactose via an α-linkage to Galβ1–4GlcNAc-R to yield Galα1–3Galβ1–4GlcNAc-R. Animals which do not express α1,3-galactosyltransferase have naturally occurring antibodies against Galα1–3Gal [14, 16]. Based on this phylogenetic relationship, Good et al. tested the ability of Galα1–3Gal versus other sugars to block binding of natural antibodies to porcine cells [11]. High concentrations (m*M*) of α-galactosyl sugars did in fact block the binding of human natural antibodies, whereas other sugars did not [11]. Consistent with the potential importance of this epitope, Sandrin et al. showed that transfection of COS cells with cDNA for α1,3-galactosyltransferase causes de novo expression of Galα1–3Gal and confers sensitivity to lysis by xenoreactive antibodies and complement [17]. Collins with the author demonstrated that elimination of the sugar from porcine cells would render the cells resistant to human xenoreactive antibodies [18]. Collins also used the phylogeny of expression of Galα1–3Gal and of antibodies specific for it to demonstrate the importance of this sugar in a xenotransplantation model [19]. All of these studies, thus suggest that to the extent that expression of Galα1–3Gal distinguishes two species, that difference and not phylogenetic distance per se is sufficient to confer susceptibility to hyperacute rejection. This is not to say that phylogeny is entirely unimportant, as it will be seen presently that susceptibility to complement mediated tissue injury is dictated by factors altogether different from antigen expression.

The antibodies responsible for provoking hyperacute rejection in pig-to-primate xenografts are for the most part IgM. Xenoreactive IgM bound to porcine endothelial cells activates complement [9, 20–22], whereas xenoreactive IgG does not [23]. These xenoreactive IgM are very much like isohemagglutinins in their functions and concentrations in the plasma [24]. Given the similarity between xenoreactive antibodies and isohemagglutinins and the similar densities of the corresponding antigens on endothelial cell surfaces, Parker has suggested that the experience of ABO-incompatible organ transplantation may be relevant for understanding xenotransplantation, the main difference being the presence in the allograft complement regulatory proteins effective against the recipient's complement but not in the xenograft [24].

Activation of the Alternative Complement Pathway

A second mechanism which might contribute to hyperacute xenograft rejection involves the activation of the complement system of the recipient via the alternative pathway on the donor organ, independently of antibody binding. The basis for this mechanism, in most cases, is the failure of factor H in the recipient's plasma to control assembly of the alternative pathway C3 convertase. In some instances, binding of xenoreactive IgG or IgA to a foreign surface might impair the interaction of that surface with factor H, contributing to same mechanism. Activation of the alternative pathway initiates hyperacute rejection of guinea pig-to-rat and rabbit-to-newborn pig xenografts and probably also in pig-to-dog xenografts [25–27]. Hyperacute rejection in these species combinations is particularly rapid and violent, and thus it is fortunate that this mechanism does not prevail in pig-to-primate xenografts. That is not to say that the alternative pathway of complement is not activated in pig-to-primate transplants, as it surely is; rather, in this case the activation of the alternative pathway is dependent on classical pathway activation, which in turn depends on antibody binding. Nor does the utilization of the alternative complement pathway as a primary mechanism of complement activation exclude a contribution of the classical pathway; in guinea pig to rat xenografts, there is good evidence for the existence of complement-fixing xenoreactive antibodies [27].

Species-Restricted Functioning of Complement Regulatory Proteins

A third mechanism which may contribute to the susceptibility to hyperacute xenograft rejection is the species-restricted functioning of cell-associated complement regulatory proteins. Several years ago, Dalmasso [4, 28] and Miyagawa [25] proposed that a xenograft might be especially susceptible to complement-mediated injury because cell membrane-associated complement regulatory proteins, such as decay accelerating factor and CD59, which protect the organ against inadvertent injury by homologous complement under physiologic conditions, might fail to control activation of heterologous complement. Based on that concept, White [29], Fodor et al. [30], and the author and colleagues [31] developed transgenic animals expressing human complement regulatory proteins, anticipating that the organs of such animals would resist injury by heterologous complement. Our recent experiments involving transplantation of organs from transgenic pigs expressing human complement regulatory proteins (decay-accelerating factor and CD59) at low levels into nonhuman primates, tested this idea [32, 33]. In most cases hyperacute rejection did not occur, demonstrating that complement regulation is indeed an important element of the susceptibility to hyperacute rejection of porcine organs by primates. Thus in pig-to-primate xenografts, discordance can be viewed as a consequence of the expression of Galα1–3Gal and the functional limitations of complement regulatory proteins in the donor and the presence of anti-Galα1–3Gal antibodies and "heterologous" complement in the recipient. The reader is referred elsewhere in this volume for further discussion of this subject.

Potential Roles of Natural Killer Cells and Antibody-Dependent Cell-Mediated Cytotoxicity

In addition to the importance of complement in hyperacute rejection, there has been interest in the possibility that natural killer (NK) cells or the mononuclear cells that mediate antibody-dependent cell-mediated cytotoxicity (ADCC) might mediate or contribute to the destruction of a discordant xenograft. This interest has been stimulated in part by Inverardi's finding that NK cells accumulate in organs perfused by xenogeneic blood and that xenoreactive IgG antibodies promote the accumulation of these cells [34]. The possibility that NK cells might contribute to tissue injury is supported on theoretical grounds by observations that these cells express receptors for major histocompatibility complex (MHC) class I antigens and under physiologic conditions the receptors deliver inhibitory signals. Presumably these MHC receptors do not recognize xenogeneic MHC molecules accounting for susceptibility to cell mediated injury. Also in favor of this idea is the observation that natural killer cells or cells mediating ADCC have immunoregulatory Fc receptors.

On the other hand, there are some important arguments against a role for NK cells. First there are no reports describing large numbers of NK cells in hyperacute rejection and there are a number of reports in which very few infiltrating cells of any type are seen. Second, the importance of NK cells in hyperacute rejection is not supported by the dramatic effects of complement inhibitors in preventing tissue injury. Finally, recent work by Magee and the authors showed that the administration of γ-globulin to primates actually prevents hyperacute rejection [23], while one might expect that this agent would enhance NK cell-mediated injury. Thus, if NK cells are important in the pathogenesis of xenograft rejection, it is probably in acute vascular xenograft rejection, rather than in hyperacute rejection.

Pathogenesis of Hyperacute Xenograft Rejection

The pathological hallmarks of hyperacute rejection include hemorrhage, widespread thrombosis, particularly involving platelets, and ischemia [7, 35]. These changes, seen within minutes of the reperfusion of a xenograft, are followed in some cases by the focal influx of neutrophils and formation of fibrin thrombi. This pathological picture, together with the immunopathology revealing deposits of antibody and complement along graft endothelium, suggest the lesions of hyperacute rejection might be brought about by global dysfunction of endothelial cells [4, 20, 36]. The question then is how activation of complement along the blood vessels of a xenograft might cause such rapid and profound changes in endothelial function.

One mechanism for the pathogenesis of hyperacute rejection might involve complement-mediated lysis of endothelial cells. The lysis of some endothelial cells would lead to the disruption of the integrity of blood vessels, loss of vascular contents and exposure of platelets to underlying matrix leading to platelet adhesion, aggregation and activation and local vasoconstriction due to loss of nitric oxide. Consistent with this possibility are recent studies showing that hyperacute rejection does not occur in C6-deficient recipients and thus presumably requires assembly of terminal complement complexes [37]. On the other hand, examination of tissue samples obtained shortly after reperfusion of xenografts, when hyperacute rejection is beginning, does not reveal widespread lysis of endothelial cells; in fact, lysis is not regularly seen until very late in the course of rejection. Thus noncytotoxic lesions are probably sufficient to cause rejection in many cases.

The author and coworkers have investigated complement-mediated changes in the function and structure of endothelial cells which might account for the pathogenesis of hyperacute rejection. As a working model, Saadi has suggested that hyperacute rejection might in fact reflect a loss of endothelial functions [36]. One potential mechanism involves the loss of heparan sulfate from endothelial cells [20]. Heparan sulfate is a protein-polysaccharide glycoconjugate which supports many endothelial functions including the barrier to cells and plasma proteins, anticoagulation, and protection from oxidants and complement [38]. A substantial amount of heparan sulfate is lost from endothelial cells within minutes of exposure to anti-endothelial cell antibodies and complement [39]. This process also occurs in vivo at a tempo that could account for some of the alteration in vascular function observed in hyperacute rejection [40].

Another mechanism by which endothelial function might be lost may involve a change in endothelial cell shape which eventuates in the formation of intercellular gaps [41]. The gaps which are formed in response to C5b67 complexes and accelerated by the membrane attack complex may explain the loss of vascular integrity and the tendency of platelets to accumulate along the junctions between endothelial cells.

The binding of natural antibodies, activation of complement or the secreted products of platelets might cause the expression of P selectin and von Willebrand factor on the endothelial cell surface [42, 43]. These changes would likely promote platelet and neutrophil adhesion and coagulation altering the coagulant posture of endothelium. The direct interaction of xenoreactive antibodies with carbohydrate epitopes on endothelial cell integrins and von Willebrand factor [22] might also affect endothelial cell functions.

Comment

Hyperacute rejection is, arguably, the most explosive and destructive type of immunologic injury. Much progress has been made in understanding the immune basis for this condition and in developing effective therapies to overcome it. The extent of this progress is reflected by the prevailing view of the immunological hurdles to xenotransplantation – while hyperacute rejection was once viewed as the major hurdle to xenotransplantation, it is no longer viewed as such by many in this field. There are now therapeutic strategies in hand that can prevent hyperacute rejection in the majority of cases and which in combination may eliminate the risk of this devastating process. Moreover, while even the smallest risk of hyperacute rejection is usually considered a contradiction to conducting a clinical allotransplant, this same risk may be less important in xenotransplantation. Allotransplants which might lead to hyperacute rejection are contraindicated in part because human organs are in short supply and as a result there is the tendency to commit organs to recipients whose risk of rejecting the organ is lowest rather than to those in greater need. Were the supply of organs unlimited, the decisions for or against transplantation could be based on the best interests of the patient.

Acknowledgments. Work in the author's laboratory summarized in this chapter was supported by grants from the National Institutes of Health (HL52297,HL50985,HL46810) and Nextran, Princeton, NJ, USA.

References

1. Calne, R.Y. Organ transplantation beween widely disparate species. Transplant. Proc. 2, 550, 1970
2. Perper, R.J.Najarian, J.S. Experimental renal heterotransplantation. I. In widely divergent species. Transplantation 4, 377, 1966
3. Hammer, C., Suckfull, M.Saumweber, D. Evolutionary and immunological aspects of xenotransplantation. Transplant. Proc. 24, 2397, 1992
4. Platt, J.L., Vercellotti, G.M., Dalmasso, A.P., et al. Transplantation of discordant xenografts: a review of progress. Immunol.Today 11, 450, 1990
5. Rose, A.G., Cooper, D.K.C., Human, P.A., Reichenspurner, H.Reichart, B. Histopathology of hyperacute rejection of the heart: experimental and clinical observations in allografts and xenografts. J.Heart Lung Transplant. 10, 223, 1991
6. Alexandre, G.P.J., Gianello, P., Latinne, D., et al. Plasmapheresis and splenectomy in experimental renal xenotransplantation. In edited by Hardy, M.A. (Ed.) Xenograft 25. Elsevier Science Publishers, New York, NY, 1989, p. 259
7. Platt, J.L., Fischel, R.J., Matas, A.J., et al. Immunopathology of hyperacute xenograft rejection in a swine-to-primate model. Transplantation 52, 214, 1991
8. Cooper, D.K.C., Human, P.A., Lexer, G., et al. Effects of cyclosporine and antibody adsorption on pig cardiac xenograft survival in the baboon. J.Heart Transplant. 7, 238, 1988
9. Dalmasso, A.P., Vercellotti, G.M., Fischel, R.J., et al. Mechanism of complement activation in the hyperacute rejection of porcine organs transplanted into primate recipients. Am.J.Pathol. 140, 1157, 1992
10. Kaplon, R.J., Michler, R.E., Xu, H., et al. Absence of hyperacute rejection in newborn pig-to-baboon cardiac xenografts. Transplantation 59, 1, 1994
11. Good, A.H., Cooper, D.K.C., Malcolm, A.J., et al. Identification of carbohydrate structures that bind human antiporcine antibodies: implications for discordant xenografting in humans. Transplant. Proc. 24, 559, 1992
12. Eckhardt, A.E.Goldstein, I.J. Isolation and characterization of a family of α-D-galactosyl-containing glycopeptides from Ehrlich ascites tumor cells. Biochem. 22, 5290, 1983
13. Galili, U., Macher, B.A., Buehler, J.Shohet, S.B. Human natural anti-α-galactosyl IgG: the specific recognition of α(1–3)-linked glactose residues. J.Exp.Med. 162, 573, 1985
14. Galili, U., Clark, M.R., Shohet, S.B., Buehler, J.Macher, B.A. Evolutionary relationship between the natural anti-Gal antibody and the Galα1–3Gal epitope in primates. Proc.-Natl.Acad.Sci.USA 84, 1369, 1987
15. Galili, U.Swanson, K. Gene sequences suggest inactivation of α-1, 3-galactosyltransferase in catarrhines after the divergence of apes from monkeys. Proc.Natl.Acad.Sci.USA 88, 7401, 1991
16. Galili, U., Shohet, S.B., Kobrin, E., Stults, C.L.M.Macher, B.A. Man, apes, and old world monkeys differ from other mammals in the expression of α-Galactosyl epitopes on nucleated cells. J.Biol.Chem. 263, 17755, 1988
17. Sandrin, M.S., Vaughan, H.A., Dabkowski, P.L.McKenzie, I.F.C. Anti-pig IgM antibodies in human serum react predominantly with Galα(1,3)Gal epitopes. Proc.Natl.Acad.S-ci.USA 90, 11391, 1993
18. Collins, B.H., Parker, W.R.Platt, J.L. Characterization of porcine endothelial cell determinants recognized by human natural antibodies. Xenotransplantation 1, 36, 1994

19. Collins, B.H., Cotterell, A.H., McCurry, K.R., et al. Hyperacute rejection of cardiac xenografts between primate species: evidence to support the significance of the α-Galactosyl determinant. J.Immunol. 154, 5500, 1995
20. Platt, J.L., Vercellotti, G.M., Lindman, B.J., et al. Release of heparan sulfate from endothelial cells: Implications for pathogenesis of hyperacute rejection. J.Exp.Med. 171, 1363, 1990
21. Parker, W.R., Bruno, D., Holzknecht, Z.E.Platt, J.L. Xenoreactive natural antibodies: isolation and initial characterization. J.Immunol. 153, 3791, 1994
22. Holzknecht, Z.E.Platt, J.L. Identification of porcine endothelial cell membrane antigens recognized by human xenoreactive antibodies. J.Immunol. 154, 4565, 1995
23. Magee, J.C., Collins, B.H., Harland, R.C., et al. Immunoglobulin prevents complement mediated hyperacute rejection in swine-to-primate xenotransplantation. J.Clin.Invest. 96, 2404, 1995
24. Parker, W., Lundberg-Swanson, K.L., Holzknecht, Z.E., et al. Isohemagglutinins and xenoreactive antibodies: members of a distinct family of natural antibodies. Hum.Immunol. 45, 94, 1996
25. Miyagawa, S., Hirose, H., Shirakura, R., et al. The mechanism of discordant xenograft rejection. Transplantation 46, 825, 1988
26. Johnston, P.S., Wang, M.-W., Lim, S.M.L., Wright, L.J.White, D.J.G. Discordant xenograft rejection in an antibody-free model. Transplantation 54, 573, 1992
27. Leventhal, J.R., Matas, A.J., Sun, L.H., et al. The immunopathology of cardiac xenograft rejection in the guinea pig to rat model. Transplantation 56, 1, 1993
28. Dalmasso, A.P., Vercellotti, G.M., Platt, J.L.Bach, F.H. Inhibition of complement-mediated endothelial cell cytotoxicity by decay accelerating factor: Potential for prevention of xenograft hyperacute rejection. Transplantation 52, 530, 1991
29. White, D.Wallwork, J. Xenografting: probability, possibility, or pipe dream? Lancet 342, 879, 1993
30. Fodor, W.L., Williams, B.L., Matis, L.A., et al. Expression of a functional human complement inhibitor in a transgenic pig as a model for the prevention of xenogeneic hyperacute organ rejection. Proc.Natl.Acad.Sci.USA 91, 11153, 1994
31. Platt, J.L.Logan, J.S. Use of transgenic animals in xenotransplantation. Transplantation Reviews 10, 69, 1996
32. McCurry, K.R., Kooyman, D.L., Alvarado, C.G., et al. Human complement regulatory proteins protect swine-to-primate cadriac xenografts from humoral injury. Nature Med 1, 423, 1995
33. Byrne, G.W., McCurry, K.R., Martin, M.J., et al. Expression of human CD59 and DAF in transgenic pigs: intrinsic regulation of complement activity. Transplantation, In Press
34. Inverardi, L., Samaja, M., Motterlini, R., et al. Early recognition of a discordant xenogeneic organ by human circulating lymphocytes. J.Immunol. 149, 1416, 1992
35. Platt, J.L. Hyperacute Xenograft Rejection. R.G. Landes Company, Austin, 1995,
36. Saadi, S., Ihrcke, N.S. and Platt, J.L. Pathophysiology of xenograft rejection. In Lieberman, R., Morris, R. (eds.) Principles of Immunomodulatory Drug Development in Transplantation and Autoimmunity. Raven Press, New York, NY, 1995.
37. Brauer, R.B., Baldwin III, W.M., Daha, M.R., Pruitt, S.K.Sanfilippo, F. Use of C6-deficient rats to evaluate the mechanism of hyperacute rejection of discordant cardiac xenografts. J.Immunol. 151, 7240, 1993

38. Ihrcke, N.S., Wrenshall, L.E., Lindman, B.J.Platt, J.L. Role of heparan sulfate in immune system-blood vessel interactions. Immunol.Today 14, 500, 1993
39. Ihrcke, N.S.Platt, J.L. Shedding of heparan sulfate proteoglycan by stimulated endothelial cells: evidence for proteolysis of cell surface molecules, J. Cell Physiol 168, 625, 1996
40. Stevens, R.B., Wang, Y.L., Kaji, H., et al. Administration of nonanticoagulant heparin inhibits the loss of glycosaminoglycans from xenogeneic cardiac grafts and prolongs graft survival. Transplant. Proc. 25, 382, 1993
41. Saadi, S.Platt, J.L. Transient perturbation of endothelial integrity induced by antibodies and complement. J.Exp.Med. 181, 21, 1995
42. Hattori, R., Hamilton, K.K., Fugate, R.D., McEver, R.P.Sims, P.J. Stimulated secretion of endothelial von Willebrand factor is accompanied by rapid redistribution to the cell surface of the intracellular granule membrane protein GMP-140. J.Biol.Chem. 264, 7768, 1989
43. Hattori, R., Hamilton, K.K., McEver, R.P.Sims, P.J. Complement proteins C5b-9 induce secretion of high molecular weight multimers of endothelial von Willebrand factor and translocation of granule membrane protein GMP-140 to the cell surface. J.Biol.-Chem. 264, 9053, 1989.

3 Role of Natural Antibody–Antigen Interactions in Xenotransplantation

J.L. Platt, W. Parker, S.S. Lin, Z. Holzknecht, and S.Saadi

Introduction

For over three decades the pathogenesis of xenograft rejection has been thought to begin with the binding of xenoreactive natural antibodies to the graft [1]. Antibody binding activates the complement system which in turn mediates tissue injury [2]. Accordingly, interrupting this series of events either by removing antibody from the recipient [1] or by depleting complement [3] prevents rejection, at least for a time. While the overall paradigm is a simple one, there are some aspects of this process which are more complex than the statement would suggest and it has been our view that the study of these processes may shed light on more fundamental scientific issues and may in the end offer insights of practical use.

Role of the Endothelial Cell in Xenotransplantation

One of our earliest contributions to this field was in advancing the concept that the endothelial cell is the target of the immune reaction leading to the rejection of a vascularized xenograft and an instrument mediating the severe tissue injury characteristic of graft rejection. As a corollary to this concept we proposed that cultured endothelial cells might offer the best model for analyzing the events associated with rejection. Thus, in 1990, we proposed that cultured endothelial cells could be used as the target for assaying xenoreactive antibodies [4] and as a model system for analyzing the cellular and biochemical responses caused by antibody binding and complement activation in a xenograft [5].

One technique we described was an immunoassay in which porcine endothelial cells cultured in microwells would be used to measure antibody binding. This assay had the advantage of providing a cellular surface which in terms of epitope composition, density and configuration may approach the circumstances prevailing in a xenografted organ. Consistent with this concept were our own recent studies which revealed that 80%–100% of the antibodies adsorbed from a serum by cultured endothelial cells are absorbed during perfusion of a xenogeneic organ and that all of the antibodies which bind specific to a xenogeneic organ also bind to the cultured cells [6].

Cultured endothelial cells have also allowed us to elucidate some of the processes which likely contribute to tissue injury and rejection of xenografts. The simplest explanation for the pathogenesis of xenograft rejection is that it results from the complement mediated lysis of graft endothelial cells. While this explanation is undoubtedly correct in some cases, it clearly fails to explain the early lesions of hyperacute rejection which include changes characteristic of vital, metabolically active cells [7, 8]. Given these observations, our first investigations in the field of xenotransplantation were aimed at elucidating noncytotoxic mechanisms of endothelial cell injury. We focused this inquiry on heparan sulfate proteoglycan, a protein polysaccharide glycoconjugate which is present on all nucleated cells and which contributes to such endothelial functions as the maintenance of endothelial integrity, anticoagulation, protection from oxidant and complement mediated injury and attachment of endothelium to underlying matrix [9]. Our initial studies revealed that, within minutes of the binding of antibodies to porcine endothelial cells and the activation of complement, heparan sulfate is shed in large amounts from the cells. The shedding of heparan sulfate proteoglycan deprives endothelial cells of the function of this molecule and, as Wrenshall with the author have shown, through interaction of the solubilized molecules with antigen presenting cells may contribute to the induction of proliferative and cytolytic T cell responses [10, 11].

Another mechanism we postulated might account for the very rapid development of hemorrhage and thrombosis in hyperacute xenograft rejection is loss of endothelial integrity allowing escape of vascular contents and exposure of circulating platelets to the underlying matrix. That this mechanism might in fact contribute to the rejection process was suggested by Saadi who demonstrated that within minutes of the formation of C5b67 complexes on endothelial cell surfaces, there occurs a change in cell shape leading to the formation of intercellular "gaps" [12]. The formation of gaps may allow the escape of components of the blood from blood vessels and bring platelets in contact with the underlying matrix.

The study of endothelial cell physiology has also contributed to understanding the pathogenic mechanisms leading to other manifestations of xenograft rejection. Leventhal with the author was the first to describe a type of lesion seen in xenografts when hyperacute rejection is averted. This lesion was called acute vascular xenograft rejection [13].

One characteristic feature of acute vascular xenograft rejection is the widespread formation of fibrin thrombi. To elucidate the mechanisms which might contribute to this process, Saadi with the author investigated the coagulant properties of endothelial cells exposed to xenoreactive antibodies and complement [14]. Formation of the membrane attack complex on porcine endothelial cells was found to cause a profound increase in the synthesis of tissue factor, a cofactor for the prothrombinase complex. Based on this and related findings, Saadi has proposed that acute vascular xenograft rejection arises in part due to the procoagulant posture of affected endothelium.

Another contribution of endothelium to xenograft rejection relates to its intrinsic susceptibility to complement. This susceptibility which is owed to the species specific functioning of cell-associated complement regulatory proteins was first pointed out by Dalmasso [15] and Miyagawa [16]. We recently carried out the first experiments testing this concept in xenotransplantation [17, 18]. Transplantation of organs from transgenic pigs with human decay accelerating factor and CD59 expressed by a variety of promoters is associated with a remarkable decrease in tissue injury and without other relevant therapies the avoidance of hyperacute rejection in most cases [18–20].

Role of the Antigenic Targets

It was our original hypothesis that the binding of xenoreactive antibodies to antigenic targets on endothelial cell surfaces might have two pathogenic roles: (1) the activation of complement, clearly an essential step in the pathogenesis of rejection and (2) the perturbation of the target molecules themselves leading to alteration in endothelial cell physiology [15, 21, 22]. It is now clear that these mechanisms may be related to the structural and functional properties of the proteins core bring antigenic epitopes.

Recent work in a number of laboratories including our own has revealed that the epitope recognized by xenoreactive natural antibodies is Galα1–3Gal. We have shown that it is to this epitope, associated predominantly with endothelial cell glycoproteins, that xenoreactive natural antibodies bind when human or non-human primate blood is passed through an organ such as a pig kidney in which Galα1–3Gal is expressed [23–25]. While it might seem on the basis of in vitro analysis that expression of the relevant carbohydrate would provide a sufficient basis for antibody binding, this supposition is in fact not supported by some of our in vivo studies.

We have found that the nature of the glycoconjugate as a whole on which an epitope is expressed has a profound impact on the binding of xenoreactive antibodies. This effect reflects in part the relatively low affinity characteristic of the interaction of single antigen combining sites on xenoreactive antibodies and the corresponding epitope. Thus xenoreactive antibodies will bind to any Galα1–3Gal in solid phase assays in which the epitopes are artificially clustered, but the antibodies seem to be more selective when binding to a cell surface. As evidence for this idea we have found that the binding of xenoreactive antibodies to the surface of cells bearing the same amount of Galα1–3Gal ranges over sevenfold in quantity [26]. Presumably, the basis for this wide range is the three-dimensional array in which the epitope is presented. As further evidence, we found that in inhibition assays, the glycoproteins bearing Galα1–3Gal extracted from cell membranes are more than one million fold more effective on a molar basis than purified sugar at inhibiting antibody binding to a cell surface. The effectiveness reflects in part the fact that the glycoproteins bear more than one epitope; however, this explanation is not by itself sufficient, as the cell membrane glycoproteins have fewer epitopes than porcine thyroglobulin; yet the cell membrane glycoproteins are more effective than thyroglobulin at blocking antibody binding. The best explanation for these observations is that the very high avidity of antibody binding to cell surfaces reflects at least in part the three-dimensional arrays in which the epitope is expressed.

The protein core on which Galα1–3Gal is expressed may also be important in determining the biological outcome of antibody binding. We have shown that human xenoreactive antibodies recognize carbohydrate substitutions on porcine endothelial cell integrins [23, 24]. Several of the integrins recognized are thought to contribute directly to endothelial integrity and thus it is possible that the binding of antibodies to these structures causes a loss of barrier function. Integrins also can transduce signals and it would seem not unlikely that the attachment of xenoreactive antibodies to endothelial cell integrins may initiate signaling that contributes to activation of endothelial cells.

Role of Xenoreactive Antibodies

Until recently, very little was known about the antibodies which initiate the rejection of xenografts. Xenoreactive antibodies can be detected by one technique or another in the serum of all mammalian species [27]; however, which of these antibodies might be important in mediating biologically relevant effects was uncertain.

One of our early observations was that xenoreactive IgM may be especially important in the pathogenesis of rejection. This idea was based on the immunopathology of rejecting xenografts which revealed that IgM of the recipient would often deposit on graft endothelium before IgG and sometimes deposition of IgG was not observed [7]. The importance of the IgM antibodies was also suggested by the finding that depletion of IgM antibodies would eliminate the ability of a human serum to cause activation of porcine endothelial cells [5] and complement-mediated cytotoxicity [28]. Recently, further evidence in support of this concept emerged from our studies in which IgG in the form of γ-globulin was administered to xenograft recipients in an effort to control complement deposition (see Chap. 31) [29]. Instead of mediating xenograft rejection, the IgG, which includes anti-Galα1-3Gal antibodies was found to prolong graft survival by diverting the activation of complement away from the graft.

When Galα1-3Gal was found to be an important epitope in xenotransplantation nearly all information concerning antibodies against that structure derived from studies of IgG [30, 31]. Parker and the author studied the properties of xenoreactive IgM antibodies which consisted predominantly of IgM specific for Galα1-3Gal [32]. The xenoreactive IgM antibodies were found to bind tightly to target cells, the effective avidity (K_{assoc}) being 10^9–10^{10} M. The high avidity presumably reflects multivalent interaction of xenoreactive IgM with the target cell surface. Of particular interest to us was the observation that the antibodies in a given serum were highly homogeneous in their binding to porcine endothelial cells, the binding resembling an oligoclonal population. Not only were the antibodies in one serum homogeneous, but the antibodies from different individuals exhibited very similar binding characteristics. Parker also found that in their origin, concentrations in serum and functional properties, xenoreactive natural antibodies are indistinguishable from isohemagglutinins, suggesting that the anti-Galα1-3Gal antibodies and anti-A and anti-B blood group antibodies are members of a family of natural antibodies [6]. Aside from the theoretical aspects of this observation there is the practical consideration that the immunological hurdle to porcine to primate xenotransplantation posed by xenoreactive antibodies may indeed resemble very closely the hurdle to ABO-incompatible transplantation, a barrier that is clinically assailable [33, 34].

Nature of Accommodation

Some years ago, the author with Chopek and Simmons made the remarkable observation that following the transplantation of an organ across a humoral ABO-blood group barrier facilitated by removal of the anti-A or anti-B antibodies from the recipient, the allograft would continue to function without evidence of tissue injury even after the anti-blood group antibodies returned to the circulation [33, 34]. Several years later the author observed a similar phenomenon in a xenograft and the phenomenon was termed accommodation [7, 15]. There are several possible explanations for accommodation, including a change in the properties of anti-donor antibodies, a change in the antigen and an acquired resistance of endothelium to humoral injury. The mechanisms underlying accommodation are still uncertain, yet there is reason to think that it may reflect in part a benefit deriving from the interaction of xenoreactive antibodies and the antigens they recognize.

Acknowledgments. The research summarized in this chapter was supported by grants from the National Institutes of Health (HL52297, HL50985 and HL46810) and from Nextran. JLP is Dorothy W. and Joseph W. Beard Professor of Experimental Surgery.

References

1. Perper, R.J.Najarian, J.S. Experimental renal heterotransplantation. I. In widely divergent species. Transplantation 4, 377, 1966
2. Gewurz, H.Clark, D.S. Participation of complement and complement-fixing antibody in the rejection of vascularized grafts. J.Lab.Clin.Med. 64, 861, 1964
3. Nelson, R.A.,Jr. A new concept of immunosuppression in hypersensitivity reactions and in transplantation immunity. Survey Ophthal 11, 498, 1966
4. Platt, J.L., Turman, M.A., Noreen, H.J., et al. An ELISA assay for xenoreactive natural antibodies. Transplantation 49, 1000, 1990
5. Platt, J.L., Vercellotti, G.M., Lindman, B.J., et al. Release of heparan sulfate from endothelial cells: Implications for pathogenesis of hyperacute rejection. J.Exp.Med. 171, 1363, 1990
6. Parker, W., Lundberg-Swanson, K.L., Holzknecht, Z.E., et al. Isohemagglutinins and xenoreactive antibodies: members of a distinct family of natural antibodies. Hum.Immunol. 45, 94, 1996
7. Platt, J.L., Fischel, R.J., Matas, A.J., et al. Immunopathology of hyperacute xenograft rejection in a swine-to-primate model. Transplantation 52, 214, 1991
8. Platt, J.L. Hyperacute Xenograft Rejection. R.G. Landes Company, Austin, 1995
9. Ihrcke, N.S., Wrenshall, L.E., Lindman, B.J.Platt, J.L. Role of heparan sulfate in immune system-blood vessel interactions. Immunol.Today 14, 500, 1993
10. Wrenshall, L.E., Carlson, A., Cerra, F.B.Platt, J.L. Modulation of cytolytic T-cell responses by heparan sulfate. Transplantation 57, 1087, 1994

11. Wrenshall, L.E., Cerra, F.B., Singh, R.K.Platt, J.L. Heparan sulfate initiates signals in murine macrophages leading to divergent biological outcomes. J.Immunol. 154, 871, 1995
12. Saadi, S.Platt, J.L. Transient perturbation of endothelial integrity induced by antibodies and complement. J.Exp.Med. 181, 21, 1995
13. Leventhal, J.R., Matas, A.J., Sun, L.H., et al. The immunopathology of cardiac xenograft rejection in the guinea pig to rat model. Transplantation 56, 1, 1993
14. Saadi, S., Holzkhecht, R.A., Patte, C.P., Stern, D.M.Platt, J.L. Complement-mediated regulation of tissue factor activity in endothelium. J.Exp.Med. 182, 1, 1995
15. Platt, J.L., Vercellotti, G.M., Dalmasso, A.P., et al. Transplantation of discordant xenografts: a review of progress. Immunol.Today 11, 450, 1990
16. Miyagawa, S., Hirose, H., Shirakura, R., et al. The mechanism of discordant xenograft rejection. Transplantation 46, 825, 1988
17. McCurry, K.R., Kooyman, D.L., Diamond, L., et al. Transgenic expression of human complement regulatory proteins in mice results in diminished complement deposition during organ xenoperfusion. Transplantation 59, 1177, 1995
18. McCurry, K.R., Kooyman, D.L., Alvarado, C.G., et al. Human complement regulatory proteins protect swine-to-primate cadriac xenografts from humoral injury. Nature Med 1, 423, 1995
19. Diamond, L.E., McCurry, K.R., Platt, J.L., et al. A human CD59 minigene encodes a biologically functional complement regulatory protein in transgenic mice. Transplant Immunol 3, 305, 1995
20. Byrne, G.W., McCurry, K.R., Martin, M.J., et al. Expression of human CD59 and DAF in transgenic pigs: intrinsic regulation of complement activity. Transplantation, In Press
21. Platt, J.L., Lindman, B.J., Chen, H., Spitalnik, S.L.Bach, F.H. Endothelial cell antigens recognized by xenoreactive human natural antibodies. Transplantation 50, 817, 1990
22. Platt, J.L. Mechanisms of tissue injury in hyperacute xenograft rejection. ASAIO J 38, 8, 1992
23. Platt, J.L.Holzknecht, Z.E. Porcine platelet antigens recognized by human xenoreactive natural antibodies. Transplantation 57, 327, 1994
24. Holzknecht, Z.E.Platt, J.L. Identification of porcine endothelial cell membrane antigens recognized by human xenoreactive antibodies. J.Immunol. 154, 4565, 1995
25. Collins, B.H., Cotterell, A.H., McCurry, K.R., et al. Cardiac xenografts between primate species provide evidence for the importance of the α-galactosyl determinant in hyperacute rejection. J.Immunol. 154, 5500, 1995
26. Alvarado, C.G., Cotterell, A.H., McCurry, K.R., et al. Variation in the level of xenoantigen expression in porcine organs. Transplantation 59, 1589, 1995
27. Landsteiner, K. The Specificity of Serological Reactions. Dover Publications, New York, NY, 1962, Ed. 2
28. Dalmasso, A.P., Vercellotti, G.M., Fischel, R.J., et al. Mechanism of complement activation in the hyperacute rejection of porcine organs transplanted into primate recipients. Am.J.Pathol. 140, 1157, 1992
29. Magee, J.C., Collins, B.H., Harland, R.C., et al. Immunoglobulin prevents complement mediated hyperacute rejection in swine-to-primate xenotransplantation. J.Clin.Invest. 96, 2404, 1995
30. Galili, U., Rachmilewitz, E.A., Peleg, A.Flechner, I. A unique natural human IgG antibody with anti-α-galactosyl specificity. J.Exp.Med. 160, 1519, 1984

31. Galili, U., Macher, B.A., Buehler, J.Shohet, S.B. Human natural anti-α-galactosyl IgG: the specific recognition of α(1–3)-linked glactose residues. J.Exp.Med. 162, 573, 1985
32. Parker, W.R., Bruno, D., Holzknecht, Z.E.Platt, J.L. Xenoreactive natural antibodies: isolation and initial characterization. J.Immunol. 153, 3791, 1994
33. Chopek, M.W., Simmons, R.L.Platt, J.L. ABO incompatible renal transplantation: initial immunopathologic evaluation. Transplant. Proc. 19, 4553, 1987
34. Bannett, A.D., McAlack, R.F., Morris, M., Chopek, M. Platt, J.L. ABO incompatible renal transplantation: a qualitative analysis of native endothelial tissue ABO antigens after transplant. Transplant. Proc. 21, 783, 1989

4 Major Carbohydrate Xenotransplantation Antigens

R. Oriol and D.K.C. Cooper

αGal Epitopes on Pig Vascular Endothelium

The main difference in carbohydrate antigens expressed at the surface of vascular endothelium, between pig and man, is the presence of human histo-blood group ABH antigens in the same location where the pig expresses αGal linear antigens [1, 2]. Humans lack α-galactosyltransferase enzyme activity and, in spite of having the same lactosamine precursor chains and similar terminal sialylated antigens, are unable to make αGal epitopes (Table 1) [3].

About 1% of the total normal human immunoglobulins are natural antibodies reacting with Galα1-3Galβ1-4GlcNac (αGal epitope), which were first described 12 years ago [3-7]. This antibody was later found to be responsible for the hyperacute vascular rejection of pig organs perfused with human blood [8, 9], because the αGal epitope is present on pig vascular endothelial cells [2, 10-12]. During hyperacute vascular rejection, endothelial cells are lysed by recipient natural antibodies and complement, leading to infiltration with neutrophils, multiple thromboses and interstitial hemorrhages [13-15]. Studies in our own laboratory indicate that the cytotoxic reaction is mediated by anti-αGal antibody and complement [16], and can be reproduced on monolayers of pig PK15 cells in culture by adding human natural antibodies and complement. Enzymatic removal of αGal epitopes from the membrane of pig cells, with coffee bean α-galactosidase, diminishes the cytotoxic effect of natural antibodies [17]. Alternatively, the cytotoxic effect of human serum on pig cells can be avoided (a) by removal of the anti-αGal antibodies from human serum using an αGal immunoabsorbent column or (b) by blocking the antibody binding sites with monovalent oligosaccharide haptens [18-20]. In this last case, the resulting antibody-hapten complex does not activate complement and consequently has no cytotoxic effect on pig cells [21]. In vitro experiments suggest that the appropriate oligosaccharide hapten, administered by the intravenous route, might be used as a treatment to prevent the in vivo hyperacute rejection of pig organs transplanted into human recipients [18, 22].

Table 1. The main oligosaccharide epitopes found on vascular endothelium of the human and porcine species

Human	Porcine
Galβ1 → 4GlcNAcβ1 → R	Galβ1-4GlcNAcβ1-R
ABH[a] → Galβ1 → 4GlcNAcβ1 → R	Galα1 → 3Galβ1 → 4GlcNAcβ1 → R
NeuAcα1 → 3Galβ1 → 4GlcNAcβ1 → R	NeuAcα2 → 3Galβ1 → 4GlcNAcβ1 → R

[a] A, GalNAcα1 → 3(Fucα1 → 2); B, Galα1 → 3(Fucα1 → 2); H, Fucα1 → 2.

Are There αGal-Negative Pigs?

A search was made to ascertain whether the pig species is genetically polymorphic for the expression of the αGal epitope and, furthermore, whether pigs devoid of the αGal epitope could be found. Unfortunately, all pigs tested (137 animals belonging to 23 different breeds) from different areas of Europe, America, Asia, and Australia expressed the αGal epitope on vascular endothelial cells [23]. The αGal epitope was also found on the vascular endothelium of wild boars (R. Oriol et al., unpublished). These observations suggest that the porcine species may be monomorphic for this antigen. However, a continuing search for αGal-negative pigs is worthwhile, because such animals might exist at very low frequency. Breeding of such αGal-negative pigs, if they are ever found, would be easier than producing αGal-negative pigs by genetic manipulation [24, 25].

Oligosaccharide Epitopes of the Vascular Compartment of Other Animal Species

Since the porcine species appears to be monomorphic for expression of αGal epitopes, other potential donors for xenotransplantation research (and clinical potential) were tested for the presence of this antigen. The Galα1–3Galβ1–4GlcNAc epitope reacts with human natural antibodies and with the isolectin I-B4 of *Griffonia simplicifolia* seeds (GSI-B4). This lectin was used to detect the presence of αGal epitopes on the vascular compartment of 23 animal species, together with the use of (a) anti-ABH human blood group antibodies, (b) peanut agglutinin lectin (PNA), which reacts with Galβ1–3GalNAc, and (c) *Lycopersicum esculentum* lectin (tomato or LEL) which reacts with polylactosamine (Galβ1–4GlcNAc)n.

Three main patterns of reactivity were found: (1) humans and Old World monkeys reacted with anti-ABH antibodies; (2) New World monkeys and lower mammals had αGal epitopes recognized by GSI-B4, in accord with previous reports [3]; (3) birds and reptiles had βGal epitopes recognized by PNA. Irrespective of the above-mentioned fluorescence patterns, all the animal species studied had positive reactions with LEL, indicating that they all have precursor poly-lactosamine chains, but each of the three groups expressed different terminal non-reducing epitopes (Table 2) [26].

Within these three main patterns, different subgroups could be distinguished, according to the specific tissue distribution of the antigens. In the first group, humans express ABH strongly on both vascular endothelium and red cells, while baboons present a clear dissociation between vascular endothelium which is positive with anti-A or anti-B, and red cells which are always negative with ABH reagents [27].

In the second group, most domestic large mammals (calf, pig, dog, sheep, goat, and rabbit) demonstrated strong expression of αGal epitopes, while other mammals (mouse, rat, hamster, gerbil, guinea pig, capybara, llama, owl monkey) and a marsupial (wallaby) had rather weak expression of αGal epitopes. The kangaroo family exhibits an upright posture, and consequently their hearts have the

Table 2. The three main patterns of carbohydrate-specific reactions identified on the vascular endothelium of different animal species

Animal Species	Fluorescent reagents			
	ABH antibodies	αGal GS1-B4	βGal PNA	βGal LEL
Humans and Old World monkeys	+	–	–	+
New World monkeys and lower mammals	–	+	–	+
Birds and reptiles	–	–	+	±

ABH, anti-human A, B, or H blood group antibodies; GSI-B4, *Griffonia simplicifolia* isolectin B4 reacting with Galα1→3Gal epitopes; PNA, peanut agglutinin reacting with Galβ1→3GalNac epitopes; LEL, *Lycopersicum esculentum* lectin (tomato) reacting with (Galβ1→4GlcNAc)n epitopes.

correct valve/muscle architecture to maintain appropriate tissue/blood pressures in the upright position. They have therefore been proposed as potential donors of hearts for human recipients [28].

Differential expression of αGal epitopes on vascular endothelium and red cells was also observed in this group. For example, rabbit red cells were strongly positive but rabbit vascular endothelium was only weakly positive. An opposite pattern, with strong vascular endothelium and weak red cells, was observed in the goat. The capybara had αGal on red cells, but was negative on vascular endothelium.

Among all the species tested, the calf had the strongest expression of αGal epitopes on both red cells and vascular endothelium. Indeed, this was the reason that the cow was selected to clone the first animal αGal transferase [29]. The mouse αGal transferase gene was independently cloned by another team [30], and taking advantage of its homology with the aforementioned genes, the pig αGal transferase gene has recently been cloned [31].

A similar heterogeneity with tissue-specific expression was observed in the group of reptiles and birds (group 3). The alligator had PNA-positive red cells and negative vascular endothelium, while the chicken and turkey had PNA-positive vascular endothelium and negative red cells. The ostrich was PNA positive on both vascular endothelium and red cells.

Natural Anti-αGal Antibodies May Protect Humans from Animal-Specific Infectious Agents

αGal epitopes are not only found in lower mammals. They have also been reported at the surface of certain parasites [32], bacteria [33], and viruses. Furthermore, the presence of αGal epitopes on some viral glycoproteins depends on the capacity of the host cells to synthesize αGal [34].

The natural anti-αGal antibodies of Old World monkeys and humans might play a role in the defense mechanisms of these species against the microorganisms carrying αGal epitopes. This could be one reason for the resistance of these species towards infection by many animal viruses [35, 36]. If this is the case, removal or blocking of anti-αGal antibodies in humans may increase their susceptibility to certain animal viruses which are normally not infectious in man. This potential risk must be kept in mind when preparing human recipients for xenotransplantation.

Oligosaccharide Epitopes of the Exocrine Compartment

Two different loci code for the human α-2-fucosyltransferase activities [37]. One produces the H antigen of the mesodermal compartment (FUT1) [38] and the other the H antigen of exocrine secretions (FUT2) [39]. These two structural genes are differentially expressed in these two body compartments due to tissue-specific regulation of expression mechanisms which have not as yet been elucidated, but which will be of crucial importance if we want to direct the expression of a new FUT gene product to the pig vascular compartment.

The human H antigen expressed in these two body compartments remains unchanged in blood group O individuals and is further transformed into A or B in the corresponding A or B histo-blood type individuals by the A or B glycosyltransferases of the ABO locus.

Almost every individual of the human species has an active FUT1 gene and expresses ABH antigens in the mesodermal compartment, with the very rare exception of Bombay individuals (<1:10 000) who have inactive FUT1 alleles and express only I or precursor chain epitopes in the mesodermal compartment. In contrast, 20 % of the Caucasian population have inactive FUT2 alleles and are therefore devoid of ABH antigens in exocrine secretions. They are called nonsecretors for this reason, but they express precursor chain or Lewis-related epitopes in exocrine secretions, and they can have normal ABH antigens on red cells and vascular endothelium.

In spite of the fact that most animal species do not express ABH antigens on the mesodermal compartment, almost all have some sort of ABH-related antigens in exocrine secretions, which are probably under the control of a gene with a function homologous to the human FUT2. The expression of this gene leads to an ABH polymorphism in the exocrine secretions of many animal species (Table 3). These "FUT2-like" genes are present in the animal genome. Therefore, it is not necessary to introduce new human FUT genes to obtain vascular endothelial expression of these genes, but rather to find the mechanisms of tissue-specific expression in order to redirect the expression of the already existing animal FUT genes to the vascular endothelial cells.

The animal ABH antigens of the exocrine compartment cannot be the main targets of the hyperacute vascular rejection of xenotransplants because they are not expressed in the vascular compartment, which is in direct and immediate contact with the antibodies of the recipient. However, in the long term they would also contribute to an immune response in transplant recipients who lack the corresponding antigens. Indeed, A-O incompatibility has previously been reported to accelerate rejection in rabbit [40] and pig [41] allograft skin models.

Table 3. Frequencies of the different ABH and I or Lewis phenotypes in exocrine secretions of selected animal species

Animal species	A	B	AB	H	I or Lewis	References
Human	32	8	3	37	20	[51, 52]
Baboon	16	50	34	<1	0	[53, 54]
Vervet (Old World monkey)	83	10	7	0	0	[53]
Pig	51	0	0	38	11	[23, 55]
Dog	45	0	0	52	3	[56, 57]
Rabbit	76	0	0	24	0	[58, 59]

The first three species (human, baboon, and vervet monkey) have fucosylated ABH antigens in both mesodermal and exocrine compartments, while the last three (pig, dog, and rabbit) express ABH antigens only in the exocrine compartment and have linear unfucosylated αGal epitopes in both mesodermal and exocrine compartments.

Humans and Old World monkeys have inactive αGal transferase pseudogenes [42, 43], which are unable to produce αGal epitopes on exocrine secretions and the mesodermal compartment. Instead, they express the ABH antigens in both body compartments (Tables 2, 4). It remains to be shown if the "knockout" of the pig αGal transferase gene will contribute to the redirection of the expression of the product of the normal pig "FUT2-like" gene [44] to pig vascular endothelial cells. Transgenic mice expressing human FUT1 in milk have been obtained [45], but to date no expression of this gene on mice vascular endothelium has been observed.

To date, the knockout of the αGal transferase gene has only been reported in the mouse [46, 47] (Chap. 51). In this species, successful competition between the expression of human FUT1 and mouse αGal gene products has also been reported [48] (Chap. 50). However, such competition experiments are anticipated to be easier in the mouse than in the pig, because the mouse expresses small numbers of αGal epitopes in the mesodermal compartment as compared to the pig.

New World monkeys and lower mammals have an active αGal transferase gene [49] and express the αGal epitope in both exocrine and mesodermal compartments, but they also express ABH and βGal antigens in exocrine secretions (Table 4).

Table 4. Main carbohydrate epitopes found in exocrine secretions of different animal species

Animal species	Fluorescent reagents			
	ABH antibodies	αGal GS1-b4	βGal PNA	βGal LEL
Humans and Old World monkeys	+	–	+	+
New World monkeys and lower mammals	+	+	+	+
Birds and reptiles	+	–	+	+

ABH, anti-human A, B, or H blood group antibodies; GSI-B4, *Griffonia simplicifolia* isolectin B4 reacting with Galα1 → 3Gal epitopes; PNA, peanut agglutinin reacting with Galβ1 → 3GalNac epitopes; LEL, *Lycopersicum esculentum* lectin (tomato) reacting with (Galβ1 → 4GlcNAc)n epitopes.

Finally, birds and reptiles lack expression of active αGal transferase genes, but they also express ABH and βGal antigens in exocrine secretions (Table 4). The absence of αGal epitopes in these species suggested that they might not be susceptible to hyperacute vascular rejection by humans or Old World primates [50]. Nevertheless, the genetic distance between birds or reptiles and humans is such that many other differences create major problems, which make these animals unlikely organ donors for the human species.

References

1. COOPER, D.K.C., KOREN, E., ORIOL, R. (1994) Oligosaccharides and discordant xenotransplantation. Immunol. Rev. 141:31
2. ORIOL, R., YE, Y., KOREN, E., COOPER, D.K.C. (1993) Carbohydrate antigens of pig tissues reacting with human natural antibodies as potential targets for hyperacute vascular rejection in pig-to-man organ xenotransplantation. Transplantation. 56:1433
3. GALILI, U., SHOHET, S.B., KOBRIN, E., STULTS, C.L.M., MACHER, B.A. (1988) Man, apes, and Old World monkeys differ from other mammals in the expression of α-galactosyl epitopes on nucleated cells. J. Biol. Chem. 263:17755
4. GALILI, U., RACHMILEWITZ, E.A., PELEG, A., FLECHNER, I. (1984) A unique natural human IgG antibody with anti-α-galactosyl specificity. J. Exp. Med. 160:1519
5. GALILI, U., MACHER, B.A., BUEHLER, J., SHOHET, S.B. (1985) Human natural anti-α-galactosyl IgG. II. The specific recognition of α(1–3) linked galactose residues. J. Exp. Med. 162:573
6. GALILI, U., CLARK, M.R., SHOHET, S.B., BUEHLER, J., MACHER, B. (1987) Evolutionary relationship between the natural anti-Gal antibody and the Galα1–3Gal epitope in primates. Proc. Natl. Acad. Sci. USA. 84:1369
7. WIESLANDER, J., MANSSON, O., KALLIN, E., et al. (1990) Specificity of human antibodies against αGal1–3Gal carbohydrate epitope and distinction from natural antibodies reacting with Galα1–2Gal or Galα1–4Gal. Glycoconjugate J. 7:85
8. GOOD, A.H., COOPER, D.K.C., MALCOLM, A.J., et al. (1992) Identification of carbohydrate structures that bind human anti-porcine antibodies: implications for discordant xenografting in humans. Transplant. Proc. 24:559
9. COOPER, D.K.C., GOOD, A.H., KOREN, E., et al. (1993) Identification of α-galactosyl and other carbohydrate epitopes that are bound by human anti-pig antibodies: relevance to discordant xenografting in man. Transplant. Immunol. 1:198
10. SAMUELSSON, B.E., RYDBERG, L., BRIEMER, M.E., et al. (1994) Natural antibodies and human xenotransplantation. Immunol. Rev. 141:151
11. SANDRIN, M.S., VAUGHAN, H.A., MCKENZIE, I.F.C. (1994) Galα(1,3)Gal as the major epitope for the pig-to-human vascularized grafts. Transplant. Rev. 8:134
12. SANDRIN, M.S., MCKENZIE, I.F.C. (1994) Galα(1,3)Gal – the major xenoantigens recognized in pigs by human natural antibodies. Immunol. Rev. 141:169
13. MAKOWKA, L., WU, G.D., HOFFMAN, A., et al. (1994) Immunohistopathologic lesions associated with the rejection of a pig to human liver xenograft. Transplant. Proc. 26:1074
14. PLATT, J.L., FISCHEL, R.J., MATAS, A.J., et al. (1991) Immunopathology of hyperacute xenograft rejection in a swine-to-primate model. Transplantation. 52:214

15. COLLINS, B.H., CHARI, R.S., MAGEE, J.C., et al. (1994) Mechanisms of injury in porcine livers perfused with blood of patients with fulminant hepatic failure. Transplantation. 58:1162
16. KOREN, E., NEETHLING, F.A., KOSCEC, M., et al. (1994) In vitro model for hyperacute rejection of xenogeneic cells. Transplant. Proc. 26:1166
17. LAVECCHIO, J.A., DUNNE, A.D., EDGE, A.S.B. (1995) Enzymatic removal of alpha-galactosyl epitopes from porcine endothelial cells diminishes the cytotoxic effect of natural antibodies. Transplantation. 60:841
18. YE, Y., NEETHLING, F., NIEKRASZ, M., et al. (1994) Evidence that intravenously administered α-galactosyl carbohydrates reduce baboon serum cytotoxicity to pig kidney cells (PK15) and transplanted pig hearts. Transplantation. 58:330
19. RIEBEN, R., VON ALLMEN, E., KORCHAGINA, E.Y., et al. (1995) Detection, immunoabsorption, and inhibition of cytotoxic activity of anti-αGal antibodies using newly developed substances with synthetic Galα1–3Gal disaccharide epitopes. Xenotransplantation. 2:98
20. NEETHLING, F., JOZIASSE, D., BOVIN, N., COOPER, D.K.C., ORIOL, R. (1996) The reducing end of αGal oligosaccharides contributes to their efficiency in blocking natural antibodies of human and baboon sera. Transplant. Int. 9:98
21. NEETHLING, F.A., KOREN, E., YE, Y., et al. (1994) Protection of pig kidney (PK15) cells from the cytotoxic effect of anti-pig antibodies by α-galactosyl oligosaccharides. Transplantation. 57:959
22. COOPER, D.K.C., YE, Y., NIEKRASZ, M., et al. (1993) Specific intravenous carbohydrate therapy. A new concept in inhibiting antibody-mediated rejection – experience with ABO-incompatible cardiac allografting in the baboon. Transplantation. 56:769
23. ORIOL, R., BARTHOD, F., BERGEMER, A.M., et al. (1994) Monomorphic and polymorphic carbohydrate antigens on pig tissues: implications for organ xenotransplantation in the pig-to-human model. Transpl. Int. 7:405
24. COOPER, D.K.C., KOREN, E., ORIOL, R. (1993) Genetically engineered pigs. Lancet. 342:682
25. GUSTAFSSON, K., STRAHAN, K., PREECE, A. (1994) Alpha 1,3 galactosyltransferase: a target for in vivo genetic manipulation in xenotransplantation. Immunol. Rev. 141:59
26. ORIOL, R., CANDELIER, J.J., TANIGUCHI, S., PETERS, L., COOPER, D.K.C. (1996) Major oligosaccharide epitopes found in tissues of 23 animal species, potential donors for organ xenotransplantation. Transplant. Proc. 28:794
27. ORIOL, R., COOPER, J.E., DAVIES, D.R., KEELING, P.W.N. (1984) ABH antigens in vascular endothelium and some epithelial tissues of baboons. Lab. Invest. 50:514
28. CAIRNS, T.D.H., TAUBE, D.H., STEVENS, N., BINNS, R., WELSH, K.I. (1991) Xenografts – future prospects for clinical transplantation. Immunol. Lett. 29:167
29. JOZIASSE, D.H., SHAPER, J.H., VAN DEN EIJNDEN, D.H., VAN TUNEN, A.J., SHAPER, H.L. (1989) Bovine α1–3 galactosyltransferase: isolation and characterization of a cDNA clone. Identification of homologous sequences in human genomic DNA. J. Biol. Chem. 264:14290
30. LARSEN, R.D., RAJAN, V.P., RUFF, M.M., et al. (1989) Isolation of a cDNA encoding a murine UDPgalactose:β-D-galactosyl-1,4-N-acetyl-D-glucosaminide-α1,3-galactosyltransferase: expression cloning by gene transfer. Proc. Natl. Acad. Sci. USA. 86:8227

31. SANDRIN„ M.S., VAUGHAN, H.A., DABKOWSKI, P.L., MCKENZIE, I.F.C. (1993) Anti-pig antibodies in human serum react predominantly with Galα(1,3)Gal epitopes. Proc. Natl. Acad. Sci. USA. 90:11391
32. ALMEIDA, J.C., KRAUTZ, G.M., KRETTLI, A.U., TRAVASSOS,L.R. (1993) Glycoconjugates of Trypanosoma cruzi: a 74 kD antigen of trypomastigotes specifically reacts with lytic anti-αGalactosyl antibodies from patients with chronic Chagas disease. J. Clin. Lab. Analysis. 7:307
33. KRIVAN, H.C., CLARK, G.F., SMITH, D.F., WILKINS, T.D. (1986) Cell surface binding site for Clostridium difficile enterotoxin: evidence for a glycoconjugate containing the sequence Galα1-3Galβ1-4GlcNAc. Infection Immunity. 53:573
34. REPIK, P.M., STRIZKI, J.M., GALILI, U. (1994) Differential host-dependent expression of α-galactosyl epitopes on viral glycoproteins: a study of eastern equine encephalitis virus as a model. J. Gen. Vir. 75:1177
35. ROTHER, R.P., FODOR, W.L., SPRINGHORN, J.P., et al. (1995) A novel mechanism of retrovirus inactivation in human serum mediated by anti-α-galactosyl natural antibody. J. Exp. Med. 182:1345
36. TAKEUCHI, Y., PORTER, C.D., STRAHAN, K.M., et al. (1996) Sensitization of cells and retroviruses to human serum by α(1,3) galactosyltransferase. Nature. 379:85
37. ORIOL, R., DANOLOVS, J., HAWKINS, B.R. (1981) A new genetic model opposing that the Se gene is a structural gene closely linked to the H gene. Am. J. Hum. Genet. 33:421
38. LARSEN, R.D., ERNST, L.K., NAIR, R.P., LOWER, J.B. (1990) Molecular cloning, sequence and expression of a human GDP-L-fucose: β-D-galactoside α-L-fucosyltransferase cDNA that can form the H blood group antigen. Proc. Natl. Acad. Sci. USA. 87:6674
39. KELLY, R.J., ROUQUIER, S., GIORGI, D., LENNON, G.G., LOWE, J.B. (1995) Sequence and expression of a candidate for the human secretor blood group α(1,2)fucosyltransferase gene (FUT2). J. Biol. Chem. 270:4640
40. ZWEIBAUM, A., BOUHOU, E. (1973) Studies on digestive groups: II. Influence of the digestive group A system on skin allografts in rabbits. Transplantation. 15:294
42. LARSEN, R.D., RIVERA-MARRERO, C.A., ERNST, L.K., CUMMINGS, R.D., LOWER, J.B. (1990) Frameshift and nonsense mutations in human genomic sequence homologous to a murine UDP-Gal:β-D-Gal(1,4)-D-GlcNAc α(1,3)galactosyltransferase. J. Biol. Chem. 265:7055
43. JOZIASSE, D.H., SHAPER, J.H., WANG JABS, E., SHAPER, N.L. (1991) Characterization of an α1-3 galactosyltransferase homologue on human chromosome 12 that is organized as a processed pseudogene. J. Biol. Chem. 266:6991
44. THURIN, J., BLASZCZYK-THURIN, M. (1995) Porcine submaxillary gland GDP-L-fucose:β-D-galactoside α-2-L-fucosyltransferase is likely a counterpart of the human secretor gene-encoded blood group transferase. J. Biol. Chem. 44:26577
45. PRIETO, P.A., MUKERJI, P., KELDER, B., et al. (1995) Remodeling of mouse milk glycoconjugates by transgenic expression of a human glycosyltransferase. J. Biol. Chem. 270:29515
46. THALL, A.D., MALY, P., LOWE, J.B. (1995) Oocyte Galα1,3Gal epitopes implicated in sperm adhesion to the zona pellucida glycoprotein ZP3 are not required for fertilization in the mouse. J. Biol. Chem. 270:21437

47. TEARLE, R.G., TANGE, M.J., ZANNETTINO, Z.L., et al. (1996) The alpha-1,3-galactosyltransferase knockout mouse – implications for xenotransplantation. Transplantation. 61:13
48. SANDRIN, M.S., FODOR, W.L., MOUHTOURIS, E., et al. (1995) Enzymatic remodeling of the carbohydrate surface of a xenogeneic cell substantially reduces human antibody binding and complement-mediated cytolysis. Nature. Med. 1:1261
49. HENION, T.R., MACHER, B.A., ANARAKI, F., GALILI, U. (1994) Defining the minimal size of catalytically active primate α1,3 galactosyltransferase: structure-function studies on the recombinant truncated enzyme. Glycobiology. 4:193
50. TANIGUCHI, S., NEETHLING, F.A., KOBAYASHI, T., et al. (1995) The ratites (ostrich, emu) as potential heart donors for humans – immunologic considerations. Transplant. Proc. 28:561
51. MOURANT, A.E., KOPEC, A.C., DOMANIEVSKA-SOBCZAK, K. (1976) In: The Distribution of the Human Blood Groups and Other Polymorphisms. Oxford University Press, Oxford, UK, p. 191 and 574
52. MARTINKO, J.M., VINCEK, V., KLEIN, D., KLEIN, J. (1993) Primate ABO glycosyltransferases – evidence for trans-species evolution. Immunogenetics. 37:274
53. SOCHA, W.W., RUFFIE, J. (1983) Blood Groups of Primates. New York, Alan R. Liss, P. 39
54. KOMINATO, Y., MENEIL, P.D., YAMAMOTO, M., et al. (1992) Animal histo-blood group ABO genes. Biochem. Biophys. Res. Commun. 189:154
55. BALANCINO, L.F., BARRA, J.L., MONTFERRAN, C.G., CUMAR, F.A. (1994) Differential interaction of Escherichia coli heat-labile toxin and cholera toxin with pig intestinal brush border glycoproteins depending on their ABH and related blood group antigen determinants. Infection Immunity. 62:1460
56. ZWEIBAUM, A., ORIOL, R., FEINGOLD, N., et al. (1974) Studies on canine secretory alloantigens (CSA). Tissue Antigens. 4:115
57. ORIOL, R., STRECKER, G., ROUSSET, M., et al. (1975) Determination of the structure of the immunodominant groups of the canine secretory alloantigens (CSA) by radioimmunoassay. Transplant. Proc. 7:523
58. ZWEIBAUM, A., BOUHOU, E. (1973) Studies on digestive groups: I. The alloantigen alloantibody system in rabbits. Transplantation. 15:291
59. VILLARROYA, H., DALIX, A.M., PARRAULT, M., ORIOL, R. (1990) Differential susceptibility to experimental allergic encephalomyelitis (EAE) in genetically defined A+ and A-rabbits. Autoimmunity. 6:47

5 Natural Antibody Polymorphism and Anti-Galα1–3Gal Antibodies

T.D.H. Cairns, J. Lee, L.C. Goldberg, B.E. Samuelsson, and D.H. Taube

Introduction – Natural Anti-carbohydrate Antibodies

The best characterized natural antibodies are anti-carbohydrate antibodies. Landsteiner described blood group A and B isoagglutinins in 1900 [1], but the original, earlier descriptions of natural antibodies were of heterophile agglutinins [2], some of which were cross-absorbable between species. Landsteiner [3] observed that species in which the target antigen of a heterophile agglutinin was absent would have naturally occurring agglutinins specific for that antigen, much as he had described individuals within a species as having A or B isoagglutinins whenever blood group A or B was absent. He regarded the presence of antigen within a species as following genera or families (although not exclusively), and the presence of heterophile agglutinin as doing likewise in a reciprocal fashion.

One such antibody, human rabbit red cell agglutinin, was identified 70 years ago [4] and was later found to reside in both IgG and IgM fractions for all of the many hundreds of normal individuals investigated [5, 6]. The dominant glycolipid in rabbit red cell membranes was found by Hakomori's group to be the pentaglycosylceramide Galα1–3Galβ1–4GlcNAcβ1–3Galβ1–4Glcβ1–1 ceramide [7], and Suzuki and Naiki identified the target epitope of human rabbit red cell agglutinins as being contained in the carbohydrate chain of this glycolipid [8]. This work was subsequently confirmed by others [9].

In parallel work, human natural IgG and IgM antibodies have been identified as binding to a variety of carbohydrates in which the terminal sugar is a galactose with an α-linkage to an unfucosylated hexose (i.e., Galα1–Hex). This was first reported by Bird and Roy [10] and later by a number of groups, some with a focus on IgG and others on IgM [9, 11]. The Galα1–Hex antigens have included Galα1–2Gal [12], Galα1–3Gal [9], and Galα1–4Gal [11]. It was found that variable fractions of antibody against such antigens would cross-react, but that some fractions bind without cross-reactivity, each to a different naturally occurring Galα1–Hex structure [11]. (Cross-reactivity to synthetic Galα1–4Hex structures may be misleading: human anti-Galα1–2Gal, for instance, cross-reacts with synthetic Galα1–3Gal-silica conjugates, but not with naturally occurring Galα1–3Gal on rabbit red cells [11].)

Galili et al. [9] found that anti-Galα1–Hex antibody isolated from individuals was polyclonal; this is in keeping with the few earlier studies on the clonality of natural anti-carbohydrate antibodies in humans [13]. It was apparent, therefore, that some anti-Galα1–Hex antibodies can have a rather simple binding requirement, and be absorbable by many different Galα1–Hex structures, but that others have a specific requirement, at least to the level of the terminal linkage and the preterminal saccharide, and that within an individual such antibody can be polyclonal, presumably accounting for the variety of fine specificities expressed.

Polymorphism of Anti-Galα1–3Gal Antibody

It is now known that the human and Old World monkey IgG and IgM anti-pig antibodies, that are dominant in pig-to-primate organ xenotransplantation, can be absorbed by rabbit red cells [14], and that they are the same heterotopic antibodies as rabbit red cell agglutinins, with target antigens that terminate in Galα1–3Gal [15]. We were interested in the possible variation in fine specificity of these antibodies, as being of particular relevance to the development of immunoadsorbents and soluble inhibitors for use in pig-to-human xenotransplantation.

Dextra Laboratories Ltd. (Reading, UK) produced four oligosaccharides based on the pentaglycosylceramide Galα1–3Galβ1–4GlcNAcβ1–3Galβ1–4Glcβ1–1 ceramide that Hakomori's group had first identified in rabbit red cells [7] and which we and our collaborators had subsequently identified in pig aorta [16].

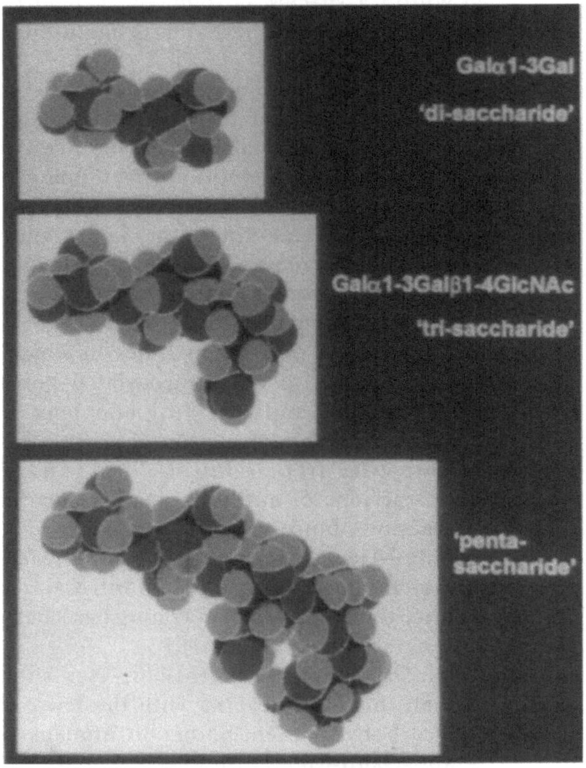

Fig. 1. Computer-derived images of three synthesized αGal antigens

The saccharides were (a) Galα1-3Gal (disaccharide), (b) Galα1-3Galβ1-4GlcNAc (type 2 trisaccharide), (c) Galα1-3Galβ1-4Glc (type 6 trisaccharide), and (d) Galα1-3Galβ1-4GlcNAcβ1-3Galβ1-4Glc (pentasaccharide) (Fig. 1). Each was provided conjugated to albumin for enzyme-linked immunosorbent assay (ELISA) and conjugated to Sepharose as an adsorbent. Although these were not necessarily representative of in vivo antigens (as described above for the different adsorbing properties of Galα1-3Gal-silica conjugates versus rabbit red cell Galα1-3Gal), it enabled the use of a panel of pure single antigens at consistent concentrations, and it was consistent with the principal aim of developing inhibitors or immunoadsorbents appropriate to the collection of anti-Galα1-3Gal antibodies.

We have tested binding of IgG and IgM to the di-, type 2 tri-, and pentasaccharide-albumin conjugates by ELISA in sera from 40 healthy humans, ten from each of the four ABO blood groups (O, A, B, and AB).

IgM Binding

IgM from 33 out of 40 individuals bound to all three saccharides. Binding to disaccharide was absent in six out of 40, and to pentasaccharide in one out of 40. Nine sera (which bound to all three saccharides) were tested further after immunoadsorption using either di- or pentasaccharide-Sepharose. In all cases, the di- and pentasaccharide Sepharoses absorbed out binding to their respective di- or pentasaccharide-albumin conjugates. However, in three out of nine cases the di-Sepharose failed to remove anti-pentasaccharide binding, and in seven out of nine the penta-Sepharose failed to remove the anti-disaccharide binding.

The penta-Sepharose revealed three adsorption patterns: (1) in two out of nine cases binding to all three saccharides was removed; (2) in three out of nine cases binding to tri- and pentasaccharide was removed, but not to disaccharide; and (3) in four out of nine cases only binding to pentasaccharide was removed.

In no case was there any binding that could not be removed by one or other saccharide Sepharose, if not both. The type 6 tri-Sepharose produced an identical absorption pattern to the penta-Sepharose.

IgG Binding

IgG binding to the three saccharides showed three distinct patterns: (1) 26 out of 40 bound to all three; (2) in eight out of 40 binding was absent to one of the three (trisaccharide in seven of eight, disaccharide in one of eight); (3) in six out of 40 there was binding to pentasaccharide only.

In the nine immunoabsorbed sera, penta-Sepharose removed all IgG activity, whereas di-Sepharose was only effective at complete absorption in two out of nine cases. Again, the type 6 tri-Sepharose produced an identical absorption pattern to the penta-Sepharose.

Our interpretation of these data is that anti-Galα1-3Gal antibody specificities vary between individuals, although there may be common patterns within populations. In addition, there is more than one anti-Galα1–3Gal specificity within an individual, as shown by the frequent requirement for more than one Galα1–3Gal-derived adsorbent.

We have also shown that these different specificities are all relevant to pig-to-human xenotransplantation, by performing serial adsorptions using the different Sepharoses so that antibodies can be eluted that react with only one of the saccharide–albumin conjugates. All such 'monoreactive', IgM are cytotoxic to pig lymphocytes, and all IgG and IgM eluates tested bind to pig tissue sections.

Comment

The possibility of such heterogeneity or polymorphism of anti-Galα1–3Gal antibody specificity has been alluded to before [17] and is consistent with the findings by isoelectric focusing followed by immune fixation of isolated anti-αGal preparations that suggested polyclonality [9]. Very similar studies of natural human Thomsen-Friedenreich antibodies using saccharides as inhibitors demonstrated that a pool of 100 sera contained Thomsen-Friedenreich antibodies that were a heterogeneous mixture of anti-carbohydrate specificities [18]. In the case of Thomsen-Friedenreich antibodies, as in the study described here and for A or B isoagglutinins, the antibodies are characterized according to their obligatory epitope requirement. However, within the family of antibodies so characterized, there are a number of different fine specificities. For anti-Galα1–3Gal antibodies, this population includes antibodies for which the isolated terminal Galα1–3Gal may be insufficient for binding, as in the case of sera in which anti-disaccharide binding is absent but anti-pentasaccharide binding present. This may represent a nonterminal carbohydrate epitope that nevertheless has a conformational requirement for the terminal residues, as has been described before for other anti-carbohydrate antibodies [19], or may be related to the effects of the terminal residues outside the antigen combining site, as described by Bundle et al. [20].

If this strategy of extracorporeal immunoadsorption of anti-Galα1–3Gal antibodies is to be utilized to induce a state of accommodation, then the consequence of this described polymorphism within the human population is a requirement for immunoadsorbent(s) sufficient to remove antibodies of all anti-Galα1–3Gal specificities.

References

1. LANDSTEINER, K. Zur Kenntis der antifermentativen, lytischen and agglutinierenden Wirkungen des Blutserums und der Lymphe. Centr. Bakt. Orig. 1900; 27:357
2. LANDOIS, L. In: Die Transfusion des Blutes. Vogel, Leipzig, 1875
3. LANDSTEINER, K. In: The Specificity of Serological Reactions. Dover, New York, 1962, p. 127

4. FRIEDBERGER, E., BOCK, G., FURSTENHEIM, A. Zur Normalantikoerkurve des Mensch durch die verschiedenen Lebensalter und ihre Bedeutung fur die Erklarung der Hautteste (Schick, Dick). Z. Immun.-Forsch. 1929; 64:294
5. TONDER, O., MILGROM, F. Studies on agglutination by macromolecular antibodies. I. Agglutination of rabbit erythrocytes by human sera. Vox. Sang. 1965; 10:708
6. TONDER, O., NATVIG, J., MATRE, R. Antibodies in human sera to rabbit erythrocytes. Immunology. 1967; 12:629
7. STELLNER, K., SAITO, H., HAKOMORI, S. Determination of aminosugar linkage in glycolipids by methylation. Aminosugar linkage of ceramide pentasaccharides of rabbit erythrocytes and of Forssman antigen. Arch. Biochem. Biophys. 1973; 155:464
8. SUZUKI, E., NAIKI, M. Heterophile antibodies to rabbit erythrocytes in human sera and identification of the antigen as a glycolipid. J. Biochem. 1984; 95:103
9. GALILI, U., MACHER, B., BUEHLER, J., et al. Human natural anti-α-galactosyl IgG. II. The specific recognition of α(1-3)-linked galactose residues. J. Exp. Med. 1985; 162:573
10. BIRD, G., ROY, T. Human serum antibodies to melibiose and other carbohydrates. Vox. Sang. 1980; 38:169
11. WIESLANDER, J., MANSSON, O., KALLIN, E., et al. Specificity of human antibodies against Galα1-3Gal carbohydrate epitope and distinction from natural antibodies reacting with Galα1-2Gal or Galα1-4Gal. Glycoconj. J. 1990; 7:85
12. AVILA, J., ROJAS, M., VELAZQUEZ-AVILA, G. Characterization of a natural human antibody with anti-galactosyl(α1-2)galactose specificity that is present in high titers in chronic Trypanosoma cruzi infection. Am. J. Trop. Med. Hyg. 1992; 47:413
13. RIEBEN, R., FRAUENFELDER, A., NYDEGGER, U. Naturally occurring ABO antibodies: long-term stable, individually distinct anti-A IgG spectrotypes. Eur. J. Immunol. 1992; 22:2129
14. HAMMELMANN, W., GRAY, D., CAIRNS, T., et al. Immediate destruction of xenogeneic islets in a primate model. Transplantation. 1994; 58:1109
15. GOOD, A.H., COOPER, D.K.C., MALCOLM, A.J., et al. Identification of carbohydrate structures that bind human antiporcine antibodies: implications for discordant xenografting in humans. Transplant. Proc. 1992; 24:559
16. SAMUELSSON, B., RYDBERG, L., BREIMER, M., et al. Natural antibodies and xenotransplantation. Immunol. Rev. 1994; 141;151
17. COOPER, D.K.C., KOREN, E., ORIOL, R. Oligosaccharides and discordant xenotransplantation. Immunol. Rev. 1994; 141:31
18. HOPPNER, W., FISCHER, K., POSCHMANN, A., et al. Use of synthetic antigens with the carbohydrate structure of asialoglycophorin A for the specification of Thomsen-Fredenreich antibodies. Vox. Sang. 1985; 48:246
19. CISAR, J., KABAT, E., DORNER, M., et al. Binding properties of immunoglobulin combining sites specific for terminal or nonterminal antigenic determinants in dextran. J. Exp. Med. 1975; 142:435
20. BUNDLE, D., EICHLER, E., GIDNEY, M., et al. Molecular recognition of a Salmonella trisaccharide epitope by monoclonal antibody Se155-4. Biochemistry. 1994; 33:5172.

6 Role of Complement in Xenograft Rejection

A.P. Dalmasso

Introduction

The immediate fate of a xenograft is largely dependent on the species relationship of the donor-host combination, which can be concordant or discordant. In a concordant combination donor and host belong to closely related species and there is no hyperacute rejection (HAR) of the transplant [1]. The recipient does not have preformed antibodies against the endothelium of the donor organ; in addition, the vascular endothelium of the donor does not directly activate recipient complement. In contrast, in a discordant combination complement activation by preexisting antibodies in the recipient or by the vascular endothelium of the donor organ causes HAR of the xenograft [2]. Biologically active fragments and protein complexes derived from complement activate and damage the endothelial cells of the graft, and recruit and activate recipient blood cells, resulting in interstitial edema, hemorrhage, and thrombosis, which ultimately destroy the graft within minutes or a few hours of revascularization.

The role of complement in HAR of a discordant xenograft is supported by early in vivo studies showing that during onset of xenograft rejection immunoglobulins and complement components accumulate in the grafted tissues. Moreover, induction of complement depletion with cobra venom factor (CVF) or use of recipients with genetic complement deficiencies resulted in prolonged survival of xenografts (reviewed in [3]). In addition to its role in HAR, complement may also be the major mediator of vascular rejection in certain concordant combinations after anti-endothelial cell antibodies are elicited in the recipient, as in hamster-to-rat heart transplants, which are rejected in a few days when sufficient anti-xenograft antibodies are produced [4].

The purpose of this chapter is to present a brief overview of the complement system and to discuss those aspects of complement that are relevant to the pathogenesis of tissue injury in xenograft rejection or that are amenable to inhibition as a potential approach to clinical xenotransplantation.

Overview of the Complement Reaction

The complement system is a major effector mechanism of various biological processes comprised of a large number of plasma and membrane-associated proteins. Complete discussion of the biochemistry and biology of complement can be found in previous publications [5–7]. The complement reaction mechanisms

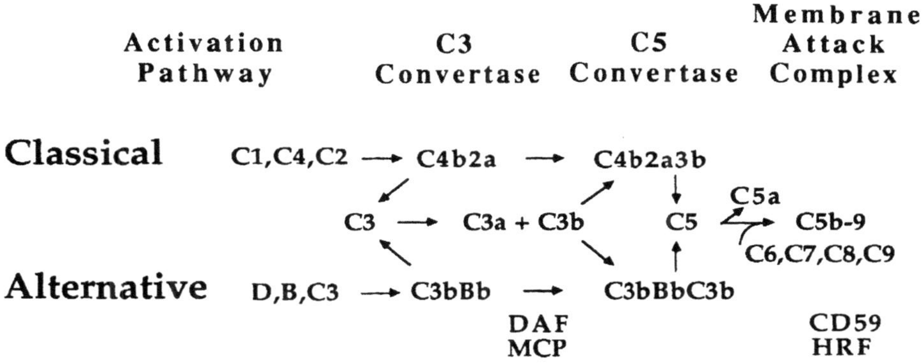

Fig. 1. Main pathways of complement activation. Also indicated are the membrane-associated complement inhibitors decay accelerating factor (*DAF*) and membrane cofactor protein (*MCP*) that inhibit the C3 and C5 convertases of both pathways, and CD59 and homologous restriction factor (*HRF*) that inhibit formation of the membrane attack complex (MAC). Soluble complement inhibitors are not shown

are activated mainly through the classical and alternative pathways (Fig. 1). Activation by either pathway results in generation of enzyme complexes that activate C3 and C5, followed by assembly of the membrane attack complex (MAC), which is shared by both pathways.

Activation Pathways

Activation of the classical pathway begins with C1, a protein complex that is composed of C1q, C1r, and C1s. Activation of C1 is accomplished mainly by IgM and IgG antibodies bound to an antigen, and requires binding of C1q by one molecule of IgM or two molecules of IgG. Activated C1s is formed, which cleaves C4 into C4a and C4b. In the presence of Mg^{2+}, C4b serves as receptor for C2, which is then cleaved by C1s into C2a and C2b. C2a remains bound to C4b, resulting in the C4b2a complex, or classical pathway C3 convertase, which cleaves C3 into C3a and C3b (Fig. 1). After removal of C3a, a highly reactive thiolester bond in C3 undergoes cleavage, which may result in covalent binding of C3b to free amino or hydroxyl groups. Of the multiple molecules of C3b that bind to a cell membrane, one binds closely to C4b2a, forming the C4b2a3b complex, which possesses C5 convertase activity. C5 is cleaved into C5a and C5b, and C5b interacts with the terminal complement proteins, resulting in assembly of the MAC.

Activation of the alternative pathway begins when modified C3 binds to certain molecules, such as bacterial polysaccharides or polymers of IgA, that protect the modified C3 from inactivation. The initial activating step involves rupture of the C3 thiolester bond, which results in a C3 product that is able to initiate activation of the alternative pathway. C3b is very effective in this regard. However, activation may also take place if the thiolester bond in C3 itself is cleaved due to its intrinsic lability, yielding the C3b-like molecule C3(H_2O). These two molecules can associate with factor B so that factor B becomes sensitive to cleavage by factor D, yielding the fragments Ba and Bb. Bb remains bound to the complex, which is known as alternative pathway C3 convertase (Fig. 1); Bb cleaves C3 into C3a and C3b, causing an amplification effect on alternative pathway activation. Addition of another C3b molecule to the C3bBb complex yields $(C3b)_2Bb$, or alternative pathway C5 convertase, that acts on C5 to produce C5a and C5b.

The assembly of the MAC begins as C5b combines with C6 and C7 to form the C5b-7 complex, which has high affinity for membrane lipid bilayers. Membrane-associated C5b-7 binds one molecule of C8, forming the C5b-8 complex, which then binds multiple molecules of C9. Membrane-bound C5b-8 can be cytotoxic, but this process is enhanced by C9. Because of the strong affinity of C5b-8 for phospholipids, the membrane bilayer is disrupted, causing increased permeability, which is further enhanced by the large channel formed by polymerized C9 [8]. The permeability changes may cause osmotic swelling and lysis of red cells. On the other hand, killing of nucleated cells by the MAC is independent of permeability changes and is associated with an increase in cellular Ca^{2+} and intracellular lipid metabolism, mitochondrial swelling, and hydrolysis of membrane lipids. In contrast to red cells, nucleated cells require multiple MAC deposition for irreversible damage to occur and are able to resist complement-mediated killing by endocytosis and exocytosis of bound MAC [9].

Control of Complement Activation

The initiation and progression of complement activation is regulated by multiple mechanisms such that every stage of the complement reaction is under control. Regulation of complement activation has evolved to protect the host against activation that occurs in inflammation and defense against microorganisms. This protection is accomplished through several plasma and membrane proteins that inhibit complement products. Control of complement activation is of major interest to xenotransplant biologists because the use of physiologic inhibitors of complement offers an opportunity for preventing complement-mediated tissue injury in xenotransplantation. Regulation of the classical pathway is provided by C1-inhibitor (C1-inh), which may bind irreversibly to activated C1r and C1s, blocking their enzymatic activity. The biological significance of C1-inh is demonstrated in patients with hereditary angioneurotic edema, a potentially life-threatening condition that is due to reduced functional activity of C1-inh [10].

Intensive control is centered around the C3 and C5 convertases of both activation pathways (see Fig. 1). There are two mechanisms that provide this control. The first is dissociation from the convertases of the enzymatic active proteins C2a and Bb. Some degree of control is due to the unstable nature of the association between the proteins of the convertases. Enhanced dissociation is provided by the interaction of the convertases with the plasma proteins C4b-binding protein and factor H, or with the membrane proteins decay-accelerating factor (DAF) and complement receptor type 1 (CR1, see Table 1) [11–13]. These inhibitors also prevent the association of C3b or C4b with Bb or C2a, respectively. The sec-

Table 1. Activities of human membrane-associated complement inhibitors

Inhibitor (synonyms)	Mechanism of inhibition	Activity in microbial infections
Decay-accelerating factor (DAF, CD55)	Dissociation of C3 and C5 convertases	Receptor for *Escherichia coli* and certain coxsackie- and echoviruses; host-derived DAF may coat HIV
Membrane cofactor protein (MCP, CD46)	Cofactor for inactivation of C3b by factor I	Receptor for measles virus and *Streptococcus pyogenes*
Complement receptor type 1 (CR1, CD35, C3b receptor)	Dissociation of C3 and C5 convertases and cofactor for inactivation of C3b by factor I	Receptor for C3b-coated *Mycobacteria*, *Leishmania*, *Legionella*, and *Babesia*
CD59 (protectin, HRF-20)	Inhibition of MAC formation	Host-derived CD59 may coat HIV
Homologous restriction factor (HRF, C8bp)	Inhibition of MAC formation	–

MAC, membrane attack complex; HIV, human immunodeficiency virus.

ond control mechanism at the C3, C5 convertase level consists of the inactivation of C3b and C4b by factor I-mediated proteolysis. This process requires that C3b or C4b first associate with a protein cofactor from plasma (factor H or C4b-binding protein) or the cell membrane (CR1 and membrane cofactor protein, MCP) (Table 1).

Another very important control mechanism consists of the inhibition of MAC formation by the proteins CD59 and homologous restriction factor (HRF) [14]. These proteins inhibit formation of the MAC through interaction with membrane-bound C5b-8 to impair the binding of C9 and with C5b-9 to block additional binding and polymerization of C9. Finally, other plasma proteins that control complement are properdin, vitronectin and clusterin. Properdin binds to and stabilizes the alternative pathway C3 convertase. Vitronectin and clusterin are multifunctional proteins that interact with late-acting complement components as complexes assemble in plasma and thus inhibit binding of the protein complex to cell membranes.

DAF, CD59, and HRF all act intrinsically, i.e., they inhibit the complement reaction only at the membrane sites where they are located. These proteins are anchored to the membrane through a glycosyl phosphatidylinositol moiety. The biological importance of these inhibitors to protect host cells against uncontrolled activation of autologous complement is shown in patients with paroxysmal nocturnal hemoglobinuria, whose erythrocytes and other cells are deficient in phosphatidylinositol-linked membrane inhibitors and show enhanced susceptibility to complement lysis [15]. This disease highlights the biological significance of these inhibitors as effective protective mechanisms for host tissues against autologous complement. MCP and CR1 are linked to the membrane through a hydrophobic peptide. Whereas MCP acts intrinsically, CR1 acts extrinsically as it is a very elongated molecule, with binding sites for C3b and C4b that are relatively remote from the cell membrane where CR1 is anchored [11]. Membrane-associated inhibitors are expressed on most cells that are in contact with blood or other biological fluids containing complement. These proteins are inhibitory to homologous complement and have little inhibitory capacity upon complement from a different species; for example, a porcine inhibitor that may be present on porcine endothelial cells probably does not inhibit human complement efficiently. Therefore, a few years ago we postulated that the presence on the xenograft endothelium of complement inhibitors of the recipient could be used to protect a xenograft [16].

Biological Role of Complement

Complement has multiple functional activities that emerge at different phases of the complement reaction and generally serve a useful purpose, mostly in defense against invading microbes [5–7]. Complement-dependent functions that contribute to this task generally promote inflammation and include increment in vascular permeability, attraction of phagocytic cells, enhancement of phagocytosis, cytotoxicity, etc. The mechanisms employed by complement in inflammation also operate in graft rejection [3, 17]. C3a and C5a cause increment in vascular permeability, contraction of smooth muscle, release of mediators from mast cells and polymorphonuclear leukocytes, and generation of oxygen radicals. C4a may also induce these effects but is a much weaker mediator than C3a and C5a. C5a is a potent chemotactic agent that promotes leukocyte adhesion and stimulates the cyclooxygenase pathway. The terminal components stimulate the conversion of arachidonic acid into various metabolic products, including prostaglandin I_2 (PGI_2), and production of oxygen radicals. The MAC also induces prothrombinase activity in platelets and endothelial cells [18].

In spite of these powerful proinflammatory effects, individuals with severe complement deficiencies do not have defective inflammatory reactions, due to the redundancy of mechanisms that promote inflammation. On the other hand, certain complement deficiencies severely compromise the ability to control certain infections, due to the significance of complement in bacterial opsonization. C3b and iC3b enhance phagocytosis of microorganisms by polymorphonuclear leukocytes and macrophages. Bb promotes macrophage spreading and enhances killing efficiency. The MAC is important to prevent dissemination of neisserial infections. C3b and C4b may neutralize virus infectivity by blocking attachment sites to host cells, and the MAC may kill certain viruses. Complement activity is of major importance in preventing the pathogenic effects of antigen–antibody complexes. Finally, several stages of complement activation participate in the regulation of the immune response, both cellular immunity and antibody formation.

Complement in Hyperacute Rejection

In HAR the xenograft is rapidly lost due to humoral mechanisms that use complement as the major effector system. Once complement is activated, biologically active protein fragments and complexes are generated from several of its components. These products are able to directly cause tissue injury and also to recruit other effector mechanisms that ultimately result in the destruction of the graft.

Pathways of Complement Activation

The initiation of complement activation during HAR may occur through the classical pathway due to binding of preexisting antibodies to the vascular endothelium of the graft or through the alternative pathway due to its direct activation by the donor endothelium.Complement activation in HAR of porcine organs transplanted into primates is initiated by deposition of IgM and activation of the classical pathway [19]. Immunohistochemistry of porcine hearts transplanted into untreated rhesus monkeys, macaques and baboons early during rejection showed deposits of classical pathway proteins along endothelial surfaces, with a distribution similar to that of IgM, and only trace deposits of alternative pathway proteins. Importantly, porcine hearts experienced no HAR upon transplantation in rhesus monkeys with normal serum complement levels but in which natural antibodies had been depleted. In cases in which the graft continued to function for several days without evidence of rejection when the animals were sacrificed, little or no complement was deposited in the surviving xenograft. Thus, in rhesus monkeys with normal complement levels, complement was not activated directly by a porcine xenograft and therefore the xenograft would not by itself trigger rejection [19].

Complement activation in discordant xenograft rejection has also been studied in an in vitro model system consisting of cultured porcine endothelial cell monolayers as targets incubated with human serum as a source of natural antibody and complement. Normal human serum was cytotoxic to porcine endothelial cells via the classical pathway. Binding of iC3b to the endothelial cells and cytotoxicity required the presence of IgM natural antibodies and components of the classical pathway; the alternative pathway did not appear to be primarily involved [19]. Recently it has been shown that xenogeneic human IgA natural antibodies bind to porcine endothelial cells in vitro, and that dimeric IgA, but not monomeric IgA, is able to activate complement via the alternative pathway [20]. Although dimeric IgA comprises a small proportion of total serum IgA, it may contain a significant amount of xenoreactive natural antibodies and, under certain conditions, might play a role in xenograft tissue injury. However, IgA does not appear to be primarily involved in HAR in pig-to-primate combinations. Recently we performed immunoabsorption of human plasma with an anti-IgM column, which caused reduction of IgM but no depletion of IgA levels. Ex vivo perfusion of swine hearts with the IgM-reduced human blood resulted in a delayed and milder form of rejection than with normal blood, in spite of preserved levels of IgA [21]. Thus IgA and activation of the alternative pathway in this model likely do not contribute substantially to tissue injury. Small amounts of residual IgM natural antibodies may have been more important than dimeric IgA natural antibodies in causing delayed loss of organ function in this model.

In certain xenograft models complement is activated via the alternative pathway. In the guinea pig-to-rat model the primary activation event may involve the alternative pathway or both pathways, depending on the strain of the recipient rat [22, 23]. In rabbit-to-newborn pig xenografts complement appears to be activated via the alternative pathway [24]. It has been recently shown that when a rat heart is transplanted into a lamb fetus HAR is mediated by activation of the alternative pathway, without participation of IgM or IgG [25].

Role of Complement in the Pathogenesis of Tissue Injury in Hyperacute Rejection

The rapid destruction of discordant xenografts that is triggered by complement activation involves the activation of the endothelial cells of the xenograft and the platelets, leukocytes and plasma proteins of the recipient. The participation of complement and the recruitment of other mediators of inflammation and coagulation result in loss of the endothelial cell barrier function, followed rapidly by interstitial edema, hemorrhage, and thrombosis, the hallmarks of HAR. Many of these processes result directly or indirectly from the biological activity of complement-derived protein fragments, as summarized in Table 2. This information has been derived in part from studies in animals that are genetically complement deficient or made hypocomplemententemic experimentally. Discordant xenografts in these animals have prolonged survival but rejection finally destroys the transplant.

Thus, in C4-deficient guinea pigs, rejection of a rat cardiac transplant occurred in 3.5 days, in contrast to 22 min in controls, and was associated with cellular infiltration [26]. The role of complement was studied by treating the recipients with CVF so that virtually complete complement deficiency would be maintained for several days. In CVF-treated rats the mean survival time of a guinea pig cardiac xenograft was prolonged from 19 min in controls to 3.7 days [27]; these rats had higher levels of anti-guinea pig antibodies than controls. These xenografts showed leukocyte margination along blood vessels, beginning at 12 h post-transplant. Progressive cell infiltration, interstitial hemorrhage,

Table 2. Pathophysiologic effects of complement fragments and complexes that may contribute to xenograft hyperacute rejection

Complement fragment or complex	Target	Pathophysiologic effect
C1q	Recipient platelets and leukocytes	Adhesion and secretion
C3a, C5a	Graft vasculature	Vasoconstriction, increased permeability
	Graft endothelium	Activation
	Recipient granulocytes and monocytes	Adhesion, chemotaxis and release of oxygen radicals and enzymes
C5a	Graft endothelium	Heparan sulfate release[a] and induction of other thrombogenic properties
iC3b	Graft endothelium	Granulocyte adhesion
C5b-7	Graft endothelium	Endothelial cell retraction and gap formation
C5b-9	Graft endothelium	Decreased anticoagulant and increased procoagulant properties; may cause cell death
	Recipient platelets	Prothrombinase activity

[a] C5a in combination with natural antibodies.

and necrosis were observed over the next 72 h. Rejected grafts showed diffuse deposition of IgM and fibrin within blood vessels and nonspecific staining for IgG, but no C3 deposition [28]. Xenograft survival of a pig heart in baboons receiving CVF alone was prolonged to 68–92 h, compared with less than 90 min in controls [27, 29]. Severe vascular rejection occurred in a xenograft lost at 68 h, and the heart that was rejected at 92 h also had areas of perivascular and interstitial mononuclear cell infiltration. There was diffuse deposition of IgM, C4 and fibrin, but no C3 or MAC. Thus, these experiments in which HAR is prevented in complement-deficient recipients suggest that a xenograft undergoes delayed rejection in 3–4 days by humoral or early cellular effector mechanisms independent of complement.

An important role for the MAC in xenograft HAR was first suggested by the prolonged survival of a xenogeneic heart in C6-deficient rabbits [30, 31]. Recent studies showed that a guinea pig heart survived for 1–2 days in C6-deficient rats, in contrast to less than 20 min in controls; rejection was associated with granulocyte and monocyte infiltrates [32]. The shorter xenograft survival in the C6-deficient rats (1–2 days) in comparison to normal rats treated with CVF (3–4 days) may be due to the ability of C6-deficient rats to generate C3a and C5a. In fact, if C6-deficient rats are given CVF to destroy C3 and C5, graft survival was prolonged to 3–4 days, with less cell infiltration [33]. Results similar to those with CVF were obtained when the C6-deficient rats were given dexamethasone [34] or recombinant neutrophil-inhibiting factor, a hookworm glycoprotein that inhibits CD11b/CD18 (Mac-1) and blocks binding of neutrophils and macrophages to endothelial cell-bound iC3b [35]. We have recently suggested that C5a and the MAC have a predominant role in HAR of a porcine heart perfused ex vivo with human blood [36]. A porcine heart perfused with unmodified human blood survived only 25 min, with histologic and immunopathologic characteristics of HAR. Addition of a monoclonal antibody against human C5 to the human blood extended heart survival in a dose-dependent manner (Fig. 2). With 200 μg anti-C5 per ml human blood, the pig heart continued to function

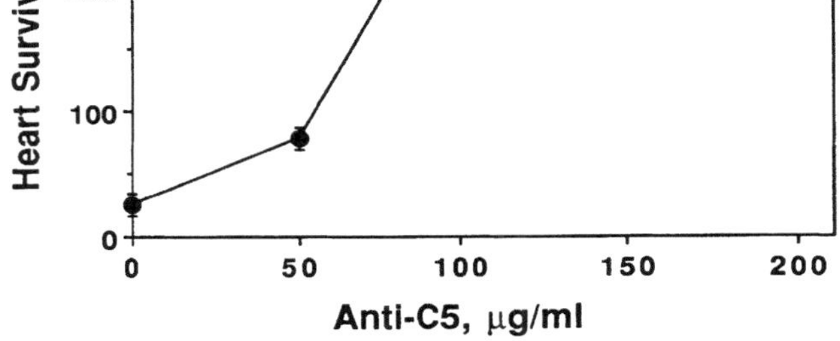

Fig. 2. Suppression by an anti-C5 monoclonal antibody of hyperacute rejection of a porcine heart perfused ex vivo with human blood. Dose-response relationship of the antibody concentration in human blood and the time to cessation of cardiac function. Results of controls with blood containing no anti-C5 are the mean ± SE of five experiments. Results of perfusions with human blood containing anti-C5 are means ± range of two experiments for each antibody concentration (from [36])

for 6 h, at which time the experiment was discontinued, without evidence of HAR and no tissue deposition of MAC. A major role for the MAC alone in HAR was supported by the ability of an anti-C8 monoclonal antibody to protect a rat heart from injury caused by perfusion with human serum [37].

In cases of discordant xenografts with intense complement activation due to high levels of IgM natural antibodies or a very effective triggering of the alternative pathway there may be sufficient MAC formation for endothelial cell killing and detachment, with exposure of the subendothelial matrix. However, before endothelial cell killing takes place or when limiting amounts of antibody or complement prevail, endothelial cell activation precedes cytotoxicity and may mediate progress toward HAR without complement-induced cytotoxicity [2]. Activation is characterized by functionally important changes in the expression of various cell constituents that may result in loss of the endothelial cell permeability barrier and anticoagulant properties and the gain of a procoagulant state. A manifestation of endothelial cell activation that may occur during HAR is the loss of heparan sulfate from porcine endothelial cells induced by human serum [38]. Heparan sulfate contributes to blood vessel barrier functions, maintenance of an anticoagulant environment, and inhibition of injury by oxygen and free radicals. We found that incubation of cultured porcine endothelial cells with natural antibody and complement in human serum caused the rapid release of a large proportion of the endothelial cell-associated heparan sulfate chains. The release preceded irreversible cell injury and was dependant upon natural antibody binding and classical complement pathway activation for generation of C5a [39]. It has recently been reported that deposition of C5b-7 on xenogeneic endothelial cells may be of major significance to the development of HAR [40]. C5b-7 was found to cause endothelial cell retraction in vitro, with formation of transient gaps between endothelial cells, through which blood cells and macromolecules could easily escape. This process may expose the subendothelium and allow platelets to adhere to collagen. The effect of C5b-7 is reversed by incorporation of C8 and C9 to C5b-7 during formation of the MAC.

Other complement-mediated changes in endothelial cell physiology could play significant roles in HAR (Table 2). Thus, after exposure to natural antibody and complement in human serum, porcine endothelial cells express membrane-bound tissue factor and lose thrombomodulin activity. C1q associated to endothelial cell-bound antibody may promote adhesion of platelets and leukocytes to the endothelium [41]. Endothelial cell-bound iC3b causes neutrophils to adhere to the endothelium through the neutrophil integrin CD11b/CD18, or CR3 [42]. Other complement fragments may participate in production of tissue pathology in HAR of a discordant xenograft. C3a and C5a may cause vasoconstriction and polymorphonuclear leukocyte adherence to the vascular endothelium. The MAC in sublytic amounts may cause Ca^{2+} influx and cell activation, resulting in release of reactive oxygen products, eicosanoids and cytokines. Among the effects of complement on endothelial cells is the release of vasoactive PGE_2 and thromboxane A_2 (TXA_2), which cause vasoconstriction and disruption of cytoskeletal actin microfilaments with widening of interendothelial junctions and increased permeability [43]. The MAC may promote thrombosis by inducing endothelial cell membrane vesiculation and assembly of the prothrombinase complex [18]. The

MAC may also contribute to injury by reducing endothelium-dependent relaxation of coronary arteries [44]. These processes may initiate injury to the grafted organ before complement-mediated endothelial cell killing takes place.

Possible Role of Complement in Delayed Xenograft Rejection

The experiments in which HAR is prevented in complement-deficient recipients showed that a xenograft is rejected after several days by humoral or early cellular effector mechanisms independent of complement [27, 28, 45]. The rejection demonstrates a morphology similar to that of vascular rejection, with infiltration of mononuclear cells but with minimal presence of T cells. This form of xenograft loss has been called delayed rejection or acute vascular rejection. In these models of delayed rejection a pathogenic role of antibodies has been considered, possibly through antibody-dependent cell cytotoxicity or other mechanisms [46, 47]. It is generally assumed that complement is not involved in delayed rejection. However, antibodies may interact with early components of the classical pathway, binding C1 and generating functionally weak but possibly significant C4a. Small amounts of C3 and C5 convertases and MAC may be formed in recipient animals treated with complement inhibitors. In experiments that use CVF to inactivate complement there is production of C3a and C5a which can activate host leukocytes, facilitating leukocyte binding and injury to xenogeneic endothelium. Complement proteins synthesized by the endothelium of the donor organ may also play a role. Antibodies alone, or with some level of complement activation, may be able to induce changes in the endothelial cells that are characteristic of an activation state, which in turn would contribute to delayed rejection [48]. Among these changes are activation of cytokine genes, expression of adhesion molecules, and changes from an anticoagulant to a procoagulant phenotype on the endothelial surface. At present little is known about the possible contribution of complement in eliciting delayed rejection of discordant xenografts.

Protection of the Xenogeneic Vascular Endothelium Against Complement

Because the vascular endothelium of the xenograft is the central target of activated complement this section focuses on strategies for protection of the endothelium from complement activation. As the blood cells of the recipient also participate in the pathogenesis of vascular rejection, often through a complement-mediated activation process, inhibition of complement activation would also prevent certain injurious effects of recipient cells on the xenograft. In recipient combinations in which HAR is triggered by natural antibodies against donor endothelial cells, such as in a primate transplanted with a porcine organ, an approach to inhibit HAR has been to remove the antibodies and use immunosuppressive therapy to maintain low antibody levels. However, it is likely that abrogation of HAR may also require inhibition of complement activation, especially in the initial post-transplant phase. The value of complement inhibition to control HAR was suggested by early observations that administration of CVF strongly suppressed HAR (reviewed in [3]). Consideration has been given to interfering with HAR by administraton of fluid phase complement inhibitors as well as by expression on xenogeneic endothelium membrane complement inhibitors of the recipient species. However, there are other possibilities that may result in protection of a xenogeneic endothelium against attack by complement that should also be considered as potential interventions for xenografting.

Antibody-Induced Endothelial Cell Protection Against Complement

Because it is possible that human natural antibodies can directly induce some form of activation of xenogeneic endothelial cells, independent of complement, we investigated whether prolonged exposure of porcine endothelial cells to anti-pig natural antibodies changed their subsequent interaction with complement [49]. We incubated porcine endothelial cells at 37 °C for 1 h or 40 h with a source of human natural antibodies. We found that, in comparison to 1 h of incubation with natural antibodies, the cells that were incubated for 40 h became markedly resistant to complement-mediated cytotoxicity. These cells processed part of the bound IgM antibodies, but not the bound IgG antibodies. They bound additional IgM antibodies, but not IgG, when re-exposed to antibody for a short period of time; thus prolonged incubation with IgM antibodies did not cause loss of endothelial cells membrane antigens. The cells incubated for 40 h showed no impairment in the ability to bind complement components. The induction of resistance to complement killing required protein synthesis and could be induced with purified human IgM but not with purified IgG (Fig. 3), and was due to the presence of anti-pig xenoreactive natural antibodies.

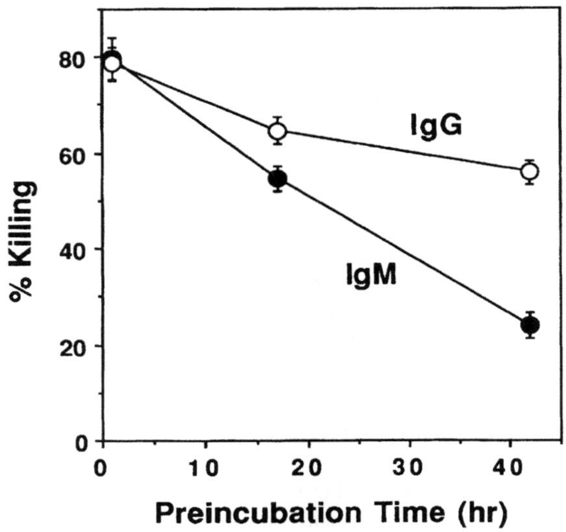

Fig. 3. Preincubation of porcine endothelial cells with purified human IgM containing anti-pig natural antibodies induces resistance of the cells to complement-mediated killing. Porcine endo-thelial cells were preincubated for various periods of time at 37 °C with purified human IgM (1.0 mg/ml) or purified human IgG (7.5 mg/ml). The cells were then incubated for 4 h at 37 °C with 40 % human serum as a source of natural antibodies and complement. Cytotoxicity was measured with a vital dye assay. IgG did not induce resistance, as the results with IgG were similar to those with medium alone (not shown). (From [49] with permission from Munksgaard International Publishers, Copenhagen, Denmark)

These observations may be of value to enhance survival of a xenograft. To the extent that the resistance of endothelial cells to complement injury was induced with anti-endothelial cell antibodies, this resistance may be analogous to accommodation that was described in a hamster-to-rat model of concordant xenografting [4]. In this model, complement depletion with CVF and suppression of cellular immunity allowed the xenograft to acquire the ability to survive when challenged by cytotoxic antibodies in the presence of normal levels of complement. Thus, in this model the presence of anti-endothelial cell antibodies may have played the critical role in induction of resistance of the graft to a subsequent exposure to antibody and complement.

Protection of Endothelial Cells Against Complement Induced by Other Modifications in the Recipient (Accommodation)

Although exposure to xenogeneic antibody may markedly reduce the response of endothelial cells to complement, this is in contrast to the induction of accommodation in allografts that was accomplished by removal of preformed antibodies in the recipient. Whether or not a condition similar to allograft accommodation can be induced in a discordant xenograft remains an open question. Accommodation is a concept that originated from observations in human renal allotransplantation across the ABO barrier. An allograft may undergo HAR when a recipient contains preformed antibodies, such as anti-A, -B, or -HLA, against antigens in the transplanted organ. In these cases, depletion of antibodies at the time of engraftment has proven critical to avert HAR. The transplant usually is not rejected when the antibody levels return a few weeks after transplantation, in spite of normal complement and persistence of donor antigen on the vascular endothelium of the graft [50, 51]. Very little is known regarding mechanisms involved in accommodation. Possibly the transplanted organ undergoes major changes in expression of critical components of its vascular endothelium; candidates include endothelial cell epitopes, membrane complement regulators, and adhesion molecules. An endothelial cell receptor may lose the ability to respond to its agonist after the initial stimulation, or the properties of the antibodies in the host may change such that they lose pathogenicity [52].

Accommodation has been induced experimentally in primates undergoing allotransplantation. Survival of organ transplants in baboons that were hyperimmunized against blood group A or B antigens was achieved by continuous administration of the specific A or B trisaccharide; when this treatment was discontinued the organ was not immediately rejected, in spite of the presence of high levels of antibodies [53]. It was also suggested that a process similar to accommodation might take place with xenografts. When xenografts in primate experiments achieved prolonged survival, it was speculated that this result might in part be explained by accommodation, as in some animals the xenograft was able to survive despite the return of antibodies [19, 54]. However, long-term accommodation has not been achieved in discordant xenotransplantation. Understanding the mechanisms that lead to induction of protection of the xenograft against immunological injury would represent a major advance for the prospect of clinical xenotransplantation.

Protection of the Xenogeneic Endothelium by Expression of Membrane-Associated Complement Regulators of the Recipient

Membrane complement inhibitors are important to protect cells from potentially harmful effects of activated autologous complement [11, 12]. However, inhibitors that may be present on vascular endothelial cells of a xenogeneic graft usually do not inhibit complement from a discordant recipient efficiently. Therefore we proposed that the expression on the xenograft endothelium of complement inhibitors of the recipient species would constitute an efficient strategy to protect a xenograft [16]. We postulated that expression of the recipient inhibitors DAF, CD46 and/or CD59 on the vascular endothelial cell membranes of a xenogeneic organ would cause inhibition of recipient complement. We demonstrated the potential for this approach by incorporating human DAF into porcine endothelial cell membranes where it protected the cells from the cytotoxic effects of human complement [16]. Nonhuman cells that were transfected with cDNA for human complement regulators expressed the corresponding proteins on the cell membrane and were also protected from attack by human complement [55–58].

Expression of Inhibitors in Transgenic Animals (see also Chaps. 47–49)

Transgenic donor animals that express human complement inhibitors have been prepared for use in experimental xenotransplantation in primates [59–64]. A positive aspect of this approach is that systemic complement activation is not impaired by localization of recipient complement regulatory proteins in the graft. This approach could potentially be used in xenotransplantation of porcine organs to humans, together with other genetic manipulations of the donor such as disabling the genes for enzymes that synthesize endothelial cell carbohydrate antigens that are the main target for natural antibodies of the recipient [65]. Methods based on genetic manipulations of the donor may provide long-term safeguard against complement-mediated rejection.

The development of transgenic animals with improved expression of human membrane complement inhibitors clearly seems to be a most fruitful area to advance preclinical xenografting. Data continue to accumulate that activation and destruction of xenogeneic endothelial cells can be inhibited with this approach. Particularly promising are technologies based on yeast artificial chromosomes that would allow the use of constructs that contain the regulatory regions as they exist in the human chromosome and the preparation of transgenic animals with one construct for expression of several inhibitors [64]. The use of promoters such as that from the ICAM-2 gene which direct expression preferentially to endothelial cells also appears to be very attractive [66]. As expected, organs from transgenic animals that express both hMCP and hDAF are better protected than organs expressing only one of the inhibitors [63]. Another approach of considerable interest is the development of chimeric complement inhibitors that act at different points in the complement reaction, as the recently developed hDAF-CD59 chimeric molecule that contains the functional domains of DAF and CD59 [67].

With regard to the production of transgenic animals, it is of interest that the expression of significant quantities of transgenic hDAF on porcine spermatozoa does not compromise the breeding potential of these animals [68]. Another consideration is that human membrane inhibitors are able to interact with certain infectious agents, often to specifically serve as receptors for microbial entry to a host cell [69], as summarized in Table 1. Thus these interactions raise the possibility that transgenic animals that express human inhibitors such as DAF, MCP, and CD59 may be susceptible to certain human pathogens. Therefore, when vaccines for the relevant pathogen are available, these animals may have to be vaccinated against those organisms.

Expression of Inhibitors Induced by In Vivo Transfection

In vivo transfection strategies to provide vascular endothelial cells with inhibitors of HAR are being considered as alternatives to transgenic animals. Thus, adenovirus-mediated transfer of hCD59 cDNA into rat endothelial cells resulted in expression of functional hCD59; however, the transduced cells showed indications of activation, with increased expression of MHC class I antigens and ICAM-1 [70]. On the other hand, in vivo hDAF gene transfection prevented tissue injury in a model of HAR of a porcine lung perfused with human blood; expression of hDAF inhibited elevations in pulmonary vascular resistance and development of pulmonary edema, and preserved gas transport [71].

Inhibitors Acquired from the Recipient

In transgenic donors that express the human complement inhibitor DAF or CD59 selectively on erythrocytes, the inhibitors may transfer to the endothelial cells of an organ like the heart [72]. Transfer may be mediated by the glycosyl phosphatidylinositol that anchors these proteins to cell membranes. When a pig heart that had acquired human inhibitors by transfer from red cells was transplanted into a baboon there was protection from HAR [59]. We therefore investigated whether porcine xenografts from unmodified donors would acquire recipient inhibitors while surviving in baboons depleted of antibodies to prevent HAR. In pig hearts or kidneys that survived up to 2 weeks we found no transfer of immunologically reactive DAF or CD59 from recipient blood cells to the vascular endothelium of the xenograft [73]. Thus protection of the xenograft appeared not to have been facilitated by a potential transfer of recipient membrane inhibitors to the endothelium of the xenograft.

Inhibition of Complement Activation with Soluble Molecules

The use of soluble complement inhibitors in xenotransplantation is of great interest, both to understand mechanisms of delayed rejection and also for potential clinical applications. The administration of a soluble inhibitor to a recipient of an organ xenograft that expresses human complement inhibitors may be important in the early period following engraftment. Most complement inhibitors of interest are directly or indirectly related to physiologic inhibitory mechanisms of complement activation. Other complement inhibitors that have been studied for use in xenotransplantation, such as FUT175 and K76, do not appear to provide sufficient inhibition to prevent HAR [74].

C1 Inhibitor and Heparin

In combinations where complement activation is mediated by the classical pathway, its selective inhibition to suppress HAR would be desirable to maintain the alternative pathway for protection of the recipient. Addition of C1-inh to human serum in vitro was found to inhibit porcine endothelial cell activation and cytotoxicity [75]. Relatively large amounts of C1-inh were needed as complete inhibition of cytotoxicity required about 40 times the C1-inh concentration of normal human serum. High concentrations are needed because C1-inh is only moderately effective when activation is triggered by strong activators like antigen-antibody complexes.

On the other hand, the effect of C1-inh is known to be enhanced by heparin. Therefore, we examined in vitro the inhibitory effect of the combination of heparin and C1-inh [76]. Deposition of C4b on pig endothelial cells exposed to human serum was strongly suppressed by addition of C1-inh plus heparin to the serum (Fig. 4), an approach that may be effective to avert HAR mediated by the classical pathway. The effect of heparin was also tested in vivo for protection against complement-mediated loss of heparan sulfate that may play a role in HAR. Non-anticoagulant heparin was tested to ascertain if it would alter the fate of heparan sulfate in guinea pig hearts radioactively labeled with [^{35}S]sulfate and

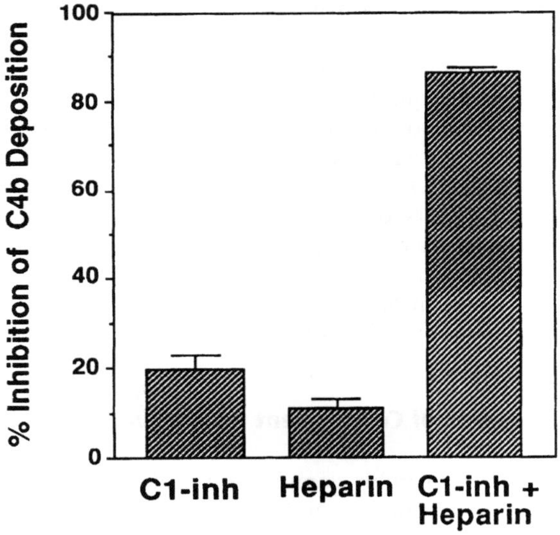

Fig. 4. Inhibitory effect of C1-inh and heparin on C4b deposition upon incubation of porcine endothelial cells with human serum as a source of natural antibodies and complement. Endothelial cells were incubated for 1 h at 37 °C with unsupplemented human serum to determine the 100 % level of C4b binding, or with human serum supplemented with 42 μ*M* C1-inhibitor (*C1-inh*), 500 μg heparin/ml, or both substances together. Binding of C4b was measured with an endothelial cell enzyme-linked immunosorbent assay (from [76])

transplanted into rats [77]. Heparin administration inhibited the release of heparan sulfate from the transplanted heart, prolonged the survival of the transplant and reduced the amount of C3b bound to the heart, in comparison to control animals.

Soluble CR1 and MCP (see also Chap. 33)

Interesting advances are being made with the use of soluble forms of membrane inhibitors that are obtained by recombinant technology using constructs without the membrane anchor region. A fluid phase complement inhibitor of great interest is the recombinant soluble form of human CR1 (sCR1), which inhibits complement in primates and other species [78]. Administration of sCR1 to rats caused a dose-dependent prolongation of the survival of a guinea pig heart transplant [79, 80]. Administration of a single dose (15 mg/kg) of sCR1 to cynomolgus monkeys prolonged the survival of a pig cardiac xenograft to 48–90 h, in comparison to rejection in less than 1 h in untreated controls [81]. Recent studies have shown that the continuous infusion of sCR1 (40 mg/kg per day) in cynomolgous monkeys maintained complement levels at less than 20 % of preinfusion values and prolonged pig heart survival to 5–7 days, while addition of immunosuppression could extend survival for several weeks [82]. The development of a modified sCR1 molecule that has a binding site for selectins to help localize the inhibitor to the site where the rejection process is taking place is of much current interest [83]. A new human recombinant complement inhibitor, soluble membrane cofactor protein, was found to be able to protect mouse endothelial cell from complement attack when present in the fluid phase [84].

Cobra Venom Factor (see also Chap. 32)

CVF is a protein analogous to C3b that binds factor B strongly but is resistant to inactivation by factor I, resulting in a very stable alternative pathway C3 convertase [85]. Therefore, administration of CVF causes inactivation of C3, C5, and terminal components. A disadvantage of CVF is that its anti-complement effect is achieved by complement activation, with generation of C3a and C5a that may be injurious to the recipient and the graft. In addition, CVF is highly immunogenic and may elicit antibodies that may render it ineffective. We have used CVF in conjunction with antibody depletion and immunosuppression to investigate the survival of a porcine cardiac xenograft in baboons [29]. Repeated administration of CVF to baboons caused marked complement depletion with minimal morbidity. One xenograft that survived 17 days had some intravascular coagulation but no clear evidence of rejection. Another xenograft functioned for 8 days, until the recipient was sacrificed, without evidence of rejection. In contrast, complement depletion alone with CVF extended graft survival to 3–4 days [29], while antibody depletion with immunosuppression prevented HAR and prolonged graft survival for several days [86]. Thus depletion of antibody and complement combined with immunosuppression achieved marked prolongation of xenograft survival.

A limitation to prolonged use of CVF and soluble CR1 in combinations in which complement is activated via the classical pathway is that these reagents also interfere with the alternative pathway that may be critical to prevent infections in immunosuppressed individuals.

Intravenous IgG (see also Chaps. 30 and 31)

IgG in large doses is an effective complement inhibitor, as a large concentration of IgG around target cells effectively competes for binding of C3b and C4b [87]. IgG has recently been shown to extend graft survival in guinea pig-to-rat [88, 89] and pig-to-human [90] combinations. When IgG was used together with conventional immunosuppression in pig-to-primate combinations graft survival was extended up to 10 days [90]. Addition of IgG in vitro to human serum reduced the binding of C3b to porcine endothelial cells, likely through decreased formation of C3 convertase on the cells [90].

Antibodies Against Complement Components

Antibodies against certain components or activation fragments of complement may have a role in protecting a xenograft, especially recombinant humanized derivatives of monoclonal antibodies [91]. We have recently demonstrated suppression of HAR with an anti-C5 monoclonal antibody in an ex vivo model of pig-to-human xenografting (Fig. 2) [36]. A monoclonal antibody against C8 protected a rat heart from damage caused by perfusion with human blood [37].

Comment

Complement continues to be actively studied with regard to its central pathophysiologic role in xenograft rejection and also as a target for inhibition in efforts to control HAR. There has been considerable progress in understanding the role of complement in the pathophysiology of HAR, with delineation of the specific involvement of various complement fragments and complexes. The prevention of HAR will probably require different interventions, including the use antibody depletion and complement inhibition. Currently, these methods have been effective to extend xenograft survival for only a few weeks.

At present, abrogation of HAR makes it possible to begin addressing issues related to mechanisms and control of delayed xenograft rejection. Further studies are needed to establish the role that complement might play in delayed xenograft rejection. In this regard current methods to avoid HAR are imperfect, and thus it is not clear whether certain phenotypic characteristics that appear in the xenograft during delayed rejection are not merely a reflection of the incomplete inhibition of complement activation in the recipient as induced by various experimental strategies.

One approach that may facilitate prolonged survival is to alter the antigenicity of the xenogeneic vascular endothelium by genetic manipulations of the donor to obtain modified expression of epitopes involved in binding of natural antibodies.

These donors would also express on their vascular endothelium membrane complement inhibitors like DAF and CD59 of the recipient species. Further work is also needed to improve methods to enhance expression of complement inhibitors in donor organs and to assure protection of the graft through continuing expression of the inhibitor. Another important area is to understand which other manipulations can be applied to the donor endothelium in order to reduce its reactivity with complement, especially if this reduction could be a part of accommodation. Evaluation of the efficacy of various approaches is hampered by the unavailability of immunosuppressive drugs of low toxicity, including drugs that are more effective for inhibition of antibody formation.

Acknowledgments. Work performed in the author's laboratory has been supported by the Department of Veterans Affairs Medical Research and the Minnesota Medical Foundation. The author is indebted to Barbara A. Benson for her assistance in the preparation of the manuscript.

References

1. Calne, R.Y. Organ transplantation between widely disparate species. Transplant. Proc. 2, 550, 1970
2. Platt, J.L., Vercellotti, G.M., Dalmasso, A.P., et al. Transplantation of discordant xenografts: a review of progress. Immunol. Today. 11, 450, 1990
3. Dalmasso, A.P. The complement system in xenotransplantation. Immunopharmacol. 24, 149, 1992
4. Hasan, R., Van den Bogaerde, J., Forty, J., et al. Xenograft adaptation is dependent on the presence of antispecies antibody, not prolonged residence in the recipient. Transplant. Proc. 24, 531, 1992
5. Dalmasso, A.P. Complement in the pathophysiology and diagnosis of human diseases. Crit. Rev. Clin. Lab. Sci. 24, 123, 1986
6. Müller-Eberhard, H.J., Complement: chemistry and pathways. In: Gallin, J.I., Goldstein, I.M., Snyderman, R., (eds.) Inflammation. Basic Principles and Clinical Correlates. Raven Press, New York, p. 33, 1992
7. Frank, M.M., Complement system. In: Frank, M.M., Austen, K.F., Claman, H.N., Unanue, E.R., (eds.) Samter's Immunological Diseases. Little, Brown and Co., Boston, p. 331, 199, 1995
8. Dalmasso, A.P. , Benson, B.A., Pore size of lesions induced by complement on red cell membranes and its relation to C5b-8, C5b-9 and poly C9. In: Podack, E.R., (ed.) Cytolytic lymphocyte clones and complement as effectors of the immune system. CRC Press, p. 207, 1988
9. Morgan, B.P., Cellular responses to the membrane attack complex. In: Whaley, K., Loos, M., Weiler, J., (eds.) Immunology and Medicine Vol. 20. Kluwer Academic Publishers, p. 325, 1993
10. Davis, A.E. C1 inhibitor and hereditary angioneurotic edema. Ann. Rev. Immunol. 6, 595, 1988
11. Hourcade, D., Holers, V.M., Atkinson, J.P. The regulators of complement activation (RCA) gene cluster. Adv. Immunol. 45, 381,1989

12. Atkinson, J.P., Oglesby, T.J., White, D., Adams, E.A., Liszewski, M.K. Separation of self from non-self in the complement system: a role for membrane cofactor protein and decay accelerating factor. Clin. Exp. Immunol. 86, S1, 1991
13. Nicholson-Weller, A., Wang, C. Structure and function of decay accelerating factor CD55. J. Lab. Clin. Med. 123, 485, 1994
14. Meri, S. Protectin (CD59). Complement lysis inhibitor and prototype domain in a new protein superfamily. The Immunologist. 2, 149, 1994
15. Rosse, W.F., Ware, R.E. The molecular basis of paroxysmal nocturnal hemoglobinuria. Blood. 86, 3277, 1995
16. Dalmasso, A.P., Vercellotti, G.M., Platt, J.L., Bach, F.H. Inhibition of complement-mediated endothelial cell cytotoxicity by decay accelerating factor. Potential for prevention of xenograft hyperacute rejection. Transplantation. 52, 530, 1991
17. Baldwin, W.M., III, Pruitt, S.K., Brauer, R.B., Daha, M.R., Sanfilippo, F. Complement in organ transplantation: Contributions to inflammation, injury, and rejection. Transplantation. 59, 797, 1995
18. Hamilton, K.K., Hattori, R., Esmon, C.T., Sims, P.J. Complement proteins C5b-9 induce vesiculation of the endothelial plasma membrane and expose catalytic surface for assembly of the prothrombinase enzyme complex. J. Biol. Chem. 265, 3809, 1990
19. Dalmasso, A.P., Vercellotti, G.M., Fischel, R.J., et al. Mechanism of complement activation in the hyperacute rejection of porcine organs transplanted into primate recipients. Am. J. Pathol. 140, 1157, 1992
20. Schaapherder, A.F.M., Gooszen, H.G., Te Bulte, M.T.J.W., Daha, M.R. Human complement activation via the alternative pathway on porcine endothelium initiated by IgA antibodies. Transplantation. 60, 287, 1995
21. Kroshus, T.J., Bolman, R.M., Dalmasso, A.P. Selective IgM reduction prolongs organ survival in an ex vivo model of pig-to-human xenotransplantation. Transplantation. 62, 5, 1996
22. Miyagawa, S., Hirose, H., Shirakura, R., et al. The mechanism of discordant xenograft rejection. Transplantation. 46, 825, 1988
23. Gambiez, L., Weill, B.J., Chereau, C., Calmus, Y., Houssin, D. The hyperacute rejection of guinea pig to rat heart xenografts is mediated by preformed IgM. Transplant. Proc. 22, 1058, 1990
24. Johnston, P.S., Lim, S.M.L., Wang, M.W., Wright, L., White, D.J.G. Hyperacute rejection of xenografts in the complete absence of antibody. Transplant. Proc. 23, 877, 1991
25. Hancock, W.W., Rajasinghe, H.A., Reddy, V.M., et al. Correction of congenital cardiac defects by fetal or neonatal discordant xenografting: initial results and key role of activation of the alternative pathway of complement. Abs. 3rd. Internat. Congr. Xenotransplant. p041, 1995
26. Jefferson, K.P., Tyerman, K.S., McLeish, M., Collier, D.S.J., Thiru, S. Donor pretreatment prolongs survival of discordant xenografts. Transplant. Proc. 23, 2280, 1991
27. Leventhal, J.R., Dalmasso, A.P., Cromwell, J.W., et al. Prolongation of cardiac xenograft survival by depletion of complement. Transplantation. 55, 857, 1993
28. Leventhal, J.R., Matas, A.J., Sun, L.H., et al. The immunopathology of cardiac xenograft rejection in the guinea pig-to-rat model. Transplantation. 56, 1, 1993
29. Leventhal, J.R., Sakiyalak, P., Witson, J., et al. The synergistic effect of combined antibody and complement depletion on discordant cardiac xenograft survival in nonhuman primates. Transplantation. 57, 974, 1994

30. Chartrand, C., O'Regan, S., Robitaille, P., Pinto-Blonde, M. Delayed rejection of cardiac xenografts in C6-deficient rabbits. Immunology. 38, 245, 1979
31. Zhow, X.J., Niesen, N., Pawlowski, I., et al. Prolongation of survival of discordant kidney xenografts by C6 deficiency. Transplantation. 50, 896, 1990
32. Brauer, R.B., Baldwin, W.M.I., Daha, M.R., Pruitt, S.K., Sanfilippo, F. Use of C6-deficient rats to evaluate the mechanism of hyperacute rejection of discordant cardiac xenografts. J. Immunol. 151, 7240, 1993
33. Johnson, E.M., Leventhal, J., Dalmasso, A.P., et al. Inactivation of C3 and C5 prolongs cardiac xenograft survival and decreases leukocyte infiltration in a model of delayed xenograft rejection. Transplant. Proc. 28, 603, 1996
34. Buchner, B., Schraa, E.O., Bonthuis, F., et al. Beneficial effect of complement depletion and treatment with dexamethasone in discordant xenografting. Abs. 3rd. Internat. Congr. Xenotransplant. p081, 1995
35. Johnson, E.M., Leventhal, J., Dalmasso, A.P., et al. Use of a novel CD11b/CD18 inhibitory agent in a C6 deficient rat to evaluate delayed xenograft rejection. Transplant. Proc. 28, 728, 1996
36. Kroshus, T.J., Rollins, S.A., Dalmasso, A.P., et al. Complement inhibition with an anti-C5 monoclonal antibody prevents acute cardiac tissue injury in an ex vivo model of pig-to-human xenotransplantation. Transplantation. 60, 1194, 1995
37. Rollins, S.A., Matis, L.A., Springhorn, J.P., Setter, E., Wolff, D.W. Monoclonal antibodies directed against human C5 and C8 block complement-mediated damage of xenogeneic cells and organs. Transplantation. 60, 1284, 1995
38. Platt, J.L., Vercellotti, G.M., Lindman, B., et al. Release of heparan sulfate from endothelial cells: implications for pathogenesis of hyperacute rejection. J. Exp. Med. 171, 1363, 1990
39. Platt, J.L., Dalmasso, A.P., Lindman, B.J., Ihrcke, N.S., Bach, F.H. The role of C5a and antibody in the release of heparan sulfate from endothelial cells. Eur. J. Immunol. 21, 2887, 1991
40. Saadi, S. , Platt, J.L. Transient perturbation of endothelial integrity induced by natural antibodies and complement. J. Exp. Med. 181, 21, 1995
41. Peerschke, E.I., Reid, K.B., Ghebrehiwet, B. Platelet activation by C1q results in the induction of alpha IIb/beta 3 integrins (GPIIb-IIIa) and the expression of P-selectin and procoagulant activity. J. Exp. Med. 178, 579, 1993
42. Vercellotti, G.M., Platt, J, Bach, F.H., Dalmasso, A.P. Neutrophil adhesion to xenogeneic endothelium via iC3b. J. Immunol. 146, 730, 1991
43. Bustos, M., Saadi, S., Platt, J.L. Modulation of endothelial metabolism by xenogenic serum: implications for vasoconstriction and permeability. Transplant. Proc. 28, 624, 1996
44. Stahl, G.L., Reenstra, W.R., Frendl, G. Complement-mediated loss of endothelium-dependent relaxation of porcine coronary arteries. Role of the terminal membrane attack complex. Circ. Res. 76, 575, 1995
45. Blakely, M.L., Van der Werf, W.J., Berndt, M.C., et al. Activation of intragraft endothelial and mononuclear cells during discordant xenograft rejection. Transplantation. 58, 1059, 1994
46. Fryer, J., Leventhal, J.R., Dalmasso, A.P., et al. Cellular rejection in a discordant xenograft when hyperacute rejection is prevented: analysis using adoptive and passive transfer. Transplant Immunol. 2, 87, 1994

47. Fryer, J.P., Leventhal, J.R., Dalmasso, A.P., et al. Beyond hyperacute rejection. Accelerated rejection in a discordant xenograft model by adoptive transfer of specific cell subsets. Transplantation. 59, 171, 1995
48. Vanhove, B., de Martin, R., Lipp, J., Bach, F.H. Human xenoreactive natural antibodies of the IgM isotype activate pig endothelial cells. Xenotransplantation. 1, 17, 1994
49. Dalmasso, A.P., He, T., Benson, B.A. Human IgM xenoreactive natural antibodies can induce resistance of porcine endothelial cells to complement-mediated injury. Xenotransplantation. 3, 54, 1996
50. Alexandre, G.P.J., Squifflet, J.P., De Bruyere, M., et al. Present experience in a series of 26 ABO-incompatible living donor renal allografts. Transplant. Proc. 19, 4538, 1987
51. Bannett, A.D., McAlack, R.F., Morris, M., Chopek, M.W., Platt, J.L. ABO incompatible renal transplantation: a qualitative analysis of native endothelial tissue ABO antigens after transplantation. Transplant. Proc. 21, 783, 1989
52. Bach, F.H., Turman, M.A., Vercellotti, G.M., Platt, J.L., Dalmasso, A.P. Accommodation: a working paradigm for progressing toward clinical discordant xenografting. Transplant. Proc. 23, 205, 1991
53. Cooper, D.K.C., Ye, Y., Niekrasz, M., et al. Specific intravenous carbohydrate therapy – a new concept in inhibiting antibody-mediated rejection: experience with ABO-incompatible cardiac allografting in the baboon. Transplantation. 56, 769, 1993
54. Fischel, R.J., Matas, A.J., Perry, E., et al. Plasma exchange, organ perfusion, and immunosuppression reduce "natural" antibody levels as measured by binding to xenogeneic endothelial cells and prolong discordant xenograft survival. Transplant. Proc. 24, 574, 1992
55. Oglesby, T.J., Allen, C.J., Liszewski, M.K., White, D.J.G., Atkinson, J.P. Membrane cofactor protein (CD46) protects cells from complement-mediated attack by an intrinsic mechanism. J. Exp. Med. 175, 1547, 1992
56. Zhao, J., Rollins, S.A., Maher, S.E., Bothwell, A.L., Sims, P.J. Amplified gene expression in CD59-transfected Chinese hamster ovary cells confers protection against the membrane attack complex of human complement. J. Biol. Chem. 266, 13418, 1991
57. Akami, T., Sawada, R., Minato, N., et al. Cytoprotective effect of CD59 antigen on xenotransplantation immunity. Transplant. Proc. 24, 485, 1992
58. Charreau, B., Cassard, A., Tesson, L., et al. Protection of rat endothelial cells from primate complement-mediated lysis by expression of human CD59 and/or decay-accelerating factor. Transplantation. 58, 1222, 1994
59. McCurry, K.R., Kooyman, D.L., Alvarado, C.G., et al. Human complement regulatory proteins protect swine-to-primate cardiac xenografts from humoral injury. Nature Med. 1, 423, 1995
60. Fodor, W.L., Williams, B.L., Matis, L.A., et al. Expression of a functional human complement inhibitor in a transgenic pig as a model for the prevention of xenogeneic hyperacute organ rejection. Proc. Natl. Acad. Sci. USA. 91, 11153, 1994
61. Rosengard, A.M., Cary, N.R.B., Langford, G.A., et al. Tissue expression of human complement inhibitor, decay-accelerating factor, in transgenic pigs: a potential approach for preventing xenograft rejection. Transplantation. 59, 1325, 1995
62. Somerville, C.A., Kyriazis, A.G., McKenzie, A., et al. Functional expression of human CD59 in transgenic mice. Transplantation. 58, 1430, 1994

63. Mulder, L.C.F., Mora, M., Lazzeri, M., et al. Human MCP and DAF double transgenic mice are completely protected from human complement attack in an in vivo model. Transplant. Proc. 28, 589, 1996
64. Langford, G.A., Cozzi, E., Yannoutsos, N., et al. Production of pigs transgenic for human regulators of complement activation using YAC technology. Transplant. Proc. 28, 862, 1966
65. Sandrin, M.S., Vaughan, H.A., Dabkowski, P.L., McKenzie, I.F.C. Anti-pig IgM antibodies in human serum react predominantly with Gal(a1-3)Gal epitopes. Proc. Natl. Acad. Sci. USA. 90, 11391, 1993
66. Cowan, P.J., Witort, E., Barlow, H., Pearse, M.J., d'Apice, A.J.F. Expression of CD59 in transgenic mice using the human ICAM-2 promoter. Abs. 3rd. Internat. Congr. Xenotransplant. p079, 1995
67. Fodor, W.L., Rollins, S.A., Guilmette, E.R., Setter, E., Squinto, S.P. A novel bifunctional chimeric complement inhibitor that regulates C3 convertase and formation of the membrane attack complex. J. Immunol. 155, 4135, 1995
68. Tucker, A.W., Davies, H.S., Carrington, C.A., et al. The fertility and breeding potential of boars expressing a functional regulator of human complement activation. Transplant. Proc. 28, 642, 1996
69. Pascual, M., French, L.E. Complement in human diseases: looking towards the 21st century. Immunol. Today. 16, 58, 1995
70. Charreau, B., Tesson, L., Quantin, B., Soulillou, J.P., Anegon, I. Adenovirus-mediated expression of human CD59 in xenogeneic endothelial cells. Abs. 3rd. Internat. Congr. Xenotransplant. p086, 1995
71. Pierson, R.N., Conary, J.T., Langford, G., et al. Targeted in vivo gene transfection modulates hyperacute rejection of pig lungs perfused with human blood. Transplant. Proc. 28, 763, 1996
72. Kooyman, D.L., Byrne, G.W., McClellan, S., et al. In vivo transfer of GPI-linked complement restriction factors from erythrocytes to the endothelium. Science. 269, 89, 1995
73. Kroshus, T.J., Bolman, R.M., Dalmasso, A.P. Studies on transfer of primate membrane-associated complement inhibitors from recipient blood to porcine donor organs. Transplant. Proc. 28, 601, 1996
74. Miyagawa, S., Shirakura, R., Matsumiya, G., et al. Prolonging discordant xenograft survival with anticomplement reagents K76COOH and FUT175. Transplantation. 55, 709, 1993
75. Dalmasso, A.P. , Platt, J.L. Prevention of complement-mediated activation of xenogeneic endothelial cells in an in vitro model of xenograft hyperacute rejection by C1 inhibitor. Transplantation. 56, 1171, 1993
76. Dalmasso, A.P. , Platt, J.L. Potentiation of C1 inhibitor plus heparin in prevention of complement-mediated activation of endothelial cells in a model of xenograft hyperacute rejection. Transplant. Proc. 26, 1246, 1994
77. Stevens, R.B., Wang, Y.L., Kaji, H., et al. Administration of nonanticoagulant heparin inhibits the loss of glycosaminoglycans from xenogeneic cardiac grafts and prolongs graft survival. Transplant. Proc. 25, 382, 1993
78. Weisman, H.F., Bartow, T., Leppo, M.K., et al. Soluble human complement receptor type 1: in vivo inhibitor of complement suppressing post-ischemic myocardial inflammation and necrosis. Science. 249, 146, 1990

79. Pruitt, S.K., Baldwin, W.M., Marsh, H.C., Jr., et al. The effect of soluble complement receptor type 1 on hyperacute xenograft rejection. Transplantation. 52, 868, 1991
80. Xia, W., Fearon, D.T., Moore, F.D., Jr., et al. Prolongation of guinea pig cardiac xenograft survival in rats by soluble human complement receptor type 1. Transplant. Proc. 24, 479, 1992
81. Pruitt, S.K., Kirk, A.D., Bollinger, R.R., et al. The effect of soluble complement receptor type 1 on hyperacute rejection of porcine xenografts. Transplantation. 57, 363, 1994
82. Pruitt, S.K., Bollinger, R.R., Collins, B.H., et al. Continuous complement (C) inhibition using soluble C receptor type 1 (sCR1): effect on hyperacute rejection (HAR) of pig-to-primate cardiac xenografts. Transplant. Proc. 28, 756, 1996
83. Ryan, U.S. Complement inhibitory therapeutics and xenotransplantation. Nature Med. 1, 967, 1995
84. Loveland, B.E., Christiansen, D., Milland, J., et al. Production and characterization of recombinant soluble CD46, an effective complement regulator in vitro and in vivo. Abs. 3rd. Internat. Congr. Xenotransplant. or58, 1995
85. Vogel, C.W. , Müller-Eberhard, H.J. The cobra venom factor-dependent C3 convertase of human complement. J. Biol. Chem. 257, 8292, 1982
86. Leventhal, J.R., Ranjit, J., Fryer, J.P., et al. Removal of baboon and human antiporcine IgG and IgM natural antibodies by immunoadsorption. Results of in vitro and in vivo studies. Transplantation. 59, 294, 1995
87. Basta, M., Fries, L.F., Frank, M.M. High doses of intravenous Ig inhibit in vitro uptake of C4 fragments onto sensitized erythrocytes. Blood. 77, 376, 1991
88. Latremouille, C., Haeffner-Cavaillon, N., Goussef, N., et al. Normal human polyclonal immunoglobulins for intravenous use significantly delay hyperacute xenograft rejection. Transplant. Proc. 26, 1285, 1994
89. Gautreau, C., Kojima, T., Woimant, G., et al. Use of intravenous immunoglobulin to delay xenogeneic hyperacute rejection. An in vivo and in vitro evaluation. Transplantation. 60, 903, 1995
90. Magee, J.C., Collins, B.H., Harland, R.C., et al. Immunoglobulin prevents complement-mediated hyperacute rejection in swine-to-primate xenotransplantation. J. Clin. Invest. 96, 2404, 1995
91. Matis, L.A., Rollins, S.A. Complement-specific antibodies: Designing novel anti-inflammatories. Nature Med. 1, 839, 1995

7 Genetic Control of Humoral Responses to Xenografts

D.V. Cramer

Introduction

The exchange of vascularized organs between most xenogeneic species stimulates an aggressive immune rejection reaction by the graft recipient. Several immunological mechanisms are thought to be involved in mediating the host response but even the most basic characteristics of these responses are incompletely understood. There is a general lack of information, for example, concerning the individual immunological components of the xenograft reaction, including the relative role of cellular and/or humoral responses, the nature of the antibody and lymphocyte subsets involved, and the structural characteristics of the antigens that serve as targets for host immune responses. This lack of a detailed understanding of many facets of the pathogenesis of the xenograft reaction has clearly limited the development of therapeutic strategies, including the generation of universal animal donors, that would prevent or avoid the rejection of these grafts.

Our recent experimental work examining the pathogenesis of the xenograft reaction has emphasized the importance of the humoral responses to the foreign grafts. The rejection of xenografts from the two species most likely to be used as donors for humans, non-human primates (particularly baboons) or pigs, is dominated in the early phases of the reaction by antibodies that precipitate the rapid loss of the graft. The use of pig xenografts in humans is limited by high levels of preformed antibody to donor tissues in most normal individuals that immediately bind to and cause a hyperacute rejection of the graft. Xenografts exchanged between species, such as the baboon-to-human combination, that do not exhibit high titers of preformed antibody, have more prolonged graft survival times. Within several days to a few weeks, however, the onset of antidonor antibody production is associated with vascular damage and failure of the new graft.

The importance of the humoral response of the host to the xenograft is the result of the severity of the damage to the graft soon after transplantation and the lack of effective forms of immunosuppression to prevent the reaction. While there are several immune mechanisms that may play important roles in rejection of the xenograft [1–3], these responses occur later in the reaction and any successful strategy for preventing xenograft rejection will first require removal of preformed anti-donor antibodies and then effective methods to prevent the production of new anti-donor antibody. To date, experiments designed to test this approach has been of limited value because of a limited understanding of the important details of the host antibody response to the grafts and a lack of effective methods to prevent antibody production. Accordingly, this chapter will review the most recent information available on the nature of humoral immune response to xenografts with the objective of providing a rational for the development of new and more specific forms of therapy.

Nature of the Humoral Response to Xenografts

The control of the early humoral immune response to xenografts is critical for providing a basis for long-term graft survival. In the pig-to-human combination, preformed antibodies found in most normal individuals can precipitate a rapid loss of a pig xenograft [4]. These preformed antibodies bind to the vascular endothelium of the graft, activate a series of inflammatory/coagulation cascades that lead to a widespread intravascular thrombosis. Other species combinations, such as the baboon-to-human, exhibit lower levels of preformed antibody and graft rejection is delayed when compared to that seen with pig donor organs [5]. In both combinations, however, long-term graft survival cannot occur without effective elimination of preformed antibody and/or the prevention of the appearance of new anti-donor antibodies induced following placement of the graft.

The importance of anti-donor antibody in the long-term survival of xenografts has been most clearly illustrated by experimental studies testing new immunosuppressive agents that prevent humoral immune responses. Traditional allograft immunosuppressive regimens are effective for preventing T cell-mediated cellular responses but they have proven to be ineffective for preventing the rejection of xenografts [1]. Recent experiments using new combinations of immunosuppressive agents have shown that it is possible to provide the conditions necessary for prolonged xenograft survival [6, 7]. This prolonged survival is permanent in selected rodent combinations and most closely correlates with suppression of antidonor antibody production. Treatment failures or withdrawal from treatment with the immunosuppressive drugs can result in rejection of the graft.

The importance of humoral responses for xenograft rejection can also be demonstrated by disrupting the activation of complement components caused by the binding of anti-donor antibody to target antigens expressed by the xenograft. Agents that prevent complement activation prolong pig-to-primate xenograft survival when repeatedly administered to the recipients [8, 9]. Graft failure after 5–7 days is seen, even with continued inactivation of complement components. The rejected grafts are characterized by the deposition of large amounts of antibody (IgM and IgG) on vascular endothelium with extensive infiltration with neutrophils and macrophages. Inclusion of immunosuppressive drugs that prevent host immune responses result in longer graft survival, suppression of antibody production, and the absence of cellular infiltration in the grafts. Of particular interest is the observation that immunosuppressive regimens that prevent host antibody production are associated with significant decreases in cellular infiltrates within the graft. Traditional immunosuppression, even with its focus on preventing the cellular components of the rejection reaction, do not effectively interfere with the cellular immune response to xenografts. This data suggests that involvement of cells in the xenograft reaction may be strongly influenced by anti-donor antibody. The appearance of neutrophils and macrophages may reflect the importance of antibody-dependent cell cytotoxicity (ADCC) as an interface between humoral and cellular responses directed at the xenogeneic grafts.

The critical issue to be addressed with regard to the nature of the humoral response to xenografts is the origin of the antidonor antibody. Antibodies are produced by at least two different pathways. The first is the traditional B cell response to antigens that depends upon T cells to drive the proliferation of B cells. T cell-driven proliferation allows for the incorporation of somatic mutations within the Ig gene variable region, thereby providing a mechanism for increasing the specificity and binding activity of the antibody [10]. The second pathway of antibody production involves a direct activation of B cells, usually with a polyvalent antigen in the absence of T cell help [11]. T cell-independent activation of B cells stimulates the production of antibodies that are expressed without substantial modification in the configuration of their Ig genes [12]. The xenograft reaction between species with preformed antibodies is generally considered to represent antibody production via T cell-independent pathways. The nature of the control of antibody production seen after exposure to the foreign graft or in species combinations for which rejection of the graft depends upon induced antibody is not known.

Natural Antibodies and the Xenograft Reaction

The sera of humans and animals normally contain antibodies that can react with multiple, apparently unrelated antigens. These antibodies recognize a variety of self and non-self antigens and can be detected at different levels in normal individuals without evidence of prior antigen exposure. These antibodies are primarily IgM immunoglobulins and they display a "polyreactive" pattern of binding in that they bind with modest levels of affinity to antigens that do not appear to share structural similarities that would account for this pattern of reactivity. The appearance of these preformed antibodies in the absence of any evidence of immunization has led to the use of the term "natural antibodies" to distinguish between these antibodies and the more common and specific antibodies produced following traditional exposure to antigen [13]. The antigens that may be recognized by natural antibodies are many different types of infectious agents, including bacteria, viruses, parasites, normal self-antigens not exposed to circulating plasma, and tissues of other (xenogeneic) species.

The natural antibodies found in the sera of normal individuals frequently react with infectious organisms, particularly bacteria [14, 15]. The reactivity of natural antibodies is characterized by binding activity directed at carbohydrate or glycoprotein epitopes, a common component of bacterial cells. The ability of natural antibodies to bind and to functionally neutralize infectious organisms suggests that many of these antibodies may be a component of a primitive, innate immune response to infectious diseases. The inactivation of infectious agents may serve as an important protective mechanism that can act early before a more specific T cell-driven antibody response is mounted by the host. This concept is consistent with the observation that there is an association between the appearance of natural antibodies to the erythrocytes of xenogeneic species and exposure to environmental antigens. Pig anti-sheep antibodies appear in the serum of piglets soon after birth unless the piglets were raised in an isolated environment [16]. Isolation of the piglets from environmental antigens, including bacteria, prevent the appearance of anti-sheep antibodies. Similarly, dogs and pig raised in gnotobiotic conditions do not develop xenoreactive antibodies to a variety of species until exposed to bacterial flora or natural foods [17].

Natural antibodies share many characteristics with antibodies produced via T cell-independent B cell pathways. The similarities in the antibodies to T cell-independent antigens and natural antibodies suggest that both sets may be produced by a common humoral immune response mechanism. Human natural antibodies to pig tissues bind to a broad spectrum of antigens in patterns like those observed for natural antibodies to infectious agents and antibodies associated with autoimmune diseases [18–20]. Natural antibodies in each of these cases are primarily IgM and apparently recognize multiple unrelated antigens, including multiple organisms, normal tissue proteins, single-stranded DNA (ssDNA), and thyroglobulin [18]. The polyreactive nature of this response has been interpreted to suggest that xenoantibodies, like those that are seen with autoimmune diseases and in response to infectious agents, may be produced by a specific subset (B-1a/B-1b) of B cells [18]. It is possible that each of these forms of antibody production are the result of the stimulation of B-1a/B-1b subsets of lymphocytes by repetitive carbohydrate antigens, such as those seen with bacterial cell walls, and this antibody inadvertently displays reactivity with xenogeneic antigens expressed as normal structures on cell surfaces. These T cell-independent antibody responses are thought to differ from the more traditional humoral response to nominal antigens in that the antibodies are produced by a distinct lineage of B cells that in adults lack a bone marrow progenitor. These cells are present as a self-replicating population of lymphocytes, primarily in the peritoneal and pleural cavities.

The broad pattern of reactivity seen with natural antibodies suggests that they may be encoded by immunoglobulin genes in a germline configuration. Antibody production by B lymphocytes can be separated into two distinct cell lineages, B-1a/1b cells and conventional B cells (or B-2 cells). B-2 cells are responsible for traditional B cell responses to antigens and are concentrated primarily in the spleen and lymph nodes. The B-2 cell response involves the participation of T cells which drive B cell proliferation to induce the generation of somatic diversity in Ig V_H and V_L genes, thereby providing the exquisite specificity of antibody recognition for foreign antigens [21]. The second lineage of cells, the B-1a/B-1b subset, is characterized by an early rearrangement of their Ig genes, either during fetal or early post-natal life, and the production of antibodies that react with multiple antigens [22, 23]. Analysis of monoclonal antibodies derived from patients with autoimmune diseases has suggested that the pattern of binding to multiple unrelated antigens may reflect a high level of variability in the CDR3 region of the V_H gene [24]. Exchanges in the D-J regions of polyreactive versus monoreactive IgM antibodies confirmed that the CDR3 region structurally most closely correlates with the characteristic of multiple antigen binding [25]. Chimerization experiments conducted with two monoclonal antibodies that react with insulin, one a polyreactive IgM autoantibody and the second a monoreactive anti-insulin IgG, has demonstrated that the Ig heavy chain variable region makes a major contribution to the polyreactivity and that this pattern of reactivity is a feature of the H chain CDR3 region and the non-mutated framework (FW1 and 3) regions of the light chain [26]. Despite the reactivity of natural antibodies with multiple antigens, the repertoire of antibody binding with self-antigens appears to be highly conserved. Analysis of natural antibodies to self- and non-self antigens in newborn infants demonstrated little variation between individuals [27]. The human neonatal IgM antibody repertoire is directed at a limited set of self-antigens and this restricted repertoire of antibody recognition persists in young, healthy adults.

Natural antibodies that react with infectious agents and self-antigens also recognize tissues and organs used for transplantation. Preformed antibodies react with a variety of normal tissue antigens, including isoagglutinins to ABO erythrocyte antigens and xenoantigens expressed by a variety of tissues from unrelated species. Transplantation of tissues or organs that express these antigens are at risk for an accelerated rejection of the graft due to the presence of these preformed antibodies [28, 29]. The ABO blood group antigens are complex carbohydrates and they are expressed on vascular endothelium in addition to erythrocytes. Anti-AB antibodies arise in individuals who lack the antigen, probably again as a result of exposure to microorganisms expressing antigens that are structurally similar to blood group antigens. Vascularized organ grafts, including kidney and hearts, are rejected in an accelerated fashion in ABO incompatible individuals due to the binding of the preformed anti-AB antibodies to the endothelium of the graft (for a review, see [30]). Circulating anti-AB antibodies is deposited on the endothelium of the graft vessels and this antibody-antigen interaction precipitates endothelial cell damage and intravascular thrombosis. Clinical transplant programs currently avoid this incompatibility by prospective tissue matching of the donor and recipient.

Preformed natural antibodies against blood group antigens share many characteristics with natural antibodies directed against xenoantigens. Normal individuals have circulating, preformed antibodies that react with a variety of tissues from different species, including swine. Perfusion of pig kidneys or livers with human blood is associated with the deposition of natural antibodies on capillary endothelium of the grafts [31, 32]. The anti-pig antibodies are considered to be similar but distinct from anti-AB isoagglutinins. There has not been evidence developed that implicates anti-AB antibodies directly in the hyperacute rejection of xenografts. There is no correlation, for example, in the level of antibody deposition with the presence or absence of antibody in AB or O blood used for perfusion [33] or differences in levels of hemagglutinating antibodies for pig erythrocytes in human plasma following absorption with selected human AB-positive erythrocytes [34].

The level of preformed natural antibody seen for a specific donor/recipient combination displays significant variation. Xenografts have traditionally been classified on the basis of the presence or absence of preformed antibodies in the serum of the recipient to the potential donor. The degree of genetic disparity between the donor/recipient species has been considered to be the prime factor in determining whether preformed antibodies are seen for individual donor/recipient pairs [35]. Recipients of xenografts from more distantly related donors are more likely to exhibit preformed natural antibodies to the donor graft. When present in significant levels, these antibodies can precipitate a rapid, hyperacute (discordant) rejection of graft within minutes or a few hours. Pig-to-human liver transplantation in the presence of preformed antibody can precipitate the loss of the xenograft within 36 h [4]. Species for which preformed antibodies are not present in high titers exhibit a less aggressive rejection reaction that may require several days to cause loss of the graft. While the pace of the reaction differs for individual donor/recipient pairs, graft rejection appears to be closely related to the level of the host antibody response to the graft. In the hamster-to-rat model, rejection of heart xenografts occurs at 4 days post-transplantation. At the time of rejection, antidonor antibody titers are rapidly increasing and passive transfer of the antibodies alone can induce hyperacute rejection in naive rat recipients of hamster heart grafts.

Preformed Versus Induced Antibody Responses

The emphasis on the importance of the presence or absence of natural preformed antibodies for xenotransplantation has led to the implicit assumption that multiple immune mechanisms may be responsible for the rejection of xenografts in different species combinations. The separation of xenograft reactions into those precipitated by preformed antibody ("discordant") and those that are not ("concordant") has been interpreted to indicate that the immune responses responsible for the different xenograft reactions are qualitatively different. The xenograft reaction responsible for discordant xenograft reactions are thought to be mediated by T cell-independent (B-1a/1b) antibody responses. The discordant reaction depends upon the presence of preformed antibody to precipitate the immediate (hyperacute) loss of the xenograft. Removal of preformed antibodies may allow for more prolonged graft survival but immune responses stimulated by placement of the graft quickly induce new antibody production. This antibody response could involve augmentation of the T cell-independent pathway responsible for the original preformed antibodies or, alternatively, may consist of a newly induced (T cell-dependent) responses to the graft antigens. The humoral response to concordant xenografts has traditionally been considered to represent the latter and consist of the exposure of the recipient to new graft antigens and the stimulation of a T cell-dependent antibody response.

The data available to support the different hypotheses explaining the nature of the humoral immune responses to xenografts is limited. A close examination of many species combinations has demonstrated that preformed anti-donor antibodies are commonly seen, even between closely related (concordant) groups of animals. Naive rats, as an example, exhibit low levels of preformed antibodies to hamsters [36] and guinea pigs [37] and mice exhibit natural antibodies to rat bone marrow cells [38]. Similar patterns of low levels of natural antibodies have also been observed among nonhuman primates [1, 39]. Western blot analysis of rat sera has clearly demonstrated the presence of preformed rat antibodies that react with hamster heart antigens. The rejection of a hamster heart xenograft is associated with the appearance of a similar but more intense pattern of antibody binding [36]. The similarities in the pattern of antigen recognition by natural rat anti-hamster antibodies before and after exposure to the graft suggests that the rapid rise in antidonor antibody is due to antibody production by a precommitted population of B cells. The same pattern of antibody binding has been reported for the guinea pig-to-rat xenograft combination [37]. The presence of preformed antibody between closely related species combinations, even in small quantities, suggests that differences in the type of xenograft rejection in "concordant" and "discordant" species combinations may be more a reflection of absolute antibody levels rather than qualitative differences in the nature of the response.

The suggestion that the humoral immune response to both "concordant" and "discordant" xenografts may be controlled by T cell-independent pathways is primarily supported by indirect data. In the pig-to-human combination, there is a substantial amount of indirect data to suggest that the early hyperacute phase of the reaction is due to the binding of preformed natural antibody produced by a B-1a/B-1b subset of B cells. Perfusion of human serum through kidney or liver xenografts depletes natural antibody cytotoxic activity directed at pig endothelial cells [32]. Antibodies eluted from these grafts are primarily IgM and display the same type of polyreactive patterns of reactivity seen for other natural and autoimmune antibodies [18, 19]. Among different individuals these antibodies may recognize a limited repertoire of target antigens. A polyreactive human anti-pig antibody expresses an idiotype that is found frequently in antibodies that bind to xenograft endothelial antigens [19].

A key unresolved issue in the reaction of human antibodies to pig xenografts is whether the antibody produced after placement of the graft is produced by the same pathway of antibody production as preformed antibody. Antibody induced by exposure to the graft could reflect augmented antibody production by precommitted B-1a/B-1b cells or the production of T cell-dependent antibodies following exposure of the recipient to new graft antigens. Patients with fulminant liver failure treated with ex vivo of pig liver perfusion to provide temporary metabolic support are clearly stimulated to produce antidonor antibodies [40, 41]. The characterization of this antibody, however, has not been of sufficient detail to address the issue of the nature of the antibody production. Increased antibody titers to donor lymphocytes and erythrocytes could be temporally correlated with perfusions of pig xenografts but this pattern of antibody reactivity could be consistent with either T cell-dependent or T cell-independent B cell responses. Of interest is the observation that the human anti-pig antibodies, like those seen for the rodent xenograft reaction, apparently bind to the same target antigens before and after ex vivo liver perfusion [41]. No new antibodies appear to be induced by exposure to the foreign organ.

Antibody responses of xenograft recipients are also incompletely characterized in primate models of xenotransplantation using pig organs. Preformed anti-pig antibodies can be removed from the serum of baboons before transplantation but anti-donor antibodies return within 48 h following cardiac xenotransplantation [42]. The recipient rapidly produces new anti-donor antibodies when the response is not modified by immunosuppressive therapy. Protocols that have been successful in preventing graft rejection have focused on preventing the host humoral immune responses and the lack of an antibody response to the graft in these experiments has made it difficult to evaluate characteristics of the response. In rodents, the rejection of heart xenografts between closely related species occurs within a few days, depending upon the species combinations. The rejection process is dominated by anti-donor antibody production, especially IgM antibodies.

Immunoglobulin Genes and the Control of Xenoantibody Responses

One approach to resolving the nature of the humoral xenograft reaction is an analysis of the structure of the immunoglobulin genes used to mediate the antibody reaction. In the hamster-to-rat model of xenotransplantation, the humoral response to heart xenografts consists of antibodies that broadly recognize several species. One of the key observations concerning this response is that B cells producing antibody to heart xenografts can be used to generate monoclonal antibodies that are capable of inducing hyperacute rejection of the hamster grafts in naive rats. These monoclonals are predominantly IgM antibodies that bind to the vascular endothelium of a wide variety of hamster organs, thymic epithelium, and small numbers of peripheral blood mononuclear cells [43]. Binding of this antibody to the endothelium causes a violent, hyperacute rejection due to activation of the traditional complement and coagulation cascades and loss of the graft due to disseminated small vessel thrombosis.

Analysis of the immunoglobulin genes that encode these monoclonal rat anti-hamster antibodies has provide some insights into the nature of the immune response between closely related (concordant) xenografts. Isolation and sequencing of the monoclonal Ig genes has demonstrated that these antibodies use selected families of germline genes in a fashion very similar to that seen for natural antibodies and autoantibodies. Comparison of the V_H and J_H genes expressed by these monoclonal antibodies with genomic DNA from newborn rat liver has demonstrated several interesting characteristics. Independent monoclonals derived from separate fusion experiments use the same V_H germline gene (Fig. 1). The V_H genes of five monoclonals differ in their nucleic acid sequence by a maximum of four residues, two of which result in an amino acid replacements. These V_H genes exhibit a high level of nucleic acid sequence identity with the V_HHAR.1 germline equivalent (99.3 % and 98.9 %, respectively). These monoclonals also use two of the four known rat J_H genes. The monoclonal J_H genes are also used in a germline configuration without evidence of a preferential association between the V_H and J_H genes. The two J_H genes used by the five monoclonals exhibit nucleotide sequence identities of 98.3 % and 100.0 % with the rat J_H1 and J_H2 germline genes, respectively. A sixth monoclonal is encoded by a closely related germline gene, with which it shares a 96.7 % nucleic acid identity (Table 1). Similar levels of homology were seen for the light chain Ig genes for one of the antibodies (HAR-1). The HAR-1V_k gene shares significant

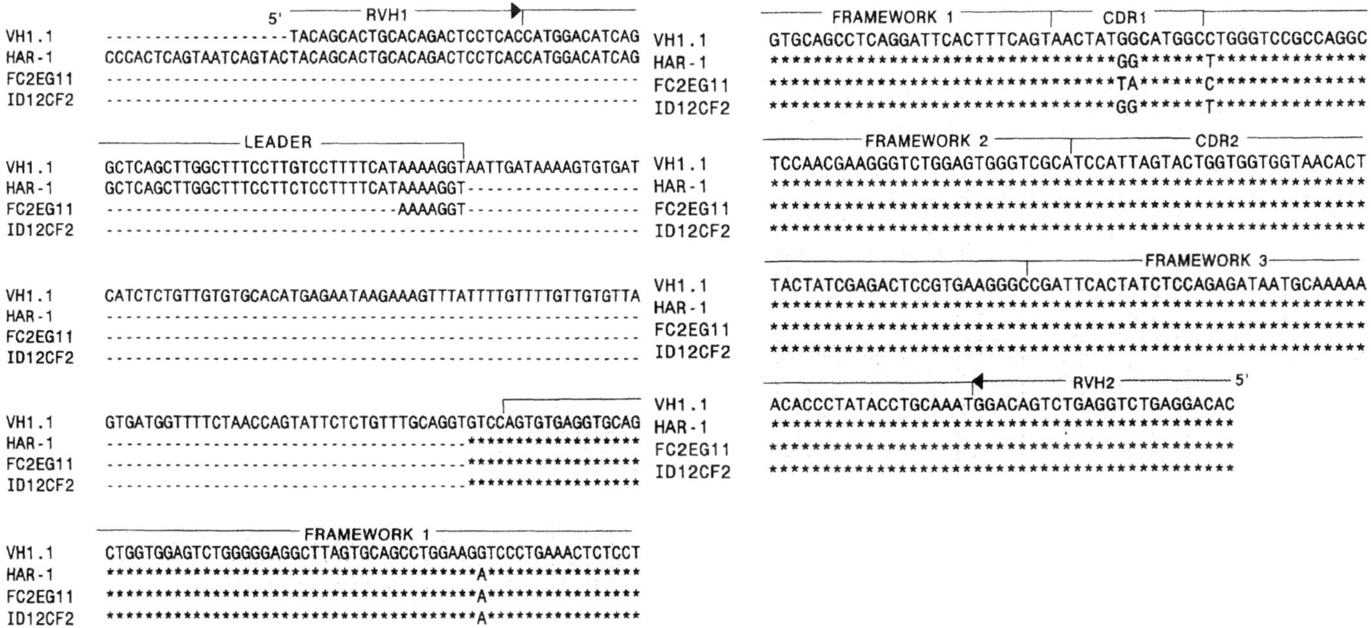

Fig. 1. Nucleic acid sequence comparisons for three independently derived monoclonal antibodies capable of causing hyperacute rejection of hamster heart xenografts to the rat germline gene V_H1.1. The three monoclonal antibodies use the same germline V_H immunoglobulin genes and two of the four rat J_H genes

Table 1. Analysis of the nucleic acid sequence data for rearranged V_H-D-V_J gene segments for rat monoclonal antibodies to hamster xenografts

mAb	V_H		D Region	J_H	
	Mutation[a]	Identity[b]		Mutation[a]	Identity[b]
HAR-1	2/0 (CDR 1/0)	V_HHAR.1 (99.3)	CATCGCGGGTATAAC	0/1	J1 (98.2)
HAR-2	2/0 (CDR 1/0)	V_HHAR.1 (99.3)	CATCGCGGGTATAAC	0/1	J1 (98.2)
HAR-ID12	2/0 (CDR 1/0)	V_HHAR.1 (99.3)	CCTTCCTATAGCAGC	0/0	J2 (100)
HAR-EG11	2/2 (CDR 1/1)	V_HHAR.1 (98.9)	GGGGAAGGC	0/0	J2 (100)
HAR-DD4	2/2 (CDR 1/1)	V_HHAR.1 (98.9)	GGGGAAGGC	0/0	J2 (100)
HAR-QG6	4/2 (CDR 2/1)	V_HHAR.2 (96.7)	CATAGG	0/1	J2 (97.8)

mAb, monoclonal antibody.
[a] Number of silent/replacement amino acid replacements; values for CDR regions done are in parentheses.
[b] Level (%) of similarity of the mAb gene to its germline equivalent.

sequence identity with the rat V_k8 gene family, a group of genes commonly used by anti-DNA antibodies. Similarly, the HAR-1J_k gene matched the first 36 nucleotides perfectly with the rat germline J_k2 gene.

The observation that antibodies capable of producing xenograft rejection share expression of Ig genes in a germline configuration led to an estimate of the in vivo usage of this gene, first in newborn and naive animals, followed by estimates of the gene frequency in rat recipients rejecting hamster xenografts. The response to hamster heart xenografts is characterized by a massive proliferation of IgM producing B cells within 4 days post-transplantation. This response, like that associated with autoantibodies, is produced by cells normally exhibiting a relatively high (1 %) frequency of a specific Ig gene in the spleens of adult animals. Polymerase chain reaction (PCR) primers specific for the germline V_HHAR.1 gene were used as probes for Ig gene specific libraries generated from splenic lymphocytes of newborn and naive adult rats and adult rats 4 and 21 days after receiving hamster heart xenografts. The newborn and adult animals express the V_HHAR.1 gene (or highly homologous members of the same family) at levels of 1.1 % and 1.0 %, respectively. The frequency of V_HHAR.1 expression rises sharply to approximately 16 % at 4 days after xenotransplantation and falls slightly to 10 % at 21 days.

The analysis of the immunoglobulin gene usage for the hamster-to-rat xenograft reaction provides support for the concept that the rejection reaction shares many features with the B-1a/1b antibody response to T cell-independent antigens and autoantibodies. A relatively high percentage (approximately 1 %) of the total Ig producing lymphocytes in the spleen of the graft recipient are involved in the antibody response to the graft. This response appears to be restricted to a small family of closely related V_H genes. The genes used for this response, like those seen for natural antibodies and autoantibodies, display a high level of nucleic acid identity with their germline progenitors. The sequence data derived from the V_H gene analysis does not exhibit any evidence of the type of somatic hypermutation that might be expected to occur due to the influence of antigen-driven selection and T cell-induced proliferation of B cells. The observation that the D and J regions of these antibodies share the same functional activity, but are structurally different from each other suggests that the CDR3 region of these molecules may not play an important role in establishing the binding characteristics of these antibodies.

The unusually small number of V_H genes involved in the hamster-to-rat xenograft reaction also suggests that the humoral response to the graft may be directed against a small number of xenoantigens. Analysis of the binding pattern of the HAR-1 monoclonal antibody indicates that this antibody reacts with a variety of carbohydrate antigens [44]. Absorption of the HAR-1 monoclonal antibody with synthetic columns representing 100 different carbohydrate epitopes allows for the identification of those antigens capable of removing the binding activity of the antibody for hamster endothelium. The carbohydrate epitope that produces that greatest removal of anti-hamster activity is the sialyl-Lewis^a antigen. The rather extensive levels of cross-reactivity with other related carbohydrates, however, also suggests that the sialyl-Lewis^a antigen may not be the only epitope capable of being recognized by this antibody. Similar observations have been reported for human preformed antibodies to pig tissues in normal individuals [45]. Careful analysis of the binding characteristics of these antibodies demonstrated relatively homogenous binding characteristics and overlapping target antigen specificity for preformed antibodies in different individuals, suggesting a restriction in the antigenic complexity of the target antigen. The results in both species are consistent with the hypothesis that xenograft target antigens in many species may be composed (at least in part) of a small number of specific carbohydrate epitopes.

The recent evidence that has accumulated on the nature of the xenograft target antigens, especially for discordant species such as the pig-to-human combination, indicate that the carbohydrate epitopes on xenograft target antigens may be expressed as a glycoprotein or glycolipid complex. One popular concept of the nature of these target epitopes is that the inactivation of the α1,3-galactosyltransferase gene in humans, apes, and Old World monkeys has led to a lack of expression of α-galactosyl epitopes and the emergence of antibodies directed at these epitopes, perhaps in response to infection of the host by microorganisms expressing similar antigens [46, 47]. This hypothesis predicts that natural anti-pig antibodies that cause the rejection of pig xenografts are directed at α1,3Gal carbohydrate epitopes expressed by antigens on the surface of pig endothelial cells.

There is a substantial amount of data demonstrating that human serum contains anti-Gal antibodies in high titers [48]. Approximately 1% of the total serum IgG is antibody that binds to α-galactosyl residues on rabbit red blood cells. Epstein-Barr virus transformed human B cells producing anti-Gal antibodies represent approximately 1% of circulating B cells and the isotypes of antibodies produced following transformation is composed of approximately equal proportions of IgG and IgM producing cells [49]. Similarly, it has been clearly demonstrated that pig cells express carbohydrate antigens, especially an unfucosylated monomorph linear B-antigen on vascular endothelial cells, that react with these anti-Gal antibodies [50, 51]. Some of these antibodies, like the natural antibodies responsible for mediating xenograft reactions, are composed of IgM antibodies and can be shown to bind to COS cells transfected with the α1,3-galactosyltransferase gene [51].

While it is clear that human serum contains substantial levels of anti-Gal antibodies and pig endothelial cells express antigens to which these antibodies may bind, it is not clear that this epitope alone or in combination with lipid and/or protein moieties functions as the target for the xenograft reaction. There is little evidence that the antibodies that react with the α-galactosyl epitopes are cytotoxic and activate complement, features of natural antibodies that appear to be the most relevant predictors of xenograft rejection. There is no evidence for the ability of these antibodies to disrupt the function of vascularized xenografts, such as ex vivo cardiac perfusion models, and controversy exists for the significance of the anti-Gal antibody binding to pig cells. Some investigators have suggested, for example, that the anti-Gal antibodies represent only a minor (<5 %) component of natural antibodies that react with pig platelets and that a majority of human natural antibodies are directed at antigens other than those detected by the anti-Gal antibodies [52]. The difficulty of clearly defining the precise specificity of low-affinity antibodies directed to carbohydrate antigens suggests that the precise nature of the target antigen(s) for natural xenoreactive antibodies will require more careful examination of the reactivity of these antibodies and their functional activity. The results of these studies will have an important influence of the selection of the therapeutic strategies to be used to prevent graft rejection. At present, however, it is not known whether these antibodies involved in the individual reactions are produced in response to a common antigenic stimulus, whether these antibodies are produced by a similar B cell pathway, or if the genes that control antibody binding activity exhibit similar levels of somatic Ig gene variation.

Comment

While a variety of immunological responses are involved in mediating the rejection of xenografts, the early phases of the reaction are dominated by host antibody responses. Preformed antibody or antibody rapidly produced in response to organ xenografts are central to the pathogenesis of the rejection reaction, precipitating either an immediate (hyperacute) or accelerated rejection of the graft secondary to widespread vascular damage and thrombosis. Recent analysis of the nature of the antibodies involved in this reaction suggests that even for widely disparate species combinations, the humoral response exhibits a set of characteristics common for a T cell-independent pathway of B cell antibody production. Preformed antibodies in humans against pig xenoantigens and antibodies in rodents produced in response to xenotransplantation share many functional and structural characteristics with a variety of natural antibodies, including those directed at infectious agents, isoagglutinins, and normal tissue proteins. These antibodies are restricted in their recognition of the targets for the xenograft reaction, suggesting they are directed at a glycoprotein or glycolipid structures with defined carbohydrate structures as part of the functional xenogeneic epitope. The restriction in the number of target specificities seen with natural antibodies and the evidence for a similar restriction in the genes responsible for mediating the antibody response to xenografts suggests that the target antigens may share important structural similarities.

These features of xenoantibody activity indicate that they may represent a component of a primitive innate immune system that is directed at preventing infections. Natural antibodies selected by environmental exposure to infectious agents can rapidly neutralize pathogens and may teleologically have predated the development of T cell-dependent mechanisms that generate more specific and higher affinity antibodies in response to infection. We have proposed that this innate immune system may be the basis for the antibody response to xenografts [53, 54]. Xenoantigens expressed by normal tissue components, such as adhesion molecules, may serve as the inadvertent target for these natural antibodies. The involvement of restricted numbers of germline genes directed at a small, but well-defined group of target antigens may provide the basis for the development of therapeutic strategies to prevent an important component of the host response to organ xenografts.

References

1. Auchincloss H, Jr. Xenogeneic transplantation: a review. Transplantation 1988; 46: 1
2. Platt JL, Bach FH. Mechanism of tissue injury in hyperacute xenograft rejection. In: Xenotransplantation. Cooper DKC, et al., eds. Heidelberg, Springer, 1991; 69
3. Makowka L, Cramer DV. The pathogenesis of the xenograft reaction. In: Advances in Transplantation, Hackel B, AuBuchon J, eds. Bethesda, Amer Assoc Blood Banks, 1993; 93
4. Makowka L, Cramer DV, Hoffman A, et al. The use of a pig liver xenograft for temporary support of a patient with fulminant hepatic failure. Transplantation 1995; 59: 1654
5. Starzl TE, Fung J, Tzakis A, et al. Baboon-to-human liver transplantation. Lancet 1993; 341: 65
6. Murase N, Starzl TE, Demetris AJ, et al. Hamster-to-rat heart and liver xenotransplantation with FK506 plus antiproliferative drugs. Transplantation 1993; 55: 701
7. Cosenza CA, Cramer DV, Tuso PJ, et al. Combination therapy with brequinar sodium and Cyclosporin A synergistically prolongs hamster-to-rat cardiac xenograft survival. J Heart Lung Transplant 1994; 13: 489
8. Pruitt SK, Kirk AD, Bollinger RR, et al. The effect of soluble complement receptor type 1 on hyperacute rejection of porcine xenografts. Transplantation 1994; 57: 363
9. Sanfilippo F. Effects of complement inhibitors on discordant rodent and pig-to-primate cardiac xenograft rejection. Proc Third Internatl Cong Xenotransplant 1995;
10. Janeway CA. The immune system evolved to discriminate infectious nonself from non-infectious self. Immunol Today 1992; 13: 11
11. Kantor AB, Herzenberg LA. Origin of murine B cell lineages. Ann Rev Immunol 1993; 11: 501
12. Casali P, Prabhakar BS, Notkins AL. Characterization of multireactive autoantibodies and identification of LEU-1+ B lymphocytes as cells making antibodies binding multiple self and exogenous molecules. Intern.Rev.Immunol. 1988; 3: 17

13. Boyden SV. Natural antibodies and the immune response. Adv Immunol 1966; 5: 1
14. Wilson GS, Miles AA. Topley and Wilson's Principles of Bacteriology and Immunity. London: Arnold, 1955
15. Shilo M. Nonspecific resistance to infections. Ann Rev Microbiol 1959; 12: 255
16. Jerne NK, Nordin AA. Plaque formation in agar by single antibody-producing cells. Science 1963; 140: 405
17. Hammer C, Hingerle M. Development of preformed natural antibodies in gnotobiotic dogs and pigs, impact of food antigens on antibody specificity. Transplant Proc 1992; 24: 707
18. Turman MA, Casali P, Notkins AL, Bach FH, Platt JL. Polyreactivity and antigen specificity of human xenoreactive monoclonal and serum natural antibodies. Transplantation 1991; 52: 710
19. Geller RL, Bach FH, Turman MA, Casali P, Platt JL. Evidence that polyreactive antibodies are deposited in rejected discordant xenografts. Transplantation 1993; 55: 168
20. Casali P, Burastero SE, Nakamura M, Inghirami G, Notkins AL. Human lymphocytes making rheumatoid factor and antibody to ssDNA belong to Leu-1+ B-cell subset. Science 1992; 236: 77
21. Berek C, Ziegner M. The maturation of the immune response. Immuol Today 1993; 14: 400
22. Chen PP, Liu MF, Sinha S, Carson DA. A 16/6 idiotype-positive anti-DNA antibody is encoded by a conserved V_H gene with no somatic mutation. Arthritis Rheum 1988; 31: 1429
23. Siminovitch KA, Mesiner V, Kwong PC, Song QL, Chen PP. A natural autoantibody is encoded by germline heavy and lambda light chain variable region genes without somatic mutation. J Clin Invest 1989; 84: 1675
24. Chen C, Stenzel-Poore MP, Rittenberg MB. Natural auto- and polyreactive antibodies differing from antigen-induced antibodies in the H chain CDR3. J Immunol 1991; 147: 2359
25. Martin T, Duffy SF, Carson DA, Kipps TJ. Evidence for somatic selection of natural antibodies. J Exp Med 1992; 175: 983
26. Ichiyoshi Y, Casali P. Analysis of the structural correlates for antibody polyreactivity by multiple reassortments of chimeric human immunoglobulin heavy and light chain V segments. J Exp Med 1994; 180: 885
27. Mouthon L, Nobrega A, Nicolas N, et al. Invariance and restriction toward a limited set of self-antigens characterize neonatal IgM antibody repertoires and prevail in autoreactive repertoires of healthy adults. Proc Natl Acad Sci USA 1995; 92: 3839
28. Starzl TE, Ishikawa M, Putnam CW, et al. Progress in and deterrents to orthotopic liver transplantation, with special reference to survival, resistance to hyperacute rejection, and biliary duct reconstruction. Transplant Proc 1974; 6: 129
29. Hume DM, Merrill JP, Miller BF, Thorn GW. Experiences with renal homotransplantation in the human: report of nine cases. J Clin Invest 1955; 34: 327
30. Alexandre GPJ, Latinne D, Carlier M, et al. ABO-incompatibility and organ transplantation. Transplant Rev 1991; 5: 230
31. Platt JL, Lindman BJ, Chen H, Spitalnik SL, Bach FH. Endothelial cell antigens recognized by xenoreactive human natural antibodies. Transplantation 1990; 50: 817

32. Tuso PJ, Cramer DV, Yasunaga C, et al. Removal of natural human xenoantibodies to pig vascular endothelium by perfusion of blood through pig kidneys and livers. Transplantation 1993; 55: 1375
33. Pozzetto U, Citterio F, Caizzi MP, et al. Humoral immune reactions to pig antigens in humans. Transplant Proc 1990; 22: 2000
34. Gautreau C, Cardoso J, Jeyaraj P, Houssin D, Weil B. Relationship between human natural anti-A, anti-B alloantibodies and anti-pig xenoantibodies. Transplant Proc 1993; 25: 389
35. Calne RY. Organ transplantation between widely disparate species. Transplant Proc 1970; 2: 550
36. Yasunaga C, Cramer DV, Cosenza CA, et al. The effect of bequinar sodium on in vivo antibody production. Transplant Proc 1993; 25 (Suppl 2): 40
37. Scherrer L, Leventhal JR, Matas AJ, Dalmasso AP. Evidence that rat xenoreactive antibodies recognize multiple protein antigens on guinea pig endothelial cells and platelets. Transplantation 1994; 58: 458
38. Aksentijevich I, Sachs DH, Sykes M. Natural antibodies against bone marrow cells of a concordant xenogeneic species. J Immunol 1991; 147: 79
39. Edwards N, Ott G, Berger C. Incidence of preformed antibodies against potential xenodonors in human serum. Transplantation 1990; 49: 1022
40. Abouna GM, Serrou B, Boehmig HJ, Amemiya H, Martineau G. Long-term hepatic support by intermittent multi-species liver perfusions. Lancet 1970; 1: 391
41. Cotterell AH, Collins BH, Parker W, Harland RC, Platt JL. The humoral immune response in humans following cross-perfusion of porcine organs. Transplantation 1995; 60: 861
42. Leventhal JR, Sakiyalak P, Witson J, et al. The synergistic effect of combined antibody and complement depletion on discordant cardiac xenograft survival in nonhuman primates. Transplantation 1994; 57: 974
43. Wu GD, Cramer DV, Kearns M, Eiras-Hreha G, Makowka L. Distribution of xenogeneic target antigens detected by a monoclonal antibody capable of inducing hyperacute rejection of hamster cardiac xenografts in rats. Transplant Proc 1994; 26: 1382
44. Cramer DV, Wu GD, Oriol R, Makowka L. Target antigen specificity of a monoclonal antibody (HAR-1) that causes the rejection of hamster heart xenografts in rats. Transplant Proc 1995; (in press)
45. Parker W, Bruno D, Holzknecht ZE, Platt JL. Characterization and affinity isolation of xenoreactive human natural antibodies. J.Immunol. 1994; 153: 3791
46. Galili U, Shohet SB, Kobrin E, Stults CL, Macher BA. Man, apes, and old world monkeys differ from other mammals in the expression of α-galactosyl epitopes on nucleated cells. J Biol Chem 1988; 263: 17755
47. Galili U. Interaction of the natural anti-Gal antibody with α-galactosyl epitopes: A major obstacle for xenotransplantation in humans. Immunol Today 1993; 14: 480
48. Galili U, Macher BA, Buehler J, Shohet SB. Human natural anti-α-galactosyl IgG. II. The specific recognition of α(1→3)-linked galactose residues. J Exp Med 1985; 162: 573
49. Galili U, Anaraki F, Thall A, Hill-Black C, Radic M. One percent of human circulating B lymphocytes are capable of producing the natural anti-gal antibody. Blood 1993; 82: 2485

50. Oriol R, Ye Y, Koren E, Cooper DKC. Carbohydrate antigens of pig tissues reacting with human natural antibodies as potential targets for hyperacute vascular rejection in pig-to-man organ xenotransplantation. Transplantation 1993; 56: 1433
51. Sandrin MS, Vaughan HA, Dabkowski PL, McKenzie IFC. Anti-pig IgM antibodies in human serum react predominantly with Gal(α1–3)Gal epitopes. Immunology 1993; 90: 11391
52. Thibaudeau K, Anegon I, Lemauff B, Soulillou JP, Blanchard D. Human natural antibodies to porcine platelets. Transplantation 1994; 57(7): 1110.
53. Wu GD, Cramer DV, Chapman FA, Oriol R, Makowka L. Genetic control of the humoral immune response to xenografts. I. Functional characterization of rat monoclonal antibodies to hamster heart xenografts. Transplantation 1995; 60: 1497
54. Borie DC, Cramer DV, Shirwan H, et al. Genetic control of the humoral immune response to xenografts. II. Monoclonal antibodies that cause rejection of heart grafts are encoded by germline immunoglobulin genes. Transplantation 1995; 60: 1504

8 Mechanisms of Delayed Xenograft Rejection[1]

D.J. Goodman, M.T. Millan, C. Ferran and F.H Bach

Introduction

The first barrier to transplantation of vascularised organs between discordant species is hyperacute rejection [1–3]. Stratagems that inhibit hyperacute rejection such as the use of cobra venom factor or soluble complement regulatory protein-1 (sCR1) have led to a delayed form of rejection which we have termed "delayed xenograft rejection" (DXR) [4] and permitted an examination of the mechanisms of DXR [5–8]. In contrast to allograft rejection, where T cells constitute greater than 90 % of infiltrating cells, the predominant cell types infiltrating the xenografts are natural killer (NK) cells (10 %–20 %) and monocytes (70 %–80 %) [8]. The infiltrating cells in delayed xenograft rejection are activated with monocytes staining positive for tumour necrosis factor (TNF)-α and interleukin (IL)-1β and NK cells staining positive for interferon (IFN)-γ [4]. DXR is also associated with endothelial cell (EC) activation, fibrin deposition and platelet aggregation [4]. In this review, we focus on the pathogenesis of delayed xenograft rejection with particular emphasis on the role of NK cells and monocytes and their potential participation in EC activation and transplant rejection. Our in vitro studies of DXR demonstrated that NK cells and monocytes activate EC by both direct cell contact and cytokine secretion resulting in the induction of a wide range of EC genes including adhesion molecules and chemoattractant molecules.

Models of Delayed Xenograft Rejection

There is a striking similarity between the histological features of DXR in guinea pig to rat [9] and pig to nonhuman primate studies [10]. The association of EC activation with an infiltrate consisting of NK cells and monocytes is a common theme [11].

Transplantation of a guinea pig heart to a rat serves as a model for discordant xenograft rejection. The inhibition of complement by cobra venom factor (CVF) results in a prolongation in cardiac graft survival from 15 min to approximately 72 h [4]. Sequential histopathological examination of cardiac transplants demonstrates infiltration of NK cells and monocytes within 12–24 h [4]. Furthermore, examination for the expression of cytokines demonstrate TNF-α and IFN-γ in

[1] D.J. Goodman and M.T. Millan contributed equally to this chapter.

association with monocytes and with NK cells, respectively. The presence of TNF-α and IFN-γ demonstrate that both cell types are activated within the rejecting organ [4]. Similar results were observed with C6-deficient rats [12], suggesting that the histopathological features of DXR are not a result of CVF treatment.

Adoptive transfer studies support a pathogenic role for monocytes in DXR. Using a guinea pig to rat heart transplant model Fryer et al. [6] demonstrated that injection of sensitised splenocytes from previously transplanted rats into xenograft recipients shortened xenograft survival. Depletion of monocytes from the splenocyte population transferred, resulted in a prolongation in xenograft survival when compared to adoptive transfer of the total splenocyte population [6]. Pig to primate studies with inhibitors of hyperacute rejection are also associated with the presence of NK cells and monocytes [10].

Endothelial Cell Activation

Type I Activation

EC activation is a prominent feature of rejecting xenografts [4, 9, 10].and plays a major role in modulating the immune response through the expression of adhesion molecules and secretion of cytokines [13]. EC activation can be divided into an early phase of EC activation which is independent of protein synthesis (type I EC activation) and a later phase, type II activation which is associated with new protein synthesis [13]. The early response to EC injury is associated with release of prostaglandin (PGE_2 and PGI_2) and endothelium-derived relaxation factor (EDRF)-nitric oxide (NO), which modulate platelet function and vascular tone (Table 1). The local expression of P selectin enhances adhesion of circulating neutrophils which may contribute further to EC injury. The release of membrane bound thrombomodulin and heparan sulphate further enhance coagulation and the loss of ecto-ADPase, which degrades ADP, presumably leads to enhanced platelet aggregation [7].

Type II Activation

Transcription of new protein is the hallmark of type II EC activation. The characteristic phenotypic features of EC activation include (Table 1), the vascular expression of adhesion molecules such as E selectin, intercellular adhesion molecule (ICAM)-1 and vascular cell adhesion molecule (VCAM)-1 and the pro-coagulant receptor for factor VII/VIIa, tissue factor [14]. The chemoattractant molecules IL-8 and monocyte chemotactic peptide (MCP)-1 are also expressed during DXR. IL-8 is a chemoattractant for neutrophils, NK cells and lymphocytes, whereas MCP-1 is a monocyte chemoattractant (109]. Both molecules are products of EC activation. We hypothesise that circulating monocytes and NK cells adhere to and activate xenogeneic endothelium [15, 16] to express adhesion receptors and secrete chemokines enhancing lymphocyte recruitment and transendothelial cell migration. In addition, activated monocytes may exacerbate the

Table 1. Classification and consequences of endothelial cell (EC) activation

EC Activation		Biological consequences
Type I	Cellular retraction	Exposure of thrombogenic subendothelium
	P selectin	PMN adhesion
	vWF release	Platelet adhesion to EC
	Heparan sulphate release	Loss of anti-thrombin III activity
	PAF release	Platelet activation
	Prostaglandin (I_2,E_2)	Vascular tone and inflammation
	Nitric oxide (NO)	Vasodilatation
	Endothelin-1	Vasoconstriction and mitogen
	Leukotriene (C_4, D_4, A_4)	vWF expression and secretion
Type II	Leukocyte–EC interactions	
	E selectin	PMN, lymphocyte, and monocyte adhesion
	ICAM-1	Leukocyte adhesion ligand for LFA-1
	VCAM-1	Leukocyte adhesion ligand for VLA-1
	MHC classes I, II	Antigen presentation to T cells
	IL-8	Chemokine
	MCP-1	Chemokine
	IL-1β	Inflammation
	Growth factors	
	M-CSF	Monocyte differentiation
	GM-CSF	Monocyte differentiation
	PDGF	Smooth muscle cell mitogen
	TGF-β	Growth regulation
	bFGF	Mitogen
	IL-6	B cell growth
	Vascular tone	
	Cyclooxygenase	Prostaglandin synthesis
	NO synthase	Synthesis of NO
	Thrombosis/matrix remodelling	
	PAI-1	Inhibition of plasminogen activator
	Plasminogen activator	Activation of plasminogen to plasmin
	Collagenase	Matrix degradation and remodelling
	Vitronectin	Extracellular matrix factor
	Tissue factor	Cofactor for extrinsic coagulation pathway
	Thrombomodulin	Regulation of aPC synthesis by thrombin

Human cytokines were added to human and porcine EC and then assayed for E selectin, MHC (SLA) class I and II antigen expression, and IL-8 secretion. SLA class I was constitutively expressed on porcine EC and was only induced with porcine IFN-γ. This demonstrates cross-species reactivity for IL-1α and TNF-α and species specificity for IL-1β and IFN-γ.
EC activation has been classified into type I activation, which occurs in the absence of new protein synthesis, and type II activation, which requires gene transcription and new protein synthesis. For each molecule described, a single example of the biological consequences has been provided. Many of the molecules have multiple functions and act on a variety of different tissues. IL, interleukin; TNF, tumour necrosis factor; IFN, interferon; MHC, major histocompatibility complex.

pro-coagulant environment by expressing tissue factor [17] and inducing EC derived plasminogen activator inhibitor (PAI)-1, which inhibits clot lysis (M.T. Millan, submitted).

Evidence for a Pathogenic Role of Natural Killer Cells in Delayed Xenograft Rejection

NK cells have been implicated in the prevention of cancer [18], inhibition of tumour metastasis [19, 20] and EC damage associated with IL-2 therapy [21]. Rare NK cell deficiency states have been reported and are associated with multiple life-threatening viral infections [22].

The role of NK cells in allograft and xenograft transplant models is undefined but several in vitro models support the concept that NK cells contribute to transplant rejection. The perfusion of rat hearts with human peripheral blood mononuclear cells resulted in the selective adhesion of NK cells, and the addition of human IgG to the cellular perfusate enhanced adhesion [23]. In addition, NK cells infiltrated the vascular wall and were associated with disruption and destruction of rat EC. Perfusion with NK cells was also associated with an increase in vascular resistance [23].

NK cells lyse target cells by at least two distinct mechanisms. NK cell-mediated cytotoxicity in the presence of antibody (antibody-dependent cell-mediated cytotoxicity) is mediated through the Fc receptor (FcγIII:CD16), which links the NK cell to the target cell. In addition, cross-linking of the CD16 receptor induces the transcription and secretion of TNF-α and IFN-γ [24]. However, the FcγIII receptor is not essential for cytotoxicity, as NK cells from FcγIII receptor deficient mice maintain the ability to adhere to and lyse NK targets [25, 26]. Direct cytotoxicity occurs in the absence of antibody and is mediated by several families of molecules which at least in part interact with major histocompatibility complex (MHC) class I molecules on the target cell surface [27]. Both ADCC and direct cytotoxicity are mediated by the release of perforin and granzymes.

Human Natural Killer Cells Activate Porcine Endothelial Cells

When we co-cultured human NK cells with porcine EC, E-selectin and IL-8 mRNA was detected after 4 h, demonstrating activation of the EC. The level of mRNA expression was maximal at effector to target (E:T) ratios of 30:1. E selectin and IL-8 mRNA expression was followed by endothelial E selectin protein expression and IL-8 secretion. E:T ratios greater than 30:1 resulted in a reduction in E selectin, IL-8 and β-actin mRNA consistent with RNA degradation due to the higher level of NK cell-mediated cytotoxicity. That it was the NK cells that activate EC was confirmed by showing that fluorescence-activated cell sorter (FACS) sorted CD56-positive cells, the NK cell clone, B22 and the FcγIII-deficient cell line, NK92 all induced the expression of E selectin and IL-8 mRNA followed by cell surface expression of E selectin and IL-8 secretion [15]. Several lines of evidence suggest that EC activation is not a consequence of EC cytotoxicity and the signals for EC activation are independent of the cytolytic machinery. Firstly, EC activation was observed at E:T ratios significantly lower than associated with detectable levels of cytotoxicity [15] and secondly, subclones of NK92 which have lost the ability to lyse EC retain the ability to activate EC (D.J. Goodman, unpublished data). In addition to the induction of E selectin and IL-8, Watson et al. have demonstrated the induction of MHC class II in Chinese hamster ovarian (CHO) cells and human umbilical EC, suggesting that human NK cells may induce MHC class II antigens in allografts and xenografts [28].

Mechanism of Natural Killer Cell-Mediated Endothelial Cell Activation

Human NK cells secrete a range of cytokines such as TNF-α, IL-1β, IFN-γ and IL-3[29] and express adhesion molecules including ICAM-1, CD11a and CD11c [29]. In order to define the mechanism of porcine EC activation by human NK cells, we studied transwell cultures where human NK cells were separated from EC by a semi-permeable membrane which permitted the passage of soluble factors, but prevented direct cell contact. NK cells failed to activate EC when separated in transwell cultures, demonstrating that cell–cell contact is essential for NK cell-mediated EC activation.

To further investigate the mechanism of NK cell-mediated EC activation and a possible role in this system for soluble mediators of EC activation, transwell cultures were prepared containing confluent EC monolayers in both the transwell and the lower chamber. The addition of NK92 cells to the upper transwell failed to induce E selectin in the lower chamber EC (Fig. 1), whereas NK cells added to the lower chamber induced E selectin in an E:T-dependent manner within 4 h.

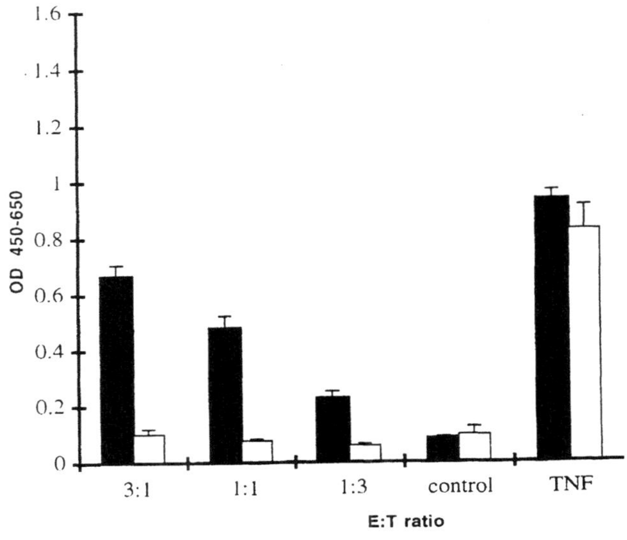

Fig. 1. Direct natural killer (NK)–endothelial cell (EC) contact is required for EC activation. EC were added to the upper and lower chambers of 96-well transwell culture plates such that media from both EC monolayers could freely communicate via a semipermeable membrane. NK92 cells were added to either the upper chamber (*white bars*) or the lower chamber (*black bars*). E selectin enzyme-linked immunosorbent assay (ELISA) was performed on the lower chamber after 4 h. Tumour necrosis factor (*TNF*) was added to either the upper or lower chambers to demonstrate membrane permeability. *E:T*, effector to target

The addition of TNF-α to the upper transwell resulted in EC activation of the lower chamber, confirming that soluble factors within the transwell can traverse the transwell membrane (Fig. 1). These data demonstrate that soluble factors from either NK cells after contact with EC or factors associated with EC activation or lysis are not primarily responsible for EC activation. Activated NK cells can express membrane-bound TNF-α and secrete TNF-α. The addition of human soluble TNF-α receptor or monoclonal mouse anti-human TNF-α antibody to co-cultures of human NK cells and porcine EC failed to inhibit the NK cell-mediated induction of E selectin or IL-8. This suggests that, in our NK–EC culture system, TNF-α did not contribute to EC activation, although the action of TNF-α at the point of cell contact between NK cells and EC cannot be ruled out.

Xenoreactive IgG Enhances Natural Killer Cell-Mediated Endothelial Cell Activation

During DXR, IgG fixed to EC can bind NK cells via the FcγIII (CD16) receptor, whereas the role of IgM appears to be less significant. In contrast, the major immunoglobulin isotype mediating complement activation during hyperacute rejection is IgM, with IgG playing a relatively minor role [2]. The addition of IgG to human NK cell–porcine EC co-cultures enhanced the level of induced E selectin at all E:T ratios studied, with the greatest augmentation occurring at the lower E:T ratios (Fig. 2). The addition of IgG also increased the level of EC cytotoxicity from 0 % to 5 % at an E:T ratio of 1:1 and from 25 % to 40 % at 30:1.

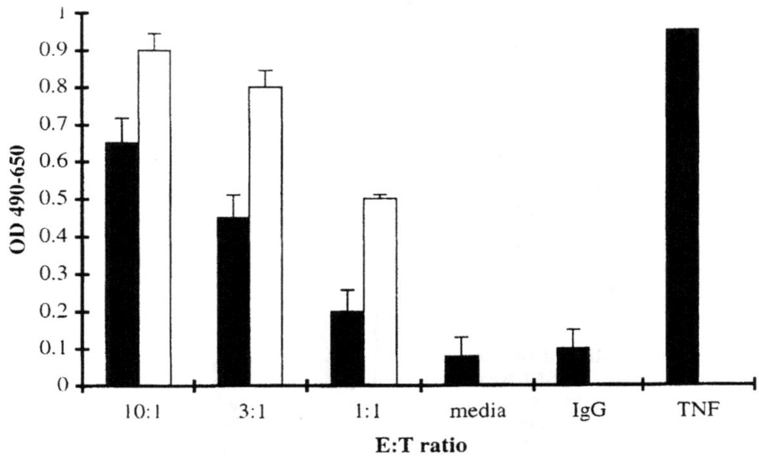

Fig. 2. Human IgG enhances natural killer (NK) cell-mediated endothelial cell (EC) activation. Human NK cells were added to porcine EC containing media (*black bars*) or media with protein G purified human IgG (*white bars*). After 4 h,E selectin enzyme-linked immunosorbent assay (ELISA) was performed. *TNF,* tumour necrosis factor; *E:T,* effector to target

Soluble factors released by NK cells do not appear to play a significant role in EC activation, and supernatants of purified human NK–EC co-cultures did not contain human TNF-α and IFN-γ. When purified human NK cells were co-cultured with porcine EC and screened by reverse transcriptase/polymerase chain reaction (RT/PCR) for the expression of human TNF-α, a weak positive signal was observed. Enzyme-linked immunosorbent assay (ELISA) for TNF-α in the supernatants failed to demonstrate TNF-α. The addition of IgG to NK–EC co-cultures resulted in a marked increase in the expression of human TNF-α mRNA and secretion of up to 47 pg TNF-α/ml over a 4-h co-culture. The biological activity of low levels of TNF-α was confirmed in vitro, with 40–50 pg TNF-α/ml activating EC to express E selectin. The co-culture supernatants were also screened for the presence of IFN-γ. In the absence of IgG, IFN-γ was not detected, and the addition of IgG resulted in human IFN-γ mRNA and 60 pg secreted IFN-γ/ml. Thus, in the presence of IgG, EC activation may be mediated by the combination of TNF-α-dependent and -independent pathways.

Endothelial Cell Activation Enhances Natural Killer–Endothelial Cell Cell Adhesion

EC activation results in the expression of multiple cell adhesion molecules such as E selectin, which contribute to NK–EC adhesion and cytotoxicity by binding sialylated Lewis^x adhesion molecules expressed on NK cells [30]. In vivo, the first EC encountered by NK cells during DXR may be activated due to prior binding of antibody and complement; we thus studied the interactions between human NK cells and pre-activated porcine EC in vitro to define if NK–EC interactions across species are influenced by prior EC activation. The CD16-deficient cell line, NK92 was studied to eliminate the possible effects of Fc-mediated adhesion and signalling. Pre-activation of EC with TNF-α or bacterial lipopolysaccharide (LPS) for 15 min did not increase NK–EC adhesion. In contrast, stimulation for 4 h resulted in a marked increase in adhesion. The enhanced adhesion after 4 h stimulation with TNF-α or LPS suggests that E selectin and ICAM-1 may play a role in NK–EC adhesion while P selectin, which is rapidly internalised does not. The increased adhesion is consistent with the concept that porcine EC activation results in the expression of adhesion molecules which bind human NK cells. Blocking antibodies to human adhesion molecules, including anti-CD11a or anti-CD18, both partially reduce adhesion and NK cellular cytotoxicity [31, 32], demonstrating that several adhesion molecules contribute to NK–EC adhesion across species.

Natural Killer Cell Target Recognition

Exciting advances in NK cell biology followed the report that NK cell activity can be modulated by MHC class I expression on the target cell and the identification of receptors for MHC class I antigen [33]. While cytolytic T cells are activated following MHC class I engagement, NK cell-mediated cytotoxicity is frequently inhibited [33]. The receptors for class I inhibition of NK cells are polymorphic and at least four specificities have been defined, two HLA-C and two HLA-B epitopes [34, 35]. The expression of NK cell receptors is heterogeneous within the NK cell population of a single donor and studies of NK cell clones have demonstrated that single clones express at least one receptor and some clones express two or more receptors.

Two questions critical to an understanding of NK–EC cell interaction across species and xenotransplantation remain unanswered: (1) Will human NK cells be inhibited by non-human MHC class I antigens and (2) will the expression of human MHC class I in porcine EC result in inhibition of NK cell-mediated cytotoxicity? Cross-species recognition of porcine class I (SLA class I) has been demonstrated with human CD8-positive T cells proliferating in response to porcine EC expressing SLA class I antigen [36]. Interestingly, the proliferative response of human T cells cultured with porcine EC is greater than the corresponding allogeneic responses to human umbilical vein EC [37]. Although suggestive of cross-species MHC class I recognition for T cells, recent evidence suggests that NK cells recognise a different epitope of the class I molecule, hence human T cells recognise SLA class I and proliferate while NK cells may not be inhibited by the same SLA class I antigen. The diversity between the MHC class I molecules especially at the regions defined to confer specificity NK cell recognition suggest that NK cell inhibition by MHC class I antigens may be confined to human and apes [33].

NK cells appear to recognise αGal1–3Gal (αGal) sugars, in addition to MHC receptors. In vitro, the addition of IgM or IgG XNA to the FcγIII-deficient cell line NK92 reduced the level of cytotoxicity (Fig. 3), consistent with work by Inverardi et al. [38], in which $F(ab)_2$ fragments reduced both adhesion and cytotoxicity of human NK cells to porcine EC. Furthermore, the binding of human NK cell to porcine EC could be competed with the same sugars which compete the binding of XNA to αGal sugars. The affinity of human NK cells to the αGal sugar epitopes expressed on porcine EC and the inhibition of NK cell adhesion and cytotoxicity with XNA may provide one explanation for the mechanism leading to prolongation in xenograft survival of guinea pig hearts transplanted to rats receiving human $F(ab)_2$ fragments prior to transplantation [39, 40].

Monocytes As Effector Cells in Delayed Xenograft Rejection

Monocytes may effect graft destruction via direct cytotoxicity, secretion of proteases and oxygen radicals, pro-inflammatory cytokines and as antigen-presenting cells (APC) leading to T cell-dependent immunologic injury. Because there are few T cells found in organs undergoing DXR [1] and nude rats, which are devoid of α/β T cells, still undergo hyperacute rejection and DXR in the same manner as normal rats [41], we will consider here the T cell-independent mechanisms by which monocytes may effect graft destruction.

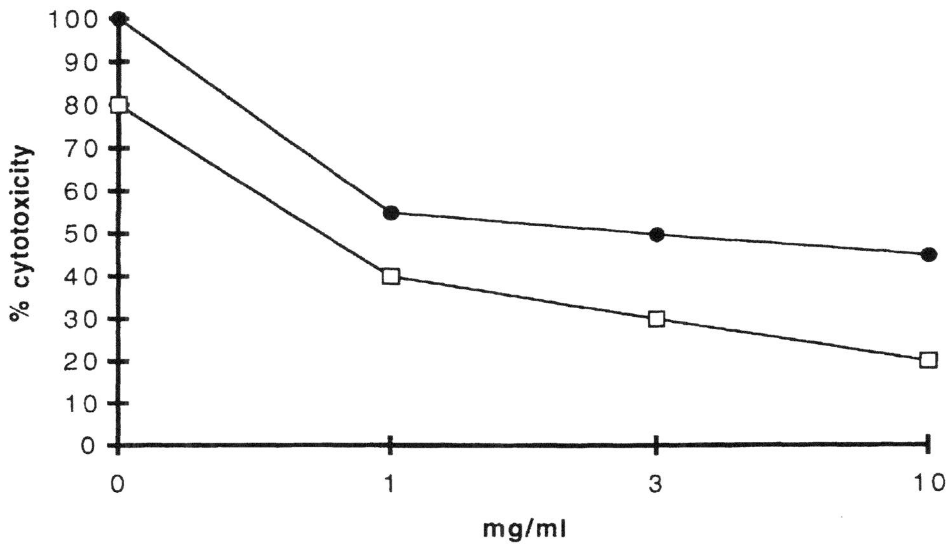

Fig. 3. Natural killer (NK) cells recognise αGal1-3Gal sugars. IgM and IgG inhibit NK92 cytotoxicity: NK92 cells were cocultured with porcine endothelial cell (EC) cultures containing either IgM (*black circles*) or IgG (*white squares*) for 4h followed by lactate dehydrogenase (LDH) release cytotoxicity assay. The immunoglobulin concentrations studied were similar to those found in human serum

Monocyte-Medicated Endothelial Cell Activation

We have reported that human monocytes are capable of directly activating porcine endothelial cells to express pro-inflammatory and pro-coagulant factors. We studied purified human monocytes or the human monocytic cell line, U937, in co-culture with porcine EC and demonstrated an increase in E selectin surface expression of (M.T. Millan, submitted).

Monocyte-mediated EC activation was also associated with the induction of the chemotactic cytokines IL-8 and MCP-1 and the pro-coagulant molecule PAI-1, an inhibitor of clot lysis (M.T. Millan, submitted). The addition of soluble (p55 or p75) TNF-α receptor to monocyte-EC co-cultures partially inhibited EC activation demonstrating both TNF-α dependant and independent mechanisms for EC activation in our monocyte-EC co-culture system (M.T. Millan et al. submitted). While IL-1α is active across the human-pig species barrier, the addition of IL-1α antagonists to monocyte-EC co-cultures failed to inhibit EC activation. As seen with NK cells, direct cell contact was essential for monocyte-mediated EC activation as transwell cultures with monocytes and EC separated by a semi-permeable membrane did not result in EC activation.

Monocyte-EC interactions result in formation of a complex cytokine network. The monocytes produce pro-inflammatory and chemotactic cytokines and also induce the EC to produce such factors [16]. Production of chemotactic cytokines by activated EC may explain the selective extravasation and activation of leukocytes and may account for the nature of the cellular infiltrate observed in rejecting discordant xenografts. Furthermore, leukocyte-EC interactions may modulate chemokine expression. For example, MCP-1 is induced during transmigration of human monocytes across human umbilical vein EC (HUVEC) monolayers [42]. We found that porcine EC also demonstrate an increase in IL-8 and MCP-1 expression when co-cultured with human monocytes (M.T. Millan, submitted). IL-8, a C-X-C chemokine, is a potent recruiter of neutrophils, NK cells, and lymphocytes while MCP-1 recruits primarily monocytes (and has recently been reported also to recruit T lymphocytes) [42]. It is still not clear whether these chemokines also demonstrate molecular incompatibility. Recent work has shown that even a single mutation in IL-8 may abrogate its angiogenic and chemotactic function; the extent to which such critical parts of the molecule and the corresponding receptor have been conserved is not clear. Kinetic studies of MCP-1 mRNA expression in monocyte–EC co-cultures demonstrated a biphasic response with an early induction after 4–6 h, not inhibited by soluble TNF-α receptor and a later peak after 24 h, which was inhibited by soluble TNF-α receptor (M.T. Millan, submitted).

Monocyte–EC interactions are not restricted to xenogeneic co-cultures as allogeneic monocytes induce EC activation and expression of MCP-1 [42] and PAI-1 [43], but these effects, even though preserved across species, may be modified due to molecular incompatibility.

Mechanisms of Monocyte–Endothelial Cell Interactions

The human monocytic cell line U937, which has not been overtly activated, approximates the adhesion behaviour of peripheral blood monocytes [44].We have shown that U937 cells adhere to quiescent porcine EC [44] and more so to activated EC [44] (M.T. Millan, submitted). It has been previously shown that adherence of human U937 cells to porcine EC under non-activated conditions is significantly greater than adherence to HUVEC [44], and EC activation results in a relatively greater increase in adhesion for the U937–HUVEC combination as compared to U937–porcine EC, which have a significantly higher level of basal adhesion. This difference does not appear to be explained by the difference between arterial and venous EC [44].

When we prevented cell contact between human monocytes and porcine EC in transwell cultures, EC activation was prevented [16]. These observations suggest that direct cell–cell interactions result in cell signalling. Signalling may occur through ligation of adhesion receptor molecules such as ICAM-1, which enhances the expression of the monocyte-derived MIP-1α in human monocute–HUVEC co-cultures [43], or the engagement of E selectin on HUVEC, which enhances the adhesive activity of the integrin CD11b/CD18 on neutrophils [45]. The literature describing allogeneic monocyte–EC adhesive interactions varies depending on the agonist, e.g. TNF, LPS, phorbol myristate acetate (PMA), duration of stimulus and the time points studied following the initial stimulus: P selectin [46–48], E selectin [49–51], ICAM-1 [52–55] and VCAM-1 [54] have all been shown to be involved in allogeneic monocyte–EC adhesion and may participate in EC activation.

Carbohydrate residues on porcine EC may be recognised by circulating monocytes and contribute to adhesion, subsequent activation and EC destruction. Russell et al. [56] have cloned and characterised a monocyte specific carbohydrate binding receptor and the level of expression is up-regulated during allograft rejection.

Monocyte–Natural Killer Cell Interactions

Although species-specific cytokines generated by activated NK cells, such as IFN-γ, will not directly stimulate porcine EC responses, IFN-γ could activate monocytes [57] within the rejecting transplant resulting in TNF-α release and further EC activation. In addition, IFN-γ stimulated monocytes secrete IL-12 [58], which can activate NK cells [58, 59]and influence the target spectrum of cytotoxic T-cells [59]. IFN-γ also synergises with IL-2 to enhance NK cell cytotoxicity [57]. IL-12 and IL-15 are generated by monocytes and can enhance NK cell-mediated cytotoxicity and synergise with IL-2. Thus NK cells and monocytes may create a cytokine network within the rejecting xenograft. The species specificity of these cytokines and their effect on EC is currently under investigation.

Molecular Incompatibility

NK cells or monocytes may secrete TNF-α, IFN-γ and IL-1α or IL-1β which activate human EC, resulting in MHC class I and II and E selectin expression [29, 57], but human IFN-γ and IL-1β are relatively species specific and in the human to pig system and do not induce the expression of MHC class II or E selectin on porcine EC [36] (Table 2). The combination of cross-species cytokine reactivity and species specificity gives rise to the concept of "molecular incompatibility" [11, 60], whereby cell–cell interactions may vary according to the molecule studied and species combination. The basis for molecular incompatibil-

Table 2. Molecular incompatibility

Human cytokine	Human EC	Porcine EC
IL-1α	+(E selectin)	(E selectin)
IL-1β	+(E selectin)	-
TNF-α	++(E selectin/IL-8)	+(E selectin/IL-8)
IFN-γ	+(MHC classes I, II)	-

EC, endothelial cell; vWF, von Willebrand factor; PAF, platelet aggregation factor; ICAM, intercellular adhesion molecular; VCAM, vascular cell adhesion molecule; MHC, major histocompatibility complex; IL, interleukin; MCP, monocyte chemotactic peptide; CSF, colony-stimulating factor; GM-CSF, granulocyte-macrophage CSF; PDGF, platelet-derived growth factor; TGF, tranforming growth factor; bFGF, basic fibroblast growth factor; PAI, plasminogen activator inhibitor; PMN, polymorphonuclear neutrophil; LFA, lymphocyte function-associated antigen; VLA, very late activation antigen; aPC, activated protein C.

ity may be attributed to either structural variation of the cytokine or cytokine receptor. In the case of IFN-γ, the species specificity resides in the structure of the IFN-γ receptor β-chain; transfection of the IFN-γ β-chain from the same species as the IFN-γ can restore IFN-γ responsiveness across species [61]. Molecular incapability is not restricted to cytokines and also includes adhesion molecules, coagulation factors and enzyme systems. The relative inefficiency of the complement regulatory proteins to inhibit complement cascade activation in discordant species combinations [3, 62, 63] has been postulated to account for the violent and immediate complement-mediated injury of discordant xenografts. The interaction of von Wilibrand factor (vWF) with platelet gpIb varies between species. In the human system sheer stress is required for platelet aggregation, but contact between porcine vWF and human platelet receptor gpIb will lead to platelet aggregation in the absence of sheer stress [11, 64]. Therefore, even if certain interactions are preserved across species, the products of these interactions may have different effects [11, 64].

Factors in Delayed Xenograft Rejection Other than Monocytes and Natural Killer Cells

Much of this review has focused on the interaction of NK cells and monocytes with EC and their subsequent role in graft rejection. In addition, the coagulation system plays a major role in vascular occlusion and graft rejection.

Coagulation

A characteristic finding in DXR is vascular thrombosis with both fibrin deposition and platelet plugging of small vessels. The interaction of tissue factor with factor VIIa appears to be the dominant interaction in determining the procoagulative effect in vitro [17]. The source of tissue factor during DXR includes the monocyte and the activated EC.

Thrombomodulin (TM) is expressed on EC and lost in response to EC injury [8]. TM binds thrombin and promotes the generation of activated protein C (aPC). Coupled with protein S, aPC splits factors Va and VIIIa, thereby inhibiting coagulation [65]. Work in our laboratory has focused on the maintenance of thrombomodulin expression on EC during inflammation and the biological functions of aPC [17]. Using retro-viral mediated gene transfer, porcine EC have been transduced with human thrombomodulin [17]. The level of the transduced human thrombomodulin is greater than that expressed on human EC and there is a parallel increased conversion of protein C to aPC in the presence of thrombin. Most importantly in these experiments, the levels of the thrombomodulin and the cofactor activity are not reduced when the EC are stimulated with an agonist. In vitro, aPC has been shown to inhibit TNF secretion by monocytes stimulated with LPS, interferon-γ and phorbol esters [65]. In vivo studies demonstrated a marked reduction in endotoxin-induced renal injury. The kidneys in aPC-treated animals displayed less fibrin deposition, mononuclear cellular infiltrate, cytokine expression and EC activation [66]. Receptors for aPC are expressed on monocytes and EC, but the biology of the actions of aPC on EC are yet to be defined [66]. Taken together, aPC is an exciting naturally occurring anti-inflammatory agent.

Platelets

Platelet aggregation is a tightly regulated dynamic process dependent on the simultaneous presence of pro- and anticoagulant factors such as EC-derived prostacycline, nitric oxide and platelet-activating factor (PAF). The initial binding of platelets to the vessel wall is dependent on the interaction of platelet GPIb with vWF present in the sub-endothelial matrix. Recent evidence suggests that the interaction between human platelets and human EC differ from the interactions of human platelets with pig EC. Most importantly, porcine vWF spontaneously interacts with the human GPIb receptor leading to platelet activation without the sheer stress needed for platelet activation following the interaction in allogeneic combinations [64]. The presence of membrane associated ecto-ADPases degrade platelet derived ADP [67], reducing platelet aggregation. Robson and colleagues in our centre have recently shown that TNF-α treatment of EC in vitro and hypoxia-reperfusion or hyperacute xenograft rejection are associated with the loss of ecto-ADPase activity [67].

Potential Therapeutic Targets

The rapid rejection of discordant vascularised xenografts has failed to be controlled with conventional immunosuppressive therapy used for allotransplantation. The more detailed understanding of the molecular and cellular biology of DXR has led to the introduction of stratagems to inhibit specific segments of the rejection process. The complexity of xenograft rejection makes it unlikely that any one therapy will be effective and ultimately combinations of therapies may be required. The tissue and organ specificity may become important factors in the evaluation of potential therapies. The involvement of NK cells and monocytes in DXR has led to modalities of treatment specifically aimed at inhibiting either monocyte or NK cell function. General inhibitors of EC activation may well be of value in xenotransplantation, an approach that Anrather, Winkler and others [68] in our laboratory have been testing.

Comment

We have described the rejection process of a discordant, immediately vascularised xenograft. The aetiology of DXR appears to be multifactorial involving NK cells, monocytes, platelets and activation of the coagulation system. Hyperacute rejection can be avoided by inhibition of complement, although it is not clear that there are not factors that contribute to hyperacute rejection that following complement inhibition will simply act later. If HAR is averted, then the graft is rejected by factors that we have grouped as constituting DXR. In this paper we have focused heavily on the role of human NK cells and monocytes as they interact with porcine EC, resulting in cellular activation, cytokine secretion and adhesion molecule expression. Interactions between infiltrating NK cells and monocytes will form local cytokine networks within the rejecting xenograft. We have briefly discussed the role of factors other than NK cells and monocytes in DXR and these have been reviewed in recent articles from our laboratory [7, 8, 11].

Stratagems will thus likely be required to inhibit EC activation, thrombosis and monocyte- and NK cell-mediated responses to achieve further prolongation in vascularised discordant xenograft survival using therapies that might be acceptable in humans. The understanding of the cellular and molecular basis for DXR coupled with novel methods of donor tissue genetic manipulation should provide transplant specific immunosuppression and prolong xenograft survival.

Acknowledgments. We thank our colleagues in the Sandoz Center for Immunobiology for their comments on this manuscript. Dr. D.J. Goodman is a Don Jacquot Travelling Fellow.

References

1. Hancock, W.W., Blakely, M.L., Vanderwerf, W., Bach, F.H. Rejection of guinea pig cardiac xenografts post-cobra venom factor therapy is associated with infiltration by mononuclear cells secreting interferon-gamma and diffuse endothelial activation. Transplant. Proc. 25: 2932, 1993
2. Platt, J.L., Lindman, B.J., Geller, R.L., et al. The role of natural antibodies in the activation of xenogenic endothelial cells. Transplantation. 52: 1037, 1991
3. Dalmasso, A.P., Vercellotti, G.M., Platt, J.L., Bach, F.H. Inhibition of complement-mediated endothelial cell cytotoxicity by decay-accelerating factor – potential for prevention of xenograft hyperacute rejection. Transplantation. 52: 530, 1991
4. Blakely, M.L., Van der Werf, W., Berndt, M.C., et al. Activation of intragraft endothelial and mononuclear cells during discordant xenograft rejection. Transplantation. 58: 1059, 1994
5. Fryer, J.P., Leventhal, J., Dalmasso, A., et al. Beyond hyperacute rejection. Transplantation. 59: 171, 1995
6. Fryer, J.P., Leventhal, J., Dalmasso, A., et al. Cellular rejection in discordant xenografts when hyperacute rejection is prevented: analysis using adoptive and passive transfer. Transpl. Immunol. 2: 87, 1994
7. Robson, S.C., Candinas, D., Hancock, W.W., et al. Role of endothelial cells in transplantation. Int. Arch. Allergy. Immunol. 106: 305, 1995
8. Bach, F.H., Robson, S.C., Ferran, C., et al. Xenotransplantation: Endothelial cell activation and beyond. Transplant Proc 27: 77, 1995
9. Leventhal, J.R., Matas, A.J., Sun, L.H., et al. The immunopathology of cardiac xenograft rejection in the guinea pig-to-rat model. Transplantation. 56: 1, 1993
10. Platt, J.L., Fischel, R.J., Matas, A.J., et al. Immunopathology of hyperacute xenograft rejection in a swine-to-primate model. Transplantation. 52: 214, 1991

11. Bach, F.H., Robson, S.C., Winkler, H., et al. Barriers to xenotransplantation. Nature Med 1: 869, 1996
12. Zhow, X-J., Nielsen, N., Pawlowski, I., et al. Prolongation of survival of discordant kidney xenografts by C6 deficiency. Transplantation. 50: 896, 1990
13. Pober, J.S., Cotran, R.S. The role of endothelial cells in inflammation. Transplantation. 50: 537, 1991
14. Esmon, C.T. Cell mediated events that control blood coagulation and vascular injury. Annu Rev Cell Biol 9: 1, 1993
15. Goodman, D.J., von Albertini, M., Wilson, A., Millan, M.T., Bach, F.H. Direct activation of porcine endothelial cells by human NK cells. Transplantation. In press
16. Millan, M.T., Ferran, C., Stuhlmeier, K.M., Geczy, C., Bach, F.H. Human monocytes activate porcine endothelial cells by direct cell contact, involving TNFα. Transplant Proc In press
17. Hofer, E., Stuhlmeier, K.M., Blakely, M.L., et al. Pathways of procoagulation in discordant xenografting. Transplant. Proc. 26: 1322, 1994
18. Pross, H.F., Lotzova, E. Role of natural killer cells in cancer. Nat. Immun. 12: 279, 1993
19. Haller, O., Hansson, M., Kiessling, R., Wigzell, H. Role of non-conventional natural killer cells in resistance against syngeneic tumor cells in vivo. Nature 270: 609, 1977
20. Talmadge, J.E., Meyers, K.M., Prieur, D.J., Starkey, J.R. Role of NK cells in tumor growth and metastasis in beige mice. Nature 284: 622, 1980
21. Kotasek, D., Ochoa, A., Vercellotti, F.M., Bach, F.H., Jacob, H.S. Lymphokine-activated killer (LAK) cells injure cultured endothelium: a possible mechanism for capillary leak syndrome in patients treated with LAK cells and interleukin-2. Trans. Assoc. Am. Physicians. 21, 1988
22. Biron, C.A., Byron, K.S., Sullivan, J.L. Severe herpes virus infection in an adolescent without natural killer cells. N. Engl. J. Med. 320: 1731, 1995
23. Inverardi, L., Samaja, M., Motterlini, R., et al. Early recognition of a discordant xenogeneic organ by human circulating lymphocytes. J. Immunol. 149: 1416, 1992
24. Anegon, I., Cuturi, M.C., Trinchieri, G., Perussia, B. Interaction of Fc receptor (CD16) interaction ligands induces transcription of IL-2 receptor (CD25) and lymphokine genes and expression of their products in human natural killer cells . J. Exp. Med. 167: 452, 1988
25. Takai, T., Li, M., Sylvestre, D., Clynes, R., Ravetch, J.V. FcRγ chain deletion results in pleitrophic effector cell defects. Cell 76: 519, 1994
26. Gong, J.H., Maki, G., Klingemann, H.G. Characterization of a human cell line (NK-92) with phenotypical and functional characteristics of activated natural killer cells. Leukemia 8: 652, 1994
27. Karre, K. Express yourself or die: Peptides, MHC molecules, and NK cells. Science 267: 978, 1995
28. Watson, C.A., Petzelbauer, P., Zhou, J., Pardi, R., Bender, J.R. Contact-dependent endothelial class II HLA gene activation by NK cells is mediated by IFN-γ-dependent and -independent mechanism. J. Immunol. 154: 3222, 1995
29. Robertson, M.J., Ritz, J. Biology and clinical relevance of human natural killer cells. Blood. 76: 2421, 1990
30. Pinola, M., Renkonen, R., Majuri, M.L., Tiisala, S., Saksela, E. Characterization of the E-Selectin ligand on NK cells. J. Immunol. 152: 3586, 1994

31. Pleass, H.C.C., Kirby, J.A., Forsyth, J.L.R., Proud, G., Taylor, R.M.R. Adhesion molecule blockade in a porcine xenograft model. Transplant. Proc. 26: 1162, 1995
32. Inverardi, L., Samaja, M., Bender, J.R., Pardi, R. Cellular early immune recognition of xenogeneic vascular endothelium. Transplant. Proc. 24: 459, 1992
33. Gumperz, J.E., Parham, P. The enigma of the natural killer cell. Science 378: 245, 1995
34. Malnati, M.S., Peruzzi, M., Parker, K.C., et al. Peptide specificity in the recognition of MHC class I by natural killer cell clones. Science 267: 1016, 1995
35. Moretta, L., Ciccone, E., Pende, D., et al. Existence of a natural killer (NK) cell repertoire for (allo)antigen recognition: definition of five distinct NK-determined allospecificities in humans. Pharmacol. Res 26 Suppl 2: 98, 1992
36. Murray, A.G., Khoudadoust, M.M., Pober, J.S., Bothwell, A.L.M. Porcine aortic endothelial cells strongly activate human T cells: Direct presentation of swine MHC antigens and effective co-stimulation by swine ligands for human CD2 and CD28. Immunity 1: 57, 1994
37. Savage, C.O.S., Hughes, C.C.W., Mcintyre, B.W., Picard, J.K., Pober, J.S. Human CD4+ T-Cells proliferate to HLA-DR+ allogeneic vascular endothelium - identification of accessory interactions. Transplantation. 56: 128, 1993
38. Inverardi, L., Clissi, B., Bender, J.R., Pardi, R. Partial overlap of carbohydrate ligands recognized by human preformed natural antibodies and natural killer cells. Transplant. Proc. In press
39. Magee, J.C., Collins, B.H., Harland, R.C., et al. Prevention of hyperacute xenograft rejection by intravenous immunoglobulin. Transplant. Proc. 27: 271, 1995
40. Latremouille, C., Haeffner-Cavaillon, N., Goussef, N., et al. Normal human polyclonal immunoglobulins for intravenous use significantly delay hyperacute xenograft rejection. Transplant. Proc. 26: 1285, 1994
41. Candinas, D., Lesnikoski, B., Grey, S.t., et al. Delayed xenograft rejection in complement depleted T-cell-deficient (nude) rat recipients of guinea pig cardiac grafts. Transplant. Proc. In press
42. Takahashi, M., Masuyama, J., Ikeda, U., et al. Induction of monocyte chemoattractant protein-1 synthesis in human monocytes during transendothelial migration in vitro. Circ. Res. 76: 750, 1995
43. Lukacs, N.W., Strieter, R.M., Elner, V.M., et al. Intercellular adhesion molecule-1 mediates the expression of monocyte-derived MIP-1a during monocyte-endothelial cell interactions. Blood. 83: 1174, 1994
44. Di Corieto, P.E., de la Motte, C.A. Characterization of the adhesion of the human monocytic cell line U937 to cultured endothelial cells. J. Clin. Invest. 75: 1153, 1985
45. Lo, S.K., Lee, S., Ramos, R.A., et al. Endothelial-leukocyte adhesion molecule 1 stimulates the adhesive activity of leukocyte integrin CR3 (CD11b/CD18, Mac-1, amb2) on human neutrophils. J. Exp. Med. 173: 1493, 1991
46. Murphy, J.F., McGregor. J.L. Two sites on P-selectin (the lectin and epidermal growth factor-like domains) are involved in the adhesion of monocytes to thrombin-activated endothelial cells. Biochem. J. 303(Pt2): 619, 1994
47. Murphy, J.F., Bordet, J.C., Wyler, B., et al. The vitronectin receptor (alpha v beta 3) is implicated, in co-operation with P-selectin and platelet-activating factor, in the adhesion of monocytes to activated endothelial cells. Biochem. J. 304(Pt2): 537, 1994
48. McEver, R.P. GMP-140: a receptor for neutrophils and Monocytes on activated platelets and endothelium. J. Cell Biochem. 45: 156, 1991

49. Hakkert, B.C., Kuijpers, T.W., Leeuwenberg, J.F., van Mourik, J.A., Roo, D. Neutrophil and monocyte adherence to and migration across monolayers of cytokine-activated endothelial cells: the contribution of CD18, ELAM-1 and VLA-4. Blood. 78: 2721, 1994
50. Leeuwenberg, J.F., Jeunhomme, T.M., Buurman, W.A. Role of ELAM-1 in adhesion of monocytes to activated human endothelial cells. Scand. J. Immunol. 35: 335, 1992
51. Rollins, S.A., Evans, M.J., Johnson, K.K., et al. Molecular and functional analysis of porcine E-selectin reveals a potential role in xenograft rejection. Biochem. Biophys. Res Commun. 204: 763, 1994
52. Conti, P., Dempsey, R.A., Reale, M., et al. Activation of human natural killer cells by lipopolysaccharide and generation of interleukin-1alpha, interleukin-1beta, tumour necrosis factor and interleukin- 6 – effect of IL-1 receptor antagonist. Immunology. 73: 450, 1991
53. Takahashi, M., Ikeda, U., Masuyama, J., et al. Involvement of adhesion molecules in human monocyte adhesion to and transmigration through endothelial cells in vitro. Atherosclerosis 108: 73, 1994
54. Weber, C., Erl, W., Pietsch, A., et al. Antioxidants inhibit monocyte adhesion by suppressing nuclear factor-kappa B mobilization and induction of vascular cell adhesion molecule-1 in endothelial cells stimulated to generate radicals. Arterioscler. Thromb. 14: 1665, 1994
55. Meerschaert, J., Furie, M.B. The adhesion molecules used by monocytes for migration across endothelium include CD11a/CD18, CD11b/CD18, and VLA-4 on monocytes and ICAM-1, VCAM-1 and other ligands on endothelium. J. Immunol. 154: 4099, 1995
56. Russell, M.E., Utans, U., Wallace, A.F., et al. Identification and upregulation of galactose/N-acetylgalactosasamine macrophage lectin in rat cardiac allografts with arteriosclerosis. J. Clin. Invest. 94: 722, 1994
57. Robertson, M.J., Ritz, J. Role of IL-2 receptors in NK cell activation and proliferation. In NK Cell-Mediated Cytotoxicity: Receptors, Signaling and Mechanism. E. Lotzova, R.B. Herberman, eds. CRC Press, Boca Raton, Florida, p. 183, 1992
58. Trinchieri, G., Kubin, M., Bellone, G., Cassatella, M.A. Cytokine cross-talk between phagocytic cells and lymphocytes – relevance for differentiation/activation of phagocytic cells and regulation of adaptive immunity. J. Cell Biochem. 53: 301, 1993
59. Robertson, M.J., Soiffer, R.J., Wolf, S.F., et al. Response of human natural killer (NK) cells to NK cell stimulatory factor (NKSF): cytolytic activity and proliferation of NK cells are differentially regulated by NKSF. J. Exp. Med. 175: 779, 1992
60. Platt, J.L., Bach, F.H. Discordant xenografting – challenges and controversies. Curr. Opin. Immunol. 3: 735, 1991
61. Hemmi, S., Bohni, R., Stark, G., Di Marco, F., Aguet, M. A novel member of the interferon receptor family complements functionality of the murine interferon g receptor in human cells. Cell 76: 803, 1994
62. Bach, F.H., Platt, J.L. Xenotransplantation – a view of issues. Transplant. Proc. 24: 49, 1992
63. Rosengard, A.M., Cary, N.R., Langford, G.A., et al. Tissue expression of human complement inhibitor, decay-accelerating factor, in transgenic pigs. A potential approach for preventing xenograft rejection. Transplantation. 59: 1325, 1995
64. Pareti, F.I., Mazzucato, M., Bottini, E., Mannucci, M. Interaction of porcine von Willibrand factor with the platelet glycoproteins Ib and IIb/IIIa complex. Br. J. Haematol. 82: 81, 1992

65. Grey, S., Tsuchida, A., Hau, H., et al. Selective inhibitory effects of the anticoagulant activated protein C on the response of human mononuclear phagocytes to lipopolysaccharide, interferon-g or phorbol ester. J. Immunol. 153: 3664, 1994
66. Hancock, W.W., Salem, H.H. Activated protein C blocks endotoxin-induced renal injury: Reduction in cytokine expression, endothelial cell activation, fibrin deposition and cellular infiltration. J Am Soc Nephrol 4: 605a, 1993
67. Robson, S.C., Siegal, J.B., Kopp, C., et al. Mechanism of abnormal thromboregulation in xenograft rejection: Loss of ecto-ADPase activity upon endothelial cell activation. Transplant Proc. In press
68. Anrather, J., Brostjan, C., Csizmadia, V., Bach, F.H., Winkler, H. Inhibition of inducible gene expression in endothelial cells. Transplant Proc. In press

9 Anti-αgalactosyl (Anti-Gal) Antibody Damage Beyond Hyperacute Rejection

U. Galili

Introduction

Xenotransplantation of pig tissues and organs into humans, or monkeys, is subjected to immunological incompatibilities greater than those encountered with rodent recipients. This is because of the ubiquitous presence of the natural anti-αgalactosyl (anti-Gal) antibody in Old World monkeys, apes and humans versus the abundant production of the α-galactosyl epitope (i.e., Galα1–3Galβ1–4GlcNAc-R) in nonprimate mammals. This carbohydrate epitope is the natural ligand for anti-Gal, and the binding of this natural antibody to the α-galactosyl epitope on the porcine cells results in the immune rejection of the xenograft [1]. Binding of anti-Gal IgM to porcine cells induces, in general, complement-mediated lysis of the cells [2–4]. Furthermore, in vivo neutralization of anti-Gal by melibiose (Galα1–6Glc) [5], or removal of serum anti-Gal by adsorption on an α-galactosyl epitope column [6], results in the elimination of hyperacute rejection.

Studies aimed to abolish hyperacute rejection have been focused primarily on the downregulation of human complement activity by raising transgenic pigs with human complement regulatory proteins, such as decay-accelerating factor (DAF) and CD59 [7, 8]. This approach, which may cope successfully with anti-Gal IgM-mediated hyperacute rejection does not resolve the detrimental effect of anti-Gal IgG binding to the α-galactosyl epitope on the porcine cells. Furthermore, the human and primate immune systems react vigorously against the porcine α-galactosyl epitope by producing an abundance of high affinity anti-Gal IgG molecules, which are likely to be detrimental to the xenograft via mechanisms other than complement-mediated lysis. This chapter includes a brief discussion of anti-Gal IgG, its specificity, evolution, production under immunologic stimulation by porcine tissues, potential role in chronic rejection of a xenograft, and possible approaches for decreasing or eliminating its detrimental effect.

Anti-Gal and the α-Galactosyl Epitope

Anti-Gal is a natural polyclonal antibody that constitutes approximately 1% of circulating immunoglobulins in humans, apes and Old World monkeys (i.e., monkeys of Asia and Africa) [9, 10]. It is mostly of the IgG isotype [9, 11], but is also found as IgM and IgA isotypes [3, 11–14]. Anti-Gal interacts specifically with the carbohydrate structure Galα1–3Galβ1–4GlcNAc-R (termed the α-galactosyl epitope), which is abundantly produced on carbohydrate chains of mammalian glycoproteins and glycolipids [15–18]. In individuals of blood type O or A, part of the anti-Gal antibodies are capable of binding also to blood group B antigen because of the structural similarity between this antigen and the α-galactosyl epitope [16]. Anti-Gal also interacts with relatively low affinity with the carbohydrates melibiose and α-methylgalactoside [9]; however, these carbohydrates are not produced by mammals.

Anti-Gal is produced in humans throughout life [9, 19] as a result of continuous antigenic stimulation by gastrointestinal bacteria [20]. Analysis of anti-Gal production by Epstein-Barr virus (EBV)-transformed human B lymphocytes has shown that as many as 1% of these lymphocytes are capable of producing the antibody [21]. Several different heavy chain immunoglobulin genes, mostly of the VH3 family, were found to encode for anti-Gal and to undergo somatic mutations [22]. This diversity in anti-Gal-producing genes is likely to be the basis for the polyclonality of this natural antibody and for the increased affinity of this antibody post-transplantation, as described below.

Evolution

Anti-Gal and the α-galactosyl epitope display a unique pattern of distribution in mammals. Anti-Gal is found only in humans, apes and Old World monkeys [10, 23]. In contrast, the α-galactosyl epitope is produced as millions of epitopes per cell in nonprimate mammals, prosimians and New World monkeys (i.e., monkeys of South America), all of which lack anti-Gal because of immune tolerance to the α-galactosyl epitope [10, 23, 24]. This distribution of anti-Gal and α-galactosyl epitope is the result of the differential activity of the glycosylation enzyme α1,3 galactosyltransferase (α1,3GT), which is constitutively active in the Golgi apparatus of cells in nonprimate mammals, prosimians and New World monkeys [23, 25], producing α-galactosyl epitope on cell surface glycolipids and glycoproteins according to the following reaction [26–28]:

$$\underset{(N\text{-acetyllactosamine})}{\text{Gal}\beta 1\text{–}4\text{GlcNAc-R} + \text{UDP-Gal}} \xrightarrow{\alpha 1,3\text{GT}} \underset{(\alpha\text{-galactosyl epitope})}{\text{Gal}\alpha 1\text{–}3\text{Gal}\beta 1\text{–}4\text{GlcNAc-R} + \text{UDP}}$$

The α1,3GT gene, which has been cloned from various nonprimate mammals [29–32] and from New World monkeys [33], was also found to be present in humans and in Old World monkeys as a nonexpressed pseudogene [29, 34–36]. The species distribution pattern of α1,3GT suggests that this enzyme appeared early in mammalian evolution before the divergence between marsupial and placental mammals and has been conserved ever since. α1,3GT has been active in primates; however, its activity was suppressed in ancestral Old World primates after they diverged from New World monkeys [24]. It is possible that ancestral Old World primates were exposed to a pathogen that was detrimental to primates and which expressed α-galactosyl epitopes. Such a pathogen was likely to exert a strong selective pressure for the evolution of primates that could suppress autologous α-galactosyl epitope synthesis, thus lose immune tolerance to it and produce antibodies (i.e., anti-Gal) as a means of defense [36, 37]. New World monkeys were not subjected to such a selective pressure because they were geographically separated from Old World primates. It is impossible to identify today the putative pathogen that induced the evolutionary selection of primates lacking the α-galactosyl epitope. However, there are many pathogens currently known to express α-galactosyl epitopes, including enveloped viruses [38–40], bacteria [20], and protozoa [41, 42].

Detailed analysis of the α1,3GT pseudogene in Old World monkeys and apes has suggested that the inactivation of α1,3GT in ancestral Old World primates occurred during a period in which monkeys and apes already existed as separate groups, i.e., less than 28 million years ago, during the Miocene period [35–37]. According to the fossil record, apes were a very successful group of primates, in terms of number and species variation, in the early Miocene. However, their numbers have gradually declined and they disappeared from the fossil record in the period of 10–5 million years ago [43]. It is, of course, impossible to determine, but tempting to speculate, that the gradual disappearance of apes in the mid- to late Miocene is related to the evolutionary selection for individuals that succeeded in the suppression of α1,3GT expression [37].

Anti-Gal-Mediated Rejection of Xenografts

The appearance of anti-Gal in Old World monkeys and apes has generated an immunologic barrier to the introduction of tissues that express α-galactosyl epitope because of the interaction of anti-Gal with these epitopes [1]. The presence of this barrier, even in primates, was recently demonstrated in the hyperacute rejection observed when a New World monkey heart was transplanted into an Old World monkey [4]. The damaging effect of anti-Gal can be induced by several mechanisms, among which the following have been experimentally demonstrated: (a) complement-mediated lysis, (b) antibody-dependent cell cytotoxicity (ADCC), and (c) activation of receptors on the xenograft cells.

Complement-Mediated Lysis

Anti-Gal IgM binding to α-galactosyl epitopes on the xenograft cells results in activation of the complement cascade and ultimately the lysis of the target cells. This was demonstrated with porcine cells in vitro [2, 44], with COS cells transfected with recombinant α1,3GT [3], and in vivo in Old World monkeys transplanted with organs from New World monkeys or pigs [4]. In vivo, rapid complement-mediated damage to the endothelial cells results in the collapse of the vascular bed of the xenograft and thus leads to hyperacute rejection.

Antibody-Dependent Cell Cytotoxicity

Hyperacute rejection occurs before other immunological mechanisms, which are capable of damaging the xenograft, are set into action. Such is the ADCC mechanism. Anti-Gal IgG molecules, which are abundant in the serum, bind to α-galactosyl epitopes on the xenograft and direct various killer cells, with

Fc receptors for IgG, to exert their cytolytic potential on the cells opsonized by the antibody [1]. Killer cells capable of binding to the Fc portion of anti-Gal include granulocytes, monocytes/macrophages, and natural killer cells. As discussed below, the efficacy of this mechanism is likely to increase posttransplantation because of the production of high-affinity anti-Gal IgG clones as an immune response to the α-galactosyl epitope on the xenograft.

Activation of Receptors on the Xenograft Cells

Most of the cell surface receptors are glycoproteins which, in cells with active α1,3GT, are likely to have α-galactosyl epitopes on part of their carbohydrate chains. Binding of anti-Gal to these epitopes may result in a continuous activation of such receptors and thus damage the physiologic activity of the cells (e.g., endothelial cells, mesangial cells, or heart muscle cells). Porcine thyroid cells may serve as an example for such a mechanism. Incubation of these cells with anti-Gal resulted in a stimulatory effect similar to that of thyrotropin (TSH), due to the binding of anti-Gal to the TSH receptors on the porcine cells [46]. It is conceivable that a similar mechanism would induce the continuous stimulation of endothelial cells and other cells of the xenograft.

Anti-Gal Production in Response to Xenografts

Hyperacute rejection mediated by anti-Gal IgM and complement has been, and still is, a formidable obstacle for xenotransplantation, which may be overcome by the generation of transgenic pigs for complement-regulatory proteins, such as DAF and CD59 [7, 8]. As indicated above, by avoiding hyperacute rejection, other mechanisms, primarily ADCC, are likely to start inducing the destruction of the xenograft in a more insidious manner. Such destruction will be exacerbated by the stimulation of the immune system to further response to the α-galactosyl epitope on the xenograft. This is because anti-Gal activity is not confined to the natural level observed in humans, but can alter significantly.

The evolution of the anti-Gal immune response in Old World primates apparently includes the ability to respond effectively against α-galactosyl epitopes on the xenograft by actively producing high-affinity anti-Gal antibody clones. These antibodies are probably highly detrimental to the graft because of their strong interaction with α-galactosyl epitopes. The production of such antibodies was clearly demonstrated in the serum of diabetic patients that received xenografts of fetal porcine islet cell clusters together with allogeneic kidney grafts [47]. The titer of anti-Gal in these patients increased by 20- to 100-fold within 7 weeks post-transplantation as a result of the immune response against the porcine α-galactosyl epitope [12, 48]. Accordingly, the affinity of the antibody was found to increase many times [12]. This immune response, which included IgG, IgM, and IgA anti-Gal antibodies, occurred in spite of the massive immunosuppressive therapy delivered to these patients [47]. These observations imply that the stimulation of the human immune system by the porcine α-galactosyl epitope is powerful enough to be effective under conditions in which the allogeneic response is suppressed. In addition, we have recently observed a similar phenomenon in monkeys. Cynomolgus monkeys, transplanted with approximately 0.5 g porcine or bovine meniscus cartilage, produced within the first 2 weeks post-transplantation anti-Gal in titers that were higher by ten- to 100-fold than the pretransplantation titers. This high activity was maintained as long as the xenograft was not removed (Galili and Stone, manuscript in preparation).

In view of the polyclonality of anti-Gal [9, 22] and the somatic mutations which occur in anti-Gal genes [22], it is probable that the introduction of porcine tissue into humans or Old World monkeys results in the stimulation of the immune system by porcine α-galactosyl epitopes, leading to the rapid selective expansion of B lymphoid clones that are capable of producing high-affinity anti-Gal antibodies, primarily of the IgG class. The increased production of high-affinity anti-Gal occurs for at least as long as the xenograft is present in the body, and is not significantly affected by immunosuppressive regimens that prevent allogeneic graft rejection. This anti-Gal immune response ought to be of great concern in xenotransplantation. Even if the detrimental effect of complement is avoided, the high-affinity interaction between these anti-Gal antibodies and the xenograft would facilitate chronic inflammatory reactions via the ADCC mechanism.

α-Galactosyl Epitope and Genetically Engineered Pigs

These considerations may be of particular relevance to the studies aimed at decreasing α-galactosyl epitope expression on porcine cells by generating transgenic pigs producing fucosyltransferase [49] (Chap. 50). In such animals, the enzyme produced by the transgene competes with α1,3GT for "capping" of the porcine cell carbohydrate chains of glycolipids and glycoproteins (with fucosyl residues) in order to generate histo-blood group H epitopes rather than α-galactosyl epitopes [49]. Since α1,3GT is extensively active in porcine cells, it is probable that such a competition will not completely eliminate, but rather decrease, the expression of α-galactosyl epitopes. The number of α-galactosyl epitopes per porcine cell usually ranges between one and 30 million [24]. Even if competition by fucosyltransferase succeeds in reducing α-galactosyl epitope expression by 95 %, the remaining $>10^5$ α-galactosyl epitopes per cell may be sufficient to induce the production of high-affinity anti-Gal and the subsequent binding of these antibody molecules to porcine cells for the effective propagation of ADCC.

These considerations are not presented to discourage the performance of studies of transgenic pigs producing various glycosyltransferases. It may be that decreasing the expression of the α-galactosyl epitope below a certain unknown threshold will be sufficient for induction of the accommodation phenomenon observed in ABO-mismatched allogeneic grafts [50]. Furthermore, a decrease in α-galactosyl epitope expression may be helpful in the induction of chimerism with porcine bone marrow or thymus [51].

Complete elimination of the α-galactosyl epitope from porcine cells is likely to resolve all the acute and chronic immune rejection processes mediated by anti-Gal. This may be achieved by genetically engineering and breeding "knockout" pigs deficient in α1,3GT. Recent reports of success in raising such knockout mice [52] (Chap. 51) implies that nonprimate mammals can develop and survive without the α-galactosyl epitope. Thus, the disruption of the α1,3GT gene in pigs and the successful growth of knockout pigs lacking α-galactosyl epitopes may be only a technical problem, dependent on obtaining appropriate embryonic stem cells. Such cells from porcine origin are not available as yet.

Comment

Overall, the information on the immune response in primates and humans that receive porcine xenografts suggests that the massive production of anti-Gal against the α-galactosyl epitope on the xenograft may be detrimental to the survival of the graft even if complement-mediated lysis is prevented. In view of this extensive immune response it is not clear whether decreasing α-galactosyl epitope expression by competition with other glycosyltransferases expressed in transgenic pigs will be sufficient to overcome the immunologic barrier provided by anti-Gal. The ultimate solution for overcoming this barrier may be the development of a pig strain that lacks the α-galactosyl epitope due to the disruption of the α1,3GT gene.

References

1. Galili U. Interaction of the natural anti-Gal antibody with α-galactosyl epitopes: A major obstacle for xenotransplantation in humans. Immunol Today 14: 480, 1993
2. Good AH, Cooper DKC, Malcolm AJ, et al. Identification of carbohydrate structures which bind human anti-porcine antibodies: Implication for discordant xenografting in man. Transplant. Proc. 24: 559, 1992
3. Sandrin M, Vaughan HA, Dabkowski PL, McKenzie IFC. Anti-pig IgM antibodies in human serum react predominantly with Galα1-3Gal epitopes. Proc. Natl. Acad. Sci. USA 90: 11391, 1993
4. Collins BH, Cotterell AH, McCurry KR, et al. Cardiac xenografts between primate species provide evidence for the importance of the α-galactosyl determinant in hyperacute rejection. J. Immunol. 154: 5500, 1995
5. Ye Y, Neethling FA, Niekrasz M, et al. Evidence that intravenously administered α-galactosyl carbohydrates reduce baboon serum cytotoxicity to pig kidney cells (PK15) and transplanted pig hearts. Transplantation 58: 330, 1994
6. Sablinski T, Monroy R, Bailin M, et al. Absorption of preformed primate anti-swine antibodies by extracorporeal perfusion through Galα(1,3)Gal column. Presented to the Third International Congress for Xenotransplantation, Boston 1995. Transplant. Proc. In press
7. Cozzi E, White DJG. The generation of transgenic pigs as potential organ donors for humans. Nature Med 1: 964, 1995

8. McCurry KR, Kooyman DL, Alvarado CG, et al. Human complement regulatory proteins protect swine to primate cardiac xenografts from human injury. Nature Med. 1: 423, 1995
9. Galili U, Rachmilewitz EA, Peleg A, Flechner I. A unique natural human IgG antibody with anti-α-galactosyl specificity. J. Exp. Med. 160: 1519, 1984
10. Galili U, Clark MR, Shohet SB, Buehler J, Macher BA. Evolutionary relationship between the anti-Gal antibody and the Galα1→3Gal epitope in primates. Proc. Natl. Acad. Sci. USA 84: 1369, 1987
11. Kujundzic M, Koren E, Neethling FA, et al. Variability of anti-αGal antibodies in human serum and their relation to serum cytotoxicity against pig cells. Xenotransplantation 1: 58, 1994
12. Galili U, Tibell A, Samuelsson B, Rydberg L, Groth CG. Increased anti-Gal activity in diabetic patients transplanted with fetal porcine islet cell clusters. Transplantation 59: 1549, 1995
13. Parker W, Bruno O, Holzkecht ZE, Platt JE. Characterization and affinity isolation of xenoreactive human natural antibodies. J. Immunol. 153: 3791, 1994
14. Hamadeh RM, Galili U, Zhou P, Griffis JM. Anti-α-galactosyl immunoglobulin A (IgA), IgG, and IgM in human secretions. Clin. Diagnost. Lab Immunol. 2: 125, 1995
15. Galili U, Macher BA, Buehler J, Shohet SB. Human natural anti-α-galactosyl IgG. II. The specific recognition of α(1→3)-linked galactose residues. J. Exp. Med. 162: 573, 1985
16. Galili U, Buehler J, Shohet SB, Macher BA. The human natural anti-Gal IgG. III. The subtlety of immune tolerance in man as demonstrated by crossreactivity between natural anti-Gal and anti-B antibodies. J. Exp. Med. 165: 693, 1987
17. Weislander J, Mannson O, Kallin E, et al. Specificity of human antibodies against Galα1–3Gal carbohydrate epitope and distinction from natural antibodies reacting with Galα1–2Gal or Galα1–4Gal. Glycoconjugate J. 7: 85, 1990
18. Galili U. Evolution and pathophysiology of the human natural anti-Gal antibody. Springer Seminars in Immunopathology 15: 155, 1993
19. Wang L, Anaraki F, Henion TR, Galili U. Variations in activity of the human natural anti-Gal antibody in young and elderly populations. J. Gerontol. (Med. Sci.) 50A: M227, 1995
20. Galili U, Mandrell RE, Hamadeh RM, Shohet SB, Griffis JM. Interaction between human natural anti-α-galactosyl immunoglobulin G and bacteria of the human flora. Infect. Immun. 56: 1730, 1988
21. Galili U, Anaraki F, Thall A, Hill-Black C, Radic M. One percent of circulating B lymphocytes are capable of producing the natural anti-Gal antibody. Blood 82: 2485, 1993
22. Wang L, Radic MZ, Galili U. Human anti-Gal heavy chain genes: Preferential use of V_H3 and the presence of somatic mutations. J. Immunol. 155: 1276, 1995
23. Galili U, Gregory CR, Morris RE. Contribution of anti-Gal to primate and human IgG binding to porcine endothelial cells. Transplantation 60: 210, 1995
24. Galili U, Shohet SB, Kobrin E, Stults CLM, Macher BA. Man, apes, and Old World monkeys differ from other mammals in the expression of α-galactosyl epitopes on nucleated cells. J. Biol. Chem. 263: 17755, 1988
25. Thall A, Etienne-Decerf J, Winand R, Galili U. The α-galactosyl epitope on mammalian thyroid cells. Acta Endocrin. 124: 692, 1991

26. Basu M, Basu S. Enzymatic synthesis of blood group related pentaglycosyl ceramide by an α-galactosyltransferase. J. Biol. Chem. 248: 1700, 1973
27. Blake DD, Goldstein IJ. An α-D-galactosyltransferase in Ehrlich ascites tumor cells: Biosynthesis and characterization of a trisaccharide (α-D-galacto(1–3)-N-acetyllactosamine). J. Biol. Chem. 256: 5387, 1981
28. Blanken WM, van den Eijnden DH. Biosynthesis of terminal Galα1–3Galβ1–4GlcNAc-R oligosaccharide sequence on glycoconjugates: Purification and acceptor specificity of a UDP-Gal: N-acetyllactosamine α1,3galactosyltransferase. J. Biol. Chem. 260: 12972, 1985
29. Joziasse DH, Shaper JH, van den Eijnden DH, Van Tunen AH, Shaper NL. Bovine α1–3galactosyltransferase: Isolation and characterization of a cDNA clone. Identification of homologous sequences in human genomic DNA. J. Biol. Chem. 264: 14290, 1989
30. Larsen RD, Rajan VP, Ruff M, et al. Isolation of a cDNA encoding murine UDP galactose: βD-galactosyl-1,4-N-acetyl-D-glucosaminide α1,3-galactosyltransferase: Expression cloning by gene transfer. Proc. Natl. Acad. Sci. USA 86: 8227, 1989
31. Sandrin MS, Dabkowski PL, Henning MM, Mouthouris E, McKenzie IFC. Characterization of cDNA clones for porcine α1,3galactosyltransferase. The enzyme generating the Galα(1,3)Gal epitope. Xenotransplantation 41: 101, 1995
32. Strahan KM, Gu F, Preece AF, et al. DNA sequence and chromosome localization of pig α1,3galactosyltransferase. Immunogenetics 41: 101, 1995
33. Henion TR, Macher BA, Anaraki F, Galili U. Defining the minimal size of catalytically active primate α1,3galactosyltransferase: Structure function studies on the recombinant truncated enzyme. Glycobiology 4: 193, 1994
34. Larsen RD, Rivera-Marrero CA, Ernst LK, Cummings RD, Lowe JB. Frameshift and nonsense mutations in a human genomic sequence homologous to a murine UDP-Galβ-D-Gal(1,4)-D-GlcNAcα(1,3) galactosyltransferase cDNA. J. Biol. Chem. 265: 7055, 1990
35. Joziasse DH, Shaper JH, Jabs EW, Shaper NL. Characterization of an α1→3-galactosyltransferase homologue on human chromosome 12 that is organized as a processed pseudogene. J. Biol. Chem. 266: 6991, 1991
36. Galili U, Swanson K. Gene sequences suggest inactivation of α1,3 galactosyltransferase in catarrhines after the divergence of apes from monkeys. Proc. Natl. Acad. Sci. USA 88: 7401, 1991
37. Galili U, Andrews P. Suppression of α-galactosyl epitopes synthesis and production of the natural anti-Gal antibody: A major evolutionary event in ancestral Old World primates. J. Human Evolution 29: 433, 1995
38. Geyer R, Geyer H, Strim S, et al. Major oligosaccharides in the glycoprotein of Friend murine leukemia virus: Structure elucidation by one and two dimensional proton nuclear magnetic resonance and methylation analysis. Biochemistry 23: 5628, 1984
39. Repik PM, Strizki JM, Galili U. Differential host dependent expression of α-galactosyl epitopes on viral glycoproteins: A study of eastern equine encephalitis virus as a model. J. General Virol. 75: 1177, 1994
40. Rother RP, Fodor WL, Springhorn JP, et al. A novel mechanism of retrovirus inactivation in human serum mediated by anti-α-galactosyl natural antibody. J. Exp. Med. 182: 1345, 1995

41. Couto AS, Conclaves MF, Colli W, deLederkremer RM. The N-linked carbohydrate chain of the 85-kilodalton glycoprotein from Trypanosoma cruzi trypomastigotes contains sialyl, fucosyl and galactosyl (α1–3) galactose units. Mol. Biochem. Parasitol. 39: 101, 1990
42. Almedia IC, Ferguson MAJ, Schenkman S, Travassos LR. Lytic anti-α-galactosyl antibodied from patients with chronic Chagas' disease recognize novel O-linked oligosaccharides on mucine-like glycosyl-phosphatidylinositol-anchored glycoproteins of Trypanosoma cruzi. Biochem. J. 304: 793, 1994
43. Andrews P. Evolution and environment in hominoidea. Nature 360: 641, 1992
44. Neethling FA, Koren E, Ye Y, et al. Protection of pig kidney (PK15) cells from the cytotoxic effect of anti-pig antibodies by α-galactosyl oligosaccharides. Transplantation 57: 959, 1994
45. Schaapherder AFM, Daha MR, LeBulte MJW, van der Woude FJ, Gooszen HG. Antibody dependent cell-mediated cytotoxicity against porcine endothelium induced by a majority of human sera. Transplantation 57: 1376, 1994
46. Winand RJ, Anaraki F, Etienne-Decerf J, Galili U. Xenogeneic thyroid-stimulating hormone-like activity of the human natural anti-Gal antibody. Interaction of anti-Gal with porcine thyrocytes and with recombinant human thyroid stimulating hormone receptors expressed on mouse cells. J. Immunol. 151: 3923, 1993
47. Groth CG, Korgsen O, Tibell A, et al. Transplantation of fetal porcine pancreas to diabetic patients: Biochemical and histological evidence for graft survival. Lancet 344: 1402, 1994
48. Satake M, Kawagishi N, Rydberg L, et al. Limited specificity of xenoantibodies in diabetic patients transplanted with fetal porcine islet cell clusters. Main antibody reactivity against α-linked galactose-containing epitopes. Xenotransplantation 1: 89, 1994
49. Sandrin MS, Fodor WL, Mouthouris E, et al. Enzymatic remodeling of carbohydrate surface of a xenogenic cell substantially reduces human antibody binding and complement mediated cytolysis. Nature Med 1: 1261, 1995
50. Alexandre GPJ, Squifflet JP, DeBruyere M, et al. Present experience in a series of 26 ABO-incompatible living donor renal allografts. Transplant. Proc. 19: 4538, 1987
51. Sykes M, Lee LA, Sachs DH. Xenograft tolerance. Immunol. Rev. 141: 245, 1994
52. Thall AD, Maly P, Lowe JB. Oocyte Galα1–3Gal epitopes implicated in sperm adhesion to the zona pellucida glycoprotein ZP3 are not required for fertilization in the mouse. J. Biol. Chem. 270: 21437, 1995

10 Human Natural Killer Cells and Natural Antibodies Recognize Overlapping Molecular Structures on Discordant Xenogeneic Endothelium

L. Inverardi and R. Pardi

Introduction

Significant progress towards an understanding of the mechanisms of recognition and rejection of xenogeneic grafts has been witnessed in the past few years. Not only has the molecular basis of discordant xenogeneic tissue recognition begun to become unveiled, but transgenic large animals have been generated that express gene products capable of efficiently interfering with some of the phenomena of immune recognition responsible for graft rejection [1, 2]. Pigs expressing human complement-regulating proteins have been successfully generated, and preclinical transplantation models in primate recipients appear promising [2, 3]. It is easy to foresee that the first clinical trials of discordant xenotransplantation will take place in the near future.

It is now well established that a major role in the immunogenicity of discordant species organs is played by carbohydrate structures expressed on the surface of selected tissues, including the vascular endothelial cell (EC), that are recognized by preformed natural antibodies of IgM and IgG class [4–6]. One such structure, which plays a crucial role as a target in the immune recognition by humans, has been defined in detail and found to be an α-galactosyl structure with α1–3 linkage, synthesized by an α1,3-galactosyltransferase [7–9], the expression of which is lost in higher species (New World monkeys and humans) due to partial deletion, nonsense or missense mutations in the coding gene affecting both alleles [10, 11]. Thus, the presence of antibodies recognizing defined carbohydrate epitopes in a given species may result from the absence of potentially tolerogenic carbohydrate epitopes during the acquisition of the immune repertoire. A very promising approach towards the modulation of the xenogeneic cell surface carbohydrate profile has been recently described that takes advantage of the competition of the human α1,2-fucosyltransferase for the same substrate used by the α1,3-galactosyltransferase (and apparently with a higher affinity), so that the introduction of the human enzyme in a xenogeneic cell expressing the galactosyltransferase functionally inactivates it [12].

Binding of human immunoglobulins to the luminal surface of vascular EC in a discordant xenogeneic organ leads to the activation of the complement cascade, to the activation of vascular EC (with consequent changes in their functional profile), to the initiation of coagulation, and eventually to massive thrombosis and intraparenchymal hemorrhage [13, 14]. Fibrin is deposited, platelets aggregate, and polymorphonuclear cells concentrate at the site of rejection. This series of events, known as hyperacute rejection, leads to functional loss of the discordant vascularized organ within minutes (or up to a few hours) from revascularization. While the role of IgM binding and complement activation represents a critical initiating event in the pathogenesis of graft rejection, there have been suggestions that additional mechanisms might also participate in causing hyperacute rejection [15, 16].

We have in the past proposed a role for early cell-mediated recognition of vascularized discordant grafts in determining the fate of a graft [17–19]. This is based on the observation of productive interaction between the vascular EC and selected lymphocyte subsets of the recipient both in ex vivo and in vitro experimental model systems. While the exact contribution of these cell-mediated recognition events in the unmanipulated recipient has been difficult to establish, it appears that when humoral hyperacute graft rejection is prevented or delayed, early cell-mediated recognition of the implanted organ might play an important role. These observations, obtained in vivo [20, 21], have led to the definition of an additional mechanism of rejection (delayed xenograft rejection, DXR) that represents a second obstacle to successful xenotransplantation across a discordant species barrier. The identification of the molecular targets of this cell-mediated recognition therefore appears to be of crucial importance for the full understanding of discordant vascularized xenotransplantation rejection.

A subsequent obstacle to successful xenotransplantation is represented by events of cell-mediated recognition similar to the ones that take place in the allogeneic setting, that have been defined as dependent mostly on the activation of $CD4^+$ T cells, and require the participation of donor-derived macrophages [22–24].

Less clear is what happens when cell or tissue (nonvascularized) transplants are performed across a discordant species barrier [25]. While studies conducted in recipient mice have suggested that T lymphocytes play the major role in determining the fate of the grafted cells (e.g., human islets of Langerhans readily engraft in the T cell-deficient nude mouse), it has been recently postulated that preformed natural antibodies might play a role also in the recognition of such cell transplants, particularly when large animals and primates are used as recipients [26–28].

Early Cellular Recognition of Discordant Xenogeneic Vascular Targets

Our interest in the past several years has been focused on defining the characteristics of the early cellular recognition of vascularized discordant grafts, by utilizing ex vivo and in vitro approaches. In the ex vivo approach, a rat heart was explanted and immediately perfused with thermostated, oxygenated buffer in a Langendorff apparatus [17, 18]. This approach allows the heart to keep beating without significantly altering its mechanical performance for several hours. Various parameters can be measured that reflect both mechanical performance (such as systolic and diastolic pressure) and other functional variables, such as vascular resistance (coronary pressure). The buffer composition can be altered by adding cells and/or immunoglobulins of any given species to partly mimic the early events of recognition of the vascularized organ that would take place if the organ were transplanted in a xenogeneic setting. The advantage of this approach is that the variables introduced in the system can be strictly controlled, making it possible to define with relative ease causal relationships between single variables and observed phenomena. The obvious disadvantage is that the introduction of artifacts, due to the limited capability of reproducing ex vivo the complexity of the in vivo situation, might lead to observations that cannot be immediately extrapolated to the in vivo situation.

Rat hearts were perfused with human peripheral blood mononuclear cells, freshly isolated from normal volunteers. The starting concentration of human peripheral blood leukocytes (PBL) was within the normal range in peripheral blood, at 10^6 cells/ml. Macrophages were removed prior to circulating the human cells through the rat organ, since nonspecific sequestration of macrophages in the apparatus (due to adhesion to the oxygenator membranes) was observed. The perfusing buffer (Krebs' Ringer Hepes) contained normal, pooled, heat-inactivated human serum at a final concentration of 2 % v/v.

Experiments were also performed in which the human serum was pretreated to eliminate IgG by means of affinity chromatography on solid phase-bound protein G. Lastly, some experiments were performed in which the IgG-depleted serum was reconstituted by the addition of purified human IgG.

Human PBL were retained in the rat heart in a time-dependent fashion. At the end of the experimental time frame (60 min), when unmanipulated whole human serum (HS) was present, approximately 30 %–40 % of the input cells could not be recovered from the recirculating perfusing buffer. When IgG-depleted HS was used, the percentage of human cell sequestration dropped to approximately 20 %. Comparison of the phenotypic profiles of the human cells before and after several cycles of perfusion suggested that particular cell subsets might be preferentially retained. In particular, cells bearing the CD16 and CD56 surface molecules – markers associated with natural killer (NK) cells – showed a marked reduction, as did cells expressing high density of the leukocyte integrin lymphocyte function-associated antigen (LFA)-1. These observations suggested that NK cells might be preferentially sequestrated in the xenogeneic organ. To formally prove that this was the case, highly enriched NK cell preparations were obtained by combined purification techniques (B and T cell depletion), and circulated in the xenogeneic organs. Negative subset selection protocols were used to avoid the possibility of activating NK cells during a positive selection procedure. When enriched NK cell preparations (routinely >90 % $CD16^+$, $CD3^-$, $CD5^-$) were circulated through the rat heart, in the presence of human IgG, up to 90 % of the cells were retained in the organ in 60 min. When IgG was removed from the serum prior to perfusion, the percentage of sequestration dropped to approximately 40 %. Add-back experiments showed that the sequestration efficiency could be causally linked to the presence or absence of IgG.

The performance of the heart was profoundly influenced by perfusion with NK cells in the presence of IgG – systolic pressure decreased, diastolic pressure increased, and the vascular resistance, as judged by coronary pressure values, increased [17]. The perfused rat heart increased substantially in volume, and became pale, likely because of interstitial edema. At the end of the experimental time, the organs were no longer rhythmically beating, mimicking to some extent an in vivo event of cell-mediated acute rejection. When human NK cells were circulated through the heart in the presence of IgG-depleted serum, although significant sequestration was still observed, no dramatic alterations in the heart performance or coronary pressure were recorded [17–19].

Similarly, perfusion of the xenogeneic organ with purified T cells did not lead to any significant alteration of either performance or vascular resistance, although some sequestration of human T cells was consistently observed (25%–30% of the input in 60 min). Interestingly, T cell sequestration rate was not influenced by the presence or absence of human IgG. Histological analysis of the hearts that had been perfused with human IgG and NK cells revealed that IgG bound to the inner surface of the vascular EC, and that NK cells were binding to the same surface, and had infiltrated the parenchyma [17] (Fig. 1). Vascular permeability was grossly altered, as suggested by the macroscopic observation of the hearts, and confirmed by the interstitial extravasation of colloidal carbon black (China ink) infused at the end of the experimental procedure. Conversely, colloidal carbon was retained in the vasculature when circulated in the control hearts (perfused with human T cells or with syngeneic or allogeneic rat cells).

Leukocyte–EC interaction is a complex multi-step process that requires the ordinate engagement of a series of receptor-ligand couples on the two cell partners. Molecular compatibility has been demonstrated in selected species combinations, including human/porcine [29], and our observations of NK cells adhering to xenogeneic EC and transmigrating into the parenchyma of the heart strongly suggest that productive interactions are taking place between the cell partners in the human/rat species combination as well, and prompted us to evaluate the possibility of interfering with such interactions to prevent adhesion and transmigration. For this reason, human NK cells were circulated through the rat heart after they had been pretreated with saturating concentrations of monoclonal antibodies specific for either the α- or the β-chain of the two leukocyte integrins expressed on human NK cells (LFA-1 and Mac-1). Inhibition of NK cell sequestration was observed when either anti-α-chain antibody was used and was maximal (80% inhibition) when an anti-β-chain antibody was used. The β-chain is shared by the two heterodimeric leukocyte integrins and, therefore, an anti-β-chain antibody targets both molecules at the same time, easily explaining the higher degree of inhibition observed [18, 19].

How do IgGs influence NK cell sequestration in the xenogeneic organ? At least two hypotheses could be postulated to explain this phenomenon: the first would suggest that IgG could, by binding to the xenogeneic EC, induce modification(s) of the EC themselves, making them a better substrate for lymphocyte adhesion. This first hypothesis is somehow weakened (although not ruled out) by the observation that T cell adhesion is uninfluenced by the presence of IgG. The second explanation of the IgG-mediated enhancement of cell sequestration could be found by hypothesizing the engagement of the receptor for the Fc fragment of IgG (FcγR III, CD16) expressed on the surface of NK cells, "bridging" the $CD16^{+}$ cells to the target structures. To ascertain whether this was the case, human NK cells were pretreated with antibodies capable of recognizing and functionally inhibiting the FcγR III, prior to perfusion through the rat heart. In keep-

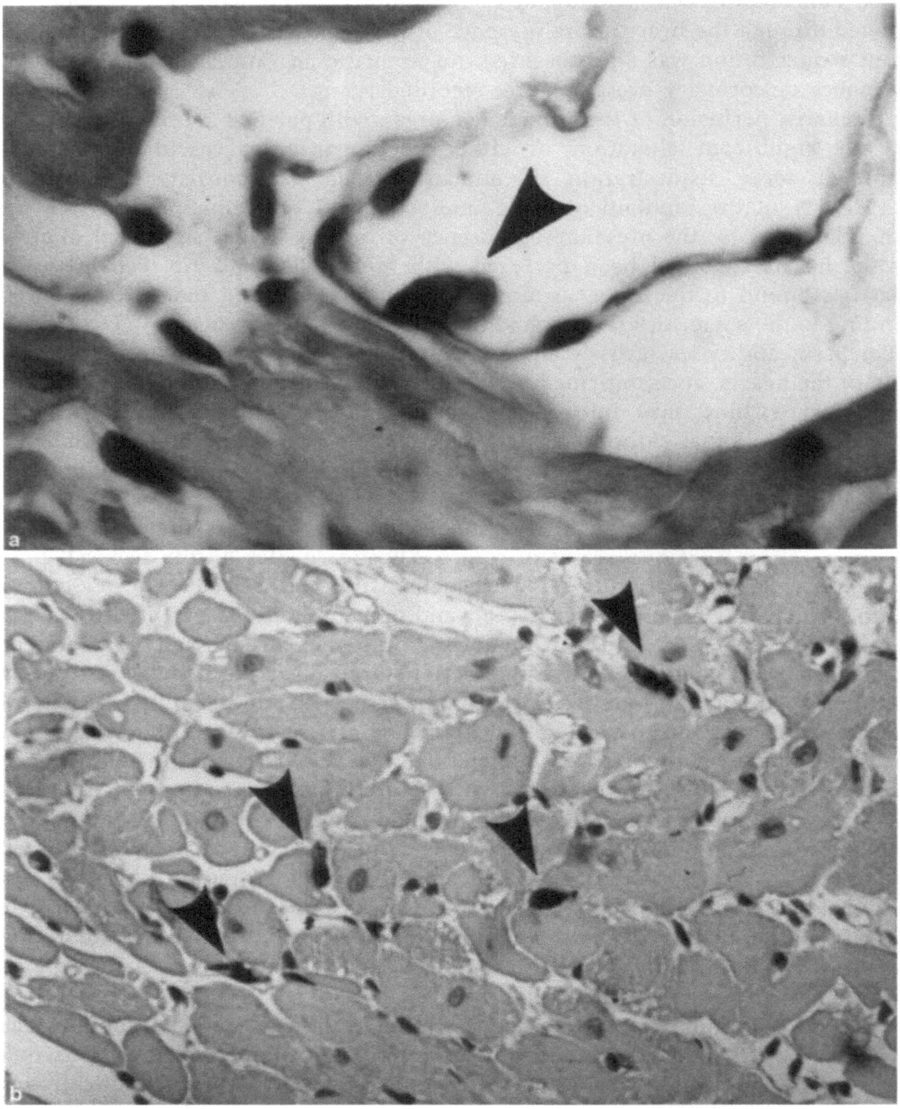

Fig. 1a,b. Human natural killer (NK) cells productively interact with a discordant xenogeneic organ ex vivo. Histological analysis of a rat heart after ex vivo perfusion with human NK cells in the presence of human IgG. **a** A small vessel of the myocardium shows the presence of a human NK lymphocyte (*arrowhead*) adhering to the endothelium. **b** Numerous NK cells are observed (*arrowheads*) infiltrating the myocardial parenchyma. In both cases, positive identification of the NK cells was obtained by immunohistochemistry using an anti-CD16 monoclonal antibody ing with the hypothesis of a crucial role of the FcγR III molecule in determining the enhancement of NK cell adhesion to xenogeneic EC in the presence of IgG, a significant inhibition of the IgG-dependent adhesion was observed.

The observations in the ex vivo system allowed us to draw the following conclusions: a productive interaction between human lymphocytes and xenogeneic endothelium takes place and is at least partly dependent on the functional integrity of leukocyte integrins; preferential interaction is observed between NK cells and EC in the xenogeneic heart, and NK cells appear capable of transmigrating into the heart parenchyma; adhesion to xenogeneic targets takes place through at least two pathways, one dependent on, the other independent of the presence of human IgG; in the presence of IgG, NK cells induce profound alterations in the heart performance and lead to increased vascular resistance and loss of selective permeability of the capillary vasculature.

In order to confirm and extend the findings obtained in the ex vivo model system, experiments were performed with purified human NK cells in vitro. Adhesion to cultured monolayers of EC obtained from various species was evaluated, as well as NK-mediated lysis of the xenogeneic EC.

Productive interaction of the enriched preparations of human NK cells was indeed confirmed in the in vitro tests and, similarly to the ex vivo system, the presence of human IgG was capable of enhancing the adhesion of NK cells to the xenogeneic EC. Also, the important role of the leukocyte integrins LFA-1 and Mac-1 was confirmed in the in vitro tests. Similar results were obtained in the experiments that used porcine, bovine, and murine EC [17–19].

The cytotoxic potential of human NK cells was also evaluated in vitro on cultured EC monolayers of different species. Consistent with the results of the ex vivo and in vitro adhesion assays, efficient lysis of the xenogeneic EC was mediated by human NK cells. Once again, lysis was more efficient in the presence of human IgG during the assay. An important role of the leukocyte integrins LFA-1 and Mac-1 could also be confirmed in the in vitro cytotoxicity assays by antibody-mediated inhibition experiments [17, 19].

Cytotoxicity is difficult to directly demonstrate in the ex vivo system, but the severely altered vascular permeability observed in the ex vivo perfusion system, together with the lytic activity observed in vitro strongly suggest that cell lysis of the vascular EC of the coronary vasculature takes place in the ex vivo perfusion experiments.

T cell subsets (also obtained freshly by negative selection techniques) of either the CD4 or the CD8 phenotype did not appear capable of mediating any significant lysis of the endothelial monolayers either in the presence or in the absence of human IgG.

These data point to a potentially important role of the NK cell subset in the early events of recognition and rejection of a discordant vascularized graft in vivo; recently, as already mentioned, results from in vivo experimental systems in which hyperacute rejection has been successfully delayed have confirmed that NK cells and other leukocyte subsets, such as macrophages, appear in the organ at the time of rejection as infiltrating elements, providing strong evidence to support a role for such populations in delayed xenograft rejection [20, 21].

While the mechanisms by which T cells recognize antigens have been characterized in detail, very little is known about NK cell-mediated recognition of the relevant targets. The definition of the xenogeneic structures recognized by NK cells therefore might not only represent an important step toward the understanding of xenograft rejection, but could also contribute to the elucidation of more general mechanisms of NK cell biology. Furthermore, the ex vivo model system could prove itself useful in the study of the early cellular events of leukocyte adhesion in a dynamic fashion.

Direct Immune Recognition of Xenogeneic Vascular and Nonvascular Tissues: Requirements for the Activation and Adhesion Steps

The earliest cell-mediated events underlying the recognition of a genetically mismatched graft by immune cells are still poorly characterized. This is mainly due to the lack of experimental settings adequate for the study of the extremely fast kinetics of cell-cell interaction in vivo. It can be assumed, however, that antigen-independent cell–cell adhesion events represent the initial trigger for subsequent inflammatory processes that contribute to the recruitment of large numbers of immunocompetent cells to the site of graft implantation. Two lines of evidence support this assumption: first, immunohistochemical analysis of biopsies taken at very early time points after implantation of the graft shows the presence of early signs of tissue damage, such as EC "swelling," but only scanty cellular infiltrates, mainly represented by polymorphonuclear cells (PMN) and macrophages, with few T lymphocytes [30]. This is not surprising, as the relative frequency of circulating T cells bearing antigen receptor complexes capable of recognizing the relevant foreign major histocompatibility complex (MHC) peptide complexes is expected to be fairly low and insufficient to account for significant recruitment of unprimed T lymphocytes into the grafted tissues. Second, experimental models of syngeneic vascular grafts show early pathologic changes in the grafted syngeneic tissue that include EC edema and polymorphonuclear cell infiltration [31, 32]. Thus, non-immune-mediated tissue damage may be the initial trigger for the inflammatory cascade leading to immune recognition of the graft.

The initial step in cell-mediated immune recognition of virtually every antigen-bearing tissue is represented by the establishment of firm intercellular adhesion between the leukocyte and the opposing cell. On the other hand, it has been demonstrated that firm adhesion of leukocytes to other cells, though required for triggering subsequent effector functions or inducing post-translational and transcriptional events associated with cell cycle progression of the leukocyte, does not occur in the absence of an initial activating stimulus acting on non adherent or loosely adherent leukocytes [33, 34]. The mechanistic explanation for the activation-dependence of leukocyte adhesion has been provided by structural and functional studies on leukocyte adhesion receptors, both of the immunoglobulin (i.e., CD31) [35] and of the integrin family (i.e., CD11a, b, c/CD18) [36]. Such studies have demonstrated that surface integrins are normally in a low avidity state for the ligand, but can be functionally upregulated by a number of activating stimuli, which transiently increase the avidity for the ligand via a poorly defined intracellular pathway.

Several molecular events, whose causal relationships and temporal sequence are as yet poorly defined, parallel the energy-dependent conversion of inactive leukocyte integrins to a ligand-binding conformation, downstream from the activating stimulus. These include protein kinase C activation and translocation [37, 38], phosphorylation on serine residues of both subunits of the heterodimer [39, 40] and acquisition of neo-epitopes by the extracellular domains of the α- and β-subunits [41–45]. In addition, energy-independent avidity shifts in integrins have been shown to occur as a consequence of changes in extracellular divalent cation concentration [42, 46], upon the release of small unsaturated lipids by activated cells [47], or upon activation-induced upregulation of surface receptor density. The activated state of leukocyte or platelet integrins is clearly accompanied by a conformational change (allosteric transition) in the extracellular domains of the heterodimer, as defined by the acquisition of neo-epitopes which are characteristic of the ligand-binding conformation of the receptor [41, 44, 45, 48]. Additionally, reversible association of the adhesion receptor to the actin-based cytoskeleton, likely to be mediated by a complex of peripheral proteins which includes talin, α-actinin and vinculin, has been shown by our [39] and other groups [49–51] to parallel the activation-induced avidity shift of leukocyte and platelet integrins (see below). Two models have been proposed to causally relate the above described phenomena. One model predicts that cell activation directly promotes a conformational change in the receptor, followed by ligand recognition, receptor clustering and cytoskeletal reorganization. Alternatively, it can be postulated that activation-induced physical association of the receptor to cytoskeletal elements precedes, and possibly promotes, conformational changes in the ligand-binding sites located in the receptor's extracellular domains, with subsequent engagement of the ligand.

Thus, direct or indirect antigen recognition is not strictly required to promote the initial adhesion of immune cells to genetically disparate tissues, provided that alternative activation pathways exist capable of upregulating the adhesive and migratory properties of circulating leukocytes. On the other hand, the recruitment of inflammatory cells such as PMN, and their subsequent activation in the local microenvironment of the grafted tissue, would lead to marked functional and structural changes of the graft vasculature, thus increasing the likelihood of potentially reactive antigen receptor-positive T cells coming in direct contact with the relevant allo- or xenogeneic MHC/peptide complexes.

What is the nature of this activating stimulus, acting at the interface between the grafted tissue and the host immune system, and capable of initiating the complex network of cellular interactions that leads to disruptive leukocyte infiltration of the graft?

Metabolic changes occurring in the grafted tissue prior to implantation may represent a major cause of pro-inflammatory reactions leading to enhanced leukocyte adhesion to the graft's vascular or nonvascular components. In a process sharing features with the ischemia-reperfusion injury, intracellular events occurring during the initial phases of reperfusion of the implanted organ (such as the conversion of xanthine dehydrogenase to xanthine oxidase, or the reduced endogenous production of nitric oxide) [52, 53] may lead to free oxygen radical-mediated changes at the level of the endothelium and of circulating leukocytes. Additionally, increased leukocyte adhesion to and transmigration through the damaged endothelium may result from upregulated expression of P selectin by vascular cells [54–56] or of specific selectin ligands by the leukocytes [57], a rapid response to injury that does not require protein synthesis. A third possibility, that emerged from our previous studies using an ex vivo model of xenograft immune recognition, is that circulating antibodies of the G class, recognizing EC surface structures, mediate upregulated EC adhesion by FcγR-expressing leukocytes, such as PMN and NK cells [17–19]. Such process would represent a special case of the Arthus phenomenon, known for a number of years and recently revisited in the context of FcγR-mediated inflammatory processes [58].

Direct Recognition of Xenogeneic Carbohydrate Epitopes by Human Natural Killer Cells

We analyzed in detail the molecular components of NK-mediated xenogeneic tissue recognition, with particular emphasis on the antibody-independent pathway, relative to XNA reactivity [59]. Our analysis was initially focused on IgG XNA, following the indication that this antibody class contributes to the early, cell-mediated recognition of xenogeneic tissues by FcγR III$^+$ leukocyte subsets. Vascular endothelium was chosen as a target tissue as it is likely to be the first and prominent xenoantigen-bearing tissue encountered in vivo by the host's immune system in a vascularized graft setting. As previously reported using whole organs or red cells from unrelated species, preabsorption experiments using vascular EC from various species indicated that human XNA, though nonreactive with homologous cells, display broad cross-reactivity across a discordant xenogeneic species barrier. Some degree of heterogeneity in the recognized antigens, however, may exist, as suggested by the variable efficiency of EC from a given species in pre-absorbing XNA directed towards unrelated species. This variability appears to involve a minority of circulating XNA whose defined specificity and potential biological significance cannot be explored by simple pre-absorption experiments and did not represent the primary focus of this study.

A large panel of carbohydrates was used to evaluate the inhibition of IgG XNA binding to xenogeneic EC to confirm and extend similar studies performed to define the specificity of IgM XNA-binding to xenogeneic EC [9]. The results of this study are shown in Table 1.

These blocking experiments show that αGal and αMan-containing mono-, di- or polysaccharides were displacing XNA binding to xenogeneic EC with relatively high efficiency, considering the demonstrated low affinity and elevated off-rate constants of carbohydrate/XNA binding in solution. Remarkable variability was observed in the IC_{50} (concentrations needed to obtain 50 % binding inhibition) of various epimeric or anomeric forms of a given monosaccharide, suggesting that the relevant XNA display fine specificities that involve the spatial orientation and accessibility of defined hydroxyl groups, rather than simple surface charge of the recognized carbohydrate epitopes. This is exemplified by the remarkable dif-

Table 1. Inhibition of XNA reactivity towards pig endothelial cells (EC) by carbohydrates in solution

Sugar	Features	IC_{50} (mM)
D-Glucose	Hexose, aldose	>100
D-Arabinose	Pentose, ketose	>100
α-D-Mannose	D-Glc epimer at C2	12.8
α-D-Galactose	D-Glc epimer at C4	10.8
D-Mannose-6P	Hexose monophosphate	15.6
D-Fructose-1P	Hexose monophosphate	>100
β-L-Fucose-6P	Methyl-hexose monophosphate	>100
N-Methyl-galactose	Methyl-hexose	18.4
Methyl-α-D-Gal*p*	Cyclic methyl-hexose	8.7
Methyl-β-D-Gal*p*	Cyclic methyl-hexose	39.9
β-D-*N*-Acetylglucosamine	*N*-Acetyl-hexose	38.2
N-Acetylneuraminate	Carboxyl-hexose	>100
Melibiose	6-α-D-Gal*p*-D-Glc	8.4
Sucrose	β-D-Fru*f*-α-D-Glc*p*	>100
Arabino-galactan	Linear polysaccharide	N.T.
Mannan	Linear polysaccharide	N.T.

Glc, glucose; Gal, galactose; Fru, fructose; *p*, pyranoside; *f*, furanoside; P, phosphate; N.T., not tested.

ference in the IC_{50} of D-glucose (>100 mM) and D-galactose (10.8 mM), that are epimers at the carbon atom in position 4 and, on the other hand, by the comparable inhibitory effects displayed by D-mannose and its phosphorylated, anionic derivative, mannose-6-phosphate. The previously reported ability of rhamnose to inhibit XNA reactivity, which we also demonstrated in our model, confirms that fine differences in the spatial orientation of hydroxyl groups may have a profound influence on XNA reactivity. Rhamnose is a 6-deoxy stereoisomer of mannose that shares identical orientation of the asymmetric carbon atoms in position 3 and 4, and displaces XNA binding with similar efficiency. Interestingly, β-L-fucose-6P and NANA, both commonly found as terminal carbohydrate residues on human cell surface glycoproteins and glycolipids, were ineffective at displacing XNA binding, despite being efficient inhibitors of lymphocyte-EC adhesion (see below). The relevant contribution of terminal αGal residues in XNA reactivity has been thoroughly established in previous studies [7–10]. Interestingly, our findings underscore the importance of mannose-containing epitopes as potential xenoantigens expressed by various discordant xenogeneic EC. Mannose-rich glycans are abundant in early eucaryotes, including common protozoa and parasites. This could explain the persistence of cross-reacting "natural" antibodies that also recognize xenogeneic mannose-containing structures.

Purified F(ab')2 fragments of pooled human IgG effectively competed whole XNA binding to pig EC, with IC_{50} observed at concentrations one order of magnitude higher than the reference 10 μM concentration of XNA used in the assay. Even lower concentrations of F(ab')2 fragments could be used by pretreating xenogeneic cells with this reagent rather than performing the competition assay at equilibrium (not shown). This suggests that a similar approach could be devised to limit primate or human XNA binding in vivo in experimental or clinical xenograft models, in an attempt to prevent Fc-dependent humoral or cell-mediated (see below) pathogenic processes leading to hyperacute rejection. The reported low affinity of XNA binding to the relevant tissue antigens, however, raises questions about the persistence of such binding in vivo for a time sufficient to achieve significant and long-lasting protection.

In an attempt to selectively define the specificity of NK cell recognition of xenogeneic EC, the same panel of carbohydrates was used in solution to interfere with binding of NK cells to xenogeneic cultured EC of porcine origin. As we have reported in previous studies [17–19], NK cells efficiently adhere to and lyse xenogeneic EC independently of EC-bound IgG XNA. To assess whether xenogeneic oligosaccharide ligands were involved in this process, adhesion assays were performed in the presence of oligosaccharides in solution. NK cell-depleted, purified T cells from the same donor were used as a specificity control. Furthermore, adhesion of NK cells and T cells to allogeneic endothelia was evaluated and compared to adhesion to xenogeneic targets, in the presence or absence of the same carbohydrates, in order to ascertain the specificity of the effects of the oligosaccharides in the recognition of xenogeneic versus allogeneic targets.

The results of such experiments, shown in Fig. 2 and Table 2, demonstrate that only a limited set of carbohydrates effectively and selectively inhibit IgG-independent adhesion of NK cells to xenogeneic targets, including melibiose and α-D-mannose; on the other hand, most inhibitory carbohydrates had limited selectivity, in that they partially inhibited adhesion to both xenogeneic and allogeneic endothelial targets; finally, and as previously reported in the literature, a limited set of oligosaccharides (such as fructose-1P, NANA, and β-L-fucose) appeared capable of mediating significant inhibition of adhesion, irrespective of the effector cell subset (NK and T cells) and the species combination (xeno- and allogeneic) examined. As previously mentioned, we have in the past reported that human NK cells adhere to xenogeneic endothelial targets via at least two pathways, one dependent on, the other independent of the presence of human IgG XNA [17–19]. It therefore appeared conceivable to hypothesize that both pathways could be inhibited by the addition of human XNA IgG F(ab')2 fragments, in view of the aforementioned overlap of the specificity of inhibition of selected carbohydrates on IgG binding and IgG-independent adhesion of human NK cells to xenogeneic EC. To test this hypothesis, F(ab')2 fragments of pooled human IgG were used to compete with the antibody-dependent and -independent adhesion of NK cells to xenogeneic EC monolayers. As controls, we utilized allogeneic EC cultures or monolayers of a human intercellular adhesion molecule (ICAM)-1-transfected murine fibroblast line that exclusively supports β_2-integrin-dependent adhesion of human NK cells

Fig. 2a–f. Selected carbohydrates inhibit human natural killer (NK) cell adhesion to xenogeneic endothelial cells. Inhibition of NK cell (*squares*) or T cell (*circles*) adhesion to pig (*black symbols*) or human (*white symbols*) endothelial cells (EC) by the indicated carbohydrates in solution, as a function of sugar concentration. **a** D-glucose. **b** Melibiose. **c** D-mannose. **d** D-mannose-6P. **e** NANA. **f** β-L-fucose-1P. Average adhesion values were 48%±11% for NK vs. pig EC, 36%±8% for NK vs. human EC, 14%±4% for T cell vs. pig EC, and 18±2 for T cell vs. human EC. Data are representative of eight separate experiments

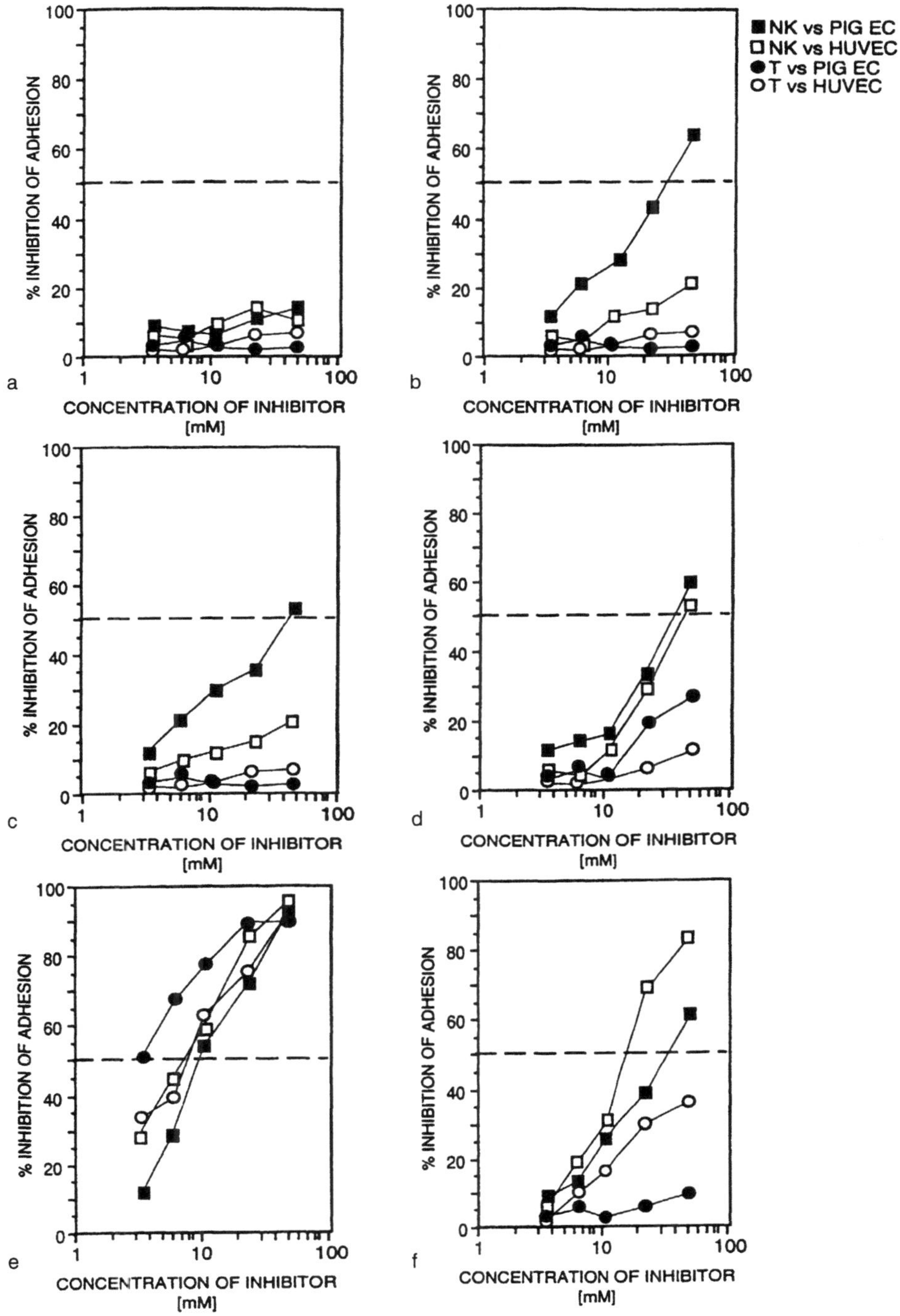
NK vs PIG EC
NK vs HUVEC
T vs PIG EC
T vs HUVEC
% INHIBITION OF ADHESION
0
20
40
60
80
100
1
10
100
CONCENTRATION OF INHIBITOR
[mM]
a
b
c
d
e
f

Table 2. Inhibition of natural killer (NK) lymphocyte adhesion to pig endothelial cells (EC) or human umbilical vein EC (HUVEC) by carbohydrates in solution

Sugar	Features	IC_{50} (m*M*)	
		Pig EC	HUVEC
D-Glucose	Hexose, aldose	>100	>100
D-Arabinose	Pentose, ketose	>100	>100
α-D-Mannose	D-Glc epimer at C2	22.7	>100
α-D-Galactose	D-Glc epimer at C4	>100	>100
D-Mannose-6P	Hexose monophosphate	18.3	29.4
D-Fructose-1P	Hexose monophosphate	12.5	8.7
β-L-Fucose-6P	Methyl-hexose monophosphate	18.6	11.4
N-Methyl-D-Galactose	Methyl-hexose	>100	>100
Methyl-α-D-Gal*p*	Cyclic methyl-hexose	31.1	>100
Methyl-β-D-Gal*p*	Cyclic methyl-hexose	>100	>100
D-*N*-Acetylglucosamine	*N*-Acetyl-hexose	>100	>100
N-Acetylneuraminate	Carboxyl-hexose	10.2	10.6
Melibiose	6-α-D-Gal*p*-D-Glc	23.8	>100
Sucrose	β-D-Fru*f*-α-D-Glc*p*	>100	>100
Arabino-galactan	Linear polysaccharide	>100	>100
Mannan	Linear polysaccharide	6.1	8.4

Glc, glucose; Gal, galactose; Fru, fructose; *p*, pyranoside; *f*, furanoside; P, phosphate.

(R. Pardi et al., unpublished). Figure 3 shows that $F(ab')_2$ fragments efficiently inhibited NK adhesion to xenogeneic EC, both in the presence and in the absence of intact xenoreactive IgG, suggesting that the hypothesized overlap of epitopes recognized by human XNA and directly by NK cells (in an antibody-independent fashion) indeed exists. NK cell adhesion to allogeneic EC or human ICAM-1^+ transfectants was unaffected by IgG $F(ab')_2$ fragments, further strengthening the hypothesis of a xenogeneic-specific mechanism of recognition.

A relevant finding in this work is the demonstration that oligosaccharide ligands appear to play a role in the antibody-independent adhesion to and destruction of xenogeneic EC by unstimulated human NK lymphocytes. Furthermore, two lines of evidence suggest that similar glycosylation patterns could be recognized by XNA and NK cells on pig vascular cells: first, the only carbohydrates displaying selective inhibition of NK cell adhesion to xenogeneic EC are D-mannose, melibiose and methyl-α-D-Gal-*p*, which also appear to be the most efficient competitors of XNA binding and, in the case of the two latter structures, have previously been shown to interfere with the recognition of the major Galα(1,3)Gal epitope by XNA on several xenogeneic tissues; second and perhaps more relevant, $F(ab')_2$ fragments of XNA effectively and selectively inhibit both adhesion to and lysis of pig EC by NK cells. These results cannot be simply explained by the persistence of FcγR-bound IgG, carried over from plasma during the NK cell purification procedure and affecting the recognition of xenogeneic cells. In fact, we were able to show that unstimulated, purified NK lym-

Fig. 3. XNA F(ab')$_2$-mediated inhibition of natural killer (NK) cell adhesion to various cell targets. Inhibition of NK cell adhesion to **a** pig endothelial cell (EC), **b** human EC, or **c** human intercellular adhesion molecule (ICAM)-1$^+$ murine NIH 3T3 transfectants by F(ab')$_2$ fragments from pooled human IgG at the indicated concentration. The assay was performed in the presence (*white symbols*) or absence (*black symbols*) of 1 μ*M* whole human IgG. Average percent adhesion values as indicated in the legend to Fig. 2 for NK vs. pig EC and NK vs. human EC, and 44%±6% for NK vs. ICAM-1+ NIH 3T3 cells. Mean ± SD of three separate experiments

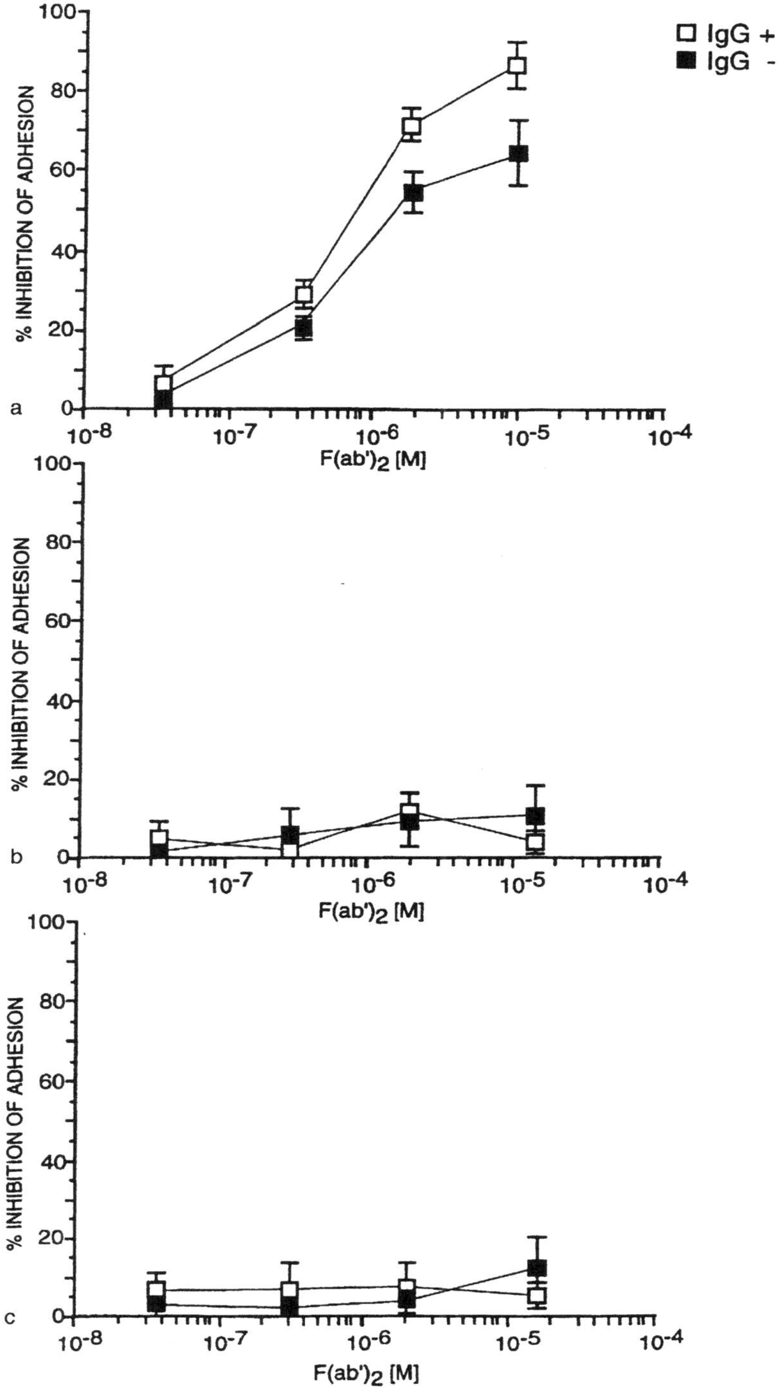

phocytes, although capable of binding monomeric or aggregated IgGs in solution, are completely devoid of preexisting, surface-bound immunoglobulins when freshly isolated and utilized in adhesion or cytotoxicity assays, as judged by indirect immunofluorescence or immunoblotting analysis [59]. We could therefore conclude that at least partial overlap exists between the target structures recognized by human XNA of G class and those recognized directly by NK cells on xenogeneic EC, based on the capability of selected soluble carbohydrates and $F(ab')_2$ fragments of human IgG XNA to inhibit NK cell-mediated direct recognition of xenogeneic EC.

The relevant contribution of lectin-carbohydrate interactions in NK/EC contact-dependent events is further stressed by the fact that several other carbohydrates, including NANA and β-L-fucose-6P, display effective inhibition of such interactions, albeit in a non-species-specific fashion. Although we cannot rule out the possibility that the observed inhibition patterns are due to xenogeneic EC membrane lectins engaging oligosaccharide ligands on NK cells, the highly selective inhibition displayed by several carbohydrates and by $F(ab')_2$ fragments suggest that the lectins involved are preferentially expressed by NK lymphocytes and recognize ligand-expressing target cells [60]. This interpretation is supported by the accumulating evidence that NK cell-specific C-type lectins are involved in essential biological functions of this lymphocyte subset, including cell activation and target cell recognition. A possible explanation of the aforementioned findings is that receptors of the selectin or NKRP-1 families, broadly expressed by NK lymphocytes, recognize highly charged, sialylated or fucosylated ligands expressed in a non species-specific fashion by vascular and non-vascular cells such as K562, whereas less characterized lectins, possibly expressed by subsets of circulating NK cells, are involved in the recognition of xenogeneic-specific oligosaccharide ligands devoid of terminal fucosylated or sialylated residues.

Several candidate receptors, whose functional significance is as yet poorly defined are indeed expressed by NK cells and could account for xenogeneic oligosaccharide ligand recognition. These include the well-known asialoglycoprotein receptor (asialoGM-1), which is specific for terminal galactose and N-acetylgalactosamine residues, but also homologues of the macrophage mannose receptor, whose expression on NK cells has been functionally demonstrated, and the NKRP-1 receptor itself, that has been shown to bind with low affinity ligands containing mannose or galactose residues. Finally, as yet uncharacterized lectin receptors, or products of the NKG-2 gene family could be involved in such a process. Parallel structural analysis of complementarity determining regions (CDR) and carbohydrate recognition domains (CRD) of xenoreactive antibodies and lectins will help clarify the structural basis of the observed common recognition patterns. Interestingly, both molecules have been reported to utilize multivalent recognition and ligand-induced clustering as means to increase the affinity and/or persistence of ligand binding.

Mammalian C-type lectins have been shown to participate in cell-cell adhesion and cellular activation processes that imply transmembrane signaling properties. Recent reports suggest that NK-specific lectins, such as the murine Ly-49 receptor, could deliver target MHC class I-dependent inhibitory signals to NK lymphocytes that would prevent them from destroying autologous tissues and would account for the acquisition of a still poorly characterized NK cell receptor repertoire during ontogeny. Our previous work indicated that integrins are the dominant adhesion receptors involved in human NK lymphocyte/xenogeneic EC cell–cell contacts.

As leukocyte integrins are normally inactive and require activation signals to be converted to a high avidity state for their ligands, we propose that lectin-mediated recognition processes could provide such activation, leading to firm adhesion of NK lymphocytes to the xenogeneic tissue and subsequent triggering of the effector cell's lytic machinery. Based on the above considerations, a comprehensive model of NK cell-dependent xenogeneic tissue destruction can be proposed: oligosaccharide ligands, displaying species-, tissue-, or differentiation stage-specific expression would be required to confer sensitivity to recognition and lysis by NK cells. The absence of relevant oligosaccharide ligands and/or the recognition of defined MHC allele products could prevent the adhesion/activation process from taking place, so that a cell displaying such a phenotype would be ignored by NK effector lymphocytes. In this context, degenerate MHC I molecules expressed by xenogeneic tissues and not recognized by their cognate receptors across species barriers would be ineffective as negative regulators of NK activation, thus rendering xenogeneic cells highly sensitive targets for human NK cell-mediated effector processes.

Natural Killer Cell Receptors: An Overview

The biological role of NK lymphocytes, which constitute a major subpopulation of lymphocytes, distinguishable from other lymphocytes by the absence of antigen receptors found on T and B cells, has remained elusive for many years and still appears somewhat controversial. The controversy stems from the very origin of the operational definition of NK cells, which was based on their ability to kill certain tumor cell lines in vitro, in the absence of prior sensitization, and by the still incomplete characterization of the existing in vivo models of deficient NK cell function [61]. At present, circumstantial evidence indicates that NK cells are closely related, functionally and ontogenetically, to cytolytic T lymphocytes (CTL), based on morphology, surface phenotype and lytic mechanisms. Several studies demonstrated an important contribution of this cell subset in the clearance of tissues which are foreign, infected by viruses or by certain protozoa, or compromised in other ways [62].

A major step forward in the understanding of the molecular mechanisms underlying target recognition by NK cells came from the observation of an inverse correlation between surface MHC class I expression by target cells and their sensitivity to lysis by NK lymphocytes. This observation led Karre et al. to propose the "missing self" hypothesis, that postulates that NK cells survey tissues for normal expression of MHC class I molecules and lyse targets when MHC class I expression is aberrant or absent, thus displaying opposing requirements compared to CTLs [63]. This hypothesis has been supported by several independent findings demonstrating that allotypic MHC class I products actually protect cells from lysis by NK cells, apparently by delivering negative regulatory signals that inhibit NK cell lytic function [64]. Further evidence in favor of the "missing self" hypothesis originated from the observation that cells from mice lacking MHC class I expression owing to disruption of the β_2-microglobulin gene, for example, are more susceptible to NK cell lysis than cells from normal mice, and the defect can be reversed by transfection with MHC class I [65, 66].

Human NK cell receptors for MHC class I have recently been cloned and found to represent a previously unknown family of type I transmembrane glycoproteins belonging to the Ig superfamily [67]. The encoded proteins (commonly known as p58 molecules) have molecular weights ranging between 58 and 70 kDa, with an extracellular portion composed of two to three Ig constant-like domains, a transmembrane region and a cytoplasmic domain of various length. The p58 family of NK cell receptors shows allelic polymorphism and mono- or oligoclonal distribution in peripheral blood NK cells. Functionally, these receptors appear for the most part to deliver an ill-defined negative signal to the expressing NK lymphocyte upon contacting the relevant MHC-peptide allotypic combination, which temporarily switches off their lytic potential.

Several alternative candidate receptors, whose functional significance is as yet poorly defined, are indeed expressed by NK cells. Interestingly, most of these receptors appear to be capable of recognizing complex carbohydrate structures on the surface of sensitive targets, and are thus functionally and/or structurally related to the C-type lectin family of receptors [68]. They include the well-known asialoglycoprotein receptor (asialoGM-1), which is specific for terminal galactose and *N*-acetylgalactosamine residues, but also homologues of the macrophage mannose receptor, whose expression on NK cells has been functionally demonstrated, and the NKRP-1 receptor itself, that has been shown to bind with low affinity ligands containing mannose or galactose residues [69]. NKRP-1 is expressed by all NK cells as a disulfide-linked homodimer. The polypeptide is a type II integral membrane protein with a deduced extracellular domain homologous to the Ca^{2+}-dependent lectin superfamily, which also include the previously cloned Ly-49 mouse receptor. The NKRP-1 receptor and related molecules appear to act as positive regulators of NK cell lytic function, unlike the typical MHC class I receptor. The only exception is represented by the Ly-49 molecule, whose function and ligand specificity appear to be similar to the p58 family of receptors, despite the fact that Ly-49 is structurally related to the C-type lectin receptor family [70]. The divergence between human and mouse NK cell receptors for MHC class I challenges the paradigm that NK cells are innate and primitive components of the vertebrate immune system [71]. Alternatively, and more likely, this apparent paradox depends on our incomplete knowledge of the mouse equivalent of the p58 family of receptors, and of the human equivalent of the Ly-49 molecules. Attractive candidates in this respect are represented by the products of the human NKG-2 gene family, which is predicted to encode for lectin-like type II membrane glycoproteins displaying limited polymorphism [72].

Natural Killer Cell Receptors for Xenogeneic Determinants?

A possible comprehensive explanation of our findings, which takes into account the existing knowledge on NK cell specific receptor molecules, is that receptors of the selectin or NKRP-1 families, broadly expressed by NK lymphocytes, recognize sialylated or fucosylated ligands expressed in a non-species-specific fashion by vascular and nonvascular cells such as K562, whereas less characterized lectins, possibly expressed by subsets of circulating NK cells, are involved in the recognition of xenogeneic-specific oligosaccharide ligands. Parallel structural analysis of CDR and CRD of xenoreactive antibodies and lectins will help clarify the structural basis of the observed common recognition patterns. Interestingly, both molecules have been reported to utilize multivalent recognition and ligand-induced clustering as a means to increase the affinity and/or persistence of ligand binding. Mammalian C-type lectins have been shown to participate in cell-cell adhesion and cellular activation processes that imply transmembrane signaling properties. The previously mentioned data suggest that NK-specific lectins, such as the murine Ly-49 receptor, could deliver inhibitory signals to NK lymphocytes that would prevent them from destroying autologous tissues expressing Class I MHC antigens and would account for the acquisition of a still poorly characterized NK cell receptor repertoire during ontogeny. Our previous work indicated that integrins are the dominant adhesion receptors involved in human NK lymphocyte/xenogeneic EC cell–cell contacts [17, 19]. As leukocyte integrins are normally inactive and require activation signals to be converted to a high avidity state for their ligands, we propose that lectin-mediated recognition processes could provide such activation, leading to firm NK lymphocyte adhesion to the xenogeneic tissue and subsequent triggering of the effector cell's lytic machinery. Based on the above considerations, a comprehensive model of NK cell-dependent xenogeneic tissue destruction can be proposed: oligosaccharide ligands, displaying species-, tissue-, or differentiation stage-specific expression would be required to confer sensitivity to recognition and lysis by NK cells. The absence of relevant oligosaccharide ligands and/or the recognition of defined MHC allele products could prevent the adhesion/activation process from talking place, so that a cell displaying such a phenotype would be ignored by NK effector lymphocytes. In this context, degenerate MHC I molecules expressed by xenogeneic tissues and not recognized by their cognate receptors across species barriers would be ineffective as negative regulators of NK activation, thus rendering xenogeneic cells highly sensitive targets for human NK cell-mediated effector processes.

References

1. Rosengard A.M., Cary N.R., Langford G.A., et al. 1995. Tissue expression of human complement inhibitor, decay accelerating factor, in transgenic pigs. A potential approach for preventing xenograft rejection. Transplantation. 59:1325
2. McCurry K.R., Kooyman D.L., Alvarado C.G., et al. 1995. Human complement regulatory proteins protect swine-to-primate cardiac xenografts from humoral injury. Nature Med. 1:423
3. White D.J, Bradley P., Dunning J., et al. 1995. Hearts from pigs transgenic for human DAF are not hyperacutely rejected when xenografted to primates. Third International Congress for Xenotransplantation. Boston, 1995
4. Platt J.L., Vercellotti G.M., Dalmasso A.P., et al. 1990. Transplantation of discordant xenografts: a review of progress. Immunol. Today. 11:450
5. Auchincloss H. Jr. 1988. Xenogeneic transplantation: a review. Transplantation. 46:1
6. Kaufman C.L., Gaines B.A., Ildstad. S.T. 1995. Xenotransplantation. Annu. Rev. Immunol. 13:339
7. Good A.H., Cooper D.K.C., Malcolm A.J., et al. 1992. Identification of carbohydrate structures that bind human antiporcine antibodies: implications for discordant xenografting in humans. Transplant. Proc. 24:559
8. Oriol R., Ye Y., Koren E., Cooper D.K.C. 1993. Carbohydrate antigens of pig tissues reacting with human natural antibodies as potential targets for vascular hyperacute rejection in pig-to-man organ transplantation. Transplantation 56:1433
9. Sandrin M.S., Vaughan H.A., Dabkowski P.L., McKenzie I.F.C. 1993. Anti-pig IgM antibodies in human serum react predominantly with Galα(1–3)Gal epitopes. Proc. Natl. Acad. Sci. USA. 90:11391
10. Galili, U. 1993. Interaction of the natural anti-Gal antibody with α-galactosyl epitopes: a major obstacle for xenotransplantation in humans. Immunol. Today. 14:480
11. Henion T.R., Macher B.A., Anaraki F., Galili U. 1994. Defining the minimal size of catalitically active primate α1,3 galactosyltransferase: structure-function studies on the recombinant truncated enzyme. Glycobiology. 4:193
12. Sandrin M.S., Fodor W.L., Mouhtouris E., et al. 1995. Enzymatic remodeling of the carbohydrate surface of a xenogeneic cell substantially reduces human antibody binding and complement-mediated cytolysis. Nature Med. 1:1261
13. Auchincloss H. Jr. 1990. Xenografting: a review. Transplant. Rev. 4:14
14. Platt J.L., Fischel R.J., Matas A.J., et al. 1991. Immunopathology of hyperacute xenograft rejection in a swine to primate model. Transplantation. 52:214
15. Thomas F.T., Marchman W., Carobbi A., et al. 1991. Immunobiology of the xenograft response: xenograft rejection in the immunodeficient rodents. Transplant. Proc. 23:208
16. Arakawa K., Akami T., Okamoto M., et al. 1994. Prolongation of heart xenograft survival in the NK-deficient rat. Transplant. Proc. 26:1266
17. Inverardi L., Samaja M., Motterlini R., et al. 1992. Early recognition of a discordant xenogeneic organ by human circulating lymphocytes. J. Immunol. 149:1416
18. Inverardi L., Samaja M., Marelli F., Bender J. R., Pardi R. 1992. Cellular early immune recognition of xenogeneic vascular endothelium. Transplant. Proc. 24:459
19. Inverardi L., Pardi R. 1994. Early events in cell-mediated recognition of vascularized xenografts: cooperative interactions between selected lymphocyte subsets and natural antibodies. Immunol. Reviews. 141:71

20. Blakely M.L., Van Der Werf W.J., Berndt M.C., et al. 1994. Activation of intragraft endothelial and mononuclear cells during discordant xenograft rejection. Transplantation. 58:1059
21. Candinas D., Lesnikoski B.A., Grey S.T., et al. Delayed xenograft rejection (DXR) in complement (c)-depleted T cell-deficient (nude) rat recipients of guinea pig cardiac grafts. Third International Congress for Xenotransplantation. Boston, 1995
22. Alter B.J., Bach F.H. 1990. Cellular basis of the proliferative response of human T cells to mouse xenoantigens. J. Exp. Med. 171:333
23. Moses R.D., Pierson R.N. III, Winn H.J., Auchincloss H. Jr. 1990. Xenogeneic proliferation and lymphokine production are dependent on CD4+ helper T cells and self antigen presenting cells in the mouse. J. Exp. Med. 172:567
24. Dorling A., Binns R., Lechler R.I. 1995. Examination of the direct human T cell xenoresponse against porcine dendritic cells and identification of inefficient SLA DR recognition. Third International Congress for Xenotransplantation. Boston, 1995
25. Satake M., Korsgren O., Ridderstad A., et al. 1994. Immunological characteristics of islet cell xenotransplantation in humans and rodents. Immunol. Reviews. 141:191
26. Hamelmann W., Gray D.W.R., Cairns T.D.J., et al. 1994. Immediate destruction of xenogeneic islets in a primate model. Transplantation. 58: 1109
27. Schachner R.D., Ricordi C., Inverardi L. 1995. Xenogeneic discordant islet transplantation: natural antibodies and complement in a human-to-rat model. Transplant. Proc. 27:3318
28. Inverardi L., Ricordi C. 1996. Transplantation of pancreas and islets of Langerhans: a review of progress. Immunol. Today. 17:7
29. Murray A.G., Khodadoust M.M., Pober J.S., Bothwell A.L.M. 1994. Porcine aortic endothelial cells activate human T cells: direct presentation of MHC antigens and costimulation by ligands for human CD2 and CD28. Immunity. 1:57
30. Rosenberg A.S., Singer A. 1992. Cellular basis of skin allograft rejection. An in vivo model of immune-mediated tissue destruction. Annu. Rev. Immunol. 10:333
31. Wanders A., Akyurek M.L., Waltenberger J., et al. 1995. Ischemia-induced transplant atherosclerosis in the rat. Art. Thromb. Vasc. Biol. 15:145
32. Wanders A., Akyurek M.L., Waltenberger J., et al. 1993. Impact of ischemia time on chronic vascular rejection in the rat: effects of angiopeptin. Transplant. Proc. 25:2098
33. Springer T.A. 1994. Traffic signals for lymphocyte recirculation and leukocyte emigration: the multistep paradigm. Cell. 76: 301
34. Pardi R., Inverardi L., Bender J.R. 1992. Regulatory mechanisms in leukocyte adhesion: flexible receptors for sophisticated travelers. Immunol. Today. 13:224
35. De Lisser H.M., Newman P.J., Albelda S.M. 1994. Molecular and functional aspects of PECAM-1/CD31. Immunol. Today. 15:490
36. Dustin L.M., Springer T.A. 1989. T cell receptor cross-linking transiently stimulates adhesiveness through LFA-1. Nature. 341:619
37. Downey G.P., Chan C.K., Lea P., Takai A., Grinstein S. 1992. Phorbol ester-induced actin assembly in neutrophils: role of protein kinase C. J. Cell Biol. 116:695
38. Hibbs M.L., Jakes S., Stacker S.A., Wallace R.W., Springer T.A. 1991. The cytoplasmic domain of the integrin lymphocyte function-associated antigen 1 β subunit: sites required for binding to intercellular adhesion molecule 1 and the phorbol ester-stimulated phosphorylation site. J. Exp. Med. 174:1227

39. Pardi R., Inverardi L., Rugarli C., Bender J.R. 1992. Antigen-Receptor complex stimulation triggers protein kinase C-dependent CD11a/CD18-cytoskeleton association in T lymphocytes. J. Cell Biol. 116:1211
40. Valmu L., Autero M., Siljander P., Patarroyo M., Gahmberg C.G. 1991. Phosphorylation of the β-subunit of CD11/CD18 integrins by protein kinase C correlates with leukocyte adhesion. Eur. J. Immunol. 21:2857
41. Diamond M.S., Springer T.A. 1993. A subpopulation of Mac-1 (CD11b/CD18) molecules mediates neutrophil adhesion to ICAM-1 and fibrinogen. J. Cell Biol. 120:545
42. Dransfield I., Cabanas C., Craig A., Hogg N. 1992. Divalent cation regulation of the function of the leukocyte integrin LFA-1. J. Cell Biol. 116:219
43. Altieri D.C. 1991. Occupancy of CD11b/CD18 (Mac-1) divalent ion binding site(s) induces leukocyte adhesion. J. Immunol. 147:1891
44. Landis R.C., Bennett R.I., Hogg N. 1993. A novel LFA-1 activation epitope maps to the I domain. J. Cell Biol. 120:1519
45. Van Kooyk Y., Weder P., Hogervorst F., et al. 1991. Activation of LFA-1 through Ca^{2+}-dependent epitope stimulates lymphocyte adhesion. J. Cell. Biol. 112:345
46. Gailit J., Ruoslathi E. 1988. Regulation of the fibronectin receptor affinity by divalent cations. J. Biol. Chem. 263:12927
47. Hermanowski-Vostaka A., van Strijp J.A.G., Swiggard W.J., Wright S.D. 1992. Integrin modulating factor-1: a lipid that alters the function of leukocyte integrins. Cell. 68:341
48. Chan B.M.C., Hemler M.E. 1993. Multiple functional forms of integrin VLA-2 can be derived from a single α2 cDNA clone: interconversion of forms induced by anti-β1 antibody. J. Cell. Biol. 120:537
49. O'Toole E.T., Katagiri Y., Faull R.J., et al. 1994. Integrin cytoplasmic domains mediate inside-out signal transduction. J. Cell. Biol. 124:1047
50. Bertagnolli M.E., Bekerle M.C. 1993. Evidence for the selective association of a subpopulation of GPIIb-IIIa with the actin cytoskeletons of thrombin-activated platelets. J. Cell Biol. 121:1329
51. Larson R.S., Hibbs M.L., Springer T.A. 1990. The leukocyte integrin LFA-1 reconstituted by cDNA transfection in a nonhematopoietic cell line is functionally active and not transiently regulated. Cell Regulation. 1:359
52. Zweier J.L., Kuppusamy P., Lutty G.A. 1988. Measurement of endothelial cell free radical generation: evidence for a central mechanism of free radical injury in postischemic tissue. Proc. Natl. Acad. Sci. USA. 85:4046
53. Seccombe J.F., Schaff H.V. 1994. Vasoactive factors produced by the endothelium: physiology and surgical implications. R.G. Landes Company, Austin TX
54. Lee W.P., Gribling P., De Guzman L., Ehsani N., Watson S.R. 1995. A P-selectin-immunoglobulin G chimera is protective in a rabbit ear model of ischemia-reperfusion. Surgery. 117:458
55. Davenpeck K.L., Gauthier T.W., Albertine K.H., Lefer A.M. 1994. Role of P-selectin in microvascular leukocyte-endothelial interaction in splanchnic ischemia-reperfusion. Am. J. Physiol. 267:622
56. Carden D.L., Young J.A., Granger D.N. 1993. Pulmonary microvascular injury after intestinal ischemia-reperfusion: role of P-selectin. J. Appl. Physiol. 75:2529
57. Kubes P., Jutila M., Payne D. 1995. Therapeutic potential of inhibiting leukocyte rolling in ischemia/reperfusion. J. Clin. Invest. 95:2510

58. Sylvestre D.L., Ravetch J.V. 1994. Fc receptors initiate the Arthus reaction: redefining the inflammatory cascade. Science. 265:1095
59. Inverardi L., Clissi B., Stolzer A., Bender J.R., Pardi R. Overlapping recognition of xenogeneic carbohydrate epitopes by human natural killer cells and preformed natural antibodies. (submitted)
60. Yokoyama W.M. 1993. Recognition structures on natural killer cells. Curr. Op. Immunol. 5:67
61. Trinchieri G. 1989. Biology of natural killer cells. Adv. Immunol. 47:187
62. Kagi D., Ledermann B., Burki K., et al. 1994. Cytotoxicity mediated by T cells and NK cells is greatly impaired in perforin-deficient mice. Nature. 369:31
63. Karre K. 1985. Role of target histocompatibility antigens in regulation of NK activity: a reevaluation and a hypothesis. In: Mechanism of Cytotoxicity by NK Cells. Herberman R.B. and Callewaert D.M. (eds), Academic Press; p. 81
64. Kaufman D.S., Schoon R.A., Leibson P.J. 1993. MHC class I expression on tumor targets inhibits NK cell-mediated cytotoxicity without interfering with target recognition. J. Immunol. 150:1429
65. Sanchez M.J., Spits H., Lanier L.L., Phillips J.H. 1993. Human natural killer thymocytes and their relation to the T-cell lineage. J. Exp. Med. 178:1857
66. Sanchez M.J., Muench M.O., Roncarolo M.G. Lanier L.L., Phillips J.H. 1994. Identification of a common T/natural killer cell progenitor in human fetal thymus. J. Exp. Med. 180:569
67. Wagtmann N., Biassoni R,. Cantoni C., et al. 1995. Molecular clones of the p58 NK cell receptor reveal immunoglobulin-related molecules with diversity in both the extra- and intracellular domains. Immunity. 2:439
68. Drickamer K. 1993. Calcium-dependent carbohydrate recognition domains in animal proteins. Curr. Op. Struct. Biol. 3:393
69. Bezouska K., Yuen C.T., O'Brien J., et al. 1994. Oligosaccharide ligands for NKR-P1 protein activate NK cells and cytotoxicity. Nature. 372:150
70. Karlhofer F.M., Ribaudo R.K., Yokoyama W.M. 1992. MHC class I alloantigen specificity of Ly 49+ IL2-activated NK cells. Nature. 358:66
71. Gumperz J.E., Parham P. 1995. The enigma of NK cells. Nature. 378:245
72. Houchins J.P., Yabe T., McSherry C., Bach F.H. 1994. DNA sequence analysis of NK-G2, a family of related cDNA clones encoding type II integral membrane proteins on human NK cells. J. Exp. Med. 173:1017

11 Hemostasis in Xenotransplantation

B.J. Hunt and K.M. Jurd

Introduction

The recent revival of interest in xenotransplantation across discordant species focused initially on immunological aspects of hyperacute rejection. More latterly, research has explored the effects of antibody and complement binding to the endothelial cell. However the ultimate end-point of hyperacute rejection (the xenograft reaction) can be considered to be microvascular thrombosis. Thus hemostasis, the complex system which maintains the fluidity of blood within a vessel, but forms a clot once the vessel wall is breached, is an obligatory component of the xenograft reaction. This chapter will cover a basic understanding of hemostasis and then discuss the relative importance of hemostatic activation in the pig-to-human xenograft reaction.

Hemostatic System

Hemostasis can be regarded as a system designed to maintain blood fluidity and vascular integrity, but also as one of the body's primary defense mechanisms along with the immune and complement systems. Its role in this context is simple. If one considers invasion by a bacterium, then the function of the hemostatic system is to immobilise it by laying down fibrin, thus allowing leukocytes and complement to act and kill the invader. Hemostasis, like the immune and complement systems, is highly complex with each hemostatic factor having multiple effects. The following account, however, has been greatly simplified.

Under physiological conditions, hemostasis is initiated by damage to the vessel wall. When a vessel is cut the release of vasoactive substances leads to vasoconstriction, thus limiting blood loss. Platelets adhere to exposed subendothelial matrix components. von Willebrand factor (vWF) is the platelet adhesion ligand [1]; it binds to subendothelial components and to specific receptors (glycoprotein Ib and IIb/IIIa) on the surface of platelets [2]. This results in platelet activation. On activation, platelets undergo a shape change, from smooth convex disc to a spiny sphere, and release the contents of dense granules rich in prothrombotic substances [3], which activate other platelets. These aggregate together by binding fibrinogen between platelet surface receptor glycoprotein IIb/IIIa, and so a platelet plug is formed [4]. Simultaneously coagulation is activated on the surface of platelets leading to the generation of thrombin and the formation of a fibrin clot which strengthens the platelet plug. Platelet activation and thrombin genera-

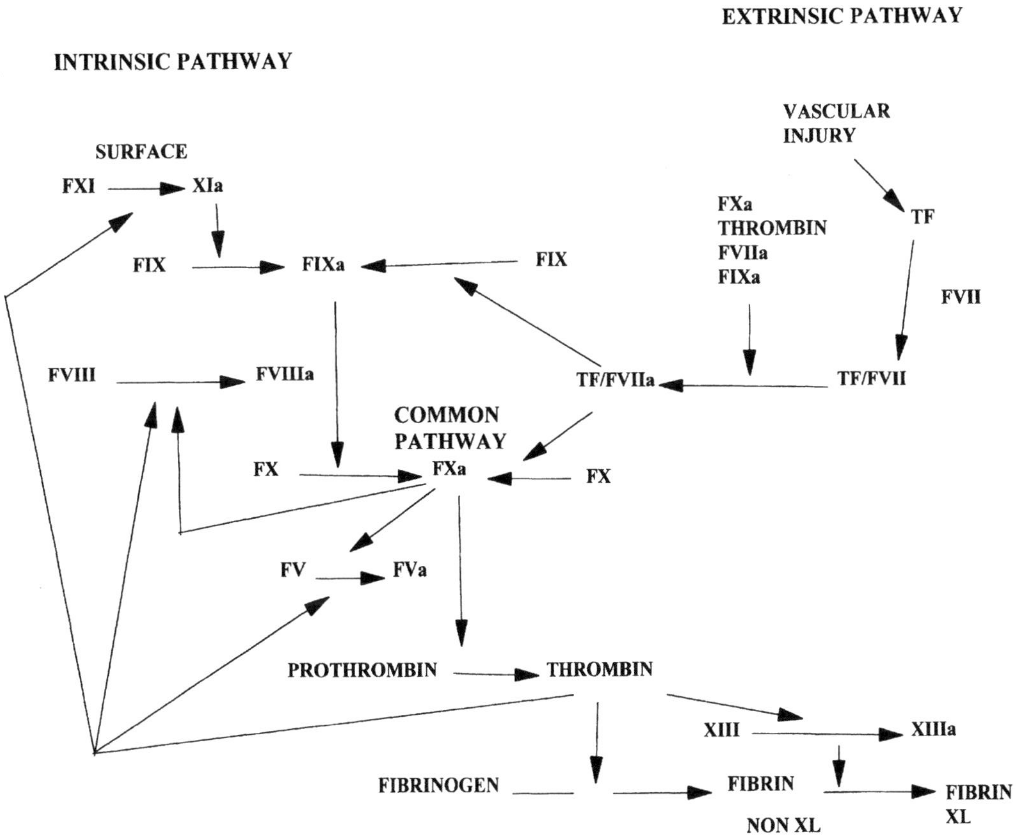

Fig. 1. Blood coagulation cascade. Physiological activation is initiated through the extrinsic pathway following vascular injury and exposure to tissue factor. The intrinsic pathway is thought to represent an amplification loop to maintain coagulation after the generation of small amounts of thrombin, which activates factor XI. Both pathways converge at the level of factor X, from which point they share a common pathway to thrombin generation and fibrin formation. Thrombin is responsible for a number of positive feedback reactions activating other coagulation factors. Activated coagulation factors (*F*) are denoted by a lower case *a*. Cross-linked fibrin (*XL*) is formed by the formation of covalent bonds between fibrin polymers. Many of the reactions require calcium ions and phospholipid, but these are omitted for simplicity. (Adapted from [10])

tion are interdependent processes. Thrombin is a potent platelet activator [5] and activated platelets accelerate thrombin generation.

The coagulation cascade is the descriptive term used to describe fibrin formation from a series of stepwise reactions involving a number of circulating blood proteins in an inactive precursor form. This complex system involves a number of zymogens: factors XII, XI, X, IX, VII and prothrombin and the pre-cofactors factors VIII and V. These are converted to the appropriate enzymes and cofactors before interacting to ultimately form fibrin. A small initiating stimulus is amplified to produce high levels of insoluble fibrin. The traditional separation of the coagulation cascade [6, 7] into the intrinsic (contact) and extrinsic (tissue factor) pathways is now outdated, since there are many interactions between the components of each pathway, such as the activation of factor IX by the tissue factor/VIIa complex [8].

Initiation of coagulation results from activation of factor VII through exposure to tissue factor [9] on the subendothelium. Tissue factor is a membrane glycoprotein present in the extravascular tissues so that when the endothelium is breached coagulation is activated. It can also be induced, by certain cytokines and thrombin, on endothelium and monocytes. The intrinsic pathway is activated by negatively charged components on the subendothelium, but is now considered to be an amplification loop of the common pathway [10], for thrombin activates factor XI [11]. Certainly patients with factor XII deficiency do not bleed excessively. A simplified interpretation of the current understanding of the coagulation mechanism is shown in Fig. 1. Many of the reactions in blood coagulation are localised to damaged procoagulant surfaces. Assembly of coagulation enzyme complexes on these surfaces results in a dramatic enhancement in reaction rate and also interferes with regulatory processes of inhibitory anticoagulant systems. Two such enzyme complexes are the X-ase and prothrombinase complexes requiring membrane-bound cofactors which serve as anchoring sites [12].

Physiological Anticoagulant Systems

In vivo there is a continuous low-grade activation of coagulation, but trace amounts of activated coagulation factors are rapidly neutralised by physiological anticoagulants, the protein C/thrombomodulin [13] (Fig. 2) and antithrombin III (ATIII)/heparan sulphate systems [14], and tissue factor pathway inhibitor (TFPI) [15].

Protein C is a plasma protein which circulates in its inactive form but, once activated, acts together with a cofactor, protein S, to inactivate factors Va [16] and VIIIa [17], thereby limiting further thrombin generation. Thrombomodulin is a glycoprotein present on the endothelial cell surface, and thrombin bound to thrombomodulin activates protein C [18]. Thus activation of protein C is dependent on thrombin and the expression of thrombomodulin. Binding to thrombomodulin also inhibits other procoagulant activities of thrombin, such as the clotting of fibrinogen, activation of factor V [19] and platelets [20].

ATIII is a glycoprotein which circulates in plasma and is the major inhibitor not only of thrombin, as its name suggests, but also the majority of activated

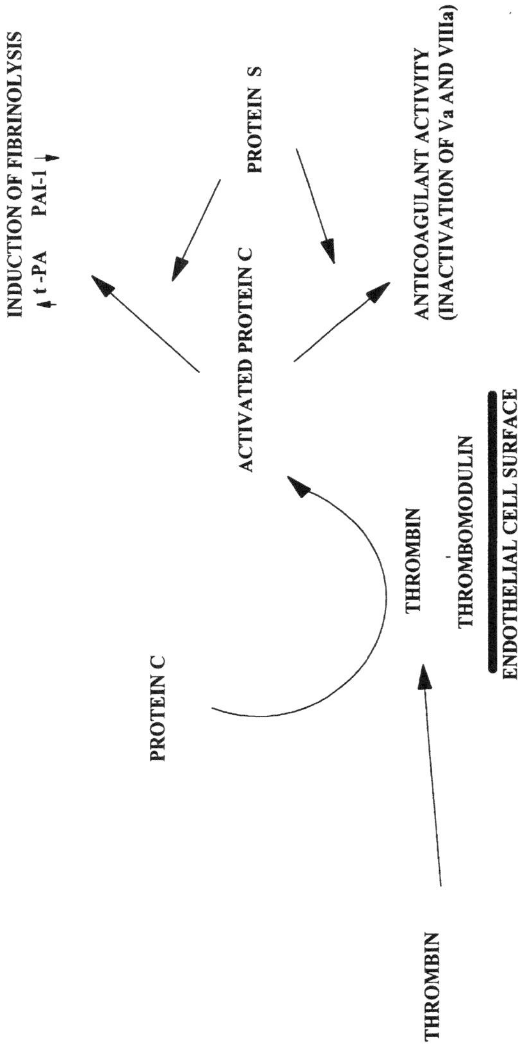

Fig. 2. Activation and function of protein C. Activated protein C inactivates factors Va and VIIIa, thereby restricting further thrombin generation. It also potentiates fibrinolysis by increasing endothelial cell synthesis and release of tissue plasminogen activator (*t-PA*) and decreasing plasminogen activator inhibitor (*PAI-1*)

intrinsic coagulation factors [21]. It is an irreversible inhibitor and its anticoagulant potential is greatly enhanced, physiologically, by heparan sulphate which coats the endothelial cell suface. A small fraction of plasma ATIII is normally bound to heparan sulphate and is thus ideally situated for inhibition of activated coagulation factors. Heparin, which is used as an anticoagulant, acts by potentiating the action of ATIII [22].

TFPI is produced by endothelial cells and is an inhibitor of the tissue factor–factor VIIa/Xa complex [15]. An increase in information regarding TFPI in recent years has established its role as an important inhibitor of small amounts of TF.

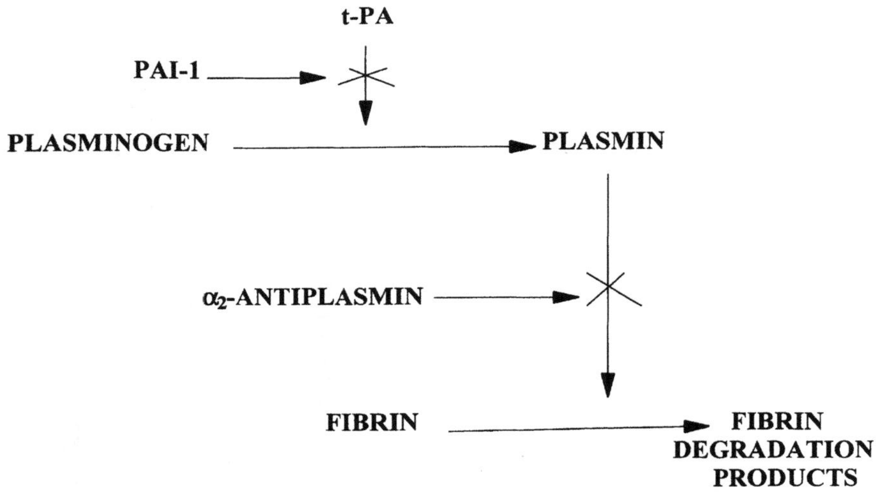

Fig. 3. Components of the fibrinolytic pathway. Plasminogen is converted to plasmin by tissue plasminogen activator (*t-PA*) bound to fibrin. Plasmin then breaks down insoluble fibrin to soluble fibrin degradation products. Plasminogen activator inhibitor (*PAI-1*) inhibits t-PA, and α_2-antiplasmin inhibits plasmin

Fibrinolysis

Clot breakdown or fibrinolysis (Fig. 3) is part of the healing process. The central protein is plasmin which, like other coagulation proteins, circulates as its inactive precursor, plasminogen. It degrades insoluble fibrin into small soluble fibrin degradation products. When fibrin is formed, plasminogen and tissue plasminogen activator (t-PA) are bound to fibrin, and plasminogen is activated by t-PA [23]. The fibrinolytic process is regulated by the inhibitors α_2-antiplasmin and plasminogen activator inhibitor (PAI)-1 [24]. PAI-1 and t-PA are both produced by the endothelium, which controls the amount of free (active) t-PA by altering the relative production of both.

Role of Endothelium

The endothelium in its quiescent state forms an antithrombotic (both anti-platelet and anticoagulant) surface to the constituents of blood. This is achieved through (a) production of prostacyclin [25] and nitric oxide [26], preventing platelet aggregation, (b) t-PA [27] promoting fibrinolysis and (c) the physiological anticoagulants thrombomodulin/protein C, heparan sulphate/ATIII and TFP1, described previously. The endothelium becomes activated under certain conditions resulting in a change of phenotype from antithrombotic to prothrombotic (Table 1). This is brought about through down-regulation of antithrombotic mechanisms and upregulation of tissue factor. The endothelium also expresses

Table 1. Hemostatic effects of endothelial cell activation

Procoagulant	Quiescent endothelium	Activated endothelium
von Willebrand factor	WP bodies	Released into plasma
P selectin	On inner lining of WP bodies	Expressed on surface
Tissue factor	Absent	Expressed on surface
Anticoagulant systems		
Thrombomodulin	Expressed on surface	Internalized
Heparan sulfate	Coats surface	Lost
TFPI	Secreted	?
Fibrinolysis		
t-PA and PAI-1	-	Upregulated PAI-1->t-PA
Anti-platelet and vasodilatory		
Nitric oxide	Released	-
Prostacyclin	Released	-
ecto-ADPase	Released	Lost
Platelet-activating factor	Released	-

WP, Weibel-Palade; TPF, tissue factor pathway inhibitor; t-PA, tissue plasminogen activator; PAI, plasminogen activator inhibitor.

binding sites for coagulation factors IX and X [28], and synthesises and expresses factor V [29]. Endothelial cell activation and its effects are described elsewhere in this volume and are therefore dealt with only briefly here.

Role of Thrombin

Thrombin functions at every level of hemostasis - at the vascular level, the cellular level and the plasma level. Thrombin possesses a central role in hemostasis in the conversion of fibrinogen to fibrin, activation of platelets [5]and other coagulation factors, such as FXI [11] FV [30], FVIII [31] and FXIII [32]. It also initiates the mechanisms for limiting both clot size and its own generation by activating the protein C system, and initiates the destruction of the clot it forms by increasing t-PA release. Thrombin also acts like a cytokine by causing both endothelial cell and monocyte activation. The effects of thrombin are depicted in Fig. 4.

Role of the Monocyte/Macrophage

Monocytes/macrophages, when activated, express tissue factor and are thus responsible for initiating hemostasis, especially in extravascular tissues. A variety of physiological and pathological stimuli, such as interleukin (IL)-1, tumour necrosis factor (TNF), lipopolysaccharide, lymphokines, immune complexes, activated complement and thrombin induce tissue factor expression on monocytes

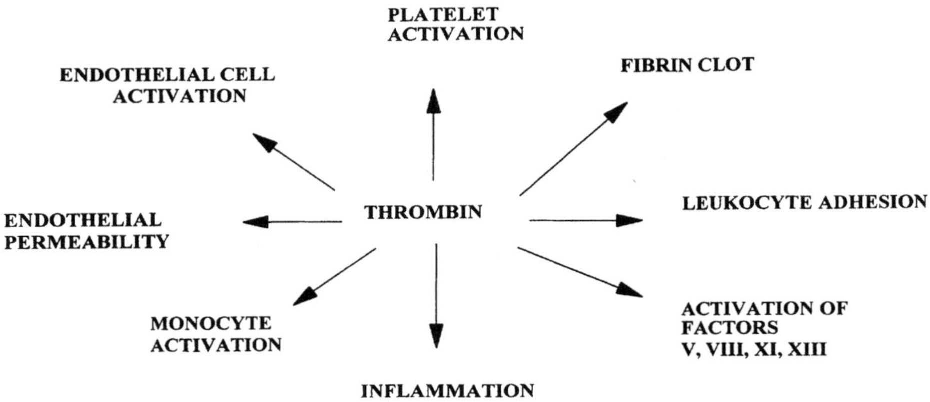

Fig. 4. Multiple effects of thrombin on hemostasis

[33]. A leukocyte adhesion molecule, Mac-1, can bind and activate factor X after monocyte exposure to ADP [34]. The significance of this activation of coagulation is uncertain.

Pathological Activation of Hemostasis

Pathological activation of hemostasis can occur under a number of circumstances. Certain bacteria can trigger coagulation by producing endotoxins, and cancerous tumours can directly activate factor X to Xa by producing a cysteine protease known as cancer procoagulant [35]. Factor X can also be directly activated by Russell's viper venom [36] whilst other snake venoms can directly defibrinate blood. Other components of coagulation, such as factor VII [37] and protein C [38], can also be directly activated by certain snake venoms. Pathological activation of prothrombin occurs by five recognised groups of exogenous prothrombin activators [39]. Some, such as the venom of *Echis carinatus*, convert prothrombin to an enzymatically active intermediate, meizothrombin, followed by autocatalysis to thrombin [40]. Others are Xa-like enzymes, have Xa and Va-like subunits or consist of thrombin-like enzymes. Prothrombin activators are also produced by certain bacteria. Some cleave peptide bonds in prothrombin, whilet others, such as staphylocoagulase, form stoichiometric complexes with prothrombin accompanied by active site exposure without proteolysis [41].

Hemostasis and Xenotransplantation

Physiological interactions between proteins in an individual may differ if the two molecules are from different species due to species differences in those proteins. As the pig is currently considered to be the most feasible donor for man [42] and is the most widely investigated, the remaining discussions of this chapter are concentrated on this area.

Complement

The current hypothesis of organ rejection in the pig-to-human xenograft reaction is that anti-pig antibodies bind to xenoantigens on the porcine endothelium, activating complement and causing subsequent hemostatic activation and thrombosis. The normal hemoastatic function of platelets can be affected by various components of the complement system. Thrombin-initiated assembly of C5b-C9 potentiates thrombin-stimulated platelet aggregation [43], and assembly of C5b-C9 on the platelet plasma membrane results in increased prothrombinase activity without lysis [44]. Complement-induced endothelial cell vesiculation results in release of membrane microparticles expressing binding sites for factor Va and increased prothrombinase activity [45]. Furthermore, xenoantibody and complement cause rapid cleavage of heparan sulphate proteoglycan from the endothelial cell surface, with 5% loss of heparan sulphate within 4 min and nearly 50% in 30 min [46]. We have shown that complement depletion with cobra venom factor delayed, but did not prevent, hemostatic activation in vitro [47]. Thus complement depletion, inhibition by soluble complement receptor 1 (sCR1) or use of an organ from a transgenic pig expressing the gene for human-accelerating factor (DAF) may prevent the immediate hemostatic activation resulting from the effects of complement, but this is only delayed.

Endothelial Cell Activation

Endothelial activation plays a role in hemostatic activation as discussed earlier, although this is not peculiar to xenotransplantation. The speed of hyperacute rejection (within a few minutes) suggests that endothelial cell activation is not responsible for immediate hemostatic activation as the expression of tissue factor takes 2–6 h to occur in vitro, but endothelial cell retraction may expose subendothelial tissue factor which would initiate coagulation. Platelet aggregation is modulated by adenine nucleotides. Quiescent endothelial cells express an ecto-ADPase that degrades ATP and ADP and thus prevents ADP accumulation. Recently, it has been found that activated porcine endothelium lost ecto-ADPase activity [48].

Interspecies Hemostatic Molecular Incompatibility

Despite removal of anti-pig antibody and complement from human blood, graft failure is only delayed and hemostatic activation still occurs, suggesting that hemostatic activation occurs independently of, or in parallel with, immunological activation. Moreover, there is the unacknowledged, but well-recognised assumption that, in situations when porcine organs are perfused with human blood, the clotting process needs to be slowed down, or inhibited, to study immunological aspects (15 units heparin/ml are required in the working pig heart and lung model; R.N. Pierson, personal communication). Human hemostatic activation has been demonstrated on passage of human blood through an ex vivo working pig heart circuit despite removal of anti-pig antibodies or complement depletion [49]. The ex vivo perfusion of a porcine liver with human blood and a pig-to-human liver xenograft have demonstrated prominent fibrin deposition on porcine endothelium associated with only weak binding of human IgM and IgG and absence of complement components [50]. Furthermore, when newborn pig hearts were transplanted heterotopically into newborn baboons, no IgM or IgG xenoantibody or complement components were present on the xenografts, but fibrin and platelet deposition were evident [51].

There are recognised molecular discordances between components of human and porcine hemostasis. Porcine vWF directly aggregates human platelets [52]. This was investigated after it was noted that hemophiliacs treated with porcine factor VIII suffered thrombocytopenia. It was found that the factor VIII concentrates contained large amounts of porcine vWF which aggregates human platelets in vivo [53]. Further studies showed that porcine vWF binds to glycoprotein Ib, and the platelet fibrinogen receptor GPIIb/IIIa is activated. Endothelial cells produce TFPI; however, activated porcine endothelium produces TFPI which,

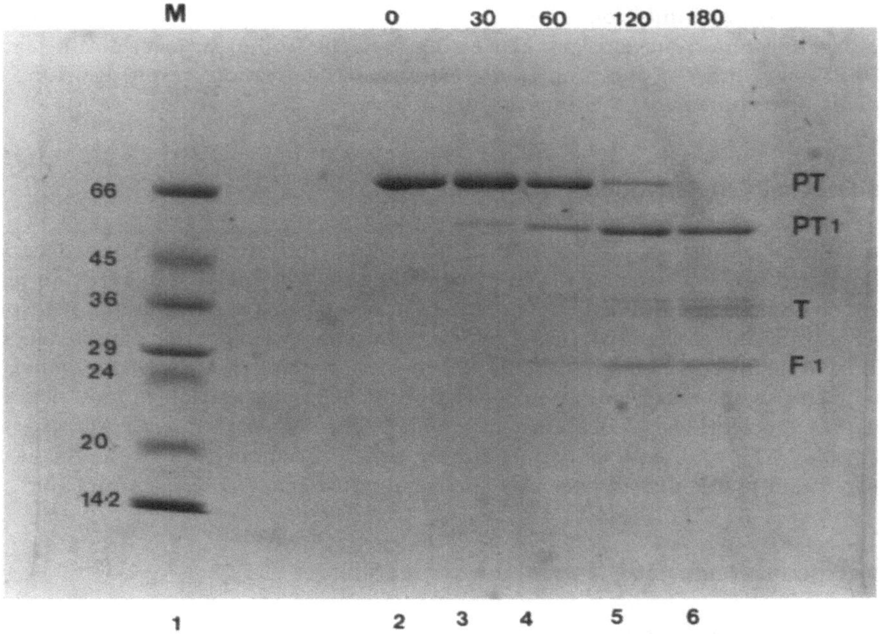

Fig. 5. Sodium dodecyl sulphate polyacrylamide gel electrophoresis (SDS-PAGE) analysis of human prothrombin activation by porcine aortic endothelial cells (PAEC). Molecular weight markers are shown in *lane 1*, marked *M*. The molecular weights are given in kilodaltons against the appropriate band. The time course of the experiment is shown along the top of the gel in minutes, at time 0 (*lane 2*), 30 (*lane 3*), 60 (*lane 4*), 120 (*lane 5*) and 180 min (*lane 6*). *PT*, prothrombin; *PT1*, prethrombin 1; *T*, thrombin; *F1*, fragment 1

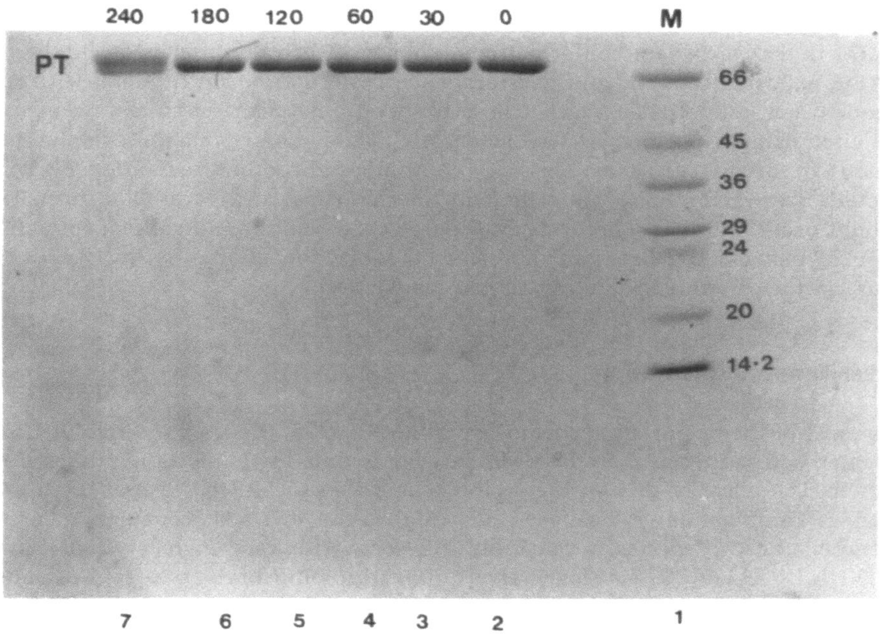

Fig. 6. Sodium dodecyl sulphate polyacrylamide gel electrophoresis (SDS-PAGE) analysis of human prothrombin activation by human umbilical vein endothelial cells (HUVEC). Molecular weight markers are shown in *lane 1*, marked *M*. The molecular weights are given in kilodaltons against the appropriate band. The time course of the experiment is given along the top of the gel in minutes, at time 0 (*lane 2*), 30 (*lane 3*), 60 (*lane 4*), 120 (*lane 5*), 180 (*lane 6*) and 240 min (*lane 7*). *PT*, prothrombin

although able to inhibit the human TF–VIIa complex, does not appear to possess anti-human Xa activity [54]. The potency of tissue factor between species is different, with porcine tissue factor less effective in human than porcine plasma [55]. Indeed, the species specificity of tissue factor is already known as mouse tissue factor is essentially ineffective in human plasma [56].

Work conducted in our own laboratory has focused on the direct activation of human hemostasis by porcine endothelium (i.e. in the absence of XNA and complement). Preliminary in vitro results suggested that as well as physiological activation of hemostasis, there may also be "pathological" or non-physiological activation of the common pathway of coagulation [57]. We thus investigated the direct activation of the common pathway by porcine endothelium by applying purified human prothrombin and factor X separately to porcine endothelium. Incubation of human prothrombin with confluent monolayers of porcine aortic endothelial cell (PAEC) resulted in its activation [58] (Fig. 5). This did not occur in the non-xenogeneic control (human umbilical vein endothelial cell, HUVEC; Fig. 6). Bovine prothrombin was not activated by PAEC and we found no evidence of direct factor X activation. In our experiments human prothrombin activation by PAEC was inhibited by the thrombin-specific inhibitor, hirudin

[59]. Thus a possible mechanism by which human prothrombin is activated by PAEC is that there is a conformational change in prothrombin upon binding to PAEC, exposing catalytic and possibly macromolecular specificity sites with subsequent autocatalytic cleavages. These observations have necessarily been made in vitro using a purified system in an attempt to dissect out the complex processes occurring in plasma. In vivo, continuous thrombin generation by PAEC would overwhelm local anticoagulant mechanisms and local clot formation would occur. Moreover, the consumption of prothrombin and subsequent activation of platelets by thrombin may lead to a bleeding diathesis; this fulfills the criteria for disseminated intravascular coagulation.

Liver Xenotransplantation

As most of the hemostatic proteins are synthesised by the liver, if a liver is transplanted across species then the recipient will assume the hemostatic profile of the donor. The effect of this on the recipient is uncertain. In the case of the pig-to-human combination, it has been shown that the levels of coagulation factors between the two species is markedly different, with very high levels of factors V, VIII, IX XI and XII and lower levels of prothrombin in the pig [55]. It is interesting to note that the Galα1,3-Gal epitope occurs in the carbohydrate chains of porcine coagulation factors. The majority of the sugar chains of porcine factor VIII contain the Galα1,3-Gal group, which is not present in human factor VIII [60]. Human fibrinogen carries four N-linked oligosaccharides with terminal NeuAcGalβ1,4GlcNAc residues [61], whereas porcine and bovine fibrinogen contain terminal Galα1,3-Galβ1,4GlcNAc [62] and is recognised by human xenoreactive antibodies [63]. The significance of this in xenotransplantation has not been studied.

The pig is currently considered to be the most likely xenotransplant donor for man. With the ever-growing information on rejection, there is increasing awareness of the importance of hemostasis in this process. Our current concern is that the molecular discordances in hemostasis between pig and man add a further layer of complexity which needs to be investigated before pig-to-human xenotransplantation becomes a clinical reality.

Acknowledgements. This work was funded by Grant no. PG/94051 from the British Heart Foundation and a grant from the Special Trustees of St Thomas' Hospital.

References

1. Girma J P, Meyer D, Verweij D L, Pannekoek J, Sixma J J. Structure-function relationship of human von Willebrand factor. Blood. 70, 605, 1986
2. Sakariassen K S, Nievelstein P F E M, Coller B S, Sixma J J. The role of platelet membrane glycoprotein Ib and IIb-IIIa in platelet adherence to human artery subendothelium. Br. J. Hematol. 63, 681, 1986

3. Holmsen H, Day H J, Stormorken H. The blood platelet release reaction. Scand. J. Hematol. Suppl. 8, 1, 1969
4. Niiya K, Hodson E, Bader R. Increased surface expression of the membrane glycoprotein IIb/IIIa complex induced by platelet activation. Relationship to the binding of fibrinogen and platelet aggregation. Blood. 70, 475, 1987
5. Harmon J T, Jamieson G A. Activation of platelets by alpha-thrombin is a receptor-mediated event. J. Biol. Chem. 261, 15928, 1986
6. Davie E W, Ratnoff O D. Waterfall sequence for intrinsic blood clotting. Science. 145, 1310, 1964
7. McFarlane R G. An enzyme cascade in the blood clotting mechanism, and its function as a biochemical amplifier. Nature. 202, 498, 1964
8. Bauer K A, Kass B L, Cate H T, Hawiger J J, Rosenberg R D. Factor IX is activated in vivo by the tissue factor mechanism. Blood. 76; 731, 1990
9. Edgington T S, Mackman N, Brand K, Ruf W. The structural biology and expression of tissue factor. Thromb. Hemostas. 66, 67, 1991
10. Davie E W, Fujikawa K, Kisiel W. The coagulation cascade: initiation, maintenance and regulation. Biochemistry. 30, 10363, 1991
11. Naito K, Fujikawa K. Activation of human blood coagulation factor XI independent of factor XII. Factor XI is activated by thrombin and factor XIa in the presence of negatively charged surfaces. J. Biol. Chem. 266, 7353, 1991
12. Mann K G, Neshiem M E, Church W R, Haley P, Krishnaswamy S. Surface-dependent reactions of the vitamin K-dependent enzyme complexes. Blood. 76, 1, 1990
13. Esmon C T. The roles of protein C and thrombomodulin in the regulation of blood coagulation. J Biol. Chem. 264, 4743, 1989
14. Marcum J A, McKenney J B, Rosenberg R D. Acceleration of thrombin-antithrombin complex formation in rat hindquarters via heparin-like molecules bound to the endothelium. J. Clin. Invest. 74, 341, 1984
15. Rapaport S I. The extrinsic pathway inhibitor: a regulator of tissue factor-dependent blood coagulation. Thromb. Hemostas. 66, 6, 1991
16. Suzuki K, Stenflo J Dahlback B, Teodorsson B. Inactivation of human coagulation factor V by activated protein C. J. Biol. Chem. 258, 1914, 1983
17. Fulcher C A, Gardiner J E, Griffin J H, Zimmerman T S. Proteolytic inactivation of human factor VIII procoagulant protein by activated protein C and its analogy with factor V. Blood. 63, 486, 1984
18. Esmon C T, Owen W G. Identification of an endothelial cell cofactor for the thrombin-catalyzed activation of protein C. Proc. Natl Acad,. Sci. 78, 2249, 1981
19. Esmon C T, Esmon N L, Harris K W. Complex formation between thrombin and thrombomodulin inhibits both thrombin-catalyzed fibrin formation and factor V activation. J Biol. Chem. 257, 7944, 1982
20. Esmon N L, Carroll R C, Esmon C T. Thrombomodulin blocks the ability of thrombin to activate platelets. J. Biol. Chem. 258, 12268, 1983
21. Bauer K A, Rosenberg R D. Role of antithrombin III as a regulator of in vivo coagulation. Seminars in Hematol. 28, 10, 1991
22. Rosenberg R D, Damus P S. The purification and mechanism of action of human antithrombin-heparin cofactor. J. Biol. Chem. 248, 6490, 1973
23. Holyaerts M, Rijken D C, Lijner H R, Collen D. Kinetics of the activation of plasminogen by human tissue plasminogen activator. J. Biol. Chem. 257, 2912, 1982

24. Collen D. On the regulation and control of fibrinolysis. Thromb. Hemostas. 43; 77, 1980
25. Moncada S. Biological importance of prostacyclin. Br. J. Pharmacol. 76, 3, 1982
26. Radomski M W, Palmer R M J, Moncada S. The anti-aggregating properties of vascular endothelium: interaction of prostacyclin and nitric oxide. Br. J. Pharmacol. 92, 639, 1987
27. Levin E G, Marzec U, Anderson J, Harker L A. Thrombin stimulates tissue plasminogen activator release from cultured endothelial cells. J. Clin. Invest. 74, 1988, 1984
28. Heimark R L, Schwartz S M. Binding of coagulation factors IX and X to the endothelial cell surface. Biochem. Biophys. Res. Commun. 111, 723, 1983
29. Cerveny T J, Fass D N, Mann K G. Synthesis of coagulation factor V by cultured aortic endothelium. Blood. 63, 1467, 1984
30. Nesheim M E, Mann K G. Thrombin-catalyzed activation of single chain bovine factor V. J. Biol. Chem. 254, 1326, 1979
31. Mann K G, Jenny R J, Krishnaswamy S. Cofactor proteins in the assembly and expression of blood clotting enzyme complexes. Ann. Rev. Biochem. 57, 915, 1988
32. Janus T J, Lewis S D, Lorand L, Shafer, J A. Promotion of thrombin-catalyzed activation of factor XIII by fibrinogen. Biochem. 22, 6269, 1983
33. Drake T A, Morissey J H, Edgington T S. Selective cellular expression of tissue factor in human tissues. Implications for disorders of hemostasis and thrombosis. Am. J. Pathol. 134, 1087, 1989
34. Altieri D C, Morrissey J H, Edgington T S. Adhesive receptor Mac-1 coordinates the activation of factor X on stimulated cells of monocytic and myeloid differentiation: an alternative initiation of the coagulation protease cascade. Proc. Natl. Acad. Sci. USA. 85, 7462, 1988
35. Gordon S G, Cross B A. A factor X activating cysteine protease from malignant tissue. J. Clin. Invest. 67, 1665, 1981
36. Khin-Ei-Han, Hutton R A. In vitro studies of Russell's viper venom on blood coagulation and fibrinolysis. Thrombosis Res. 46, 363, 1987
37. Nakagaki T, Lin P, Kisiel W. Activation of human factor VII by the prothrombin activator from the venom of Oxyuranus scutellatus (Taipan snake). Thrombosis Res. 65, 105, 1992
38. Kisiel W, Choi E, Kondo S. Isolation of protein C activator from Southern copperhead venom. Biochem. Biophys. Res. Commun. 143, 917, 1987
39. Rosing J, Tans G. Inventory of exogenous prothrombin activators. Thrombosis Hem. 65, 627, 1991
40. Kornalik F Blomback B. Prothrombin activation induced by Ecarin – a prothrombin converting enzyme from Echis carinatus venom. Thromb. Res. 6, 57, 1975
41. Hendrix H., Lindhout T., Mertens K., Engels W., Hemker H. C. Activation of human prothrombin by stoichiometric levels of staphylocoagulase. J. Biol. Chem. 258, 3637, 1983
42. Cooper D K C, Ye Y, Rolf L L Jr, Zuhdi N. The pig as potential organ donor for man. In: Xenotransplantation (First edition). Cooper D K C, et al. (eds). Springer, Heidelberg, 1991, p. 481
43. Polley M J, Nachman R L. Human complement in thrombin-mediated platelet function. Uptake of the C5b-C9 complex. J Exp. Med. 150, 633, 1979
44. Weidmer T, Esmon C T, Sims P J. Complement proteins C5b-9 stimulate procoagulant activity through platelet prothrombinase. Blood. 68, 875, 1986

45. Hamilton K K, Hattori R, Esmon C T, Sims P J. Complement proteins C5b-C9 induce vesiculation of the endothelial plasma membrane and expose catalytic surface for assembly of the prothrombinase enzyme complex. J. Biol. Chem. 265, 3809, 1990
46. Platt J L, Vercellotti G M, Lindman G J, et al. Release of heparan sulphate from endothelial cells. J. Exp. Med. 171, 1363, 1990
47. Jurd K M, Lee J, Cairns T, Hunt B J. Effect of Galα1,3Galβ1,4GlcNAc and complement depeletion on hemostatic activation in an in vitro model of the pig to human xenograft reaction. Transplant. Proc. (in press)
48. Robson S C, Siegel J B, Kopp C, et al. Mechanism of abnormal thromboregulation in xenograft rejection: loss of ecto-ADPase activity upon endothelial cell activation. Transplant. Proc. (in press)
49. Hunt B J, Duning J J, Segal H, et al. Pig-to-human xenograft reaction: is hemostatic activation dependent on the presence of anti-pig antibodies or complement? Transplant. Proc. 26, 1156, 1994
50. Makowka L, Cramer D V, Hoffman A, Sher L, Podesta L. Pig liver xenografts as a temporary bridge for human allografting. Xeno. 1, 17, 1993
51. Michler R E, Xu H, O'Hair D P, et al. Newborn discordant cardiac xenotransplantation: potential application to human. Transplant. Proc. (in press)
52. Pareti F I, Mazzucato M, Bottini E, Mannucci P M. Interaction of porcine von Willebrand factor with the platelet glycoproteins Ib and IIb/IIIa complex. Br. J. Haematol. 82, 81, 1992
53. Forbes C D, Prentice C R M. Aggregation of human platelets by purified porcine and bovine antihemophilic factor. Nature: New Biology. 241, 149, 1973
54. Kopp C W, Robson S C, Hancock W W, Bach F H, Geczy C. Porcine endothelial tissue factor pathway inhibitor antagonises human tissue factor but not factor Xa. Transplant. Proc. (in press)
55. Reverdiau-Moalic P, Watier H, Vallee I, et al. Comparative study of porcine and human blood coagulation systems: possible relevance in xenotransplantation. Transplant. Proc. (in press)
56. Janson T L, Stormorken H, Prydz H. Species specificity of tissue thromboplastin. Hemostasis. 14, 440, 1984
57. Jurd K M, Cairns T, Hunt B J. Activation of hemostasis in an in vitro model of the pig-to-human xenograft reaction. Transplant. Proc. 26,1159, 1994
58. Jurd K M, Gibbs R V, Hunt B J. Activation of human prothrombin by porcine aortic endothelial cells – a potential barrier to xenotransplantation. Blood Coagulation Fibrinol, 7, 336, 1996
59. Stone S R, Hofsteenge J. Kinetics of the inhibition of thrombin by hirudin. Biochemistry. 25, 4622, 1986
60. Hironaka T, Furukawa K, Esmon C T, et al. Structural study of the sugar chains of porcine factor VIII – tissue and species-specific glycosylation of factor VIII. Arch. Biochem. Biophys. 307, 316, 1993
61. Townsend R R J. Biol. Chem. 257, 9704, 1982
62. Thall A, Galili U. Distribution of Galα1,3Galβ1,4GlcNAc residues on secreted mammalian glycoproteins (thyroglobulin, fibrinogen, and immunoglobulin G) as measured by a sensitive solid-phase radioimmunoassay. Biochemistry. 29, 3959, 1990
63. Blanchard D, Thibaudeau K, Soulillou J P. Porcine antigenic targets for human natural antibodies. Xeno. 3, 68, 1995

12 Mechanism of Cellular Xenograft Rejection

R.D. Moses and H. Auchincloss, Jr.

Introduction

While less is known about xenogeneic cell-mediated immune responses in comparison with allogeneic responses, the gap in understanding is becoming smaller. Since earlier reviews of this topic just a few years ago [1, 2], many previously generated hypotheses have been confirmed and expanded, and new insights have come to light. However, recent data have caused us to seriously re-examine one important hypothesis, namely that the xenogeneic cellular immune response might be weaker and more easily controlled than the allogeneic response [2]. This hypothesis was based primarily on the observation from in vitro studies that the induction phase of the xenogeneic cellular response was weak in unprimed hosts [2]. Furthermore, the induction phase depended on $CD4^+$ helper T cells recognizing xenoantigens indirectly as peptides in association with self major histocompatibility complex (MHC) molecules, rather than directly as in alloantigen recognition [3]. While these in vitro observations generally still hold true, it is now known that these indirectly reactive helper T cells uniformly mediate brisk in vivo xenograft rejection, even in murine responders with impaired in vitro responses. How such indirectly xenoreactive helper T cells can mediate powerful in vivo responses remains a subject of intense speculation and study.

The purpose of the present chapter is to review current understanding of cellular immunity to xenoantigens. The material is organized as follows: (a) general considerations regarding xenogeneic cell-mediated immunity; (b) in vitro studies of the cellular, antigenic, and molecular requirements of the xenogeneic cellular response, and the question of direct versus associative (indirect) recognition of xenoantigens – matters that will be addressed separately for the helper and effector phases of the response; (c) observations on nonclassical (non-cytotoxic T cell-mediated) effector pathways; (d) in vivo studies of xenogeneic cell-mediated immunity; (e) mechanisms and control of cell-mediated xenograft rejection; (f) conclusions; and (g) speculation on future directions of inquiry.

Xenogeneic Celluar Immunity – General Considerations

Early in vivo studies showed that cell-mediated immunity has a role in xenograft as in allograft rejection [4, 5]. In vitro studies established that T cells have a central role in xenogeneic cellular immune responses [6, 7], and adhesion studies revealed that T cell adhesion to target cells showed species specificity [8], a process now known to be mediated by cell surface accessory molecules. These and other early observations set the stage for the current rapid proliferation in knowledge about xenogeneic cellular responses. Factors contributing to this expansion of knowledge include a better understanding of T cell and other mononuclear cell subsets involved in allogeneic responses, the availability of a wide array of monoclonal antibodies, the use of transfection and transgenic techniques, and the use of exon-shuffling techniques to create hybrid cell surface molecules. The results of these studies will be reviewed, first for the helper and then for the effector phase of the xenogeneic cellular response. Attention will be focused on the results of in vitro studies, from which most current knowledge of the cellular, antigenic, and molecular requirements of the xenogeneic cellular response has been obtained. The extent to which these results can (or cannot) be extrapolated to in vivo xenograft rejection will be discussed thereafter.

In Vitro Xenogeneic Cellular Immunity – Helper Phase

Strength of the Helper Response

A general question that arises is the overall strength of the xenogeneic response. For the helper phase of the response, studies have examined proliferation and interleukin (IL)-2 production in xenogeneic mixed leukocyte reaction (MLR) assays and have yielded conflicting results. Several studies found weak or no primary xenogeneic MLR for a range of responder species, including the human [9–11], sheep [12, 13], goat [12], guinea pig [13, 14], duck [13], goose [13], pigeon [13], rat [12, 13, 15–17], and mouse [3, 18, 19]. In contrast, others found the primary xenogeneic MLR to be equal in magnitude to [20–44] or even stronger than [45, 46] the allogeneic MLR. Many of the reports of intact primary responses were recent studies examining the human anti-pig MLR [33–42, 44, 46]. Several groups examined xenogeneic IL-2 production, again with conflicting results. Some investigators reported intact primary xenogeneic IL-2 production by human T cells in response to stimulation by mouse or pig cells [21, 34, 47]. In contrast, we found weak or no IL-2 production by naive mouse T cells in response to stimulation by monkey, pig, or human stimulator cells [3]. Another group reported diminished human anti-pig IL-2 production [48]. A small number of recent studies have examined xenogeneic helper responses quantitatively by limiting dilution analysis (LDA). Two studies reported responses at allogeneic levels, including human anti-pig [46] and human anti-mouse [49] responses. In contrast, one study of human anti-pig proliferative responses reported LDA precursor frequencies tenfold lower than those seen in allogeneic responses, although bulk MLR responses were nearly equivalent [48].

The decreased helper xenogeneic responses found in some studies cannot be attributed to an inhibitory effect of the xenogeneic cells in culture, since brisk secondary in vitro responses have been a uniform finding. How then can the discrepancy in results be explained? There are three likely (and not mutually exclusive) explanations. First, several of the reports of intact primary xenogeneic helper responses involved phylogenetically close species combinations, including human–chimpanzee [26], sheep–goat [12, 25], duck–chicken [13], and rat–mouse [27, 28, 30, 43]. In these cases, the close relationship may make the response more like an allogeneic reaction. Second, differences in xenogeneic responsiveness may exist among species. Many of the intact primary responses were reported for human responders [21, 22, 24–27, 32–42, 44, 46, 49]. Finally, some intact primary responses, including human anti-mouse [39, 47], human anti-pig [40], and mouse anti-human [20], were found to be dependent on the presence of responder antigen-presenting cells (APC), suggesting indirect recognition of the xenoantigens in association with responder MHC molecules. Why there should be a primary response to xenogeneic MHC peptides in association with self MHC molecules and one to similarly presented MHC alloantigens [50] but not one to processed nominal antigens is not known. One possibility is that the intact responses reflect prior sensitization by cross-reactive environmental antigens [15]. Whichever of these possibilities is most pertinent to a given xenogeneic situation, the bulk of evidence indicates that in vitro helper responses to xenoantigens are frequently weaker than responses to alloantigens in unprimed hosts. This is particularly true as the phylogenetic disparity between responder and stimulator increases. The intact primary human anti-pig helper response is an exception of potential clinical significance. Furthermore, in vivo studies, irrespective of in vitro results, consistently show brisk helper-mediated responses to xenografts (see below).

Cellular and Antigenic Requirements of the Helper Response

The induction phase of the xenogeneic cellular response has generally been found to be dependent on Lyt-1$^+$ or CD4$^+$ helper T cells [3, 18, 20, 21, 33, 35, 39, 41, 44, 47, 48, 51]. This has been the case for both human [21, 33, 35, 39, 41, 44, 47, 48] and mouse [3, 18, 20, 51] responses. This differs from the finding that both CD4$^+$ and CD8$^+$ cells can generate both in vitro [52] and in vivo [53] helper responses in MHC-disparate allogeneic combinations. Two recent reports of intact CD8$^+$ T cell proliferation in vitro, both involving human anti-pig responses [35, 46], are exceptional cases reminiscent of allogeneic-like responses. Unlike allogeneic responses, it would appear that the T_h2 subset of helper T cells is stimulated by xenoantigens preferentially over the T_h1 subset [54]. It has been suggested that this T_h2 predominance occurs early in the time course of the response [43], offering a possible explanation for the observation that xenogeneic proliferative responses generally peak later in vitro than do allogeneic responses. As in allogeneic responses, xenogeneic helper T cell responses require stimulation by APC [3, 18, 20, 32, 38, 41, 44, 47, 55, 56], a topic that will be discussed further in the section on direct versus associative recognition. Several recent reports reveal that vascular endothelial cells, serving as APC, can stimulate brisk proliferative responses of human lymphocytes to pig [33, 35, 40, 42, 46] and mouse [39] xenoantigens.

Xenogeneic class II MHC antigens have been found to be the principal target antigens recognized by xeno-specific helper T cells [18, 20, 21, 33, 35, 39, 41, 44,

46, 48, 49, 55]. One report [55] also described weak helper T cell responses to xenogeneic class I MHC and *Mls* antigens, and the two recent studies describing human CD8$^+$ responder T cells found the responses to be directed against class I xenoantigens based on antibody-blocking experiments [35, 46]. Human and rat helper T cell responses to mouse xenoantigens were found to be specific for the same polymorphic determinants of the mouse MHC (H-2) as recognized by mouse allogeneic helper T cells [9, 21, 30, 32, 55, 56]. Other responses, including mouse anti-monkey [3], mouse anti-human [18, 20], and human anti-dog [24], were found to be specific for monomorphic determinants of xenogeneic class II MHC molecules. In one study involving human anti-pig helper T cell clones, some clones were found to recognize polymorphic pig class II determinants, while others appeared to recognize monomorphic or possibly non-MHC determinants [44]. It is important to note, however, that the dominant role of class II MHC molecules as the target antigens of xenoreactive helper T cells does not imply direct recognition of those antigens in all cases. In fact, many of the responses appear to involve recognition of the MHC antigens after processing and presentation in association with self MHC molecules (see below). This raises the possibility that processed non-MHC xenoantigens are also recognized as target peptides by xenoreactive helper T cells in some cases.

In summary, the cellular and antigenic requirements of xenogeneic helper responses are characterized by a predominant role of CD4$^+$ helper T cells recognizing monomorphic or polymorphic determinants of xenogeneic class II MHC antigens presented by APC, similar in many respects to the requirements for allogeneic responses. Primary differences from allogeneic responses include the minimal role of the CD8$^+$ helper subset in most xenogeneic combinations, the preferential activation of T_h2 rather than T_h1 cells early in the time course, and the recognition, in some xenogeneic combinations, of monomorphic rather than polymorphic determinants of class II MHC molecules and perhaps of peptides of non-MHC molecules.

Cell Surface Molecule Requirements of the Helper Response

Proper T cell function is dependent on the appropriate interaction of several types of cell surface molecules present on the responder and target populations (see Table 1). Diminished helper T cell xenogeneic responses could then result from defective interaction of one or more of these cell surface molecules across species differences.

T Cell Receptor

One possible explanation for diminished helper T cell xenogeneic responses might be a defect in T cell receptor (TCR) recognition of xenoantigen. This could arise either through a genetic deficiency in the TCR repertoire for xenogeneic MHC molecules or to an acquired failure of generation of TCR's with affinity for xenoantigens during thymic education. Several recent studies of helper responses suggest that, at least for mouse anti-human responses, TCR recognition of xenoantigen is intact. This has been shown in two studies involving mice carrying a human class II transgene in which human MHC (HLA)-restricted helper responses [57, 58] and HLA-specific tolerance [58] were found to be intact. A contradictory result was found in a similar study in which mouse T cells did not proliferate in response to syngeneic stimulators expressing a transfected HLA class II antigen [59]. However, the latter result could equally be explained by a deficiency of CD4 interaction across species differences (see below).

In order to eliminate any confounding effects of CD4 interactions, two studies examined helper responses to exon-shuffled hybrid MHC class II molecules in which the CD4 ligand (the β2 domain of MHC class II) was syngeneic to the responder cell, whereas the TCR ligand (the α1/β1 domains) was xenogeneic. In both experiments, appropriate thymic deletion of autoreactive T cell clones and MHC-restricted nominal antigen-specific proliferative responses were found to be intact in mice carrying such exon-shuffled transgenic HLA class II molecules [60, 61]. Furthermore, human T cell proliferative responses to mouse H-2 antigens were restored by the expression of exon-shuffled hybrid MHC class II molecules in which the CD4 ligand region was of human origin and the TCR ligand region was of mouse origin [62]. In another line of study, mouse proliferative responses to HLA class II antigens expressed as transgenic products on mouse stimulator cells were restored, albeit partially, by the expression of transgenic human CD4 on the responder cells [63]. Taken together, these studies indicate that mouse and human helper T cells do acquire a TCR repertoire for xenogeneic MHC molecules during normal thymic education. Further support for this conclusion comes from the demonstration of a remarkable homology of the hypervariable regions of MHC molecules across species differences, even, in some instances, to a greater degree than that observed among alloantigens [64].

CD4

Another possible defect might occur in the interaction of the CD4 molecule of the T cell with its ligand, namely, the β2 domain of the xenogeneic MHC class II molecule. This interaction has been studied recently using several different model systems. In one line of investigation, the in vitro proliferative response of human lymphocytes to mouse [11] and pig [37, 44, 46] class II xenoantigens was blocked by anti-human CD4 monoclonal antibody, indicating that the human CD4 molecule can interact with mouse and pig MHC class II molecules. The ability of human CD4 to interact with mouse class II xenoantigens has also been shown in numerous studies in which the response of mouse T cells deficient in native CD4 to mouse class II antigens was enhanced by the presence of human CD4 molecules on the responder cells. The latter were added to the responders either through transfection [65, 66] or transgenic [58, 63, 67, 68] techniques. Enhanced responses were documented for IL-2 production [65, 66], proliferation [63, 67, 68], help for antibody production [58, 67, 68], and cytotoxic T cell (CTL) induction [58]. In addition, the presence of transgenic human CD4 molecules restored the development of mature CD4+ T cells in CD4-knockout mice [58, 67, 68]. In contrast, two studies found diminished proliferation of human $CD4^+$ responders to exon-shuffled hybrid class II molecules containing both human and mouse domains when the CD4 ligand portion of the MHC molecule was of mouse rather than human origin [62, 69]. However, the negative results in the latter two studies probably reflect a special defect in human CD4-mouse I-E interaction rather than a defect in interactions with mouse class II molecules generally [49].

In contrast to the intact human CD4-mouse class II interaction, most studies have shown a defect in the mouse CD4-human class II interaction. This defect has been shown in studies utilizing CD4 transfection [70], CD4 transgenic [63], and xenogeneic class II transgenic [71] techniques. Outcome parameters included cell adhesion [70], proliferation [63], and thymic T cell deletion [71], utilizing both human [70] and mouse [63, 71] responders. Similarly, two studies utilizing transfected exon-shuffled hybrid class II molecules containing both human and mouse domains [72, 73] and one study utilizing transfected hybrid CD4 molecules [74] showed diminished cell adhesion [72, 74], IL-2 production [72, 74], and proliferation [73] with mouse CD4 on the responder population and human class II on the target population. One study did show intact nominal antigen-specific HLA class II-restricted proliferation of mouse $CD4^+$ T cells to mouse stimulators expressing transgenic human class II molecules [75]. However, since the requirement for accessory molecules such as CD4 can be low or absent in instances of very high TCR affinity for xenoantigen, an occasional discrepant result might not be unexpected.

Thus, while a few discrepant results have been reported, the evidence overwhelmingly favors the conclusion that human CD4-mouse class II and human CD4-pig class II interactions are intact, and that a defect exists in mouse CD4-human class II interactions.

Accessory Molecules

A potential defect could also reside in the interaction of accessory cell surface molecules across species differences. Examples of such accessory molecule interactions include lymphocyte function-associated antigen (LFA)-1 with intercellular adhesion molecule (ICAM)-1 (or ICAM-2 or ICAM-3), CD2 with LFA-3, CD28 with B7-1 (or B7-2 or B7-3), and very late activation antigen (VLA)-4 with vascular cell adhesion molecule (VCAM)-1 (see Table 1). Experiments to test this possibility for helper responses have shown varying results. A study in which TCR triggering was achieved by crosslinking with an anti-CD3 monoclonal antibody showed that various mouse and primate APC could induce proliferation of purified human T cells [76]. This finding suggests intact accessory molecule (and lymphokine) interaction between human T cells and mouse and primate stimulator cells. Additionally, studies examining proliferative responses of human lymphocytes to mouse [11] and pig [35, 46] stimulators have demonstrated blocking of those responses by monoclonal antibodies directed against human LFA-1 [11, 35], CD2 [35], and CD28 [11, 46]. These results suggest intact interaction between human LFA-1 and CD28 and their mouse and pig ligands, and between human CD2 and its pig ligand. In similar studies, proliferative responses of mouse lymphocytes to human stimulators were blocked by monoclonal antibodies directed against human ICAM-1 [77, 78] and mouse LFA-1 [77], suggesting intact interaction of mouse LFA-1 with its human ligand. On the other hand, proliferation was not blocked by monoclonal antibodies directed against mouse CD2 or human LFA-3 [77], implying that the interaction of mouse CD2 with its human ligand is defective. Also, blocking studies have revealed a defect in interaction of human CD2 with its respective mouse ligand [79]. The latter result was also found in a study demonstrating enhancement of human anti-mouse proliferative responses by the transfection of human LFA-3 into the mouse stimulator cells [49]. However, in that same study, transfected human ICAM-1 also enhanced proliferation [49], suggesting defective human LFA-1 interaction with mouse ICAM-1 and contrasting with the previously mentioned finding of intact interaction of human LFA-1 with its mouse ligand [11]. We described experiments in which absent mouse proliferative responses to alloantigens expressed on transfected human APC were not reconstituted by exogenous mouse lymphokines, suggesting defective accessory molecule interactions between mouse responders and human stimulators [80].

Further information has been gained from monoclonal antibody blocking studies in cell adhesion assays, suggesting intact interaction of human LFA-1 with its mouse [81] and pig [82, 83] ligands and human VLA-4 with its pig ligand [82, 83]. In contrast, these same studies suggested defective interaction of mouse LFA-1 with its human ligand [81] and human CD2 with its pig ligand [83]. Finally, the demonstration that rat pancreatic islet graft survival was prolonged in mice by the in vivo administration of monoclonal antibodies directed against mouse CD2 suggests intact interaction of mouse CD2 with its rat ligand [84].

Thus, despite a few discrepancies among studies, one can conclude from these helper T cell and adhesion assays that human T cell accessory molecules generally do function well across species differences, whereas mouse T cell accessory molecules often do not, particularly as the phylogenetic disparity increases. Furthermore, LFA-1–ICAM-1 interactions seem to be largely preserved across species differences, whereas CD2–LFA-3 interactions are more frequently defective. Initial reports suggest intact interactions of human CD28 and VLA-4 with their respective ligands for certain stimulator species. Interestingly, initial results suggest that most of the above accessory molecule interactions (LFA-1, CD28, and VLA-4 with their respective ligands) are intact for the human anti-pig response. The human CD2 interaction with its pig ligand may be a case of defective interaction of potential clinical importance, in that the CD2 molecule serves not only an adhesion but also a signalling function for T cells. Further studies will be needed to define the interaction of adhesion molecules that bind multiple ligands, such as the CD28 interaction with B7–1, B7–2, and B7–3. This could have clinical implications, since the different ligand interactions can have different effects on T cells.

Lymphokines

Finally, defective lymphokine interaction across species differences could play a role in diminished helper T cell xenogeneic responses. Results of experiments to test this possibility have been conflicting. Two studies showed that highly purified, unprimed human T cells failed to proliferate in response to stimulation by mouse APC [32, 56]. The addition of either autologous human APC [32, 56] or exogenous human IL-1 [32, 56] or human IL-2 [32] to the culture reconstituted the proliferative response. At first glance, these results would seem to indicate a defect in the interaction of mouse IL-1 or IL-2 with human receptors. However, the possibility that the reconstitution of the proliferative responses resulted from incomplete responder APC depletion rather than correction of a lymphokine defect was not rigorously excluded in these studies. This alternative explanation is suggested by a similar study examining responder APC-depleted human anti-mouse T cell responses [47]. The latter study showed that xenoantigen was recognized indirectly as peptides on responder APC and that exogenous lymphokines failed to reconstitute the response. We have also been unable to restore primary mouse T cell-proliferative responses to monkey or human stimulators by exogenous recombinant mouse IL-1, IL-2, IL-4, or interferon (IFN)-γ [80]. This implies more than simply a lymphokine interaction defect underlying diminished xenogeneic proliferative responses. Furthermore, the study referred to earlier [76], in which T cell receptor triggering was achieved by crosslinking with an anti-CD3 monoclonal antibody, showed that various mouse and primate APC could induce proliferation of purified human T cells. This suggests intact lymphokine function across species barriers. On the other hand, one study showed that exogenous guinea pig but not mouse mitogen-stimulated supernatant in the MLR culture reconstituted primary guinea pig anti-mouse cell-mediated lympholysis (CML) activity [12], suggesting a xenogeneic lymphokine defect presumably at the induction phase in that species combination. Recent studies suggest defects in human granulocyte-macrophage colony-stimulating factor (GM-CSF) activity on murine APC [11] and in human IFN-γ activity on porcine endothelial cells [85].

Thus the data regarding lymphokine interactions across species differences for helper T cell xenorecognition are conflicting and incompletely studied. The bulk of evidence suggests that lymphokine interaction defects are probably not the principal factor underlying diminished in vitro helper xenogeneic responses.

Direct Versus Associative Recognition of Xenoantigens by Helper Cells

It is evident from the material reviewed thus far that the weak helper T cell xenogeneic responses observed in primary in vitro assays for certain xenogeneic combinations can result from any of several defects in molecular interactions between T cells and xenogeneic stimulator cells. Since such defects would be expected to interfere with direct T cell recognition of xenoantigens on xenogeneic APC, the question arises as to whether T cells preferentially recognize xenoantigens as processed peptides in association with self MHC molecules on host cells, in the manner of recognition of nominal antigens. The answer to this question has important implications regarding mechanisms of cell-mediated xenograft rejection.

Once again, discrepant results have been reported in the literature. Utilizing responder and/or stimulator APC-depleted cultures, we found that mouse anti-monkey helper T cell responses were strictly dependent on the presence of responder (mouse) APC and were blocked by anti-H-2 class II antibody [3]. Similar results have been found by others for mouse anti-human [18, 20] and human anti-mouse [39, 47] helper responses, both indirectly by blocking with anti-host MHC class II antibodies [18, 20, 39] and directly by APC depletion [47]. These findings have been demonstrated for both primary [20, 39, 47] and secondary [3, 18] in vitro helper responses, and for experimental protocols describing either intact [20, 39, 47] or absent [3, 18] primary responses. In the human anti-mouse helper T cell responses [47], chloroquine treatment of responder APC, which interferes with the processing of exogenous antigens, and paraformaldehyde treatment of stimulator cells, which prevents shedding of xenoantigens, each abrogated the generation of xenospecific CTL, presumably by blocking the response at the induction phase. Only one study, examining the response of human $CD4^+$ helper T cells to mouse stimulators transfected with exon-shuffled hybrid MHC class II molecules containing mouse variable regions and human constant regions, showed direct xenorecognition [49]. This was shown by the efficacy of anti-H-2 class II but not anti-HLA class II monoclonal antibody in blocking the proliferative response. The latter result notwithstanding, the bulk of evidence suggests that, for mouse–human interactions, helper T cells recognize disparate xenoantigens primarily after processing and presentation of those antigens in association with self class II MHC molecules on host APC rather than through direct recognition.

Contrasting with these results, one study examined the APC requirements of human helper T cell responses to a range of species less disparate than the mouse [47]. This study showed that human anti-pig proliferation could occur in the absence of human APC [47]. Furthermore, the generation of human CTL specific for the xenoantigens of a range of species, including the rhesus, pig, rabbit, and even rat, was found to be dependent on the presence of stimulator and not responder APC during the bulk MLR culture [47]. These results suggest that human helper T cells can recognize xenoantigens less disparate than the mouse directly on xenogeneic APC. This finding was corroborated by several subsequent studies of human anti-pig helper T cell responses, in which direct xenorecognition was shown by class II monoclonal antibody blocking studies [37, 41, 46] or by APC manipulations [38, 41]. A single conflicting study, examining human helper proliferative responses to porcine endothelial cells, suggested indirect recognition based on APC depletion and class II blocking techniques [40]. A recent study, involving similar experimental techniques, revealed that both pathways could be utilized in the recognition of pig antigens by human helper T cells, with direct recognition appearing to be the dominant pathway [44]. Thus the preponderant evidence favors primarily direct recognition by human helper T cells of xenoantigens from a range of stimulator species (including the pig) less disparate than the mouse.

In Vitro Xenogeneic Cellular Immunity – Effector Phase

Strength of the Effector Response

For the effector (cytotoxic) phase of the response, in vitro xenogeneic CML assays using both bulk cultures and LDA have been performed. Results from bulk assays have again been conflicting. Many studies reported diminished xenogeneic CML activity, either as an isolated finding [86–89] or in direct comparison with allogeneic responses [90–93]. This was observed for human [88, 90, 92], rat [86], and mouse [87–91, 93] responders. In contrast, a smaller number of studies reported human [21, 33, 47, 48, 94], guinea pig [12], rat [12, 95, 96], and mouse [12] xenogeneic CML responses to be at the level of allogeneic responses. Among the latter studies, the human anti-pig response has consistently been found to be intact by bulk CML assay [33, 47, 48, 94]. On the other hand, when examined quantitatively by LDA, the large majority of studies examining both human anti-pig [97, 98] and primary [99–101] and secondary [100, 102–105] mouse anti-human xenogeneic CML responses have shown lower precursor frequencies than those usually observed for allogeneic responses. A report of intact primary mouse anti-human CML examined by LDA represents an exceptional case [106]. Another exception is the report of human anti-pig CTL precursor frequencies measured by LDA to be five- to eightfold greater than those observed for allogeneic responses [48]. Thus, the preponderant evidence suggests that in vitro xenogeneic CML responses frequently are weaker than allogeneic responses. However, for the potentially clinically relevant human anti-pig response, bulk CML responses are intact, and quantitative responses as measured by LDA have been diminished in only some studies.

Cellular and Antigenic Requirements of the Effector Response

For the effector phase of the xenogeneic response, most studies of xenogeneic CML activity in vitro have shown a central role for T cells [6, 7, 34, 107, 108]. The majority of studies have shown that T cell-mediated cytotoxicity resides overwhelmingly in the $CD8^+$ subset [21, 47, 48, 94, 109–112]. This was observed for responses not only to xenogeneic class I MHC antigens [21, 110–112] but also to class II antigens [109–111]. The cytotoxic response against class II antigens was not blocked by anti-CD8 monoclonal antibody [109]. Recent reports of CD4+ mouse anti-rat CTL [51] and $CD4^+$ class II-specific human anti-pig CTL [44] represent exceptional cases. Interestingly, in the latter study, one of the class II-specific human anti-pig CTL clones was found to be $CD8^+$ [44]. The nearly exclusive role of the $CD8^+$ subset in studies of T cell-mediated xenogeneic cytotoxicity differs somewhat from the allogeneic situation in the mouse, where $CD4^+$ T lymphocytes can mediate cytotoxic responses to class II MHC alloantigens [50]. The likely role of potent non-classical effector mechanisms of xenograft rejection will be discussed below.

Several studies have examined the nature of the target antigens recognized by xeno-specific CTL. Responses have uniformly been found to be specific for MHC antigens [21, 86, 88, 107–111, 113, 114], similar to allogeneic responses. While some groups have found CML activity to be directed solely against class I MHC antigens [21, 86, 88, 107, 112–114], others have found the responses to be distributed between class I and class II antigens [108, 110, 111] or even exclusively against class II antigens [44, 109]. An unusually high incidence of MHC class II-specific CTL might be explained by poor CD8 molecule function across species differences (see below). This would result in a failure to channel CTL toward recognition of xenogeneic class I antigens. Although a few studies have reported mouse CTL to be specific for monomorphic determinants of both class I and II MHC xenoantigens [88, 91, 100, 110], the majority of studies have found xenogeneic responses to be directed predominantly or exclusively against the polymorphic regions of those antigens [12, 21, 56, 86, 88, 94–96, 106, 107, 110–116]. The fine specificity of several human anti-mouse CTL lines has been mapped to the identical polymorphic determinants of mouse class I molecules recognized by allospecific CTL [116].

In summary, many of the cellular and antigenic requirements of the effector phase of in vitro xenogeneic responses are similar to those of allogeneic responses. Some differences include the nearly exclusive use of the $CD8^+$ subset for CTL-mediated xenogeneic responses, the tendency toward CTL recognition of class II as well as class I MHC xenoantigens, and the recognition, in some cases, of monomorphic rather than polymorphic determinants of MHC xenoantigens. Finally, a difference of potential importance is the likelihood of nonclassical effector pathways for xenoantigens (see below).

Cell Surface Molecule Requirements of the Effector Response

CTL activity depends on the appropriate interaction of several types of cell surface molecules present on the effector and target populations (Table 1). Diminished xenogeneic cytotoxicity could then result from defective interaction of these cell surface molecules across species differences, as discussed for helper responses.

T Cell Receptor

As for helper xenogeneic responses, diminished xenogeneic cytotoxicity might result from a defect in TCR recognition of xenoantigen. This could arise either through a genetic deficiency in the TCR repertoire for xenogeneic MHC molecules or to an acquired failure of generation of TCR's with affinity for xenoantigens during thymic education. To examine these possibilities, one approach has been to measure xenogeneic CML responses of transgenic mice expressing an HLA class I antigen in the thymus. If the diminished TCR xenorepertoire were an acquired phenomenon, the presence of a xenogeneic MHC molecule during thymic education might correct this defect. CTL from such mice were found to recognize viral antigens in association with the HLA molecule in a restricted fashion [117] and not to lyse MHC-identical mouse cells transfected with the HLA molecule encoded by the transgene [118]. These results point to a role for

Table 1. Examples of cell surface molecule interactions that may be involved in T cell–xenogeneic cell interactions

Type of interaction	Responder cell surface molecule	Xenogeneic cell surface molecule
Antigen recognition	T cell receptor	MHC molecule α1/α2 (cl I) or α1/β1 (cl II) domains
Accessory molecule	CD4	Monomorphic class II MHC β2 domain
	CD8	Monomorphic class I MHC α3 domain
	LFA-1 (CD11a/CD18)	ICAM-1 (CD54), ICAM-2 (CD102), or ICAM-3 (CD50)
	CD2	LFA-3 (CD58)
	CD28 or CTLA-4	B7–1 (CD80), B7–2 (CD86), or B7–3
	VLA-4 (CD49d)	VCAM-1 (CD106)
Lymphokine	IL-1 receptor	IL-1
	TNF-α	TNF receptor
	IFN-γ	IFN receptor

LFA, lymphocyte function-associated antigen; VLA, very late activation antigen; IL, interleukin; TNF, tumor necrosis factor; IFN, interferon; MHC, major histocompatibility complex; ICAM, intercellular adhesion molecule; VCAM, vascular cell adhesion molecule.

the xenogeneic MHC molecule in positive and negative selection, respectively. However, the HLA-restricted viral responses were much weaker than those restricted by native H-2 molecules [93], and CML responses against human xenoantigens were no greater in the transgenic mice than in nontransgenic mice in most [99, 103, 105] but not all [119] studies. The latter findings imply that the presence of a xenogeneic MHC molecule in the thymus only weakly influences the TCR repertoire for xenoantigens. These results could be interpreted as showing a defect in TCR-xenogeneic MHC molecule interaction. However, in view of the important role of the CD8 molecule in the thymic selection of class I-restricted T cells [120–122], these results could equally be explained by a defect in CD8-xenogeneic MHC molecule interaction during thymic selection.

In order to eliminate any confounding effects of CD8 interactions across species differences, transgenic mice were generated that expressed exon-shuffled hybrid class I molecules containing human domains in the TCR ligand region (α1 and α2 domains) and a mouse domain in the CD8 ligand region (α3 domain). Such mice were found to mount appropriate HLA-restricted nominal antigen [123] and HLA-allogeneic [124] cytotoxic responses. Thus, there does not appear to be a genetic deficiency in the mouse CTL repertoire for xenogeneic MHC molecules. In another approach, transgenic mice expressing the human CD8 molecule were tested for anti-human CML responses [125]. Cytotoxic responses against HLA class I antigens, as measured both by bulk CML assay and LDA, were restored to levels seen against H-2 alloantigens by the presence of the human CD8 transgene [125]. Furthermore, HLA class I-restricted nominal antigen responses were restored in animals also expressing a transgenic HLA class I antigen, which would then be available for T cell education in the thymus [125]. Also, mouse anti-human xenogeneic cytotoxic responses were restored when the targets cells were transfected with exon-shuffled hybrid MHC molecules containing a mouse domain in the CD8 ligand region [87, 126]. Taken together, these results strongly suggest that mouse CTL do acquire a TCR repertoire for xenogeneic MHC molecules during normal thymic education.

CD8

Transfection and transgenic models have been used to examine the possibility of a defect in TCR/CD8 interactions with xenogeneic MHC molecules by CTL. In one type of experiment, mouse CTL primed against a human or pig class I MHC xenoantigen were tested in vitro for killing of mouse cells expressing the specific xenoantigen either by transfection or transgenic techniques. Since the targets were of mouse origin, accessory molecule and lymphokine interactions would be expected to be intact. Any deficiency in cytotoxicity should then only result from deficiencies of TCR and/or CD8 interactions with the xenoantigens. Although some such studies reported relatively intact killing [106, 127, 128], the large majority of studies [89, 99–101, 104, 105, 129–131] reported weak CML activity. Given the demonstration that TCR interactions with xenoantigens are probably intact (see above), the likely explanation for these results is a defect in mouse CD8 interaction with human or pig class I MHC molecules.

In order explicitly to distinguish between TCR and CD8 defects, cytotoxic responses to exon-shuffled hybrid MHC molecules containing mouse $\alpha1$ and $\alpha2$ domains and a human $\alpha3$ domain, or human $\alpha1$ and $\alpha2$ domains and a mouse $\alpha3$ domain, have been investigated. While one such study found that the precursor frequency of mouse CTL specific for an HLA class I xenoantigen transfected onto a mouse target cell was not enhanced by the presence of a human $\alpha3$ domain [102], three other studies have demonstrated that the primary defect resided in the CD8-xenogeneic $\alpha3$ domain interaction [87, 126, 132]. Among the latter investigations, one study [132] showed that alloprimed human and mouse CML responses against targets transfected with the appropriate allogeneic MHC molecules were diminished by the presence of a xenogeneic $\alpha3$ domain (mouse and human, respectively) in the transfected molecules. A second study [87] showed that xenoprimed mouse anti-human CML responses against targets transfected with the appropriate xenogeneic MHC molecule were enhanced by the presence of a mouse $\alpha3$ domain in the transfected molecule. Finally, both the latter [87] and a third study [126] showed that the induction of mouse allogeneic [126] and anti-human xenogeneic [87, 126] CML responses depended on the presence of a mouse rather than a xenogeneic (human) $\alpha3$ domain in the transfected stimulating antigens. The latter observations were made for both in vivo [126] and in vitro [87] stimulations. Another group of investigators reported diminished mouse CML responses to a transfected MHC alloantigen when expressing a human rather than a mouse α3 domain [133], although they attributed this to an alteration in the configuration of the α1 and α2 domains by the xenogeneic α3 domain rather than to a defect in CD8-xenogeneic α3 domain interaction.

Further support for defects in CD8 interactions across species differences come from studies involving transgenic mice alluded to earlier [123, 124]. In one study, HLA-transgenic mouse T cells educated to mount HLA class I-restricted nominal antigen-specific CML responses were found to lyse targets more efficiently when the targets expressed exon-shuffled hybrid MHC class I antigens containing a mouse rather than a human domain in the CD8 ligand region [123]. In another study, HLA-transgenic mouse T cells were found to mount stronger anti-HLA class I-specific "allogeneic" cytotoxic responses when the HLA transgene contained a mouse domain in the CD8 ligand region [124]. The latter finding presumably reflects more effective thymic education to the HLA molecule in the thymus after correction of the defect in CD8 interaction across species differences.

Taken together, the evidence strongly suggests a defect in CD8 interactions for mouse anti-human, mouse anti-pig, and human anti-mouse CTL responses. Interestingly, although examined in proliferative rather than cytotoxic assays, human $CD8^+$ T cells have been shown to mount a proliferative response to pig endothelial cells [35, 46], and this response is blocked by anti-CD8 monoclonal antibodies [46]. This suggest that the CD8 interaction for the human anti-pig combination is intact.

Accessory Molecules

A series of experiments has addressed the question of a defect in accessory molecule interactions by examining the ability of HLA class I-specific alloreactive CTL to lyse mouse tumor cell targets transfected with the target HLA class I molecule. Several studies using transfected mouse L cell and other mouse targets showed a failure of target lysis whether or not human β_2-microglobulin was supplied either exogenously or by cotransfection [92, 134–138]. These results were initially attributed to a defect in accessory molecule interaction across species differences or possibly to a defect in expression of appropriate human self peptides in association with the transfected HLA class I molecules [138]. However, these interpretations were questioned following the demonstration that mouse L cells generally do not express ICAM-1 [139]. It was subsequently shown that ICAM-1-expressing mouse P815 tumor cells [88, 140–142] and an unusual ICAM-1-expressing mouse L cell variant [143] were lysed well when transfected with the appropriate xenogeneic class I MHC molecules. The latter results implied that human LFA-1 could indeed interact with mouse ICAM-1. This conclusion was further supported by the observations that human anti-mouse [88, 140], human anti-monkey [92], and mouse anti-human [109] CML responses were blocked by anti-responder LFA-1 antibody. A recent report showed that human $CD16^+$ natural killer (NK) cell binding to rat endothelial cells was blocked by anti-human LFA-1 antibody, suggesting intact LFA-1 function for that species combination. On the other hand, a second major accessory molecule pathway, namely, CD2 on the T cell interacting with LFA-3 on the target cell, has been shown not to function in the human anti-mouse combination [92, 140, 143, 144], although it does function in human anti-monkey [92] and mouse anti-rat [84] responses.

These observations from investigations of effector responses corroborate the conclusions derived from studies of helper responses. Thus human T cell accessory molecule interactions across species differences are more preserved than those of murine T cells, and LFA-1 interactions across species differences are generally intact. Effector studies suggest that CD2 does function when species differences are small (human–monkey and mouse–rat) but not when they are disparate (human–mouse).

Direct Versus Associative Recognition of Xenoantigens by Effector Cells

Analogous to the situation for helper T cells, given the likely presence of one or more defects in cell surface molecule interactions across species differences, the question arises: Do CTL preferentially recognize xenoantigens as processed peptides in association with self MHC molecules on host cells, or do they recognize those antigens directly on xenogeneic target cells? The answer to this question also has important implications regarding mechanisms of cell-mediated xenograft rejection.

Virtually every study of the effector phase of the response has shown some ability of CTL to lyse xenogeneic targets and therefore to recognize xenoantigens directly. However, as described earlier, features of this interaction are unusual, including the nearly exclusive use of the $CD8^+$ CTL subset even for recognition of class II MHC xenoantigens, the defective function of the CD8 accessory molecule for many species combinations, and the relatively even distribution of responses directed against class I and class II MHC xenoantigens. This can be explained partly by the general observation that accessory molecule requirements across species differences decrease following CTL activation. These observations also suggest that the xeno-reactive T cells measured in these assays might represent relatively rare CTL clones that do not require CD8 molecule function because of very high TCR affinity for xenoantigens. This raises the possibility that xenogeneic CTL may more frequently recognize xenoantigens in association with self MHC molecules. In order to study this question, a series of experiments was performed utilizing mouse T cells primed against human or pig xenoantigens. CML responses of the mouse T cells against xenogeneic (or allogeneic) targets were compared to responses against H-2-identical mouse targets expressing the appropriate xenogeneic class I antigen by transfection or transgenic techniques [89, 99–101, 103, 104, 106, 128–130, 145]. The latter targets would present xenoantigens not only in native form but also as peptides in association with host (mouse) MHC molecules. While some studies [89, 101, 106, 128] favored direct over associative recognition of xenoantigens, a larger number of studies [99, 100, 103, 104, 129, 130, 145] demonstrated predominantly or exclusively associative recognition. The evidence for associative recognition included significantly greater lysis of transfected mouse targets than xenogeneic targets [99, 100, 129, 130, 145], blocking of the lysis of transfected targets by anti-host H-2 antibodies [99, 100, 103, 129, 145], and lysis of transfected mouse targets coexpressing self but not allogeneic H-2 molecules [100, 103, 104, 129]. The identification of the specific oligopeptides of the xenogeneic class I MHC antigens recognized in association with self MHC molecules by the xenoreactive CTL [104, 146] provided further confirmation of the existence of an associative recognition pathway. Thus the evidence is mixed regarding direct versus associative recognition of xenoantigens by CTL but does show a substantial role for associative recognition of xenoantigens by CTL.

Nonclassical (Non-Cytotoxic T Lymphocyte-Mediated) Effector Pathways

The possibility of a non-T cell-mediated effector mechanism of xenograft rejection, involving either NK cells, macrophages, or antibody-dependent cell-mediated cytotoxicity (ADCC) was raised in some early studies [7, 147–151]. A few years ago, our colleagues characterized a population of helper-dependent Thy-1$^+$ CD4$^-$ CD8$^-$ NK1.1$^+$ NK-like effector cells with potent xenogeneic cytotoxic activity in bulk mouse anti-rat MLR cultures (D. Doody and H.J. Winn, personal communication). These NK-like cells were not generated in allogeneic cultures and did not lyse allogeneic targets. Thus they may constitute a non-T cell cytotoxic effector population unique to xenogeneic responses. Another group described a population of CD4$^-$ CD8$^-$ MHC-nonspecific γ/δ T cells cytotoxic for rat targets in a mouse anti-rat CML assay [112]. We consistently observed a population of non-T cell, HLA-nonspecific, NK-like effectors with potent cytotoxicity in bulk rhesus peripheral blood lymphocyte anti-human B lymphoblastoid cell line CML assays (R.D. Moses and R.E. Gress, unpublished observations).

More recently, a number of studies have suggested the capacity of human NK cells to mediate xenograft damage in vitro. Several studies described the generation of potent NK lytic activity in human anti-pig MLR cultures [33, 34, 37, 152, 153]. Enhancement of target lysis by exogenous IL-2 suggested lymphokine-activated killer (LAK) activity in the effector population [152]. NK cell effectors seem to be preferentially generated over classical CTL when vascular endothelial cells are the stimulator population [153]. An ADCC mechanism of target lysis has also been demonstrated in human anti-pig cultures against mononuclear cell [152] and endothelial cell [154] targets. The effectors in the latter study were characterized as CD16$^+$ NK cells [154]. Human NK cells mediating lytic damage have also been demonstrated in an ex vivo study of rat hearts perfused with human lymphocytes [155] and in a study of adherence of human lymphocytes to rat and bovine endothelial cells [156].

While the results of in vitro studies strongly suggest an ability of nonclassical effector cells to mediate xenograft damage, the data supporting a role for nonclassical effector mechanisms of xenograft rejection in vivo has, at least thus far, been more limited. Some studies have suggested a role for NK cells [157–159], ADCC [158], macrophages [160], or unconventional Thy-1$^-$ sIg$^-$ lymphoid cells [161] in murine models of skin [157], heart [157–159, 161], and pancreatic islet [160] xenograft rejection. Interestingly, a pure delayed-type hypersensitivity mechanism was found not to play a role in a murine model of islet xenograft rejection [162]. These in vivo studies will be discussed further in the next section.

Thus numerous studies suggest the ability of NK cells and possibly macrophages, ADCC effectors, γ/δ T cells, and/or other unconventional lymphoid cells to mediate potent in vitro cytotoxic responses against xenogeneic targets. Of potential importance, NK cells have been shown to mediate brisk cytotoxic responses in human anti-pig assays. The extent to which these effector populations play a role in xenograft rejection in vivo remains incompletely studied.

In Vivo Studies of Xenogeneic Cellular Immunity

While in vitro studies can provide qualitative and quantitative information on the cellular, antigenic, and molecular aspects of the cell-mediated xenogeneic response, in vivo models have the capacity to reveal the biologically relevant mechanisms operational in xenograft rejection. With antibody blocking or depletion techniques and various genetic manipulations of the donor or host, in vivo studies can also provide information at the cellular and molecular level as well.

In a series of experiments involving skin and heart xenograft rejection in mice with varying combinations of genetically deficient T, B, and NK/K cell function, indefinite survival was consistently found whenever a T cell deficiency was present [157]. These studies point to a central role for T cells in this murine model of xenograft rejection. We showed that the CD4+ T cell subset, in particular, is of central importance in xenograft rejection. This was based on the demonstration that CD4-specific, but not CD8-specific immunosuppression in vivo significantly prolonged both xenogeneic [163] and pig class I-transgenic syngeneic [164] but not whole MHC-disparate allogeneic skin graft survival in the mouse. The central role of $CD4^+$ T cells in xenograft rejection was further demonstrated by the ability of $CD4^+$ T cells adoptively transferred into severe combined immunodeficiency (SCID) SCID mice to mediate xenogeneic skin graft rejection following in vivo depletion and/or blocking of $CD8^+$ T cells, B cells, and NK cells [165]. This and other observations in murine models of pancreatic islet [166–173], heart [161, 172, 174, 175], and skin [172] xenograft rejection point to a central role for $CD4^+$ T cells in the mediation of xenograft rejection in murine hosts.

While $CD4^+$ T cells clearly play the dominant role in mediating xenograft rejection, $CD8^+$ T cells have been shown to have an ancillary role. In studies alluded to earlier, we demonstrated greater prolongation of xenogeneic skin graft survival in the mouse with in vivo depletion of both $CD4^+$ and $CD8^+$ cells in comparison with depletion of $CD4^+$ cells alone [163]. Furthermore, studies have demonstrated the ability of a mouse anti-rat CTL line [176] and a human anti-mouse CTL clone [177] to mediate xenospecific pancreatic islet rejection and dermal tissue injury, respectively, when adoptively transferred to the appropriate xenogeneic host. At least one study has shown the ability of adoptively transferred primed $CD8^+$ T cells to induce rat skin xenograft rejection in T cell-deficient mice [178].

With respect to nonclassical effector pathways, one study alluded to earlier utilizing mice genetically deficient in the function of various lymphocyte subsets suggested an ancillary role for NK/K cells in xenograft rejection [157]. A role for NK cells has also been suggested by the demonstration of prolonged survival of hamster hearts in either NK-deficient rats [159] or T cell-deficient rats treated with anti-NK cell antibody [158]. An additional role for ADCC was suggested in the latter study by the efficacy of primed serum to induce prompt heart graft rejection in complement-deficient rats [158]. The intriguing finding that macrophages were the predominant cell type infiltrating rejected pig islet grafts in rats, whereas T cells predominated in rejected allografts, raises the possibility that macrophages are a principal effector in some forms of xenograft rejection [160]. Finally, a study alluded to earlier showed that pig or rat pancreatic islet cells, transplanted as mixed cell suspensions along with syngeneic islets, were selectively rejected, whereas the syngeneic islets were spared (despite an intense surrounding infiltrate) [162]. This finding argues against a pure delayed-type hypersensitivity mechanism of rejection, i.e., one involving nonselective graft destruction mediated by soluble factors alone. The extent to which the latter result, involving xenogeneic pancreatic islet rejection, can be extrapolated to the rejection of solid organ xenografts remains to be determined.

Mechanisms and Control of Cell-Mediated Xenograft Rejection

In nearly all the above studies, utilizing models in which the humoral rejection process played a minor or no role, cell-mediated xenograft rejection was uniformly brisk. $CD4^+$ T cells, in particular, appear to mount powerful rejection responses to xenografts in vivo [179]. Furthermore, only a paucity of studies, utilizing immunosuppressive strategies directed against cell-mediated responses, have shown prolonged xenograft survival in direct comparison with allograft survival [163, 164, 180]. How then does one reconcile the difference between the generally weak helper and effector responses to xenoantigens observed in vitro and the strong cell-mediated responses seen in vivo? Given our current level of knowledge, one can only speculate as to the underlying causes, although it is likely that several mechanisms contribute to the vigorous responses observed in vivo.

In order to conceptualize better the possible rejection mechanisms involved, two separate schemes of cell-mediated xenograft rejection have been considered. One scheme is based on the so-called three-cell model of CTL activation [181]. According to the three-cell model, the activation of CTL by helper T cells requires intimate physical contact between the two types of T cells bound to the same APC. One can then envision four potential mechanisms of rejection, depending on the utilization of direct versus indirect recognition of xenoantigen at both the helper and effector phases of the response (Fig. 1).

In mechanism A, both helper T cells and CTL are postulated to recognize xenoantigens directly on xenogeneic cells. In this case, a classical allograft-like CTL-mediated mechanism of rejection would be expected. Based on the data reviewed earlier, this mechanism would be expected for phylogenetically close host–donor species combinations and for the human anti-pig response, two situations in which direct xenorecognition has been demonstrated in vitro.

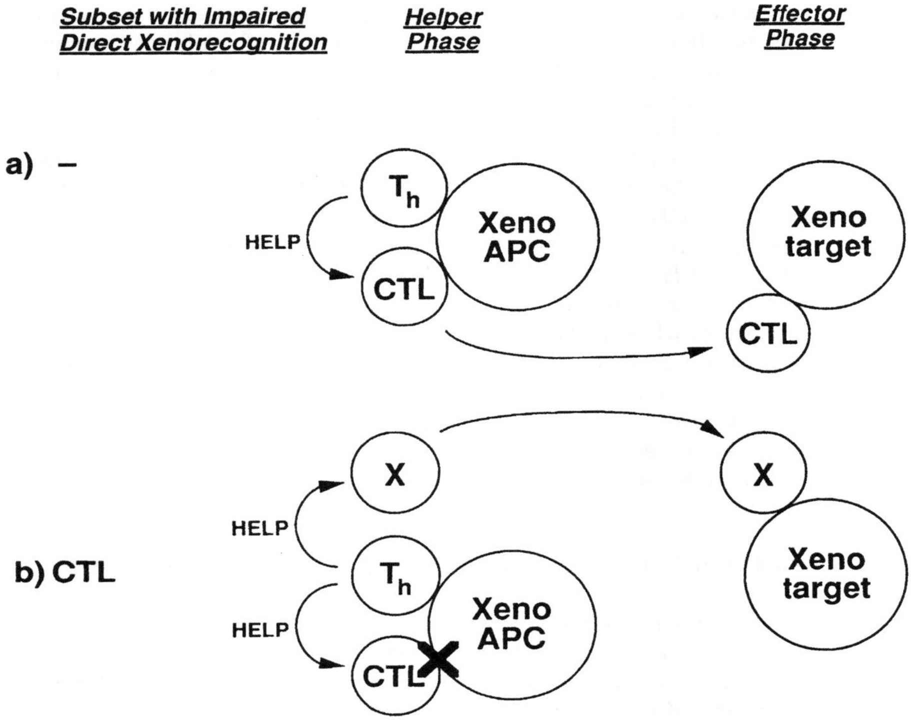

In mechanism B, direct xenorecognition is postulated to be intact for helper T cells but not for CTL. In this case, one could envision the activation of a nonclassical effector pathway mediated by any of the MHC antigen-nonspecific effectors discussed earlier, such as NK cells, macrophages, ADCC effectors, or atypical lymphoid cells (designated "X" in Fig. 1). The recent demonstrations that such xenoreactive effectors exist, that they are potent in vitro, and that they may be preferentially activated when direct CTL xenorecognition is impaired [34] suggest that this rejection mechanism may play a role in vivo. The exact effectors involved, the mechanisms of effector activation, and the xenoantigens recognized remain to be elucidated.

In mechanism C, direct xenorecognition is postulated to be intact for CTL but not for helper T cells. In this nonclassical scenario, indirectly reactive helper T cells, responding to xenoantigens after processing and presentation as peptides in association with self MHC molecules on host APC, would activate directly reactive CTL. If such activation of classical CTL by indirectly reactive helper T cells is eventually shown to occur in xenograft rejection, as appears to be the case for allograft rejection [182], it could help to explain (along with mechanism D below) the discrepancy between weak primary helper T cell xenoresponses in vitro and brisk rejection responses in vivo.

Finally, in mechanism D, neither helper T cells nor CTL can recognize xenoantigens directly. In this case, as in mechanism C, helper T cells would respond to

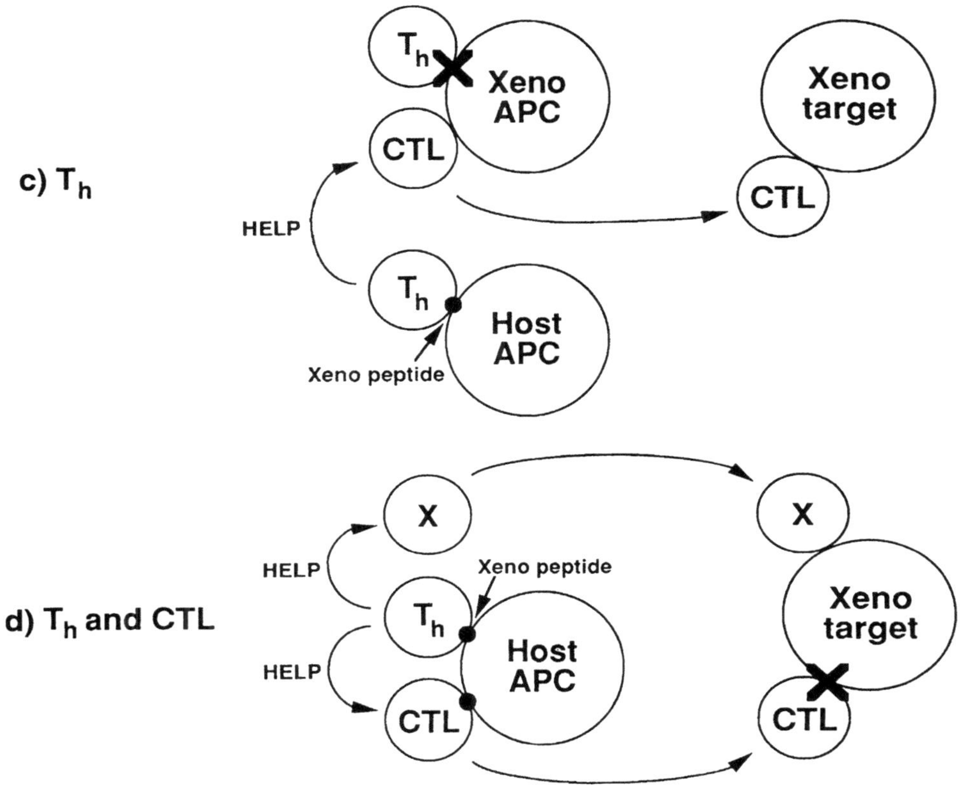

Fig. 1A–D. Implications of impaired direct recognition of xenoantigens on mechanisms of xenograft rejection in the context of the three-cell model of cytotoxic T cell (*CTL*) activation [181]. **A** If both helper T cells (T_h) and CTL can recognize xenoantigens directly on xenogeneic cells, then T_h will activate CTL specific for the antigens expressed on the somatic cells of the xenograft, and the graft will be rejected by a classical CTL-mediated mechanism. **B** If T_h but not CTL are able to recognize xenoantigens directly on xenogeneic cells, then it is postulated that T_h will induce population X of antigen-nonspecific cytotoxic effector cells, e.g., natural killer (NK) cells or macrophages, to mediate graft rejection by a nonclassical CTL-independent mechanism. **C** If CTL but not T_h are able to recognize xenoantigens directly on xenogeneic cells, then it is possible (albeit contrary to conventional theory) that T_h, responding to xenogeneic peptides on host antigen-presenting cells (*APC*), might induce graft rejection by a quasi-classical CTL-mediated mechanism. **D** If neither T_h nor CTL can recognize xenoantigens directly, then it is postulated that T_h, responding to xenogeneic peptides on host APC, will induce population X of antigen-nonspecific cytotoxic effector cells to mediate graft rejection by a nonclassical CTL-independent mechanism

xenogeneic peptides presented on host APC. As in mechanism B, such helper T cells might then induce nonclassical effectors to mediate xenograft destruction in an MHC-nonspecific fashion. This pathway would not be hindered by a defect in direct xenorecognition by helper T cells and could explain (along with mechanism C) the brisk responses seen in vivo despite the weak primary helper responses often observed in vitro. It should be noted that these four hypothetical mechanisms would not necessarily be mutually exclusive, given the nonhomogeneous populations of cells mediating immune responses in a given host.

An alternative scheme of cell-mediated xenograft rejection focuses on the scenario described in Fig. 1C (directly xenoreactive CTL, indirectly xenoreactive helper T cells) and is based on the so-called four-cell model of CTL activation [182]. According to the four-cell model, it is postulated that both B cells and CTL recognize xenogeneic class I MHC molecules directly on xenogeneic APC. It is further postulated that helper T cells recognize xenogeneic peptides in association with self class II MHC molecules expressed on host B cells, the latter serving as APC. A four-cell cluster would then form in which indirectly xenoreactive helper T cells could induce graft rejection by a classical CTL-mediated mechanism (Fig. 2). This scheme of xenograft rejection is consistent with the evidence from many in vitro studies, which show that helper T cells frequently recognize xenoantigens indirectly whereas CTL commonly use the direct pathway of xenorecognition. Furthermore, the four-cell model has some theoretical appeal over the analogous three-cell model (mechanism C above) in that the former entails an intimate approximation of helper T cells and CTL.

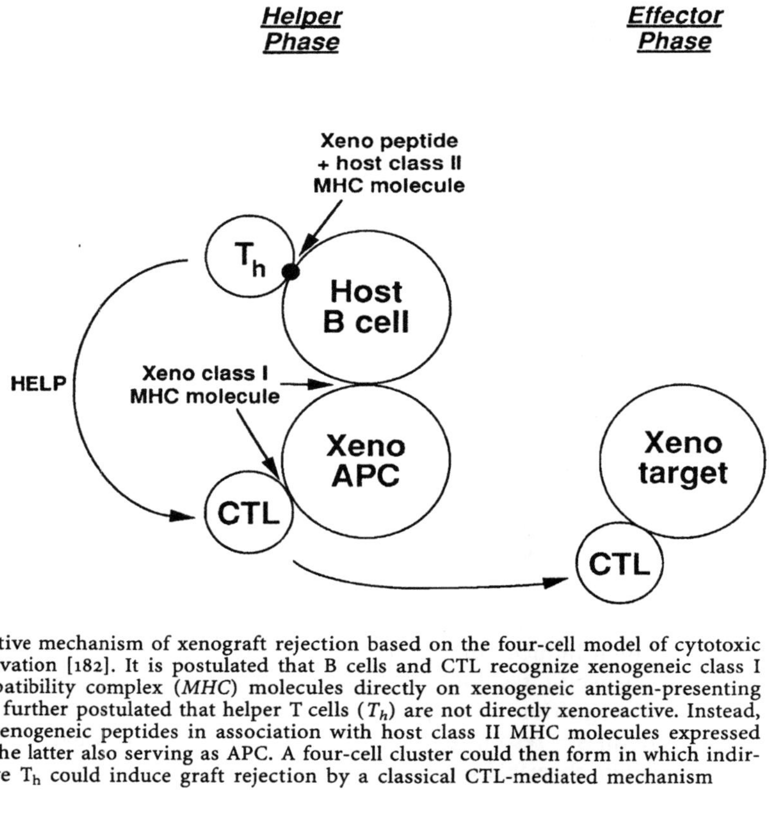

Fig. 2. An alternative mechanism of xenograft rejection based on the four-cell model of cytotoxic T cell (*CTL*) activation [182]. It is postulated that B cells and CTL recognize xenogeneic class I major histocompatibility complex (*MHC*) molecules directly on xenogeneic antigen-presenting cells (*APC*). It is further postulated that helper T cells (T_h) are not directly xenoreactive. Instead, they recognize xenogeneic peptides in association with host class II MHC molecules expressed on host B cells, the latter also serving as APC. A four-cell cluster could then form in which indirectly xenoreactive T_h could induce graft rejection by a classical CTL-mediated mechanism

Thus, several not mutually exclusive pathways of xenograft rejection can be postulated, supported by recently acquired knowledge of nonclassical effector mechanisms and the characterization of species combinations with intact direct xenorecognition. Which mechanism or mechanisms are operational in a given xenografting situation remain to be elucidated.

Based on these observations, we continue to support the notion that cell-mediated xenograft rejection is highly dependent on the helper phase of the response and thus susceptible to modification by immunosuppression directed against $CD4^+$ helper T cells. However, in light of newly acquired knowledge of effector mechanisms, cellular xenograft rejection, once activated, would be expected to be stronger than allograft rejection. Furthermore, our current knowledge of human anti-pig responses suggests that any of the effector mechanisms discussed above could potentially contribute to xenograft destruction. Thus, cellular xenograft rejection in the clinical setting would be expected to be, if anything, more difficult to control than allograft rejection.

Comment

Current knowledge of xenogeneic cell-mediated immune responses can be summarized as follows:

1. Helper T cell and CTL responses to xenoantigens are often weaker in vitro than to alloantigens. This results from diminished frequencies of xenoreactive helper T cell and CTL precursors in unprimed hosts and is manifested by decreased or undetectable responses in primary in vitro MLR, IL-2 production, and CML assays. These responses are particularly weak for phylogenetically disparate responder-stimulator combinations and for murine responders. In vitro human responses to xenoantigens, on the other hand, are either intact or only mildly diminished for most stimulator species, notably including the pig.
2. Helper xenogeneic responses are mediated almost exclusively by $CD4^+$ T cells recognizing monomorphic or polymorphic determinants of MHC class II molecules. Preliminary evidence suggests a preferential activation of the T_h2 subset early in the time course of the response. Vascular endothelial cells appear to be a particularly potent APC stimulating the xenogeneic helper response.
3. CTL-mediated xenogeneic responses are mediated almost exclusively by $CD8^+$ T cells recognizing monomorphic or polymorphic determinants of MHC class I and, suprisingly, class II molecules. The even distribution of class I- and class II-specific CTL probably reflects a deficiency of CD8 interaction across species differences with a resultant lack of channeling of CTL solely to class I-positive targets.
4. In vitro studies have demonstrated potent non-classical effector pathways of xenogeneic cellular immunity mediated by NK cells, macrophages, ADCC, and/or atypical lymphoid cells. Preliminary evidence suggests a potential role for such effectors in xenograft rejection in vivo, although qualitative and quantitative aspects of this response remain poorly understood. Interestingly, a strong human NK cell-mediated response to pig xenoantigens has been

demonstrated in vitro, particularly when tested against vascular endothelial cell targets.

5. The weakness of xenogeneic T cell responses observed in vitro results from defects in molecular interactions at the cell surface between T cells and xenogeneic cells. The number and severity of defective interactions (see Table 1) increase as the phylogenetic disparity increases and correlate with the degree of deficiency of helper T cell and CTL-mediated responses in vitro. Although the available information is incomplete, there is clear evidence for defective CD2, CD4, and CD8 interactions across disparate species differences and for murine responders. There are probably additional, albeit less well characterized, defects in lymphokine interactions. There is little evidence for a major defect in LFA-1 function across species differences or in the TCR repertoire for xenoantigens at either the genetic or the acquired level. Interestingly, cell surface molecule interactions appear to be largely intact for the human anti-pig response, not only for the above-mentioned molecules but also for CD28 and VLA-4 interactions with their ligands.
6. For those cases where cell surface molecule interactions are defective, T cells more easily recognize xenoantigens indirectly as peptides in association with host MHC molecules (in the manner of recognition of nominal antigens) rather than directly on xenogeneic cells (in the manner of recognition of MHC alloantigens). This phenomenon applies to both helper T cells and CTL and has been most clearly demonstrated for disparate species combinations and for murine responses to xenoantigens. On the other hand, the bulk of evidence to date suggests that human T cells can recognize pig xenoantigens directly on pig cells and thus would not be expected to utilize the indirect pathway preferentially for recognition of those antigens.
7. Despite the weak in vitro T cell responses to xenoantigens seen in some species combinations, in vivo xenograft rejection is uniformly brisk. This discrepancy remains poorly understood. One can speculate that helper T cells recognizing xenoantigens indirectly on host APC can mount a potent rejection response by either of two possible mechanisms. One such possibility is that indirectly xenoreactive helper T cells recruit either nonclassical effector cells, which then mediate graft destruction in an MHC-nonspecific fashion (Fig. 1D), or directly xenoreactive CTL, which mediate MHC-specific graft destruction (Fig. 1C). The other possibility is that indirectly xenoreactive helper T cells bound to directly xenoreactive B cells recruit directly xenoreactive CTL bound to xenogeneic APC in a four-cell cluster (Fig. 2). These various hypothetical effector pathways would result in rejection responses at least as potent as those mediated by classical CTL-mediated rejection of allografts. In addition to nonclassical effector mechanisms, classical CTL-mediated rejection, possibly including $CD4^+$ effector cells, would be expected to contribute to xenograft rejection in those species combinations where direct T cell recognition of xenoantigens is intact. The human response to pig xenografts will likely be an example of this "double-jeopardy" situation.
8. Despite the potent effector mechanisms operating against xenografts, the induction phase does appear to be highly dependent on $CD4^+$ helper T cells. This raises the possibility that cellular xenograft rejection might be suscepti-

ble to control with CD4-specific immunosuppresion. This has been shown in murine models by the efficacy of in vivo CD4-specific immunosuppression in prolonging the survival of skin, pancreatic islet, and heart xenografts but not whole MHC-disparate allografts. However, whether this approach can be extrapolated to the clinical setting, where, for example, the human anti-pig response seems to be largely allogeneic-like, remains to be proven. Thus, with the new knowledge now available, we must moderate previous conclusions and express concern that cell-mediated xenograft rejection may be more difficult to control than allograft rejection. Indeed, immunosuppressive strategies may have to be directed against not only allogeneic-like rejection mechanisms but also those unique to xenografting, including rejection mechanisms mediated by non-classical effector pathways.

Future Directions

1. While some cell surface molecule interactions have been well characterized across certain species differences, a number of interactions, particularly those involving lymphokines as well as certain adhesion, activation, and down-regulatory molecules, remain poorly defined. Examples include the interactions of CD28, VLA-4, CD40, and Fas with their ligands. Future studies should characterize these interactions in more detail and should concentrate on the clinically relevant human anti-pig response.
2. The suggestion that T_h2 cells are preferentially activated against xenoantigens should be explored further with attention to the possibility of new immunosuppressive strategies based on this property of the xenogeneic response.
3. If vascular endothelial cells are found to play an important role in graft rejection in vivo, attention should be focused on characterizing cell-mediated responses to xenogeneic endothelial cells. Indeed, recent studies suggest that they are potent stimulators of nonclassical effector populations.
4. Further study of nonclassical effector mechanisms of xenograft rejection is needed. Attention should be directed to defining the effector cell populations involved, the target antigens recognized (perhaps glycoproteins and/or αGal), and the mechanisms of effector cell activation (perhaps deinhibition by lack of human class I molecule expression).
5. While xenogeneic responses have been examined extensively in vitro, there remains a paucity of information regarding the induction and effector phases of xenograft rejection in vivo. Studies should be designed to elucidate further the in vivo rejection process.
6. Finally, while much effort has been directed towards characterizing the human anti-pig response, it may be worthwhile to examine human responses to other potential donor species in the hope of finding an alternative species stimulating weaker cell-mediated immune responses than those observed against the pig.

References

1. Auchincloss H Jr. Xenogeneic transplantation. A review. Transplantation 1988; 46: 1
2. Moses RD, Auchincloss H Jr. Mechanism of cellular xenograft rejection. Xenotransplantation. The Transplantation of Organs between Species 1991; 101
3. Moses RD, Pierson RNI, Winn HJ, Auchincloss H Jr. Xenogeneic proliferation and lymphokine production are dependent on CD4+ helper T cells and self antigen-presenting cells in the mouse. J. Exp. Med. 1990; 172: 567
4. Lance EM, Medawar PB. Survival of skin heterografts under treatment with antilymphocytic serum. Lancet 1968; 1: 1174
5. Manning DD, Reed ND, Shaffer CF. Maintenance of skin xenografts of widely divergent phylogenetic origin on congenitally athymic (nude) mice. J. Exp. Med. 1973; 138: 488
6. Newlands ES, Roitt IM. Evidence for two cell populations involved in the rejection of a xenograft in mice. Transplantation 1975; 20: 13
7. Dennert G. Effector mechanisms of cell-mediated immunity to xenogeneic cell antigens. J. Immunol. 1974; 113: 201
8. Galili U, Galili N, Vanky F, Klein E. Natural species-restricted attachment of human and murine T lymphocytes to various cells. Proc. Natl. Acad. Sci. USA 1978; 75: 2396
9. Asantila T, Vahala J, Toivanen P. Response of human fetal lymphocytes in xenogeneic mixed leukocyte culture: phylogenetic and ontogenetic aspects. Immunogenetics 1974; 1: 272
10. Hersh EM. Blastogenic responses of human lymphocytes to xenogeneic cells in vitro. Transplantation 1971; 12: 287
11. Lucas PJ, Bare CV, Gress RE. The human anti-murine xenogeneic cytotoxic response. II. Activated murine antigen-presenting cells directly stimulate human T helper cells. J. Immunol. 1995; 154: 3761
12. Woolnough JA, Misko IS, Lafferty KJ. Cytotoxic and proliferative lymphocyte responses to allogeneic and xenogeneic antigens in vitro. Aust. J. Exp. Biol. Med. Sci. 1979; 57: 467
13. Lafferty KJ, Jones MAS. Reactions of the graft-versus-host (GVH) type. Aust. J. Exp. Biol. Med. Sci. 1969; 47: 17
14. Greineder DK, Rosenthal AS. Macrophage activation of allogeneic lymphocyte proliferation in the guinea pig mixed leukocyte culture. J. Immunol. 1975; 114: 1541
15. Wilson DB, Fox DH. Quantitative studies on the mixed lymphocyte interaction in rats: VI. Reactivity of lymphocytes from conventional and germfree rats to allogeneic and xenogeneic cell surface antigens. J. Exp. Med. 1971; 134: 857
16. Wilson DB, Nowell PC. Quantitative studies on the mixed lymphocyte interaction in rats: IV. Immunological potentiality of the responding cells. J. Exp. Med. 1970; 131: 391
17. Nielsen HE. Reactivity of lymphocytes from germfree rats in mixed leukocyte culture and in graft-versus-host reaction. J. Exp. Med. 1972; 136: 417
18. Viguier M, Lotteau V, Charron D, Debré P. Xenogeneic recognition of soluble and cell surface HLA class II antigens by proliferative murine T cells. Eur. J. Immunol. 1987; 17: 1540
19. Gill RG. The role of direct and indirect antigen presentation in the response to islet xenografts. Transplant. Proc. 1992; 24: 642
20. Yoshizawa K, Yano A. Mouse T lymphocyte proliferative responses specific for human MHC products in mouse anti-human xenogeneic MLR. J. Immunol. 1984; 132: 2820

21. Swain SL, Dutton RW, Schwab R, Yamamoto J. Xenogeneic human anti-mouse T cell responses are due to the activity of the same functional T cell subsets responsible for allospecific and major histocompatibility complex-restricted responses. J. Exp. Med. 1983; 157: 720
22. Peck AB, Alter BJ, Lindahl KF. Specificity in T cell mediated lympholysis: identical genetic control of the proliferative and effector phases of allogeneic and xenogeneic reactions. Transplant. Rev. 1976; 29: 189
23. Shons AR, Najarian JS. Xenograft rejection in human beings. Rev. Surg. 1975; 32: 70
24. Hirshberg H, Rankin B, Thorsby E. Specificity of human lymphocytes proliferating in response to allogeneic and xenogeneic cells in vitro. Transplantation 1974; 17: 593
25. Shons AR, Kromrey C, Najarian JS. Xenogeneic mixed leucocyte response. Cell. Immunol. 1973; 6: 420
26. Bach FH, Engstrom MA, Bach ML, Sell KW. Histocompatibility matching. VII. Mixed leukocyte cultures between chimpanzee and man. Transplant. Proc. 1972; 4: 97
27. Widmer MB, Bach FH. Allogeneic and xenogeneic response in mixed leukocyte cultures. J. Exp. Med. 1972; 135: 1204
28. Knight SC, Thorbecke GJ. Ontogeny of cellular immunity: development in rat thymocytes of mixed lymphocyte reactivity to allogeneic and xenogeneic cells. Cell. Immunol. 1971; 2: 91
29. Rudolph RH, Hered B, Epstein RB, Thomas ED. Canine mixed leukocyte reactivity and transplantation antigens. Transplantation 1969; 8: 141
30. Hollander N, Ginsburg H, Feldman M. In vitro generation of memory lymphocytes reactive to transplantation antigens. J. Exp. Med. 1974; 140: 1057
31. Toivanen P, Asantila T. Ontogeny of allogeneic and xenogeneic cell recognition. II. Studies on fetal lamb [Abstr]. Scand. J. Immunol. 1974; 3: 891
32. Alter BJ, Bach FH. Cellular basis of the proliferative response of human T cells to mouse xenoantigens. J. Exp. Med. 1990; 171: 333
33. Elsen M, Soares M, Latinne D, Cornet A, Bazin H. Role of activated natural killer and CD4+, CD8+ cells in the cellular rejection of a discordant xenograft. Transplant. Proc. 1993; 25: 447
34. Satake M, Korsgren O, Ridderstad A, et al. Immunological characteristics of islet cell xenotransplantation in humans and rodents. Immunol. Rev. 1994; 141: 191
35. Rollins SA, Kennedy SP, Chodera AJ, et al. Evidence that activation of human T cells by porcine endothelium involves direct recognition of porcine SLA and costimulation by porcine ligands for LFA-1 and CD2. Transplantation 1994; 57: 1709
36. Ulrichs K, Eckstein V, Muller-Ruchholtz W. Xenogeneic T-cell-mediated immune reactivity in the model of pig-to-humans: first findings with native stimulator cells. Transplant. Proc. 1994; 26: 1045
37. Kirk AD, Li RA, Kinch MS, et al. The human antiporcine cellular repertoire. In vitro studies of acquired and innate cellular responsiveness. Transplantation 1993; 55: 924
38. Heiser A, Ulrichs K, Eckstein V, Muller-Ruchholtz W. Xenogeneic cellular response of human lymphocytes to porcine lymphocytes and isolated porcine pancreatic islets. Transplant. Proc. 1992; 24: 2881
39. Haisch CE, Lodge PA, Huber SA, Thomas FT. The vascular endothelial cell acts as the primary stimulus of T-lymphocyte proliferation in the in vitro xenogeneic response (XIR). Transplant. Proc. 1991; 23: 212

40. Vallee I, Watier H, Thibault G, et al. Evidence of noninvolvement of swine MHC class II in the in vitro proliferative response of human lymphocytes to porcine endothelial cells. Transplantation 1995; 59: 897
41. Yamada K, Sachs DH, DerSimonian H. Direct and indirect recognition of pig class II antigens by human T cells. Transplant. Proc. 1995; 27: 258
42. Bravery CA, Rose ML, Yacoub MH. Proliferative responses of highly purified human CD4+ T cells to porcine endothelial cells. Transplant. Proc. 1994; 26: 1157
43. Wren SM, Wang SC, Thai NL, et al. Evidence for early Th2 T cell predominance in xenoreactivity. Transplantation 1993; 56: 905
44. Yamada K, Sachs DH, DerSimonian H. Human anti-porcine xenogeneic T cell response. Evidence for allelic specificity of mixed leukocyte reaction and for both direct and indirect pathways of recognition. J. Immunol. 1995; 155: 5249
45. Widmer MB, Sondel PM, Bach FH. Responsiveness of germfree mice in mixed leukocyte culture: re-examining the nature of the responding unit. J. Exp. Med. 1972; 136: 398
46. Murray AG, Khodadoust MM, Pober JS, Bothwell AL. Porcine aortic endothelial cells activate human T cells: direct presentation of MHC antigens and costimulation by ligands for human CD2 and CD28. Immunity 1994; 1: 57
47. Lucas PJ, Shearer GM, Neudorf S, Gress RE. The human antimurine xenogeneic cytotoxic response: I. Dependence on responder antigen-presenting cells. J. Immunol. 1990; 144: 4548
48. Kumagai-Braesch M, Satake M, Korsgren O, Andersson A, Moller E. Characterization of cellular human anti-porcine xenoreactivity. Clin. Transplantation 1993; 7: 273
49. Batten P, Heaton T, Fuller-Espie S, Lechler RI. Human anti-mouse xenorecognition. Provision of noncognate interactions reveals plasticity of T cell repertoire. J. Immunol. 1995; 155: 1057
50. Golding H, Mizuochi T, McCarthy SA, Cleveland CA, Singer A. Relationship among function, phenotype, and specificity in primary allospecific T cell populations: identification of phenotypically identical but functionally distinct primary T cell subsets that differ in their recognition of MHC class I and class II allodeterminants. J. Immunol. 1987; 138: 10
51. Matsumiya G, Shirakura R, Miyagawa S, et al. Assessment of T-cell subsets involved in antibody production and cell-mediated cytotoxicity in rat-to-mouse cardiac xenotransplantation. Transplant. Proc. 1994; 26: 1214
52. Mizuochi T, Ono S, Malek TR, Singer A. Characterization of two distinct primary T cell populations that secrete interleukin 2 upon recognition of class I or class II major histocompatibility antigens. J. Exp. Med. 1986; 163: 603
53. Sprent J, Webb SR. Function and specificity of T cell subsets in the mouse. Adv. Immunol. 1987; 41: 39
54. Morris CF, Simeonovic CJ, Fung MC, Wilson JD. Intragraft expression of cytokine transcripts during pig proislet xenograft rejection and tolerance in mice. J. Immunol. 1995; 154: 2470
55. Lindahl KF, Bach FH. Genetic and cellular aspects of xenogeneic mixed leukocyte culture reaction. J. Exp. Med. 1976; 144: 305
56. Brunswick M, Lake P. Functional interactions of human and murine lymphoid cells. I. Analysis of primary and secondary responses. Cell. Immunol. 1986; 103: 441

57. Altmann DM, Douek DC, Frater AJ, et al. The T cell response of HLA-DR transgenic mice to human myelin basic protein and other antigens in the presence and absence of human CD4. J. Exp. Med. 1995; 181: 867
58. Yeung RS, Penninger JM, Kundig TM, et al. Human CD4-major histocompatibility complex class II (DQw6) transgenic mice in an endogenous CD4/CD8-deficient background: reconstitution of phenotype and human-restricted function. J. Exp. Med. 1994; 180: 1911
59. Hagihara M, Shimura T, Tsuchida F, et al. Xenogeneic iso-, allo-, and xeno-MLR and CML assay using HLA-DP and -DQ transgenic mice. Transplant. Proc. 1994; 26: 1319
60. Woods A, Chen HY, Trumbauer ME, et al. Human major histocompatibility complex class II-restricted T cell responses in transgenic mice. J. Exp. Med. 1994; 180: 173
61. Lawrance SK, Karlsson L, Price J, et al. Transgenic HLA-DR alpha faithfully reconstitutes IE-controlled immune functions and induces cross-tolerance to E-alpha in E-alpha-0 mutant mice. Cell 1989; 58: 583
62. Ramesh P, Barber L, Batchelor JR, Lechler RI. Structural analysis of human anti-mouse H-2E xenorecognition: T cell receptor bias and impaired CD4 interaction contribute to weak xenoresponses. International Immunol. 1992; 4: 935
63. Barzaga-Gilbert E, Grass D, Lawrance SK, et al. Species specificity and augmentation of responses to class II major histocompatibility complex molecules in human CD4 transgenic mice. J. Exp. Med. 1992; 175: 1707
64. Gustafsson K, Germana S, Hirsch F, et al. Structure of miniature swine class II DR beta genes: Conservation of hypervariable amino acid residues between distantly related mammalian species. Proc. Natl. Acad. Sci. USA 1990; 87: 9798
65. von Hoegen P, Miceli MC, Tourvieille B, Schilham M, Parnes JR. Equivalence of human and mouse CD4 in enhancing antigen responses by a mouse class II-restricted T cell hybridoma. J. Exp. Med. 1989; 170: 1879
66. von Hoegen P, Miceli MC, Tourvieille B, Schilham M, Parnes JR. Equivalence of human and mouse CD4 in enhancing antigen responses by a mouse class II-restricted T cell hybridoma. J. Exp. Med. 1989; 170: 1879
67. Law YM, Yeung RS, Mamalaki C, et al. Human CD4 restores normal T cell development and function in mice deficient in murine CD4. J. Exp. Med. 1994; 179: 1233
68. Killeen N, Sawada S, Littman DR. Regulated expression of human CD4 rescues helper T cell development in mice lacking expression of endogenous CD4. EMBO J. 1993; 12: 1547
69. Lombardi G, Barber L, Aichinger G, et al. Structural analysis of anti-DR1 allorecognition by using DR1/H-2Ek hybrid molecules. Influence of the beta-2 domain correlates with CD4 dependence. J. Immunol. 1991; 147: 2034
70. Clayton LK, Sieh M, Pious DA, Reinherz EL. Identification of human CD4 residues affecting class II MHC versus HIV-1 gp120 binding. Nature 1989; 339: 548
71. Nishimura Y, Iwanaga T, Inamitsu T, et al. Expression of the human MHC, HLA-DQw6 genes alters the immune response in C57BL/6 mice. J. Immunol. 1990; 145: 353
72. Vignali DA, Moreno J, Schiller D, Hammerling GJ. Species-specific binding of CD4 to the beta-2 domain of major histocompatibility complex class II molecules. J. Exp. Med. 1992; 175: 925
73. Konig R, Huang LY, Germain RN. MHC class II interaction with CD4 mediated by a region analogous to the MHC class I binding site for CD8. Nature 1992; 356: 796

74. Lamarre D, Ashkenazi A, Fleury S, et al. The MHC-binding and gp120-binding functions of CD4 are separable. Science 1989; 245: 743
75. Yamamoto K, Fukui Y, Esaki Y, et al. Functional interaction between human histocompatibility leukocyte antigen (HLA) class II and mouse CD4 molecule in antigen recognition by T cells in HLA-DR and DQ transgenic mice. J. Exp. Med. 1994; 180: 165
76. Uren S, Bolcevic Z, Hwang LR, Boyle W. Accessory cell signals need not be species restricted in xenogeneic activation. Transplant. Proc. 1992; 24: 208
77. Tsunetsugu-Yokota Y, Mizuochi T, Hashimoto H, et al. Analysis of function of a human antigen-presenting cell by xenogeneic interaction with mouse T cells. Immunol. Letters 1994; 40: 73
78. Zeng Y, Gage A, Montag A, et al. Inhibition of transplant rejection by pretreatment of xenogeneic pancreatic islet cells with anti-ICAM-1 antibodies. Transplantation 1994; 58: 681
79. Miller GT, Hochman PS, Meier W, et al. Specific interaction of lymphocyte function-associated antigen 3 with CD2 can inhibit T cell responses. J. Exp. Med. 1993; 178: 211
80. Moses RD, Winn HJ, Auchincloss H Jr. Evidence that multiple defects in cell-surface molecule interactions across species differences are responsible for diminished xenogeneic T cell responses. Transplantation 1992; 53: 203
81. Johnston SC, Dustin ML, Hibbs ML, Springer TA. On the species specificity of the interaction of LFA-1 with intercellular adhesion molecules. J. Immunol. 1990; 145: 1181
82. Birmele B, Thibault G, Watier H, et al. Human peripheral blood lymphocyte adhesion to xenogeneic porcine aortic endothelial cells: preferential adhesion of CD3-CD16+ NK cells. Transplant. Proc. 1994; 26: 1150
83. Pleass HC, Kirby JA, Forsythe JL, Proud G, Taylor RM. Adhesion molecule blockade in a porcine xenograft model. Transplant. Proc. 1994; 26: 1162
84. Chavin KD, Lau HT, Bromberg JS. Prolongation of allograft and xenograft survival in mice by anti-CD2 monoclonal antibodies. Transplantation 1992; 54: 286
85. Watier H, Vallee I, Thibault G, et al. Effect of human inflammatory cytokines on porcine endothelial cell MHC molecule expression: unique role for TNF-alpha in MHC class-II induction. Transplant. Proc. 1994; 26: 1152
86. Burakoff SJ, Dorf ME, Benacerraf B. Specificity of rat xenogeneic cell-mediated cytolysis for the products of the K and D loci of the mouse H-2 complex. J. Immunol. 1977; 118: 1795
87. Irwin MJ, Heath WR, Sherman LA. Species-restricted interactions between CD8 and the alpha3 domain of class I influence the magnitude of the xenogeneic response. J. Exp. Med. 1989; 170: 1091
88. Achour A, Begue B, Gomard E, et al. Specific lysis of murine cells expressing HLA molecules by allospecific human and murine H-2-restricted anti-HLA T killer lymphocytes. Eur. J. Immunol. 1986; 16: 597
89. Bluestone JA, Pescovitz MD, Frels WI, Singer DS, Hodes RJ. Cytotoxic T lymphocyte recognition of a xenogeneic major histocompatibility complex antigen expressed in transgenic mice. Eur. J. Immunol. 1987; 17: 1035
90. Stejskal V, Holm G, Perlmann P. Differential cytotoxicity of activated lymphocytes on allogeneic and xenogeneic target cells. I. Activation by tuberculin and by staphylococcus filtrate. Cell. Immunol. 1973; 8: 71

91. Burakoff SJ, Ratnofsky SE, Benacerraf B. Mouse cytolytic T lymphocytes induced by xenogeneic rat stimulator cells exhibit specificity for H-2 complex alloantigens. Proc. Natl. Acad. Sci. USA 1977; 74: 4572
92. Mentzer SJ, Barbosa JA, Strominger JL, Biro PA, Burakoff SJ. Species-restricted recognition of transfected HLA-A2 and HLA-B7 by human CTL clones. J. Immunol. 1986; 137: 408
93. Dill O, Kievits F, Koch S, Ivanyi P, Hammerling GJ. Immunological function of HLA-C antigens in HLA-Cw3 transgenic mice. Proc. Natl. Acad. Sci. USA 1988; 85: 5664
94. Dunham DM, Hahn EC. Characterization of porcine xenoreactive cytotoxic T lymphocytes. Veterinary Immunol. Immunopathol. 1992; 34: 209
95. Berke G, Ax W, Ginsburg H, Feldman M. Graft reaction in tissue culture: II. Quantification of the lytic action on mouse fibroblasts by rat lymphocytes sensitized on mouse embryo monolayers. Immunology 1969; 16: 643
96. Ginsburg H. Graft versus host reaction in tissue culture: I. Lysis of monolayers of embryo mouse cells from strains differing in the H-2 histocompatibility locus by rat lymphocytes sensitized in vitro. Immunology 1968; 14: 621
97. Newberg MH, Ridge JP, Vining DR, Salter RD, Engelhard VH. Species specificity in the interaction of CD8 with the alpha-3 domain of MHC class I molecules. J. Immunol. 1992; 149: 136
98. Cunningham AC, Butler TJ, Kirby JA. Demonstration of direct xenorecognition of porcine cells by human cytotoxic T lymphocytes. Immunology 1994; 81: 268
99. Barra C, Perarnau B, Gerlinger P, et al. Analysis of the HLA-Cw3-specific cytotoxic T lymphocyte response of HLA-B7×human beta2m double transgenic mice. J. Immunol. 1989; 143: 3117
100. Holterman MJ, Engelhard VH. HLA antigens expressed on murine cells are preferentially recognized by murine cytotoxic T cells in the context of the H-2 major histocompatibility complex. Proc. Natl. Acad. Sci. USA 1986; 83: 9699
101. Kievits F, Wijffels J, Lokhorst W, Ivanyi P. Recognition of xeno-(HLA, SLA) major histocompatibility complex antigens by mouse cytotoxic T cells is not H-2 restricted: A study with transgenic mice. Proc. Natl. Acad. Sci. USA 1989; 86: 617
102. Engelhard VH, Le AT, Holterman MJ. Species-specific structural differences in the alpha1 and alpha2 domains determine the frequency of murine cytotoxic T cell precursors stimulated by human and murine class I molecules. J. Immunol. 1988; 141: 1835
103. Hammerling GJ, Hunt T, Dill O, Moreno J. Cytotoxic T lymphocyte recognition of HLA-A2 antigens in normal and HLA-Cw3-transgenic mice. Eur. J. Immunol. 1989; 19: 599
104. Pala P, Corradin G, Strachan T, et al. Mapping of HLA epitopes recognized by H-2-restricted cytotoxic T lymphocytes specific for HLA using recombinant genes and synthetic peptides. J. Immunol. 1988; 140: 871
105. Le AT, Bernhard EJ, Holterman MJ, et al. Cytotoxic T cell responses in HLA-A2.1 transgenic mice. Recognition of HLA alloantigens and utilization of HLA-A2.1 as a restriction element. J. Immunol. 1989; 142: 1366
106. Kievits F, Boerenkamp WJ, Lokhorst W, Ivanyi P. Specificity and frequency of primary anti-HLA cytotoxic T lymphocytes in normal and HLA-B27.2-, HLA-B27.5-, and HLA-Cw3-transgenic mice. A transgenic model for MHC xenoantigen recognition. J. Immunol. 1990; 144: 4513

107. Carnaud C, Fadai-Ghotbi M, Lesavre P, Bach JF. Education of human lymphocytes against mouse cells: specific recognition of H-2 antigens. Eur. J. Immunol. 1977; 7: 81
108. Burakoff SJ, Engelhard VH, Kaufmann J, Strominger JL. Induction of secondary cytotoxic T lymphocytes by liposomes containing HLA-DR antigens. Nature 1980; 283: 495
109. Greenstein JL, Foran JA, Gorga JC, Burakoff SJ. The role of T cell accessory molecules in the generation of class II-specific xenogeneic cytolytic T cells. J. Immunol. 1986; 136: 2358
110. Engelhard VH, Benjamin C. Isolation and characterization of monoclonal mouse cytotoxic T lymphocytes with specificity for HLA-A, -B, or -DR alloantigens. J. Immunol. 1982; 129: 2621
111. Engelhard VH, Kaufman JF, Strominger JL, Burakoff SJ. Specificity of mouse cytotoxic T lymphocytes stimulated with either HLA-A and -B or HLA-DR antigens reconstituted into phospholipid vesicles. J. Exp. Med. 1980; 152: 54S
112. Okumura C, Suto R, Furukawa K, et al. Induction of murine gamma-delta T cells cytotoxic for xenogeneic rat cells. J. Immunol. 1995; 154: 1114
113. Lindahl KF, Bach FH. Human lymphocytes recognise mouse alloantigens. Nature 1975; 254: 607
114. Engelhard VH, Benjamin C. Xenogeneic cytotoxic T-cell clones recognize alloantigenic determinants on HLA-A2. Immunogenetics 1983; 18: 461
115. Berke G, Clark WR, Feldman M. In vitro induction of a heterograft reaction: immunological parameters of the sensitization of rat lymphocytes against mouse cells in vitro. Transplantation 1971; 12: 237
116. Gress RE, Nathenson SG, Lucas PJ. Fine specificity of xenogeneic antigen recognition by human T cells. Transplantation 1989; 48: 93
117. Kievits F, Ivanyi P, Krimpenfort P, Berns A, Ploegh HL. HLA-restricted recognition of viral antigens in HLA transgenic mice. Nature 1987; 329: 447
118. Bernhard EJ, Le AT, Barbosa JA, Lacy E, Engelhard VH. Cytotoxic T lymphocytes from HLA-A2 transgenic mice specific for HLA-A2 expressed on human cells. J. Exp. Med. 1988; 168: 1157
119. Barra C, Gournier H, Garcia Z, et al. Abrogation of H-2-restricted CTL responses and efficient recognition of HLA-A3 molecules in DBA/2 HLA/A24 responder mice. J. Immunol. 1993; 150: 3681
120. Smith L. CD4+ murine T cells develop from CD8+ precursors in vivo. Nature 1987; 326: 798
121. Kisielow P, Bluthmann H, Staerz UD, Steinmetz M, von Boehmer H. Tolerance in T-cell-receptor transgenic mice involves deletion of nonmature CD4+8+ thymocytes. Nature 1988; 333: 742
122. Sha WC, Nelson CA, Newberry RD, et al. Selective expression of an antigen receptor on CD8-bearing T lymphocytes in transgenic mice. Nature 1988; 335: 271
123. Vitiello A, Marchesini D, Furze J, Sherman LA, Chesnut RW. Analysis of the HLA-restricted influenza-specific cytototxic T lymphocyte response in transgenic mice carrying a chimeric human-mouse class I major histocompatibility complex. J. Exp. Med. 1991; 173: 1007
124. Kalinke U, Arnold B, Hammerling GJ. Strong xenogeneic HLA response in transgenic mice after introducing an alpha-3 domain into HLA B27. Nature 1990; 348: 642

125. LaFace DM, Vestberg M, Yang Y, et al. Human CD8 transgene regulation of HLA recognition by murine T cells. J. Exp. Med. 1995; 182: 1315
126. Samberg NL, Scarlett EC, Stauss HJ. The alpha3 domain of major histocompatibility complex class I molecules plays a critical role in cytotoxic T lymphocyte stimulation. Eur. J. Immunol. 1989; 19: 2349
127. Epstein H, Hardy R, May JS, Johnson MH, Holmes N. Expression and function of HLA-A2.1 in transgenic mice. Eur. J. Immunol. 1989; 19: 1575
128. Rocca A, Degos L, Pla M. Analysis of primary HLA-specific cytotoxic T cell response in graft-draining lymph nodes – a transgenic mouse model for in vivo recognition of human MHC antigens. Transplantation 1991; 52: 1062
129. Maryanski JL, Accolla RS, Jordan B. H-2 restricted recognition of cloned HLA class I gene products expressed in mouse cells. J. Immunol. 1986; 136: 4340
130. Chamberlain JW, Nolan JA, Gromkowski SH, et al. Cell surface expression and alloantigenic function of a human class I MHC heavy chain gene (HLA-B7) in transgenic mice. J. Immunol. 1988; 140: 1285
131. Taurog JD, Lowen L, Forman J, Hammer RE. HLA-B27 in inbred and non-inbred transgenic mice. Cell surface expression and recognition as an alloantigen in the absence of human beta2-microglobulin. J. Immunol. 1988; 141: 4020
132. Maziarz R, Allen H, Strominger JL, et al. Recognition of interspecies hybrid class I histocompatibility antigens by antigen-specific cytolytic T lymphocytes. Proc. Natl. Acad. Sci. USA 1985; 82: 6276
133. Maziarz RT, Burakoff SJ, Bluestone JA. The alpha-3 domain of class I MHC proteins influences cytotoxic T lymphocyte recognition of antigenic determinants located within the alpha-1 and alpha-2 domains. J. Immunol. 1988; 140: 4372
134. Barbosa JA, Mentzer SJ, Minowada G, et al. Recognition of HLA-A2 and -B7 antigens by cloned cytotoxic T lymphocytes after gene transfer into human and monkey, but not mouse, cells. Proc. Natl. Acad. Sci. USA 1984; 81: 7549
135. Bernabeu C, Finlay D, van de Rijn M, et al. Expression of the major histocompatibility antigens HLA-A2 and HLA-B7 by DNA-mediated gene transfer. J. Immunol. 1983; 131: 2032
136. van de Rijn M, Bernabeu C, Royer-Pokora B, et al. Recognition of HLA-A2 by cytotoxic T lymphocytes after DNA transfer into human and murine cells. Science 1985; 226: 1083
137. Bernabeu C, Maziarz R, Spits H, et al. Coexpression of the human HLA-A2 or HLA-B7 heavy chain gene and human beta2-microglobulin gene in L cells. J. Immunol. 1984; 133: 3188
138. Bernhard EJ, Le AT, Yannelli JR, et al. The ability of cytotoxic T cells to recognize HLA-A2.1 or HLA-B7 antigens expressed on murine cells correlates with their epitope specificity. J. Immunol. 1987; 139: 3614
139. Golde WT, Kappler JW, Greenstein J, et al. Major histocompatibility complex-restricted antigen receptor on T cells. VIII. Role of the LFA-1 molecule. J. Exp. Med. 1985; 161: 635
140. Koller TD, Clayberger C, Maryanski JL, Krensky AM. Human allospecific cytolytic T lymphocyte lysis of a murine cell transfected with HLA-A2. J. Immunol. 1987; 138: 2044

141. Maryanski JL, Moretta A, Jordan B, et al. Human T cell recognition of cloned HLA class I gene products expressed on DNA transfectants of mouse mastocytoma P815. Eur. J. Immunol. 1985; 15: 1111
142. Gomard E, Begue B, Sodoyer S, et al. Murine cells expressing an HLA molecule are specifically lysed by HLA-restricted antiviral human T cells. Nature 1986; 319: 153
143. Cowan EP, Coligan JE, Biddison WE. Human cytotoxic T-lymphocyte recognition of an HLA-A3 gene product expressed on murine L cells: the only human gene product required on the target cells for lysis is the class I heavy chain. Proc. Natl. Acad. Sci. USA 1985; 82: 4490
144. Barbosa JA, Mentzer SJ, Kamarck ME, et al. Gene mapping and somatic cell hybrid analysis of the role of human lymphocyte function-associated antigen-3 (LFA-3) in CTL-target cell interactions. J. Immunol. 1986; 136: 3085
145. Engelhard VH, Powers GA, Moore LC, Holterman MJ, Correa-Freire MC. Cytotoxic T lymphocyte recognition of HLA-A/B antigens introduced into EL-4 cells by cell-liposome fusion. J. Immunol. 1984; 132: 76
146. Maryanski JL, Pala P, Corradin G, Jordan BR, Cerottini J. H-2-restricted cytolytic T cells specific for HLA can recognize a synthetic HLA peptide. Nature 1986; 324: 578
147. Escobar MR, Sigel MM. Effects of lymphoid cells and serum on target cells in xenogeneic cell-culture systems. Proc. Soc. Exp. Biol. Med. 1970; 134: 744
148. Grant CK, Avis PJ, Hall JG, Alexander P. Evidence for the role of antibody in the cytotoxic action of lymph cells on xenogeneic target cells. Transplantation 1971; 11: 356
149. Harding B, MacLennan ICM. The distribution of antibody and antibody-producing cells after immunization with xenogeneic cells. Immunology 1972; 23: 35
150. Moller G, Svehag SE. Specificity of lymphocyte-mediated cytotoxicity induced by in vitro antibody-coated target cells. Cell. Immunol. 1972; 4: 1
151. Chaussy C, Hammer C, Pongratz H, et al. Prolongation of graft survival in rats and dogs by a specific antimacrophage serum (AMS). Transpl. Proc. 1975; 7: 779
152. Chan DV, Auchincloss H Jr. Human anti-pig cell-mediated cytotoxicity in vitro involves non-T as well as T cell components. Xenotransplantation 1996; 3: 158
153. Inverardi L, Pardi R. Humoral and cellular recognition of discordant xenogeneic Langerhans islets. Transplant. Proc. 1994; 26: 1034
154. Schaapherder AF, Daha MR, te Bulte MT, van der Woude FJ, Gooszen HG. Antibody-dependent cell-mediated cytotoxicity against porcine endothelium induced by a majority of human sera. Transplantation 1994; 57: 1376
155. Inverardi L, Samaja M, Motterlini R, et al. Early recognition of a discordant xenogeneic organ by human circulating lymphocytes. J. Immunol. 1992; 149: 1416
156. Inverardi L, Samaja M, Marelli F, Bender JR, Pardi R. Cellular early immune recognition of xenogeneic vascular endothelium. Transplant. Proc. 1992; 24: 459
157. Thomas FT, Marchman W, Carobbi A, et al. Immunobiology of the xenograft response: xenograft rejection in immunodeficient animals. Transplant. Proc. 1991; 23: 208
158. Lin Y, Sobis H, Vandeputte M, Waer M. Natural killer cells, antibody-dependent cellular cytotoxicity, and complement synthesis by the xenograft itself play a role in xenograft rejection. Transplant. Proc. 1995; 27: 286
159. Arawaka K, Akami T, Okamoto M, et al. Prolongation of heart xenograft survival in the NK-deficient rat. Transplant. Proc. 1994; 26: 1266

160. Wallgren AC, Karlsson-Parra A, Korsgren O. The main infiltrating cell in xenograft rejection is a CD4+ macrophage and not a T lymphocyte. Transplantation 1995; 60: 594
161. Sakakibara N, Click RE, Sakakibara K, et al. Unconventional lymphocytes involved in rejection of xenogeneic heart grafts. Lab. Invest. 1990; 62: 481
162. Korsgren O, Jansson L. Characterization of mixed syngeneic-allogeneic and syngeneic-xenogeneic islet-graft rejections in mice. Evidence of functional impairment of the remaining syngeneic islets in xenograft rejections. J. Clin. Invest. 1994; 93: 1113
163. Pierson RN, Winn HJ, Russell PS, Auchincloss H Jr. Xenogeneic skin graft rejection is especially dependent on CD4+ T cells. J. Exp. Med. 1989; 170: 991
164. Auchincloss H Jr, Moses R, Conti D, et al. Rejection of transgenic skin expressing a xeno-class I antigen is CD4-dependent and CD8-independent. Transplant. Proc. 1990; 22: 1059
165. Wecker H, Winn HJ, Auchincloss H Jr. CD4+ T cells, without CD8+ or B lymphocytes, can reject xenogeneic skin grafts. Xenotransplantation 1994; 1: 8
166. Ricordi C, Lacy PE, Sterbenz K, Davie JM. Low-temperature culture of human islets or in vivo treatment with L3T4 antibody produces a marked prolongation of islet human-to-mouse xenograft survival. Proc. Natl. Acad. Sci. USA 1987; 84: 8080
167. Kaufman DS, Kong CS, Shizuru JA, Gregory AK, Fathman CG. Use of anti-L3T4 and anti-Ia treatments for prolongation of xenogeneic islet transplants. Transplantation 1988; 46: 210
168. Wilson JD, Simeonovic CJ, Ting JHL, Ceredig R. Role of CD4+ T-lymphocytes in rejection by mice of fetal pig proislet xenografts. Diabetes 1989; 38 (Suppl 1): 217
169. Lacy PE, Ricordi C, Finke EH. Effect of transplantation site and anti-L3T4 treatment on survival of rat, hamster, and rabbit islet xenografts in mice. Transplantation 1989; 47: 761
170. Kawai M, Gotoh M, Monden M, et al. Effect of L3T4 and Lyt-2 monoclonal antibodies on islet xenograft (rat to mouse) rejection. Transplant. Proc. 1989; 21: 2709
171. Gill RG, Wolf L, Daniel D, Coulombe M. CD4+ T cells are both necessary and sufficient for islet xenograft rejection. Transplant. Proc. 1994; 26: 1203
172. Thomas F, Araneda D, Henretta J, Pittman K, Marchman W. Extended and expanded studies of xenograft rejection in immunodeficient animals. Transplant. Proc. 1994; 26: 1224
173. Desai NM, Bassiri H, Kim J, et al. Islet allograft, islet xenograft, and skin allograft survival in CD8+ T lymphocyte-deficient mice. Transplantation 1993; 55: 718
174. Sakakibara N, Click RE, Condie RM, Jamieson SW. Rejection/acceptance of xenografts. Transplant. Proc. 1989; 21: 524
175. Sakakibara N, Jamieson SW, Wolf P, Weisberg D, Click RE. Rejection of rat cardiac xenografts by mouse CD4 or CD8 T cells. Transplant. Proc. 1995; 27: 264
176. Wolf L, Gill RG. Xenoreactive T-cell lines initiate pancreatic islet graft destruction in vivo. Transplant. Proc. 1993; 25: 440
177. Gress RE, Katz SI, Lucas PJ. Human CD8+ xenoreactive T cells mediate tissue injury in vivo. Transplantation 1993; 56: 484
178. Click RE, Weisberg D, White J, Reichenbach D, Jamieston SW. Rejection of rat skin xenografts by either murine CD4 or CD8 T cells. Transplantation 1994; 58: 1020
179. Auchincloss H Jr. Why is cell-mediated xenograft rejection so strong? Xeno 1995; 3: 19–22

180. Lenschow DJ, Zeng Y, Thistlethwaite JR, et al. Long-term survival of xenogeneic pancreatic islet grafts induced by CTLA4Ig. Science 1992; 257: 789
181. Mitchison NA, O'Malley C. Three-cell-type clusters of T cells with antigen-presenting cells best explain the epitope linkage and noncognate requirements of the in vivo cytolytic response. Eur. J. Immunol. 1987; 17: 1579
182. Lee RS, Grusby MJ, Glimcher LH, Winn HJ, Auchincloss H Jr. Indirect recognition by helper T cells can induce donor-specific cytotoxic T lymphocytes in vivo. J. Exp. Med. 1994; 179: 865

13 Human T Cell Response to Porcine Tissues

M.L. Rose

Introduction

The human cellular response to alloantigens is exceedingly strong, both in terms of the numbers of T cells recognizing foreign alloantigens and the cytokine profile of activated T cells. Before describing the human response to porcine antigens it is necessary to understand two recent concepts which have advanced our understanding of the vigour of the host anti-allograft response. The first is the significance of direct presentation; the second is the molecular requirements for cells to cause direct stimulation of allogeneic T cells.

Direct and Indirect Antigen Presentation

In recent years there has been a growing interest in the relative role of direct and indirect antigen presentation as mechanisms of causing allograft rejection. Direct antigen presentation or allo-restricted recognition is a molecular cross-reaction. Host T cells, educated to recognize complexes formed between self peptides and self-allelic forms of major histocompatibility complex (MHC) molecules, cross-react with complexes of nonself (or self) peptides and allogeneic forms of MHC which are expressed on cells of the foreign graft. This cross-reaction leads to the situation whereby a large proportion of T cells in a nonimmunized host (1/500) recognize foreign allogeneic MHC molecules. Indirect presentation or self-restricted presentation is when foreign or graft-derived peptides are processed by host antigen-presenting cells (APC) and presented to T cells within self MHC molecules. In this case, recognition within a non-immunized host is by relatively small numbers (1/100 000–1/10^6) of peptide-specific T cells. The proportion of T cells recognizing antigens derived from an allograft in this case will be similar to the number recognizing other foreign peptides.

It is usually assumed that the rapid nature of cell-mediated allograft rejection is a result of direct presentation of allo-MHC molecules. There is increasing experimental evidence that indirect presentation of allo-MHC molecules also leads to allograft rejection [1], albeit at a slower tempo. Crossing the species barrier by presenting xenoantigens to human T cells should not hinder indirect presentation. There seems no reason why human T cells should not recognize peptides derived from pig or mice, provided they are presented complexed to self MHC on the surface of host APC. However, such a response would not be expected to lead to the vigorous cellular rejection commonly encountered in non-immunosuppressed recipients of allografted organs. The interesting question to those wishing to predict the nature of the cellular response following engraftment of pig tissues into man is whether human T cells directly recognize pig MHC molecules.

Human Endothelial Cells as Antigen-Presenting Cells

Expression of allogeneic molecules is not sufficient to activate T cells. It is now known that the signals provided by interaction between peptide–MHC complex and the antigen-specific T cell receptor are too weak to initiate interleukin (IL)-2 synthesis by T cells. Dendritic cells and cells of the monocyte/macrophage series are potent stimulators of allogeneic T cells, but fibroblasts, epithelial cells and smooth muscle cells, despite expressing MHC molecules, do not stimulate allostimulation [2]. Full activation of resting T cells requires costimulatory molecules as well as MHC expression. Examples of costimulatory molecules present on APC are B7.1 and B7.2, which signal through T cell CD28, and lymphocyte function-associated antigen (LFA)-3 (CD58) and CD59, which signal through T cell CD2.

Although dendritic cells historically have been considered to be the most important cell initiating allograft rejection [3], more recently attention has focused on the endothelial cells as performing a similar role (for a review, see [2]). The reason for this is that in humans (and pigs) microvascular endothelial cells constitutively express MHC class II antigens [4, 5]. This is unlike rodents, where the only MHC class II-positive cells in hearts or kidneys are dendritic cells. It has been shown by a number of groups that cultured human umbilical vein endothelial cells (HUVEC), once induced to express MHC class II by interferon (IFN)-γ, cause allostimulation of resting $CD4^+$ T cells [6], and one of the costimulatory molecules is LFA-3 [6]. Thus human endothelial cells, unlike other stromal cells, can act as APC and cause direct presentation of alloantigens to resting T cells.

This information, plus the observation that endothelial cells are the first cells to be seen by the immune system, has focused attention on whether porcine endothelial cells can act as APC for human T cells. In particular, it has focused attention on whether porcine endothelial cells are directly recognized by human T cells (i.e., without participation of human APC) and whether porcine endothelial cells have the necessary costimulatory molecules to cause full activation of T cells.

Expression of Major Histocompatibility Complex and Accessory Molecules on Porcine Endothelial Cells

Early work from Sachs' laboratory [5] , using monclonal antibodies (mAbs) raised against murine class II and immunocytochemistry on frozen sections, showed in situ staining of SLA class II antigens on endothelial cells from renal and aortic tissue from miniature swine. More recently, we have confirmed the

Table 1. Expression of major histocompatibility complex (MHC) molecules and B7 receptors on porcine endothelial cells: effect of treatment with species-specific interferon (IFN)-τ

mAb	(*n*)	Specificity	PAEC untreated (% positive)	(*n*)	PAEC +rpoIFN-τ (% positive)
Control	11	No first antibody	1.1± 0.8	13	1.1± 0.8
PT85A	11	SLA class I	99.4± 0.9	13	98.6± 3.1
L243	4	HLA-DR	2.1± 1.3	4	1.3± 1.3
L227	3	Common determinants HLA class II	14.1±10.8	4	67.0±56.9
DA6.231	11	Common determinants HLA class II	29.2±21.0	12	95.8±10.0
MSA-3	7	SLA-DR	18.7±16.2	8	96.9± 0.9
TH16B	11	SLA-DwQ	28.0±25.1	12	98.5± 2.2
mCTLA-4-Ig	9	Mouse/human B7	2.3± 1.5	9	31.5±19.0
MAC323	3	Pig CD45	1.1± 0.6	4	0.7± 0.2

From [7].
PAEC, pig aortic endothelial cells; mAb, monoclonal antibody.

constitutive expression of SLA class II on the microvasculature of pig heart and the microvascular and luminal endothelial cells of pig aorta [7], using a variety of mAbs raised against human or swine MHC class II antigens. Thus mAbs DA6.231 (HLA-DRβ), L227 (common determinant HLA class II), TH16B (SLA-DQ), and MSA3 (SLA-DR) all stain porcine cardiac endothelial cells [7].

Flow cytometric analysis of cultured and passaged pig aortic endothelial cells (PAEC) reveals that, in our hands, variable numbers of PAEC constitutively express SLA class II molecules (Table 1). In some cases substantial numbers of PAEC expressed class II; thus DA6.231 detected between 4% and 49% positive cells from 12 preparations; mAbs against porcine determinants (MSA3, Th16) also stained substantial numbers of PAEC (18.7% ± 16.2% and 28% ± 25.1%, respectively) . The constitutive expression of SLA class II on frozen sections of pig aorta and the persistence of expression on variable numbers of cells after several weeks in culture contrasts with the absence of MHC class II expression on HUVEC, detected in situ [8] or in culture. This species difference in constitutive expression of class II probably accounts for the differences in ability to stimulate resting T cells (see below). Basal expression of SLA class II on passaged PAEC has not been found by all workers [9, 10]. The differences are presumably accounted for by the source of pig (ours are outbred) or possibly culture conditions.

Effect of Cytokines on Expression of Major Histocompatibility Complex, Accessory, and Adhesion Molecules

In the allograft it is known that amplification of the cellular response (i.e., maturation of effector cells, migration of effector cells into the graft) depends on local release of inflammatory cytokines – tumor necrosis factor (TNF)-α, IL-1β, IL-4, IFNγ – and their effect on the local endothelium. As part of our understanding of the human cellular response to xenografted pig tissue, it is necessary to know whether human cytokines can promote inflammatory changes in pig endothelial cells. We have tested the effect of human TNF-α, IL-1β, IL-4, and IFN-γ on expression of MHC, accessory and adhesion molecules by porcine endothelial cells and used a porcine recombinant IFN-γ as a positive control.

HUVEC, which are constitutively negative for MHC class II antigens, can be induced to express class II by treatment with recombinant human IFN-γ (rhIFN-γ) . It can be seen from Table 1 that porcine IFN-γ induces SLA class II molecules on PAEC; thus the numbers of cells staining with L227, DA6.231, MSA-3, and TH16B increased considerably (>95 % positive) after 5 days of treatment with rpoIFN-γ. Similar results were reported by Watier et al. [11]. In con-

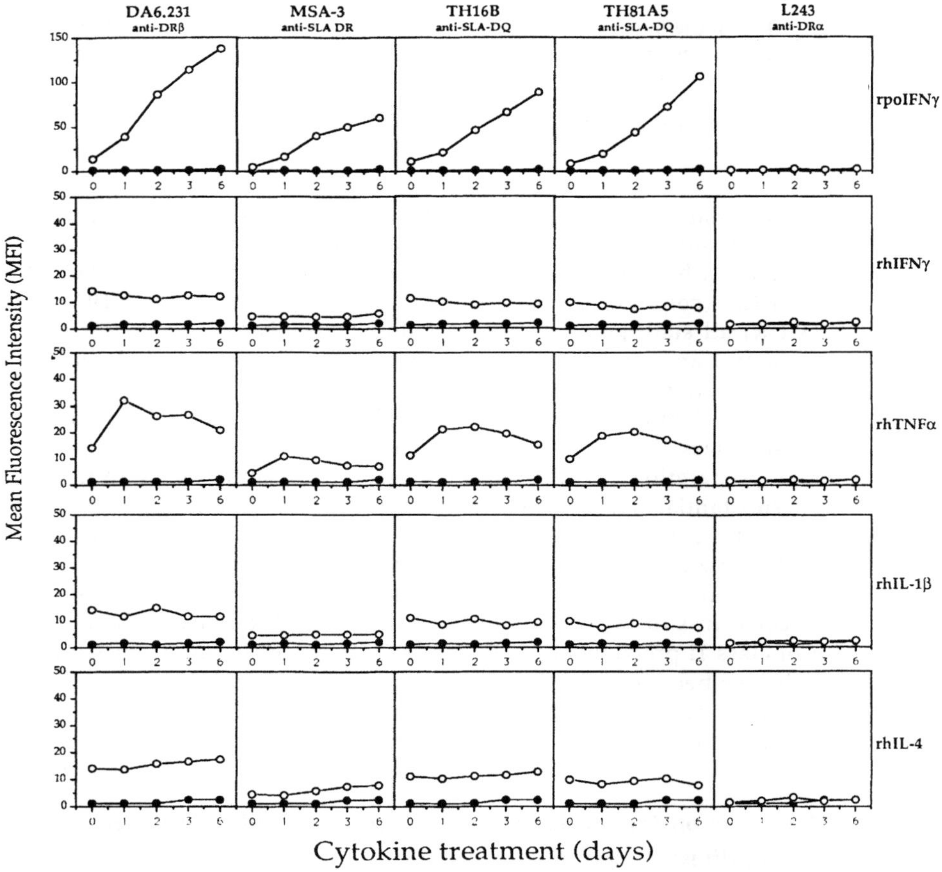

Fig. 1. Pig aortic endothelial cells (PAEC) were incubated with different cytokines – rpo interferon (*IFN*)-γ, rhIFNγ, rh tumor necrosis factor (*TNF*)-α, rh interleukin (*IL*)-1β, rhIL-4 – for 0–6 days and samples removed at 24-h intervals for flow cytometric analysis. The results are expressed as mean fluorescence intensity (MFI, arbitrary units) . The monoclonal antibodies (mAb) used to detect class II were: DA6.231 (anti-DRβ), MSA-3 (anti-SLA-DR), TH16B (anti-SLA-DQ), TH81A5 (anti-SLA-DQ), and L243 (anti-DRα). *Black circles*, negative control; *white circles*, antibody. Representative of three experiments. (From [12], with permission)

trast, and also reported by Watier et al. [11], human recombinant IFNγ had no effect (data not shown). In further experiments, a time-course experiment compared the abilities of rpoIFN-γ, rhIFN-γ, and human recombinant TNF-α, IL-1β, and IL-4 to upregulate MHC class II expression on PAEC (Fig. 1). In this particular experiment, increase in intensity of expression of class II was investigated. The only cytokines able to induce/upregulate class II expression were rpoIFN-γ and rhTNF-α. Further experiments showed that rhTNF-α also increases numbers of class II-positive cells [12]. The surprising ability of human TNF-α to increase class II expression confirms the earlier observation of Watier et al. [11]. In humans, only IFN-γ is able to induce class II expression [13]. That this effect is truly mediated via TNF, and not a contaminant, was proven by the observation that the effect of TNF was inhibited by anti-TNF antibody [12].

Important accessory molecules, at least for dendritic cell stimulation of an alloreaction, are B7.1 and B7.2 [14]. These molecules interact with T cell CD28 or CLTA-4. In order to asses whether porcine endothelial cells express B7 molecules, PAEC were cultured with fluorosceinated CTLA-4-Ig, a fusion protein with very high affinity for B7 [7, 12]. It can be seen from Table 1 that resting PAEC bind small but significant quantities of CTLA-4-Ig, and this value is significantly increased by rpoIFN treatment. We have also found that human TNF-α, but not human IFN-γ, IL-1β or IL-4, significantly increases binding of CTLA-4-Ig to PAEC [12] (Fig. 2).

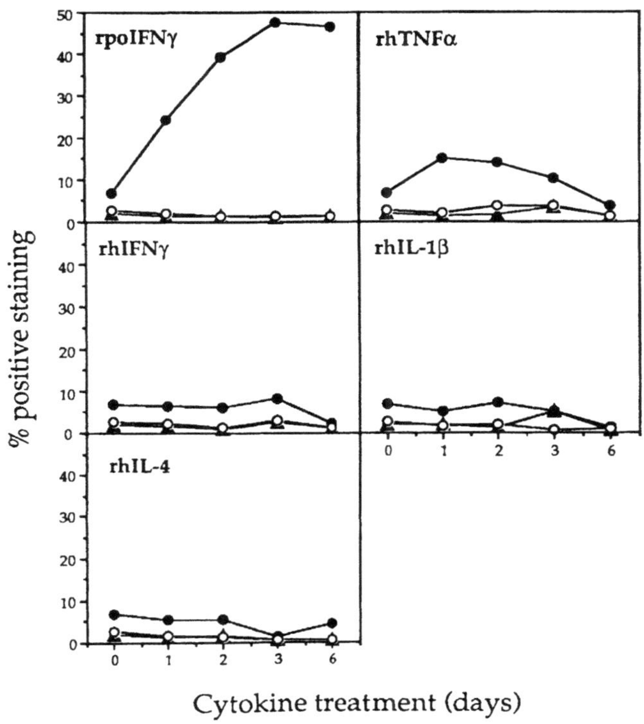

Fig. 2. Pig aortic endothelial cells (PAEC) were either untreated or treated with rpo interferon (*IFN*)-γ, rhIFN-γ, rh tumor necrosis factor (TNF)-α, rh interleukin (IL)-1β, and rhIL-4 for 0–6 days, and flow cytometric analysis was used to assess the percentage of cells binding CTLA-4-Ig (*black circles*) or control Ig (*white circles*). *Black triangles,* negative control. Representative of three experiments. (From [12], with permission)

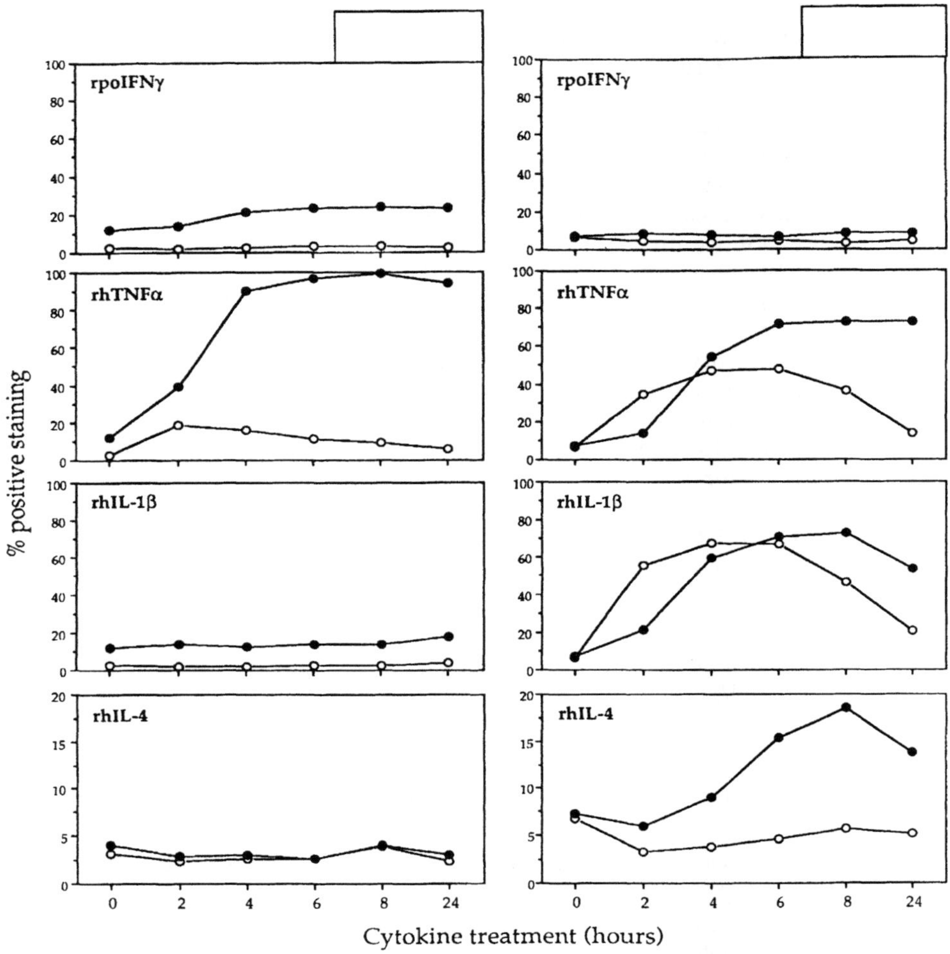

Fig. 3. Comparison of vascular cell adhesion molecule (VCAM)-1 (*black circles*) and E selectin (*white circles*) expression on pig aortic endothelial cells (PAEC, *left*) and human umbilical vein endothelial cells (HUVEC, *right*) in response to stimulation by human cytokines. PAEC and HUVEC were either untreated or treated with rpo interferon (*IFN*)-γ, rh tumor necrosis factor (*TNF*)-α, rh interleukin (*IL*)-1β, and rhIL-4 over a period of 24h; samples were taken at 2-h intervals up to 8h, and at 24h. Flow cytometric analysis was carried out, and the results are expressed as the percentage of positive cells binding monoclonal antibody (mAb). The mAbs used were: 8.1F8 (anti-porcine VCAM-1), 1.4C3 (anti-human VCAM-1), and 1.2B6 (anti-porcine/human E selectin). Representative of three experiments. (From [12], with permission)

Expression of endothelial leukocyte adhesion molecule (ELAM)-1 and vascular cell adhesion molecule (VCAM)-1 is essential for adhesion of neutrophils and mononuclear cells to endothelial cells, respectively. These antigens are not constitutively expressed on human endothelial cells but are unregulated by TNF-α, IL-1β (in the case of ELAM-1) and TNF-α, IL-1β, and IL-4 (in the case of

VCAM-1; Fig. 3). The only human cytokine found to upregulate porcine ELAM-1 and VCAM-1 was again TNF-α [12] (Fig. 3).

The consistent finding of our studies has been that rhuTNF-α, but not human IL-1β, IL-4, or IFN-γ, cause upregulation of SLA class I and class II molecules, upregulation of B7 receptors, and induction of VCAM-1 and ELAM-1. It appears, therefore, that PAEC do not have receptors for human cytokines IFN-γ, IL-1β, and IL-4, and that TNF-α is likely to be the most important inflammatory cytokine in relation to a xenograft. The cross-reactivity of human TNF with porcine tissues is not surprising; comparison of nucleotide sequences of the human and porcine gene show 85% sequence homology [15], and a number of studies have shown effects of rhTNF-α on pig vasculature after infusion in vivo [16] and on porcine smooth muscle cells in vitro [17]. Transfection experiments [18] have shown that p55 is the active component of the TNF receptor on PAEC.

There are good reasons to believe that upregulation of these molecules has functional consequences. Tsang et al. [19] have shown 71% nucleotide homology between porcine and human E selectin, and that a porcine E selectin immunoglobulin chimeric molecule binds to both porcine and human neutrophils. Similarly, the porcine VCAM-1 molecule identified using mAb 8.1F8 (Fig. 3) has been shown to have 77% homology with human VCAM-1 [20]. Mueller et al. [21] have shown that porcine VCAM -1 is a ligand for human VLA-4 found on human monocytes and lymphocytes.

T Cell Response to Porcine Endothelium

As explained above, it is to be expected that porcine xenoantigens can be recognized *indirectly*, i.e., when presented in recipient APC to recipient T cells. It is therefore not surprising that coculture of human peripheral blood mononuclear cells (PBMC), a mixture of lymphocytes and monocytes, and porcine endothelium results in proliferation of PBMC [7, 22]. Much more important is whether highly purified T lymphocytes, in the absence of recipient monocytes, proliferate in response to porcine endothelial cells. In this laboratory, we have stringently purified human $CD4^+$ and $CD8^+$ T cells using positive selection on antibody-coated magnetic beads [7]; residual DR^+ cells are then removed by complement-mediated cytolysis using anti-DR antibody. The cells are shown to be free of contaminating monocytes by flow cytometry and by the absence of proliferation to the monocyte-dependent mitogen phytohemagglutinin. For comparison with human endothelial cells, our laboratory has used the human endothelial cell line Eahy.926.

Human PBMC, $CD4^+$, and $CD8^+$ T cells were cocultured with untreated and species-specific IFN-γ-treated PAEC or human endothelial cells for 3–8 days. T cell proliferation was assessed every day by uptake of [^{3}H]thymidine [7] (Fig. 4). The endothelial cells had been pretreated with mitomycin C to prevent them proliferating in vitro. It can be seen that, as expected, PBMC proliferated in response to both treated and untreated endothelial cells. Interestingly, $CD4^+$ T cells gave a strong proliferative response to PAEC regardless of whether they had been pretreated with rpoIFN-γ. In contrast , but as previously reported

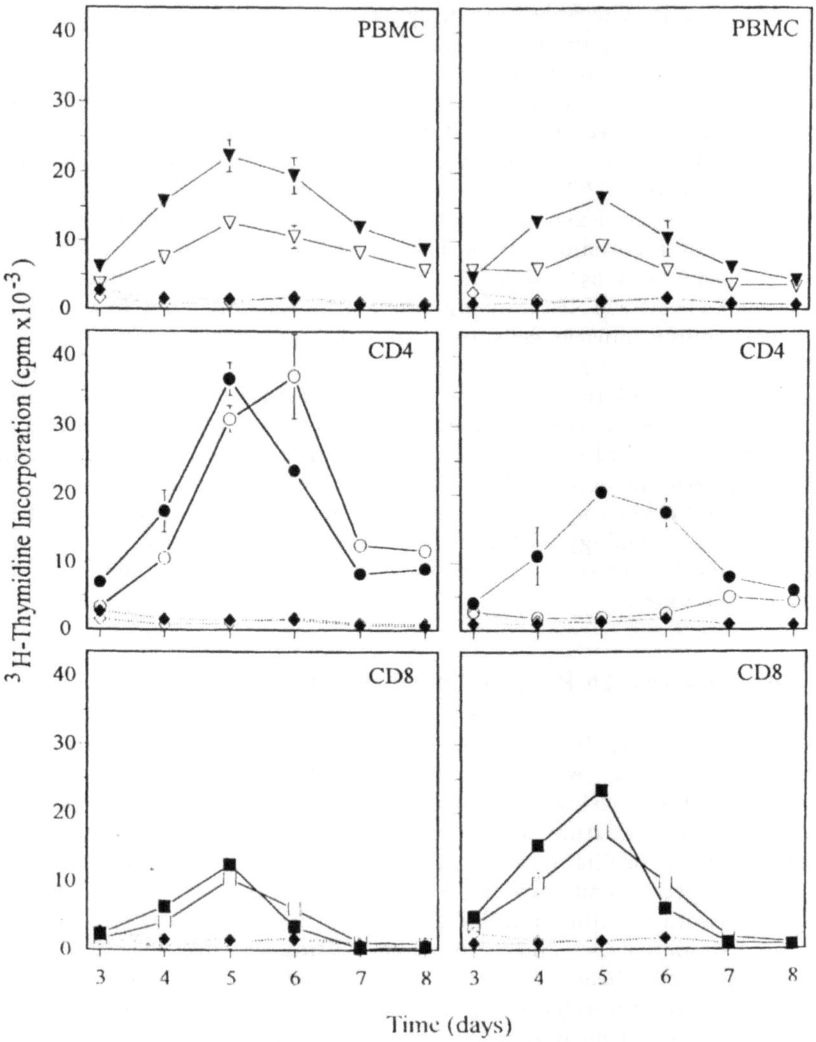

Fig. 4. Proliferative response of peripheral blood mononuclear cell (*PBMC, triangles*), $CD4^+$ T cells (*circles*), and $CD8^+$ T cells (*squares*) to untreated (*open symbols*) and rpo interferon (IFN)-γ-treated (*closed symbols*) xenogeneic pig aortic endothelial cells (PAEC, *left*) and untreated (*open symbols*) and rhuIFNγ-treated (*closed symbols*) allogeneic EAhy.926 (*right*). Background proliferation of stimulators alone (*diamonds*) is shown on each graph. Proliferation of responders alone never exceeded 600 cpm. Responders at 2×10^5 cells/well, and all stimulators at 5×10^4 cells/well. Proliferation was measured by uptake of [^{3}H]thymidine on days 3–8 after initiation of culture. Results are expressed as mean cpm of triplicate wells ± standard deviation. Representative of five experiments. (From [7], with permission)

[6], $CD4^+$ T cells only proliferate to rhuIFN-γ-treated endothelial cells. $CD8^+$ T cells also proliferated in response to untreated and IFN-γ-treated PAEC.

That the strong response of $CD4^+$ T cells to untreated PAEC was due to constitutive expression of SLA class II antigens was supported by experiments which showed proliferation to untreated (and rpoIFN-γ-treated) PAEC was significantly inhibited by mAbs DA6.231, Th16B, and MSA3, all of which bind to pig SLA class II molcules [7] (Fig. 5). In contrast, L243 (specific for HLA-DR) , which fails to bind to PAEC, did not inhibit human T cell proliferation to PAEC. Rollins et al. [22] also demonstrated that highly-purified CD4 and $CD8^+$ T cells proliferated to untreated PAEC, and that the $CD8^+$ T cell response was inhibited by mAbs to MHC class I antigens. This is in contrast to Murray et al. [6], who required treatment of PAEC with species-specific IFN-γ to cause proliferation. That the $CD4^+$ T cell proliferation was inhibited by anti-SLA class II [7, 10] supports the concept of direct recognition of SLA class II by human T cells. There is also evidence of indirect recognition. Valee et al. [9], using PAEC which do not constitutively express class II reported a strong proliferative response by PBMC, which is reduced when monocytes are removed. The proliferative response of T cells to PAEC is accompanied by massive secretion of IL-2 [7, 10]. Interestingly , the levels secreted are approximately ten times more than elicited by human endothelial cells.

Secondary Signals

An important difference between the T cell response to porcine and human endothelial cells is the dependence of the costimulatory molecules CD28/CTLA-4. Despite being an essential molecule for the allogeneic mixed lymphocyte response [14], human endothelial cell have no known B7 receptors [10, 23]. It was therefore surprising to discover that CTLA-4-Ig does inhibit, significantly but partially, the proliferative response of CD4+T cells to PAEC [7] (Fig. 6). However, this is consistent with the results showing expression of B7 or B7-like receptors on untreated and IFN-treated PAEC [7, 10]. Restifo et al. (24) have also concluded that human T cells react with xenogeneic B7 receptors, and showed the response of human T cells to porcine PBL was inhibited by CTLA-4-Ig. That the proliferative response and IL-2 production are only partially inhibited by high concentrations of CTLA-4-Ig [12] suggests that other secondary signals must be involved. Inhibitory studies using antibodies against CD2 and LFA-1 [10, 22] show these to be important secondary interactions.

Response of Human T Cells to Porcine Monocytes/Macrophages

The classical mixed lymphocyte response, whereby PBMC from one individual are mixed with PBMC or splenocytes from another individual, has been reproduced using human PBMC mixed with porcine PBMC or splenocytes [25–30]. All agree that there is a vigorous human anti-pig proliferative response, which is inhibited by mAbs against porcine DR and DQ antigens [25, 26], the kinetics

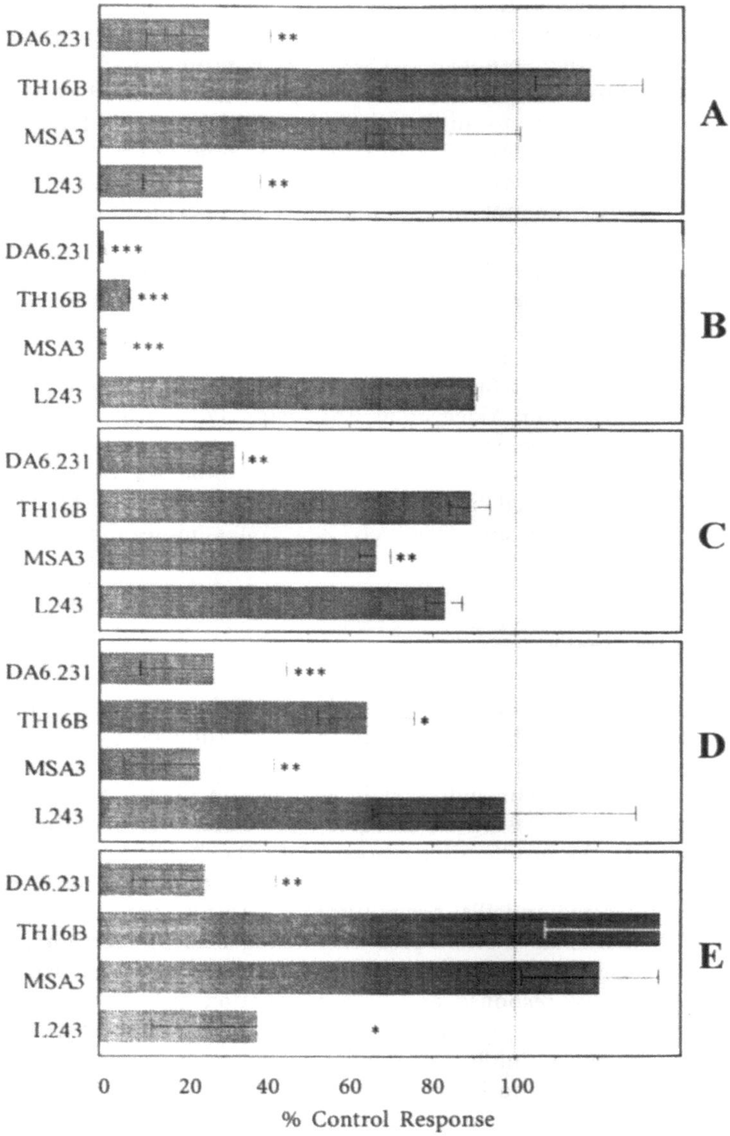

Fig. 5. Proliferative response of CD4$^+$ T cells to **A** human spleen, **B** pig spleen, **C** untreated pig aortic endothelial cells (PAEC), **D** rpo interferon (IFN)-γ-treated PAEC, and **E** rhuIFNγ-treated human umbilical vein endothelial cells (HUVEC). Human and pig splenocytes were plated at 10^5 cells/well, endothelial cells at 5×10^4 cells/well. Responder cells were added at 2×10^5 cells/well. Proliferation measured at day 6 by uptake of [^{3}H]thymidine. Wells either contained no monoclonal antibody (mAb) during this culture period or were cultured in the presence of DA6.231 (at 1:300 and 1:150), TH16B (final concentration, 2 μg/ml), MSA3 (final concentration, 2 μg/ml), or L243 (at 1:50). Counts from experimental triplicate wells are expressed as a percentage ± standard deviation of those found in control (no mAb) triplicate wells. Representative of three experiments . ***$p \leq 0.001$, **$p \leq 0.01$, *$p \leq 0.05$. (From [7], with permission

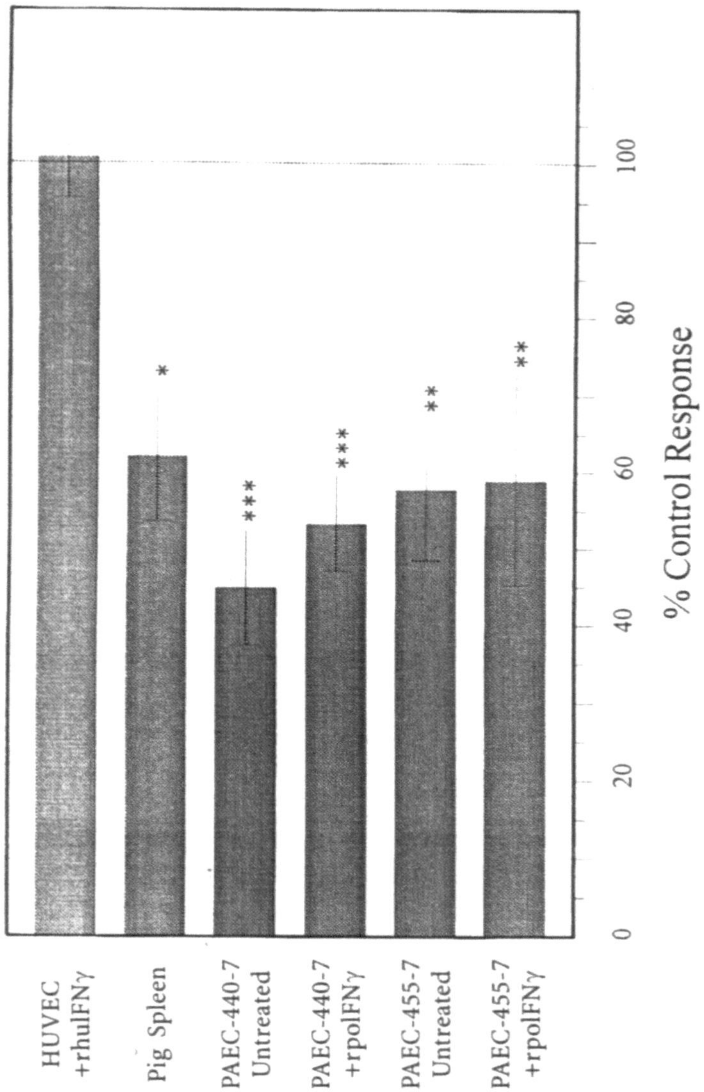

Fig. 6. Effect of CTLA-4-Ig on day 6 proliferative response of $CD4^+$ T cells to rhu interferon (*IFN*)-γ-treated human umbilical vein endothelial cells (*HUVEC*), pig splenocytes, untreated or rpoIFNγ-treated pig aortic endothelial cells (*PAEC*; two lines, PAEC-440-7 and PAEC -455-7). CTLA-4-Ig or control Ig were added at the start of coculture. Counts from experimental wells are expressed as a percentage ± standard deviation of those found in wells containing control Ig. $^{***}p \leq 0.001$, $^{**}p \leq 0.01$, $^{*}p \leq 0.05$. Representative of four experiments. (From [7], with permission)

and strength of the response being similar to the allogeneic MLR [28]. The relative contribution of direct and indirect pathways has been assessed by depleting responder and/or stimulator populations of APC [26, 30, 31]; Yamada [26] found that if APC were depleted from both responder and stimulator, there was no response. APC in the stimulator alone caused direct recognition, whereas APC in the responder alone allowed indirect recognition. Herlinger and Plaess [30, 31] also concluded that both pathways allowed responsiveness of human T cells to porcine xenoantigens.

Dorling and colleagues [32–34] have used porcine alveolar dendritic cells as a method of assessing the relative contributions of direct and indirect recognition to T cell responsiveness. They found that freshly prepared alveolar cells (expressing low levels of SLA antigens and no B7 receptors) are unable to directly stimulate purified T cells, but in the presence of responder APC, 1/24 000–1/150 000 T cells recognize processed xenoantigens. In contrast, when the cells are allowed to mature overnight, they upregulate SLA class I and class II antigens, become positive for CTLA-4-Ig, and now produce vigorous proliferation of purified T cells , with a high frequency of 1/3500–1/13 000 T cells directly recognizing SLA-DR antigens. It is likely that this response is dependent on B7 receptors.

As with porcine endothelial cells, a number of different molecules on human T cells (CD2, ICAM-1 , and CD28) appear to interact with their respective ligands on porcine APC (LFA-1, LFA-3, B7 receptors) to give the secondary signal necessary for proliferation [24, 27, 30]. As yet , there is no discrimination between different molecules controlling direct and indirect recognition. The human anti-pig mixed leukocyte response results in cytokine release including IL-2 [29, 31], Il-4 and IFN-γ [29] in similar quantities to that produced from allostimulation.

Cytotoxicity

Coculture of human PBL with porcine PBL or splenocytes results in production of primed cytotoxic T cells which can lyse 51 Cr-labeled porcine target cells [35, 36]. However, unprimed PBL also lyse porcine PBL [25, 35], and this has been shown to be due to NK activity.

Comment

Human T cells recognize porcine xenoantigens present on endothelial cells and dendritic cells, resulting in vigorous cell proliferation and secretion of cytokines. Recognition occurs through direct and indirect pathways. Thus, when SLA class II is constitutively present on endothelial cells, direct recognition of these antigens occurs. Alternatively, porcine endothelial antigens can be processed and presented indirectly by autologous human monocytes . There is evidence for cross-species reactivity between some human cytokines (in particular TNF-α) and ligands (human CD28) for receptors on pig cells. It is likely that transplantation of vascularized porcine grafts into humans will result in a vigorous T cell response, equivalent in vigour to allogeneic graft rejection.

References

1. Benichou G, Takizawa PA, Olson CA, McMillan M, Sercarz EE. Donor major histocompatibility complex (MHC) peptides are presented by recipient MHC molecules during graft rejejection. J.Exp.Med., 1992, 175: 305
2. Pober JS, Orozz C, Rose ML, Savage CO. Overview: can graft endothelial cells initiate a host antigraft response? Transplantation, in press
3. Lechler RI, Batchelor JR. Restoration of immunogenicity to passenger cell depleted kidney allografts by the addition of donor strain dendritic cells. J. Exp. Med. 1982, 155: 31
4. Rose ML, Coles MI, Griffin RJ, Pomerance A, Yacoub MH. Expression of class I and class II major histocompatibility antigens in normal and transplanted human heart. Transplantation, 1986, 41: 776
5. Pescovitz MD, Sachs DH, Lunney JK, Hsu SM. Localisation of class II MHC antigens on porcine renal vascular endothelium. Transplantation, 1983, 37: 627
6. Savage COS, Hughes CCW, McIntyre BW, Picard JK, Pober JS. Human CD4+ T cells proliferate to HLA DR+ allogeneic vascular endothelium: identification of accessory interactions. Transplantation, 1993, 56: 128
7. Bravery CA, Batten P, Yacoub MH, Rose ML. Direct recognition of SLA and HLA-like class II antigens on porcine endothelium by human T cells results in T cell activation and release of IL-2. Transplantation, 1995, 60:1024
8. Page CS, Rose ML, Yacoub MH, Pigott R. Antigenic heterogeneity of vascular endothelium. Am J Pathol. 1992, 141: 673
9. Vallee I, Watier H, Thibault G, et al. Evidence of noninvolvement of swine MHC class II in the in vitro proliferative response of human lymphocytes to porcine endothelial cells. Transplantation1995, 59: 897
10. Murray AG, Khodadoust MM, Pober JS, Bothwell ALM. Porcine aortic endothelial cells activate human T cells: direct presentation of MHC antigens and costimulation by ligands for human CD2 and CD28. Immunity 1994, 1: 57
11. Watier H, Vallee I, Thibault G, et al. Effect of human inflammatory cytokines on porcine endothelial cell MHC molecule expression: Unique role for TNFα in MHC class II induction. Transplant Proc 1994, 26: 1152
12. Batten P, Yacoub MH, Rose ML. Effect of human cytokines (IFNγ, TNFα, IL-1β, Il-4) on porcine endothelial cells: induction of MHC and adhesion molecules and functional significance of these changes. Immunology 1996, 87:127
13. Collins T, Korman AJ, Wake CT, et al. Immune interferon activates multiple class II major histocompatibility complex genes and the associated invariant chain in human endothelial cells and dermal fibroblasts. Proc. Natl. Acad. Sci USA. 1984, 81: 4917
14. June CH, Bluestone JA, Nadler LM, Thompson CB. The B7 and CD28 receptor families. Immunology Today, 1994, 15: 321
15. Pauli U, Beutler B, Petrhans E. Porcine tumour necrosis factor alpha; cloning with the polymerase chain reaction and determination of the nucleotide sequence. Gene, 1989, 81: 185
16. Kruse-Elliott KT, Pino VM, Olson NC. Effect of PAF receptor antagonism on cardiopulmonary alterations during coinfusion of TNFα and IL-1α in pigs. Am J Physiol, 1993, 264: 175

17. Shibano T, Vanhoutte PM. Induction of NO production by TNFα and lipopolysaccharide in porcine coronary arteries without endothelium. Am.. J Physiol, 1993, 263: 403
18. Ferran C, Cooper JT, Brostjan C, et al. Expression of a truncated form of the human p55 TNF-receptor in bovine aortic endothelial cells renders them resistant to TNF. Presented at the Third International Congress of Xenotransplantation, Boston, 1995
19. Tsang YTM, Stephens PE, Licence ST, et al. Porcine E-selectin: cloning and functional characterisation . Immunology 1995, 85: 140
20. Tsang YTM, Haskard DO, Robinson MK. Cloning and expression kinetics of porcine vascular cell adhesion molecule. Biochem Biophys Res Comm 1994, 201: 805
21. Mueller J., Evans M, Matis L, Elliot E. Porcine vascular cell adhesion molecule mediates endothelial cell adhesiveness to human T cells. Presented at the Third International Congress for Xenotransplantation, Boston, 1995
22. Rollins SA, Kennedy SP, Chodera AJ, et al. Evidence that activation of human T cells by porcine endothelium involves direct recognition of porcine SLA and costimulation by porcine ligands for LFA-1 and CD2. Transplantation 1994, 57: 1709
23. Page C, Thompson C, Yacoub MH, Rose ML. Human endothelial stimulation of allogeneic T cells via a CTLA-4 independent pathway. Transpl Immunol 1994, 2: 342
24. Restifo AC, Woodward MA, Tran HM, et al. Cross-species binding of murine CTLA4-Fc and potential for the study of cross-species CD29-B7 interactions. Presented at the Third International Congress for Xenotransplantation, Boston, 1995
25. Kirk AD, Li RA, Kinch MS, et al. The human antiporcine cellular repetoire. Transplantation 1993, 55: 924
26. Yamada K, Sachs DH, DerSimonian H. Direct and indirect recognition of pig class II antigens by human T cells. Transplant Proc. 1995, 27: 258
27. Xu Y, White-Schaf ME, Latinne D, et al. Induction of human anti-porcine T cell hyporesponsiveness by pertubation of human CD2. Presented at the Third International Congress for Xenotransplantation, Boston, 1995.
28. Saetre AM, Lillevang ST, Kemp E, Kristensen T. In vitro comparison of human xenogeneic and allogeneic cellular immune responses using serum free media. Presented at the Third International Congress for Xenotransplantation, Boston, 1995
29. Heiser A, Breitkreuz A, Sun Y, Muller-Ruchholtz W. In vitro studies of IL-2, IL-4 and IFNγ and their receptors on human lymphocytes stimulated with xenoeneic porcine lymphocytes. Presented at the Third International Congress for Xenotransplantation, Boston, 1995
30. Herrlinger K, Eckstein V, Muller-Ruchholtz W, Ulrichs K. Human T cell activation is mediated predominantly by direct recognition of porcine SLA and involves accessory molecule interaction of ICAM-1/LFA-1 and CD2/LFA3. Presented at the Third International Congress for Xenotransplantation, Boston, 1995
31. Plaess HCC, Kirby JA, Forsythe JLR, Proud G, Taylor RMR. An investigation of porcine xenoantigen recognition. Presented at the Third International Congress for Xenotransplantation, Boston, 1995
32. Dorling A, Binns R, Lechler RI. Significant indirect recognition of porcine xenoantigens in the primary xenogeneic MLR. Apparant priming of adult humans against pig antigens. Presented at the Third International Congress for Xenotransplantation, Boston, 1995

33. Dorling A, Binns R, Lechler RI. Examination of the direct human T cell xenoresponse against porcine dendritic cells and identification of inefficient SLA-DR recognition. Presented at the Third International Congress for Xenotransplantation, Boston, 1995
34. Dorling A, Binns R, Lechler RI. Isolation of porcine dendritic cell population for use in assessment of human T cell anti-pig xenoresponses. Presented at the Third International Congress for Xenotransplantation, Boston, 1995
35. Cunningham, AC, Butler TJ, Kirby JA. Demonstration of direct xenorecognition of porcine cells by human cytotoxic T lymphocytes. Immunology 1994, 81: 268
36. Chan DV, Auchincloss H. Human anti-pig cell mediated cytotoxicity in vitro may have as many as three different components. Presented at the Third International Congress for Xenotransplantation, Boston, 1995

14 Cellular Interactions in Discordant Xenotransplantation

S.A. Rollins and L.A. Matis

Introduction

The advent of effective strategies to eliminate the hyperacute rejection of porcine organs has placed greater focus on the human anti-porcine cellular interactions that may contribute to discordant xenograft rejection. A better understanding of these issues will facilitate the development and implementation of therapeutic approaches to achieve long-term xenograft survival.

Adhesion Molecules and the Acute Inflammatory Response

The molecular interactions that occur between donor organ vascular endothelium and circulating recipient leukocytes are key to the initiation of acute cellular graft rejection. In the allotransplant setting, the adhesion molecules expressed by vascular endothelium are well characterized and have provided valuable insight for the identification of homologous molecules on porcine endothelium. Leukocyte adhesion to allograft vascular endothelium is mediated by several adhesion molecules including E selectin, P selectin, vascular adhesion molecule (VCAM)-1, intercellular adhesion molecule (ICAM)-1, and CD58 [1, 2]. A three-step model of leukocyte adhesion to endothelium in vivo has been proposed (for a review, see [2]). The initial binding event involves interactions between endothelial cell selectins (E selectin and P selectin) and their ligands on leukocytes. These interactions allow leukocytes to roll on the endothelium, but do not support firm adhesion. The second step involves the activation of rolling leukocytes by chemokines or cell surface proteins such as CD31. Finally, stable leukocyte adhesion to endothelium is mediated by interactions between leukocyte lymphocyte function-associated antigen (LFA)-1, very late activation antigen (VLA)-4 and their respective ligands, ICAM-1 and VCAM-1, on vascular endothelium.

The importance of these adhesive interactions in the cellular rejection of allotransplants has been demonstrated in vivo (for a review, see [2]). For example, treatment of recipients with a combination of blocking monoclonal antibodies to LFA-1 and ICAM-1 leads to long-term survival of mouse heart allografts as well as tolerance induction [3]. Similar results have been achieved using functionally blocking antibodies against VCAM-1 [4]. Additionally, clinical trials with human allogeneic kidney grafts suggest that monoclonal antibodies directed against the adhesion pair LFA-1/ICAM-1 may significantly attenuate cellular allograft rejection [5].

Recent experiments exploring potential pig-to-human xenotransplantation suggest that many of the receptor–ligand interactions between leukocytes and endothelial cells that mediate cellular allograft rejection may also play a key role in cellular xenograft rejection. These studies demonstrate that porcine homologues of human endothelial cell adhesion molecules retain the capacity to bind to human leukocytes, and therefore may account for the significant leukocyte infiltrates that are observed during the earliest stages of hyperacute and acute xenograft rejection.

The first study to examine the adhesive interactions between human leukocytes and porcine endothelial cells revealed that activation of human complement on the surface of porcine aortic endothelial cells (PAEC) resulted in the deposition of iC3b, which mediates adhesion via interaction with the human leukocyte antigen CD11b/CD18 [6]. More recently, we have extended these studies to examine the relative contribution of early (iC3b) and late (C5b-9) complement component deposition to leukocyte adhesion [7]. These studies revealed that activation of human complement on the surface of PAEC rapidly (15–30 min) induced human neutrophil adhesion. This binding was, in part, mediated by surface-bound C3b; however, 50 % of the binding was found to be C5b-9 dependent. Additionally, C5b-9-dependent adhesion was blocked by the treatment of neutrophils with sialidase, suggesting that human C5b-9 deposition results in the expression of a P selectin homologue on the PAEC surface.

P Selectin

P selectin is an inducible endothelial cell surface glycoprotein that mediates the adhesion of neutrophils, monocytes, eosinophils, natural killer (NK) cells, and a subset of T cells to activated endothelium [8]. Structurally, P selectin belongs to a family of adhesion molecules termed "selectins" that also includes E selectin and L selectin [8]. These molecules are characterized by common structural features, such as an NH_2 terminal lectin-like domain, an epidermal growth factor (EGF) domain, and a discreet number of complement repeat modules (approximately 60 amino acids each) similar to those found in certain complement-binding proteins. Surface expression of P selectin is induced on human endothelium in response to histamine, thrombin, and the terminal complement proteins, C5b-9 [8]. Recently, the human leukocyte receptor for human P selectin has been identified and found to contain sialic acid (sialyl Lewis^x, and sialyl Lewis^a) as a necessary component for interaction with the P selectin protein [9].

There are several lines of evidence that point to P selectin as a likely contributor to leukocyte adhesion during hyperacute xenograft rejection. First, in vivo models of lung inflammation have demonstrated that intravascular complement activation leads to rapid expression of P selectin on platelets and endothelium and that blockade of P selectin-mediated adhesion decreases neutrophil binding and pulmonary damage [10]. Second, xenogeneic organs transplanted into C6-deficient recipients are not hyperacutely rejected and leukocyte infiltration is significantly delayed, suggesting that the inability to generate C5b-9 in this setting prevents the rapid upregulation of P selectin and therefore leukocyte adhesion

[11]. Finally, in vivo studies in a discordant rodent xenotransplant model have shown that, within minutes of revascularization, P selectin is expressed on donor organ vascular endothelium in concert with activated complement components [12].

In order to functionally characterize the porcine P selectin homologue, the full-length porcine P selectin cDNA was isolated [7]. The molecule contained an open reading frame encoding 646 amino acids with 81% identity to human P selectin. Transfection of COS cells with the porcine P selectin cDNA resulted in surface expression of the protein and markedly increased the binding of human neutrophils to these cells. As was demonstrated for the C5b-9-dependent binding of PAEC, the binding of both purified soluble and COS-expressed porcine P selectin to human neutrophils was blocked by edetic acid (EDTA) or treatment of human leukocytes with sialidase. Finally, treatment of PAEC with whole human serum, but not C8-deficient human serum, resulted in the rapid expression of porcine P selectin on the cell surface. Taken together, these data show that porcine P selectin mediates the binding of human neutrophils to PAEC in vitro. Further, these data suggest that deposition of C5b-9 during hyperacute rejection results in the expression of porcine P selectin which may, in addition to iC3b, contribute to the rapid adhesion of neutrophils to porcine xenografts.

E Selectin

In addition to P selectin, a second selectin, E selectin, may also play a role in xenograft rejection. E selectin is a cytokine-inducible endothelial cell surface glycoprotein that mediates the adhesion of neutrophils, monocytes, eosinophils, NK cells, and a subset of T cells to activated endothelium [13]. The expression of E selectin is induced on human endothelium in response to interleukin (IL)-1, tumor necrosis factor (TNF)-α, or bacterial lipopolysaccharide (LPS) through transcriptional upregulation [14]. Recently, the human leukocyte receptor for human E selectin has also been identified [15]. As was demonstrated for P selectin, these studies revealed that this receptor contained sialic acid (sialyl Lewis^x, and sialyl Lewis^a) as a necessary component for interaction with the E selectin protein. In addition, E selectin expression is selectively upregulated on the vascular endothelium of renal and cardiac tissue during acute rejection [16]. E selectin expression correlates with the early course of cellular rejection and corresponds to the migration of inflammatory cells into the graft tissue. Taken together, these studies provide evidence that cytokine-induced expression of E selectin on donor organ endothelium may contribute to the binding and subsequent transmigration of inflammatory cells into the graft tissue, and thereby play an important role in acute cellular allograft rejection.

In order to define whether E selectin may play a role in the human anti-porcine cellular response, porcine E selectin was cloned and characterized [17]. Isolation of the porcine E selectin cDNA revealed an open reading frame encoding 485 amino acids with 75% identity to human E selectin. Northern blot analysis showed that untreated or human IL-1 treated PAEC did not express detectable levels of porcine E selectin mRNA, while treatment of PAEC with human

TNF-α resulted in high levels of porcine E selectin mRNA. Expression of porcine E selectin on the surface of COS cells resulted in a tenfold increase in binding to human neutrophils. As was demonstrated for neutrophil-PAEC adhesion, pretreatment of human neutrophils with sialidase or EDTA completely blocked adhesion to porcine E selectin-transfected COS cells, confirming that this interaction was divalent cation-dependent and that sialic acid is a necessary component of the porcine E selectin receptor on human leukocytes. Taken together, these data establish that porcine E selectin mediates adhesive interactions between PAEC and human leukocytes. Further, these experiments suggest that release of human TNF-α during the inflammatory response to porcine xenografts may promote cellular interactions that contribute to xenograft rejection.

Vascular Cell Adhesion Molecule

In addition to the porcine selectins, we have cloned and functionally characterized the porcine homologue of vascular cell adhesion molecule or VCAM [18]. VCAM is a cytokine-inducible adhesion molecule that is predominantly expressed on endothelial cells [19]. VCAM interacts with VLA-4, a β_1-integrin found on all peripheral blood leukocytes except neutrophils [20]. Under normal conditions, VCAM expression is minimal or absent and can be induced by cytokines such as TNF-α or IL-1 [19]. Thus VCAM plays a role in the adhesion of leukocytes to endothelium during inflammatory responses.

The role of VCAM in allograft rejection is well established. In murine cardiac allograft models, functionally blocking antibodies against VCAM have significantly attenuated the cellular immune response resulting in prolonged graft survival [4]. To determine whether porcine VCAM retains the capacity to bind to VLA-4 on human leukocytes, porcine VCAM was functionally characterized [18]. Both soluble and surface-expressed forms of recombinant porcine VCAM were capable of binding to VLA-4 on human lymphoid cells. Moreover, functionally blocking monoclonal antibodies (mAbs) raised against the recombinant porcine molecule were able to block the adhesion of human lymphoid cells to cytokine-activated porcine endothelial cells. These data suggest that porcine VCAM retains the capacity to interact with human VLA-4 and therefore could play a role in the human anti-porcine cellular immune response.

In summary, we have identified and characterized three porcine endothelial cell adhesion molecules (P and E selectin, VCAM) that retain the capacity to interact with their respective ligands on human leukocytes. Our data, when viewed in light of the role of these molecules in allograft rejection, suggest that these molecules could play a critical role in the initial attachment, adhesion and transmigration of leukocytes into a porcine xenograft, and therefore represent attractive targets for therapeutic intervention.

Cellular Immunity in Xenotransplantation

Strength of the Cellular Response

Consideration of the various components of a cellular immune response initially led to the speculation that xenogeneic cellular reactivity would prove to be substantially weaker than corresponding allogeneic responses [21]. First, the strength of a primary alloreactive response is thought to directly reflect the fact that the T cell receptor repertoire is selected to recognize syngeneic major histocompatibility complex (MHC) molecules. Thus a population of receptors with intrinsic specificity for intraspecies MHC molecules would consequently manifest less cross-reactivity with more distantly related xenogeneic MHC molecules, resulting in a lower precursor frequency of T cells specific for xenogeneic MHC. Second, in addition to T cell receptor engagement, activation of T lymphocytes requires appropriate costimulation via cell surface receptors such as CD4, CD8, CD28, CD2, and LFA-1. In this light, xenogeneic responses could be attenuated due to the inability of such costimulatory molecules to interact with their homologous ligands across the species barrier. Similarly, T cell responses are further enhanced and magnified following the elaboration by antigen-presenting cells (APCs) of various cytokines (e.g., IL-12). The failure of such soluble factors to signal T cells of a disparate species could further diminish the magnitude of the resulting cellular response.

Studies examining the strength of xenogeneic cellular responses in a variety of T cell/APC species combinations have yielded mixed results, probably reflecting differential engagement of the various components required to elicit such responses [21]. It is clear, however, that for some species combinations, including the clinically relevant human anti-porcine response, primary cellular xenoreactivity is at least as potent as that observed for the corresponding alloreactive response.

In vitro studies of the primary human anti-porcine xenogeneic immune response have suggested that, as for allografts, acute cellular rejection of porcine xenografts will be mediated predominantly by MHC-specific T lymphocytes. Results from several groups of investigators have clearly demonstrated potent xenogeneic mixed lymphocyte responses (MLRs) when human T cells are cultured in the presence of porcine APC populations – either endothelial cells or peripheral blood APCs [22–26]. Analysis of the human anti-porcine mixed lymphocyte reaction has been performed using pig peripheral blood APCs, purified dendritic cell populations, or endothelial cells as a source of stimulator cells. Such studies have uniformly demonstrated that human T cells, both CD4 and CD8 subsets, can be directly activated by porcine APCs [23–25]. Detailed examination of the components of this response have shown remarkable preservation of virtually all intercellular molecular interactions across the species barrier. Thus, evidence has shown that human CD4, CD8, CD2, LFA-1, VLA-4, and CD28 all functionally engage porcine ligands; in turn, blockade of these pathways can inhibit human anti-porcine cellular interactions [22–26]. Similarly, human TNF appears competent to activate porcine endothelial cells, although human IL-1 and interferon-γ do not.

Pathways of the Cellular Response

Following transplantation of any organ graft to a recipient, two distinct pathways of host cellular response may ensue. The first, or "direct", pathway refers to the activation of responding host T cells following direct recognition of graft MHC and non-MHC antigens. This pathway has generally been considered to predominate in the acute cellular rejection phase of an allograft. The second, or "indirect", pathway is activated as a result of processing of donor graft-derived peptides (which may be of either MHC or non-MHC origin), which in turn are "re-presented" by MHC molecules on recipient APCs. Given the sheer number of potential peptide epitopes that may be derived from the numerous polymorphic proteins expressed on a xenograft, it has been speculated that the indirect pathway would play a particularly important role in xenograft rejection. For example, the indirect pathway could still serve as the mode of in vivo xenograft rejection in those species combinations where molecular mismatches impair the direct activation of host T cells by donor APCs.

A number of studies have illustrated the complexity of in vivo mechanisms of graft rejection, and shown that both pathways may play a role in mediating rejection of both allografts and xenografts. For example, the rapid rejection of donor organs from MHC knockout mice transplanted into allogeneic recipients allowed Auchincloss and colleagues to conclude that the indirect pathway may play a significant role even in allograft rejection, and thus this pathway is not likely to represent a unique feature of cellular rejection of xenografts [21]. Nor, conversely, will the indirect pathway necessarily predominate in xenograft rejection. For example, Lenschow et al. [27] showed that rejection of xenogeneic islets by mice could be prevented by antibodies recognizing only donor B7 molecules, thus blocking only direct recognition of the islet graft by the recipient.

Moreover, evidence has been reported that the direct pathway can lead to xenograft rejection even in species combinations where a direct xeno-MLR response in vitro is weak or absent [21]. For example, although murine anti-porcine $CD4^+$ T cell-dependent MLRs are very weak in vitro, pig skin grafts are rapidly rejected by recipient mice in a CD4-dependent fashion, even in mice with no endogenous class II MHC expression, thus ruling out re-presentation of xenogeneic peptides on host MHC molecules as the mechanism of such in vivo rejection [21]. Thus, outcomes of in vivo transplant experiments cannot invariably be predicted from in vitro mixed lymphocyte reactions.

Analyses of the human anti-porcine xenogeneic response suggest that both direct and indirect pathways of recognition will have a role in the patient's cellular response to a pig organ. Studies with purified human T cell populations, including T cell clones, have clearly shown direct recognition of porcine class II and class I MHC molecules involving both T cell receptors and CD4 and CD8 molecules, and activation of these cells by porcine APCs. Although some conflicting data have been reported, several groups have found that the precursor frequency of human anti-porcine T cells equals, or even exceeds that of a corresponding allogeneic MLR [23]. On the other hand, clear evidence for a primary role of the indirect pathway in the human anti-porcine MLR has also been independently obtained. In one recent study, comparison of the magnitude of the human anti-porcine primary xeno MLR in the presence or absence (no indirect presentation) of class II-bearing human APCs suggested that approximately 25 % of the primary human anti-porcine response was due to the indirect pathway [25]. Others have observed that a strong primary component of the indirect pathway in the human anti-porcine xeno MLR is seen in T cells from adult individuals but not in peripheral T cells from umbilical cord blood [28]. This suggests that priming to pig antigens either directly or through cross-reactive determinants occurs throughout life, and would therefore be reflected in the cellular immune response to a porcine xenograft. The fact that the indirect response is mediated primarily by $CD4^+$ T cells suggests one reason why they play such a prominent role in cellular xenograft rejection.

Potential Immunosuppressive Mechanisms

Similarities between various aspects of the human anti-pig xeno MLR and a human allogeneic MLR suggest that immunosuppressive mechanisms that have proven so successful in clinical allogeneic organ transplantation might have similar utility in suppressing the acute cellular rejection of discordant xenografts. However, experience has repeatedly shown that extrapolation from preclinical in vitro analysis to the in vivo setting is often problematic. In fact, limited experience to date with organ transplant models across species barriers has indicated that prevention of cellular rejection with standard immunosuppressive modalities has proven to be difficult and may reflect more complex mechanisms than suggested by the experience with allografts [21]. For instance, there appears to be a uniquely critical role for the CD4 subset of T cells in xenograft rejection [21]. In addition, given the large number of polymorphic proteins expressed by a xenograft relative to an allograft, the induced humoral immune response may play an especially prominent role in xenograft rejection, requiring the implementation of strategies to inhibit host B cell responses. Finally, transplants across discordant species barriers may elicit an NK cell response to the graft, which is normally not a component of allogeneic transplantation. NK cells have clearly been observed in tissue sections of rejecting discordant xenografts. The recent identification of immunoglobulin-like receptors on human NK cells, whose class I MHC recognition on species homologous cells is required for appropriate down-regulation of NK function, offers the opportunity to rationally examine the potential activity of human NK cells in the setting of a porcine xenograft by testing whether such human NK receptors can recognize the appropriate homologous porcine class I MHC molecules [29].

Nevertheless, the xenograft setting also offers some unique therapeutic opportunities for ameliorating host anti-graft cellular immunity. For example, we have developed monoclonal antibodies specific for porcine adhesion molecules that block the interaction of human leukocytes with porcine endothelial cells or monocytes [18]. Clinically, such antibodies could be used to prevent leukocyte migration into the graft as well as subsequent activation. Furthermore, because such antibodies would recognize ligands expressed only on cells within the graft and not on host tissue, they represent a potential therapeutic modality to specifically block anti-graft immunity without any impairment of the host's immune response to other antigens. This would be a highly selective form of immunosuppression that is uniquely applicable to xenotransplantation.

Comment

Addressing the cellular components of the host response to a porcine xenograft will be critical for making xenotransplantation a clinical reality. With the anticipated near-term availability of organs resistant to hyperacute rejection [30], it should soon be possible to examine these issues more definitively using appropriate porcine-to-primate in vivo transplant models.

References

1. Bevilacqua M.P. (1993) Endothelial-leukocyte adhesion molecules. Ann. Rev. Immunol. 11:767
2. Inverardi L., Socci, C., Pardi, R. (1993) Leukocyte adhesion molecules in graft recognition and rejection. Xeno 1:35
3. Isobe M., Yagita, H., Hokumora, K., Ihara, R. (1992) Specific acceptance of cardiac allograft after treatment with antibodies to ICAM-1 and LFA-1. Science 255:1125
4. Orosz C.G., Ohyne, R.G., Pelletier, R.P., et al. (1993) Treatment with anti-vascular adhesion molecule-1 monoclonal antibody induces long term murine cardiac allograft acceptance. Transplantation 56:453
5. Le Mauff B., Hourmant, M., Rougier, J.P., et al. (1991) Effect of anti-LFA-1 (CD11a) monoclonal antibodies on acute rejection of human kidney transplants.Transplantation 52:291
6. Vercellotti G.M., Platt, J.L., Bach, F.L., Dalmasso, A.P. (1991) Neutrophil adhesion to xenogeneic endothelium via iC3b. J. Immunol. 146:730
7. Rollins S.A., Matis, L.A., Johnson, K.K., Li, L., Rother, R.P. (1996) Porcine P-selectin and surface bound C3b mediate human leukocyte binding to procine endothelium: Implications for hyperacute rejection. Submitted for publication
8. Bevilacqua M.P., Nelson, R.M. (1993) Selectins. J. Clin. Invest. 91:379
9. Asa D., Raycroft, L., Ma, L., et al. (1995) The P-selectin glycoprotein ligand functions as a common human leukocyte ligand for P and E-selectins. J. Biol Chem. 270:11662
10. Mulligan M.S., Paulson, J.C., Frees, S.D., et al. (1993) Protective effects of oligosaccharides in P-selectin-dependent lung injury. Nature 364:149
11. Brauer R.B., Baldwin, W.M., Daha, M.R., Pruitt, S.K., Sanfilippo, F. (1993) Use of C6-deficient rats to evaluate the mechanism of hyperacute rejection of discordant xenografts. J. Immunol 151:7240
12. Blakely M.L., Van Der Werf, W.J., Berndt, M.C., et al. (1994) Activation of intragraft endothelial and mononuclear cells during discordant xenograft rejection. Transplantation 58:1059
13. Bevilacqua, M.P., Stengelin, S., Gimbrone, M.A., Seed, B. (1989) Endothelial leukocyte adhesion molecule 1: An inducible receptor for neutrophils related to complement-regulatory poteins and lectins. Science 243:1160

14. Montgomery K.F., Osborn, L., Hession, C., et al. (1991) Activation of endothelial-leukocyte adhesion molecule-1 (ELAM-1) gene transcription. Proc. Natl. Acad. Sci. USA 88:6523
15. Berg E.L., Robinson, M.K., Mansson, O., Butcher, E.C., Magnani, J.L. (1991). A carbohydrate domain common to both sialyl Lea and sialyl Lex is recognized by the endothelial cell leukocyte adhesion molecule (ELAM-1). J. Biol. Chem. 23:14869
16. Allen M.D., T.O. McDonald, V.E. Himes, et al. (1993) E-selectin expression in human cardiac grafts with cellular rejection. Circulation88:243
17. Rollins S.A., Evans, M.J., Johnson, K.K., et al. (1994) Molecular and functional analysis of porcine E-selectin reveals a potential role in xenograft rejection. Biochem. Biophys. Res. Comm. 204:763
18. Mueller J.P., Evans, M.J., Cofiell, R., et al. (1995) Porcine vascular cell adhesion molecule (VCAM) mediates endothelial cell adhesion to human T cells.Transplantation 60:1299
19. Osborn L., Hession, C., Tizard, R., et al. (1989) Direct expression cloning of vascular cell adhesion molecule 1 (VCAM-1), a cytokine induced endothelial cell protein that binds to lymphocytes. Cell59:1203
20. Elices M.J., Osborn, L., Takada, Y., et al. (1990) VCAM-1 on activated endothelium interacts with leukocyte VLA-4 at a site distinct from the VLA-4/fibronectin binding site. Cell60:577
21. Auchincloss, H., Jr. (1995) Why is cell-mediated xenograft rejection so strong? Xeno 3: 19
22. Kirk, A. D., Li, R. A., Kinch, M. S., et al. (1993) The human antiporcine cellular repertoire. In vitro studies of acquired and innate cellular responsiveness.Transplantation 55: 924
23. Murray, A. G., Khodadoust, M. M., Pober, J. S., Bothwell, A. L. (1994) Porcine aortic endothelial cells activate human T cells: direct presentation of MHC antigens and costimulation by ligands for human CD2 and CD28. Immunity 1: 57
24. Rollins, S.A., Kennedy, S.P., Chodera, A.J., et al. (1994) Evidence that activation of human T cells by porcine endothelium involves direct recognition of porcine SLA and costimulation by porcine ligands for LFA-1 and CD2. Transplantation 57: 1709
25. Yamada, K., Sachs, D. H., DerSimonian, H. (1995) Human anti-porcine xenogeneic T cell response. Evidence for allele specificity of mixed leukocyte reaction and for both direct and indirect pathways of recognition. J. Immunol. 155: 5249
26. Matis, L. A., Elliott, E. A., Evans, M. J., et al. (1995) The molecular basis of human anti-porcine cellular interactions. Xeno. In press
27. Lenschow, D. J., Zeng, Y., Thistlethwaite, J. R., et al. (1992) Long-term survival of xenogeneic pancreatic islet grafts induced by CTLA4lg. Science 257: 789
28. Dorling, A., Binns, R., Lechler, R. I. (1995) Significant in direct recognition of porcine xenoantigens in the ‚primary' xenogeneic MLR. Apparent priming of adult humans against pig antigens (Abstract). Presented at the Third International Congress for Xenotransplantation, Boston. Transplant. Proc.In press
29. Gumperz, J. E., Parham, P. (1995) The enigma of the natural killer cell. Nature 378: 245
30. Sandrin, M. S., Fodor, W. L., Mouhtouris, E., et al. (1995) Enzymatic remodelling of the carbohydrate surface of a xenogeniec cell substantially reduces human antibody binding and complement-mediated cytolysis. Nature Med. 1: 1261

15 Immunoprivileged Sites for Allo- and Xenotransplantation

J.H. Dinsmore

Introduction

The existence of sites in the body in which allogeneic or xenogeneic transplants survive for extended periods (sometimes indefinitely) have been recognized for many years and have been designated "immunologically privileged sites." A list of privileged sites include the brain, the eye (anterior chamber and cornea), certain endocrine organs (prostate, adrenal cortex, testis, ovary) [1], the pregnant uterus [2], the thymus [3], hair follicles, and the hamster cheek pouch [1]. In particular, the brain, anterior chamber of the eye, and testis have been shown to provide a protective environment against immune attack for cells transplanted to these sites.

The immune responses elicited by an allograft or xenograft are the result of a complex interaction between various antigens and antigen-presenting cells (APC) of the graft and subsets of host lymphocytes and host APC. The effector elements generated by the host immune system that mediate graft rejection are composed of various lymphocytes and/or antibodies, depending on the type of graft involved. The mechanisms underlying immune privilege have been the subject of numerous studies. From early studies, the idea emerged that antigens present in immunoprivileged locations were simply not seen by the immune system and were sequestered in some way [1]. This idea stemmed in part from the observation that many of these sites (eye, brain, hamster cheek pouch) appeared to lack lymphatic drainage, thereby restricting proper efferent flow of antigens to the host immune system. While poor lymphatic drainage may account in part for the existence of immune privileged sites, there is clearly sufficent lymphatic drainage from all privileged sites to allow for host sensitization to occur. Thus, the mechanisms for the establishment and maintenance of immune privilege are multifaceted and will likely vary depending on the particular site.

Recent data have emerged that highlight the supposition that multiple mechanisms provide immune protection at privileged sites. Specifically, the involvement of CD-95 or Fas and Fas ligand (FasL) in conferring immune privilege in the eye and testis has been revealed [4, 5]. For the purposes of this review, a brief listing and description of known immunoprivileged sites wil be given, followed by a more detailed discussion of what is known about the mechanisms for immune privilege in three sites: the brain, the eye, and the testis.

Immunoprivileged Sites: An Overview

Hamster Cheek Pouch

Syrian hamsters have paired, highly distensible cheek pouches that extend back beneath the skin of the shoulders and are lined by buccal mucous membrane. These pouches function in food storage and can be easily accessed in the anesthetized animal for implantation of tissue. The cheek pouch as such provides a hospitable environment for extended survival of allografts and in some cases xenografts. Presently, data indicate that the immune privilege exhibited within the cheek pouch is due to the absence or paucity of lymphatic vessels in this tissue as well as due to the lack of APC [6]. The lack of lymphatic drainage from the cheek pouch has been demonstrated by a number of measures, including a graft-versus-host (GVH) lymph node assay [7] that affords a sensitive means of determining which lymph nodes drain a particular tissue. When such a lymph node GVH assay was performed, there were no nodes detected in the vicinity of the cheek pouch [8].

Endocrine Organs: Prostate and Adrenal Cortex

The immune privileged status of the prostate has come under question [9, 10]. Originally, the prostate was thought to lack lymphatic drainage. However, detailed studies have shown that there are small lymphatics within the connective tissue lying between glandular elements [9]. Likewise, dye injected into the rat prostate did pass to draining lymph nodes, but more slowly than dye injected into other sites such as the bladder [8]. Finally, survival of allografts in the prostate was only marginally prolonged in comparison to survival of allografts placed in other sites [9]. These combined data cast doubt on whether the prostate is an immunoprivileged site.

The adrenal gland is another endocrine tissue that has been shown to provide protection for transplanted tissues. Parathyroid tissues transplanted to the adrenal cortex survive for extended times when compared to transplants placed in other peripheral sites [11, 12]. Local synthesis of immunosuppressive factors, such as corticosteroid hormones, may be responsible for the immunoprivilege observed in the adrenal cortex. Consistent with this hypothesis, corticosteroids have been shown to possess anti-inflammatory and immunosuppressive properties [13].

Pregnant Uterus

The embryo contains major histocompatibility complex (MHC) antigens derived from both maternal and paternal sources and, therefore, mechanisms exist to inhibit immunologic rejection of the fetus by the maternal immune system. The maternal immune system does recognize fetal alloantigens during pregnancy as antibodies to paternal antigens are produced in the pregnant female. The immune protection afforded the fetus appears to be the result of local factors produced at the maternal-placental interface. Tissues transplanted to the non-pregnant uterus do not show prolonged survival [14], whereas tissues placed at the maternal fetal interface do show prolonged survival [2]. Release of cytokines, immune suppressive factors (e.g., transforming growth factor-α, TGF-α), prostaglandins, and the presence of high concentrations of glycosaminoglycans (GAGs) on placental tissues all appear to play a role in regulating the immune response in the pregnant uterus [2, 15].

Thymus

Recently, the extended survival of allogeneic transplants to the thymus have been demonstrated [3]. When pancreatic islets were transplanted to the thymus of rats, islets survived long term and a state of systemic donor specific unresponsiveness was induced in the transplant recipient [3]. The long-term survival of islets in the thymus has been attributed to thymic deletion or suppression of islet reactive T cells. Further, studies have shown that intrathymic injection of islets into neonatal BB rats results in the inhibition of autoimmune diabetes [16]. Although transplantation of cells to the thymus of rodents has been effective for protecting cells against rejection and for inducing tolerance, the applicability of this technique to larger animals is uncertain because the thymus of larger animals is involuted and difficult to find.

Brain

The brain has been shown to be an immunologically privileged site for the transplantation of many different tissues of both allogeneic and xenogeneic sources [17–25]. However, that privilege is not absolute. In general, allografts in the brain do not require immunosuppression for long-term survival whereas xenotransplants do require some form of immunosuppression [22, 26]. The nature of the immunologic privilege within the brain is multifaceted, and it is the multidimensional aspects of immune privilege that make it an easier location to obtain long-term graft survival.

Because any inappropriate immune response in the brain would be highly deleterious, multiple mechanisms to restrict immune responses in the brain exist. Components providing immune protection in the brain include the following: (a) the blood-brain barrier (BBB), (b) the lack of both MHC I and II expression on brain cells, (c) the paucity of APCs, (d) the limited lymphatic flow to the brain, and (e) the presence of local factors, such as TGF-α capable of inhibiting T cells (for a review, see [18, 26]). The BBB restricts the access of both humoral (i.e., antibody and cytokine) and cellular immune responses [27]. Thus the BBB is an important component of immune privilege in the brain, and the relative success of any grafting procedure will depend on whether or not the BBB is restored after engraftment [28–31]. As a rule, only neural tissue has the capacity to form a proper BBB, and therefore, all other tissue types transplanted to the brain will be more susceptible to eventual rejection [29].

For optimal success with grafting to the brain, there are several factors which must be considered. The type of cell used for transplant will impact eventual survival, although many different cell types have been successfully maintained after transplantation into the brain [17, 20, 29, 32, 33]. Whether cell suspensions or whole tissue pieces are transplanted is important [29, 34]. When intact tissue is transplanted, a hybrid vascular network is formed in the graft with vascular elements being derived from both the donor and recipient [29]. In this situation, foreign antigens on the donor vasculature act as targets for the host immune system, and additionally, the donor vasculature is exposed to harmful natural antibodies present in some xenograft combinations. In contrast, dissociated cell suspensions grafted to the brain are vascularized by the host, with little or no contribution from the donor [29, 34].

The location to where tissue is transplanted is another variable. Lymphocytes and antibodies have greater access to cerebrospinal fluid (CSF) than to brain parenchyma [27, 35]; grafts placed in the ventricles are subject to a more vigorous immune attack than those placed in the parenchyma [36, 37]. Further, there are regions of the brain (circumventricular organs, pituitary) where the BBB is not complete [38], making these targets less attractive for transplantation.

Finally, the method by which tissues or cells are placed within the brain can affect graft survival. Generally, the more destructive the transplant procedure, the greater the risk of rejection. Therefore, stereotactic transplantation with the smallest bore cannula compatible with the tissue to be transplanted will provide for optimal chances of success [39].

Eye and Testis: Involvement of Fas

Both the anterior chamber of the eye and the testis are remarkable immune privileged sites, known for their ability to support allogeneic and xenogeneic transplants [2, 11, 40, 41]. Immune privilege at these site is mediated by multiple mechanisms functioning coordinately. Both the anterior chamber of the eye and the testis have diminished lymphatic flow. However, there is sufficient lymphatic flow such that this one mechanism alone is not sufficient to provide immune privilege at these sites. Additional factors involved are locally produced factors that create a regional inhibition of immune responses. Locally produced factors that are known to inhibit immune responses include the following: (a) TGF-α (eye and testis), (b) neuropeptides (eye), (c) complement inhibitors (eye), and (d) corticosteroids (testis) [42].

Finally, recent work has now shown that there is an additional element to immune privilege in both the eye and testis, FasL-induced apoptosis [4, 5]. FasL is expressed in both the eye and testis and does provide immune privilege at these sites [4, 5]. Apoptotic cell death is induced when FasL, a cell surface molecule with homology to tumor necrosis factor, binds to its receptor Fas. Various cells and tissues such as thymus, liver, heart, lung, kidney, and ovary express Fas, but only relatively few cells (activated T cells, Sertoli cells, and cells in the eye) express FasL [4, 5, 43]. In the immune system, Fas and FasL function to downregulate immune reactions and are used by T cells to induce target cell death. Thus, FasL expression in immune privileged sites would act to inhibit any immune responses by inducing the apoptotic cell death of invading immune cells.

Comment

The discovery of FasL expression in immune privileged sites is exciting, and it will be interesting to determine if the Fas system is involved in immune privilege at other sites, such as the brain. Additionally, there is the potential for conferring immune privilege to tissues transplanted to non-privileged sites via FasL expression. The outcome of such experiments using FasL expression to promote immune protection for transplanted tissues will have important implications for transplantation research.

References

1. Barker, C.F., Billingham, R.E. (1977). Immunologically privileged sites. Advances in Immunology 25: 1
2. Streilein, J.W., Wegman, T.G. (1987). Immunologic privilege in the eye and the fetus. Immunol. Today 8: 362
3. Posselt, A.M., Barker, C.F., Tomaszewski, J.E., et al. (1990). Induction of donor-specific unresponsiveness by intrathymic islet transplantation. Science 249: 1293
4. Bellgrau, D., Gold, D., Selawry, H., et al. (1995). A role for CD95 ligand in preventing graft rejection. Nature 377: 630
5. Griffith, T.S., Brunner, T., Fletcher, S.M., Green, D.R., Ferguson, T.A. (1995). Fas ligand-induced apoptosis as a mechanism of immune privilege. Science 270: 1189
6. Bergstresser, P.R., Fletcher, C.R., Streilein, J.W. (1980). Surface densities of Langerhans cells in relation to rodent epidermal sites with special immunologic properties. J. Invest. Dermatol. 74: 77
7. Levine, S. (1968). Local and regional forms of graft-versus-host disease in lymph nodes. Transplantation 6: 799
8. Head, J.R., Billingham, R.E. (1985). Immunologically privileged sites in transplantation immunology and oncology. Perspectives in Biology & Medicine 29: 115
9. Neaves, W.B., Billingham, R.E. (1979). The lymphatic drainage of the rat prostate and its status as an immunologically privileged site. Transplantation 27: 127
10. Shridhar, P. (1979). The lymphatics of the prostate gland and their role in the spread of prostatic carcinoma. Ann R Coll Surg Engl 61: 114
11. Whitmore, W.F., Gittes, R.F. (1978). Intratesticular grafts: the testis as an exceptional immunologically privileged site. Trans Am Assoc GU Surg 70: 76–80
12. Kukreja, S.C., Johnson, P.A., Ayala, G., Bowser, E.N., Williams, G.A. (1979). Allotransplantation of rat parathyroid glands: effects of organ culture and transplantation into the adrenal gland. Experientia 35: 559

13. Compton, M.M., Caron, L.M., Cidlowski, J.A. (1987). Glucocorticoid action on the immune system. J. Steroid Biochem 27: 201
14. Sakonju, I., Taura, Y., Nakaichi, M., Nakama, S., Kagabu, S. (1994). Intrauterine transplantation of isogenic pancreatic islets in experimental diabetic rats. J Vet Med Sci 56: 729
15. Wilbanks, G.A., Streilein, J.W. (1992). Fluids from immune privileged sites endow macrophages with the capacity to induce antigen-specific immune deviation via a mechanism involving transforming growth factor-beta. Eur J Immunol 22: 1031
16. Posselt, A.M., Naji, A., Roark, J.H., Markmann, J.F., Barker, C.F. (1991). Intrathymic islet transplantation in the spontaneously diabetic BB rat. Ann Surg 214: 363; discussion 371
17. Tze, W.J., Tai, J. (1984). Intracerebral allotransplantation of purified pancreatic endocrine cells and pancreatic islets in diabetic rats. Transplantation 38: 107
18. Widner, H., Brundin, P. (1988). Immunological aspects of grafting in the mammalian central nervous system. A review and speculative synthesis. Brain Res 472: 287
19. Bjorklund, A. (1991). Neural transplantation–an experimental tool with clinical possibilities. Trends in Neurosciences 14: 319
20. Lee, H.C., Ahn, K.J., Lim, S.K. et al. (1992). Allotransplantation of rat islets into the cisterna magna of streptozotocin-induced diabetic rats. Transplantation 53: 513
21. Deacon, T.W., Pakzaban, P., Burns, L.H., Dinsmore, J., Isacson, O. (1994). Cytoarchitectonic development, axon-glia relationships, and long distance axon growth of porcine striatal xenografts in rats. Exp. Neurol. 130: 151
22. Pakzaban, P., Isacson, O. (1994). Neural xenotransplantation: reconstruction of neuronal circuitry across species barriers. Neuroscience 62: 989
23. Garcia, A.R., Deacon, T.W., Dinsmore, J., Isacson, O. (1995). Extensive axonal and glial fiber growth from fetal porcine cortical xenografts in the adult rat cortex. Cell Transplantation 4: 515
24. Isacson, O., Deacon, T.W., Pakzaban, P., et al. (1995). Transplanted xenogeneic neural cells in neurodegenerative disease models exhibit remarkable axonal target specificity and distinct growth patterns of glial and axonal fibres. Nature Med 1: 1189
25. Pakzaban, P., Deacon, T.W., Burns,, L.W., Dinsmore, J., Isacson, O. (1995). A novel mode of immunoprotection of neural xenotransplants: masking of donor major histocompatibility complex class I enhances transplant survival in the central nervous system [published erratum appears in Neuroscience 1995;66:761]. Neuroscience 65: 983
26. Sloan, D.J., Wood, M.J., Charlton, H.M. (1991). The immune response to intracerebral neural grafts. Trends in Neurosciences 14: 341
27. Cserr, H.F., Knopf, P.M. (1992). Cervical lymphatics, the blood-brain barrier and the immunoreactivity of the brain: a new view. Immunol. Today 13: 507
28. Young, M.J., Rao, K., Lund, R.D. (1989). Integrity of the blood-brain barrier in retinal xenografts is correlated with the immunological status of the host. J Comp Neurol 283: 107
29. Broadwell, R.D., Charlton, H.M., Ebert, P., et al. (1990). Angiogenesis and the blood-brain barrier in solid and dissociated cell grafts within the CNS. Prog. Brain Res. 82: 95
30. Pollack, I.F., Lund, R.D. (1990). The blood-brain barrier protects foreign antigens in the brain from immune attack. Exp Neurol 108: 114

31. Bertram, K.J., Shipley, M.T., Ennis, M., Sanberg, P.R., Norman, A.B. (1994). Permeability of the blood-brain barrier within rat intrastriatal transplants assessed by simultaneous systemic injection of horseradish peroxidase and Evans blue dye. Exp. Neurol. 127: 245
32. Tze, W.J., Tai, J. (1988). Allotransplantation of dispersed single pancreatic endocrine cells in diabetic rats. Diabetes 37: 383
33. Ortega, J.D., Sagen, J., Pappas, G.D. (1992). Short-term immunosuppression enhances long-term survival of bovine chromaffin cell xenografts in rat CNS. Cell Transplantation 1: 33
34. Giest, M.J., Maris, D.O., Grady, M.S. (1991). Blood-brain barrier permiability is not altered by allograft or xenograft fetal neural cell suspension grafts. Exp. Neurol. 111: 166
35. Hickey, W.F., Hsu, B., Kimura, H. (1991). T-lymphocyte entry into the central nervous system. J. Neurosci. Res. 28: 254
36. Mason, D.W., Charlton, H.M., Jones, A.J., et al. (1986). The fate of allogeneic and xenogeneic neuronal tissue transplanted into the third ventricle of rodents. Neuroscience 19: 685
37. Sloan, D.J., Baker, B.J., Puklavec, M., Charlton, H.M. (1990). The effect of site of transplantation and histocompatibility differences on the survival of neural tissue transplanted to the CNS of defined rat strains. Prog. Brain Res. 82: 141
38. Broadwell, R.D., Charlton, H.M., Balin, B.J., Salcman, M. (1987). Angioarchitecture of the CNS, pituitary gland, and intracerebral grafts revealed with peroxidase cytochemistry. J. Comp. Neurol. 260: 47
39. Lindvall, O., Widner, H., Rehncrona, S., et al. (1992). Transplantation of fetal dopamine neurons in Parkinson's disease: one-year clinical and neurophysiological observations in two patients with putaminal implants. Ann Neurol 31: 155
40. Selawry, H.P., Whittington, K.B., Forster, H.G. (1988). Intratesticular islet xenograft survival in relation to tissue cyclosporine levels. Am J Med Sci 295: 497
41. Ar'Rajab, A., Dawidson, I.J., Harris, R.B., Sentementes, J.T. (1994). Immune privilege of the testis for islet xenotransplantation (rat to mouse). Cell Transplantation 3: 493
42. Streilein, J.W. (1995). Unraveling immune privilege. Science 270: 1158
43. Nagata, S., Golstein, P. (1995). The Fas death factor. Science 267: 1449

16 Immunobiology of Xenotransplantation in Rodents

F.T. Thomas, W. Marchman, A. Carobbi, J. Contreras, J. George, E. Larkin, K. Pittman, C. Haisch, and J.M. Thomas

Introduction

Rodents have always been the favored species for laboratory research. The animals are inexpensive, their lodging and care are simple and cost-effective, and they can be bred in a well-controlled environment to develop pure strains with known histocompatibility. The recent futuristic developments in transgenic mice creates the potential for selectively and discretely manipulating virtually every subset and element of the immune system for transplant research. Rodent use in organ transplantation research has previously been limited by their small size. Recently, the development of microsurgery has permitted the performance of a large number of whole-organ grafts in rodents, including kidney, pancreas, spleen, liver, lung, and heart. The utility of rodents in skin grafting is legendary. One of the most useful papers on skin grafting technique was published by Billingham over 45 years ago using rodents, and this remains a recommended up-to-date reference on experimental skin grafting [1]. Perhaps the most important factor in the utility of these animals is the ability to perform large numbers of solid-organ grafts in a cost-effective manner consistent with modern concerns for animal welfare.

Over the past 10 years, our group has worked extensively with over 3000 rodents in xenograft studies [2–32]. This chapter summarizes our experience and that of others using rodent models to develop effective immunosuppression (IS) for preventing xenograft rejection (XR) and to generate insights into mechanisms of XR. In this respect, experimental modeling using rodents has yielded critically important results with xenografts. To date, rodent models have arguably yielded the majority of basic information on XR. It quickly became apparent that conventional immunosuppressive agents, including cyclosporine, were ineffective in xenografting [2]. Emphasis was therefore shifted to newer immunosuppressive modalities, including FK506, 15-deoxyspergualin (DSG), quality-controlled rabbit antithymocyte globulin (RATG), and total lymphoid irradiation (TLI) [4–6, 8]. More recently, exciting new drugs like mycophenolate mofetil, leflunomide, brequinar sodium and others have been tested in rodent xenografts (Chaps. 44–46). Importantly, rodent models, especially the genetically controlled immunodeficient models [9, 10] and transgenic mice [3, 26, 29], have been used to develop a better understanding of the mechanisms of XR.

Studies of infiltrating cells in rejecting xenografts were utilized in an attempt to explain the basic processes of humoral and cell-mediated immunity in XR. Antibody studies were utilized to determine the effect of xenograft anti-donor antibody, as well as to study blocking of antibody formation by immunosuppressive drugs, the role of antibodies in hyperacute rejection, and delayed xenograft rejection as well as in facilitation and tolerance of xenografts.

Important insights were gained into the basic nature of XR by studies in genetically immunodeficient rodent strains [9, 10, 16]. The immunodeficient models have included the X-linked immunodeficiency (XID) mouse (native and reconstituted), nude (*Nu*) mouse, beige (*Be*) mouse, and mice having various combinations of these genetic mutations, as well as the nude rat. We have utilized the model of a primarily vascularized heart graft in these immunodeficient mice to study mechanisms of XR. Some of these studies were among the first to establish that the endothelial cell epitopes were the major stimulus to development of in vitro xenogeneic reactivity in rodents [7, 15]. Another of these studies demonstrated that T cell immunity, as well as antibody-dependent cellular cytotoxicity (ADCC) and lymphokine-activated killer (LAK) cell activity were developed against the endothelial cell by xenogeneic cells [15]. Extraordinary opportunities to dissect XR have recently become available with development of transgenic (TG) animals. We have studied XR in class I and II major histocompatibility complex (MHC)-deficient mice as well as the so-called RAG, uMT, and other transgenic strains [19, 26, 29].

An Overview of Xenograft Models

A wide variety of animal species have been used in xenograft studies. The array of experimental models is nearly as kaleidoscopic as the animal kingdom itself! They include the following: (a) primates, (b) large domesticated animals such as pigs, goats, and dogs, (c) a host of rodent xenograft models involving primarily the rat, mouse, hamster, and guinea pig, and even (d) studies of lower amphibians and other non-mammalian species. Our experience, to be reviewed here, primarily involves three rodent species – the mouse, rat, and hamster.

Mouse

The excellent insights into the mouse MHC and the recent availability of transgenic mice are important reasons for choosing the mouse in transplant studies. However, a casual perusal of literature reveals a provocative number of papers in which the reason for choosing the mouse is not obvious. Especially when salubrious results are obtained, scepticism is inevitable. Often the issue is complex. For example, the plethora of successful schemes for prolonging islet xenograft survival in the mouse makes one wonder whether science might best be served by searching for an immunomodulation system that does *not* prolong islet xenografts in the mouse – this would truly be a scientific curiosity! However, who doubts the value of the NOD mouse in islet grafting? The model is elegant, and prolonging islet xenografts in this recipient mouse is indeed difficult. A number of authors have dealt with the problem of "user-friendly" mouse models recently [18, 35, 39, 40, 41]. Perhaps some modeling concepts could be agreed upon, such as encouraging the well-published investigator to repeat his system using a rat recipient (especially the Lewis rat). A progressive ascension up the evolutionary scale – mouse to dog to primate to man – seems a productive scheme and has certainly worked well in recent tolerance studies [3].

Skin Grafting in the Rodent

Early in our experience, it became clear that the rodent skin graft was an excellent model for studying xenograft immunity and IS drug potency and toxicity. To begin with, the elegant genetic controls possible in these animals, especially the mouse, provided an immunological milieu with a uniform pattern and tempo of rejection. In vivo studies demonstrated a vigorous, well-defined, and rapid progression of mouse, rat, and hamster skin rejection, often complete within 24–48 h of the first indication of impending rejection.

Equally consistent was the inability of immunosuppressive agents currently used to effect a delay in XR. Every IS drug studied, when used as monotherapy, failed to significantly modify survival of these xenografts, with the exception of RATG, which slightly prolonged skin grafts. Therapy with two or three drug combinations, however, produced some significant improvements in skin graft survival, with delay of rejection beyond 30–40 days in some cases [2, 4].

In general, the skin xenograft models showed patterns of rejection and prolongation which closely mimicked other xenograft models (such as the heterotopic cardiac xenograft and pancreas islet xenografts). There was a similar tempo and vigor of rejection between the organ grafts tested. Interestingly, cyclosporine, even at toxic doses of 25–50 mg/kg per day, did not produce significant prolongation of graft survival or modification of the basic histological pattern of XR. Similar results were obtained with other conventional IS drugs when used as monotherapy or together. However, combinations of RATG and splenectomy with FK506 and DSG produced significant prolongation of both the heart and skin graft. The ineffectiveness of TLI and cyclosporine has been a consistent finding in our studies and in studies of other groups using the heart and other organ xenograft models [2, 5, 6, 13, 14, 42, 43].

Thus, there is high concordance of graft survival and prolongation in these two models despite the use of different donor organs. We view the skin test as a "screening assay" to permit rapid, inexpensive testing of a wide variety of suppressive agents. Agents shown to be suppressive in screening assays then receive more definitive confirmation of their potency in heart or pancreas islet xenografting. Despite the utility and relevance of skin grafting, formidable limitations of skin graft models came to light in studies of transgenic animals [26, 29]. Class I and II MHC "knockout" mice rejected skin grafts normally, but showed marked prolongation of heart grafts. Thus skin graft results cannot be indiscriminately utilized in graft rejection studies.

The skin xenograft has another advantage – the ability to access drug toxicity in a relatively pure form, unfettered by vagaries of microsurgery and anesthesia involved in other, more stressful, xenograft models. In contrast to xenografts of solid, primarily vascularized organs such as heart, kidney, pancreas, and liver, the anesthesia and transplant morbidity and mortality for skin grafts approaches 0 %. With only a few months experience, most researchers can perform literally hundreds of skin xenografts without technical morbidity or mortality. In this situation, it is possible to accurately ascribe morbidity, and especially mortality, to the effects of immunosuppressive drugs.

Drug Toxicity

Studies from our laboratory and others have established that virtually all agents with the ability to prolong xenograft survival are associated with significant morbidity and mortality in rodents. It therefore behooves the xenograft investigator to accurately and carefully look for morbidity and mortality associated with these toxic immunosuppressive agents. A number of publications in the literature imply, for example, that doses of 20–50 mg cyclosporine/kg can be given with no significant toxicity. Mortalities of up to 80 % can be seen but are often not attributed to toxicity associated with these agents. Deaths after skin xenografting have been described as due to "technical complications." Our studies suggest that this is not a plausible explanation, and that deaths in animals following skin grafting done by skilled personnel are almost certainly attributable to the IS agent, if anesthetic toxicity is excluded. There can be little meaningful discussion of immunosuppression for xenografting without careful attention to the potential or actual toxicity of potent new immunosuppressive agents, since toxicity is so frequently present at the doses necessary to prolong xenografts.

Effects of Vascularization on Xenograft Rejection

Rodent xenograft models have exhibited analogies to allotransplantation and also illustrate novel immunobiologic principles. Xenografts that can be either primarily vascularized or secondarily vascularized, like islets and skin grafts, have shown that the mouse skin xenograft is variably resistant to antibody-mediated attack during its residence in the host. Interestingly, recent studies in our laboratory demonstrate that the islet allograft, which has a similar secondary vascularization, has an entirely different susceptibility to antibody rejection. It seems that such models, studied in a more detailed manner, might yield important results in understanding XR.

Vascular Endothelial Cell

Studies of the xenogeneic response to the vascular endothelial cell (VEC) [7, 15] showed that mouse VECs isolated in vitro induce high levels of xenogeneic T cell responses as well as ADCC and complement-dependent cytolysis compared to the xenogeneic reaction with splenocytes. These findings with the VEC are provocative since they correlate well with the in vivo xenograft rejection reaction, which is much stronger than alloreactivity. Later studies elegantly demonstrated that a carbohydrate epitope (αGal1–3Gal) was the primary inducer of this strong anti-VEC xenogeneic response. Transgenic animals with α1,3-galactosyltransferase knockout induce weak xenogeneic responses [23].

Pancreatic Islet Transplantation

The pancreatic islet deserves special mention as a rodent xenograft model (Chap. 41). The islet, like the skin graft, undergoes a type of secondary neovascularization and survives for the first few days in the host without primary vascular connections with the host circulation. A number of investigators have suggested that the islet is susceptible to an almost immediate 24- to 48-h hyperacute-type rejection [44]. This rejection has been termed primary nonfunction in that the grafts fail to lower blood sugar at any time in the post-transplant period. Though primary failure of the xenograft may be due to early severe accelerated rejection, a number of authors have attributed early islet failure to deficiencies of isolation and culture techniques which impair islet viability. A factor of great interest is the ability to virtually eliminate this unique and early islet rejection in the xenograft [21, 22, 24, 33] with effective IS drugs. In our own group's series, discordant pig islets had a mean survival of >200 days – one of the best survivals recorded for discordant xenografts. Most importantly, these survivals were obtained without chronic immunosuppression and as such represent an operational tolerance. Thus, islet xenotransplants may be a favored graft among the various organ xenografts.

Recent studies in rodents with type II diabetes (non-insulin-dependent diabetes mellitus, NIDDM) have suggested a unique potential application of xenotransplants in reversing type II diabetes [33]. This entity has long been thought to be due to a primary metabolic lesion variously referred to as "insulin resistance," "post-receptor insulin defects," etc. Our group's studies in the classic model of NIDDM, the Zucker rat, however, strongly suggest that insufficient islet insulin secretion is a central factor in NIDDM, and the insulin resistance usually reverses when this insulin secretory abnormality is corrected by islet xenotransplantation. Since there are about ten times as many humans with NIDDM compared to type I diabetes, this may be a fruitful area.

Xenograft Studies in Immunodeficient Rodents

A number of rodent models with specific immune deficiencies, including the nude mouse (T cell-deficient and athymic, the beige mouse [killer (K) and natural killer (NK) cell-deficient, specifically], the xid mouse (excellent immunodeficiency showing B cell and antibody deficiencies), and SCID mouse (severe combined immunodeficiency mouse, with both T and B cell deficiencies and normal K and NK cells), and genetic combinations of these four animals have recently become available [45]. Animals with specific immune deficiencies, including complement deficiencies and other dysfunctions of the immune system are also available, but have not been utilized widely in definitive xenograft experiments to date. This section will focus on the best studied mutations in mice, the *scid* mutation, the nude (*Nu*) mutation, the beige (*Be*) mutation, and the *xid* animals, and combinations of these mutants, as well as the nude rat. Over 30 single-gene mutations leading to immunodeficiency have been characterized and inbred. In addition, ten mice strains with multiple mutations of immunodeficiency have been described, as well as rat, guinea pig, and hamster mutants [45–47, 49–53].

Nude Rodent

The nude (*Nu*) genetic aberration has been described in both the mouse and the rat [9, 10, 16, 19, 28, 35, 37, 46, 47, 49, 50, 51]. The nude mouse was one of the earliest animals studied for T cell immunodeficiency. The nude rat developed as a mutation in a group of animals in Scotland, and separately in New Zealand.

Using the basic Rowlett nude rat and backcrossing it with outbred strains, including Lewis, Buffalo and Wistar Furth, National Institutes of Health (NIH) staff have developed a nude rat which is herein referred to as the NIH nude rat. The animal in the homozygous state is hairless, athymic, and known to have marked T cell deficiencies. Animals used should be younger than 8–10 weeks old, since older animals show development of T cell expansion and differentiation [45]. The young animals show severe depletion of lymphocytes in the thymus-dependent pericortical area of lymph nodes, as well as in the thymus-dependent splenic periarteriolar sheaths. Peyer's patches are small, and lymphocyte counts (presumably B cells) are high. Antigen retention by the follicular dendritic cells is essentially normal. NK activity is normal-to-increased in nude rats, as it is in nude mice.

In the thoracic duct, B cells are normal or increased, but T cells are markedly reduced (<5 %). T cells in the peripheral lymph node tissues are less than 2 % of total lymphocytes in young animals, up to age 4–8 weeks. Markedly deficient T cell function is seen as measured by alloreactivity in mixed lymphocyte cultures (MLC), development of cytotoxic cells, development of helper cells producing interleukin-2 (IL-2), and responses to phytohemagglutinin (PHA) and concanavalin A (ConA).

In short, the nude rat is an elegant model of an athymic pure T cell defect [45, 46]. One of the most critical insights into XR was the independent reports of two laboratories [10, 56] of the normal to heightened XR in these animals despite their T cell deficiency. These results significantly changed our concepts of XR which was previously felt to be heavily dependent on T cell activity. In addition, more recent studies have demonstrated that even concordant xenografts are rejected primarily by B cell and antibody responses. Finally, studies just completed demonstrate that contrary to accepted concepts, T cell-independent antibodies are critical to XR, and even long-term XR does not depend on T cells. The recent demonstration of the CD4 epitope on some macrophages makes it possible that some observed effects of CD4 on xenografts ascribed to T cells may be related to $CD4^+$ macrophages.

Beige Mouse

The beige (*Be*) mutant is a light-colored variant of the C57B1/6J mouse. These animals show hypopigmentation, and the genetic mutant has arisen in a number of different laboratories [52]. The phenotypic manifestations resemble the Chediak-Higashi syndrome in humans. The animals have a basically intact T cell system but have a selective impairment of NK cell function. NK cells do not mount an antibody-dependent or antibody-independent cytolysis of tumor cells in vivo. The animals apparently have LAK cell precursors and presumably normal LAK cell activity. In short, this is an elegant model for studying isolated K and NK cell activity as it might relate to XR and/or tumor growth.

Results of Xenografting in Immunodeficient Rodents

Our group has now studied xenograft rejection in a wide variety of genetic immunodeficient strains. Results are summarized in Fig. 1. In these studies, heart xenografts were placed in selectively immunodeficient animals and their rejection times recorded. In addition, biopsies of the grafts were examined for the nature and degree of infiltrating cells.

Control heart grafts survived 5.4±3.6 days. The striking and unexpected observation that the nude rat rejects tissue xenografts in a normal manner and tempo, as previously noted, has been a seminal finding. Heterotopic cardiac allografts (not shown here) survived indefinitely, thus confirming the total functional T cell deficiency of these animals.

Another striking finding was the delay of rejection of both allografts and xenografts in the beige animals which have defective NK and K cell function.

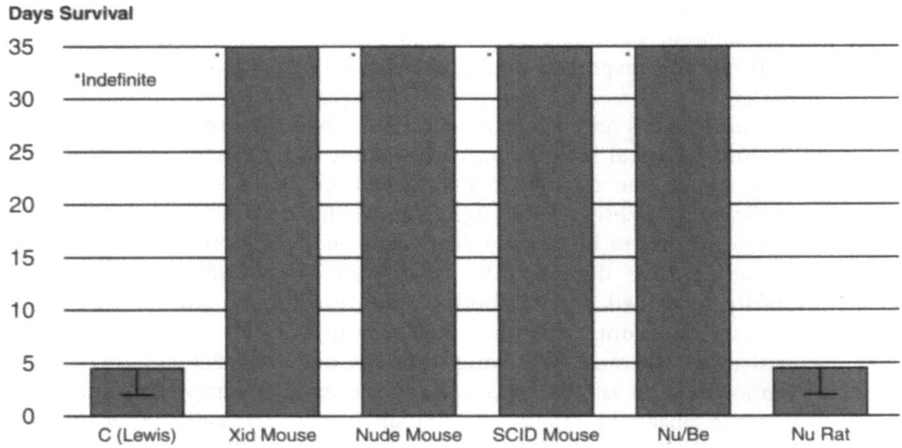

Fig. 1. Survival of xenografts in immunodeficient rodents. *C*, control

Since B and T cell function appear to be normal in these animals, it would appear that NK and K cell activity is involved in the early acute rejection of allografts and in XR. Further studies by our group, however, have failed to implicate NK or K cells in XR.

The xid mutation is a marked deficiency in T cell-independent B cell immunity [47]. Our group has previously reported that the xid animals rejected their xenografts in a normal manner. Studies of this animal colony showed discrepancies in B cell response related to backcrosses. A stable, better defined, xid colony was obtained and thoroughly tested. This colony had a stable and severe B cell deficiency. When cardiac xenografts were done in these animals (xid-2), indefinite survival was obtained. This is one of the strongest lines of evidence that the B cell is central to XR.

The SCID animals maintained their skin grafts for an indefinite period and showed a marked blunting of the xenogeneic response in histopathologic sections. However, SCID animals reconstituted with purified CD4 cells obtained by fluorescence-activated cell sorter (FACS) and bead separation rejected skin grafts in 14 days but still did not reject vascularized heart grafts [35]. The striking difference between rejection of these two grafts in rodents is yet another example of organ differences in XR. Interestingly, animals reconstituted with purified B cells rejected xenografts in a normal manner at 6.8 ± 1.6 days. Of extraordinary interest was the lack of requirement for T cells and failure of intensification of rejection with T cell and B cell reconstitution. These results suggest (as have other experiments) that antibody XR involves T-independent antibodies. These overall results, obtained from immunodeficient animals, have done more, perhaps than any other results, in outlining some basic concepts of XR with scientific precision. These results were contrary to many accepted dogmas of XR, and established beyond doubt that B cell reactivity and antibody effector systems which are T cell-independent are the primary reactors in XR. Most importantly, this concept goes far in explaining empirical results which did not make sense by traditional concepts. The weakness of T cells in in vitro xenogeneic reactivity (the MLC, for example) and the poor ability of strong anti-T cell IS agents like cyclosporine to suppress XR is entirely compatible with and supportive of a strong B cell role in XR. Recent studies in our laboratory have demonstrated a primary role for B cell reactivity even in concordant xenografts, a concept which has been vigorously rejected to date. This issue deserves critical analysis. Interestingly, the strong block of XR by ATG seemed enigmatic to this concept until the recent demonstration that polyclonal ATG in fact contains far more non-T cell monoclonal specificities than those for T cell epitopes. In addition, the non-T cell specificities are found at far greater titers, and thus the ability of ATG to block XR is an expected finding based on the important concepts from these studies in immunodeficient animals. Similarly, the importance of non-MHC targets of XR (endothelial carbohydrate epitopes) would be expected since T cell reactivity is strongly directed to MHC epitopes.

Studies of the Immunobiology of Xenografts

In early studies, our group looked at some basic immunobiologic principles of xenograft rejection in rodents. These studies were designed as one part of a comprehensive overview of xenografting in an attempt to develop more rational perspectives of XR.

Strain Specificity

One of the first areas we explored was the question of strain specificity in xenografts. Previous authors have maintained that XR can be highly dependent upon the strain of the species utilized in xenograft experiments in mice [48]. One experiment we designed as a stringent test of this concept was to compare the survival of cardiac xenografts in the weak allograft responder ACI rat recipient to survival of cardiac xenografts in the high responder Lewis strain. The ACI strain is known for its low responsiveness and will accept a number of fully allogeneic cardiac allografts with only minimal immunological manipulation maintained for short periods of time.

Despite these differences, hamster-to-rat cardiac xenograft survival was similar (3.8 ± 1.2 versus 4.1 ± 0.6 days, respectively) in Lewis versus ACI recipients. In a like manner, skin grafts done between a hamster and the ACI versus the Lewis rats showed no difference in graft survival or in histopathological infiltrate of rejected grafts [18].

Our conclusion from this study is that rat strain differences exert minor, if any, effects on xenograft survival, despite earlier findings. Either of these concepts could have practical implications in future clinical xenografting. Other recent studies indicate that MHC antigens are not primary targets of XR, a finding which fits well with the lack of strain specificity recently found.

Anti-donor Antibodies

An area of great interest is the role of antibodies in xenograft rejection. The failure of skin grafts to hyperacutely reject is a curious phenomenon since in many of the donor-recipient xenograft models studied a high level of anti-donor cytotoxic antibody was present in the recipient. Furthermore, investigations have demonstrated a relative ease of induction of the skin analog of hyperacute rejection in allografts, the so-called "white graft." However, the hamster heart placed in the Lewis rat, and also the hamster liver, do not hyperacutely reject despite high levels of anti-hamster antibody in Lewis sera. The cardiac xenograft findings also stand in stark contrast to the relative ease of induction of allogeneic hyperacute rejection in cardiac allografts in the rat, as shown by Forbes, Guttman, and others [36].

A common explanation for the failure of rats to develop hyperacute rejection is the low level of complement seen in these animals. It was striking for us, therefore, to observe in some other experiments a hyperacute rejection pattern in the

Lewis rat in 15–20 min, with classical rejection patterns of massive swelling, epicardial ecchymoses, a dilated and cyanotic heart, and a cessation of heart beat.

Using a plasmapheresis technique developed in our laboratory with multiple centrifugation of the plasmapheresed aliquots, we were able to show that plasmapheresis of 10 ml blood daily for 2 consecutive days pretransplant was able to markedly prolong the guinea pig heart graft to 2–3 h. At the end of this time, the heart looked completely normal without any signs of hyperacute rejection, but the experiment had to be terminated because of blood leakage at the suture line, presumably due to defects in clotting factors removed during plasmapheresis.

The guinea pig studies were important in showing that the Lewis rat can exhibit normal complement-dependent cytotoxicity and a vigorous hyperacute rejection of a xenografted heart without deliberate induction of preformed anti-donor antibody. Interestingly enough, there was no significant difference between anti-guinea pig antibody levels in the Lewis rat and the anti-hamster antibody levels, irrespective of the failure of the Lewis rat to generate an effective hyperacute rejection of the hamster, but not the guinea pig, heart. While there is much reason to believe that antibody is the primary effector in this model, there are a large number of observations leading to the conclusion that levels of antibodies do not show a direct positive correlation with rejection in many situations. Thus it seems highly possible that factors other than complement-dependent antibody (e.g., NK cell, antibody-dependent cellular cytotoxicity, LAK cells, platelets) may interact with humoral antibody to produce effector mechanisms generating hyperacute rejection.

The xenograft rodent models can be very useful in dissecting out the basic elements of hyperacute rejection seen in discordant xenografts. Previous studies of hyperacute rejection in xenografts (especially pig-to-dog) have outlined roles for platelets, polymorphonuclear neutrophils (PMNs), leukocytes, hemagglutinating red blood cells, complement, and anti-donor antibody. Our studies in rodents, as well as those of others, also suggest that multiple mechanisms may be involved since humoral antibody and/or complement alone do not seem sufficient to explain the disparate results seen.

Humoral Antibody, Xenograft Rejection, and Humoral Accommodation

The immediate problem in discordant XR is a hyperacute rejection pattern which is even more robust than allograft hyperacute rejection. This XR has been identified as primarily related to preformed natural antibodies and complement activation. Unfortunately, despite over 30 years of intensive study, little progress has been made. Rodent models are quite useful in these studies, and recently the use of a soluble complement receptor (sCR_1) has prolonged guinea pig xenografts from hours to a few days. The same results can be achieved by cobra venom factor (CVF) which has been used for 30 years in xenograft models. Blocking secondary reactions, such as platelet activation, also helps but only for a short time (minutes to hours).

In this author's opinion, basic concepts are badly needed in this area. For example, guinea pig hearts are rejected with little evidence of strong preformed antibodies. It has been suggested that the alternative pathway of complement is involved. This hypothesis needs further exploration. Similarly, a host of articles suggests that natural antibodies are not important because a single plasmapheresis has only a mild effect on hyperacute rejection. It is known, however, that antibody rebound is quick following a single pheresis, and multiple phereses need to be done. Studies with single pheresis should be viewed skeptically.

The expansion of a newly described basic concept into elegant derivatives was beautifully demonstrated with humoral antibody systems and XR. Once the importance of HA in XR was defined, many studies focussed and expanded this area. White's group established that even long-surviving xenografts were mostly vulnerable, but occasionally resistant to HA directed against their antigens. Murase, et. al., in a strikingly energetic study, demonstrated that IS agents with known anti-B cell activity effectively blocked XR beyond the degree seen with anti-T cell agents. Marchman et al. demonstrated the tight correlation of early XR and antibody titers. Carobbi et al. showed the critical role of splenectomy in blocking development of anti-xenograft titers and preventing early XR. In fact, there are few IS measures which can impact XR to the great degree that splenectomy does.

Perhaps the most positive and conceptually critical studies of the role of antibody in the long survival of xenografts are the serial studies of patterns of CDC and ADCC reported in a seminal study by our group [20] and expanded and extended in a number of subsequent publications [19, 20, 25, 27, 30, 31, 34, 35]. This study demonstrated basic correlates of anti-donor CDC and ADCC with XR. Basically independent of the IS drugs given, the classical hamster heart-to-Lewis rat model demonstrated clear patterns of HA associations with XR. In xenorecipients with early (day 1–14) rises in CDC and ADCC, acute and severe XR occurred, usually by 1 week post-transplantation. Histopathology demonstrated clear-cut patterns of severe humoral antibody-mediated rejection, including severe small vessel vasculitis, small and large vessel occlusion with infarction, interstitial hemorrhage, massive tissue edema and extravasation. The correlation of antibody titers and XR was excellent ($r=0.92$, $p<0.05$). In xenografts surviving 20–40 days or so, CDC and ADCC levels also correlated well with XR ($r=0.87$, $p<0.05$), and histopathology was predominantly a vascular rejection pattern, although mononuclear cell infiltrates were more prominent than in early rejectors. Of interest, however, was a basic similarity in CDC and ADCC antibody titers between these two groups at the time of rejection.

Early studies in immunodeficient rodents support this concept since animals with marked deficiencies in T cells (such as nude rats) can reject xenografts in a rapid, vigorous manner with apparently normal patterns of cellular reactivity. In addition, xenograft rejection in the hamster-to-Lewis rat heart model is apparent at 24–48 h and peaks by 72 h. This accelerated destruction of grafts occurs far before development of significant T cell cytotoxicity at 7–10 days. LAK cell activity is easily inducible in 48–72 h with sufficient levels of IL-2 in culture. Thus the early in vivo cytotoxicity seen in these rodent xenograft models is probably a non-T cell type cytotoxicity, most likely LAK and/or ADCC killing. Patselas et al., however, were unable to detect LAK killing in xenograft rejection even when the recipients were given rIL-2 to maximumly elevate IL-2 levels.

Immunodeficient models which show a marked delay in XR (or even indefinite survival of xenografts), such as the SCID model, the *xid/Nu/Be* model, and the *Nu/Be* model, all have defects in LAK killing. In contrast, animals with LAK killing intact or relatively normal, all reject xenografts normally. NK defects will lead to a slight prolongation of xenograft models from 7–14 days, as shown by our group in the Be mouse. These findings are highly reproducible and suggest that LAK cell killing is a possible primary mechanism of XR.

Another fascinating aspect of these findings is that they would go far to explain the reason why agents with strong anti-T helper cell activity, such as RATG and anti-L3T4 monoclonal antibodies, are potent blockers of xenogeneic responses. A similar explanation for the effectiveness of TLI in blocking xenograft survival seems appropriate and rational. Since this agent also blocks LAK cell cytotoxicity, identification of afferent and efferent arms of xenogeneic reactivity would seem to be critical in developing a basic understanding of this immune response. Our group directly accessed the role of NK cells in XR with negative results, but these studies need to be repeated.

Recent studies of the so-called xid deficiency may provide insight into the role of B cell activity in xenograft rejection since these animals have now been convincingly demonstrated to lack xenoreactivity. Cardiac grafts in these animals are prolonged indefinitely. These animals have normal T cell, NK and LAK activity. While the results of these studies need to be confirmed and expanded by immunological reconstitution experiments, the early findings are provocative. Hopefully, these findings in rodents will permit a better understanding of the mechanism of xenograft rejection which may permit the development of better techniques for immunomodulation of the xenograft response.

A recent finding of major interest is the discovery that nude rats with marked T cell deficiency reject cardiac xenografts in a completely normal tempo and fashion [9, 10]. In addition to this striking finding, further studies demonstrated that splenectomy partially ablated this response and prolonged graft survival to a mean of 28 days without IS. These results demonstrate that T cell-deficient animals can have normal xenogeneic rejection responses which are partially dependent upon the spleen and surely based on B cell rejection mechanisms. More recent studies clearly demonstrate that the antibodies involved are T cell-independent, probably directed at carbohydrate epitopes on the xenograft endothelium.

Role of the Spleen in Xenograft Rejection

Because antibody responses are known to be important in XR, it seemed logical to us that the spleen, important in the antibody response to intravenously injected antigens, might well be important in xenoantibody responses. Therefore, we performed splenectomy in a number of animals, both pretransplant and at the time of transplantation, and measured xenograft survival [11, 19, 28, 31, 35].

In the hamster-to-Lewis rat heart recipient, splenectomy produced a decrease in the humoral antibody response but no significant prolongation of graft survival. Splenectomy plus 15 mg cyclosporine/kg, however, produced a rather marked mean xenograft prolongation to nearly 22 days in this model. Of even greater interest, however, was the ability of FK506, when used in combination with splenectomy, to prolong graft survival to a mean of 40 days. Splenectomy and DSG given at 2.5 mg/kg also prolonged graft survival up to 87 days, and this, too, was highly significant. These graft survivals were some of the longest survivals seen to-date in over 1000 hamster-to-Lewis rat cardiac xenografts. Recently, our group has attained essentially indefinite survival with splenectomy and a variety of immunosuppressive agents in this model.

All prolongations were associated with decreased antibody titers in the responding animals. The most effective decrease in antibody titers was produced by splenectomy plus DSG. These results clearly demonstrate that splenectomy can act with suppressive drugs in a synergistic manner and suggests that splenectomy may be important in xenografting, despite its poor ability to prolong either primary or secondary allografts.

The most recent studies in our laboratory indicate that the effects of splenectomy on xenograft rejection may be independent of blockade of T cell-independent antibody production by the spleen. There was a poor correlation of T cell-dependent antibody block by splenectomy and xenograft prolongation [35]. These findings suggest that splenectomy may act to prolong xenograft survival by blocking of T cell-independent antibody formation. Finally, some current studies suggest that the splenic microenvironment may be important in bringing together essential cells in XR which cannot act as effectively when they are not geographically proximate.

Histopathology of Xenograft Rejection

One of the most poorly understood areas of xenograft rejection is the histopathology of xenograft rejection (Chaps. 17–21). There have been only a few reports on this subject, and a large number of these were prior to the modern era of immunobiologic sophistication, including monoclonal antibody markers of infiltrating cells. Our studies began with standard histopathology obtained with hematoxylin and eosin stains in hamster hearts removed after rejection by Lewis rat recipients [12, 13].

The early lesions of the accelerated rejection model with preformed antibodies were a vasculitis with endothelial disruption, pyknosis, swelling, and overall disruption of endothelial integrity. Associated with this, there was often a severe hemorrhagic infiltrate, high numbers of PMNs but little myocyte necrosis. Most of the myocyte necrosis seemed to be secondary to infarcts, which appeared in stage II xenograft rejection in this model. In this stage, there were multiple microinfarcts and multiple areas of obstruction of the vessels and plugging by platelet–thrombin–fibrin complexes with intermeshed cells. In a milder stage of xenograft rejection seen in immunosuppressed animals at a later time, there was a more marked infiltrate of cells into the interstitium and myocardial swelling and myocyte necrosis which was more uniform, suggesting a direct and local attack upon the cells and not an ischemic necrosis as suggested by the earlier phase of vasculitis and thrombosis within the blood vessels.

Some studies were performed with monoclonal antibody stains and showed infiltrates of T cells, a high percentage of macrophages in the infiltrate, as well as cells resembling large granular lymphocytes (presumably K, NK, or LAK cells). We performed FACS analyses of infiltrating cells using antibodies. In most early humoral rejection (up to 10 days), no significant cellular infiltrate was seen. In the later rejections, in animals treated with DSG and/or FK506, a significant cellular infiltrate was observed. This infiltrate, by FACS analysis, was composed of 10%–40% T cells with T helper cells slightly predominating over T cytotoxic/suppressor cells. A significant portion of the T helper cell population was double labeled, and two-color florescence demonstrated a macrophage and T helper cell phenotype. These findings are supported by recent studies of Moeller's group demonstrating a similar pattern. These results suggest that macrophage infiltrates may be even more prominent than early studies suggested. Hancock et al. have recently characterized this as "delayed xenograft rejection," suggesting a major role for macrophages and NK cells in this reaction.

In addition to vasculitis, early xenograft rejection is characterized by small vessel thrombosis. Microinfarcts are often seen in the adjacent tissues. More commonly, the interstitium shows a hemorrhagic pattern with edematous, separated intermyocyte spaces. The major hallmark of discordant xenografts is, thus, a severe vasculitis with clotting infarction and disruption of endothelial integrity. This process, undoubtedly mediated by humoral antibody, can be blocked by some suppressive agents, especially DSG, cyclophosphamide and methotrexate.

Operational Tolerance to Xenografts in Rodents

Immune tolerance has come to the forefront of clinical and experimental transplantation in recent years. The inexorable loss of grafts to chronic rejection and the unacceptable morbidity and mortality of chronic IS have forced the conclusion that a system developing a more favorable host environment for the graft, hopefully to the degree that some or all of the chronic IS drugs could be abandoned, must be fostered. In addition to systems deliberately focused on donor-specific tolerance induction, conventionally treated graft recipients have developed drug-induced tolerance which permits long-term graft survival even when IS drugs are decreased or discontinued. Recently, xenograft systems producing a similar result, which must be labeled "operational tolerance," have been described. For example, discordant pig islet xenografts have functioned up to 8 months without chronic IS [21] and other discordant islet models with long-surviving grafts (200 days or more) after discontinuance of immunosuppression have been described [20, 22, 28, 30, 31, 34]. Studies of these operationally tolerant xenografts suggest that the tolerance is specific to the transplanted islets and not easily demonstrable with second grafts, a point of immunology which is both puzzling and disconcerting to many immunologists, but perhaps of lesser interest to the surgeon since his primary goal of graft acceptance without chronic IS has been apparently achieved.

In rodents, recent studies from at least three laboratories have established the capability of achieving long-term survival of disparate heart grafts (hamster-to-rat) with discontinuance of suppression. More detailed reports of these animals should be most informative, but some emerging concepts have already been studied. In the case of White's group, long-term survival was obtained with a cyclosporine-based regimen (incorporating adjuvant anti-B cell agents) but was a bit unstable in that cyclosporine discontinuance at a late date could lead to rejection. Murase et al. (Pittsburgh) achieved impressive long-term survival but required B cell blockade also. These authors documented that graft survival occurred despite some evidence of anti-graft humoral immunity. Unfortunately, serial studies of humoral immunity were not correlated with graft survival. Quarantillo et al. studied both CDC and ADCC antibodies serially and established that a tight correlation between early titers of antibody and xenograft rejection was clearly evident. Most striking, however, was the loss of this tight correlation with reversion to a noncorrelative relationship after 40–60 days of graft residence. Later, almost without exception, long-term graft survival without rejection was seen despite high antibody titers.

These results are strong support for the "humoral accommodation theory" of Platt and Bach [54]. If this concept is correct, long-term xenograft survival may be expected on a regular basis in the near future. Most importantly, the xenograft recipient may not require chronic immunosuppression, an important achievement since the dose and toxicities of most agents required for xenografting are probably unacceptable on a long-term basis.

Study of Immunosuppressive Modalities in Rodent Xenografts

There is reasonable cause to believe that the single major impediment to application of clinical xenografting in the near future is the problem of short- and long-term rejection of the xenogeneic graft accentuated because of the great disparity of xenoantigens between the donor and host. Ten years ago, our group began a comprehensive study of IS in xenografting using rodents. Rodents were selected deliberately because we felt from preliminary studies that a number of new drugs given in varying doses would have to be screened in order to obtain effective suppression of the xenograft response. Furthermore, we knew that these drugs are quite toxic in almost every instance, both because of the need for such a vigorous blocking of the immune system and also because so many of the drugs are effective only at high doses. The many difficult variables suggested at the time that rodent studies were done would be important as a beginning point.

Early studies of IS to prevent XR were discouraging. At the Xeno 25 meeting in 1988, our group reported the use of a variety of IS agents in skin grafting and with the reproducible but difficult Syrian hamster-to-Lewis rat cardiac xenograft [2]. Unfortunately, the results in both of these systems using a variety of IS agents were very discouraging. In most cases, only a few days prolongation of grafts was seen. One or two studies reported spectacular results, but these could not be reproduced [6, 42] by other laboratories. Hsu et al. [4] reported prolongation of discordant skin xenografts to 20–25 days using ATG combined with DSG or FK506. In 1992, Carobbi et al. [11] reported prolongation of hamster-to-Lewis rat grafts using splenectomy combined with FK506 or DSG. White's group prolonged this graft also by combining long-term cobra venom factor therapy with cyclosporine and/or cyclophosphamide [26]. Following the description of the close association of antibody development and XR by Marchman et al. [8, 12], two groups simultaneously and independently reported normal XR in markedly T cell-deficient animals [10, 55]. These studies set the stage for fruitful empirical study of xenograft IS since they established that B cell and antibody reactivity was the primary factor in XR.

In xenografting as in allografting, many of the contributions to the immunobiology of graft rejection and acceptance have been made by rodent studies. In the case of xenografting, the development and availability of selectively bred, genetically stable, immunodeficient animals has allowed development of seminal observations, such as the role of B cells in XR, the lack of T cell importance in XR, the role of humoral accommodation in graft prolongation, and the ability to generate tolerance in a variety of xenografts. Similarly, the contributions of transgenic mice to the understanding of XR are legion. For example, the xenografting of solid organs in mice lacking class I and class II antigens (the class I and class II knockout mice) clearly demonstrated that solid organ xenografts were not rejected by an immune mechanism directed against class I and class II antigens. This observation was not unexpected given the prior knowledge that T cell reactivity was not at the core of XR and that strain specificity had little to do with XR. These observations continue to be of importance, however, because the concept of a T cell-mediated immune cell response presumably directed at MHC antigens is still being considered as a primary mechanism of XR. Observations of graft rejection in the αGal1-3Gal-deficient rodents has also led to the critical observation that this epitope would appear to be among the strongest of all epitopes against which XR is induced.

In terms of future observations, transgenic rodents will no doubt be critically important in demonstrations of the role of antigen responses of endothelial cells. In XR it is possible that xenograft reactivity is a result of an afferent effector mechanism involving antigen presentation by endothelial cells and development of reactivity at this level, or that XR is primarily related to a reaction initially developed at the level of the endothelial cell antigens, with the later development of a systemic component leading to an efferent immune response involving damage and cytotoxicity of the xenogeneic endothelial cells. Development of both efferent and afferent endothelial cell reactivity in XR has been previously demonstrated, but further studies to more clearly define elements of this reaction have not, to date, been well reported. The role of antigen presenting cells would seem to be critically important since the endothelial cell is known to be clearly capable of antigen presentation. This, too, may prove to be an important area for study using transgenic animals which could illuminate the basic factors in antigen presentation involved in xenograft reactivity.

Comment

Notable progress has been made in the understanding of the immunobiology of XR since the first edition of this volume was published about five years ago. The central role of B cells and antibodies interacting with a vigorous complement-dependent immune effector system has been established and the secondary role of T cells in XR delineated. The critical importance of endothelial cell epitopes, including the αGal1-3Gal epitope, in inducing xenograft immunity has been established, and a variety of immunosuppressive techniques have been developed to block humoral antibody responses, strong complement responses, and ancillary pro-inflammatory reactivity. In the first decade or so of solid scientific xenograft investigations, prolonged survival of disparate xenografts has been established, thus permitting the observation of serial, long-term xenoreactivity. As a corollary of these observations, the insightful and novel theory of humoral accommodation has been, for the first time, empirically demonstrated in animal strains with long-term graft survival by serial studies of CDC and ADCC.

Finally, the demonstration of what is best described as "operational tolerance," with long-term xenograft survival unsurpassed in many models using only short and discontinuous immunosuppression with no long-term chronic drug therapy, is perhaps the most optimistic of all the findings in disparate xenografts to-date. It does not seem unreasonable to predict that the xenograft barrier may be broken in the near future using available suppressive agents.

References

1. Billingham, R.E., Medawar, P.B. Free skin grafting in mammals. J. Exper. Biol. 28, 385, 1951
2. Thomas, F.T., DeMasi, R.J., Daniel, H., et al. Comparative immunosuppression for xenografting. In: Xenograft 25. Hardy, Mark A. (ed.), Elsevier, Amsterdam, 1989, p. 55
3. Thomas, F.T., Thomas, J.M., Ganghoff, O., Gross, U. Mechanisms of cell-mediated rejection. In: Kidney Transplant Rejection. Williams, G.M., Burdick, J.F., and Solez, K. (eds.) Marcell Dekker, Inc., New York and Basel, 2nd Edition. In press, 1996
4. Hsu, S., Daniel, H., Thomas, J.M, Thomas, F.T. Synergism of FK-506 and rabbit antithymocyte globulin (RATG) in prolongation of xenografts (XG). Surg. Forum, 39, 374, 1988
5. Thomas, F.T., DeMasi, R., Araneda, D., et al. Comparative efficacy of immunosuppressive drugs in xenografting. Transplant. Proc. 22, 1083, 1990
6. DeMasi, R., Alqaisi, M., Araneda, D., et al. Re-evaluation of total lymphoid irradiation (TLI) and cyclosporine therapy in the Syrian hamster to Lewis rat cardiac xenograft model. Transplantation. 49, 639, 1990
7. Haisch, C., Lodge, A., Huber, S., Thomas, F.T. In vitro human versus murine xenogeneic reactions. Transplantation. 50, 528, 1990
8. Marchman, W., Araneda, D., DeMasi, R., et al. Combination therapy with 15-deoxyspergualin and total lymphoid irradiation prolongs xenograft survival in the hamster-to-rat cardiac xenograft model. Transplantation 53:30, 1992
9. Marchman, W., Thomas, F.T., Araneda, D., Carobbi, A., Thomas, J.M. Xenograft rejection in immunodeficient mice. Surg. Forum. 41, 376, 1990
10. Thomas, F.T., Marchman, W., Carobbi, A., et al. Immunobiology of the xenograft response: xenograft rejection in immunodeficient animals. Transplant. Proc. 23, 308, 1991

11. Carobbi, A., Araneda, D., Patselas, T., Thomas, J.M., Mosca, F. Effect of splenectomy in combination with FK-506 and 15-deoxyspergualin on cardiac xenograft survival. Transplant. Proc. 23, 549, 1991
12. Marchman, W., Araneda, D., DeMasi, R., et al. Therapy of total lymphoid irradiation and 15-deoxyspergualin prolongs survival in the hamster-to-rat xenograft model. Transplant. Proc. 23, 201, 1991
13. DeMasi, R., Araneda, D., Gross, U., et al. Improved xenograft survival with continued infusion deoxyspergualin and RATG. J. Invest. Surg. 4, 59, 1991
14. DeMasi, R., Araneda, D., Gross, U., Daniel, H., Thomas, F.T. 15-Deoxyspergualin (DOSP) is a potent immunosuppressive agent in xenografting. Eur. Surg. Res. 21, 35, 1989
15. Haisch, C., Lodge, A., Huber, S., Thomas, F.T. The vascular endothelial cell is central to xenogeneic immune reactivity. Surgery. 108, 306, 1990
16. Patselas, T., Thomas, F.T., Araneda, D., Thomas, J.M. Vascularized heart transplantation in immunodeficient mice. Curr. Surg. 1990, In press
17. Thomas, S., Moon, S., Thomas, F. Techniques of chronic plasmapheresis and antibody depletion in small animals. Transplant Proc. 26, 1333, 1994
18. Araneda, D., Moon, S., Pittman, K., Thomas, F. Considerations of the validity of mouse-to-rat xenograft combinations in xenograft testing. Transplant Proc. 26, 1228, 1994
19. Thomas, F., Araneda, D., Henretta, J., Pittman, K., Marchman, W. Extended and expanded studies of xenograft rejection in immunodeficient animals. Transplant Proc. 26, 1224, 1994
20. Thomas, F., Araneda, D., Quarantillo, P. Long-term survival of disparate cardiac xenografts: induction of tolerance and humoral accommodation. Transplant Proc. 26, 1220, 1994
21. Henretta, J., McFadden, T., Pittman, K., Thomas, J., Thomas, F. Six- to eight-month survival of discordant pig islet xenografts documented by differential species, insulin, and C-peptide in animals given short-term immunosuppression. Transplant Proc. 26, 1138, 1994
22. Pittman, K., Henretta, J., Thomas, J., Thomas, F. Use of discordant islet xenografts for the treatment of type II diabetes. Transplant Proc. 26, 1135, 1994
23. Tearle, R.G., Tange, M.J., Zannettino, Z.L., et al. The α1,3-galactosyltransferase knockout mouse. Transplantation 61, 13, 1996
24. Henretta, J., Pittman, K., McFadden, T., Thomas, F. Successful discordant pancreatic islet xenotransplantation by prevention of primary nonfunction graft rejection and autoimmune disease recurrence. Transplant Proc. 26, 1133, 1994
25. Thomas, F., Pittman, K., Ljung, T., Cekada, E. Deoxyspergualin is a unique immunosuppressive agent with selective utility in inducing tolerance to pancreas islet xenografts. Transplant Proc. 27, 417, 1995
26. Henretta, J., Araneda, D., Pittman, K., Thomas, J., Thomas, F. Studies of Class I and Class II antigens, CD4+ and CD8+ T lymphocytes in allograft and xenograft rejection. Surg. Forum. 45, 428, 1994
27. Quarantillo, P., Araneda, D., Cekada, E., et al. Marked prolongation of cardiac xenograft survival by adaptive transfer of xenoactivated cells. Surg. Forum. 45, 452, 1994
28. Araneda, D., Thomas, F., Ljung, T., Cekada, E., Pittman, K. The primacy of humoral antibody (CDC and ADCC) in concordant xenograft rejection (CXR). Transplant Proc. 27, 268, 1995

29. Henretta, J., Araneda, D., Pittman, K., Thomas, J.M., Thomas, F.T. Studies of Class II (CII) antigen and CD4 cells in allograft and xenograft rejection by use of transgenic animals. J Surg Research. Submitted for publication
30. Quarantillo, P., Thomas, F.T., Araneda, D., Thomas, J. Humoral accommodation as a basis for cardiac xenograft tolerance. Proceedings of Tolerance Induction. (eds. W. Alexander, G. Rood) R. G. Landes Company/Springer, Austin, 1996, p. 193
31. Carobbi, A., Thomas, F.T., Quarantillo, P., Thomas, J. Crucial role of splenectomy (SPLX) in induction of xenograft tolerance (XT). Proceedings of Tolerance Induction. (eds. W. Alexander, R. Good) R.G. Landes Company/Springer, Austin, 1996, p. 189
32. Patselas, T., Thomas, F., Araneda, D., Marchman, W. Role of natural killer and killer cells in concordant xenograft rejection. Transplant Proc. 27, 262, 1995
33. Thomas, F.T., Ljung, T., Henretta, J., Pittman, K., Thomas, J. Reversal of Type II (NIDDM) diabetes by pancreas islet transplantation: an emerging new concept in pathophysiology of an enigmatic disease. Transplant Proc. 27, 3167, 1995
34. Thomas, F.T., Pittman, K., Thomas, J.M. Induction of functional xenograft tolerance of pig islets in the autoimmune NOD mouse. Transplant Proc. 27, 3323, 1995
35. Thomas, F., Thomas, J., Pittman, K., et al. An overview of xenograft studies in immunodeficient animals. Xeno. In press, 1996
36. Forbes, R.D.C., Kuramochi, T., Guttmann, R.D. A controlled sequential morphologic study of hyperacute cardiac allograft rejection in the rat. Lab. Invest. 33, 280, 1975
37. Thomas, F., Cekeda, E., Llung, T., Thomas, J. Rejection of skin and cardiac allo- and xenografts in reconstituted scid mice. Xeno. Submitted for publication, 1996
38. Araneda, D., Moon, S., Pittman, K., Thomas, F. Considerations of the validity of mouse-to-rat xenograft combinations in xenograft testing. Transplant Proc. 26, 1228, 1994
39. Brayman, K.L., Morel, P., Field, J., et al. A comparison of mice and rats as recipients for canine islet xenografts. Transplant Proc. 24, 651, 1992
40. Sawyer, G., Gustaffson, K., Fabre, J.W. Vascularized mouse-to-rat heart grafts: an unexpectedly difficult model of xenotransplantation. Transplant. Proc. 27, 309, 1995
41. Nicolae, M., Ketchum, R.J., Jahr, H., Janoff, H., Brayman, K.L. Islet xenografts in mice and rats: I. Exocrine tissue is detrimental to engraftment and survival of human islet xenografts. Transplant Proc. 26, 774, 1994
42. Steinbruchel, D.A., Madsen, H., Neilson, B., Larsen, S. Total lymphoid irradiation, cyclosporine-A, and a monoclonal anti-T cell antibody in hamster-to-rat heart transplantation. Transplant. Int. 3, 36, 1990
43. Steinbruchel, D.A., Madsen, H.H., Neilson, B., et al. Graft survival in a hamster-to-rat heart transplantation model after treatment with total lymphoid irradiation, cyclosporine-A, and a monoclonal anti-T cell antibody. Transplant. Proc. 22, 1088, 1990
44. Kaufman, D.B., Rabe, F.L., Dunn, D.L., Sutherland, D.E.R. Effect of host immunomodulation on the prevention of islet allograft primary nonfunction in a murine model. Transplant. Proc. 22, 857, 1990
45. Gershwin, M.E., Merchant, B. (eds.) Immunologic Defects in Laboratory Animals. New York, Plenum, Vol. 1, 1981
46. de Jong, W.H., Steerenberg, P.A., Ursem, P.S., et al. The athymic nude rat. III. Natural cell-mediated cytotoxicity. Clin. Immunol. Immunopathol. 17, 193, 1980

47. Sprent, J., Bruce, J. Physiology of B cells in mice with X-linked immunodeficiency (xid) III. Disappearance of xid B cells in double bone marrow chimeras. J. Exp. Med. 160, 711, 1984
48. Jooste, V., Winn, H. Strain variations in the responses of mice to xenografts of skin. Transplant. Proc. 9, 375, 1977
49. Festing, M.F.W., May, D., Connors, T.A. An athymic mutation in the rat. Nature. 274, 365, 1978
50. Mjaaland, S., Fossum, S. Ag processing normal in nude rats. Scand. J. Immunol. 26, 141, 1987
51. Rygaard, J., Paulsen, C. Xenogeneic tumors grow in nude mice. Actu. Pathol. Microbiol. Immunol. Scand. (A). 77, 758, 1969
52. Roder, J., Duwe, A. The beige mutation in the mouse selectively impairs natural killer cell function. Nature. (London). 278, 451, 1979
53. Dorshkind, K., Pollack, S., Bosma, M., Phillips, R. NK cells are present in SCID mice. J. Immunol. 134, 3798, 1985
54. Bach, F.H., Robson, S.C., Winkler, H., et al. Barriers to xenotransplantation. Nature Med. 1, 869, 1995
55. Lim, S.M.L., Li, S.Q., Wee, A., et al. Normal xenograft rejection in immunodeficient rats. Transplant Proc. 23, 581, 1991
56. Lim, S.M.L., Li, S.Q., Wee, A., et al. Both concordant and discordant heart xenografts are rejected by athymic (nude) rats with the same tempo as in T cell competent animals. Transplant. Proc. 23, 581, 1991

… Bruce, J. [illegible]
… The appearance of [illegible]
… 86, … 1964 [illegible]
… R., Wirth, H., Stat… [illegible]
… dent. Proc. 9, 373 … [illegible]
… M…, Alex, P., [illegible]
… S., Forbes, S. [illegible]
… L., Nielsen, [illegible]
… Scand. … [illegible]
…, Dowe, A.: The … [illegible] … neural
… Nature (London) … [illegible]
…, R., Pollack, S., [illegible]
… 1968 [illegible]
… H., Johnson, S.C., … [illegible]
… 1969 [illegible]
… S.Q., … [illegible]
… Transplant. Proc. … [illegible]
… L., … S.Q., We… [illegible]
… period by … [illegible]
… Transplant. Proc. … [illegible]

III Pathology of Xenograft Rejection

17 Histopathology of Kidney Xenograft Rejection

S. Larsen and H. Starklint

Introduction

The morphological and immunological changes developing in the renal graft, evaluated qualitatively as well as quantitatively, depend on the genetic relationship between donor and recipient. Based on the genetic differences, five transplantation systems can be defined:

1. *Isogeneic.* Tissue transplanted from one individual to another individual with an identical genetic constitution (monovular twins)
2. *Autogeneic.* Tissue transplanted from one place to another in the same individual
3. *Allogeneic.* Tissue transplanted from one individual to another of the same species
4. *Xenogeneic (concordant).* Tissue transplanted to an individual of a closely related species (e.g., chimpanze to man)
5. *Xenogeneic (discordant).* Tissue transplanted to an individual of a distantly related species (e.g., pig to man)

Based on knowledge of the morphological changes that occur in human kidney graft biopsies, mainly obtained in situations with impaired renal graft function [1], and from studies on experimental xenografting, the lesions attributed to transplantation may be divided into two basic groups: (1) lesions caused by histoincompatibility specific for the transplant situation and (2) lesions due to noxious influences (physical, infectious, or side effects of medical treatment, including immunosuppressants).

The histoincompatibility-mediated lesions are traditionally divided into three types of rejection: (1) hyperacute (humoral), (2) acute (cellular), and (3) chronic. However, sometimes no sharp limits exist between these conditions; a clear-cut distinction is difficult, morphologically as well as immunologically, because more than one type of rejection may be present simultaneously. Furthermore, changes secondary to noxious influences may modify any of the histoincompatibility-related lesions, both quantitatively and qualitatively.

The morphology of xenografts varies with the animals used and with the discrepancy between the species. The mechanisms behind these variations are largely unknown. However, in some xenografted organs the morphological manifestations are very much like those found in human allografts, implicating the possibility of similar pathogenetic mechanisms, which is why we use the descriptive terminology as applied in clinical transplantation.

The pathogenesis of hyperacute rejection is known to be mediated by complement activation [2]. The development of pigs being transgenic for human decay-accelerating factor (hDAF), inhibiting the formation of classical and alternative pathways and C5 convertase [3], may in the future result in clinical trials of suitable organs from these animals. The progress in modifying donor organs for human transplantation will most probably modify the morphological changes seen in hyperacute rejection and, furthermore, may mimic the acute rejection seen in human allografts.

With this in mind, a group of renal pathologists, nephrologists and transplant surgeons (who met in Banff, Canada, in August 1991) has developed a schema for international standardization of nomenclature and criteria for the histological diagnosis of renal allograft rejection [4, 5]. According to this classification, tubulitis and intimal arteritis are regarded as the principal lesions indicative of acute rejection. Tubulitis is also found in hyperacute rejection, but in this situation is completely "masked" by the pronounced tubular necrosis. In the acute allograft rejection, tissue damage is limited to a degree where the phenomenon of tubulitis is easily seen.

The purpose of this chapter is to illustrate the morphological patterns that create a spectrum of lesions as seen in concordant and discordant renal xenografts, and, furthermore, to illustrate the changes found in kidneys perfused in vitro with xenogeneic blood. Our personal experience is based on studies on transplantation of kidneys from different species (about 500 animals), and on isolated kidneys after perfusion with human blood (whole blood, platelet-poor, or leukocyte-poor) and plasma, and also with blood from other animals. Details of the results of these experiments have been published previously [6–23].

From our material (obtained mainly from untreated animals) some patterns have become clear and these will be illustrated by typical examples. In the legends to each figure, comment will be made of other situations where similar appearances have been documented. The lesions seen in various experimental models are summarized in Tables 1–3, which demonstrate the light microscopic "patterns" found in different xenotransplant situations.

Methods

The macroscopic changes that occurred in the donor kidneys were described by the colleagues who performed the transplantations and hemoperfusions. The results were recorded, but were not made available to the two pathologists who received biopsies. One of us (S. Larsen) received match-like pieces the size of needle-biopsies, whereas the other (H. Starklint) received median frontal slices of the whole kidney.

For light microscopy, the tissue was fixed in buffered formalin. Paraffin sections were stained with hematoxylin and eosin (H&E) supplemented with methenamine-silver for basement membranes and with periodic acid–Schiff (PAS) and Frazer-Lendrum's stains for platelets and fibrin, respectively.

For electron microscopy, cortical tissues were "teased" into small fragments and fixed in 2.5 % glutaraldehyde in a modified Tyrode buffer. Following postfixation in osmium tetraoxide, specimens were treated conventionally, and ultrathin sections were stained with uranyl acetate/lead citrate.

Table 1. Experimental renal xenografting in the hare-to-rabbit concordant model

Group	*n*	Treatment/immune modulation	Longest graft survival	Histopathology[a]	Reference
1	10	Control	6 days	Thrombocyte aggregation, vascular endothelial hyperplasia, interstitial mononuclear cell infiltration, vascular wall necrosis, thrombosis	[8]
2	5	Steroids, cytostatic agents	6 days	Thrombocyte aggregation, vascular wall necrosis, thrombosis	[8]
3	10	CSA	98 days	Mesangial cell hyperplasia, glomerular endocapillary hyperplasia, interstitial mononuclear cell infiltration, tubular necrosis	[8]
4	3	CSA (10 mg/kg per day)	10 days	Thrombocyte aggregation	[15]
5	7	CSA (15 mg/kg per day)	91 days	Mesangial cell hyperplasia, thrombocyte aggregation	[15]
6	8	Presensitized with blood or skin grafts	60 min	Mesangial cell hyperplasia, glomerular endocapillary hyperplasia, thrombocyte aggregation, glomerular thrombosis	[20]
7	28	Leflunomide, CSA, and splenectomy	72 h	Medullary tubular necrosis	[23]

CSA, cyclosporine.
[a] No immune deposits were detected on the rejected kidney, except in group 6, where goat anti-rabbit polyglobulin and goat anti-rabbit C3 were present, and in group 7, in which IgM was consistently demonstrated after 24 h in the glomerular capillary wall and tubular capillaries.

Table 2. Experimental renal xenografting in discordant models

Group	Donor/ recipient	*n*	Treatment	Longest graft survival	Histopathology[a]	Reference
1	Rabbit/cat	16	Steroids, cytostatic agents, cobra venom factor	72 h	Vascular endothelial hyperplasia, tubular necrosis	[16]
2	Rabbit/cat	40	Steroids, cytostatic agents	10 min	Thrombocyte aggregation, thrombosis	[16]
3	Rabbit/cat	5	Ticlopidine[b], cyclosporine, cobra venom factor	4 days	Tubular necrosis	[14]
4	Pig/rabbit	5	Dazoxiben	40 min	Thrombocyte aggregation	[12]
5	Pig/rabbit	5	Control	60 min	Thrombocyte aggregation	[12]
6	Rabbit/pig	5	Control	45 min	Thrombocyte aggregation	[14]
7	Rabbit/pig	5	Control	60 min killed	Thrombocyte aggregation	[14]
8	Rabbit/cat	13	Cobra venom factor	7 days	Tubular necrosis	[13]
9	Rabbit/cat	50	Various agents (no cobra venom factor)	60 min	Thrombocyte aggregation	[13]

[a] Immune deposits on the rejected kidney were not looked for in group 3 and were undetectable in the other groups.
[b] An antiplatelet agent.

Table 3. Experimental hemoperfusion of rabbit kidneys using human blood (discordant model)

Group	*n*	Treatment	Longest graft survival (min)	Histopathology[a]	Reference
1	5	Control	30	Thrombocyte aggregation, vascular wall inflammation, tubular necrosis (on electron microscopy, the endothelium was seen to be loosened)	[10]
2	5	Control	24	Thrombocyte aggregation	[13]
3	5	Platelet-poor human blood	60	Thrombocyte aggregation	[13]
4	5	Prostacyclin	60 min	Thrombocyte aggregation	[13]

[a] Rabbit anti-human IgM and IgG were detected on the kidney in all groups, and rabbit anti-human C3 was detected in groups 2–4.

Tissue for immunofluorescence microscopy was frozen using dry ice and blocked in Tissue-Teck® gelatine (Ames Laboratory) before 1–2 μm sections were cut at −24 °C. The sections were mounted on clean slides and treated by a direct fluorescent technique [20].

Types of Lesions (Tables 1–3)

Definitions of Lesions (Light Microscopy)

1. *Mesangial cell hyperplasia* (Fig. 1). Increased number of cells localized to the mesangium.
2. *Glomerular endocapillary hyperplasia* (Fig. 2). Increased number of intralumenal cells, which may be of endothelial origin or inflammatory mononuclear cells. Often a combination of mesangial cell and endocapillary cell hyperplasia is seen in the same glomerulus (endomesangial hyperplasia).
3. *Thrombocyte aggregation* (Fig. 3). Presence of thrombocytes localized to the lumena, focally or disseminated, as small clots or occluding aggregates in the arterial vessels, juxtaglomerular arterioles, and capillary loops of the glomeruli.
4. *Vascular endothelial hyperplasia* (Fig. 4). Increased number of endothelial cells resulting in a reduction or occlusion of vascular lumena.
5. *Interstitial mononuclear cell infiltration* (Fig. 5). The cells in interstitial infiltrates are mainly mononuclear cells, i.e., small and large lymphocytes, macrophages and, to a lesser degree, plasma cells.
6. *Arteritis* (Fig. 6). The lesions are most severe in medium-sized and small arteries where the endothelial cells are slightly hyperplastic with hydropic degeneration and often piled up in two layers. The intima is thickened due to edema, and accumulation of mononuclear cells is often present. Fibrin may cover parts of the lumenal surface or is seen as droplets in the thickened intima. The media is often infiltrated by mononuclear cells.

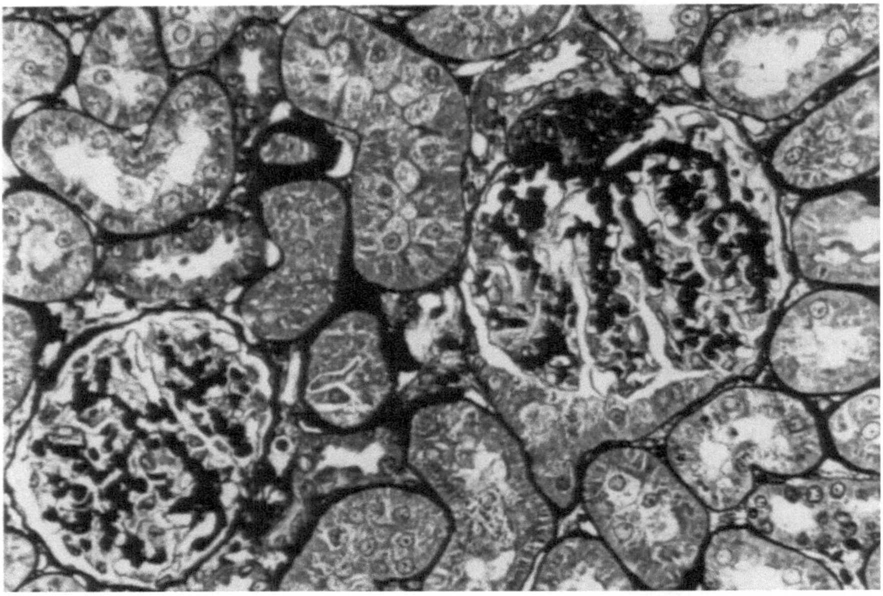

Fig. 1. Diffuse and global mesangial widening and hyperplasia in a hare kidney transplanted into a rabbit. ×830, methenamine-silver

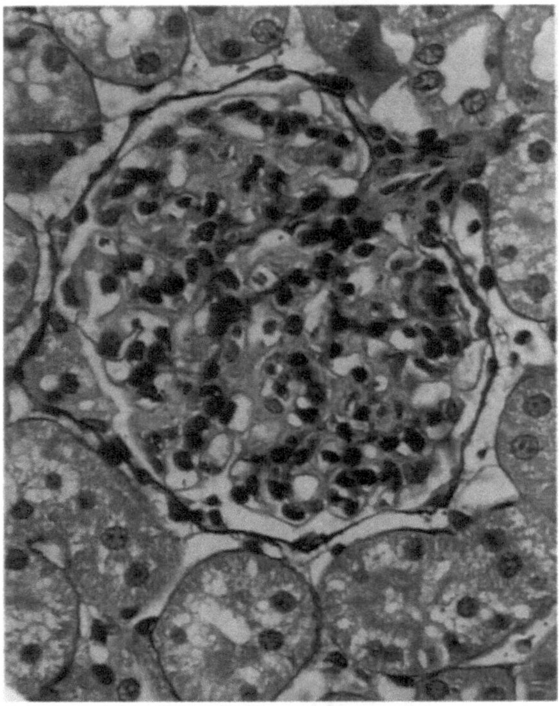

Fig. 2. Focal proliferation of mesangial and endothelial cells with accentuated mesangium at the vascular pole in a hare kidney transplanted into a rabbit (×400, H&E). Glomerulonephritis-like appearances were especially found in the hare-to-rabbit model, but were also seen in (a) rabbit kidneys autotransplanted following perfusion with human blood, (b) hare kidneys transplanted into splenectomized rabbits, and (c) rabbit kidneys flushed with human whole blood or plasma

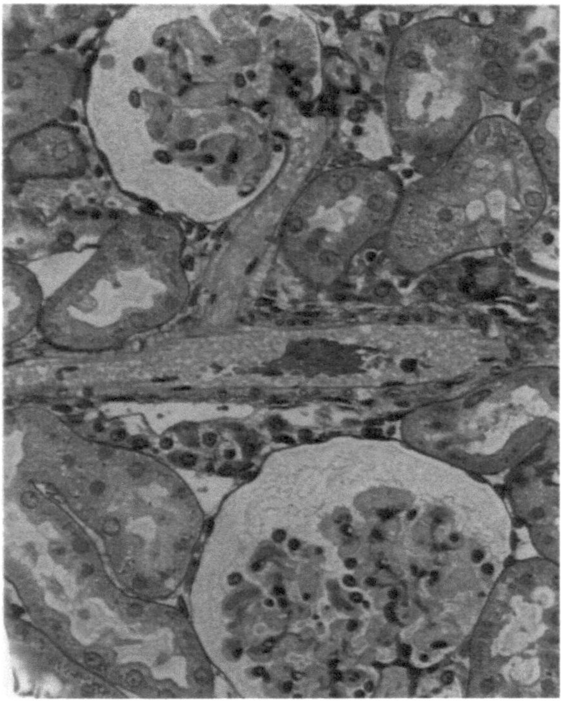

Fig. 3. Tightly packed platelets in the glomerular capillary tuft, the efferent arterioles, and an interstitial arteriole. The section is from a rabbit kidney transplanted into a cat, without treatment. ×300, H&E–PAS

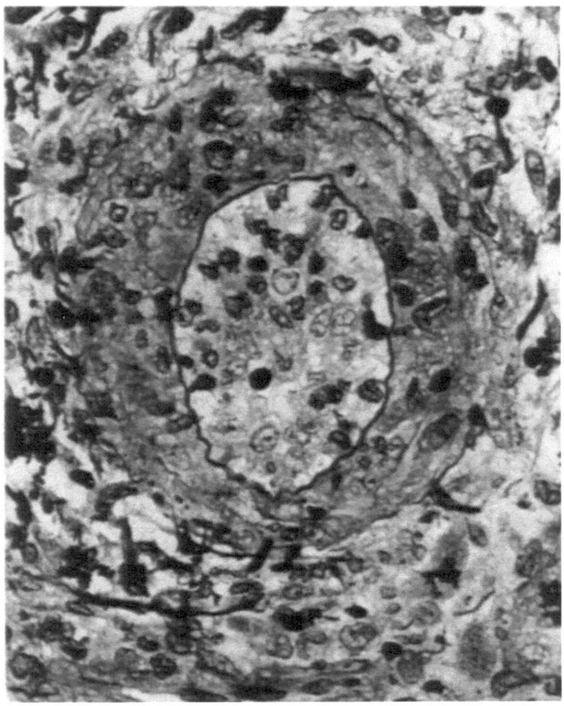

Fig. 4. Acute rejection of a kidney transplanted from hare to rabbit. The interlobular artery shows an intense endothelial proliferation, and the surrounding mononuclear infiltrate is pleomorphic with blasts and lymphocytes (×480, H&E–PAS). These findings were seen almost exclusively in xenotransplants between hare to rabbits, but were also observed on a few occasions in autotransplanted rabbit kidneys after they had been perfused with human blood

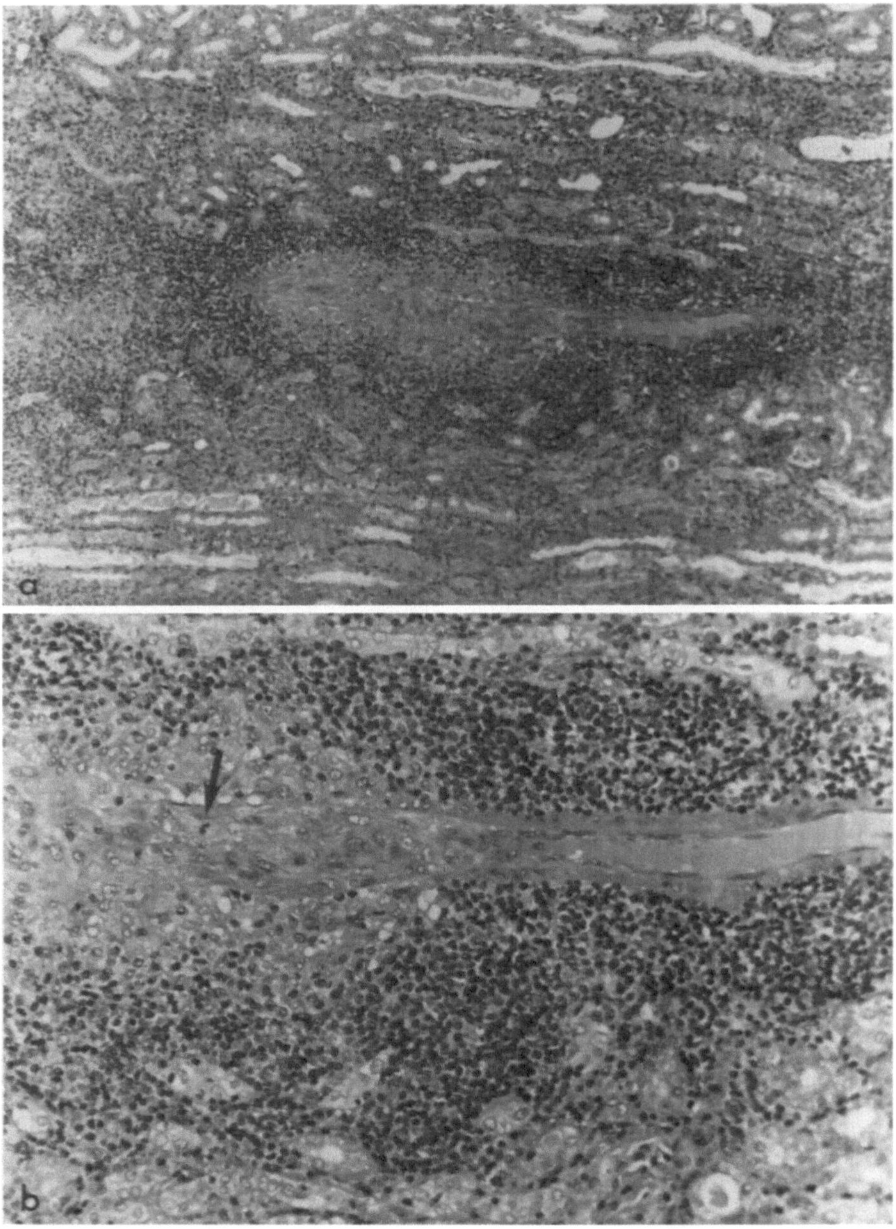

Fig. 5a,b. Acute rejection of kidney transplanted from hare to rabbit. **a** The kidney tissue is fairly well preserved. A mantle of mononuclear cells is seen around the vessels (×63, H&E). **b** A severe endothelial proliferation exists, segmentally blended, which obscures the different components of the vessel wall. The mitotic figure is in an endothelial cell (*arrow*). ×125, H&E

Fig. 6. a Interlobar artery with a nearly empty lumen showing a loosened endothelium surrounded by granulocytes (including eosinophils) and mononuclear cells present in the intima and media (×240, H&E).

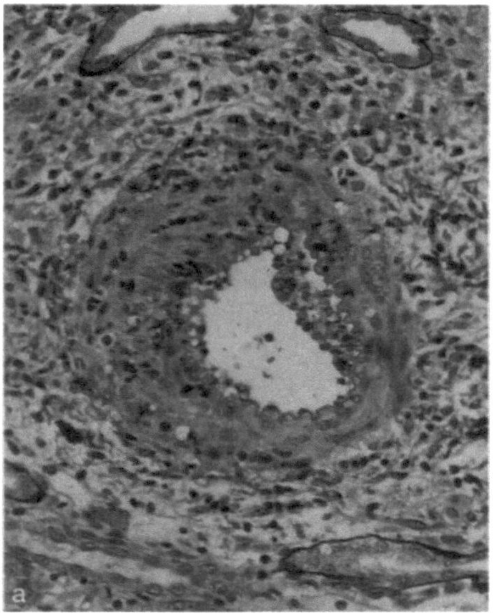

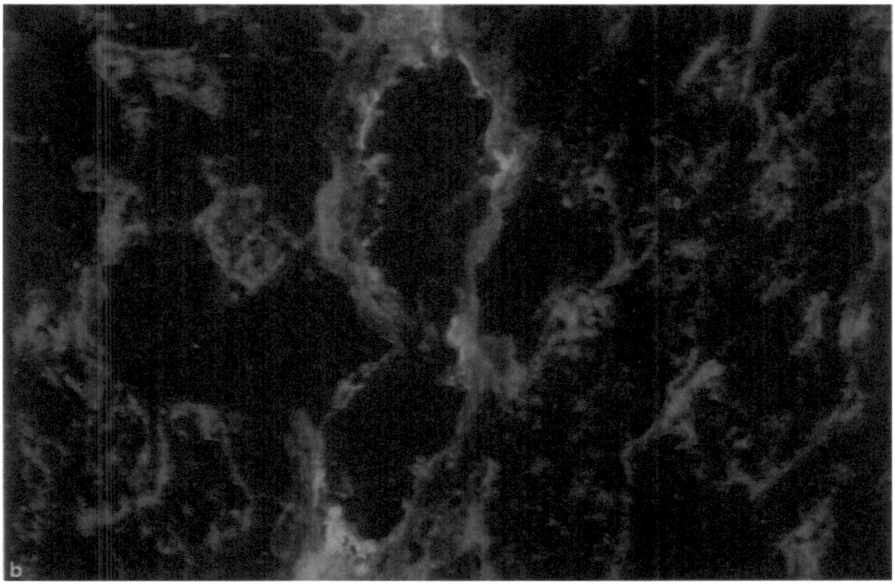

b Immunofluorescence microscopy illustrating an interlobar artery with granular deposits of rabbit anti-human IgM localized to the endothelium, which in small areas is loosened. An equal pattern and distribution were shown using anti-human fibrin/fibrinogen and C3. Inflammatory reactions related to the endothelial lining (intima and/or media) showed a wide spectrum of morphological alterations in different experiments, but also in different kidneys in the same experimental model. It was found in perfusion and flush experiments using rats, rabbits, and pigs as donors and humans (blood and plasma), rabbits, and cats as recipients. It could also be seen when kidneys from hares and pigs were transplanted into presensitized rabbits

7. *Vascular wall necrosis* (Fig. 7). The lesion is often fibrinous in its staining quality. Initially, the inner part of the media is involved. Larger areas with destruction of the internal elastica and intima may be seen in later stages. If arterial necrosis is accompanied by leukocyte infiltration in the media, the use of the term "arteritis" may be justified.
8. *Tubular necrosis* (Fig. 8). Partial tubular necrosis, most often subcapsular, is seen in a few tubular profiles or as small areas surrounded by groups of preserved tubules. Necrosis may affect single tubular cells, small groups, or the total tubular epithelium. The nuclei show pyknosis; later on, all cytologic details may disappear. Calcification of necrotic proximal tubular cells may be seen.
9. *Tubulitis* (Fig. 9). Infiltration of tubular epithelium by leukocytes, usually lymphocytes.
10. *Thrombosis* (Fig. 10). Arterial vessels or glomerular capillary loops where lumena are partially or totally occluded with fibrin material containing red blood cells and/or thrombocytes and/or granulocytes.

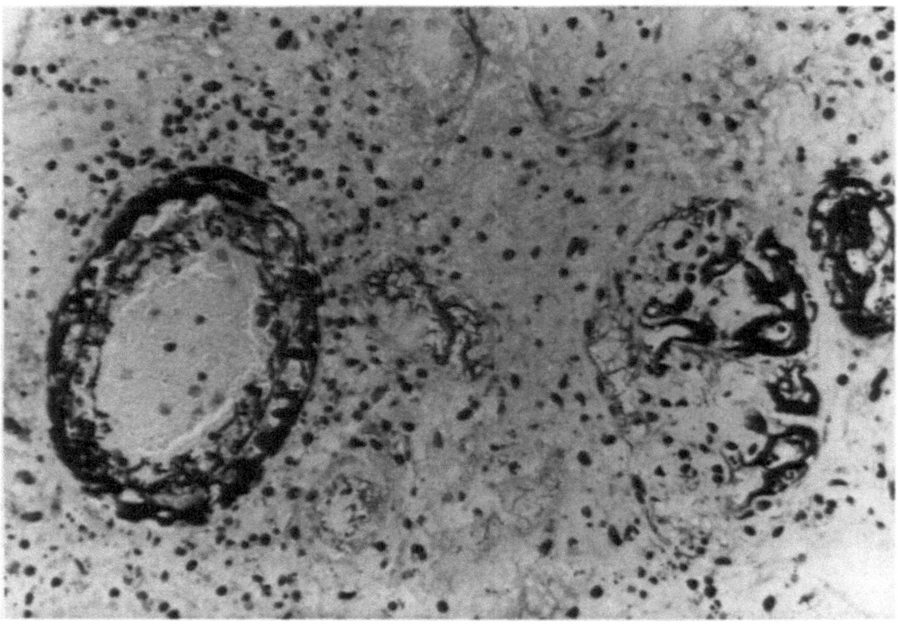

Fig. 7. Hyperacute rejection of a kidney transplanted from hare to rabbit. *Left*, an interlobular artery shows necrosis and deposition of fibrin in its wall. *Right*, a typical glomerulus contains fibrin that tapers and occludes the capillary lumen. The tubules are severely damaged by ischemia with heavy interstitial edema and few inflammatory cells. This pattern was nearly exclusively found in the hare-to-rabbit model. A few examples were seen when rabbit kidneys were autotransplanted following perfusion with human blood. ×830, Frazer Lendrum

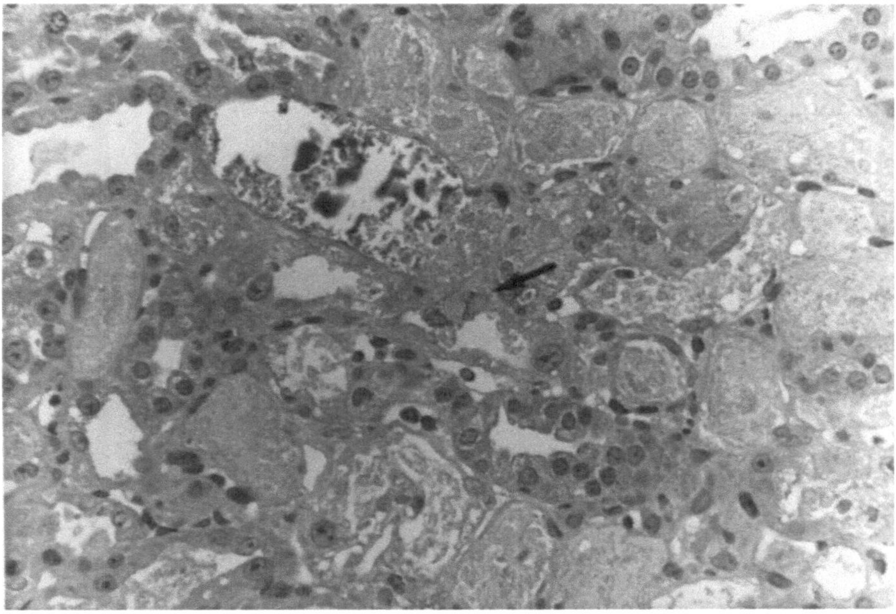

Fig. 8. Subcapsular area in a rabbit kidney transplanted into a cat, which survived for 1 week while receiving cobra venom factor once every day. Totally and partially necrotic tubules, some calcified, are seen. A few mitotic figures (*arrow*) suggest some capacity for regeneration. Tubular necrosis was found in many xenografted models, but was most frequent and extensive in cats treated with cobra venom factor (Table 2). This suggests that this compound is tubulotoxic, as are certain other snake poisons. However, in other experimental groups, small areas demonstrated necrosis of what appeared to be proximal tubules. Such changes were observed in hare-to-rabbit transplants, and following perfusion of goat kidneys with blood from rabbits, cats, and man. Many of the transplanted animals received cyclosporine, usually in dosages of approximately 15 mg/kg per day, which in our experience is not toxic to the tubules to the extent seen in the experiments [22]. x830, H&E

Results

From a technical point of view, most of the investigated tissues were satisfactorily preserved. Some of the experimental situations, however, led to heavy tissue damage, making detailed interpretation difficult or even impossible. Methenamine-silver stain for basement membranes, which is of great importance for diagnosis in the human kidney, was often difficult to interpretate in the experimental animals. The "staining window" between good visualization of peripheral membranes and overstaining, especially of the mesangial area, is very narrow. Therefore, in doubtful cases we recommend the use of series of impregnation times in order to ensure a clear picture of the different structures. The main purpose of the electron microscopic studies was to verify the presence of platelets and to evaluate both their granularity and relation to endothelial cells.

The morphological features seen can be summarized under the following diagnostic headings.

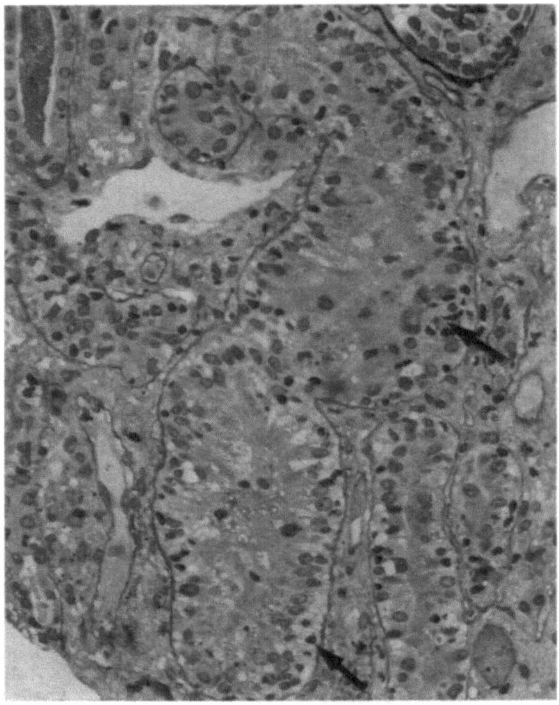

Fig. 9. Tubulitis. Longitudinal section of a tubule. Note the clear space that usually separates lymphocyte nuclei (*arrows*) from adjacent cells. ×240, methenamine-silver

Morphological Conditions Seen Mainly in Concordant Xenograft Rejection (Table 1)

1. *Hyperacute rejection.* A widespread glomerular microthrombosis was found, i.e., not confined to a single area of the kidney and thus presumably not related to infarction of the transplanted organ (Fig. 7).
2. *Acute rejection.* Perivascular and interstitial infiltrates of lymphoid cells accompanied by varying degrees of endothelial proliferation were found (Figs. 4, 5). The composition of the infiltrates varied with the maturity and differentiation of lymphocytes, some exhibiting a great number of plasma cells.
3. *Mixed-picture hyperacute and acute rejection* (Fig. 10). This was seen in some cases and was related to accelerated rejection.
4. *Chronic rejection of glomerular type* (Fig. 11). Glomerular cellular proliferations and membranous-like patterns were found in long-term survivors accompanied by immune complex deposition diagnosed by immuno fluorescence.

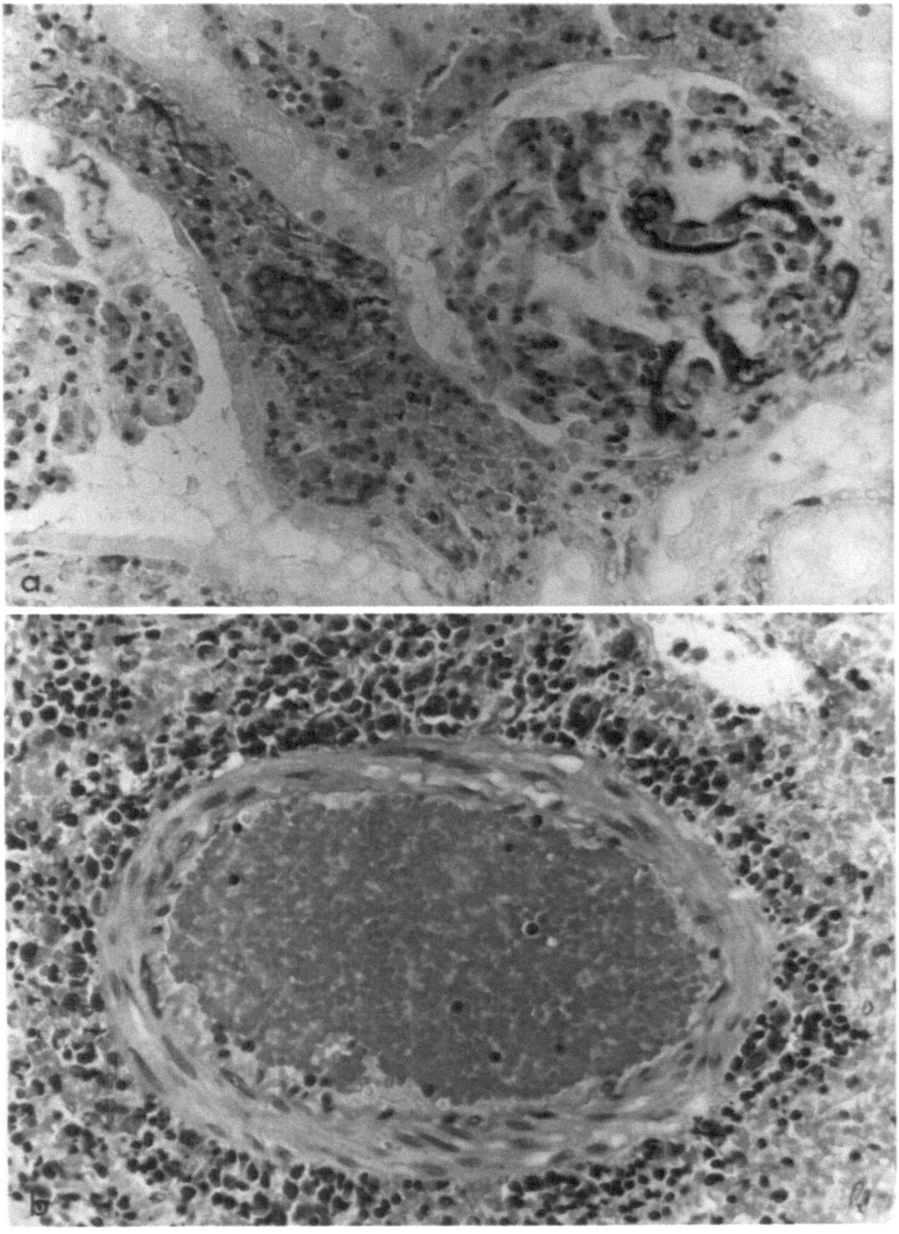

Fig. 10a,b. In some cases of hare-to-rabbit concordant xenotransplantation, a mixed picture of hyperacute and acute rejection was seen. **a** The glomerulus contains fibrin along the capillary walls, but this was not seen in all glomeruli. Apart from the presence of edema and interstitial bleeding the tissues are rather well preserved. ×240, Frazer-Lendrum. **b** A great number of parenchymal vessels showed mantles of mononuclear cells. ×240, H&E. This mixed picture was solely found in the hare-to-rabbit kidney transplantations

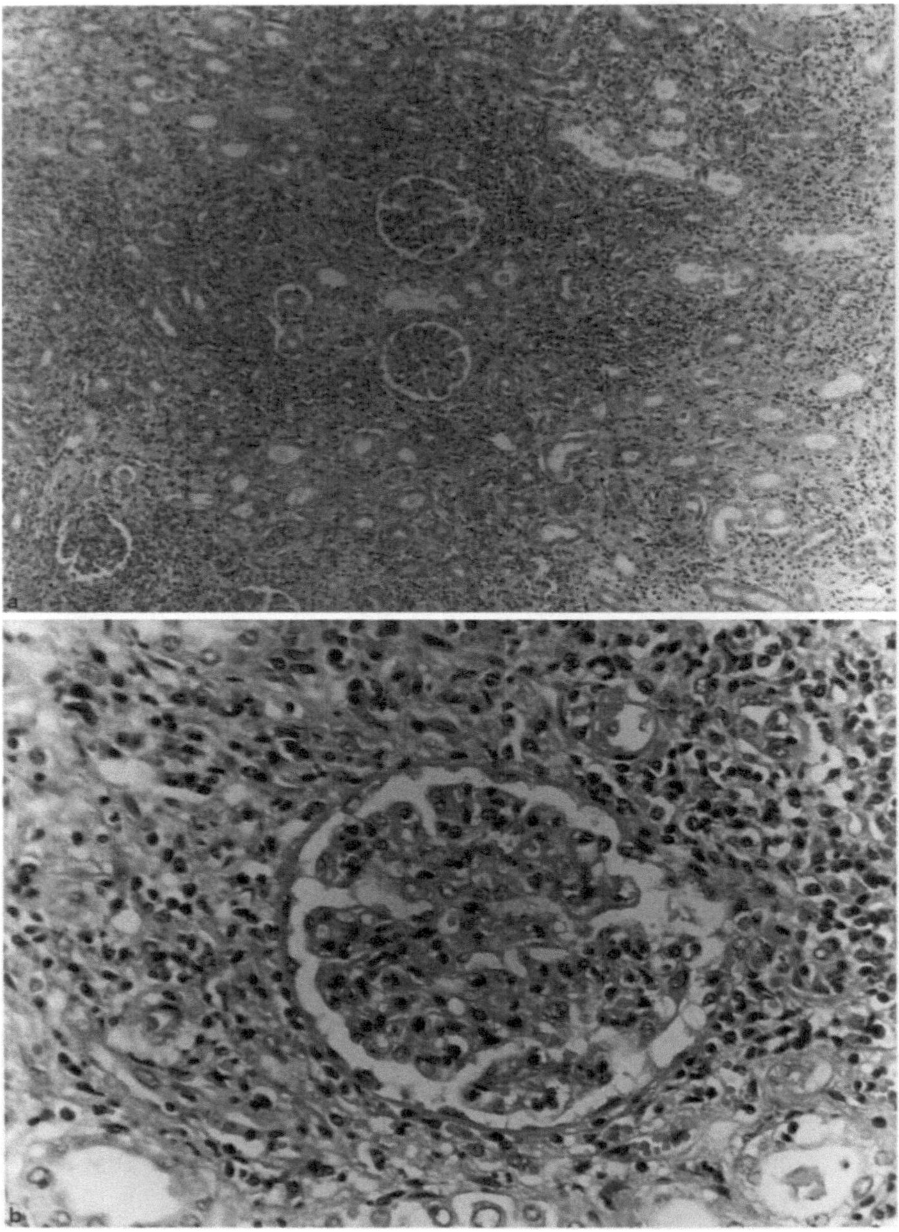

Fig. 11a,b.

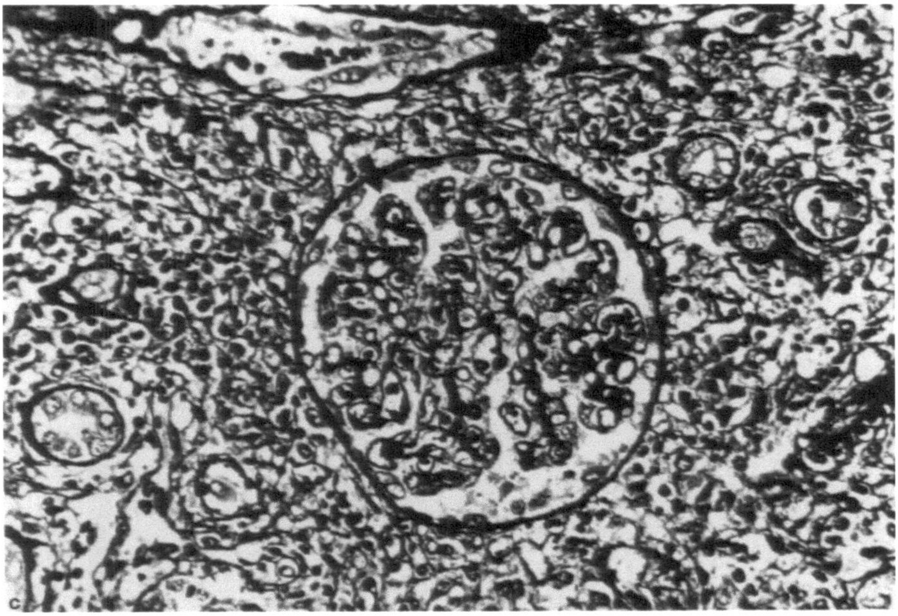

Fig. 11a–c. Chronic glomerular rejection was diagnosed in a few long-term surviving nephrectomized rabbits transplanted with a hare kidney. **a** Some interstitial fibrosis and mononuclear cell infiltration can be seen. ×63, H&E. **b** A slight glomerular hypercellularity and thickened peripheral basement membranes. ×200, H&E. **c** These membranes are duplicated in some loops (*arrow*). ×200, methenamine-silver. These were rare findings, seen only in rabbits transplanted with hare kidneys and who had received cyclosporine (15 mg/kg per day i.m.) for 30 days, the animals surviving 9–13 weeks

5. *Glomerulonephritis-like alterations.* This was observed in cases with either focal segmental or diffuse global mesangial cell hyperplasia and/or endocapillary hyperplasia (Figs. 1, 2). Not all of these were accompanied by immune deposits. Differentiation from the chronic rejection of glomerular type (as described in point 4) was certainly problematic and mainly related to graft survival time. Glomerulonephritis-like alterations were found more frequently than chronic rejection of glomerular type.
6. *Venous endothelium paved with neutrophile granulocytes.* The classical light-microscopic picture of the inflammatory response was found in untreated hamster-to-rat kidneys from day 3 in parenchymal veins and peritubular capillaries not accompanied by platelet aggregation or fibrin thrombi. Polyreactive xenoantibodies increased rapidly at the same time (Figs. 12–15).

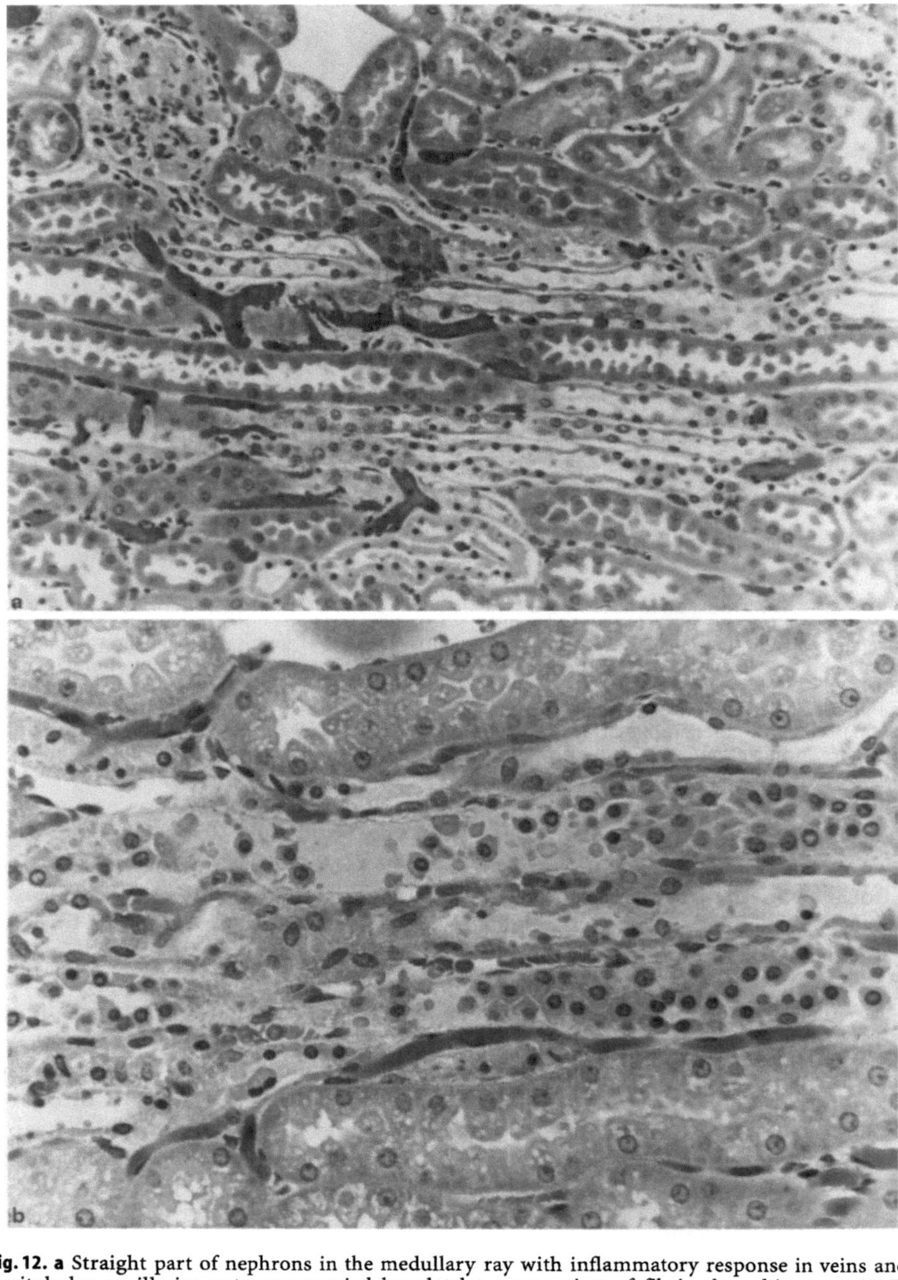

Fig. 12. a Straight part of nephrons in the medullary ray with inflammatory response in veins and peritubular capillaries not accompanied by platelet aggregation of fibrin thrombi. ×120, H&E. **b** Extensive pyknosis and loosening of the epithelial cells. ×240, H&E. This phenomenon has only been met after perfusion of rabbit kidneys with human blood. It is not clear whether it is the result of a technical problem or a feature of ischemia secondary to platelet aggregation

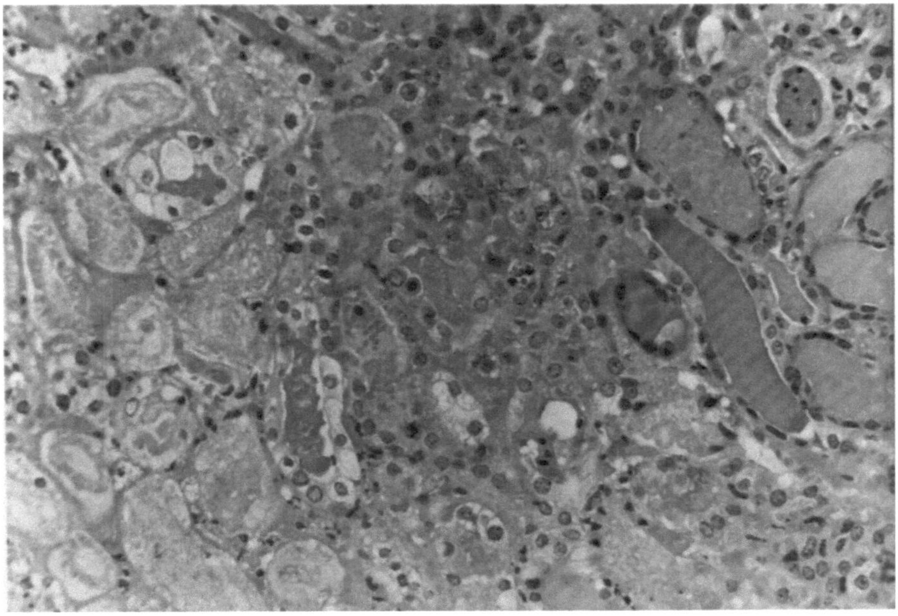

Fig. 13. Necrotic tubular profiles in the outer medulla of a hamster kidney transplanted to a Lewis rat (after 24 h). The alterations were followed by a few, scattered single necroses of cortical tubules, not differing from those found in syngeneic controls (surgical trauma). ×220

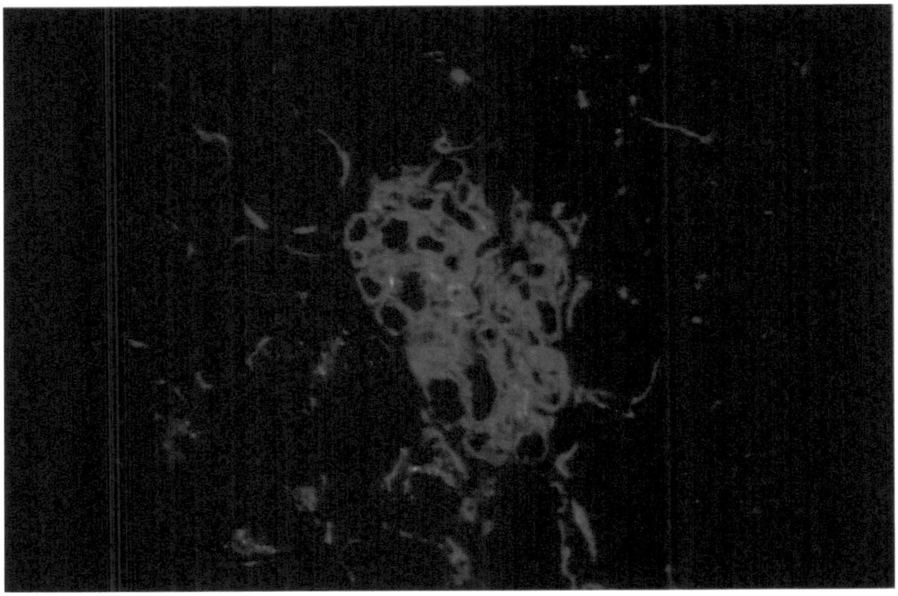

Fig. 14. Same kidney as seen in Fig. 13. After 24 h, immunofluorescence showed IgM antibodies along the glomerular basement membrane and in the wall of the peritubular capillaries. The intensity increased until 36 h, which is shown in this figure. After 48 h, polyreactive xenoantibodies were rapidly increasing, as measured by a hemolytic assay

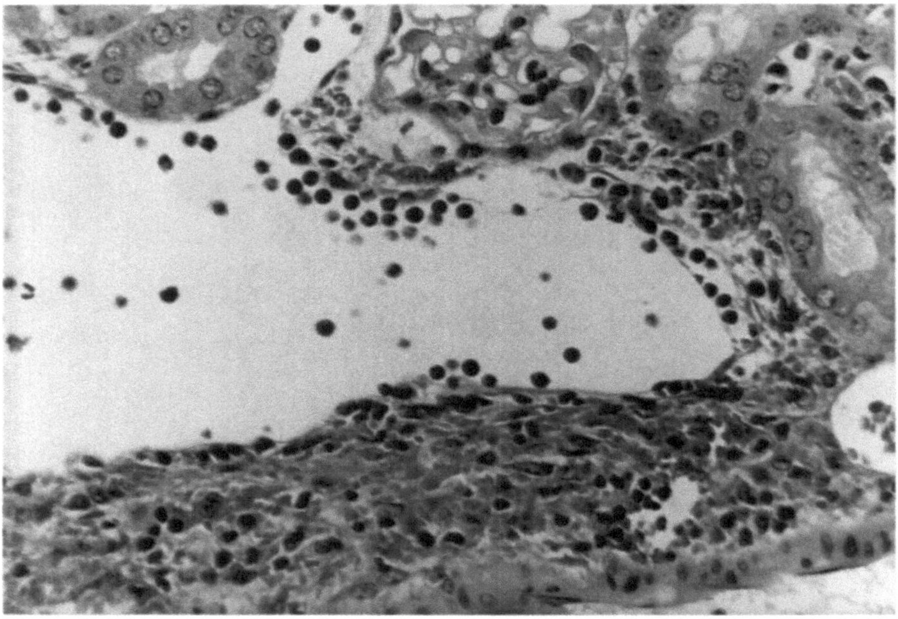

Fig. 15. Same kidney as seen in Figs. 13 and 14. Parenchymal veins with preserved endothelial lining paved with neutrophil granulocytes. A similar picture was found in the peritubular capillaries. The kidney structure was preserved with the exception of extensive tubular necrosis of the outer medulla. On day 5, the kidneys were completely necrotic. ×220

Morphological Conditions Seen Mainly in Discordant Xenograft Rejection (Tables 2, 3)

1. *Tubular necrosis.* Necrotic and desquamated epithelium was seen in proximal tubules, and not attributed to infarction. The basement membranes of the necrotic tubules were intact. No inflammatory reaction was found. A possible sequel, in the form of calcified tubular epithelium, was a frequent finding in all animals, especially rabbits (Fig. 8).
2. *Platelet aggregation.* Diagnosed by light microscopy or, preferably, ultrastructurally (Figs. 3, 16), platelets were found in glomerular capillaries and sometimes in parenchymal arteries. Aggregation could be accompanied by fibrin deposits and the presence of either neutrophils or, especially in the rabbits, eosinophilic granulocytes. The number of platelets varied with the experimental design and the species used. The significance of these findings remains unclear. Platelets could demonstrate preserved granules or be degranulated; the significance of this difference remains uncertain. Pseudopodia could be found in relation to the surfaces of endothelial cells, without apparent reaction

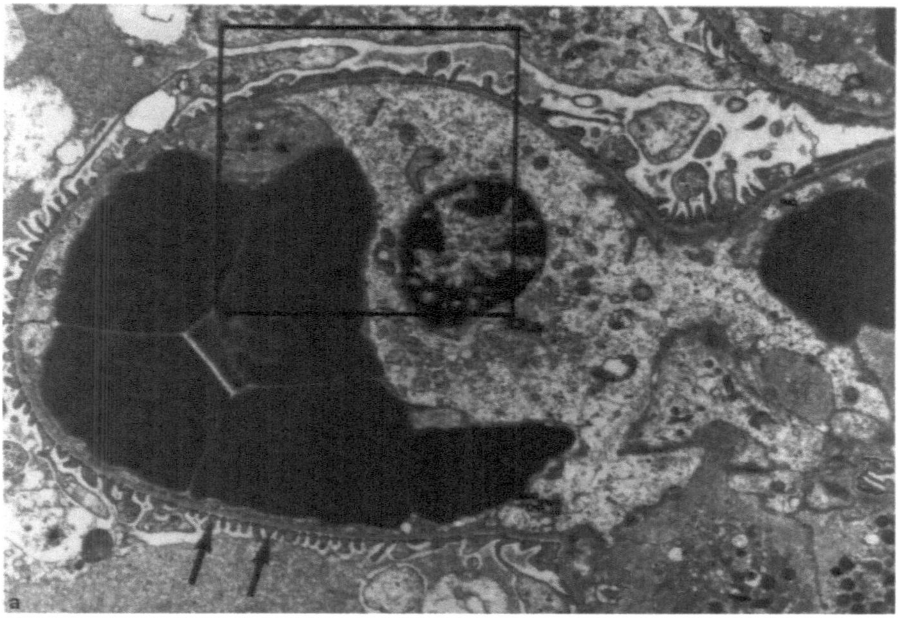

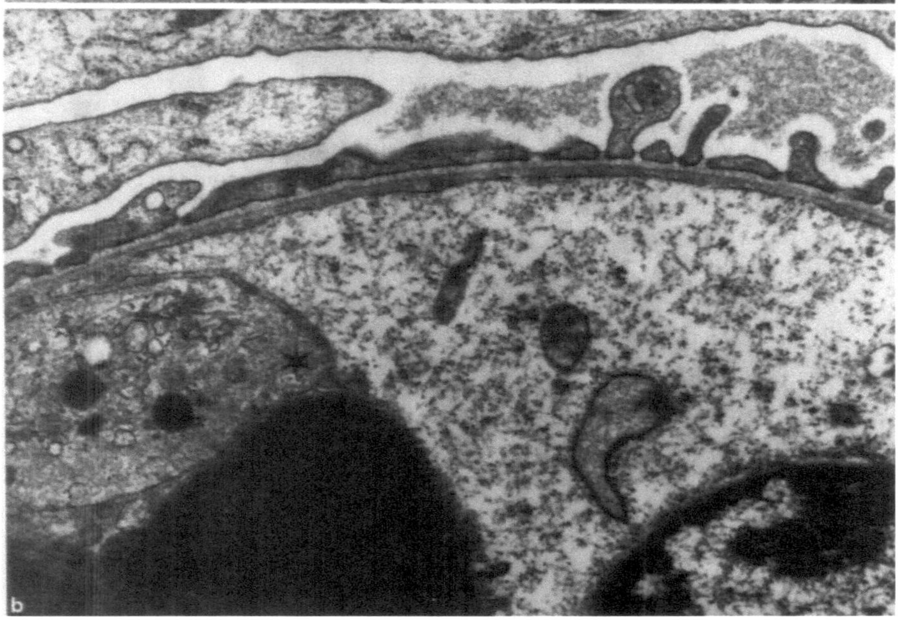

Fig. 16a–c. Electron micrographs from glomerular capillary loops in a rabbit kidney transplanted into a cat. **a** The endothelial cell in the center is edematous but preserved, as is the fenestrated endothelial cytoplasm peripheral to the erythrocytes (*arrows*). ×5960, uranyl-lead. **b** The *framed area* in **a** showing the contact between a platelet (*asterisk*) and an endothelial cell. ×17 520. c Basement membranes from two neighbouring capillary walls. *Left*, endothelial cell cytoplasm with edema and proximity to red blood cells. *Right*, fenestrated and preserved endothelial cytoplasm in apposition to platelets; the foot-process in between (*asterisks*) is flattened. ×26 700

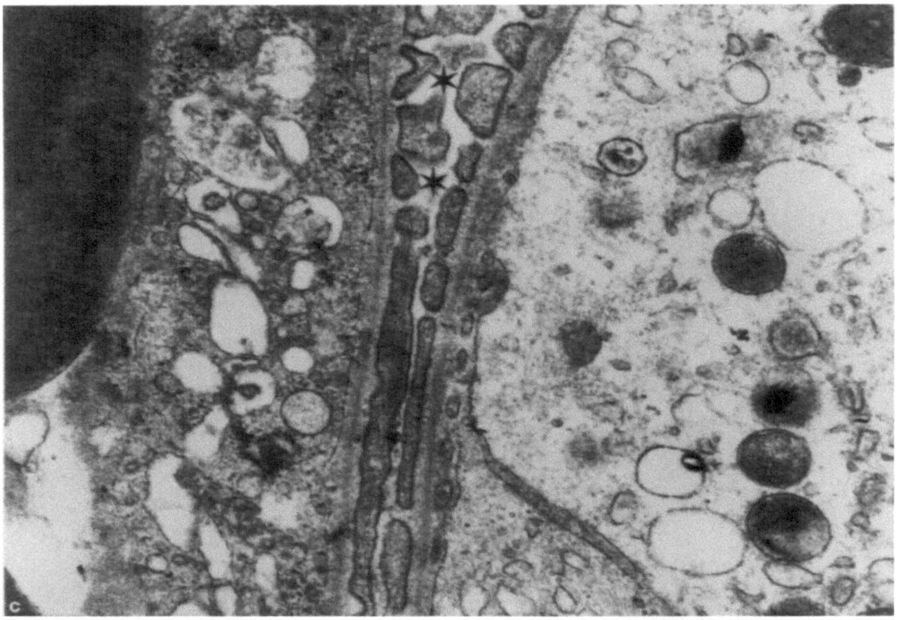

Fig. 16c.

in the latter (Figs. 17–19). Platelet aggregation was sometimes accompanied by damage and/or removal of endothelial cells, and in such cases the platelets were frequently found together with granulocytes. This could occur in glomerular capillaries and/or parenchymal arteries (Fig. 6, 20, 21).

3. *Glomerular microthrombosis.* This consisted mainly of fibrin, but was often accompanied by granulocytes and, in the parenchymal arteries, by thrombosis and granulocytic adhesion to endothelial cells, the latter often showing degeneration and/or necrosis (Fig. 22).
4. *Distinct tubular pyknosis.* This was presumably located in the straight part of the proximal tubules or the thick ascending part of the distal tubules, and was found in the medullary ray with well-preserved collecting tubules (Fig. 12). This condition was seen exclusively in the hemoperfusion experiments (Table 3).

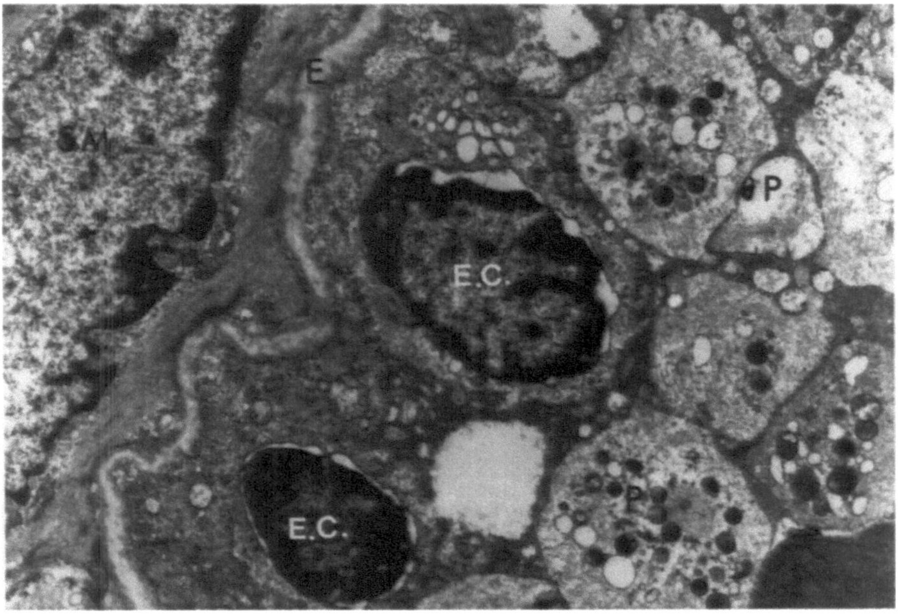

Fig. 17. Parenchymal artery from rabbit kidney transplanted into a nephrectomized cat without treatment. The endothelial cells (*E.C.*) are intact in spite of close apposition to partly degranulated platelets (*P.*). *E*, elastic lamina; *SM*, smooth muscle cell. This appearance, with severe aggregation of platelets in vessels without morphological damage to the endothelium and with no inflammatory response apart from edema, was seen in (i) rabbit kidneys transplanted into cats, (ii) rabbit kidneys transplanted into baby pigs that were presumed to be antibody free, and (iii) following perfusion of rabbit, rat, and goat kidneys with human blood. ×8960, uranyl-lead

Comment

Light, electron, and immunofluorescence microscopy alone have demonstrated significant morphological results. However, these methods are restricted to structural alterations and are of limited value in giving us a detailed understanding of graft rejection. The multifactorial influences on the graft and the complexity of the mechanisms involved in the immune response are major factors making the interpretation of histological findings difficult.

The application of methods that detect changes at the macromolecular level has proved valuable in further enlightening problems in human allografting.

DNA technological methods, e.g., northern blotting, Southern blotting, in situ hybridization, polymerase chain reaction (PCR), and immunochemical techniques, e.g., immunohistochemistry, enzyme-linked immunosorbent assay (ELISA), have provided valuable information concerning gene expression and the presence of human complement inhibiting proteins.

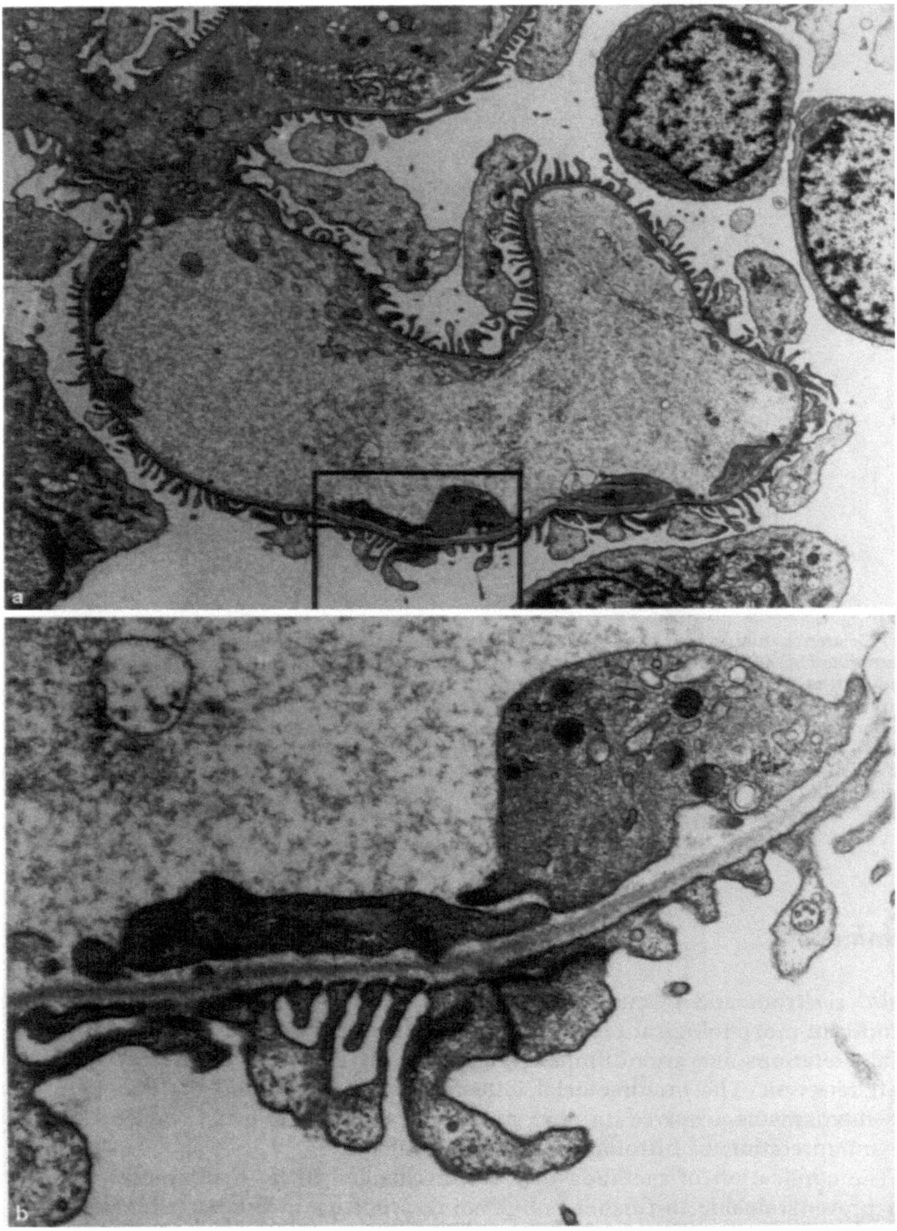

Fig. 18. a Glomerular loop with a few platelets sticking to the denuded basement membrane of a rabbit kidney after perfusion with human plasma. ×3900, uranyl-lead. **b** The *framed area* in a showing nearly completely degranulated platelets. The structure of the basement membrane and the overlying podocytes is normal. ×17520, uranyl-lead

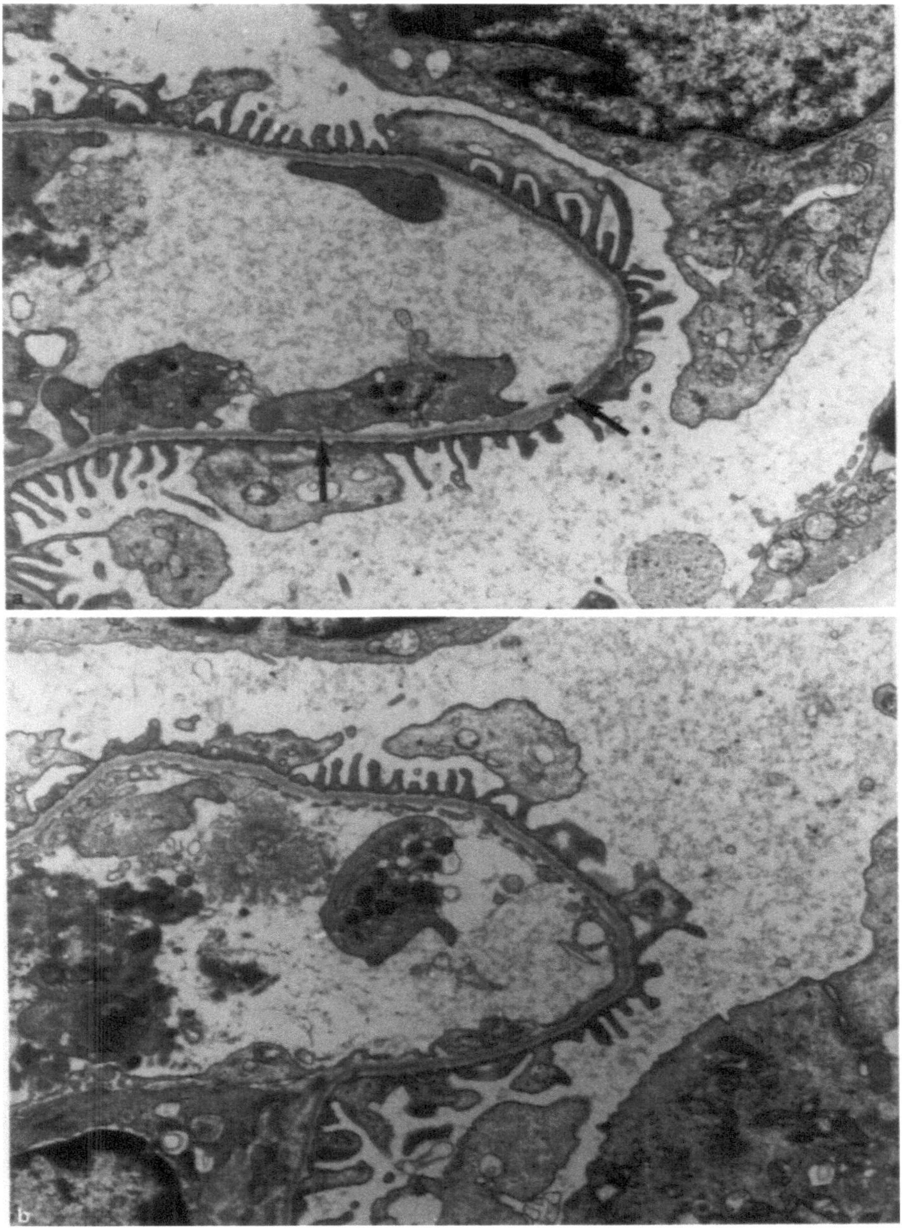

Fig. 19a,b. Two capillary loops from the same glomerulus in a rabbit kidney perfused with human plasma. **a** Denuded basement membrane with possible residuals of endothelial cytoplasm (*arrows*). ×8960). **b** Preserved endothelium with granulated platelets and sparse fibrin (*asterisk*) in the lumen. ×8960, uranyl-lead. Accumulation of platelets with endothelial damage, but without significant inflammatory response (with initially granulocytes, but also fibrin) was found mainly in perfusion experiments simulating discordant xenografting. It was also seen following transplantation of hare kidney to rabbits presensitized with repeated skin grafts or transfusions

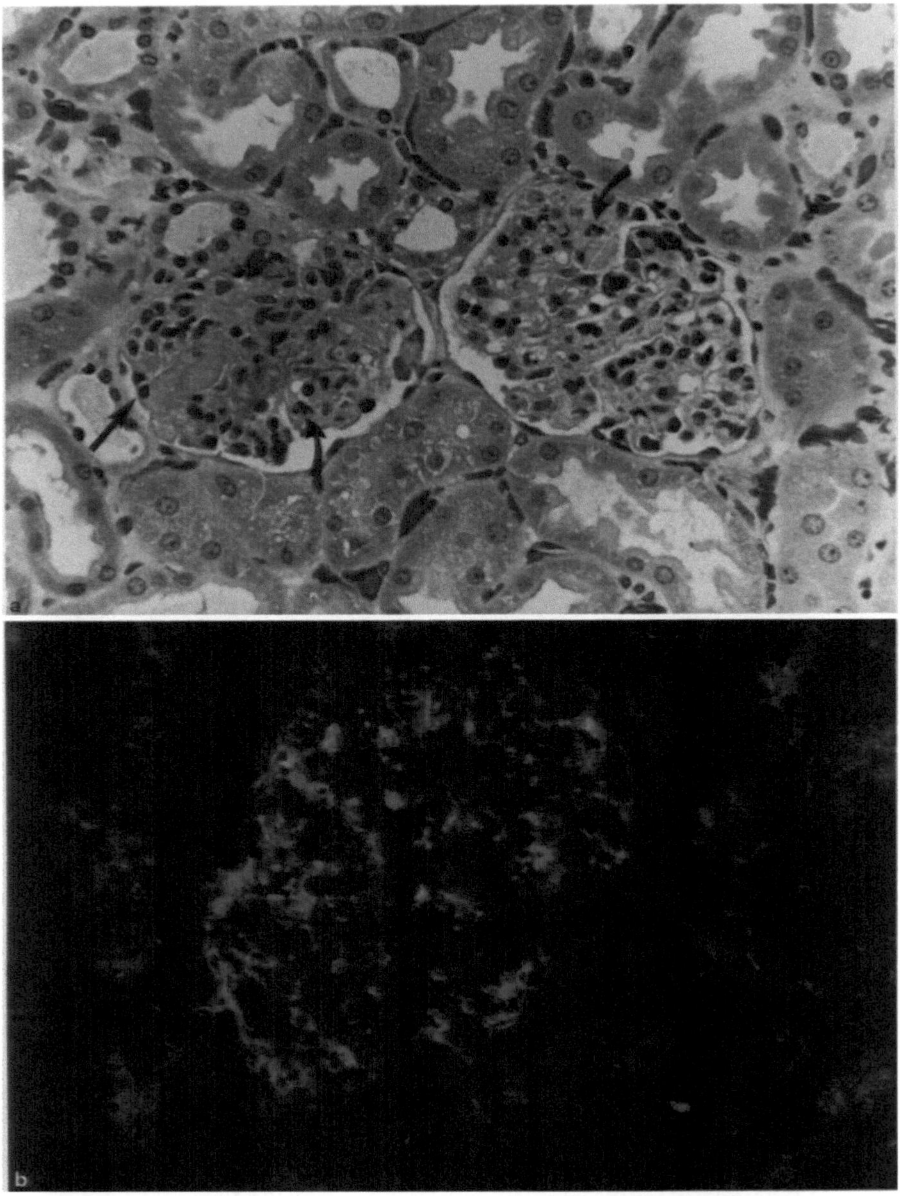

Fig. 20a,b. Rabbit kidney perfused with human blood. **a** Two glomeruli containing platelets (*straight arrow*) and a few granulocytes (*curved arrows*) in the capillary lumena. ×200, H&E). **b** Immunofluorescence microscopy showing a glomerulus with deposits of rabbit antihuman IgG in a granular pattern along the basement membranes in the capillary loops and to a lesser degree in the mesangium

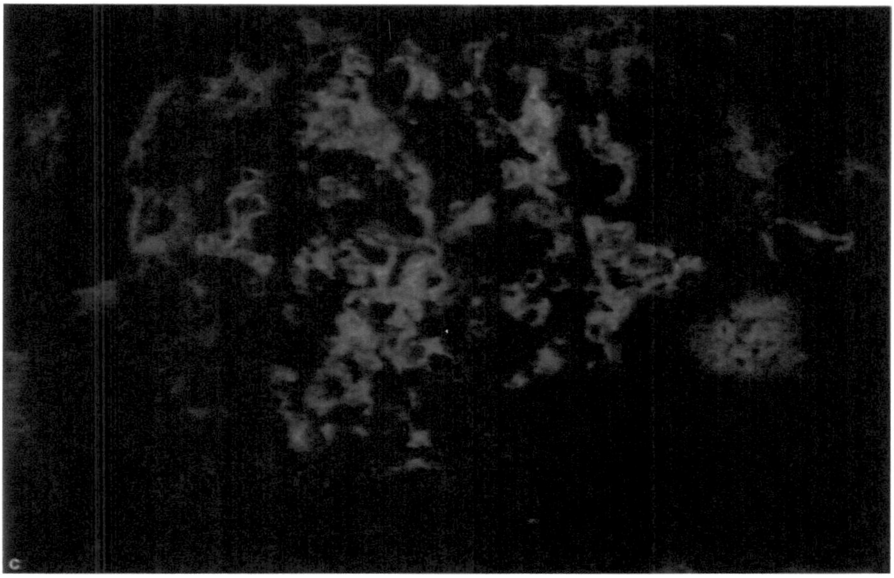

Fig. 20c. A glomerulus (from the same experiment as **b**) shows granular pattern and distribution of rabbit antihuman C3 very similar to that of rabbit antihuman IgG

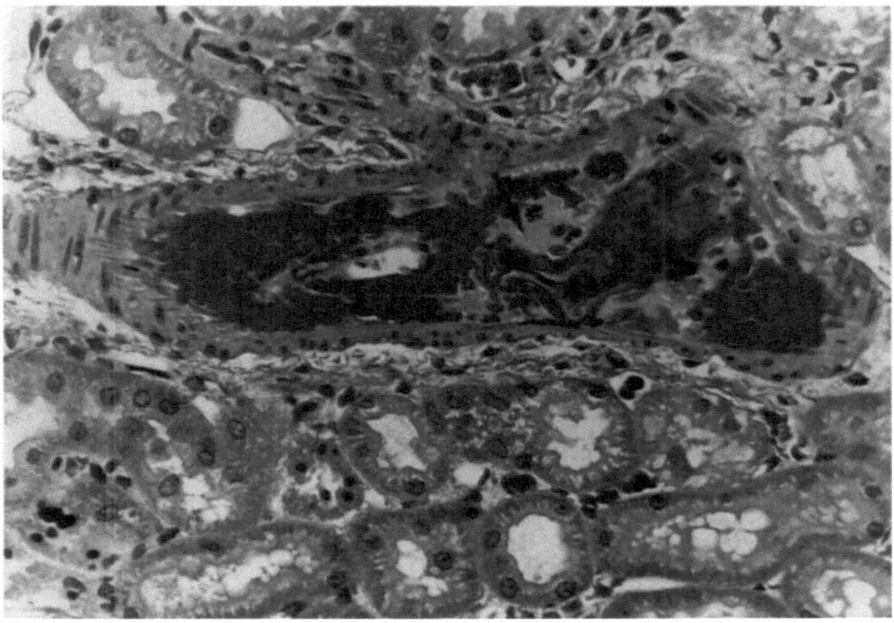

Fig. 21. Arcuate artery from rabbit kidney perfused with human blood. *Left*, in the partially obliquely cut lumen, there are red blood cells; *middle*, platelets (*arrow*); *right*, fibrin. ×200, H&E

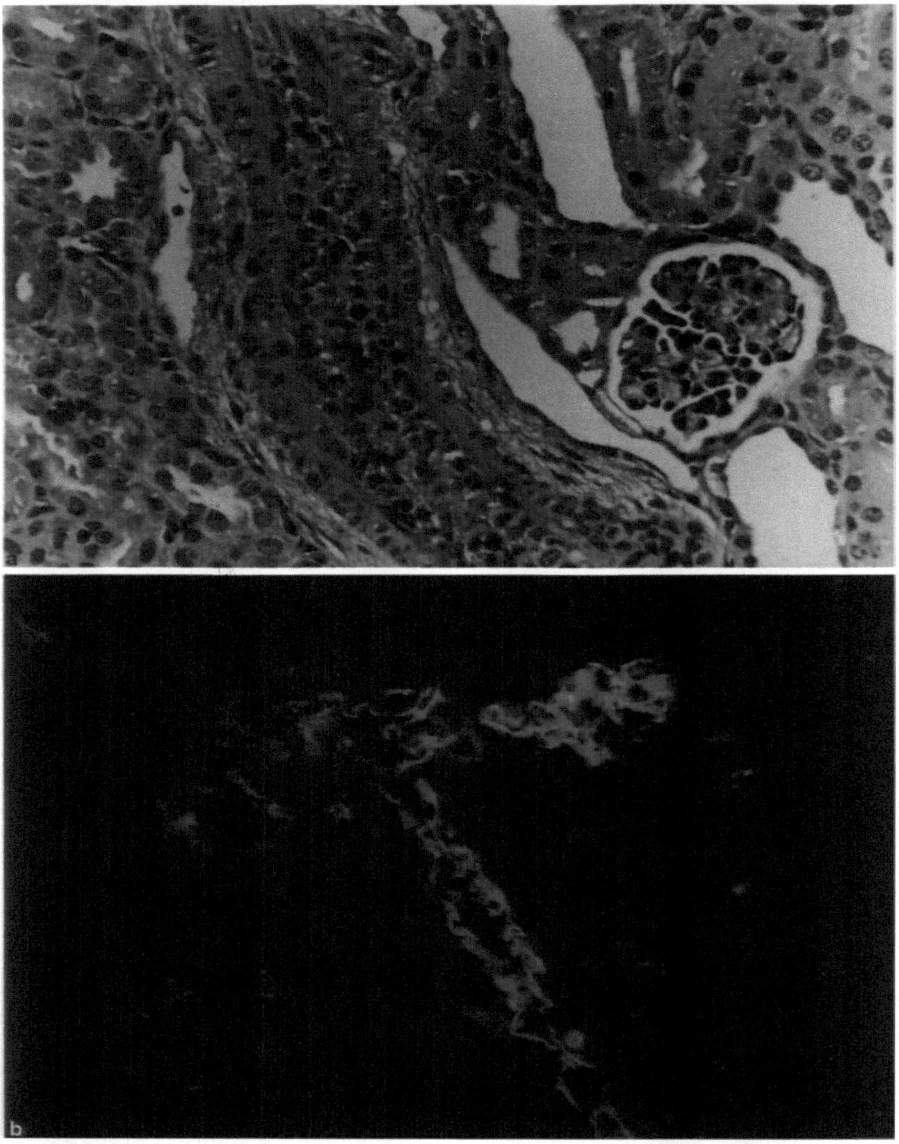

Fig. 22a,b. Baby pig kidney flushed with human blood. **a** The partly immature glomerulus contains a moderate number of platelets. In the interlobular artery, the lumen is stuffed with neutrophils, platelets and sparse fibrin. ×200, H&E. **b** Immunofluorescence microscopy illustrating rat antihuman IgG localized along the endothelial parts of the arterioles and the capillary loops in the glomeruli

Further research is needed employing these methods in vitro and in vivo, with special regard to the cellular constituents - e.g., phenotypes, receptors, signal hormones (cytokines), major histocompatibility complex (MHC) system (Ia antigens), adhesion molecules - involved in the activation and effectuation of the immune response. These methods, together with standardized histological examination [5], will increase our understanding and treatment of rejection. Appropriate treatments for the various pathogenetic types of rejection may then be achieved.

References

1. Brun, C., Olsen, S. Atlas of Renal Biopsy. Munksgaard, Copenhagen, 1981
2. Dalmasso, A.P. The complement system in xenotransplantation. Immunopharmacology, 24, 149, 1992
3. Rosengard, A.M., Cary, N.R.B., Langford, G.A., et al. Tissue expression of human complement inhibitor, decay-accelerating factor, in transgenic pigs. Transplantation, 59, 1325, 1995
4. Solez, K., Axelsen, R.A., Benediktsson, H, et al. International standardization of criteria for the histologic diagnosis of renal allograft rejection: The Banff working classification of kidney transplant pathology. Kidney Internat. 44, 411, 1993
5. Bogman, M.J.J.T., Dooper, I.M.M. Banff classification for the histological diagnosis of renal graft rejection: what are the advantages? Nephrol Dial Transplant 10, 1291, 1995
6. Dieperink, H., Steinbrüchel, D., Starklint, H., Larsen, S. Kemp, E. Improvement in hare-to-rabbit kidney transplant survival. Transplant Proc 19, 1140, 1987
7. Green, C.J., Kemp, E., Kemp, G., et al. Prolongation of concordant renal xenografts in rabbit recipients by a short course of cyclosporin A treatment. In Cyclosporin A. D.J.G. White (ed.), Elsevier, Amsterdam, 1982, p. 155
8. Jørgensen, K.A., Kemp, E., Olsen, T.K., et al. Activation of fibrinolysis during xenoperfusion. Thrombosis Res. 46, 473, 1987
9. Jørgensen, K.A., Kemp, E., Barfort, P., et al. Xeno- and auto-perfusion of rabbit kidney. Machine perfusion with blood at 37 °C. Acta. Path. Microbiol. Immunol. Scand. (Sect. A) 93, 305, 1985
10. Jørgensen, K.A., Kemp, E., Barfort, P., et al. On the role of platelets and leucocyte in renal xenoperfusion. Acta Path. Microbiol. Immunol. Scand. (Sect. A) 94, 223, 1986
11. Jørgensen, K.A., Kemp, E., Barfort, P., et al. The survival of pig to rabbit renal xenografts during inhibition of thromboxane synthesis. Thrombosis Res. 32, 585, 1983
12. Jørgensen, K.A., Kemp, E., Barfort, P., et al. Platelet aggregation is not essential for xenograft rejection. Thrombosis Res., 43, 87, 1986
13. Kemp, E., Kemp, G., Starklint, H., Larsen, S. Immunosuppression with cobra venom factor, anti-platelet-aggregator and cyclosporin A in renal xenotransplantation. Transplant Proc. 14, 116, 1982
14. Kemp, E., Kemp, G., Larsen, S., Starklint, H., Green, C.J. Xeno-banking. In Organ Preservation, Present and Future. D.E Pegg, J.A. Jacobsen, N.A. Halasz (eds.). MTP Press Ltd., London, p. 291, 1982

15. Kemp, E., Kemp, G., Larsen, S. Survival of discordant renal xenografts up to 3 days: assessment of function, light and immunofluorescent microscopy. Scand J. Urol. Nephrol. (Suppl.) 54, 150, 1980
16. Kemp, E., Starklint, H., Larsen, S., Dieperink. H. Cyclosporine in concordant renal hare-to-rabbit xenotransplantation: prolongation and modification of rejection, and adverse effects. Transplant Proc. 17, 1351, 1985
17. Kemp, E., Steinbrüchel, D., Starklint, H., et al. Renal xenograft rejection: prolonging effect of captopril, ACE-inhibitors, prostacyclin, and cobra venom factor. Transplant Proc. 19, 4471, 1987
18. Kemp, E., White, D., Dieperink, H., et al. Delayed rejection of rabbit kidneys transplanted into baby pigs. Transplant Proc. 19, 1143, 1987
19. Larsen, S., Starklint, H., Dieperink, H., Kemp, E. Immunofluorescence microscopy in experimental renal allo-and xenografts. Transplant Proc. 22, 1061, 1990
20. Larsen, S. Immunofluorescent microscopy findings in minimal or no change-disease and slight generalized mesangioproliferative glomerulonephritis. Acta Path. Microbiol. Scand. (Sect. A), 86, 531, 1978
21. Starklint, H., Larsen, S., Jørgensen, K.A., Dieperink, H. Kemp, E. Flush perfusion of rabbit kidneys with auto-, allo-and xenogeneic blood. Scand J Urol Nephrol 25, 45, 1991
22. Dieperink, H. Cyclosporin A nephrotoxicity. Dan. Med. Bull. 36, 235, 1989
23. Salomon, S., Steinbrüchel, D.A., Nielsen, B., Lillevang, S., Kemp, E. The effect of leflunomide, cyclosporine and splenectomy in two different organ systems of concordant xenotransplantation in rats. Transplant Proc., in press

18 Histopathology of Cardiac Xenograft Rejection

A.G. Rose

Introduction

The establishment of cardiac transplantation as a routine treatment for end-stage cardiac failure has placed ever-increasing demands upon human organ donation. Despite increased public acceptance of organ donation, human sources of transplanted hearts are insufficient to meet the demand. While formidable problems, particularly that of hyperacute rejection (HAR), stand in the way of cross-species organ transplantation, the great shortage of human donor hearts has led to renewed interest in xenotransplantation and, consequently, in finding a means of preventing HAR.

While the pathology of both acute and chronic cardiac allograft rejection has been well documented [1, 2] the morphology of hyperacute (antibody-mediated, vascular, humoral) rejection is less well known. Cardiac xenografts have been used in isolated instances in humans in attempts to save the life of a patient for whom no human donor heart was immediately available [3–5] (Chap. 56). Many experiments have been performed to try and further understanding of the etiology and pathogenesis of humoral rejection [6–41]. Present knowledge of the pathology of hyperacute rejection is mainly based upon the findings in experimental animals.

HAR is believed to be initiated by the presence of preformed antibodies which have resulted from prior antigenic stimulation by blood transfusions, pregnancy, or previous tissue allografts, or to be associated with ABO blood group incompatibility or cross-species differences. The latter is presently not a clinical problem, since cardiac xenografts are not used to treat patients, but may become one in the future. Pathologists may encounter HAR where cross-species experimental transplants have been performed. There are no significant morphologic differences between the HAR that occurs in allografts and that which occurs in discordant xenografts.

Varying levels of antibody may be present in one species against a closely related species. In general, the greater the phylogenetic disparity of the two species, the greater will be the titer of species-specific antibody. Antibody-mediated rejection usually takes place rapidly within a few minutes or hours and usually within 24 h following an organ being transplanted between widely disparate species. The process may take several days to develop in more closely related species. There is increasing evidence that even when transplantation is between closely related species, the presence or development of antibodies plays a significant role in the development of rejection. Although immunosuppression may delay the changes of antibody-mediated rejection beyond the initial 24-h period following the transplant, from the perspective of light microscopy the process appears to be the same. The term "delayed vascular rejection" is sometimes used to cover this type of rejection response when it occurs later than 24 h post-grafting.

While neutrophils have been regarded as an important component of HAR (analogous to their role in the Arthus phenomenon), hyperacute cardiac xenograft rejection in the rat model shows the usual pattern of vascular myocardial damage in the absence of neutrophils. In personal experience with hyperacutely rejected xenografts [24–34, 36, 42, 43, 46], in which extensive interstitial hemorrhage was the predominant feature, a significant number of neutrophils accompanied the interstitial hemorrhage. However, the ratio of white to red blood cells was the same as that encountered in the peripheral blood. Forbes et al. [17] do not exclude the possibility that neutrophils may play a role in the production of myocardial injury in the *later* stages of humoral rejection.

Others have focused upon the role that various components of complement may play in the pathogenesis of HAR [23]. Experiments in C6-deficient rabbits show that activity of the sixth component of complement is needed for HAR to occur. Likewise in studies on recipient hemolytic C3 activity, it has been shown that complement activation by graft-bound antibody is an important effector mechanism for humoral rejection in an inbred rat model [35]. Depletion of the third component of complement by cobra venom factor has also led to prolonged survival of xenografts [42, 43]. Rats with a hereditary platelet function defect are able to effect HAR [17]. The role of antibody to the vascular endothelial cells in early rejection in patients undergoing cardiac transplantation is receiving attention [44, 45].

Macroscopic Appearances of the Donor Heart During Hyperacute Rejection

Heterotopically transplanted hearts, whether from closely related or widely disparate donor species, usually begin beating satisfactorily in sinus rhythm either spontaneously or after electrical defibrillation. The hyperacutely rejecting heart initially becomes swollen and distended with blood over a period of only a few minutes. The normal pink-colored myocardium is replaced by a dusky, cyanotic hue. The observed macroscopic changes are compatible with a venous type infarction of the heart. Shortly after these changes develop, graft function becomes seriously compromised.

Histopathology of Xenograft Rejection

Longer-surviving concordant xenografted hearts, when heavily immunosuppressed with pharmacologic agents (Table 1) undergo typical cellular rejection. In our experience, however, unmodified cellular rejection is uncommon in non-immunosuppressed cardiac xenograft models, since antibody-mediated rejection is so common.

Table 1. Histopathology of rejection and survival periods of selected heterotopic cardiac allografts and xenografts in the baboon

Group	*n*	Type of rejection[f]				Graft survival	
		Vascular	Mixed	Cellular	None	Mean (days)	SD
Allografts (baboon-to-baboon)							
1. No IS	10	0	0	10	0	11.0	5.6
2. ABO-incompatible, no IS	9	2	2	5	0	12.4	11.7
3. CSA, MP	10	0	0	1	9 (1)	>30.0	–
4. ABO-incompatible, CSA, MP	8	2	1	4 (1)	1	22.5	12.0
Concordant xenografts (vervet monkey-to-baboon)							
5. No IS	9	5	4	0	0	10.3	5.2
6. ABO-incompatible, no IS	9	3	2	4	0	73	5.6
7. CSA, AZA, MP	6	1	0	5 (2)	0	13.0	8.2
8. ABO-incompatible, CSA, AZA, MP	5	1	1	3 (1)	0	11.4	11.2
9. CSA, AZA, MP } i.v. MP	5	1	0	3	1 (1)	19.0	21.8
10. RATG, CSA, AZA, MP } therapy for } rejection	6	1	0	2	3 (3)	43.3	18.5
11. 15-DS, CSA, ZA, MP } episodes	7	1	0	2	4 (4)	20.1	11.5
12. 15-DS, CSA, MP}	5	0	3	1	1 (1)	35.6	14.2
13. TLI, CSA, AZA, MP}	5	0	1 (1)	3 (3)	1 (1)	16.2	9.8
14. ABO-incompatible, TLI, CSA, AZA, MP	5	2 (1)	0	1 (1)	2 (1)	17.8	10.5
Discordant xenografts (pig-to-baboon)							
15. No IS[a]	4	4	0	0	0	–	–
16. Splenectomy[b]	3	3	0	0	0	–	–
17. CSA, AZA, MP[c]	5	5	0	0	0	–	–
18. Antibody adsorption[d]	7	7	0	0	0	–	–
19. Antibody adsorption, CSA, AMA, MP[e]	4(1)	4	0	0	0	–	–

IS, immunosuppressive therapy; CSA, cyclosporine; AZA, azathioprine; MP, methylprednisolone; 15-DS, 15-deoxyspergualin; TLI, pretransplant total lymphoid irradiation; RATG, rabbit antithymocyte globulin.
[a] Individual experiments: 40, 60, 180, 480 min.
[b] Individual experiments: 30, 350, 480 min.
[c] Individual experiments: 15, 15, 40, 75 min, 5 days.
[d] Individual experiments: 360, 480 min, 0.5, 4, 4, 4, 4, 5 days.
[e] Individual experiments: 480 min, 0.5, 1, 4 days
[f] Figures in parentheses denote number of recipients that died.

Fig. 1. a Thrombosis occludes a tributary (*top right*) of a subepicardial vein. The deeper myocardium (*bottom*) shows focal hemorrhages, while the superficial myocardium appears edematous (pig-to-baboon). H&E, ×10. **b** High-power view of thrombosis in venule seen in **a**. Interfascicular edema is present in the surrounding myocardium (pig-to-baboon). H&E, ×50

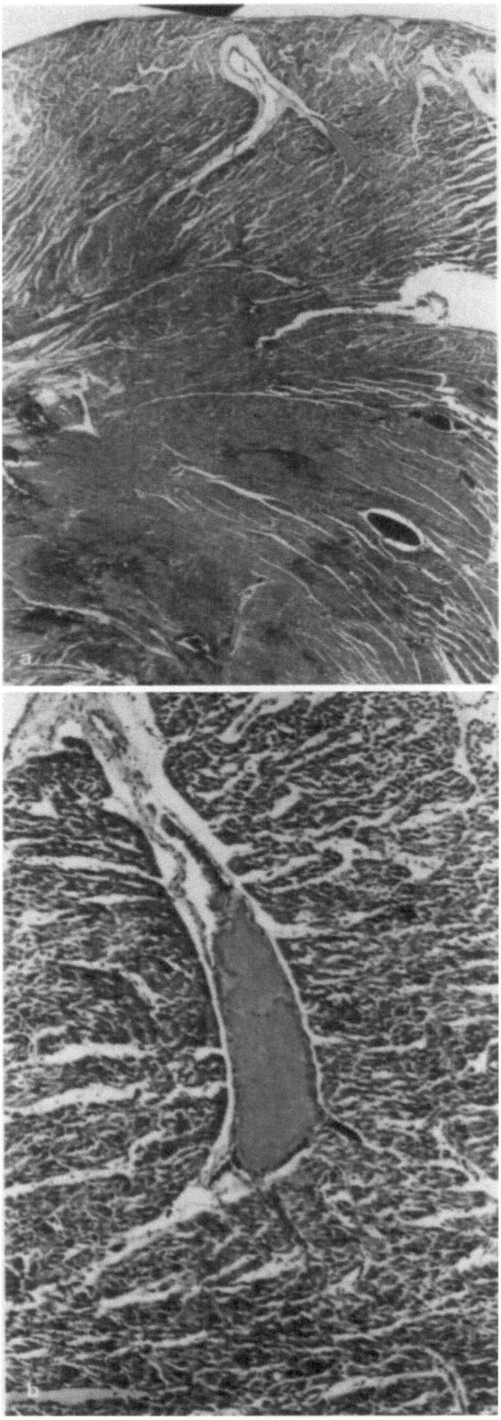

Antibody-Mediated (Hyperacute, Vascular, Humoral) Rejection

The classical concept is that, if the antibody titer is high enough, one may have antibodies coming into immediate contact with the donor heart vascular endothelium, and, in association with complement deposition, this may cause direct injury or destruction of the endothelial lining cells. Recent experimental work suggests that the humoral rejection response may be suppressed in some closely related animal models for as long as days, weeks or months by a combination of certain drugs, some of which are not yet available for clinical use [32, 36]. Surviving endothelial cells may show prominent mitotic activity in an attempt to re-endothelialize the vessel; such attempts are usually inadequate.

The earliest thrombi are noted within venules (Fig. 1a,b) both draining into the epicardium and in smaller tributaries lying within the myocardium. Swelling and activation of capillary endothelial lining cells is also noted. This is soon followed by severe capillary congestion (Fig. 2) involving most of the myocardium. Interfascicular edema of the myocardium also becomes prominent. This is followed by subendocardial, interstitial hemorrhage, which initially may be focal (Fig. 3), but soon becomes extensive, and may extend to involve the inner half of the myocardium (Fig. 4). The outer half of the myocardium usually shows edema only (Fig. 5). The capillary destruction is thus zonal, and this suggests that hemodynamic forces on the capillaries secondary to venous thrombosis, rather than a direct antibody effect, is important with regard to the changes in the capillaries. HAR pathologically has features suggestive of a venous infarct of the heart. Secondary degenerative changes, including contraction band necrosis may become evident in the myocytes. In severe cases, the graft may ultimately become totally necrotic.

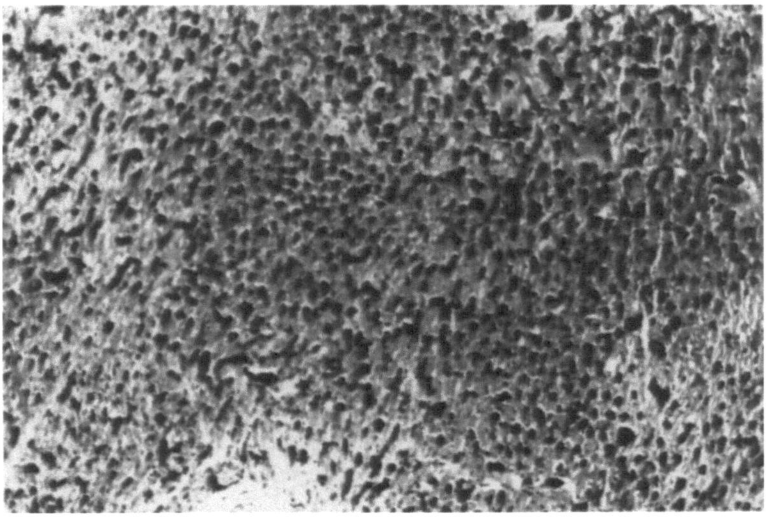

Fig. 2. Severe capillary congestion in early hyperacute rejection of a cardiac xenograft (pig-to-baboon). H&E, ×150

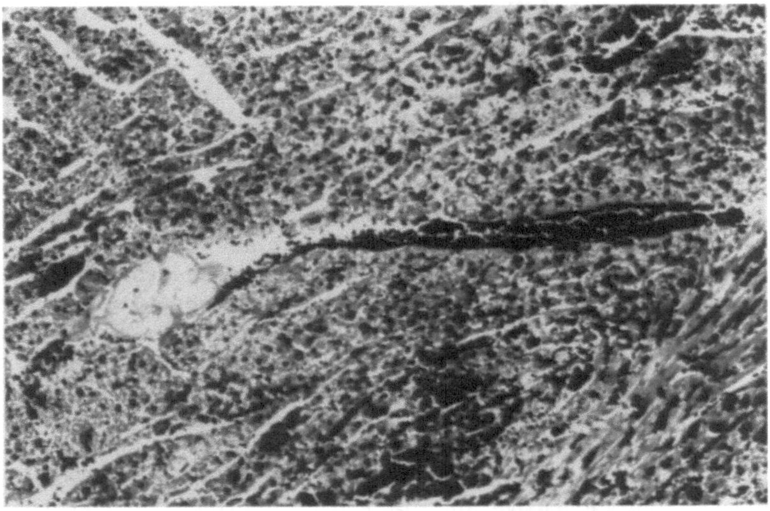

Fig. 3. Focal interstitial hemorrhage (*bottom*) is associated with thrombosis and congestion of a venule (*middle*) and surrounding capillary congestion (pig-to-baboon). H&E, ×150

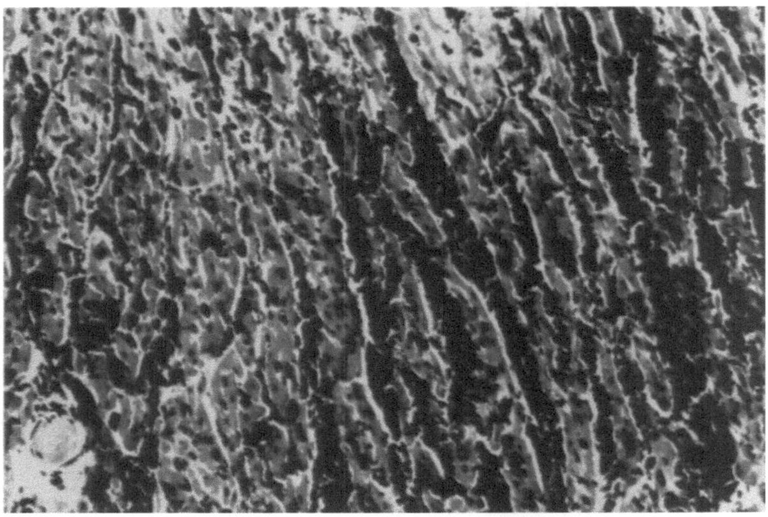

Fig. 4. Diffuse, severe (subendocardial) interstitial hemorrhage is noted in this hyperacutely rejected cardiac xenograft (pig-to-baboon). H&E, ×200

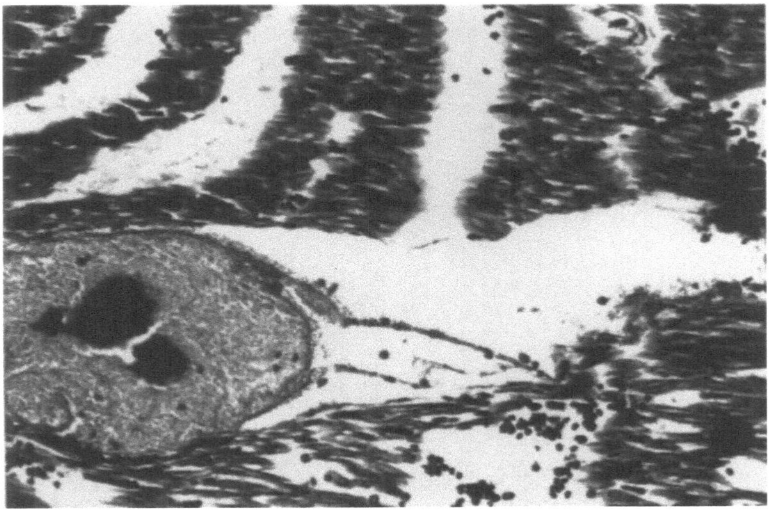

Fig. 5. Severe interfascicular edema separates fascicles of myocytes around a thrombosed venule (pig-to-baboon). H&E, ×280

Mixed Cellular and Antibody-Mediated Rejection

Mixed cellular and antibody-mediated rejection [34] (Figs. 6, 7) is characterized by prominent focal perivascular collections of lymphocytes which extend in a limited fashion between adjacent myocytes. Elsewhere the myocardium shows typical features of antibody-mediated rejection as detailed earlier. The modest number of lymphocytes present does not appear to be sufficient to explain very extensive microvascular damage or myocyte necrosis on the basis of acute cellular rejection alone. Lymphocytic infiltration is not a characteristic feature of pure antibody-mediated rejection.

Modification of Xenograft Rejection by Pharmacological Immunosuppression in Concordant Xenografts (Vervet Monkey-to-Baboon)

Survival of vervet monkey hearts transplanted into ABO-compatible non-immunosuppressed baboons (Table 1) did not differ significantly from that of allografts. HAR or mixed cellular and antibody-mediated rejection was seen in all cases. Rejection occurred in one animal within 24 h. When xenografting was performed between ABO-incompatible pairs, mean survival time was reduced, mainly through the occurrence of HAR (sometimes occurring within 1 h) in a third of cases. Post-transplant immunosuppression with cyclosporine (CSA), azathioprine (AZA), and methylprednisolone (MP) did not significantly prolong cardiac xenograft survival in either ABO-compatible or ABO-incompatible pairs, and there were still instances of HAR, particularly in the ABO-incompatible

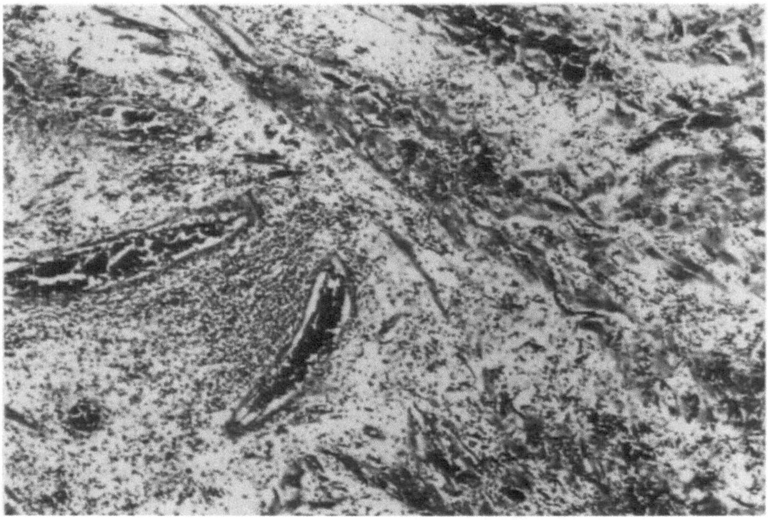

Fig. 6. Mixed cellular and antibody-mediated rejection is characterized by massive interstitial edema and hemorrhage, leading to wide separation of bundles of myocytes plus focal collections of lymphocytes mainly around small blood vessels (vervet monkey-to-baboon). H&E, ×80

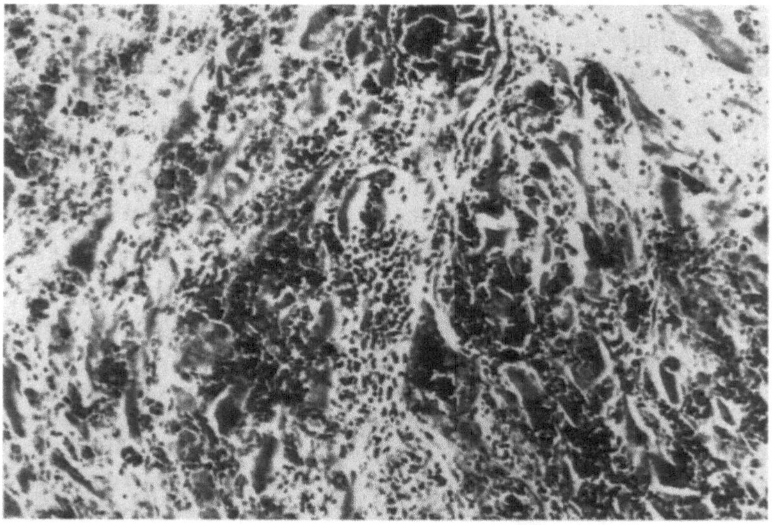

Fig. 7. High-power view of mixed cellular and antibody-mediated rejection with focal (centrally situated) groups of lymphocytes surrounded by severely edematous, hemorrhagic myocardium (vervet monkey-to-baboon). H&E, ×150

group. When rejection episodes were treated by bolus MP therapy, graft survival was significantly extended. The addition of rabbit antithymocyte globulin to the induction immunosuppressive regimen and antirejection therapy (in the form of bolus MP) extended graft survival significantly, but there was a 50 % recipient mortality due to infection, diarrhea and other side effects. When maintenance CSA, AZA, and MP therapy was combined with 15-deoxyspergualin, and rejection episodes were again treated with bolus MP, graft survival was prolonged, but four of the seven recipients (57 %) died of treatment-related complications. If 15-deoxyspergualin was combined with maintenance CSA and MP only, and MP used for acute rejection episodes, there was a reduction in the treatment-related mortality to 20 % and a prolongation of xenograft survival.

In the myocardial biopsies taken from grafted hearts in these four groups, acute cellular and mixed rejection predominated, but HAR was still seen in some cases. The mean number of rejection episodes seen in these groups ranged from 0.8 to 2.5 episodes per animal.

Rejection in Discordant Xenografts (Pig-to-Baboon)

Discordant xenografting between pig and unmodified baboon resulted in histopathological features of hyperacute rejection in every case. Neither splenectomy nor pharmacological immunosuppression increased mean survival time of the grafts, but pretransplant hemoperfusion of donor pig kidneys by the recipient baboon (to absorb out the preformed antibodies on the kidneys before exposing the heart) increased graft survival significantly in four of seven hearts. Nevertheless, all four hearts eventually showed typical features of delayed vascular rejection at the time that function ceased even though cessation of function took 4–5 days to occur. The addition of pharmacologic immunosuppression to pretransplant hemoperfusion did not lead to any further prolongation of graft survival. Discordant xenografts treated with cobra venom factor and pharmacologic immunosuppression (with or without pretransplant splenectomy), however, have survived for <25 days [42, 43], although delayed vascular rejection gradually developed during this period.

Grading of Antibody-Mediated Rejection

If future attempts to introduce xenografting into clinical practice prove successful, it will be essential to have a clinically relevant, reproducible grading system for antibody-mediated rejection. Rose and Cooper [46] have proposed a grading system for antibody-mediated rejection which may be used in both experimental studies and in the clinical situation. The grading system has the following two major categories: *grade A* (unmodified antibody-mediated rejection) and *grade B* (mixed antibody-mediated and acute cellular rejection). Both grades A and B are subcategorized into mild, moderate, or severe subgrades.

Grade A: Unmodified Antibody-Mediated Rejection

1. *Mild.* This initial mild phase shows venous thrombi and swelling and activation of capillary endothelial cells. Myocytes appear normal and capillaries are intact.
2. *Moderate.* In addition to the features described above, congestion of capillaries followed by interfascicular edema are seen. Sludging of red blood cells occurs with the development of occasional thrombi within capillaries. Focal interstitial hemorrhage develops in the inner layers of the myocardium.
3. *Severe.* In addition to the features noted above, disruption of capillaries, often subtended by thrombosed venules, is noted. Interstitial hemorrhage may be widespread throughout all layers of the myocardium, but is maximal in the inner half of the myocardium. Focal myocyte necrosis may develop, and this may become extensive. Vascular thrombosis becomes obtrusive in venules, capillaries, and in some arteries. In delayed vascular rejection, some thrombi may show signs of organization.

Grade B: Mixed Antibody-Mediated and Acute Cellular Rejection

This may show any of the three above-described grades of antibody-mediated rejection plus interstitial lymphocytic infiltration (i.e., acute cellular rejection). Such mixed rejection is usually not seen within the first 7–10 days following grafting. Delayed vascular rejection is superimposed upon acute cellular rejection. Focal aggregates of lymphocytes are present within the edematous, hemorrhagic myocardial interstitium.

Ultrastructure of Antibody-Mediated Cardiac Rejection

Electron microscopy [6, 7, 13, 17, 20, 48, 49] of hyperacutely rejecting cardiac xenografts (Figs. 8–12) may yield either few pathologic alterations or evidence of severe graft destruction, depending upon (a) the stage at which the biopsy is taken and (b) the layer within the myocardium from which the biopsy is obtained (for example, interstitial hemorrhage is rarely seen away from the subendocardium). The major described features, namely varying combinations of capillary occlusion due to platelet and fibrin thrombi (Figs. 8–12) and endothelial cellular swelling, may not be obvious in many cases of HAR.

In experimental studies [50], platelet thrombi were more frequently seen in porcine xenografts in dogs than in baboons. Electron microscopy findings should always be cautiously interpreted in the light of the clinical data and light microscopy.

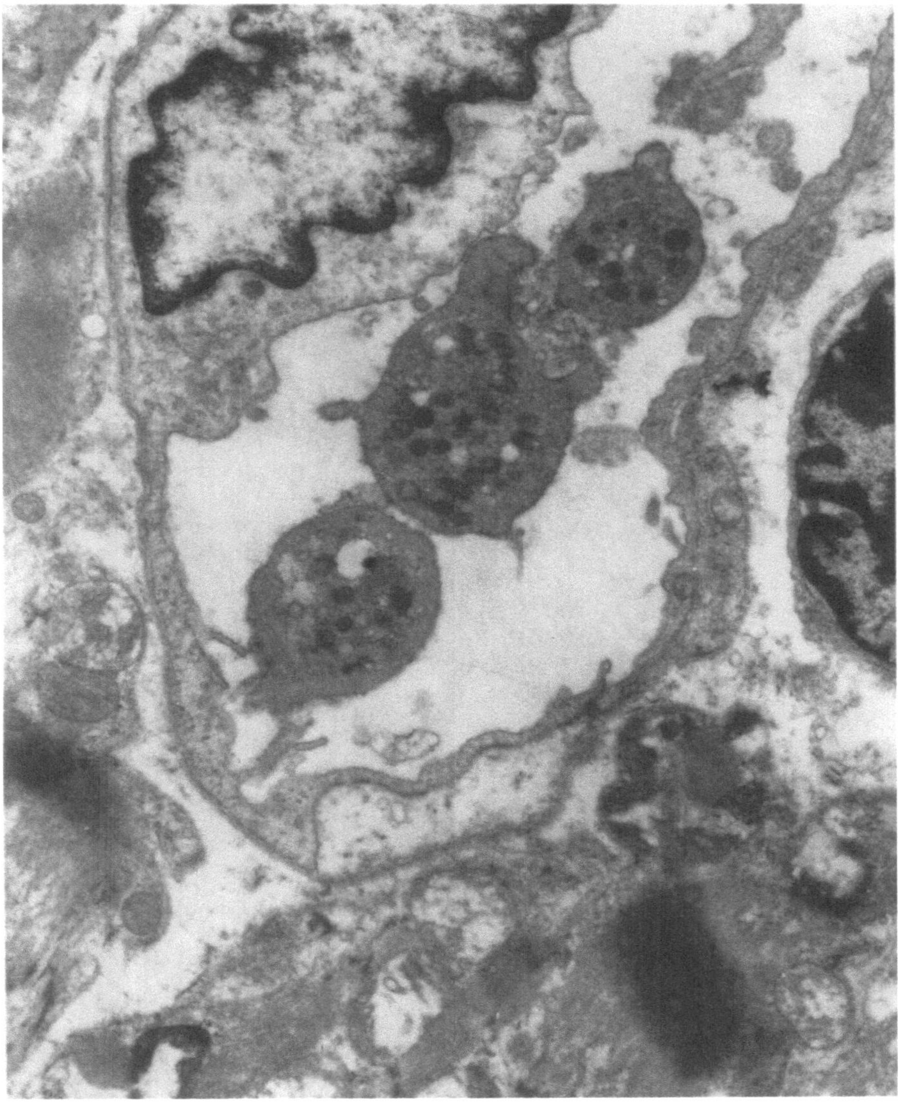

Fig. 8. Electron photomicrograph showing early platelet aggregation within a capillary of a hyperacutely rejecting cardiac xenograft (pig-to-dog). Original magnification, ×18 000

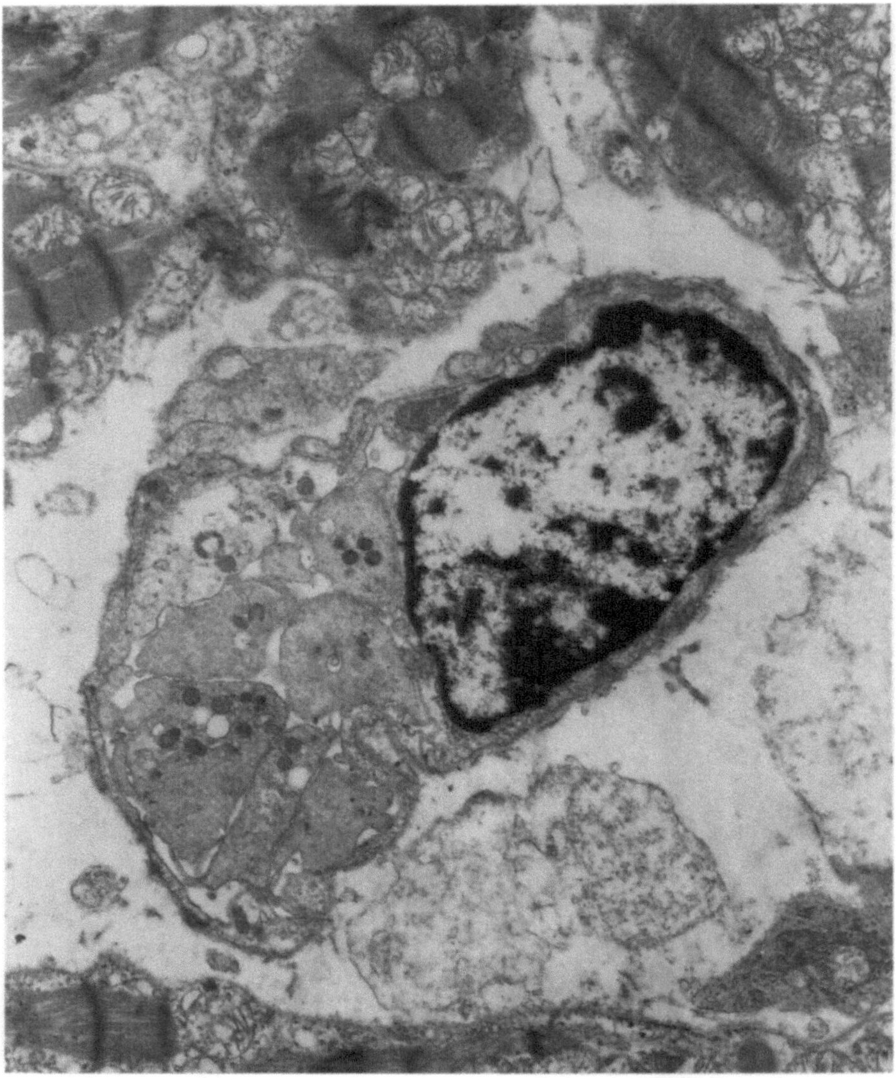

Fig. 9. Electron photomicrograph showing hyperacute rejection of a pig heart 10 min after transplantation into a dog. Aggregated platelets can be seen within a capillary, which also shows a prominent endothelial cell nucleus. Original magnification, ×12 000

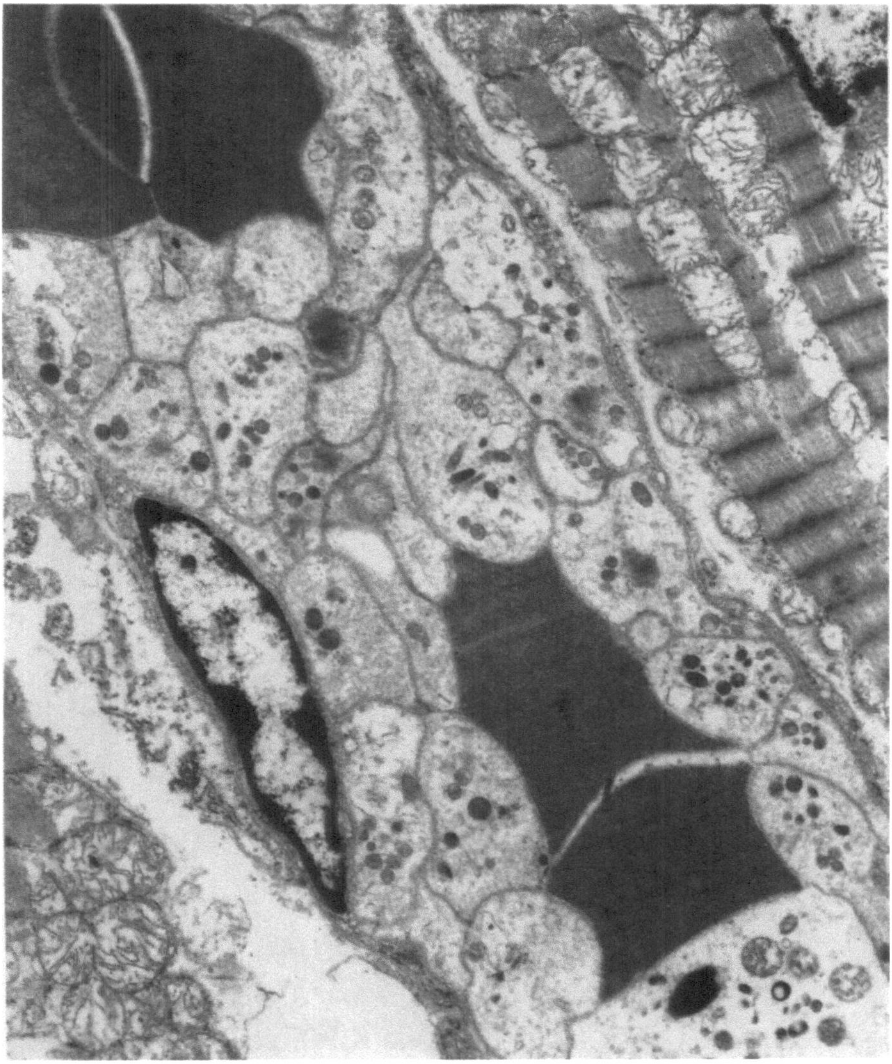

Fig. 10. Electron photomicrograph showing severe capillary luminal obstruction due to aggregation of platelets, many of which appear degranulated (pig-to-dog). Original magnification, ×12 000

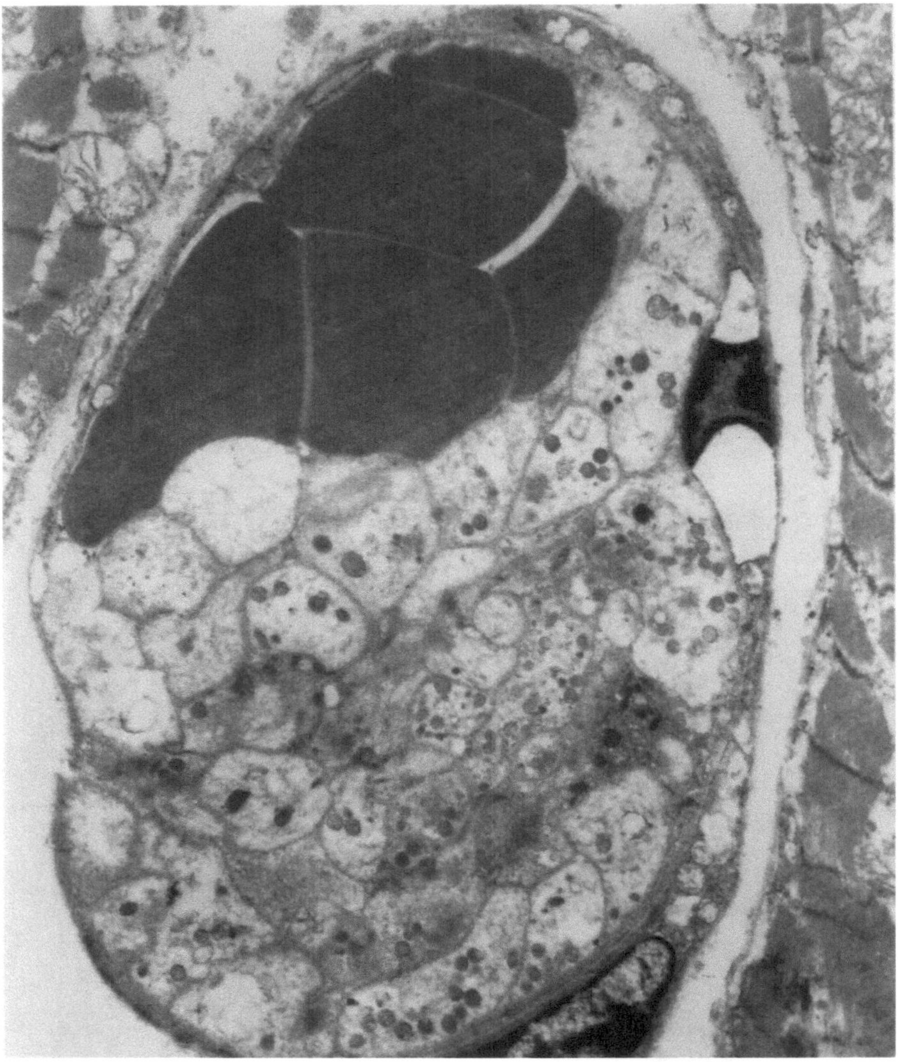

Fig. 11. Electron photomicrograph showing degranulated aggregated platelets occluding most of the lumen of a capillary in a hyperacutely rejecting porcine cardiac xenograft in a canine recipient 13 min after transplantation. Original magnification, ×12 000

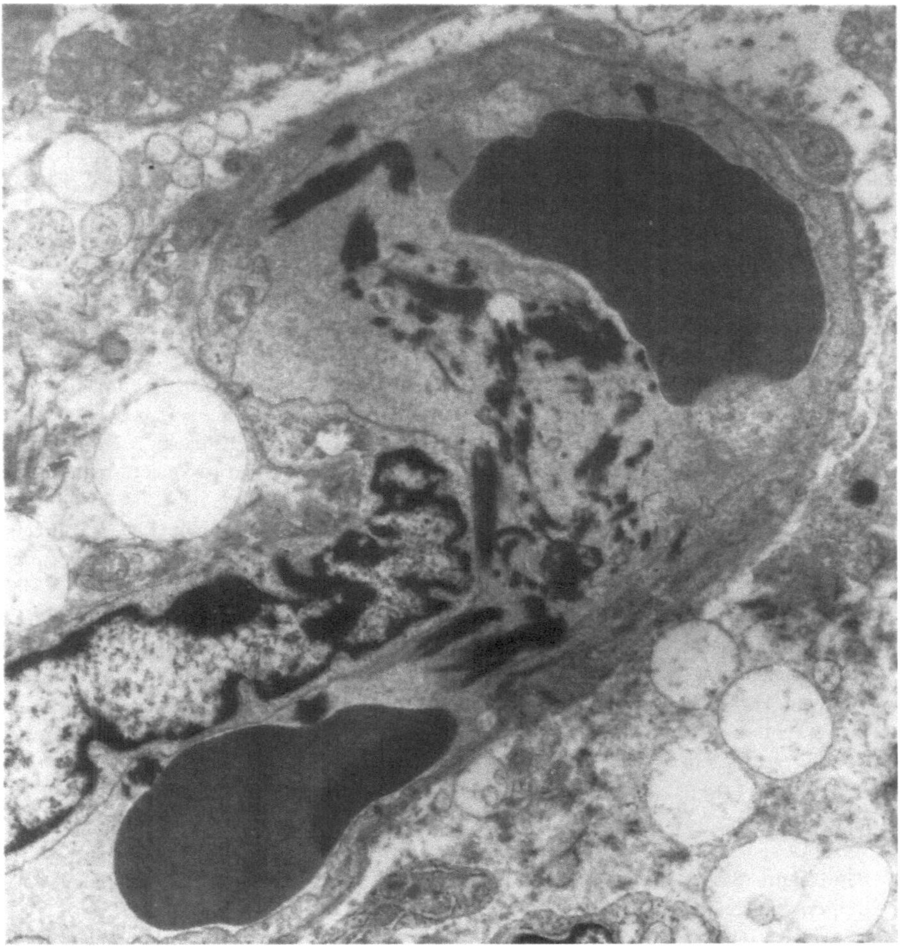

Fig. 12. Electron photomicrograph shows the lumen of a capillary to be occupied by dark-staining fibrin strands which lie between two erythrocytes. Hyperacute rejection of porcine cardiac xenograft in a baboon at 3 h. Original magnification, ×15 000

References

1. Rose, A.G., Uys, C.J. Pathology of acute rejection. In: D.K.C. Cooper and D. Novitzky (eds.) The Transplantation and Replacement of Thoracic Organs. Kluwer; Dordrecht, 1990, p.115
2. Rose, A.G., Uys, C.J. Pathology of graft atherosclerosis (chronic rejection). In: D.K.C. Cooper and D. Novitzky (eds.) The Transplantation and Replacement of Thoracic Organs. Kluwer; Dordrecht, 1990. p.161
3. Hardy, J.D., Chavez, C.M., Kurrus, F.E., et al. Heart transplantation in man: development studies and report of a case. J. Amer. Med. Assoc. 188, 1132, 1964
4. Barnard, C.N., Wolpowitz, A., Losman, J.G. Heterotopic cardiac transplantation with a xenograft for assistance of the left heart in cardiogenic shock after cardiopulmonary bypass. S. Afr. Med. J. 52, 1035, 1977
5. Bailey, L.L., Nelson-Cannarella, S.L., Concepcion, W., Jolley, W.B. Baboon-to-human cardiac xenotransplantation in a neonate. J. Amer. Med. Assoc. 254, 3321, 1985
6. Forbes, R.D.C., Guttmann, R.D., Kuramochi, T., Klassen J., Knaack, J. Non-essential role of neutrophils as mediators of hyperacute cardiac allograft rejection in the rat. Lab. Invest. 34, 229, 1976
7. Forbes, R.D.C., Kuramochi T., Guttmann, R.D., Klassen J., Knaack, J.A. A controlled sequential morphologic study of hyperacute rejection in the rat. Lab. Invest. 33, 280, 1975
8. Forbes, R.D.C., Guttmann, R.D. Mechanisms of humoral mediated cardiac allograft rejection in vivo: controlled comparative morphological studies utilizing inbred rat models. J. Heart Transplant. 1, 196, 1982
9. Sharma, H.M. , Rosenweig, J., Chatterjee S., Moore S., De Champlain, M.L. Platelets in hyperacute rejection of heterotopic cardiac allografts in presensitized dogs. Am. J. Pathol. 70, 155, 1973
10. Caves, P.K., Dong, E., Morris, R.E. Hyperacute rejection of orthotopic cardiac allografts in dogs following solubilized antigen pre-treatment. Transplantation. 16, 252, 1973
11. Guttmann, R.D. Genetics of acute rejection of rat cardiac allografts and a model of hyperacute rejection. Transplantation. 17, 383, 1974
12. Kuwahara, O., Kondo, Y., Kuramochi, T., et al. Organ specificity in hyperacute rejection of canine heart and kidney allografts. Ann. Surg. 180, 72, 1974
13. Cattell, V., Jamieson, S.W. Hyperacute rejection of guinea-pig to rat cardiac xenografts. I. Morphology. J. Pathol. 115, 183, 1975
14. Corry, R.J., Kelly, S.E. Survival of cardiac xenografts. Effect of antithymocyte serum and enhancing heteroserum. Arch Surg. 110, 1143, 1975
15. Jamieson, S.W. Modification of the hyperacute reaction in the rat by sulphinylpyrazone. Thromb. Diath. Haemorrh. 30, 349, 1975
16. Whittum, J.A., Lindquist, R.R. Mechanism of cardiac allograft rejection in the inbred rat: the effect of complement depletion by cobra venom factor on hyperacute cardiac allograft rejection. Transplantation. 24, 26, 1977
17. Forbes, R.D., Guttmann, R.D., Bazin H. Hyperacute rejection of cardiac allografts in a rat strain with a hereditary platelet function defect. Lab. Invest. 37, 158, 1977

18. Guttmann, R.D. In vitro correlates of rejection. I. Suppressive effect and specificity in mixed lymphocyte interaction of alloantiserum producing hyperacute rejection. Transplant. Proc. 9, 755, 1977
19. Forbes, R.D., Guttmann, R.D., Kuramochi, T. Controlled studies of the pathogenesis of hyperacute cardiac allograft rejection in actively immunized recipients. Transplant. Proc. 9, 301, 1977
20. Forbes, R.D., Guttmann, R.D., Pinto-Blonde, M. A passive transfer model of hyperacute rat cardiac allograft rejection. Lab. Invest. 41, 348, 1979
21. Guttmann, R.D., Bazin H. Lack of significance of allograft differences in hyperacute rejection of rat cardiac allografts. Transplantation. 28, 155, 1979
22. Coleman, D.A., Eichwald, E.J. Hyperacute rejection of allografted murine hearts and the white graft reaction. Transplantation. 26, 355, 1978
23. O'Regan, C.C., Robitaille, P., Pinto-Blonde, M., Chartrand, C. Delayed rejection of cardiac xenografts in C6-deficient rabbits. Immunology 38, 245, 1979
24. Lexer, G., Cooper, D.K.C., Rose, A.G., et al. Hyperacute rejection in a discordant (pig-to-baboon) cardiac xenograft model. J. Heart Transplant. 5, 411, 1986
25. Lexer, G., Cooper, D.K.C., Wicomb, W.N., et al. Cardiac transplantation using discordant xenografts in a non-human primate model. Transplant. Proc. 19, 1153, 1987
26. Cooper, D.K.C., Lexer, G., Rose, A.G., et al. Cardiac allograft survival in ABO blood group incompatible baboons. Transplant. Proc. 19, 1036, 1987
27. Cooper, D.K.C., Human, P.A., Reichart, B. Prolongation of cardiac xenograft (vervet monkey-to-baboon) function by a combination of total lymphoid irradiation and immunosuppressive drug therapy. Transplant. Proc. 19, 4441, 1987
28. Cooper, D.K.C., Human, P.A., Rose, A.G. Is ABO compatibility essential in xenografting between closely related species? Transplant. Proc. 19, 4437, 1987
29. Reemtsma, K., Pierson, R.N., Marboe, C.C., et al. Will atherosclerosis limit clinical xenografting? Transplant. Proc. 19 (4 Suppl 5), 108, 1987
30. Cooper, D.K.C., Human, P.A., Lexer, G., et al. Effects of cyclosporine and antibody adsorption on pig cardiac xenograft survival in the baboon. J. Heart Transplant. 7, 238, 1988
31. Cooper, D.K.C., Rose, A.G., Lexer, G., et al. Cardiac allotransplantation across major blood group barriers in the baboon. J. Med. Primatol. 17, 333, 1988
32. Reichenspurner, H., Human, P.A., Boehm, D.M., et al. Optimalization of immunosuppression after xenogeneic heart transplantation in primates. J. Heart Transplant. 8, 200, 1989
33. Cooper, D.K.C., Human, P.A., Rose, A.G., et al. The role of ABO blood group compatibility in heart transplantation between closely related animal species. J. Thorac. Cardiovasc. Surg. 97, 447, 1989
34. Rose, A.G., Cooper, D.K.C., Human, P.A., Reichenspurner, H., Reichart, B. Histopathology of hyperacute rejection of the heart - experimental and clinical observations in allografts and xenografts. J. Heart Lung Transplant. 10, 223, 1991
35. Forbes, R.D., Pinto-Blonde, M., Guttmann, R.D. The effect of anticomplementary cobra venom factor on hyperacute rat cardiac allograft rejection. Lab. Invest. 39, 463, 1978.
36. Reichenspurner, H., Human, P.A., Rose, A.G., Reichart, B., Cooper, D.K.C. Effect of pharmacologic immunosuppression on donor heart survival in a closely related non-human primate xenograft model. Transplant. Proc. 22, 1086, 1990

37. Bahar, R.H., Mohammed, M.M., Dayern H.A. Detection of infection of a cardiac xenograft by thallium - 67 scan. Internat. J. Cardiol 13, 88, 1986
38. Tufveson, G., Roos-Engstrand, E., Gannedahl, G., Fellstrom, B., Larson, E. Heterotopic cardiac xenograft transplantation from mouse to rat. Transplant. Proc. 22, 139, 1990
39. O'Hair, D.P., McManus, R.P., Johnson, C.P., Scott, J.P. The role of antiendothelial antibody in primate cardiac xenograft rejection. Transplant. Proc. 24, 506, 1992
40. Leventhal, J.R., Mathas, A.J., Sun, L.H., et al. The immunopathology of cardiac xenograft rejection in the guinea pig-to-rat model. Transplantation 56, 1, 1993
41. Brauer, R.B., Lam, T.T., Wang, D., et al. Intrahepatic systems of C. in the rat is sufficient for complement -mediated hyperacute rejection of a guinea pig cardiac xenograft. Transplantation 59, 1073, 1995
42. Kobayashi, T., Taniguchi, S., Ye, Y., et al. Prolongation of graft survival following pig-to-baboon heart transplantation by cobra venom factor without natural antibody depletion. Submitted for publication
43. Rose, A.G., Kobayashi, T., Kosanke, S., White, D.J.G., Cooper, D.K.C. Histopathology of delayed vascular (humoral) rejection in C3-depleted discordant (pig-to-baboon) cardiac xenografts treated with cobra venom factor (CVF) - prominent role of venular thrombosis. Submitted for publication
44. Trento, A., Hardesty, R.L., Griffith, B.P., et al. Role of the antibody to vascular endothelial cells in hyperacute rejection in patients undergoing cardiac transplantation. J. Thorac. Cardiovasc. Surg. 95, 37, 1988
45. Hammond, E.H., Yowell, R.L., Numoda, S., et al. Vascular (humoral) rejection in heart transplantation: pathologic observations and clinical implications. J. Heart Transplant. 8, 430, 1989
46. Rose, A.G., Cooper, D.K.C. An histopathologic grading system of hyperacute (humoral, antibody mediated) cardiac xenograft and allograft rejection. J. Heart Lung Transplant. 15, 804, 1996
47. Rose, A.G., Cooper, D.K.C. Ultrastructure of hyperacute rejection in cardiac xenografts. In Cooper, D.K.C., et al. (Eds). Xenotransplantation. (First edition) Heidelberg, Springer, 1991, p 243
48. Mullerworth, M.H., Lixfield, W., Rachkewich, R.A., et al. Hyperacute rejection of heterotopic heart allografts in dogs. Transplantation 13, 570, 1972
49. Forbes, R.D., Guttmann, R.D. Evidence for complement-induced endothelial injury in vivo: a comparative ultrastructural tracer study in a controlled model of hyperacute rat cardiac allograft rejection. Am. J. Pathol. 106, 378, 1982
50. Debault, L., Ye, Y., Rolf, L.L., et al. Ultrastructural features in hyperacutely rejected baboon cardiac allografts and pig cardiac xenografts. Transplant. Proc. 24, 612, 1992

19 Mechanism of Discordant Cardiac Xenograft Rejection – An Alternative View Based on Ultrastructural Observations

S. Aziz, K. Suzuki, and D. Thorning

Introduction

In contradistinction to organ transplants between closely related (concordant) species, where rejection appears to be mediated largely by cellular immune reactions, rejection following transplantation involving widely disparate (discordant) species appears to be mediated largely by humoral mechanisms [1, 2]. Pigs are a potential source of donor organs for human xenotransplantation, and various experimental models have been used to study pig organ rejection after such procedures [3].

The heterotopic guinea pig-to-rat cardiac transplant model was first described by Jamieson [4], and histologic observations of intravascular thrombi and interstitial hemorrhage have been reported as evidence of typical humoral rejection in this model [5–9]. The events initiating rejection have not been fully elucidated and have been the subject of debate. Anti-guinea pig cytotoxic antibodies have been detected in rat serum prior to transplantation, and it has generally been assumed that these react with antigens in the grafts and initiate an immunoinflammatory reaction. Available evidence suggests that this reaction injures endothelial cells, activates obstructive intravascular thrombosis, and thereby induces ischemic injury in the grafts.

A pig heart-to-rhesus monkey model of xenograft rejection demonstrated IgM deposition on donor endothelium and IgG extravasation similar to albumin. These observations suggested that IgM deposition was involved in initiating rejection, that loss of normal vascular permeability was a secondary feature, and that IgG distribution was a reflection of altered vascular permeability [10, 11].

Many investigators have focused on the donor vascular endothelial cell surface as the initial target of natural antibodies and the site of injurious reaction that leads to graft rejection. Despite this focus, the exact mechanisms underlying rejection remain unknown. Normal endothelial cell surfaces have an anticoagulant activity that tends to inhibit local intravascular coagulation, although various stimuli can alter this activity and, indeed, activate procoagulant activity on the same endothelial cell surfaces [12].

We have used the heterotopic guinea pig-to-rat cardiac model and transmission electron microscopy to evaluate the structural alterations in myocardial tissue that occur after hyperacute rejection. Our observations will be presented and their possible significance discussed.

Experimental Model

Donor guinea pigs (375–475 g) and recipient Lewis rats (250–275 g) were anesthetized by intraperitoneal injections of pentobarbital (50 mg/kg). The donors were given intravenous heparin (1000 units) prior to harvesting their hearts.

Explantation involved transecting the great vessels via the transverse sinus and tying off the venae cavae and then all pulmonary veins en masse. The explanted heart was placed in 4 °C saline and protected with topical cold saline during implantation. Intra-abdominal transplantation was effected by anastomosing the donor aorta to the recipient infra-renal aorta and the donor pulmonary artery to the recipient inferior vena cava. These end-to-side anastomoses were made with 8/0 prolene. The xenograft ischemic period ranged from 23 to 30 min.

Of a total of 14 cardiac xenografts, four were excised "early" at 4 min after reperfusion, and ten were removed "late" after cessation of myocardial contractions (at a mean of 6.80 ± 1.51 min). The apical segments of each of these hearts were minced with razor blades into 5-mm cubes and then immersed in 5 % glutaraldehyde fixative. Fixed tissue samples were processed for thick-section transmission light microscopy (TLM) and thin-section transmission electron microscopy (TEM) as follows:

1. Minced tissue samples were postfixed in 2 % osmium tetroxide in 0.2 *M* syn-collidine buffer, dehydrated in a graded series of ethanol (35 % → 70 % → 95 % → 100 %), infiltrated with propylene oxide, and embedded in polymerized medcast resin.
2. Each block of embedded tissue was trimmed, then cut into 0.1-µm "thick" sections, which were stained with methylene blue-azure II and examined by TLM to select samples for further processing.
3. Selected sample blocks (at least one from each heart) were trimmed to appropriate size and cut into about 75-nm "thin" sections, which were placed on grids and stained with uranyl acetate and Millonig's lead acetate.
4. Stained tissue samples on grids were examined with a Jeol JEM-100s electron microscope.

Microscopic evaluation was conducted by a diagnostic pathologist who knew that the heart tissue samples had been obtained after hyperacute rejection but was otherwise unaware of the details of the experiment. TLM revealed qualitatively similar, but quantitatively variable, changes in the myocardium of all samples. These changes included myocyte hypercontraction, microvascular congestion/(perhaps) thrombosis, and some combination of interstitial edema and hemorrhage. There was no specific evidence of interstitial leukocyte infiltration. At least one sample from each heart was selected for study by TEM, the selection process being guided by the "most characteristic" tissue alterations in each heart. Evaluation was conducted as follows:

1. One grid from each selected sample was surveyed to find the "most characteristic" tissue changes (as identified previously by TLM); these changes were readily identified in every sample.
2. The most representative tissue alteration in one grid space of each sample was recorded on film in a series of overlapping images at ×3000 magnification.

3. The film was developed, prints were made at ×2.9 magnification, and these prints were used to construct a montage from each heart sample for final study.

Transmission Electron Microscopy Observations (Figs. 1–12)

The TEM study confirmed the TLM observations of myocyte hypercontraction, microvascular congestion, and interstitial edema with and without erythrocyte extravasation. There was no specific evidence of intravascular thrombosis, i.e., no intravascular fibrin, in any sample, although a few wisps of fibrin were rarely noted in the interstitium. There was no evidence of intravascular leukocyte margination, interstitial leukocyte infiltration, or immune complex deposition in or around the microvasculature.

Protein-rich interstitial edema was the principal alteration from normal. Whereas the normal, nonfibrous, extracellular cardiac matrix has an appearance on TEM that is essentially clear with only barely perceptible proteoglycans, the interstitial fluid in these hyperacutely rejected donor hearts not only distended the space (edema) but also contained an increased concentration of plasma-like proteins. While these changes were already identifiable in the hearts removed 4 min after implantation, they were far more prominent in the hearts removed after cessation of contractions, at which time the edema fluid protein density was generally similar to that of condensed plasma in adjacent microvascular channels.

Interstitial edema was accompanied by microvascular congestion and patchy erythrocyte extravasation into the interstitial space (microvascular hemorrhages). These changes were identified in every sample; however, they were more prominent and extensive in the hearts removed after cessation of contractions. In the latter hearts, the congested vessels were distended by compact aggregates of erythrocytes without the usual amount of associated plasma (condensation). In a few samples, occasional microvascular channels contained marginated platelets, and others contained platelet aggregates; however, there was no evidence of platelet degranulation (release of stored products).

Despite plasma fluid and protein extravasation, multifocal microvascular congestion and erythrocyte aggregation, intravascular platelet aggregation (uncommon), and erythrocyte extravasation, *there was no concomitant structural evidence of endothelial cell injury.* The normally attenuated and intact endothelial cell forms were never swollen or necrotic, although a few appeared to be more condensed that adjacent counterparts. Their overlapping cell–cell contact regions had essentially normal appearances, although the actual occluding cell–cell junctions (tight junctions) in these regions could not be specifically evaluated. The endothelium, in general, remained normally attached to its basement membrane, which defines the outer microvascular boundary and connects these channels to the fibrous interstitial framework. In one sample, there was a single break in the otherwise intact endothelial basement membrane, and this break occurred at the site of maximum erythrocyte extravasation.

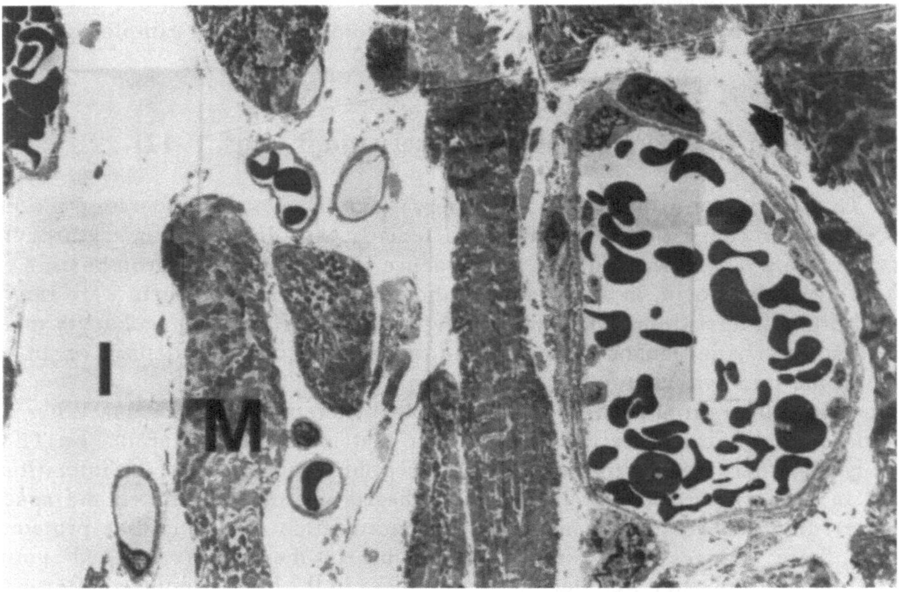

Fig. 1. Transmission electron microscope (TEM) montage of myocardium of a heart removed after 4 min. The interstitial space (*I*, interstitium) between myocytes (*M*) and microvascular channels appears to be distended by fluid. This fluid is relatively electronlucent without excess protein and therefore resembles normal interstitial fluid. One myocyte (*arrowhead*) shows nonspecific hypercontractile change. The various-sized microvascular channels contain erythrocytes and platelets suspended in a usual amount of plasma. All of the various myocardial tissue cell types appear intact

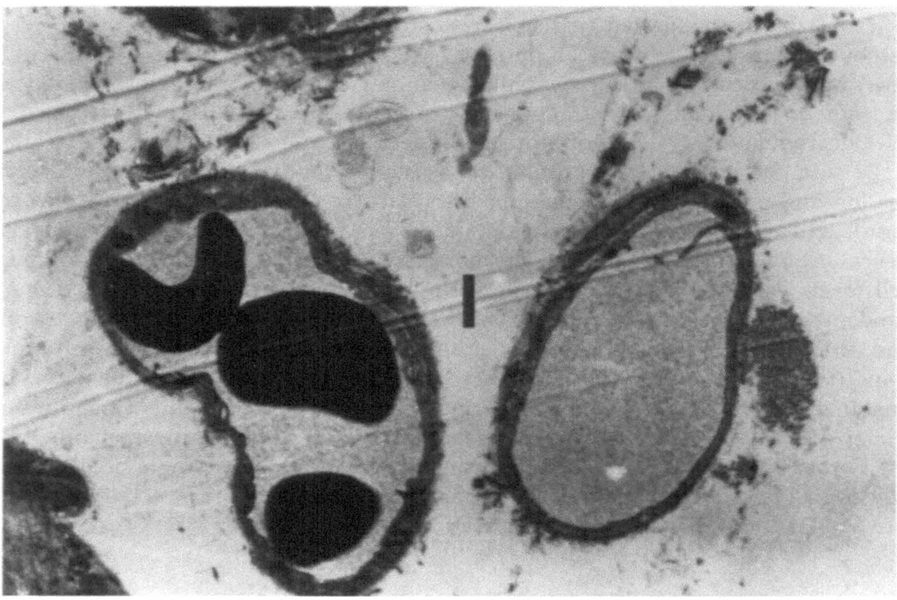

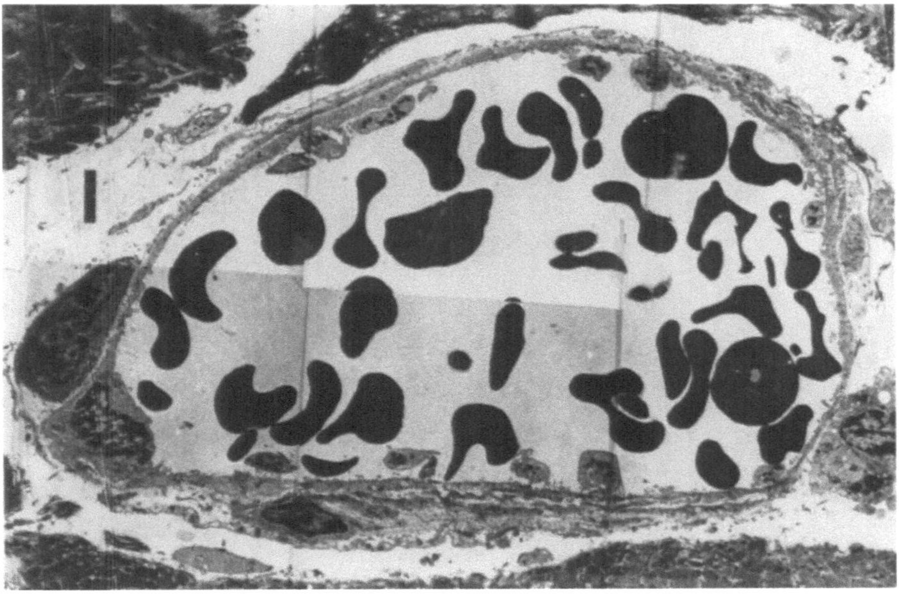

Fig. 3. Magnified transmission electron microscope (TEM) view of the microvascular venule seen in Fig. 1. The venular lumen is normally distended by blood components, including erythrocytes and platelets, separated by granular-appearing plasma proteins. Most of the platelets are located along the endothelial aspect and may be "marginated;" they are not aggregated nor degranulated. The endothelium is intact. Note the nucleus and perinuclear cytoplasm of one endothelial cell on the *left* side of the figure. There are intact pericytes in the otherwise thin wall, as well as thin layers of fibrocytic cytoplasm apposed to the interstitial aspect of the intact (but not appreciable) venular basement membrane. The interstitium (*I*) is similar to that seen in Fig. 2

Fig. 2. Magnified transmission electron microscope (TEM) view of microvascular capillaries seen in Fig. 1. The capillary lumina are normally distended by blood components, including erythrocytes, separated by granular-appearing plasma proteins. The endothelium is intact. Note the flap-like protrusion of endothelial cytoplasm at the overlapping cell-cell junction. There is a small amount of fibrous extracellular matrix proteins apposed to the interstitial aspect of the intact endothelial basement membrane (outer boundary of capillary wall not specifically appreciated at this magnification). The interstitium (*I*) has slightly more nonfibrous protein concentration, but this is only barely appreciable

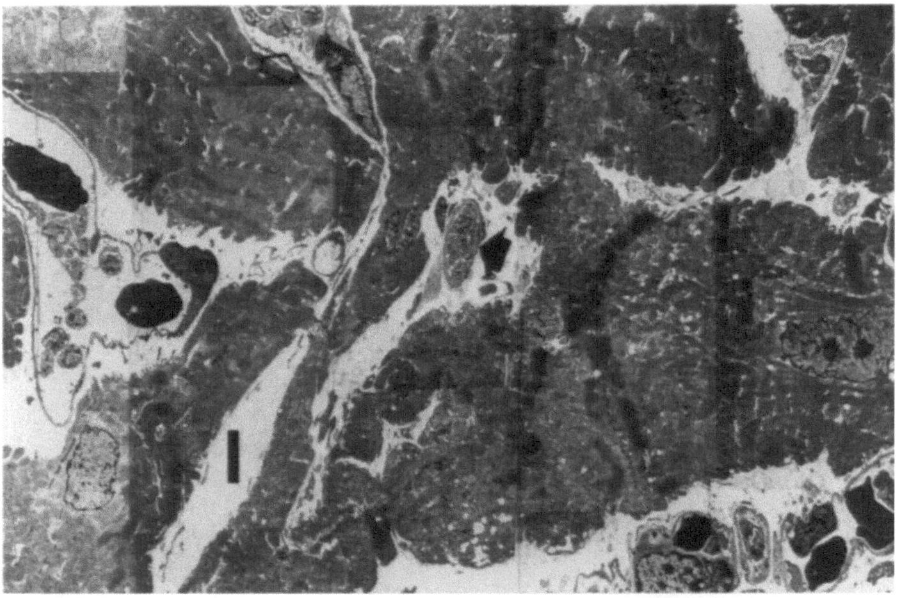

Fig. 4. Transmission electron microscope (TEM) montage of myocardium from another heart removed after 4 min. The interstitium (*I*) is essentially similar to that illustrated in Figs. 1–3. Several myocytes show nonspecific myofibrillar hypercontractions, creating irregular, variably thick, band-like densities. These changes were observed focally in all samples. The intact microvascular channels contain erythrocytes and platelets suspended in a usual amount of plasma, although several channels (*arrowheads*) have apparent platelet aggregates with less than usual intervening plasma volume

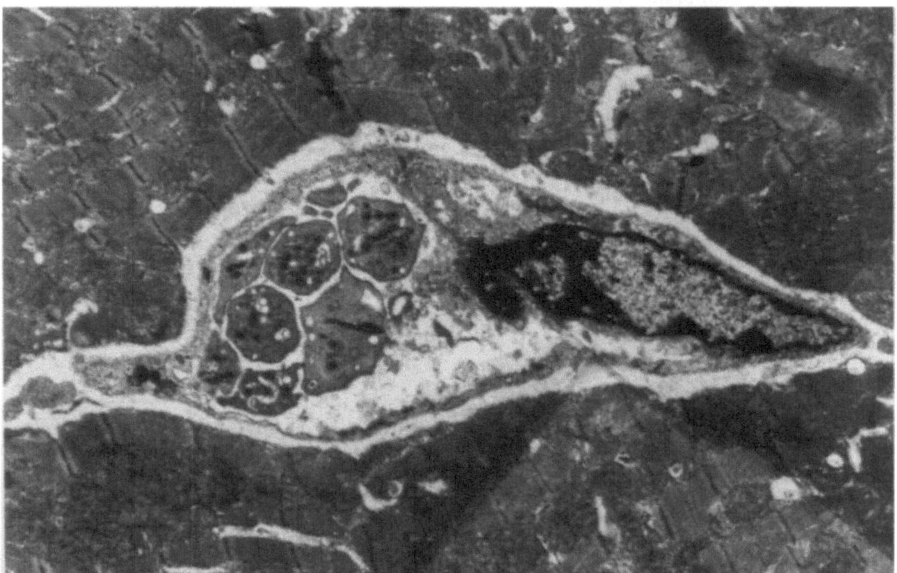

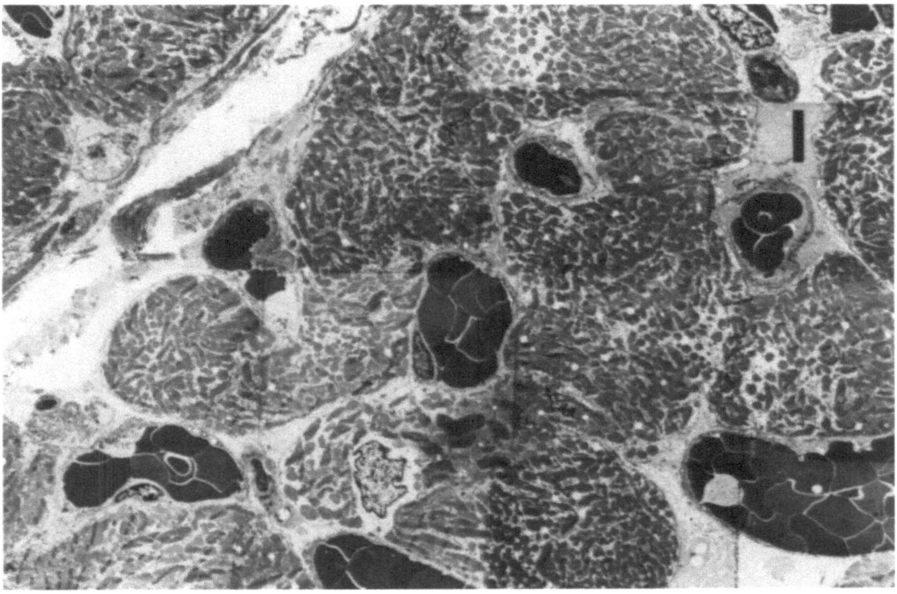

Fig. 6. Transmission electron microscope (TEM) montage of myocardium from a heart removed after cessation of contractions. The interstitium (*I*) now has a readily apparent increase in granular protein density. Myocytes are essentially intact. The microvascular channels are packed with erythrocytes and also show a relative decrease in plasma volume. There are no extravasated erythrocytes

Fig. 5. Magnified transmission electron microscope (TEM) view of a platelet aggregate seen in Fig. 4. There is no evidence of platelet degranulation or intravascular fibrin formation. The capillary endothelium is intact. Note some of the hypercontracted myofibrils in adjacent myocytes

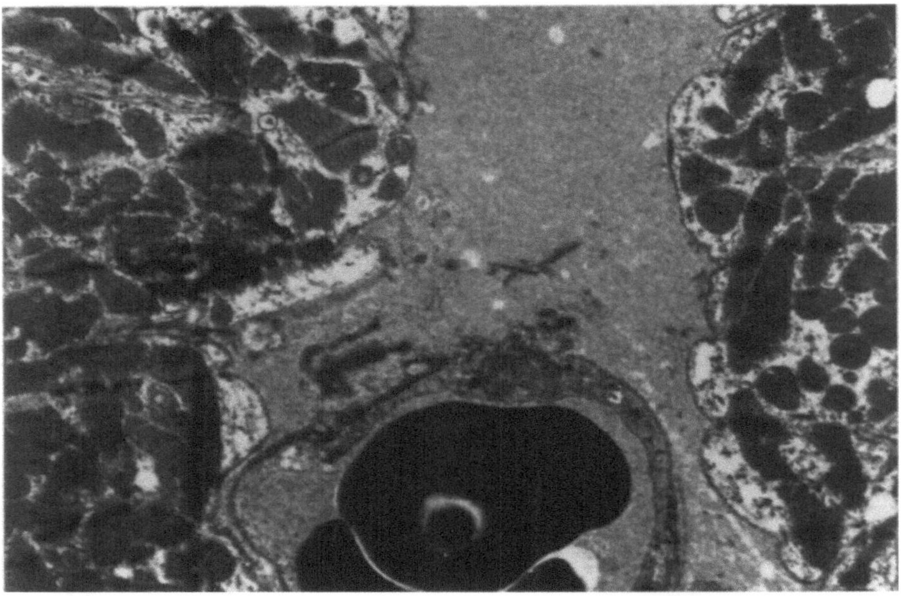

Fig. 7. Magnified transmission electron microscope (TEM) view of a microvascular capillary seen in Fig. 6. The vascular lumen contains erythrocytes and plasma; note the granular protein density of this plasma and compare it with the more normal density seen in Figs. 2 and 3. Note also the same granular protein density of the extravascular interstitial fluid, which is similar to that of nearby plasma and remarkably different from the more normal appearing fluid seen in Fig. 2. This observation indicates a marked alteration in normal endothelial permeability, resulting in protein-rich interstitial edema. The endothelium appears intact although one endothelial cell which is overlapped by the cytoplasmic process of an adjacent one appears unusually condensed. There is no evidence of intravascular fibrin formation, although there are several wispy interstitial filaments that could represent fibrin formation from extravasated fibrinogen. Note that there is some variation in apparent protein density within the interstitial fluid; this may reflect variation in local lymphatic clearance of excess fluid and/or protein

Fig. 9. Transmission electron microscope (TEM) montage of myocardium from another heart removed after cessation of contractions. The interstitium (*I*) has a readily apparent increase in granular protein density. Myocytes are essentially intact. Most microvascular channels are packed with erythrocytes and also show a relative decrease in plasma volume. There are a few extravasated erythrocytes

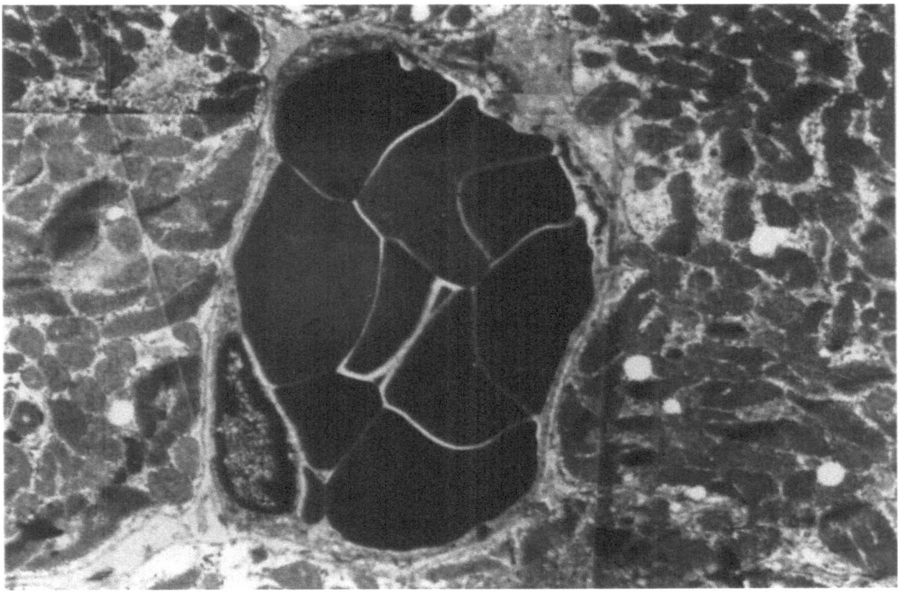

Fig. 8. Magnified transmission electron microscope (TEM) view of another microvascular capillary seen in Fig. 6. The vascular lumen is packed with otherwise intact erythrocytes, there is little appreciable plasma, and the endothelium is intact. There is no evidence of intravascular fibrin formation

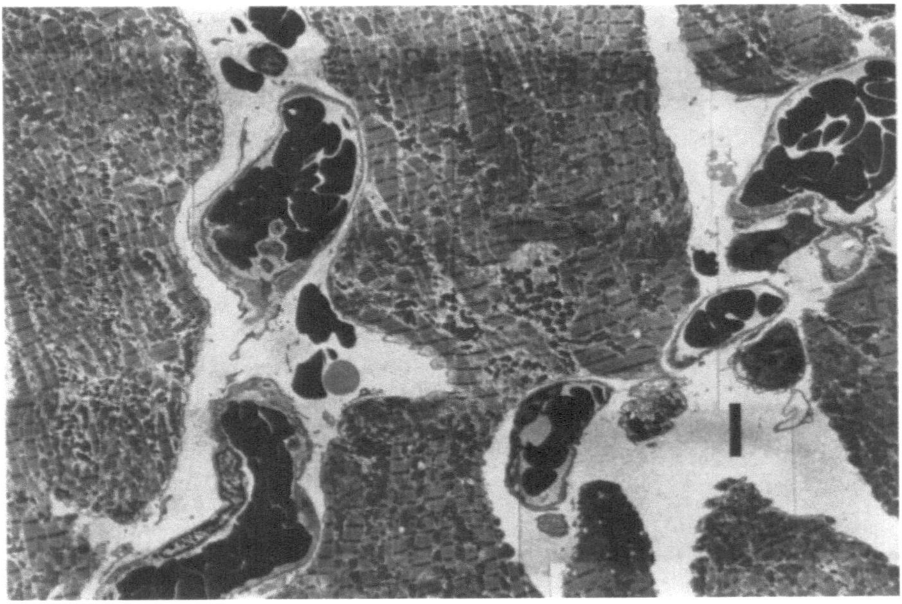

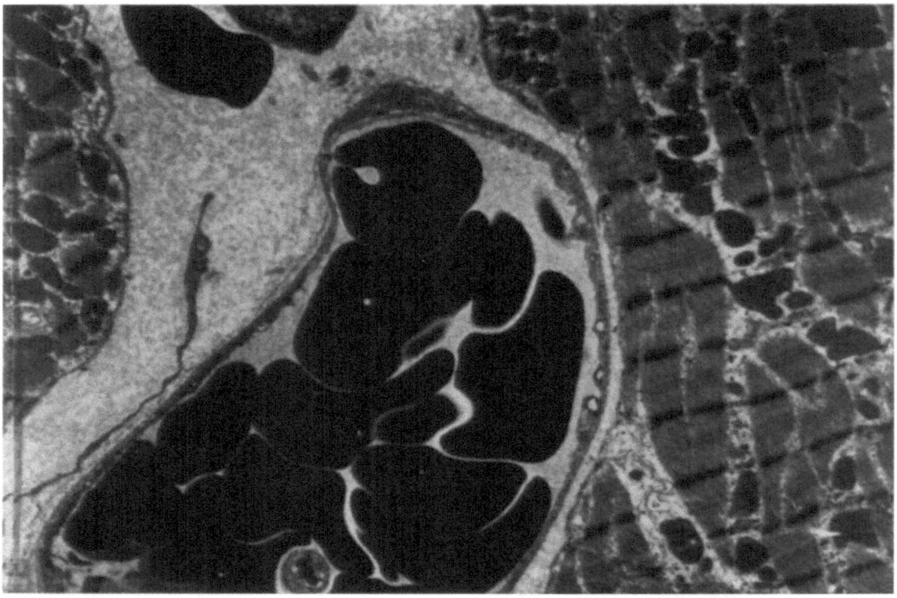

Fig. 10. Magnified transmission electron microscope (TEM) view of a microvascular capillary seen in Fig. 9. The vascular lumen is packed with intact erythrocytes, and the endothelium appears normal and intact. There is no evidence of intravascular fibrin formation. Note that the granular protein densities in plasma and interstitial fluid are similar, again indicating protein-rich interstitial edema

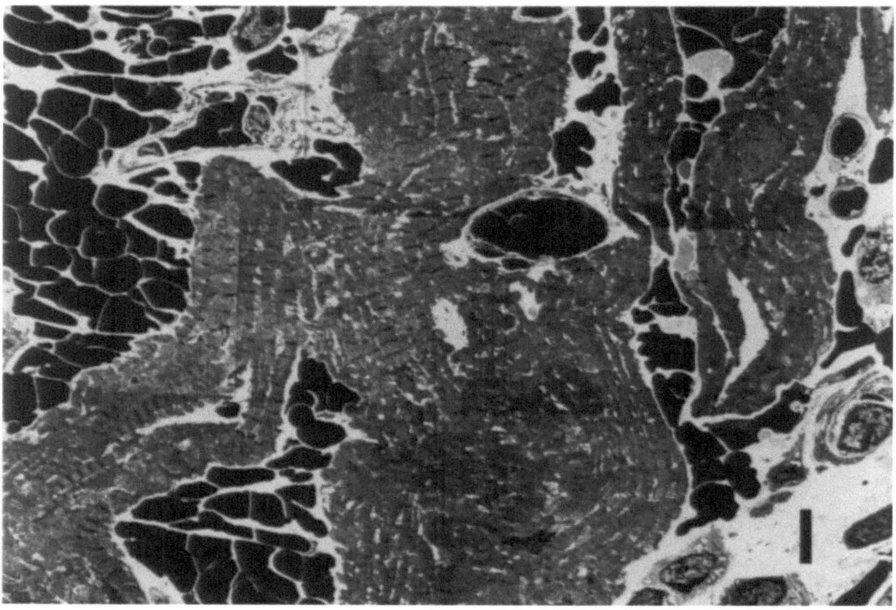

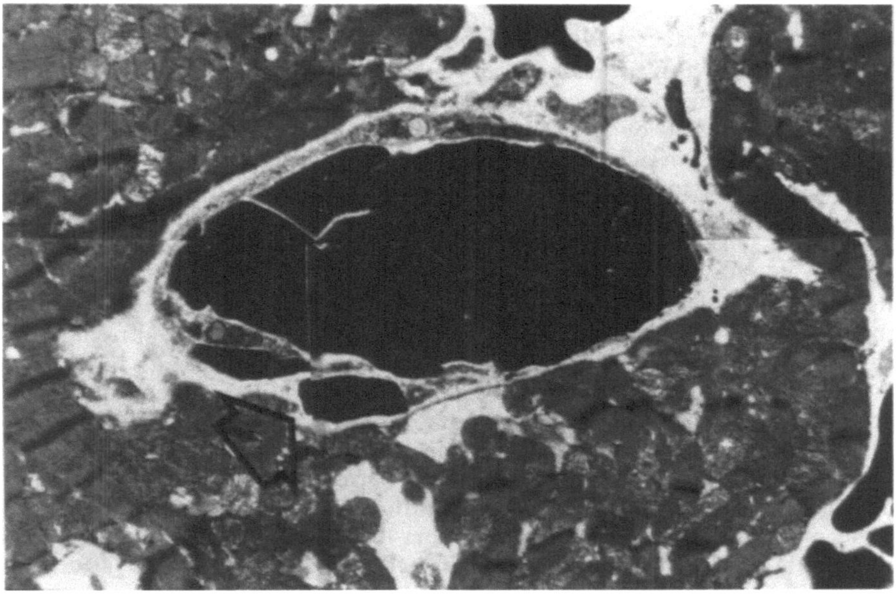

Fig. 12. Magnified transmission electron microscope (TEM) view of a microvascular capillary seen in Fig. 11. The vascular lumen is packed with intact erythrocytes, and the endothelium generally appears intact; however, there is an apparent defect (*arrowhead*) in the capillary wall (endothelium plus basement membrane), allowing passage of erythrocytes from the lumen into the interstitium. This was the only such defect identified in all of the sites photographed

Fig. 11. Transmission electron microscope (TEM) montage of myocardium from another heart removed after cessation of contractions. The interstitium (*I*) in this selected site contains a large number of extravasated erythrocytes. Myocytes are essentially intact, and at least one microvascular channel is packed with erythrocytes. There are a few extravasated erythrocytes

Comment

The lack of donor organs has been an impetus for research on discordant transplantation, and rejection has emerged as a major barrier to the success of this procedure. The results of studies using various animal models have focused interest on the donor vascular endothelium, which is the initial site of interaction between donor organ and recipient circulation. It has been proposed that (a) preformed antibodies in the recipient bind to antigens on the luminal surfaces of donor vascular endothelial cells, (b) this interaction activates circulating complement, (c) these combined interactions alter endothelial surfaces in a manner that inhibits their usual anticoagulant activity and promotes a procoagulant state (endothelial activation), and (d) local intravascular thrombosis and resultant tissue ischemia occur. Based on this proposed mechanism, various investigators have focused on preventing vascular endothelial activation as a key to clinically successful xenotransplantation [13].

Our TEM study of hyperacute rejection of guinea pig hearts in rat recipients demonstrates loss of normal microvascular permeability as the only consistent and characteristic myocardial tissue alteration. This alteration allows flooding of the myocardial interstitium with plasma-like fluid with or without extravasated erythrocytes. The fluid loss from the microvasculature causes local hemoconcentration evidenced by erythrocytes packed in distended lumina. We could find no evidence of intravascular coagulation, i.e., there were no intravascular fibrin aggregates, and there was only meager evidence of extravascular fibrin formation in rare sites in occasional heart samples. There were occasional intravascular platelet aggregates, but none of the observed platelets showed any evidence of degranulation. Finally, with the exception of a single site of apparent endothelial basement membrane rupture (Fig. 12), the microvascular endothelium *remained intact* and attached to its respective basement membrane and demonstrated no morphologic evidence of cell injury.

Our TEM observations are somewhat at variance with those of others. Cattell and Jamieson [5], using the same model, examined tissue samples from hearts removed at 4, 8, and 12 min postimplantation and tissue samples from one heart biopsied at 1.5, 2, 3, 4, 5, and 6 min postimplantation. They reportedly observed microvascular congestion, platelet aggregation, and endothelial cell detachment from the basement membrane; they did not observe neutrophilic leukocytes, "prominent" fibrin formation, or plasma protein extravasation into the interstitium. They concluded that "endothelial activation" induced platelets to aggregate and release their granular contents and that these platelet products initiated endothelial damage and fibrin formation.

Rose and Cooper [14], using outbred Landrace pigs as donors and either mongrel dogs (n=3) or Chacma baboons (n=3) as recipients, examined tissue samples from hearts removed after hyperacute rejection and cessation of contraction. In the three hearts removed from dog recipients, they observed varying quantities of platelet thrombi with intact endothelium. In the three hearts removed from baboon recipients, they observed that one was "too badly damaged to evaluate," one had intact endothelium with no evidence of "widespread platelet thrombi," and one showed "endothelial cell swelling" with no evidence of "widespread platelet thrombi." In both sets of animals, they observed variably extensive fibrin deposition and myocyte hypercontraction, but did not report protein-rich interstitial edema or specific evidence of intravascular thrombosis.

Debault et al. [15] also reported vascular endothelial changes in pig cardiac xenografts transplanted into dogs, as evidenced by vacuoles in the endothelium, with platelet adherence to the vascular walls, and intraluminal fibrin thrombi. Vascular wall injury was evidenced by disrupted endothelium and hemorrhage. Increased extravascular fluid was apparent.

TLM and TEM observations of rejecting and rejected cardiac xenografts have consistently noted myocyte hypercontractions and various microvascular alterations, and all have supported to some extent the proposed mechanism of rejection, as outlined above. Previous TEM observations have focused attention on the presence and importance of platelet aggregation, intravascular coagulation, and endothelial damage as principal and interrelated pathogenetic events. In contrast, our own TEM observations have focused attention on an alteration of microvascular permeability and plasma fluid/protein extravasation as principal and interrelated pathogenetic events. Most notably, our observations did not provide any evidence of platelet degranulation (release), intravascular thrombosis (fibrin formation), or specific endothelial cell injury.

We have no explanation for the disparities between these TEM observations. In accordance with the proposed mechanism of hyperacute rejection, our observations would be consistent with the notions that (a) preformed antibodies in the recipient bind to antigens on the luminal surfaces of donor vascular endothelial cells, (b) this interaction activates circulating complement, and (c) these combined interactions alter the vascular endothelial cells in some manner. They would not support any role for intravascular coagulation. Although we commonly observed erythrocyte "plugs" in the microvasculature, none of these was associated with fibrin, and we attribute them to stasis and hemoconcentration following loss of intravascular fluid. Although we observed no morphologic evidence of endothelial cell injury or physical displacement, we suspect the loss of plasma fluid/proteins reflects a major alteration in the function of occluding (tight) endothelial cell–cell junctions. Such alteration could involve structural and/or functional changes that could not be assessed by our TEM study.

The basic ultrastructural findings associated with the hyperacute rejection of cardiac xenografts would seem to require additional study by independent investigators. We believe that the possibility of a major change in endothelial permeability suggests new and potentially significant avenues for further investigation and therapeutic approaches.

References

1. Calne RY. Organ transplantation between widely disparate species. Transplant. Proc. 2; 550,1970
2. Auchincloss H Jr. Xenografting: a review. Transplant. Rev. 4; 4, 1990
3. Platt JL, Bach FH. The barrier to xenotransplantation. Transplantation. 52; 937, 1991

4. Jamieson SW. Xenograft hyperacute rejection. A new model. Transplantation. 17; 533,1974
5. Cattell V, Jamieson SW. Hyperacute rejection of guinea pig-to-rat cardiac xenografts. I. Morphology. J. Path. 115; 183,1975
6. Marino IR, Celli S, Ferla G, et al. Histopathological, immunofluorescent, and electron-microscopic features of hyperacute rejection in discordant renal xenotransplantation. In Xenotransplantation (First edition). DKC Cooper, et al. (eds), Springer, Heidelberg, 1991, p. 207
7. Ito S, Camussi G, Tetta C, Milgrom F, Andres G. Hyperacute renal allograft rejection in the rabbit. The role of platelet-activating factor and of cationic proteins derived from polymorphonuclear leukocytes and from platelets. Lab. Invest. 51; 148, 1984
8. Forbes RD, Guttmann RD. Histopathology and mechanism of rejection in xenotransplantation. In Xenograft 25. MA Hardy, ed., Excerpta Medica, New York, 1989, p. 133
9. Forbes RD, Kuramochi T, Guttmann RD, Klassen J, Knaack J. A controlled sequential morphologic study of hyperacute cardiac allograft rejection in the rat. Lab. Invest. 33; 280, 1975
10. Platt JL, Fischel RJ, Matas AJ, et al. Immunopathology of hyperacute xenograft rejection in a swine-to-primate model. Transplantation. 52; 214, 1991
11. Bach FH, Dalmasso, G, Platt JL. Immunoglobulins involved in xenotransplantation. Histological staining. Transplant. Rev. 6; 1, 1992
12. Verrier ED. The vascular endothelium: friend or foe. Ann. Thorac. Surg. 55; 818, 1993
13. Bach FH, Blakely ML, van der Werf W, et al. Discordant xenografting: a working model of problem and issues. Xeno. 1; 8, 1993

20 Histopathology of Liver Xenotransplantation in the Nonhuman Primate

Y. Luo, L. Mieles, S.D. Kosanke, and D.K.C. Cooper

Introduction

Early studies of liver xenotransplantation in the nonhuman primate were carried out by Calne et al. in the 1960s and 1970s [1, 2] (Tables 1, 2). Starzl et al. performed a small number of clinical liver xenotransplants at that time [3–6] and again more recently [7–9] (Chap. 58), and Makowka et al. carried out one clinical auxiliary pig liver transplant in 1993 [10, 11]. There remains little research in this field, although a small number of groups have explored liver xenotransplantation in nonhuman primate models [12–17] (Tables 1, 2). Porter [6] and Wight [19] have reviewed the histopathological features of hepatic xenograft rejection.

Our own studies, details of which have been reported fully elsewhere [16–18], will be briefly reviewed.

Experimental Protocols

Liver transplantation was performed in five groups (Table 3). In group 1, liver allografting was performed in baboons. Concordant liver xenografting (between vervet monkeys and baboons) was carried out in groups 2 and 3, and discordant

Table 1. Experiences with concordant liver xenotransplantation in nonhuman primates

Donor	Recipient	Type of transplant	n	Immunosuppressive therapy	Survival (days)	Reference
Cynomolgus monkey	Rhesus monkey	OLT	3	ALS	<1–20	[2]
Vervet monkey	Baboon	OLT	13	CyA+AZA+steroids+ splenectomy	2 to >360	[12, 13]
Vervet monkey	Baboon	HLT	8	CyA+CPP+steroids	20–123	[16–18]
Vervet monkey (ABO-incompatible)	Baboon	HLT	6	CyA+CPP+steroids	28–45	[16–18]
Baboon	Vervet monkey	OLT	6	CyA+CPP+steroids	<1 (n=4), 93 (n=1), >1000 (n=1)	[15]

OLT, orthotopic liver transplantation; HLT, heterotopic liver transplantation; ALS, antilymphocyte serum; CyA, cyclosporine; AZA, azathioprine; CPP, cyclophosphamide.

Table 2. Experiences with discordant liver xenotransplantation in nonhuman primates

Donor	Recipient	Type of transplant	*n*	Immunosuppressive therapy	Survival (h)	Reference
Pig	Baboon	OLT	7	None/steroids/steroids+AZA	6–84	[1]
Pig	Rhesus monkey	OLT	3	ALS	<12	[2]
Pig	Chimpanzee	OLT	1	None	8	[2]
Pig	Cynomolgus monkey	OLT	4	WBI+TI+ATG+BM+ECP	2–72	[14]
Pig	Baboon	OLT	2	WBI+TI+ATG+BM+ECP	2–72	[14]
Pig	Rhesus monkey	OLT	6	None/steroids+CyA+Dashen	2–5.5	[17, 18]
Pig	Baboon	HLT	2	CPP+CyA+steroids	2	[17, 18]

OLT, orthotopic liver transplantation; HLT, heterotopic liver transplantation; AZA, azathioprine; WBI, whole body irradiation; TI, thymus irradiation; ATG, antithymocyte globulin; BM, bone marrow transfusion; ECP, extracorporeal plasmapheresis; CyA, cyclosporine; Dashen, a Chinese traditional medicine; CPP, cyclophosphamide.

xenografting between pigs and either baboons or rhesus monkeys in groups 4 and 5.

The operative technique of heterotopic liver transplantation in the baboon (used in groups 1–4) has been described by Mieles et al. [16] and was based on that introduced clinically several years ago [20]. The technique of orthotopic liver transplantation (group 5) was also based on the standard clinical technique [21].

All recipient baboons and all donor animals were ABO blood typed (using saliva in nonhuman primates and blood in pigs). Baboons and vervet monkeys were also typed for simian blood groups (Dr. W.W. Socha, Laboratory for Experimental Medicine and Surgery in Primates, New York University, New York, USA).

Table 3. Summary of histopathological changes of liver allografts and xenografts

Group	Total (*n*)	Studies (*n*)	Early vascular rejection	Acute cellular rejection	Reversibility of acute cellular rejection by methylprednisolone therapy	Periportal fibrosis
Heterotopic transplants in the baboon						
1. Allografts (baboon-to-baboon)	8	5	–	+	+	–
2. Concordant ABO-compatible (vervet monkey-to-baboon)	8	5	+	++	±	+
3. Concordant ABO-incompatible (vervet monkey-to-baboon)	6	3	++	+++	–	++
4. Discordant (pig-to-baboon)	2	2	+++			
Orthotopic transplants in the rhesus monkey						
5. Discordant (pig-to-rhesus monkey)	6	4	+++			

From [18].

Simian blood type crossmatching was negative in all cases (groups 1–3). Lymphocytotoxic crossmatching between donor and recipient was also performed in all experiments in groups 1–3, and was negative in all cases.

All recipient baboons received intravenous (i.v.) pharmacologic immunosuppression including (a) continuous cyclosporine infusion (to maintain a whole blood level at >2000 ng/ml) [16] begun 2–7 days before liver transplantation, (b) cyclophosphamide (1–2 mg/kg per day), also begun 2–7 days before transplantation, and (c) methylprednisolone (500 mg on the day of operation, with a tapering dose to 2 mg/kg per day), as detailed elsewhere [16]. Three of the rhesus monkey recipients received no immunosuppressive therapy, and three received (a) cyclosporine (10 mg/kg per day), (b) methylprednisolone (500 mg/day i.m.), both begun 2 days before operation, and (c) dashen (a traditional Chinese medicine), which is believed to provide some protection of the vascular endothelium and also has an anticoagulant effect (at 5 mg/kg i.v. during operation).

Liver biopsies (under direct vision) were obtained at the time of excision of the liver from the donor and at intervals of several days post-transplantation. If the macroscopic appearance of the liver suggested hyperacute rejection (i.e., the liver was cyanotic and swollen), a biopsy was taken 30 min after reperfusion. At the time of euthanasia or spontaneous death, all animals were necropsied with most or all viscera, including the transplanted liver, being examined.

The liver biopsies were stored in 10 % neutral-buffered formalin, placed into paraffin blocks, sectioned, and stained with (a) hematoxylin and eosin (H&E) and (b) phosphotungstic acid hematoxylin (PTAH). The following histopathological features were studied: (a) cellular infiltrates (neutrophils, lymphocytes, eosinophils), (b) blood vessels (congestion, hemorrhage, fibrin aggregation, and venulitis or arteritis), (c) hepatocytes (vacuolation, necrosis), (d) bile ducts (inflammation, necrosis), and (e) interstitial tissue (fibrosis). Special attention was paid to the portal zone and central vein. (Immunohistopathological studies are underway but the results are not yet available for reporting.)

Of the 30 experiments performed, the histopathological features outlined below are based on 19 experiments in which technical complications were excluded and where the liver functioned for at least 1 h to 123 days before the recipient was either electively euthanized or died spontaneously (Table 3).

Macroscopic Appearances

Allografts and Concordant Xenografts (Groups 1–3)

The appearances of the allografts (group 1) and concordant xenografts (groups 2 and 3) were similar in the early stages in all experiments. Hyperacute rejection was not observed. The grafted livers became congested and slightly edematous during the first 30–60 min after reperfusion. Bile was secreted in all cases within 2 h. Within the first month, the grafted livers became covered by a thick, fibrous envelope, and their consistency became firmer in some cases though never obviously cirrhotic. Despite frequent episodes of acute cellular rejection, concordant xenografts functioned adequately for elective periods of up to 4 months [16].

Discordant Xenografts (Groups 4 and 5)

After reperfusion, discordant auxiliary liver xenografts (group 4) became cyanotic and swollen within 30–60 min. No bile was produced. Following orthotopic transplantation (group 5), the discordant grafts initially appeared less cyanotic and swollen than the auxiliary grafts. Bile was produced in all cases. Cyanosis and edema of the liver slowly increased. Graft failure or recipient death occurred within 5.5 h in all cases.

Microscopic Findings

Allografts (Group 1)

Histopathological changes consistent with hyperacute or acute vascular rejection were absent in all instances. Acute cellular rejection occurred in some cases, generally within the first 10 days, but was usually mild or moderale (Fig. 1), consisting mainly of lymphoid and eosinophil cell infiltration in the portal zones. When acute rejection became more severe it was associated with vasculitis and bile duct damage (Fig. 2). The acute cellular rejection could be reversed with i.v. methylprednisolone therapy (Fig. 3). No fibrosis developed during follow-up periods of a maximum of 62 days.

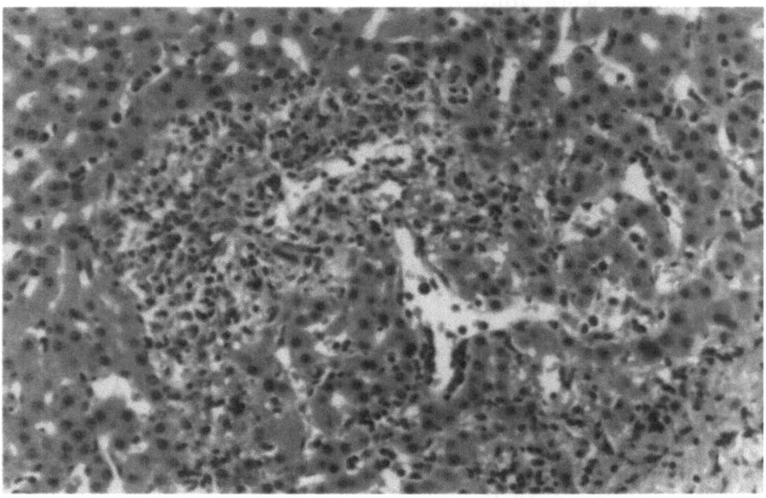

Fig. 1. Moderale acute cellular rejection of a group 1 allograft at 13 days, demonstrating a periportal lymphoid cellular infiltrate. H&E, ×200

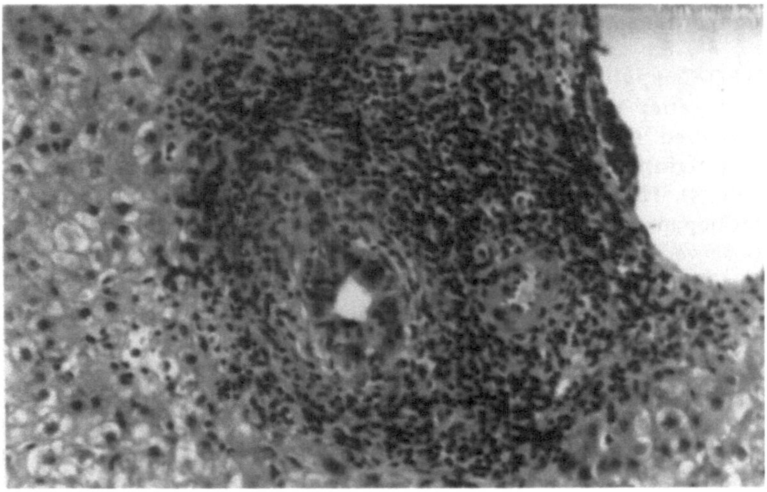

Fig. 2. Same allografted liver as in Fig. 1. Acute cellular rejection at 20 days, consisting of an intense periportal lymphoid cellular infiltrate, bile duct inflammation and vasculitis. H&E, ×200

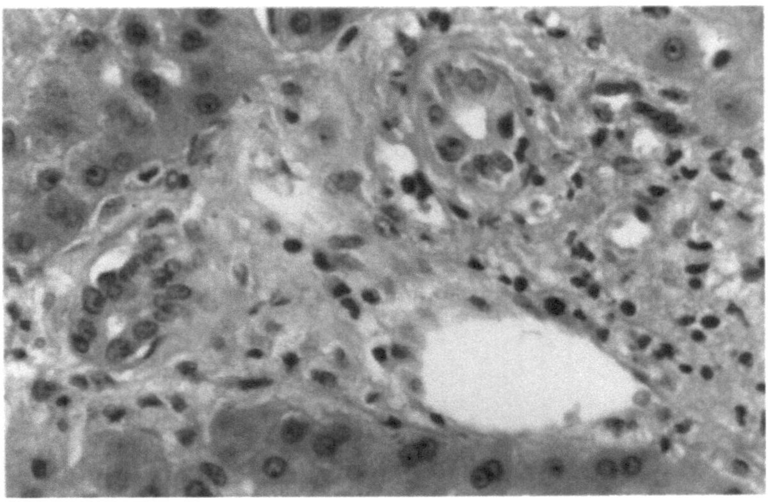

Fig. 3. Same allografted liver as in Figs. 1 and 2 at 30 days (after a course of intravenous methylprednisolone) showing reversal of acute cellular rejection. H&E, ×400

Concordant Xenografts (Groups 2 and 3)

ABO-Compatible Xenografts (Group 2). Mild congestion was frequently observed early after reperfusion (Fig. 4). Hemorrhage and fibrin aggregation were not observed. Cellular infiltration occurred, as in the allografts, consisting of portal zone lymphoid cell and eosinophil infiltration, vasculitis and bile duct damage (Fig. 5). The eosinophil infiltrate was more intense than in the allografts. Periportal hepatocellular necrosis and diffuse lobular lymphoid cell infiltration were also observed in severe cases, and were generally more obvious than after allografting. Episodes of acute cellular rejection were reversible by i.v. methylprednisolone in some baboons, but low-grade rejection usually persisted (Fig. 6), resulting in the gradual development of periportal or interstitial fibrosis beginning around 30–60 days post-transplantation (Fig. 7).

ABO-Incompatible Xenografts (Group 3). Hyperacute rejection was not observed. However, mild post-reperfusion congestion was again present, though hemorrhage and fibrin aggregation were generally absent. Acute cellular rejection, including lymphoid cell and eosinophil infiltration, bile duct damage, as well as vasculitis, occurred earlier and was more severe than that seen in the ABO-compatible group (Fig. 8). Moderately severe rejection often occurred within 7 days and, even with i.v. methylprednisolone therapy, was never fully reversible. Periportal fibrosis was seen, and in one baboon it appeared as early as 10 days post-transplantation (Fig. 9). Severe lymphoid cell infiltration, fibrosis and parenchymal necrosis were end-stage events in irreversible rejection (Figs. 10, 11).

Discordant Xenografts (Groups 4 and 5)

The histopathologic changes were similar in both discordant groups investigated, with the changes developing earlier in the heterotopic pig-to-baboon model (group 4). Severe congestion and hemorrhage were the dominant features (Figs. 12, 13), occurring within 30–60 min after reperfusion, although fibrin aggregation was rarely seen. Some intravascular neutrophil accumulation and arteritis were present, but lymphoid cell infiltration was minimal (Figs. 14, 15).

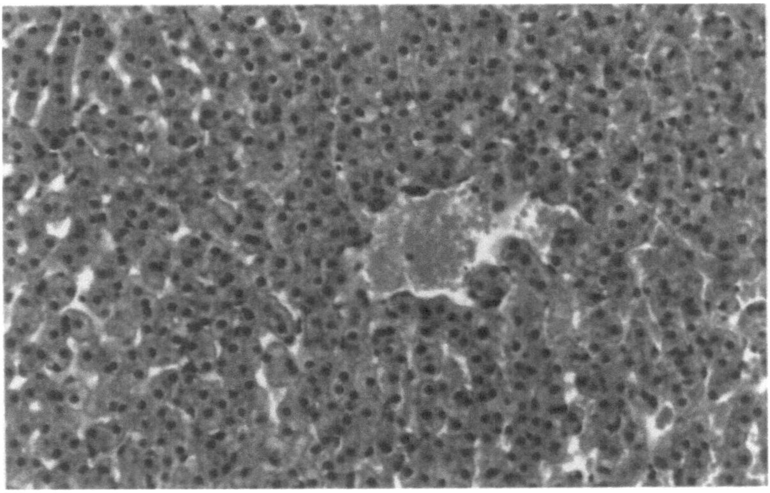

Fig. 4. Group 2 ABO-compatible concordant xenograft 1 h after reperfusion showing mild congestion. H&E, ×200

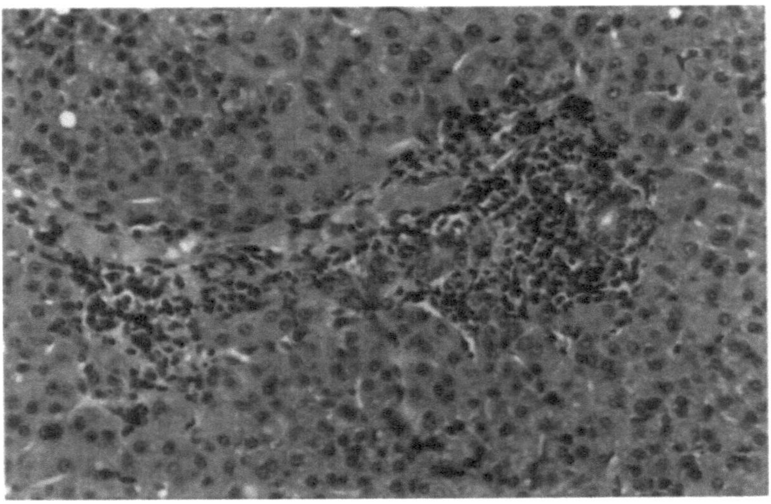

Fig. 5. Group 2 ABO-compatible concordant xenograft at 7 days, revealing moderate acute cellular rejection consisting of a periportal lymphoid cellular infiltrate. H&E, ×200

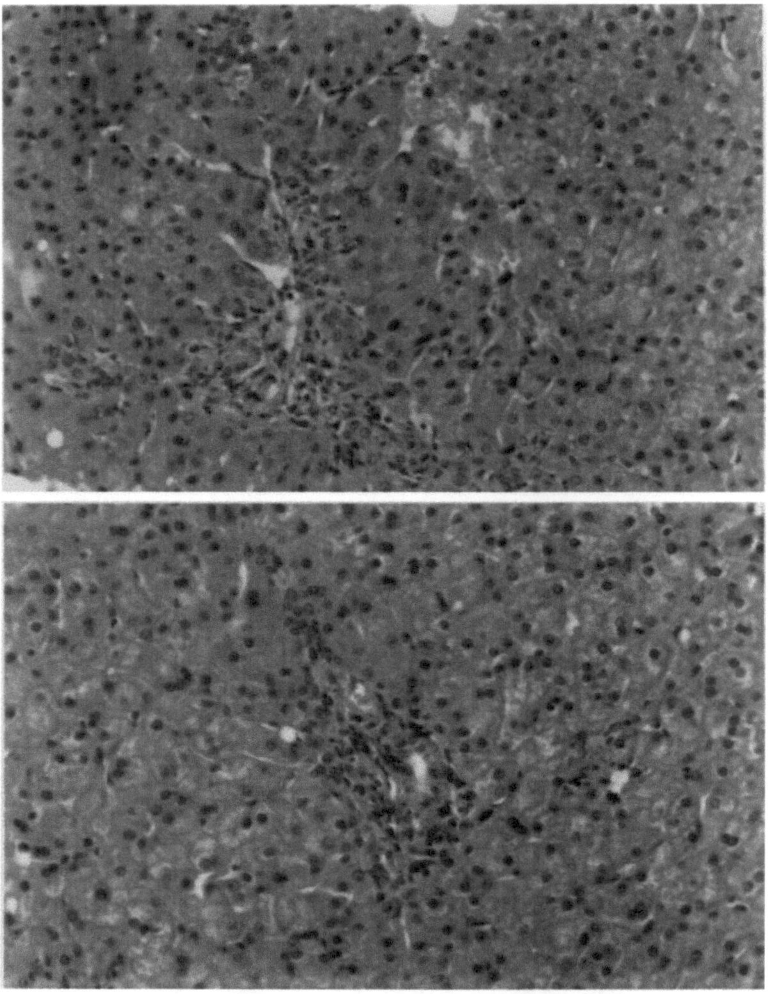

a

b

Fig. 6a,b. Same liver as in Fig. 5 at **a** 20 and **b** 50 days, showing significant resolution, but some persistence of cellular rejection after a course of intravenous methylprednisolone therapy. H&E, ×200

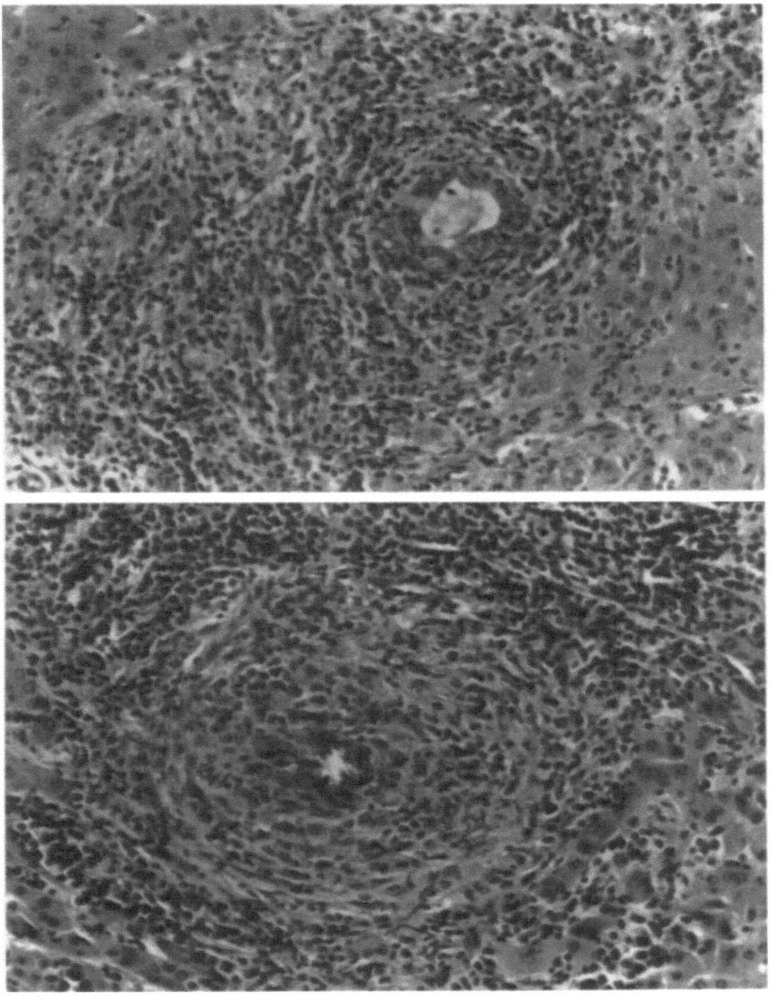

a

b

Fig. 7a,b. Group 2 ABO-compatible concordant xenograft at **a** 30 and **b** 60 days, showing a lymphoid cell infiltrate and peribiliary fibrosis in the portal zone. H&E, ×200

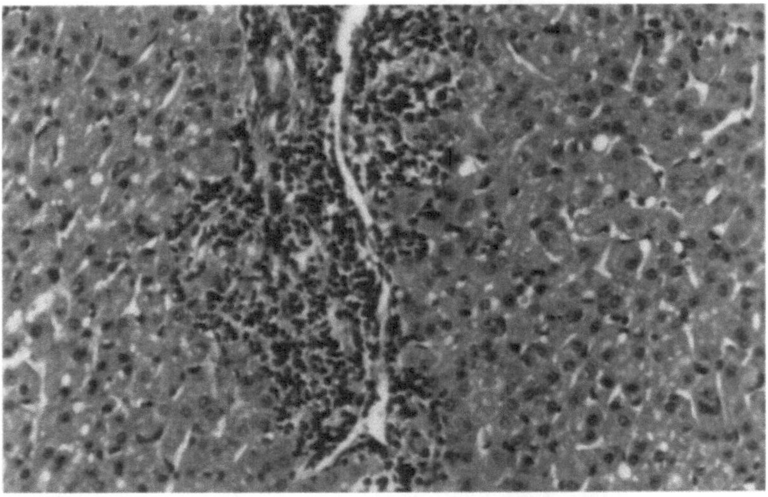

Fig. 8. Group 3 ABO-incompatible concordant xenograft at 10 days, demonstrating moderate acute cellular rejection, consisting predominantly of lymphocytes with a few eosinophils, and venulitis. H&E, ×200

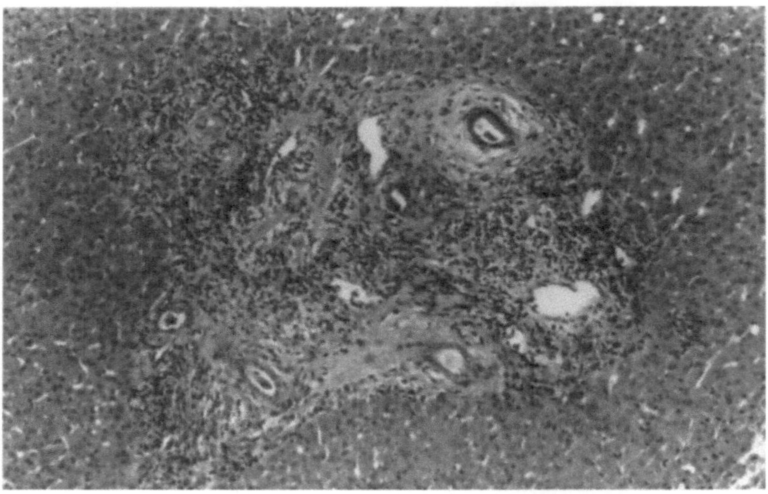

Fig. 9. Group 3 ABO-incompatible concordant xenograft at 10 days, revealing a lymphoid cell infiltrate and peribiliary fibrosis. H&E, ×100

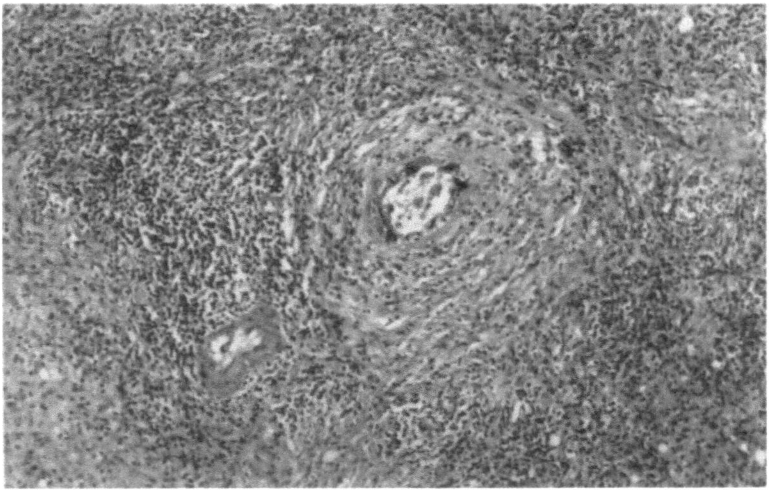

Fig. 10. Group 3 ABO-incompatible concordant xenograft at 45 days, characterized by an intense diffuse cellular infiltration and peribiliary fibrosis. H&E, ×100

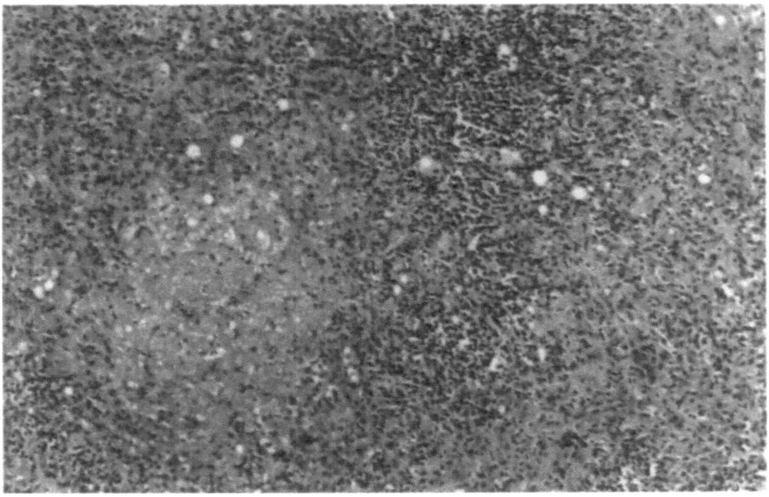

Fig. 11. Group 3 ABO-incompatible concordant xenograft at 45 days, with an intense diffuse cellular infiltration and hepatocellular necrosis. H&E, ×100

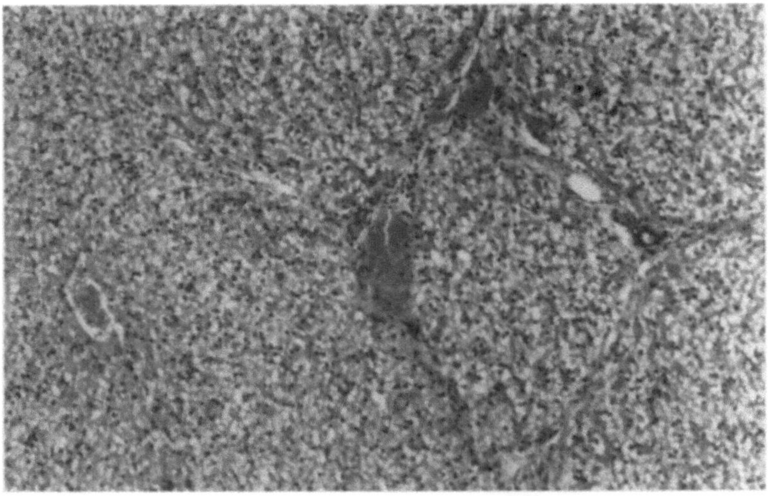

Fig. 12. Group 4 discordant xenograft at 1 h, with a hyperacute vascular reaction consisting primarily of severe congestion. H&E, ×100

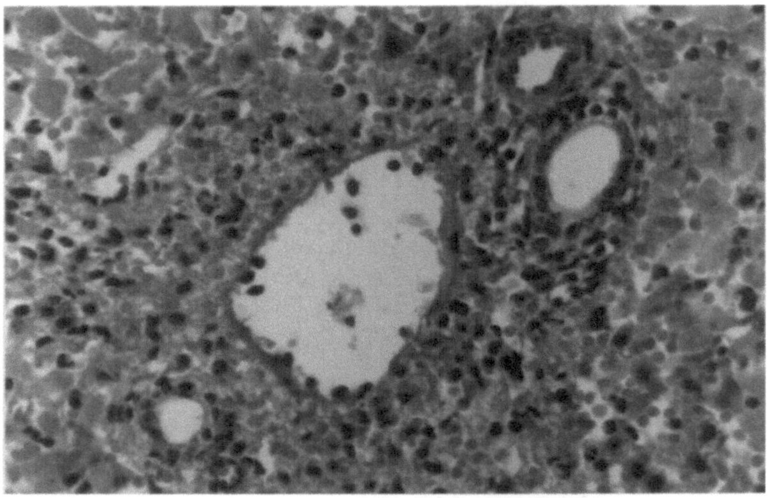

Fig. 13. Group 5 discordant xenograft at 2 h, with interstitial hemorrhage but minimal lymphoid cell infiltration. H&E, ×400

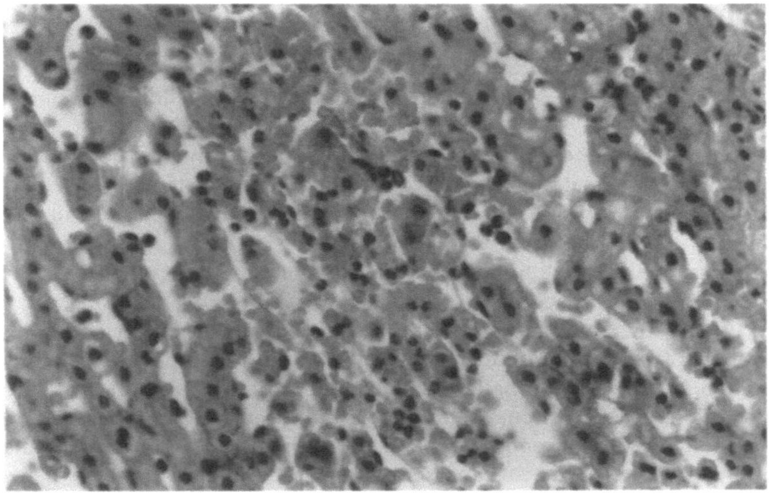

Fig. 14. Group 5 discordant xenograft at 2 h, with evidence of hemorrhage and neutrophil accumulation. H&E, ×400

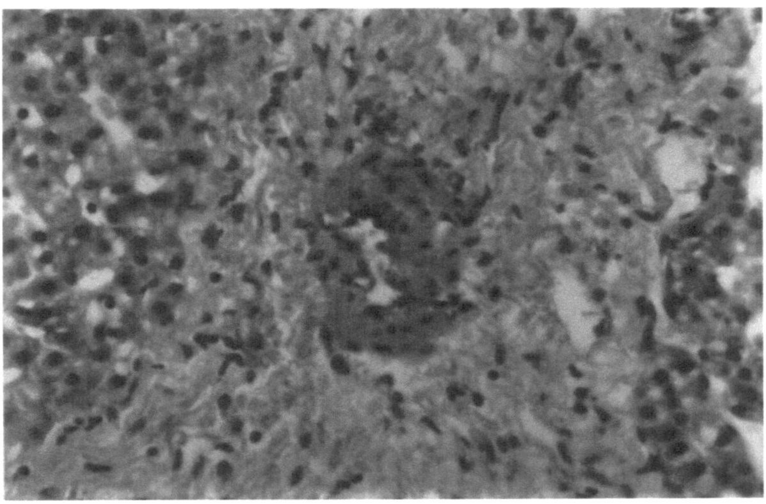

Fig. 15. Group 5 discordant xenograft at 2 h, showing arteritis (H&E×400).

Comment

Two potential donor candidates for hepatic xenotransplantation are the pig [22] and baboon [23]. Both have anatomy and physiology relatively similar to humans.

The histopathologic features seen in our study in vervet monkey-to-baboon and pig-to-primate liver xenotransplantation models are consistent with findings in concordant [7] and discordant [10] liver xenotransplantation in humans and in animal models reported from other centers [1, 2, 12, 13]. Acute lymphoid cell infiltration is the predominant feature in concordant grafts, and hemorrhage and congestion in discordant grafts. A spectrum in the timing and severity of acute cellular rejection and hyperacute vascular rejection could be distinguished, ranging from (a) allografting through (b) ABO-compatible concordant xenografting to (c) ABO-incompatible concordant xenografting, and, finally, to (d) discordant xenografting. Acute cellular rejection developed earlier and was more severe in the concordant xenografts than in the allografts, and hyperacute rejection was seen only in the discordant xenografts. The effectiveness of conventional pharmacologic immunosuppression became less successful as the disparity between donor and recipient increased (Table 3).

In our concordant groups, peribiliary fibrosis was quite common, though cholestasis was not observed. The cause of the fibrosis remains unclear; whether it resulted from an immunological process (e.g., chronic rejection) or from some other pathologic mechanism (e.g., nutritional or physiological disturbance) requires further investigation. In our discordant groups, neither intravascular fibrin aggregation nor occlusive thrombosis was identified. We are unable to explain this significant difference when compared with the reported results from other centers.

With the currently available immunosuppressive therapy, concordant liver xenotransplantation in nonhuman primates proved relatively successful. Cellular rejection was more severe than following allografting, and was followed by increasing periportal fibrosis, beginning at a relatively early stage, particularly in the ABO-incompatible concordant xenografts. From our results we would predict that, as a biological bridge to allografting, concordant liver xenotransplants could be expected to support patients with end-stage liver disease for periods of days, weeks, or occasionally months, but are unlikely to function satisfactorily if inserted as permanent transplants.

Although conventional immunosuppressive therapy (cyclosporine, steroids, and cyclophosphamide or azathioprine) prolongs survival of concordant liver xenografts in nonhuman primates, this therapy (in the absence of procedures to deplete anti-pig antibodies and/or complement) was, as anticipated, unsuccessful in preventing hyperacute rejection of discordant liver xenografts. Although hyperacute rejection related to the presence of donor-specific lymphocytotoxic antibodies or ABO antibodies very rarely occurs following liver allotransplantation [24, 25] (probably because of the role of Kupffer cells, sinusoidal cells, and the dual blood supply [26]), the liver would not, therefore, appear to be an immunologically "privileged" organ following discordant xenotransplantation.

Immunofluorescent studies have not yet been completed in our own experiments, but will be published in due course. Donato et al. [13], however, performed immunohistologic studies on liver allografts and vervet monkey xenografts in baboons. Cellular infiltration components were similar in the two groups, with mainly $CD4^+$ and $CD8^+$ lymphocytes, B lymphocytes, and plasma cells, suggesting that the same cellular mechanisms were involved. IgG and IgM linear sinusoidal deposition was also observed in both groups during rejection episodes. To our knowledge, there are no reports in the literature to-date on the immunohistopathology of discordant liver xenotransplants in nonhuman primates, although there is one report following pig liver transplantation in a human patient [10, 11].

The heterotopically-placed discordant liver xenografts (group 4) were rejected more quickly than the orthotopically placed grafts (group 5). As most complement is generated in the liver, the removal of the recipient liver (in orthotopic liver xenotransplantation) may be beneficial in removing the production of native host complement and thus reducing the severity of complement-based hyperacute rejection [27].

References

1. CALNE, R.Y., WHITE, H.J.O., HERBERTSON, B.M., et al. Pig-to-baboon liver xenografts. Lancet. 1968; 1:1176
2. CALNE, R.Y., DAVIS, D.R., PENA, J.R., et al. Hepatic allografts and xenografts in primates. Lancet. 1970; 1:103
3. STARZL, T.E. Experience in Hepatic Transplantation. W.B. Saunders, Philadelphia, 1969, p. 408
4. GILES, G.R., BOEHMIG, H.J., AMEMIYA, H., HALGRIMSON, C.G., STARZL, T.E. Clinical heterotransplantation of the liver. Transplant. Proc. 1970; 2:506
5. STARZL, T.E., ISHIKAWA, M., PUTNAM, C.W., et al. Progress in and deterrents to orthotopic liver transplantation, with special reference to survival, resistance to hyperacute rejection, and biliary stump reconstruction. Transplant. Proc. 1974; 6:129
6. PORTER, K.A. Pathology of the orthotopic homograft and heterograft. In: Experience in Hepatic Transplantation. Starzl, T.E. (ed), W.B. Saunders, Philadelphia, 1969, p. 422
7. STARZL, T.E., FUNG, J., TZAKIS, A., et al. Baboon-to-human liver transplantation. Lancet. 1993; 341:65
8. STARZL, T.E., TZAKIS, A., FUNG, J.J., et al. Human liver xenotransplantation. Xeno. 1993; 1:4
9. STARZL, T.E., TZAKIS, A., FUNG, J.J., et al. Prospects of clinical xenotransplantation. Transplant. Proc. 1994; 26:1082
10. MAKOWKA, L., CRAMER, D.V., HOFFMAN, A., et al. The use of a pig liver xenograft for temporary support of a patient with fulminant hepatic failure. Transplantation. 1995; 59:1654
11. MAKOWKA, L., WU, G.D., HOFFMAN, A., et al. Immunohistopathologic lesions associated with the rejection of a pig-to-human liver xenograft. Transplant. Proc. 1994; 26:1074

12. GRIDELLI, B., GATTI, S., PIAZZINI, A., et al. Xenogeneic orthotopic liver transplantation in nonhuman primates. Transplant. Proc. 1993; 25:457
13. DONATO, M.F., AROSIO, E., BERTI, E., et al. Immunopathology of liver allograft and xenografts in nonhuman primates. Transplant. Proc. 1993; 25:850
14. POWELSON, J., COSIMI, A.B., AUSTEN, W., et al. Porcine-to-primate orthotopic liver transplantation. Transplant. Proc. 1994; 26:1353
15. ZHONG, R., TUCKER, J., BARCIA, B., et al. The long-term survival and functional tolerance of baboon-to-monkey kidney and liver xenografts – a preliminary report. Presented to the Third International Congress for Xenotransplantation, Boston, 1995. Transplant. Proc. In press
16. MIELES, L., YE, Y., LUO, Y.E, et al. Auxiliary liver allografting and xenografting in the nonhuman primate. Transplantation. 1995; 59:1670
17. LUO, Y., KOSANKE, S., MIELES, L., et al. Histopathology of concordant and discordant liver xenotransplants in the nonhuman primate (Abstract). Hepatology. 1995;22(4,Pt.2):213A
18. LUO, Y., KOSANKE, S., MIELES, L., et al. Comparative histopathology of hepatic allografts and xenografts in the nonhuman primate. In press
19. WIGHT, D.G.D. Histopathology of liver xenograft rejection. In: Xenotransplantation. Cooper, D.K.C., et al. (eds), Springer, Heidelberg, 1991, pp. 253
20. TERPSTRA, O.T. Heterotopic liver transplantation. In: Atlas of Liver, Pancreas and Kidney Transplantation. Kremer, B., Broelsch, C.E., Henne-Bruns, D. (eds). Thieme, New York, 1994, p. 95
21. KREMER, B. Standard techniques in orthotopic liver transplantation. In: Atlas of Liver, Pancreas and Kidney Transplantation. Kremer, B. Broelsch, C.E., Henne-Bruns, D. (eds). Thieme, New York, 1994, p. 36
22. COOPER, D.K.C., YE, Y., ROLF, L.L., ZUHDI, N. The pig as potential organ donor for man. In: Xenotransplantation. Cooper, D.K.C., et al. (eds), Springer, Heidelberg, 1991, pp. 481
23. LUO, Y., TANIGUCHI, S., KOBAYASHI, T., NIEKRASZ, M., COOPER, D.K.C. Screening of baboons as potential organ donors for humans. Xenotransplantation. 1995; 2:244
24. GORDON, R.D., IWATSUKI, S., ESQUIVEL, C.O., et al. Experience with primary liver transplantation across ABO blood groups. Transplant. Proc. 1987; 19:4575
25. DEMETRIS, A.J. Perioperative immune events. In: Liver Transplantation, a 31 Year Perspective. Starzl, T.E., Demetris, A.J. (eds). Current Problems in Surgery, Year Book Medical Publishers, Chicago, 1990, p. 61
26. KROM, R.A.F., KONDO, M., MOORE, S.B. Liver transplantation and the lymphocyte crossmatch. Transplant. Rev. 1995; 9:207
27. VALDIVIA, L.A., FUNG, J.J., DEMETRIS, A.J., et al. Donor species complement after liver xenotransplantation. Transplantation. 1994; 57:918

21 Immunopathology of Discordant Xenograft Rejection

W. W. Hancock

Introduction

The response of a vertebrate to a vascularized xenograft from a distant (discordant) species can involve essentially all of the components of innate and adaptive immunity, and their combined effects on the graft are explosive, typically resulting in hyperacute rejection (HAR) within several minutes. Thus, the host reaction to a discordant xenograft is one of the most violent and powerful immune responses known. Moreover, when HAR is avoided by removal or depletion of xenoreactive natural antibodies (XNA) and/or complement (C), xenografts are still rejected within several days in a second wave of immune injury, termed delayed xenograft rejection (DXR) [1, 2], which is T cell-independent [3]. Even survival beyond this initial few days post-transplant (post-Tx) is not sufficient to ensure long-term survival, since a third wave of the immune response is evoked, involving T cell-dependent reactions.

Given this multifaceted and complex series of immunologic obstacles, at least the second of which (DXR) has so far received only scant attention, it is little wonder that successful transplantation of discordant xenografts is still in its infancy, and there are many avenues for productive research. Indeed, it is easy in the field of discordant xenotransplantation to find innumerable, sometimes quirky, phenomena to study, since one is basically studying the effects of an inflammatory response on a large, multicellular organ with its attendant vasculature, parenchymal cells and connective tissues.

This chapter takes a somewhat more restricted focus, emphasizing events or pathways (a) whose interruption or suppression has been shown experimentally to be of therapeutic benefit or (b) based upon extrapolation from other transplant responses, are likely to result in graft destruction if the xenograft has not already succumbed beforehand to another process. (In the same way that considerable "redundancy" is recognized in the field of cytokines, based upon multiple proteins with overlapping functions, there is considerable redundancy in the xenoresponse such that thwarting one pathway only leads to challenge by another.) The current state of the field is to try to understand the priming and pathogenesis of these responses. Tolerance induction or, in less abstract terms, avoiding these responses is as yet only an immunologist's dream, rather than an established biologic phenomenon.

This chapter complements recent reviews of the topic [4–6] and, given the likely future clinical application of discordant xenografts, focuses primarily on analysis of intragraft events occurring during rejection of vascularized xenografts, particularly cardiac grafts performed across phylogenetically disparate (i.e., discordant) combinations, such as pig-to-primate in which HAR is regularly observed.

Immunopathology of Hyperacute Rejection

Xenoreactive Natural Antibodies and Complement

The classical morphologic features of HAR are macroscopic engorgement and discoloration of the organ and, on light microscopy, interstitial hemorrhages with platelet microthrombi. In contrast to accelerated allograft rejection, HAR is so rapid that neutrophil accumulation is not seen, and large vessels are uninvolved. Immunohistologic analysis of pig-to-primate xenografts shows typically dense deposition of immunoglobulins and C components throughout the vascular bed, consistent with the presence of host XNA directed against carbohydrate moieties on endothelial and other cells, and activation of C through the classical pathway. Though early studies emphasized the predominance of IgM deposition [7], recent studies have established that deposition of IgG and IgA also occur [8, 9]. This is more than a trivial point since the presence of IgA antibodies provides a mechanism for activation of the alternate pathway of C, in addition to classical pathway activation by IgM and IgG. The alternate pathway components, including properdin and factor B, can be shown to colocalize with intragraft IgA during development of HAR [9]. Similarly, the presence of IgG can provide a ready means for recruitment and activation of leukocytes bearing Fc receptors (fcR) (CD16, CD32, CD64; as will be considered later).

Platelets

Though far less studied than XNA and C, HAR also features activation and degranulation of platelets, potentially as a result of local generation of C fragments (C5b-C9); C3a and C5a-induced mast cell degranulation, histamine and serotonin release, with local generation of platelet-activating factor (PAF); FcR signaling upon exposure to deposited XNA; or ischemic injury and endothelial cell retraction with platelet GP1b interaction with subendothelial matrix-bound von Willebrand factor (vWF). Even in the absence of C activation, therefore, there are multiple signals to stimulate platelets. An additional factor may include the very rapid loss of endothelial ecto-ADPase which normally maintains a non-thrombogenic state at the endothelial surface; loss of ecto-ADPase expression occurs as a result of ischemia/reperfusion injury, C activation, and other factors [10]. Though the extent of platelet microthrombi formation may not be great enough to cause rapid graft dysfunction through purely physical disruption of blood perfusion through the microvasculature, platelet aggregation and activation lead to fibrin deposition. In addition, as detailed in the section on DXR, if HAR is avoided, subsequent development of DXR can be linked to platelet activation in the very early post-Tx period. Targeting of platelets with an anti-P selectin antibody [11], PAF antagonist [11], or GPIIb/IIIa antagonist [12] significantly prolongs survival of guinea pig-to-rat cardiac xenografts.

Coagulation

There is rapid assembly of coagulation factors on the platelet surface through several related events. Receptors for factor V are upregulated upon platelet activation, and platelet membrane phospholipids are exposed as a result of microparticle formation, facilitating the binding and assembly of a prothrombinase complex. Platelets also degranulate, resulting in high local concentrations of fibrinogen and other coagulation factors present in alpha granules. Lastly, the trigger to platelet aggregation provided by thrombin or collagen results in release of ADP and serotonin. The combined effects of local platelet aggregation and activation are activation of coagulation and dense fibrin deposition, causing graft ischemia and rapid, progressive loss of organ function. A key role for coagulation, as powerful as that of C, was recently demonstrated in an ex vivo perfusion system [13], and studies of targeting thrombin in vivo are underway.

Type I Endothelial Activation

Our knowledge of endothelial responses during HAR is limited, whereas considerably more is known of the effects of XNA, C, and thrombin on cultured endothelial cells [4]. Endothelial responses during HAR do not involve gene activation or protein synthesis, and are therefore examples of what may be termed endothelial cell (EC) stimulation or type I EC activation. It is known that within minutes of revascularization, P selectin is translocated from cytoplasmic Weibel-Palade bodies to the membrane surface, where it persists for several hours (longer than predicted by in vitro studies wherein P selectin expression typically lasts only minutes) [11]. P selectin upregulation in vivo can occur as a result of EC stimulation by thrombin, histamine or the membrane attack complex of C (C5b-9). Additional events reported include loss of membrane ecto-ADPase [10], contributing to platelet aggregation, and, based upon in vitro data, C5a-induced loss of heparan sulfate [14, 15], and exposure of foreign carbohydrates such as sulfatides [16] which can activate the contact system of coagulation.

Summary of Hyperacute Rejection

Immediately upon revascularization of a discordant xenograft, C activation begins to occur on the surface of endothelial cells. The anaphylatoxins C3a and C5a are generated and act locally on basophils and mast cells to release histamine and cause degranulation of platelets, including serotonin. Within seconds, histamine, and serotonin bind to receptors on endothelial cells, stimulate surface expression of PAF and P selectin, and cell contraction. PAF causes a dramatic increase in vascular permeability and endothelial cells contraction, resulting in sludging of platelets and RBC within the microcirculation. Endothelial cell retraction exposes underlying vWF, basement membranes and collagen to plasma components, including platelets and the contact activator, Hageman factor. Together, these responses result in stasis, platelet aggregation, and interstitial hemorrhages, which rapidly reduce compliance, such that a cardiac xenograft heart fails within minutes.

Immunopathology of Delayed Xenograft Rejection

If HAR is avoided by depleting XNA or by blocking the action of C, xenografts are rejected in days instead of minutes to hours, by a process referred to as DXR [1, 2]. DXR occurs in large [17] and small animal [2] models of discordant xenograft rejection. Serial analysis of cardiac xenografts in C-depleted recipients shows that the grafts undergo progressive infiltration by mononuclear cells, and after several days develop focal infarcts and interstitial hemorrhages, widespread activation of coagulation within the microvasculature and cessation of graft function. Considerable mechanistic insights have been obtained through manipulations in the guinea pig-to-rat model, and the important points will be reviewed. However, it is important to remember that although HAR and DXR can be clearly defined, they represent parts of a continuum. Some of the components of HAR, such as platelet activation or immunoglobulin deposition, do not typically result in HAR if C activation is avoided, and yet these responses, as well as activation of coagulation and endothelial cell responses, may contribute to development of DXR.

Platelets

Platelet exposure to PAF, thrombin or C fragments stimulates membrane expression of P selectin. If xenografts are not subject to HAR, surface P selectin provides a tethering point for adhesion of leukocytes, especially monocytes. In addition, platelets contain chemokines which are expressed upon activation, a key example is RANTES [17, 18]. Thus local platelet aggregation and activation results in release of potent chemotactic signals which attract monocytes. Monocytes responding to such signals adhere to newly expressed P selectin on platelets and endothelial cells and undergo activation, e.g., P selectin ligation on the monocyte membrane causes tissue factor induction [19], as well as production of further chemokines, including RANTES and monocyte chemotactic peptide (MCP)-1.

Leukocytes

Over 75 % of intragraft leukocytes are mononuclear phagocytes, with additional contributions from NK cells (10 %–20 %) and only very small numbers (approximately 5 %) of T cells (i.e., bearing classical TCR-α/β) until at least several days post-Tx. The presence of T cells or XNA is not essential for DXR in C-depleted rats [3], but it has been difficult to determine the actual roles of macrophages and NK cells. Infiltrating macrophages produce large amounts of tumor necrosis factor (TNF)-α and interleukin (IL)-1β during xenograft rejection, as well as IL-7, IL-12, inducible isoform of nitric oxide synthase (iNOS), and various chemokines. Some monokines, such as IL-1β and IL-6 are likely to act only on host cells, e.g. contributing to systemic fever and acute phase response. Others, such as TNF-α, appear to act across species, and the upregulation of adhesion molecules (see below) is consistent with such effects. TNF-α also has direct toxic effects on myocardial cells. IL-7 and IL-12 are relevant to NK cell recruitment and activation, with IL-12 playing a key role in induction of interferon (IFN)-γ production; xenografts display extraordinarily dense IFN-γ expression during development of DXR. However, the extent to which IFN-γ acts across species is controversial and appears to depend upon the species combinations involved. Guinea pig hearts do show upregulation of MHC class II, but incubation of guinea pig leukocytes with recombinant rat IFN-γ does not induce class II (W.W. Hancock, unpublished observations). Nevertheless, since IFN-γ is the most potent activator of macrophages known, regardless of direct effects across species barriers, the action of IFN-γ on host macrophages is likely to be dramatic. Though notoriously difficult to deplete, transfer of macrophages from C-depleted rats sensitized with a guinea pig xenograft to a naive, C-depleted recipient results in acceleration of DXR, indicating a role for macrophages in the pathogenesis of DXR [20]. There are no data as yet concerning the results of NK cell depletion in discordant models.

FcR-Dependent Leukocyte Recruitment During Delayed Xenograft Rejection

There are several mechanisms which could explain the recruitment of macrophages and NK cells which occurs from an early stage following engraftment in C-depleted recipients; these include immune adherence via FcR, lectin binding, and the actions of chemokines. Both leukocyte populations express FcR (CD16/FcγRIII, CD32/CD16/FcγRII), and macrophages also express CD64 (CD16/FcγRI). Such FcR are important to the development of ADCC, cell activation and phagocytosis. However, binding via FcR may not be critical since depletion of IgG-XNA to less than 5% of normal rat serum through plasmapheresis and B cell-directed immunosuppression has no effect on cellular infiltration or the tempo of DXR [3].

Lectin Expression and Delayed Xenograft Rejection

Macrophages and NK cells express lectins recognizing a variety of carbohydrate residues. There are no data as to the in vivo significance of recently identified NK cell lectins [21], though intragraft rat NK cells do express the NKR-P1 lectin [2]. In some animal models of tumor immunity and chronic allograft rejection, induction of macrophage lectin expression can provide a novel means for macrophage recruitment, activation and development of cell cytotoxicity. We have investigated macrophage lectin involvement in DXR by synthesizing peptide sequences based on the recently cloned rat C-type macrophage lectin and preparing mouse anti-rat hybridomas [22]. Five monoclonal antibodies were identified based upon lack of binding to normal guinea pig or rat tissues and positive binding to macrophage lectin by enzyme-linked immunosorbent assay (ELISA). Comparison of serial guinea pig-to-rat xenografts with rat cardiac allografts showed selective and dense expression by infiltrating macrophages within xenografts; labeling was present by 12 h and peaked at 4–5 days with complete destruction of xenografts, whereas corresponding allografts lacked more than trace macrophage lectin labeling. Moreover, comparable induction of macrophage lectin on activated rat macrophages was seen in nude or XNA-depleted xenograft recipients, and upon incubation of rat macrophages with guinea pig cells in vitro. These studies show that (a) rat macrophage undergo activation upon exposure to xenogeneic cells, (b) macrophage lectin expression is a key early feature of DXR, even in the absence of host T cells or XNA, and, thus, (c) targeting of macrophage lectin with specific monoclonal antibodies (mAbs) or administration of specific sugars to saturate the membrane molecule may be a new approach to blocking macrophage infiltration and activation during development of DXR.

Chemokines and Leukocyte Recruitment in Delayed Xenograft Rejection

A third and probably key means for mononuclear cell recruitment is the intragraft expression of chemokines. Our initial studies focused on a role for MCP-1 since, in vitro, MCP-1, is the most potent chemotactic factor for macrophage known. We analyzed guinea pig xenografts in Lewis rats depleted of C by use of cobra venom factor (CVF). Small numbers of rat macrophage were detected adjacent to vessels in guinea pig transplants (Tx) at 12 h and peaked at the time of rejection, when they constituted more than 75 % of intragraft leukocytes. Macrophages were activated as shown by dense labeling for IFN-γ, TNF-α, and IL-1β. Labeling for MCP-1 was detected from 12 h post-Tx in association with macrophage, and increased thereafter. By 48 h, double labeling studies showed that more than 50 % of intragraft macrophage, plus focal endothelial cells and smooth muscle cells, were MCP-1 positive. Labeling was specific as shown by absorption studies with rMCP-1. In vitro, rat macrophage lacked MCP-1 expression under baseline conditions, or after stimulation with IL-1β, IL-2, IL-6, or TNF-α, whereas at 12 hours and later, more than 75 % of cells were MCP-1 positive upon exposure to rIFN-γ. These data showed that MCP-1 expression is (a) a consistent and specific feature of xenograft rejection, (b) associated with activated macrophage, and (c) likely induced by IFN-γ production from NK cells. Given MCP-1 can itself recruit and activate NK cells, xenograft rejection in C-depleted recipients may be the result of a complex and cytokine-dependent recruitment and activation of host macrophage.

These studies provided new insights and suggested likely therapeutic strategies for leukocyte recruitment and activation during DXR, but before pursuing use of anti-MCP-1 mAbs in vivo, we tested the extent of chemokine expression in pig-to-primate cardiac xenografts, again in the context of C depletion [17]. As illustrated in Fig. 1, cardiac xenografts in which HAR was prevented by host therapy with the decomplementing agent, CVF, showed the key features of DXR described in small animals [2]. Importantly for consideration of potential targeting strategies, macrophage began to accumulate around P selectin-positive (activated) platelets by 4 h. These platelets expressed RANTES, which was detectable from within minutes of platelet activation in the early post-Tx period. By 4 h, additional C-C chemokines such as MCP-1, MCP-2, and macrophage inflammatory protein (MIP)-1β were present in considerable amounts. Given that the latter cytokines recruit and activate macrophage and NK cells [18], and that grafts by day 5 showed dense accumulation of activated macrophages and lesser numbers of NK cells, it is likely that no single chemokine is responsible for mononuclear cell entry into rejecting xenografts. It remains to be tested whether intragraft chemokine expression can be blocked or diminished by targeting very early events. It is known from rodent models that use of a GPIIb/IIIa antagonist to block platelet activation significantly improves graft survival, at least in part by decreasing intragraft mononuclear cell recruitment [12], but, as intragraft inflammation develops, a multitude of cell types can produce these chemokines, thereby rendering successful targeting unlikely when using this strategy alone.

Endothelial Responses During Delayed Xenograft Rejection

Analysis of serial samples from small [2]and large animal models [17] has demonstrated considerable evidence of endothelial cell activation during discordant xenograft rejection. Endothelial responses include the following: (a) shift to a procoagulant state, with downregulation of surface thrombomodulin and induction of tissue factor, consistent with dense local fibrin deposition, (b) induction of leukocyte adhesion molecules, including, progressively, E selectin and intercellular adhesion molecule (ICAM)-1, (c) production of chemokines, such as MCP-1, and other cytokines. The significance of endothelial activation in DXR is controversial. On the one hand, these are "downstream" events which are present in essentially any inflammatory response, albeit to a more florid extent than usual. On the other hand, the ability to genetically engineer the donor animal suggests the potential for modulating endothelial responses by genetic approaches, e.g., by regulated targeting of NFkB-dependent endothelial cell pathways [4, 6]. This Center has the unifying concept that in lieu of dense T cell-directed immunosuppression, with additional targeting of complement, coagulation, and host macrophage and NK cells, modulation at the graft level by such genetic approaches will be important to the development of clinical xenotransplantation as a practical solution to the lack of organ donors; testing in vivo in small animals is underway.

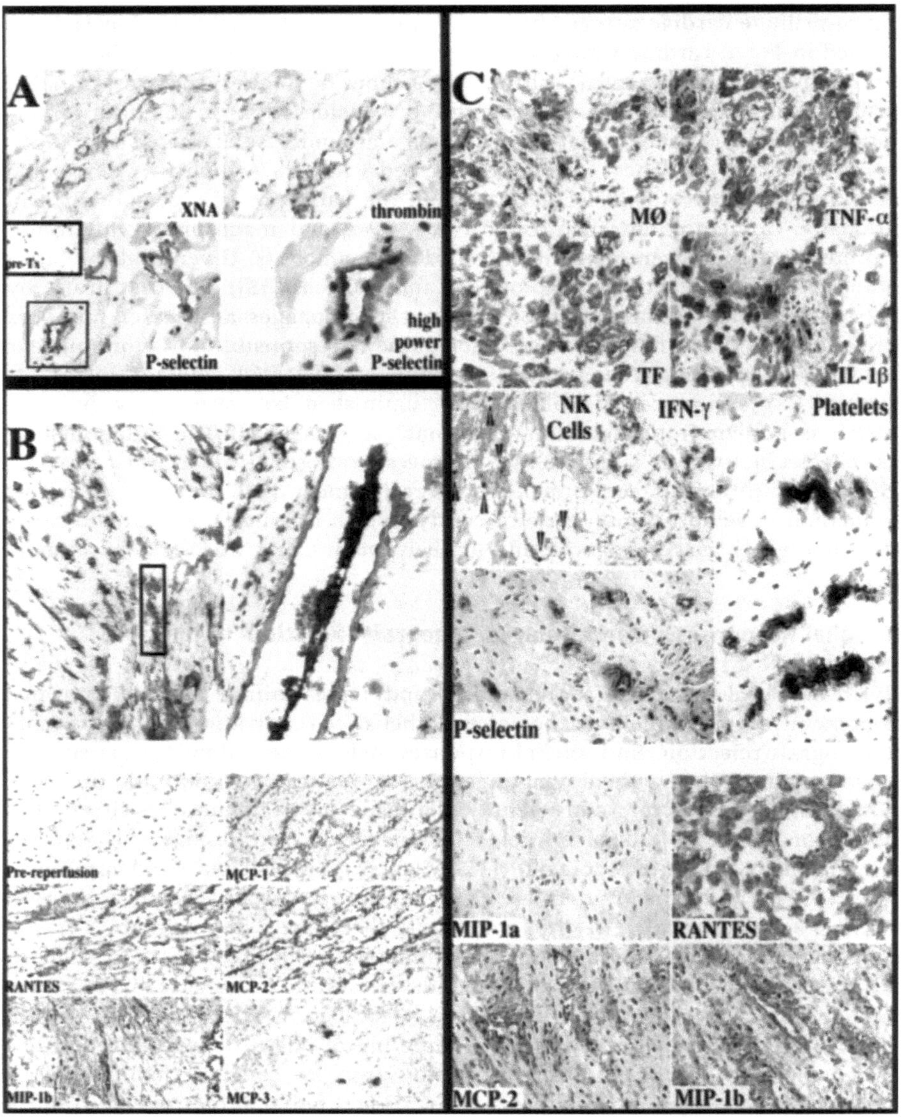

Fig. 1A–C. Immunoperoxidase analysis of cryostat sections of serial biopsies from a pig cardiac xenograft transplanted into a baboon which was treated with cobra venom factor (CVF) to block development of hyperacute rejection (HAR); photomicrographs are from three consecutive periods post-transplantation to document some of the key features of delayed xenograft rejection (DXR) in large animals. A Vascular deposition of IgM and thrombin on penetrating branches of the coronary arteries and associated veins, with labeling for P selectin below. The antibody used recognizes a conformational determinant such that pretransplantation (*pre-Tx*) vessels are unlabeled (*inset*), whereas widespread vascular labeling is seen by the time of initial biopsy (7 min post-revascularization). The area indicated by the *square* at the *lower left* is shown at high power on the *right* to demonstrate the strong membrane labeling of arteriolar endothelial cells (type I endothelial activation). *XNA*, xenoreactive natural antibodies. **B** Selected events at 4 h post-transplantation. *Upper left*, dense labeling of platelets and graft endothelial cells for P selectin. The area indicated by a *rectangle* is shown at high power on the *right*, to demonstrate the attachment of host macrophage to platelet microthrombi. Below this, a composite of chemokine expression is shown. Though no *RANTES* is present pre-reperfusion, widespread expression by platelets and endothelium is seen at 4 hours post-transplantation, in addition to expression of monocyte chemotactic peptide (*MCP*)-1, MCP-2, and to a lesser extent macrophage inflammatory protein (*MIP*)-1β, whereas only minor labeling for MCP-3 was observed. These chemokines principally attract and activated macrophage and, to some extent, natural killer (*NK*) cells. **C** Events at day 5 post-transplantation when essentially no primate T cells were present. Grafts show dense infiltration by large inflammatory macrophages ($CD14^+$) whose activation is demonstrated by their labeling for tumor necrosis factor (*TNF*)-α, tissue factor (*TF*), and interleukin (*IL*)-1β. In addition to activated macrophages, interferon (*IFN*)-γ-producing NK cells (*arrowheads*) and vascular plugging by P selectin-positive platelets (the latter also $GPIIb^+$) are seen. Consistent with ongoing macrophage and NK cell recruitment, dense labeling of macrophages and endothelium for RANTES is present, in addition to lesser amounts of MCP-2 and MIP-1β, but not MIP-1α. Additional sections (not shown) documented widespread endothelial cell activation and fibrin deposition

Comment

Our data indicate that once HAR is overcome by CVF treatment, xenografts undergo a series of steps involving mononuclear and endothelial cell activation, cytokine expression, platelet and fibrin deposition, and rejection within a few days. Logically, DXR may be caused by (a) infiltrating mononuclear cells, (b) consequences of endothelial cell activation, or (c) combination of (a) and (b). NK cells could be present secondary to direct "recognition" of xenogeneic endothelial cells, and either cell type could be present through FcR binding of IgG bound to endothelial cells, lectin interactions, or chemokine production. Aspects of direct binding and activation of endothelial cells by macrophages [23] and NK cells [24] are reviewed elsewhere in this volume (Chap. 8). Once present and activated, mononuclear cell products, including cytokines and tissue factor, contribute to coagulation, damage surrounding endothelial cells, and depress myocardial contractility. The factors that result in activation of endothelium in DXR are not well defined. XNA binding to pig endothelial cells in vitro causes upregulation of IL-1, IL-8, and plasminogen activator inhibitor (PAI)-1 [4], though the in vivo relevance of this finding is not established. Following stimulation, activated endothelial cells contribute to inflammation and thrombosis. most likely scenario in our opinion is that DXR is based on a combination of the effects mediated by activated mononuclear *and* endothelial cells. In this schema, any one event that leads to activation of either the donor organ endothelium or host mononuclear cells would likely become amplified via the multiple interactive circuits between inflammation and coagulation. As NK cells are stimulated, they release IFN-γ, which promotes macrophage activation, cytokine production and other responses. Release of TNF-α from activated mononuclear cells could activate endothelial cells, causing a further recruitment of leukocytes through induction of adhesion molecules, as well as stimulation of a procoagulant state through upregulation of tissue factor and downregulation of thrombomodulin and angiotension (AT)-III. Downregulation of thrombomodulin expression, resulting in a markedly reduced capacity of endothelial cells to bind thrombin and activate protein C may further enhance macrophage cytokine production, since activated protein C appears to have a key role in inhibition of macrophage activation in vivo and in vitro [25, 26]. The cumulative effect of fibrin generation and local hypoxia, the toxic effects of TNF, IL-1, and other cytokines, and a potential direct effect of mononuclear cell binding to endothelial cells may suffice to cause DXR. The extent to which T cell activation contributes to this process if DXR is prolonged further remains to be determined.

References

1. Hancock, W.W., Blakely, M.L., Van der Werf, W., Bach, F.H. 1993. Rejection of guinea pig cardiac xenografts post-cobra venom factor therapy is associated with infiltration by mononuclear cells secreting interferon-gamma and diffuse endothelial activation. Transplant. Proc. 25:2932
2. Blakely, M.L., Van der Werf, W.J., Berndt, M.C., et al. 1994. Activation of intragraft endothelial and mononuclear cells during discordant xenograft rejection. Transplantation. 58:1059
3. Candinas, D., Bach, F.H., Hancock, W.W. 1996. Delayed xenograft rejection (DXR) in complement-depleted T cell-deficient (nude) rat recipients of guinea pig cardiac xenografts. Transplant. Proc. 28:678
4. Bach, F.H., Robson, S.C., Ferran, C. et al. 1994. Endothelial cell activation and thromboregulation during xenograft rejection. Immunol. Rev. 141:5
5. Hancock, W.W., Bach, F.H. 1994. The immunopathology of discordant xenograft rejection. Xeno 2:68
6. Bach, F.H., Winkler, H., Ferran, C., et al. 1995. Endothelial activation is a barrier to xenotransplantation. Nature Med 1:869
7. Platt, J.P., Fischel, R.J., Matas, A.J., et al. 1991. Immunopathology of hyperacute xenograft rejection in a swine-to-primate model. Transplantation. 52:214
8. Leventhal, J.R., John, R., Fryer, J.P., et al. 1995. Removal of baboon and human antiporcine IgG and IgM natural antibodies by immunoadsorption - Results of in vitro and in vivo studies. Transplantation. 59:294
9. Kobayashi, T., Neethling, F.A., Koren, E., et al. 1996. In vitro and in vivo investigation of the anti-complement agents, FUT-175 and K76COOH, in the prevention of hyperacute rejection following discordant xenotransplantation in a non-human primate model. Transplant. Proc. In press
10. Robson, S.C., Candinas, D., Lesnikoski, B.A., et al. 1996. Glomerular ecto-ADPase activity is inhibited with reperfusion injury and cobra venom factor administration. Transplant. Proc. 28:536
11. Coughlan, A.F., Berndt, M.C., Dunlop, L.C., Hancock, W.W. 1993. In vivo studies of P-selectin and platelet-activating factor during endotoxemia, accelerated allograft rejection, and discordant xenograft rejection. Transplant. Proc. 25:2930
12. Candinas, D., Lesnikoski, B.A., Hancock, W.W., et al. 1996. Inhibition of platelet integrin GPIIb/IIIa prolongs survival of discordant cardiac xenografts. Transplantation. 62:1
13. Robson, S.C., Young, V.K., Cook, N.S., et al. 1996. Thrombin inhibition in an ex vivo model of porcine heart hyperacute rejection. Transplantation. 61:862

14. Platt, J.L., Vercellotti, G.M., Lindman, B.J., et al. 1990. Release of heparan sulphate from endothelial cells: Implications for pathogenesis of hyperacute rejection. J. Exp. Med. 171:1363
15. Platt, J.L., Dalmasso, A.P., Lindman, B.J., Ihrcke, N.S., Bach, F.H. 1991. The role of C5a and antibody in the release of heparan sulfate from endothelial cells. Eur. J. Immunol. 21:2887
16. Hunt, B.J., Rosenberg, R.D. 1993. The essential role of haemostasis in hyperacute rejection. Xeno 1:16
17. Hancock, W.W., Kobayashi, T., Cooper, D.K.C. 1996. Chemokine expression and mononuclear cell activation during development of delayed xenograft rejection in pig-to-primate cardiac xenografts. (In preparation)
18. Hancock, W.W. 1996. Chemokines and the pathogenesis of T cell-dependent immune responses. Am. J. Pathol. 148:681
19. Celi, A., Pelligrini, G., Lorenzet, R., et al. 1994. P-selectin induces the expression of tissue factor on monocytes. Proc. Natl. Acad. Sci. USA. 91:8767
20. Fryer, J.P., Leventhal, J.R., Dalmasso, A.P., et al. 1995. Beyond hyperacute rejection – Accelerated rejection in a discordant xenograft model by adoptive transfer of specific cell subsets. Transplantation. 59:171
21. Duchler, M., Offterdinger, M., Holzmuller, H., et al. 1995. NKG2-C is a receptor on human natural killer cells that recognizes structures on K562 target cells. Eur J Immunol 25:2923
22. Hancock, W.W., Russell, M.E., Sayegh, M.H. 1996. Induction of macrophage lectin during development of delayed xenograft rejection (DXR). Transplantation. In press
23. Millan, M.T., Ferran, C., Stuhlmeier, K.M., Geczy, C., Bach, F.H. 1996. Direct activation of porcine endothelial cells by human NK cells. Transplant. Proc. In press
24. Goodman, D.J., von Albertini, M., Wilson, A., Millan, M.T., Bach, F.H. 1996. Direct activation of porcine endothelial cells by human NK cells. Transplantation. In press
25. Grey, S., Tsuchida, A., Hau, H., et al. 1994. Selective inhibitory effects of the anticoagulant activated protein C on the responses of human mononuclear phagocytes to LPS, IFN-γ or phorbol ester. J. Immunol. 153:3664
26. Grey, S.T., Hancock, W.W. 1996. A physiologic anti-inflammatory pathway based upon thrombomodulin expression and generation of activated protein C by human mononuclear phagocytes. J. Immunol. 156:2256

IV Experimental Xenotransplantation Between Closely Related Species

22 Experimental Concordant Kidney Xenotransplantation in Primates

J.A. Myburgh, J.A. Smit, and J.H. Stark

Introduction

To our knowledge there have been no reports on experimental concordant kidney xenotransplantation in primates since the last edition of this volume apart, from those of the Johannesburg group in 1994 [1, 2]. The data in these reports were presented at the Second International Congress for Xenotransplantation in Cambridge, England, in 1993, and additional unpublished studies have been performed since then.

These studies were based on the extensive experience of the Johannesburg group with the use of a modified regimen of total lymphoid irradiation (TLI) in kidney and liver allotransplantation in the baboon [3, 4]. In brief, the optimal regimen of TLI which evolved in these studies consisted of a cumulative dose of irradiation of 800 cGy administered to a wide field in fractions of 80 or 100 cGy twice a week. The wide field included the whole torso from the base of the skull downwards, and the proximal ends of the humeri and femora. With this regimen, durable operational tolerance, defined as normal graft function in a healthy recipient for more than 1 year after transplantation, was attained on average in one third of recipients. The tolerance was specific in that skin grafts from the original donor baboons were accepted indefinitely whereas skin and kidneys from third party baboons placed more than 6 months after the original transplantation were rejected in an unmodified acute fashion. It must be stressed that these results were not obtained when a narrower field, similar to the mantle and inverted-Y fields used clinically in patients with Hodgkin's, was employed.

Bone marrow injection from the kidney donor was not necessary for tolerance induction, and was in fact counterproductive, whether whole bone marrow or T cell-depleted marrow was used. Attempts to increase the tolerant fraction obtained, by brief peritransplant courses of cyclosporine (CyA), prednisone, rabbit anti-human thymocyte globulin (RATG), or mycophenolate mofetil (MM), were unsuccessful, and in the case of CyA counterproductive. Similarly, the addition of two fractions of TLI after transplantation virtually abolished tolerance production. These findings suggested the involvement of active mechanisms of tolerogenesis, which could be opposed or abolished by additional immunosuppressive maneuvers.

In vitro studies in the tolerant baboons showed three patterns of mixed lymphocyte responsiveness (MLR): (1) donor specific hypo- or unresponsiveness in five of 12 baboons studied up to 4.5 years after transplantation, (2) broad nonspecific hyporesponsiveness to both donor and third-party baboons in five of 12 baboons, and (3) donor responsiveness with a nonspecific suppressor factor in the serum of two tolerant baboons [5]. This suppressor factor was also demonstrated in the serum of three other baboons with hyporesponsiveness. Nonspecific non-T cell suppressor cells, expressing myeloid-associated antigens CD 11b and CD 38, were demonstrated by add-in MLR experiments [6, 7].

Baboon-To-Monkey Kidney Xenotransplantation

The species used were Chacma baboons (*Papio ursinus orientalis*; mean weight, 14.4 kg; range, 12.2–16.6 kg), and vervet monkeys (*Cercopithecus aethiops*; mean weight, 5.9 kg; range, 5.5–6.8 kg). Baboons were used as the kidney donors for monkeys in seven groups. Donors and recipients were red blood cell-compatible and were selected for absence of preformed complement-dependent cytotoxic antibodies (CDC).

Graft survivals are given in Table 1. Untreated animals (group 1) survived for 7, 8, and 9 days. Serum creatinine levels rose precipitously from day 4, and histologic examination of the grafts showed features of acute cellular and marked humoral rejection with hemorrhage, necrosis, and vasculitis.

The optimal regimen of TLI for baboon kidney allografts, namely a cumulative dose of 800 cGy given as fractions of 100 cGy twice a week to a wide field, was used for the monkey recipients in group 2. Three monkeys rejected their grafts acutely on days 11, 15, and 21. Histologically, the first of these showed evidence of mixed cellular and humoral rejection, and the latter two showed acute cellular rejection. A fourth monkey developed hemorrhagic enteritis on day 16 and was killed. Serum creatinine was normal, and the graft, although macroscopically normal, showed patchy round cell infiltration. The final two monkeys survived for 365 and 550 days. In these animals the serum creatinine levels remained normal for approximately 11 months after transplantation, after which they rose gradually. Histological examination of the graft surviving for 365 days showed severe acute cellular and humoral rejection with extensive interstitial hemorrhage superimposed on changes of chronic vascular rejection in the form of a mild-to-moderate degree of intimal proliferation in some of the interlobular and arcuate ves-

Table 1. Baboon-to-monkey kidney xenotransplantation graft survival

Group		Survival (days)
Group 1	Controls	7, 8, 9
Group 2	TLI alone	11, 15, 16, 21, 364, 550
Group 3	TLI + RATG 10 mg/kg days -1 and 0	21, 84, 289, 293
Group 4	TLI + intrathymic spleen cells day -7	4, 5, 5, 6, 17, 29
Group 5	MM 100 mg/kg per day	7, 8, 14, 31
Group 6	TLI + MM 70 mg/kg day 0	11, 12, 14
Group 7	TLI + MM 50 mg/kg days 0–9	15, 24, 27, >97

TLI, total lymphoid irradiation; RATG, rabbit anti-human thymocyte globulin; MM, mycophenolate mofetil.

sels. The graft surviving for 550 days also showed acute cellular rejection and extensive interstitial hemorrhage, but no chronic vascular changes were noted.

The monkeys in group 3 received the same regimen of TLI and, additionally, 10 mg rabbit anti-human thymocyte globulin/kg on the day before and the day of transplantation. In the monkeys surviving for 289 and 293 days, the serum creatinine levels were normal until days 251 and 255, respectively, after which a gradual rise occurred. Histologically, all four grafts showed features of cellular rejection. There were no obliterative vascular features of chronic rejection. The monkeys in group 4 received TLI plus intrathymic injection of donor baboon spleen cells on day 7. There were no long survivors (range, 4–29 days), and all grafts showed evidence of acute cellular and hemorrhagic vascular rejection. The effects of intrathymic donor spleen cell injection in this group of primate xenografts were similar to those seen in baboon kidney allografts, namely sensitization of the recipients and abrogation of the effect of TLI [8].

MM alone (100 mg/kg per day by mouth; group 5) had a modest effect on graft survival, with two of the four monkeys surviving longer than untreated controls, namely 14 and 31 days. The addition of MM (70 mg/kg on the day of transplantation) to 800 Cgy of TLI pretransplantation (group 6) appeared to abrogate the effect of TLI, with graft survival being only 11, 12, and 14 days. In the group which received 800 cGy TLI pretransplantation and 50 mg MM/kg per day from day 0 to day 9 (group 7), one baboon is still alive with normal graft function 3 months after transplantation and may achieve operational tolerance, but the overall results in this group will not be as good as those with TLI alone.

Immunologic Studies in Baboon-to-Monkey Xenografts

In the two long-surviving monkeys in group 2, low levels of nonspecific cytotoxic antibodies against baboon, but not monkey, lymphocytes (15 %–20 % cell lysis by ^{51}Cr release CDC assays) developed 3 weeks after transplantation, and persisted until 3 months after transplantation. Reduction of the sera with dithiothreitol confirmed that most of the cytotoxicity was due to IgM. Antibody-dependent cellular cytotoxicity (ADCC), with the use of normal monkey lymphocyte effectors at an effector target ratio of 50:1, paralleled CDC activity (20 %–30 % cell lysis). Lymphocyte-mediated cytotoxicity was present transiently during the antibody-positive period, with peak lysis of donor lymphocytes (28 % and 34 %, respectively) 2 months after transplantation. TLI obliterated the proliferative response of monkey lymphocytes to interleukin (IL)-2, concanavalin A, and phytohemagglutinin. MLR to baboon cells was markedly reduced after TLI, with a slow recovery towards pre-TLI levels 5 months after transplantation. TLI inhibited mitogen-induced IL-2 synthesis to below measurable levels (10 fmol/ml) for 2 months. Synthesizing ability for IL-2 recovered fully by 5 months after transplantation without any immediate deterioration of graft function. Sera collected 32 days after transplantation blocked one-way donor-specific and nonspecific MLR using cryopreserved, pre-TLI recipient lymphocytes as responders.

Open wedge biopsies from these two grafts 3 months after transplantation revealed occasional periglomerular and interstitial foci of chronic inflammatory cells and a focal glomerulopathy, with about one in ten glomeruli affected by areas of subtle but unequivocal mesangial thickening. The intrarenal vasculature was entirely normal. Immunofluorescence staining revealed focal glomerular deposits of IgM and IgG, but no complement. The monkey which died of rejection 15 days after transplantation developed IgM cytotoxic antibodies with 49 % specific cell lysis 10 days after transplantation.

Monkey-To-Baboon Kidney Xenotransplantation

The graft survival data for kidney xenotransplantation in the reciprocal combination are given in Table 2. The mean weight of the monkey donors was 6.3±1.5 kg and of the baboon recipients was 16.3±1.5 kg. The animals were again red blood cell-compatible and there were no preformed anti-monkey lymphocytotoxic antibodies in the sera of the recipient baboons.

The median graft survival of the untreated controls (4 days; group 1) was one half of that in the baboon-to-monkey combination. Histologic examination of the rejected grafts showed acute cellular rejection in three grafts and a combination of cellular and humoral rejection in one graft. The same regimen of TLI which resulted in long-term survival in two of six monkey recipients of baboon kidneys had no effect at all on the survival of monkey kidneys in baboon recipients (group 2). The only difference from the untreated controls was a histological pattern of typical acute cellular rejection and little if any evidence of humoral rejection.

In group 3, unilateral donor nephrectomy was performed 6 weeks before transplantation. This resulted in a mean increase in the weight of 48 % of the donor kidneys. The rationale of this experiment was to assess the possible beneficial effect of an increase in the size of the transplanted nephron mass on graft survival. However, this maneuver had no effect on graft survival, the median being 5 days. In the final group (group 4), intrathymic injection of donor monkey spleen cells 7 days before transplantation, in combination with pretransplant TLI, did not improve graft survival and, as in our experience in baboon renal allografting, this maneuver resulted in evidence of sensitization in that two of the six grafts showed histologic features of hyperacute rejection (graft survival, 3 days) and a third graft showed features of combined acute cellular and humoral rejection.

Table 2. Monkey-to-baboon kidney xenotransplantation graft survival

Group		Survival (days)
Group 1	Control	3, 3, 5, 5
Group 2	TLI 800 cGy	3, 3, 4, 4, 6, 6
Group 3	TLI 800 cGy[a]	4, 4, 5, 5, 5, 8
Group 4	RLI + IT spleen cells day -7	3, 3, 5, 5, 6, 8

[a]Unilateral donor nephrectomy 6 weeks pretransplantation.

Immunological Studies in Monkey-To-Baboon Xenotransplantation

The sera of baboon recipients surviving for 5 or more days after transplantation of monkey kidneys were studied for the presence of anti-monkey lymphocytotoxic antibodies in ^{51}Cr release CDC assays. These were consistently negative, including the cases in which the graft showed hemorrhagic rejection.

Comment

The prolongation of baboon-to-monkey kidney xenograft survival by TLI is remarkably similar to that obtained in baboon allotransplantation – 1 year and 18 months in two of six monkeys receiving TLI alone, and nearly 10 months in two of four monkeys receiving TLI and two perioperative injections of RATG. These animals did not quite attain our definition of operational tolerance established with TLI in baboon kidney allotransplantation, namely indefinite graft survival with normal function more than 1 year after transplantation. In all four monkeys, graft function started to deteriorate before the end of the year and the grafts were eventually lost to rejection. Nevertheless, the demonstration that TLI can produce at least partial tolerance in concordant renal xenotransplantation in primates is tremendously encouraging.

As with the use of TLI in baboon renal allotransplantation, there is an indication that the concomitant use of a brief course of immunosuppressive drug therapy in concordant xenotransplantation tends to counteract the tolerogenic effect of TLI alone. This has not been the finding in other studies with different species and organs.

The group at Duke University [8] found that in heterotopic cardiac transplantation from Syrian hamsters to Lewis rats TLI alone resulted in only minimal, albeit significant prolongation of graft survival, whereas the combination of TLI plus moderate-to-high doses of CyA produced exceptional prolongation of more than 100 days. Similarly, a combination of TLI, splenectomy, and CyA resulted in the best hamster-to-rat liver xenograft survival. The reasons for the differences may be species related, and it should be noted that the irradiation fields used involved shielding of the head, lungs, limbs, and tail. The same group also studied heterotopic cardiac xenografts from rhesus to cynomolgus monkeys [9]. Untreated controls had graft survival rates of 7, 11, and 14 days. The three monkeys that received TLI (total dose, 1500 cGy), splenectomy, and daily CyA (to maintain a whole blood trough level of 200 ± 100 ng/ml) had graft survival rates of 152, 174, and more than 474 days [8]. Unfortunately, the study did not include a group receiving CyA and splenectomy without TLI.

Roslin et al. [10] have also recently reported a longer than 1-year graft survival in two of six heterotopic cervical hearts from cynomolgus monkeys to baboons. They used our regimen of 800 cGy wide-field TLI in combination with CsA and prednisolone after transplantation. TLI alone resulted in graft survival of 28, 29, and 30 days compared with 6 and 7 days in untreated controls. Their immunologic studies led them to hypothesize that TLI induced a state of B cell unresponsiveness to monkey xenoantigens, but was insufficient to induce long-term inhibition of T cell responses, which were, however, suppressed by CyA therapy. Although these studies involved different species of baboon and monkey from those in the Johannesburg experiments, namely *Papio anubis* versus *Papio ursinus*, and cynomolgus versus vervet monkeys, it is perhaps relevant that we also were unable to produce long-term graft survival with TLI alone in the monkey-to-baboon combination.

It would be interesting to have data of heterotopic graft survival in the reciprocal combination, namely baboon-to-cynomolgus monkey. The phenomenon of widely different graft survival patterns is well recognized in reciprocal transplants between certain rat strains. It would seem that there are also "easy" and "difficult" concordant primate xenograft combinations, as illustrated by the diametrically opposed results obtained in baboon-to-monkey and monkey-to-baboon renal transplantation. However, these studies did not reveal strong serological or histological evidence of an earlier or greater antibody/complement component in the monkey-to-baboon combination than in the baboon-to-monkey combination to account for the inability of TLI to prolong graft survival in the former combination.

In terms of potential clinical applicability to baboon-to-human kidney transplantation, it remains to be established whether the effect of TLI will resemble that seen in baboon-to-monkey transplantation or that seen in monkey-to-baboon transplantation. The six baboon-to-human kidney transplants reported by Starzl escaped hyperacute rejection and functioned for 6–60 days [12]. At the end they developed fierce cellular rejection, and the key histopathologic finding was occlusive endothelialitis that had choked of much of the arterial supply. No less important is the question whether the much smaller kidneys of even the largest male baboons will be large enough for adult humans not only in physiological terms, but also in terms of the mounting evidence that alloantigen-independent factors, including a reduced nephron mass, are important in chronic attrition of graft survival after renal transplantation [13].

References

1. MYBURGH, J.A., SMIT, J.A., STARK, J.H. Transplantation tolerance following total lymphoid irradiation in baboon-to-vervet monkey kidney xenotransplantation. Transplant. Proc. 26, 1080, 1994
2. SMIT, J.A., STARK, J.H., MYBURGH, J.A. Immunologic responses of two monkeys tolerating baboon renal xenografts after total lymphoid irradiation. Transplant. Proc. 26, 1063, 1994
3. MYBURGH, J.A. SMIT, J.A., BROWDE, S., STARK, J.H. Current status of total lymphoid irradiation. Transplant. Proc. 15, 659, 1983
4. MYBURGH, J.A. Total lymphoid irradiation and transplantation tolerance. In: Progress in Transplantation. Morris, P.J., Tilney, N.L. (eds). Churchill Livingstone, Edinburgh, 1985, p. 16
5. STARK, J.H., SMIT, J.A., MYBURGH, J.A. Nonspecific mixed lymphocyte culture inhibitory antibodies in sera of tolerant transplanted baboons conditioned with total lymphoid irradiation. Transplantation. 57, 1103, 1994

6. SMIT, J.A., STARK, J.H., MYBURGH, J.A. Mechanisms of immunological tolerance following total lymphoid irradiation. Transplant. Proc. 19, 490, 1987
7. GRAY, C.M. Characterization of TLI-induced peripheral blood suppressor cells after transplantation. In: Total Lymphoid Irradiation, Kidney Transplantation and Cellular Immunity. PhD thesis. University of the Witwatersrand, Johannesburg, 1985, p. 137
8. SMIT, J.A., STARK, J.H., MYBURGH, J.A. Intrathymic donor antigen in baboon kidney transplantation. Afr. J. Health Sci. 2, 1995 (in press)
9. HALPERIN, E.C., KNECHTLE, S.J., HARLAND, R.C., et al. Irradiation for xenogeneic transplantation. Radiother. Oncol. 18, 29, 1990
10. BOLLINGER, R.R., FABIAN, M.A., HARLAND, R.C., et al. Total lymphoid irradiation for cardiac xenotransplantation in nonhuman primates. Transplant. Proc. 23, 587, 1991
11. ROSLIN, M.S., TRANBAUGH, R.E., PANZA, A., et al. One-year monkey heart xenograft survival in cyclosporine-treated baboons. Transplantation. 54, 949, 1992
12. STARZL, T.E., VALDIVIA, L.A., MURASE, N., et al. The biological basis of and strategies for clinical transplantation. Immunol. Rev. 141, 213, 1994
13. TULLIUS, S.G., TILNEY, N.L. Both alloantigen-dependent and -independent factors influence chronic allograft rejection. Transplantation. 59, 313, 1995

23 Experimental Concordant Liver Xenotransplantation in Nonhuman Primates

B. Gridelli, S. Gatti, M.F. Donato, P. Andreani, L.R. Fassati, and D. Galmarini

Introduction

The limited supply of cadaveric liver grafts and the recurrence of B and C viral hepatitis in the transplanted liver has led to the consideration of baboons as a potential source of liver xenografts for transplantation into humans. In the early 1960s, Starzl obtained survival of up to 2 months of baboon kidneys transplanted in patients with end-stage renal failure [1] and showed that the xenografts were rejected by a mixture of humoral and cellular mechanisms and that the cellular component was stronger than that observed in allotransplantation [2]. The liver is more resistant than the kidney to humoral rejection, and the discovery of cyclosporine and other immunosuppressants, such as FK506 (tacrolimus), has improved the control of cellular rejection. Extensive research on the role of preformed antibodies and complement activation in rejection of organs transplanted between different species has opened the path to new therapeutic strategies to prevent humoral xenograft rejection [3]. It seems that long-term survival of concordant liver xenografts is within our grasp, although the two most recent cases of baboon-to-human liver xenotransplantation performed in Pittsburgh failed 70 and 26 days after the transplant [4] (Chap. 58).

Experimental Models of Concordant Organ Xenotransplantation

The chimpanzee is phylogenetically closer to humans than other primates [5] but, being an endangered species, few chimpanzees are available for biomedical (mainly virological) research. This limitation conditions the choice of an experimental model for concordant liver transplantation. The survival of cynomolgus monkey-to-baboon xenografts has been reported to be similar to allograft survival and it seems that this combination is a good experimental model for the chimpanzee-to-human donor/recipient combination [6, 7]. The vervet monkey-to-baboon combination has been used by Cooper et al. [8] to study the outcome of concordant heart xenotransplantation. Their results showed that, in spite of vigorous immunosuppression, graft survival beyond a few weeks was impossible to obtain and, at histology, it was evident that heart xenografts had been rejected by a mixture of humoral and cellular mechanisms [8–10]. These observations indicate that the vervet monkey-to-baboon model can be categorized as a "difficult" combination, as opposed to the cynomolgus-to-baboon which seems to be an "easy" combination. White et al. [11] suggested that it is appropriate to study the mechanisms of concordant xenograft rejection in "difficult" species combinations.

By comparing the outcome and the histological findings reported by Cooper in his experiments and by Starzl in his baboon-to-human kidney cases it seems that the vervet monkey-to-baboon is an appropriate preclinical model to use to generate information that can be relevant to the baboon-to-human situation.

Liver Xenotransplantation

In 1990 we started a research project on vervet monkey-to-baboon orthotopic xenogeneic liver transplantation with the objective of studying the outcome of concordant liver xenografts in nonhuman primates receiving an immunosuppressive protocol similar to the one used clinically, with the adjunct of splenectomy [11]. Valdivia had shown that in the hamster-to-rat model, splenectomy was crucial in prolonging the survival of hepatic xenografts [12].

Our nonhuman primates were caught in the wild in South Africa and selected for experiments on the basis of virological and immunological studies. The donor–recipient combinations were chosen on the basis of negative lymphocytotoxic crossmatch and identical or compatible blood groups. The immunosuppressive regimen was based on the association of steroids, azathioprine, cyclosporine, and a 5-day course of rabbit antithymocyte globulin (ATG). The baboons were splenectomized at the time of transplantation. Cyclosporine was administered intravenously and then intramuscularly to maintain a target blood level of 600–900 ng/ml (by radioimmunoassay, RIA) which was similar to the target blood level that we used clinically.

Two baboons survived 340 and 420 days with an orthotopically transplanted vervet monkey liver, demonstrating that long-term survival of concordant liver xenografts is possible. However, in these baboons and others that died earlier, mainly for technical reasons, it was evident that rejection was not completely controlled. Rejection was poorly controlled also in a group of baboon-to-baboon liver allotransplants which received the same immunosuppressive regimen.

In a subsequent study, we showed that baboon lymphocytes need four times more cyclosporine than human lymphocytes to be inhibited when stimulated. In contrast, FK506 was effective at the same concentrations on baboon and human lymphocytes [13]. This is a very important finding to consider whenever baboons are used for transplantation studies. In order to obtain the degree of cyclosporine-based immunosuppression that is currently utilized clinically, the target blood level should be four times higher in the baboon than in humans. In our experience, such high levels of cyclosporine do not induce nephrotoxic effects in baboons [13].

Two liver xenografts were hyperacutely rejected and upon a retrospective analysis it was shown that the recipient baboons had some preformed antibodies directed against vervet monkey antigens [14]. On electron microscopy, the sinusoidal cell lining of the hyperacutely rejected liver xenografts was completely destroyed. IgG, Clq, and C3 granular deposits were evident at immunopathology

[15]. The immunopathology study of liver biopsies of the long-term surviving baboons showed that the cellular infiltrates were mainly composed of $CD4^+$ cells and indicate the presence of some IgG deposits. No major difference between allografts and xenografts was evident; however, after xenotransplantation cellular immune reactions appeared stronger and more persistent. In the xenografts, lobular T and B cell infiltrates and Kupffer cell and endothelial cell activation indicated poorly controlled rejection activity [15].

We did not conduct sophisticated studies on the functional competence of the monkey liver in the xenogeneic environment, but showed that long-term surviving animals had normal levels of albumin and coagulation factors [14]. However, signs of vitamin B_{12} deficiency became evident around 1 year after the transplant in spite of appropriate diet. One animal died of vitamin B_{12} deficiency and the other was rescued with high parenteral dose of vitamin B_{12} administration but died several weeks later of chronic rejection [11]. It is possible that the carrier protein synthesized by the monkey liver was ineffective in transporting the vitamin to the xenogeneic targets. This indicates that even in a concordant combination functional donor/recipient incompatibility of liver xenografts is possible.

The vervet monkey-to-baboon model of liver xenotransplantation has been recently used by Mieles et al. [17] to explore the possibility of using baboon livers as auxiliary bridge xenografts in patients with acute liver failure. Mieles used the higher cyclosporine doses that we suggested and, although the presence of the native baboon liver rendered the functional data difficult to evaluate, it was confirmed that concordant liver xenografts can function in the xenogeneic environment. Since the baboons were electively euthanized between 35 and 120 days after xenotransplantation, no conclusive information on the effect of the higher doses of cyclosporine used to control rejection can be derived from this study.

A presentation at the Third International Congress for Xenotransplantation reported long-term survival of one baboon-to-monkey liver xenotransplant in which immunosuppression was based on the association of cyclosporine and cyclophosphamide [18]. The monkey was reported to be alive over 2 years after the procedure by which time all immunosuppression had been discontinued, indicating that the phenomenon of liver graft survival without immunosuppression reported following allotransplantation can occur in xenotransplantation as well.

Comment

The experimental data on concordant liver xenotransplantation in nonhuman primates are still limited, but some important conclusions can be made:

1. Liver xenografts in nonhuman primates are immunologically privileged, attaining longer survival than heart xenografts.
2. Although liver xenografts are more fiercely rejected than allografts, it seems that, in properly matched pairs, the same immunologic mechanisms are operative.
3. Some degree of functional incompatibility may exist, but it is clear that the liver in a concordant xenogeneic environment can sustain normal life.

4. When the baboon or other nonhuman primate is used to generate clinically relevant information on immunosuppressive drugs, it is important to test in vitro the effect of such drugs on lymphocytes.

Many objections have been raised to the concept of using nonhuman primates as donors for organ or cellular clinical xenotransplants and these need to be properly addressed [19]. If these obstacles can be overcome, future clinical trials of baboon-to-human liver xenotransplantation should be preceded by adequate testing of immunosuppressive protocols in nonhuman primates. It seems that the vervet monkey-to-baboon combination can provide an excellent preclinical model in which to evaluate immunosuppressive strategies and gain some insight on liver xenograft functional compatibility.

Acknowledgments. This work was supported in part by grants from CNR Target Project "Biotechnology and Bioinstrumentation" and "Ricerca finalizzata trapianto di fegato sperimentale tra primati". It was also supported by the Association for Research on Transplantation (ART).

References

1. STARZL, T.E., MARCHIORO, T.L., PETERS, G.N., et al. Renal heterotransplantation from baboon-to-man: experience with 6 cases. Transplantation. 2:752, 1964
2. PORTER, K.A. Pathological changes in transplanted kidneys. In: Experience in Renal Transplantation. T.E. Starzl (ed), W.B. Saunders, Philadelphia, 1964
3. BACH, F.H., AUCHINCLOSS, H., ROBSON, S.C. Xenotransplantation. In: Transplantation Immunology. F.H. Bach, H. Auchincloss (eds), Wiley-Liss, New York, 1995
4. STARZL, T.E., FUNG, J.J., TODO, S., et al. Prospect of clinical xenotransplantation. Transplant. Proc. 26:1082, 1994
5. HAMMER, C. Evolutionary considerations in xenotransplantation. In: Xenograft 25. M.A. Hardy (ed), Excerpta Medica, Amsterdam, 1989
6. KURLANSKY, P.A., ROBBINS, R.C., SMITH, C.R., et al. Comparable survival of intraspecies and cross-species primate cardiac transplants. Transplant. Proc. 19:1067, 1987
7. SADEGHI, A.M., ROBBINS, R.C., SMITH, C.R., et al. Cardiac xenograft survival in baboons treated with cyclosporine in combination with conventional immunosuppression. Transplant. Proc. 19:1149, 1987
8. COOPER, D.K.C., HUMAN, P.A., ROSE, A.G., et al. The role of ABO blood group compatibility in heart transplantation between closely-related animal species. J. Thorac. Cardiovasc.Surg. 97:447, 1989
9. COOPER, D.K.C., HUMAN, P.A., REICHART, B. Prolongation of cardiac xenograft (vervet monkey-to-baboon) function by a combination of total lymphoid irradiation and immunosuppressive drug therapy. Transplant. Proc. 19:4441, 1987
10. ROSE, A.G. Histopathology of cardiac xenograft rejection. In: Xenotransplantation. D.K.C. Cooper, E. Kemp, K. Reemtsma, D.J.G. White (eds), Springer, Heidelberg, 1991
11. WHITE, D.J.G., VAN DER BOGARDE, J., LIM, S.M.L. The immunology of xenotransplantation. Ann. Acad. Med. 20:770, 1991
12. GRIDELLI, B., GATTI, S., PIAZZINI, A., et al. Xenogeneic orthotopic liver transplantation in nonhuman primates. Transplant. Proc. 25:457, 1993

13. VALDIVIA, L.A., MONDEN, M., GOTOH, M., et al. Hepatic xenografts from hamster-to-rat. Transplant. Proc. 19:1158, 1987
14. STARK, J.H., SMIT, J.A., GRIDELLI, B. Sensitivity of baboon lymphocytes to cyclosporin A and FK506: relative resistance of allo-activated cell to CyA. Transplant. Int. 7:372, 1994
15. GRIDELLI, B., GATTI, S., PIAZZINI, A., et al. Orthotopic liver xenotransplantation in the baboon. Transplantationsmedizin. 6(S):148, 1994
16. DONATO, M.F., AROSIO, E., BERTI, E., et al. Immunopathology of liver allografts and xenografts in nonhuman primates. Transplant. Proc. 25:850, 1993
17. MIELES, L., LE, Y., LUO, Y., et al. Auxiliary liver allografting and xenografting in the nonhuman primate. Transplantation. 59:1670, 1995
18. ZHONG, R., TUCKER, J., GARCIA, B., et al. The long-term survival and functional tolerance of baboon-to-monkey kidney and liver xenografts - a preliminary report. Transplant. Proc. In press
19. TRAVIS, J. The xeno-solution. Perils and promise of transplanting animal organs into people. Science News. 148:298, 1995

24 Use of Tacrolimus (FK506) and Antimetabolites as Immunosuppressants for Xenotransplantation Across Closely Related Rodent Species

L.A. Valdivia, N. Murase, A.S. Rao, A.J. Demetris, J.J. Fung, and T.E. Starzl

Introduction

In the present chapter, we will review our studies of the potential role of tacrolimus in xenotransplantation based largely on experiments in which rats were recipients of vascularized organs from either hamsters or mice. Because these xenografts after transplantation elicit a strong humoral response and are rejected within a few days, these models were considered until the last few years to be moderately difficult [1–10], more so than the sheep-to-goat combination of Perper and Najarian [11] or the wolf-to-dog model of Hammer et al. [12].

Hamster-to-Rat Model

This model was added to the transplant research armamentarium by Clyde Barker and Rupert Billingham at the University of Pennsylvania [1]. However, 16 years passed before significant progress was made in breaking down this xenogeneic barrier. Then, Knechtle et al. [13] reported extended survival of hamster hearts in rat recipients treated with total lymphoid irradiation followed by cyclosporine. However, a precise explanation for this limited success was not evident. The advent of tacrolimus, a more potent T cell-directed immunosuppressant [14–21] has permitted better insight into the mechanisms of xenograft rejection in this model, especially when it has been combined with other agents that disrupt the xenogeneic immune reaction at a different site. The use of such drug combinations has consistently led to indefinite survival in the hamster-to-rat and other closely related rodent organ xenotransplant models as will be described in the following pages. We will also discuss how these experiments have cast light on the mechanisms of xenograft rejection.

Humoral Responses

Using complement-dependent cytotoxicity assays, low titers (1:16–1:32) of preformed anti-hamster cytotoxic antibodies have been demonstrated in the sera of naive Lewis rats [22]. Isotyping studies using flow cytometric analysis invariably reveal a greater preponderance of IgM rather than IgG antibodies. Rejection of liver xenografts is accompanied by astronomical elevations of antihamster cytotoxic antibodies and massive enlargement of the spleen in untreated recipients [23]. Within the spleen, this is associated with marked stimulation of $IgM^{++ bright}/IgD^{+ dull}$ B cells, which in the rat are preferentially localized in the marginal zone and red pulp. Given its marked diminution following tacrolimus therapy, this response has appeared to be at least partially T cell dependent [22]. Nevertheless, the localization and phenotypic profile of the responding recipient splenocytes also have suggested the involvement of a subpopulation of B cells which are mediators of a T-independent immune response [22, 24]. Since the host's primitive defense against blood-borne polysaccharide antigens is mediated by B cells of similar phenotype [25], it is therefore tempting to speculate that splenic IgM^{++}/IgD^{+} B cells in the rat studied by Langer et al. [22] are analogues of human $CD5^{+}$and mouse Ly 1^{+} B cell subsets [26]. These cells have also been implicated to play a seminal role in the generation of destructive xenoreactive antibodies in other models [27], although recent experiments by Pitre et al. [28] contradict this assumption.

Fate of Different Organs

Heart

Hamster hearts are rejected by antibody-mediated mechanisms within 3–4 days [1–10]. There is evidence for progressive platelet and fibrin deposition in the microvasculature and margination of neutrophils in larger vessels, with accompanying endothelial cell hypertrophy and focal denudation. There is also evidence for increased deposition of IgM, IgG, and C3 in both the endothelium of the larger vessels and in that of the microvasculature [22]. These events lead to widespread hemorrhagic necrosis precipitating xenograft loss. The use of tacrolimus (1–2 mg/kg per day until rejection) alone does not significantly prolong graft survival nor does it alter the histopathological or immunofluorescence observations detailed above [5, 7, 22]. It also fails to attenuate the gradually increasing xenospecific cytotoxic antibody titers in the recipients lending further credence to earlier contentions that the generation of xenoantibodies by a T cell-independent mechanism, along with complement, serve as main effectors in this model [29]. Further corroboration of this assertion is obtained when an increase in the titers of anti-hamster antibodies is noted in T cell-deficient nude rats receiving hamster heart xenografts [30–32]. In addition, Van den Bogaerde et al. [29] have shown that inhibition of recipient complement by cobra venom factor results in prolonged survival of hamster heart xenografts only when combined with a T-cell immunosuppressant like cyclosporine, pointing out the duality of the humoral and cellular mechanisms of xenograft rejection.

In an attempt to abate cardiac xenograft rejection, thereby prolonging survival, Murase et al. [7] have also tested tacrolimus in combination with antimetabolites such as cyclophosphamide, methotrexate, brequinar sodium (BQR) and RS-61443. Of the antimetabolites used, cyclophosphamide, a purine antimetabolite with pronounced B cell specificity [33], and BQR, which inhibits de novo pyrimidine [34], consistently allow for protracted heart xenograft survival (Table 1). More prolonged graft survival is witnessed when cyclophosphamide plus tacrolimus immunosuppression therapy is used. Similarly, when RS-61443, a purine synthesis inhibitor [35], is used in combination with tacrolimus a dramatic prolongation in xenograft survival is observed [7]. When used alone, mizorbine, an inhibitor of purine synthesis [36], and deoxyspergualin (DSG), an analogue of the antitumor antibiotic spergualin [37], have no discernible effect on cardiac xenograft survival, which is, however, prolonged with the addition of tacrolimus to the immunosuppressive regimen (Table 1). Methotrexate when used alone leads to modest prolongation of survival; however, when used in combination with tacrolimus results in indefinite graft survival. Interestingly, the use of tacrolimus alone in splenectomized recipients also results in indefinite survival of subsequently transplanted cardiac xenografts [38].

Table 1. Survival of hamster heart, liver, and kidney xenografts in Lewis rats immunosuppressed with tacrolimus and antiproliferative agents

Organ	Treatment	Dose (mg/kg per day)	Median survival (days)
Heart [7]	None	–	3.0
	FK506	2.0	4.0
	BQR	4.5	>42.0
	RS-61443	40.0	7.0
	Cyclophosphamide	15.0	56.0
	Methotrexate	0.5	13.0
	Mizorbine	7.5	4.0
	DSG	5.0	4.0
	FK506 + BQR[a]	1.0 + 4.0	>100.0
	FK506 + RS-61443[a]	2.0 + 20.0	>100.0
	FK506 + cyclophosphamide[a]	2.0 + 7.5	>100.0
	FK506+methotrexate[a]	2.0 + 1.0	>100.0
	FK506 + mizorbine[a]	2.0 + 7.5	>52.5
	FK506 + DSG[a]	2.0 + 5.0	>100.0
	FK506 + cyclophosphamide[b]	2.0 + 80.0	>100.0
	Splenectomy [38]	-	5.0
	FK506 + splenectomy [38]	2.0	>100.0
Liver [7]	None	-	7.0
	BQR	3.0	12.0
	RS-61443	20.0	7.0
	Cyclophosphamide[a]	7.5	9.0
	FK506 + BQR[a]	1.0 + 3.0	>100.0
	FK506 + RS-61443[a]	1.0 + 20.0	>100.0
	FK506 + cyclophosphamide[a]	1.0 + 7.5	>100.0
	FK506 + cyclophosphamide[b]	1.0 + 80.0	>100.0
Kidney [67]	None	–	6.0
	FK506	2.0	6.0
	Cyclophosphamide	7.5	8.0
	FK506 + cyclophosphamide[a]	2.0 + 10.0	11.5
	FK506 + cyclophosphamide[a]	1.0 + 15.0	79.0

BQR, brequinar sodium; DSG, deoxyspergualin.
[a]Antimetabolites were given in either 14- or 30-day course.
[b]Cyclophosphamide was given as a single injection 10 days before organ transplantation.

Consistent with the findings of Kumararatne et al. [39], we also observed that a single dose of cyclophosphamide (500 mg/m^2, i.p.) results after 10 days in the depletion primarily of the IgM^{++}/IgD^{+} cells normally residing in the marginal zone of the spleen [22]. To elucidate the role played by these B cells in xenograft rejection, hamster hearts were transplanted into rats with or without tacrolimus therapy 10 days after a single bolus injection of cyclophosphamide. Although slight prolongation of xenograft survival is observed in animals pretreated with cyclophosphamide alone, the addition of tacrolimus nevertheless results in indefinite graft survival (Table 1). These observations suggest that splenic B cells of this distinct phenotype may mediate an important effector function culminating in xenograft rejection in this model. However, there is a T cell-mediated mechanism of graft injury which neither cyclophosphamide nor splenectomy, when used alone (23, 38, 40, 41), are able to attenuate. Accordingly, the use of strategies which allow for inhibition of both B and T cell function provides an optimal means to control xenograft rejection in this model [6, 7].

Liver

Unlike heart xenografts, hamster livers are acutely rejected by untreated Lewis rat recipients in 7 days by a composite humoral and cell-mediated immunity [5, 7, 22, 23]. The early deposition of anti-hamster antibodies in the sinusoids and portal tracts is followed by cellular infiltration in these areas composed largely of recipient CD8^{+} T and few natural killer cells. This histopathological finding differs from that witnessed during liver allograft rejection, where the initial cellular infiltrate is localized primarily in the portal or perivenular areas [42]. These findings provide support for a role of antibody-mediated cellular cytotoxicity in xenograft rejection [43–45]. When tacrolimus is used alone, it significantly prolongs xenograft survival with 10 %–30 % of the recipients surviving indefinitely [5, 7, 46]. Single drug therapy using either BQR, RS-61443 or cyclophosphamide has minimal impact on graft survival, whereas the addition of tacrolimus to BQR, RS-61443, or cyclophosphamide-treated recipients leads to their indefinite survival (Table 1). As with hearts, pretreatment of liver xenograft recipients with a single bolus injection of cyclophosphamide 10 days prior to organ transplantation also results in their indefinite survival (Table 1) [7, 22].

Despite its moderate efficacy in prolonging liver xenograft survival, tacrolimus when used alone does not mitigate the extreme elevation of xenospecific cytotoxic antibody titers in the recipient serum, which reach a peak around day 7 post-transplantation. However, by day 30 post-transplantation, these antibodies become undetectable in tacrolimus-treated recipients, the majority of whom nevertheless succumb to late graft failure subsequent to biliary obstruction [22]. We have hypothesized that this outcome represents a delayed manifestation of humoral injury which may have transpired early during the period following transplantation [47]. This assertion is further substantiated by the obvious lack of biliary complications and long-term survival of tacrolimus-treated recipients who had received a short perioperative course of BQR or RS-61443; both of which are known to partially abate the initial peak antibody response [7].

Although tacrolimus does not have an effect on xenoantibody production when therapy starts on the day of transplantation, Tsugita et al. [48] have shown that this immunosuppressant not only abrogates the hyperacute liver xenograft rejection induced by pretransplant infusion of hamster hepatocytes or liver nonparenchymal cells (NPC, which include liver sinusoidal cells), but also prolongs graft survival beyond that achieved by pretransplant treatment with tacrolimus alone. The interesting observation is that, although the cytotoxicity (IgM) of the recipient's serum against hamster lymphocytes remains high despite tacrolimus therapy, that against hamster-specific NPC is blunted. Similarly, we have shown recently that T cell-deficient nude rats that receive hamster whole blood 1 week prior to transplantation with a hamster heart never reject the graft in a hyperacute fashion. Indeed, the heart xenografts survive indefinitely in most of the cases [49]. These observations indicate the importance of T cell help in the induction of xenosensitization and hyperacute rejection in this xenograft model.

Our achievement of long-term survival in liver xenograft recipients has afforded us the opportunity to study several physiological and immunological features uniquely associated with this organ. We have specifically investigated the metabolic and coagulatory changes [50, 51] that occur in the liver xenograft recipients and the cellular events that lead to the induction of donor-specific tolerance [46]. Rats who accept hamster liver xenografts exhibit species-specific unresponsiveness to subsequently transplanted donor organs. It must be emphasized that while they retain donor-specific tolerance, the liver recipients are fully capable of rejecting organs from other animal species [46].

This species-specific immunological unresponsiveness, afforded best by the liver but also witnessed after heart xenotransplantation as reported by Tanaka et al. [52], may be ascribed to the establishment of chimerism, which has been shown to play a seminal role in the induction of donor-specific tolerance [53–56]. Additionally, it is also well known that given their species-specific restriction, certain membrane-associated complement (C) regulatory proteins, such as decay-accelerating factor (DAF), membrane cofactor protein (MCP), and CD59 antigen, among others, play an important role in protecting autologous or homologous tissues from collateral damage that may be prompted by C activation [57–62]. Therefore, the production by the liver of species-specific circulating C proteins may provide yet another mechanism by which this organ may exert its observed protective effects.

Further credence to the latter hypothesis is provided by exhaustive experiments in rats in which species-specific tolerance is successfully achieved by prior hamster liver xenotransplantation [63, 64]. The intravenous administration of C-depleted (but not enriched) rat anti-hamster hyperimmune serum into these tolerant animals has no deleterious effect on simultaneously transplanted hamster hearts which enjoy prolonged survival. These observations underscore the pernicious nature of heterologous C which, following xenotransplantation of organs other than livers, may play a major role in mediating the antibody-dependent rejection [65]. In view of this it would be reasonable to predict that clinical transplantation of organs, other than livers, from transgenic pigs expressing human C regulatory proteins on their endothelium would prevent hyperacute rejection as has already been demonstrated by White et al. [66]. Of concern, however, is the potential risk to the liver recipient of heterologous C secreted by the xenografted organ, whose uninhibited activity may precipitate an autoimmune-like syndrome. This is an area of research which warrants further investigation.

Kidney

Similar to our observations for hearts, Miyazawa et al. [67] have reported that hamster kidney xenografts are rejected by untreated rat recipients in 5–6 days predominantly by a humoral response. The use of tacrolimus alone does not prolong graft survival nor has any appreciable effect on the generation of rat anti-hamster IgM antibodies. Although the additional use of cyclophosphamide along with tacrolimus extends xenograft survival, the results are not as dramatic and consistent as those obtained with heart and liver xenografts (Table 1). Attempts to deplete heterospecific antibodies by pre-transplant perfusion of recipient's blood through donor-strain kidneys or livers, as well as the use of the anti-complementary agent K76 [68, 69], result in marginal prolongation of survival of subsequently transplanted kidney xenografts in tacrolimus/cyclophosphamide-treated rat recipients (Table 1). Interestingly, Ye et al. [70] have observed that the majority of kidney xenograft recipients develop severe polyuria which is not corrected by restriction of water intake. Since the minimal histopathological changes in the kidney xenografts cannot account for the de novo development of diabetes insipidus witnessed in this model, it is speculated that there might be a functional incompatibility between transporter proteins expressed on cells in hamster kidney with that of their ligands in the rats. Attempts are underway to provide substantial evidence for the latter postulate.

Mouse-to-Rat Model

Similar to our observations in the hamster-to-rat model, mouse hearts when transplanted into unmodified rat recipients are rejected by antibody-mediated mechanisms within 2–3 days [71–73]. However, Pan et al. [73] have shown that liver xenografts when transplanted into untreated Lewis rats survive for approximately 7 days, succumbing eventually to combined antibody and cell-mediated rejection (Table 2). Although no appreciable difference in mouse heart xenograft

Table 2. Survival of B10.BR mouse hearts and livers xenografted into Lewis rat recipients with or without tacrolimus immunosuppressive therapy

Organ	Tacrolimus	Graft survival (days)	Median survival (days)
Heart	No	2, 2, 2, 2, 2, 2, 3, 3	2.7±1.7
Heart[a]	Yes	2, 2, 3, 3, 3	2.8±0.8
Liver	No	7, 7, 7, 7, 7	7.0
Liver[b]	Yes	18, 18, 28, 37, 61, 82, 93, 107, 110, 111, 117, 133, 203, 207, 221	103.9±64.7

[a] 1 mg/kg per day, i.m.
[b] 1 mg/kg per day ×30 days followed by 0.5 mg/kg every other day for the next 70 days.

survival is observed following tacrolimus administration, it does however, improve the outcome in mouse liver graft recipients, 50% surviving beyond 100 days. Despite the presence of elevated xenospecific antibodies, the observation of long-term liver xenograft survival in this model further emphasizes the inherent resistance of this organ to antibody-mediated injury. The donor-specific protective effect afforded by the transplanted liver following hamster-to-rat xenotransplantation is also witnessed in this model. This effect appears to be species-specific but non-major histocompatibility complex (MHC) restricted, allowing for transplanted mouse hearts obtained from donors of varying MHC phenotype to be equally protected, whereas hearts obtained from hamster are promptly rejected [74].

Comment

Our studies have demonstrated that the interdiction of the initial B cell proliferative response is the critical first step towards successful xenotransplantation in closely related species. Once the antibody barrier is breached, the need for the antiproliferative drugs apparently diminishes with tacrolimus-based monotherapy being sufficient to maintain graft function. The manipulation of the donor and/or the recipient with novel agents such as phosphatidic acid inhibitors [75] and the creation of chimeric donors [76, 77] are some of the more contemporary approaches that are currently being employed in our laboratory to make xenotransplantation a clinical reality.

Acknowledgments. This work was aided by Project Grant No. DK29961 from the National Institutes of Health, Bethesda, MD, USA.

References

1. Barker, C. F., Billingham, R. E. Histocompatibility requirements of heart and skin grafts in rats. Transplant Proc 3: 172, 1971
2. Kakita, A., Blanchard, J., Fortner, J. G. Hamster-to-rat cardiac xenografts: a useful model for transplantation studies. J Surg Res 19: 99, 1975
3. Homan, W. P., Williams, K. A., Fabre, J. W., Millard, P. R., Morris, P. J. Prolongation of cardiac xenograft survival in rats receiving cyclosporin A. Transplantation 31: 164, 1981
4. Valdivia, L. A., Monden, M., Gotoh, M., et al. Evidence that deoxyspergualin prevents sensitization and first-set cardiac xenograft rejection in rats by suppression of antibody formation. Transplantation 50: 132, 1990
5. Valdivia, L. A., Fung, J. J., Demetris, A. J., Starzl, T. E. Differential survival of hamster-to-rat liver and cardiac xenografts under FK-506 immunosuppression. Transplant Proc 23: 3269, 1991
6. Hasan, R., Van Den Bogaerde, J. B., Wallwork, J., White, D. J. G. Evidence that long term survival of concordant xenografts is achieved by inhibition of antispecies antibody production. Transplantation 54: 408, 1992

7. Murase, N., Starzl, T. E., Demetris, A. J., et al. Hamster to rat heart and liver xenotransplantation with FK506 plus antiproliferative drugs. Transplantation 55: 701, 1993
8. Leventhal, J. R., Matas, A. J. Xenotransplantation in rodents: A review and reclassification. Transplant Rev 8: 80, 1994
9. Makowka, L., Cramer, D. V. The pathogenesis of xenograft rejection. Clin Transplantation 8: 145, 1994
10. Starzl, T. E., Valdivia, L. A., Murase, N., et al. The biological basis of and strategies for clinical xenotransplantation. Immunol Rev 141: 213, 1994
11. Perper, R. J., Najarian, J.S. Experimental renal heterotransplantation. II. Closely related species. Transplantation4: 700, 1966
12. Hammer, C., Chaussy, C., Weber, H., et al. Exceptionally long survival time in xenogeneic organ transplantation. Transplant Proc 13: 881, 1981
13. Knechtle, S. J., Halperin, E. C., Bollinger, R. R. Xenograft survival in two species combinations using total-lymphoid irradiation and cyclosporine. Transplantation 43: 173, 1987
14. Goto, T., Kino, T., Hatanaka, H., et al. Discovery of FK-506, a novel immunosuppressant isolated from Streptomyces Tsukubaensis. Transplant Proc 19: 4, 1987
15. Kino, T., Hatanaka, H., Miyata, S., et al. FK-506, a novel immunosuppressant isolated from a streptomyces. II. Immunosuppressive effect of FK-506 in vitro. J Antibiot 40: 1256, 1987
16. Ochiai, T., Nakajima, K., Nagata, M., et al. Effect of a new immunosuppressive agent, FK-506, on heterotopic cardiac allotransplantation in the rat. Transplant Proc 19: 1284, 1987
17. Murase, N., Todo, S., Lee, P-H., et al. Heterotopic heart transplantation in the rat receiving FK-506 alone or with cyclosporine. Transplant Proc 19: 71, 1987
18. Todo, S., Demetris, A. J., Ueda, Y, et al. Canine kidney transplantation with FK-506 alone or in combination with cyclosporine and steroids. Transplant Proc 19: 57, 1987
19. Todo, S., Ueda, Y., Demetris, A. J., et al. Immunosuppression of canine, monkey, and baboon allografts by FK 506 with special reference to synergism with other drugs, and to tolerance induction. Surgery 104: 239, 1988
20. Starzl, T. E., Todo, S., Fung, J., et al. FK 506 for human liver, kidney and pancreas transplantation. Lancet 2: 1000, 1989
21. Todo, S., Fung, J. J., Starzl, T. E., et al. Liver, kidney, and thoracic organ transplantation under FK 506. Ann Surg 212: 295, 1990
22. Langer, A., Valdivia, L. A., Murase, N., et al. Humoral and cellular immunopathology of hepatic and cardiac hamster-into-rat xenograft rejection - Marked stimulation of $IgM^{++bright}/IgD^{+dull}$ splenic B cells. Am J Pathol 143: 85, 1993
23. Valdivia, L. A., Monden, M., Gotoh, M., et al. Prolonged survival of hamster-to-rat liver xenografts using splenectomy and cyclosporine administration. Transplantation 44: 759, 1987
24. Liu, Y. J., Zhang, J., Lane, P. J. L., Chan, E. Y. T., MacLennan, I. C. M. Sites of specific B cell activation in primary and secondary responses to T-cell dependent and T cell-independent antigens. Eur J Immunol 21: 2951, 1991
25. Janeway, C. A. The immune system evolved to discriminate infectious nonself from noninfectious self. Immunol Today 13: 11, 1992
26. Herzenberg, L. A., Stall, A. M., Lalor, P. A., et al. The Ly-1 B cell lineage. Immunol Rev 93: 81, 1986

27. Bach, F. H., Dalmasso, A. P., Platt, J. L. Xenotransplantation: A current prospective. Transplant Rev 6: 163, 1992
28. Pitre, J., Müller, E., Satake, M. Human xenoreactive natural antibodies against Gala(1–3) pig terminal residues are not produced by $CD5^+$ B lymphocytes. Transplant. Proc. 28:545, 1996
29. Van den Bogaerde, J., Aspinall, R. Wang, M-W, et al. Induction of long-term survival of hamster heart xenografts in rats. Transplantation 52: 15, 1991
30. Lim, S. M. L., Whee, A., Chung, I., White, D. J. G. An analysis of xenograft rejection in the nude rat model. Transplant Proc 23: 581, 1990
31. Thomas, F. T., Marchman, W., Carobbi, A., et al. Immunobiology of the xenograft response: xenograft rejection in immunodeficient animals. Transplant Proc 23: 308, 1991
32. Tsugita, M., Valdivia, L. A., Woo, J., et al. The effect of splenectomy on cardiac and liver xenografts in the Nude rat. Transplant Proc 26: 1210, 1994
33. Putnam, C. W., Halgrimson, C. G., Groth, C. G., et al. Immunosuppression with cyclophosphamide in the dog. Clin Exp Immunol 22: 323, 1975
34. Chen, S. F., Ruben, R. L., Dexter, D. L. Mechanism of action of the novel anticancer agent 6-fluoro-2-(2′-fluoro-1,1′-biphenyl-4-yl)-3-methyl-4-quinolinecarboxylic acid sodium salt (NSC368390): Inhibition of de novo pyrimidine nucleotide biosynthesis. Cancer Research 46: 5014, 1986
35. Nelson, P. H., Eugui, E., Wang, C. C., Allison, A. C. Synthesis and immunosuppressive activity of some side-chain variants of mycophenolic acid. J Med Chem 33: 833, 1990
36. Hayashi, M., Hirano, T., Yaso, M., Mizuno, K., Ueda, T. Studies on bredinin. III. Chemical synthesis of bredinin (A novel imidazole nucleoside). Chem Pharm Bull 23: 245, 1975
37. Takeuchi, T., Iinuma, H., Kunimoto, S., et al. A new antitumor antibiotic, spergualin: Isolation and antitumor activity. J Antibiotics 34: 1619, 1981
38. Celli, S., Valdivia, L. A., Fung, J. J., et al. Long-term survival of heart and liver xenografts with splenectomy and FK 506. Transplant Proc 25: 647, 1993
39. Kumararatne, D. S., Gagnon, R. F., Smart, Y. Selective loss of large lymphocytes from the marginal zone of the white pulp in rat spleens following a single dose of cyclophosphamide. Immunol 40: 123, 1980
40. Valdivia, L. A., Monden, M., Gotoh, M., et al. An important role of the spleen in rejection of hamster-to-rat xenografts. Transplant Proc 20: 329, 1988
41. Carobbi, A., Araneda, D., Patselas, T., Thomas, J. M., Mosca, F. Effect of splenectomy in combination with FK506 and 15-deoxyspergualin on cardiac xenograft survival. Transplant Proc 23: 549, 1991
42. Demetris, A. J., Qian, S., Sun, H., et al. Early events in liver allograft rejection. Am J Pathol 138: 609, 1991
43. Thomas, F., Araneda, D., Henretta, J., Pittman, K., Marchman, W. Extended and expanded studies of xenograft rejection in immunodeficient animals. Transplant Proc 26: 1224, 1994
44. Arakawa, K., Akami, T., Okamoto, M., et al. Prolongation of heart xenograft survival in the NK-deficient rat. Transplant Proc 26: 1266, 1994
45. Nielsen, B., Lillevang, S., Salomon, S., Steinbrüchel, D. A., Kemp, E. Hamster hearts transplanted to normal Lewis rats and rnu/rnu rats ("Nude rats") are rejected at the same tempo but by different mechanisms. Transplant Proc 26: 1189, 1994

46. Valdivia, L. A., Demetris, A. J., Fung, J. J., et al. Successful hamster-to-rat liver xenotransplantation under FK506 immunosuppression induces unresponsiveness to hamster heart and skin. Transplantation 55: 659, 1993
47. Nakamura, K., Murase, N., Becich, M. J., et al. Liver allograft rejection in sensitized recipients: observations in a clinically relevant small animal model. Am J Pathol142: 1383, 1993
48. Tsugita, M., Valdivia, L. A., Celli, S., et al. Prevention of sensitization and hyperacute rejection in liver and heart xenografts by FK 506 plus donor antigens. Transplant Proc 27: 277, 1995
49. Tsugita, M., Rao, A. S., Sun, H., et al. Pretreatment of recipients (Nude rat) with donor antigens leads to prolonged survival of hamster heart xenografts. Transplant Proc 28: 706, 1996
50. Valdivia, L. A., Lewis, J. H., Celli, S., et al. Hamster coagulation and serum proteins in rat recipients of hamster xenografts. Transplantation56: 489, 1993
51. Celli, S., Valdivia, L. A., Kelly, R. H., et al. Functional cooperation of xenoproteins after hamster-to-rat liver transplantation: With particular reference to hamster C3 and secretory component for rat IgA. Xenotransplantation 2: 46, 1995
52. Tanaka, M., Murase, N., Nomoto, M., et al. Tacrolimus (FK506)-dependent tolerance after liver and heart xenotransplantation: Inhibition of humoral response and acceptance of donor organs. Transplant Proc 28: 679, 1996
53. Starzl, T. E., Demetris, A. J., Murase, N., et al. Cell migration, chimerism, and graft acceptance. Lancet 339: 1579, 1992
54. Starzl, T. E., Demetris, A. J., Trucco, M., et al. Cell migration and chimerism after whole organ transplantation: The basis of graft acceptance. Hepatology 17: 1127, 1993
55. Starzl, T. E., Demetris, A. J., Trucco, M., et al. Chimerism and donor specific nonreactivity 27 to 29 years after kidney allotransplantation. Transplantation 55: 1272, 1993
56. Starzl, T. E., Murase, N., Demetris, A. J., et al. Drug development and testing in relation to cell migration and chimerism. Transplant Proc 25: 469, 1993
57. Hourcade, D., Holers, V. M., Atkinson, J. P. The regulators of complement activation (RCA) gene cluster. Adv Immunol 45: 381, 1989
58. Nicholson-Weller, A., Burge, J. Isolation of a human erythrocyte membrane glycoprotein with decay-accelerating activity for C3 convertases of the C system. J Immunol 129: 184, 1982
59. Seya, T., Turner, J. R., Atkinson, J. P. Purification and characterization of a membrane protein (gp 45–70) that is a cofactor for cleavage of C3b and C4b. J Exp Med 163: 837, 1986
60. Schoenermark, S., Rauterberg, E. W., Shin, M. L., et al. Homologous species restriction in lysis of human erythrocytes: a membrane-derived protein with C8-binding capacity functions as an inhibitor. J Immunol 136: 1772, 1986
61. Zalman, L. S., Wood, L. M., Mueller-Eberhard, H. J. Isolation of a human erythrocyte membrane protein capable of inhibiting expression of homologous complement transmembrane channels. Proc Natl Acad Sci USA 83: 6975, 1986
62. Rollins, S. A, Zhao, J., Ninomiya, H., Sims, P. J. Inhibition of homologous complement by CD59 is mediated by a species-selective recognition conferred through binding to C8 within C5b-8 or C9 within C5b-9. J Immunol 146: 2345, 1991

63. Valdivia, L. A, Fung, J. J., Demetris, A. J., et al. Donor species complement after liver xenotransplantation: The mechanism of protection from hyperacute rejection. Transplantation 57: 918, 1994
64. Starzl, T. E., Murase, N., Tzakis, A., et al. Clinical xenotransplantation. Xenotransplantation 1: 3, 1994
65. Platt, J. L, Bach, F. H. The barrier to xenotransplantation. Transplantation 52: 937, 1991
66. White, D. J. G., Braidley, P., Dunning, J., et al. Hearts from pigs transgenic for human DAF are not hyperacutely rejected when xenografted to primates. The Third International Congress for Xenotransplantation. September 27–October 1, 1995. Boston, MA, USA
67. Miyazawa, H., Murase, N., Demetris, A. J., et al. Hamster to rat kidney xenotransplantation - Effects of FK506, cyclophosphamide, organ perfusion, and complement inhibition. Transplantation 59: 1183, 1995
68. Miyazaki, W., Tamaoka, H., Shinohara, M., et al. A complement inhibitor produced by Stachybotrys complementi, nov. sp. K-76, a new species of Fungi Imperfecti. Microbiol Immunol 24: 1091, 1980
69. Starzl, T. E., Tzakis, A., Fung, J. J. Prospects of clinical xenotransplantation. Transplant Proc 26: 1082, 1994
70. Ye, Q., Murase, N., Tanaka, M., et al. Possible functional incompatibility and adaptation of hamster kidney graft in xenogeneic rat environment. Transplant Proc 28: 694, 1996
71. Jeekel, J., de Putter, C., Lameyer, L. D. F., Westbroek, D. L. The survival of mouse skin and heart heterografts in rats treated with xenogeneic hyperimmune anti-donor antiserum. Transplantation 17: 605, 1974
72. Nakajima, K., Sakamoto, K., Ochiai, T., et al. Prolongation of cardiac xenograft survival in rats treated with 15-deoxyspergualin alone and in combination with FK506.Transplantation 45: 1146, 1988
73. Pan, F., Valdivia, L. A., Tsugita, M., et al. FK 506 prolongs survival of liver but not heart mouse-to-rat vascularized xenografts. Transplant Proc 26: 1211, 1994
74. Valdivia, L. A., Pan, F., Tsugita, M., et al. The protection from humoral rejection given by a liver xenograft is species-specific and non-MHC restricted. Transplant Proc27: 270, 1995
75. Valdivia, L. A., Murase, N., Rao, A. S., et al. Perioperative treatment with phosphatidic acid inhibitor (lisofylline) leads to prolonged survival of hearts in the guinea pig → rat xenotransplant model. Transplant Proc 28: 749, 1996
76. Valdivia, L. A., Sun, H., Rao, A. S., et al. Prolonged survival of hearts obtained from chimeric donors in a mouse → rat xenotransplant model. Transplant Proc 28: 744, 1996
77. Beschorner, W. E., Qian, Z., Mattei, P., et al. Induction of human chimerism and functional suppressor cells in fetal pigs. Feasibility of surrogate tolerogenesis for xenotransplantation. Transplant Proc 28: 648, 1996

V Experimental Xenotransplantation Between Widely Disparate Species

25 Roles of Anti-αGal Antibody and Oligosaccharide Therapy in Xenotransplantation

F.A. Neethling, S. Taniguchi, S.F. Li, E. Koren, R. Oriol, R.D. Cummings, and D.K.C. Cooper

Introduction

It is now generally agreed that the hyperacute rejection (HAR) of pig organs by both human and nonhuman primates is related to the presence of preformed "natural" antibodies in the host [1–4]. The true origin of these antibodies is speculative, but they develop within a few weeks after birth, probably as soon as the neonate's gastrointestinal tract becomes colonized by microorganisms [5, 6]. The antibody-antigen reaction that takes place on the surface of the vascular endothelium stimulates the complement cascade and "activates" the endothelial cells [7], leading to endothelial cell damage with capillary disruption and interstitial hemorrhage [8], resulting in rapid destruction of the tissues with loss of function.

Concept of Accommodation

There is evidence from both clinical [9–11] and experimental [12–15,16] studies of allografting across the ABO histo-blood group barrier that if anti-A or anti-B antibodies can be depleted (or otherwise inhibited) for a relatively short period of time (days rather than weeks) then an ABO-incompatible organ transplanted during this "window" will not be hyperacutely rejected despite the subsequent return of normal levels of antibody and complement. This concept, first demonstrated in clinical ABO-incompatible kidney transplantation by Alexandre et al. [9, 10], has variously been termed anergy, adaptation, or accommodation [17]. The mechanism by which accommodation occurs remains unclear, but there is some evidence that the target antigens are masked or capped, possibly by blocking antibody [12].

It should not be overlooked that "accommodation" occurs spontaneously with no specific therapeutic intervention in approximately one third of patients who receive an ABO-incompatible heart [18], kidney [19, 20] or liver [21] allograft. Long-term graft survival has been documented in this group of patients despite the continuing presence of anti-A and/or anti-B antibodies. The remaining two thirds reject their organ allografts either hyperacutely (in the case of the heart and kidney) or in an accelerated manner (in the case of the liver). The reasons and mechanisms whereby antibody-mediated rejection does not occur in one third of recipients of ABO-incompatible organs remain unknown.

A similar situation has been demonstrated in the baboon, but in this species spontaneous accommodation occurs in approximately two thirds of recipients [22] as opposed to only one third in humans.

After the demonstration that accommodation could occur after ABO-incompatible organ transplantation, the phenomenon was initially explored in discordant xenotransplantation by both the Cape Town group using the pig-to-baboon cardiac model [23] and by the Bruxelles group using the pig-to-baboon renal model [24]. Although truly long-term accommodation has not been achieved following the transplantation of a discordant xenograft, some prolongation of survival of both hearts (for periods of days to weeks) [23, 25–28] and kidneys (for a period of up to 22 days) [24] has been reported, and further investigation seems warranted.

Transplantation of ABO-Incompatible Allografts – A Paradigm of Discordant Xenotransplantation

The histo-blood group A and B epitopes, against which anti-A and anti-B antibodies are directed, are carbohydrates, the structures of which have been accurately defined (Fig. 1) [29–33]. Furthermore, these trisaccharides can be synthesized [33, 34] and, when attached to a solid support, act as highly efficient immunoaffinity columns. Plasma or blood repeatedly passed through such a column is rapidly depleted of the respective antibody, as first demonstrated by Bensinger et al [35–37] and Bannett et al. [11].

Following successful preliminary studies by Romano and his colleagues [38–40], in 1987 we began an exploration of the possibility of preventing hyperacute rejection of ABO-incompatible baboon cardiac allografts by the intravenous (i.v.) infusion of the specific A or B trisaccharide against which the anti-A or anti-B antibodies were directed. When the trisaccharide is infused continuously

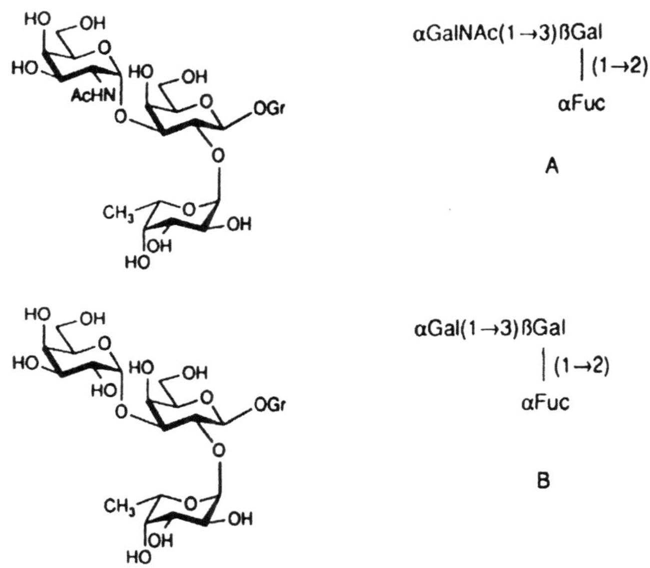

Fig. 1. A Trisaccharide ethyl ester (*top*) and B trisaccharide ethyl ester (*bottom*)

into the host's circulation, the specific antibodies bind to the trisaccharide and are thus "neutralized," i.e., they are no longer freely available to "attack" the transplanted ABO-incompatible organ [12,14,15,16]. As the trisaccharide is a small molecule, a hapten-like effect results, leading neither to immunogenicity nor complement activation. The trisaccharide is rapidly excreted in the urine and bile, immune complexes are not formed, and therapy in baboons is totally innocuous.

In the anti-A or anti-B *hypersensitized* baboon receiving both trisaccharide infusion and conventional pharmacologic immunosuppressive therapy (cyclosporine, azathioprine or cyclophosphamide, and corticosteroids), survival of ABO-incompatible cardiac allografts was extended from a mean of *19 min* in control experiments to more than *28 days*. Accommodation was clearly achieved in several cases; in one baboon the graft functioned for >30 days after cessation of trisaccharide infusion.

Identification of Human Anti-Pig Antibodies as Anti-αGal Antibodies

The results of these ABO-incompatible studies suggested to us that similar techniques of antibody adsorption or inhibition would be possible if the antibody (or antibodies) that initiated discordant xenograft destruction also proved to be directed against a carbohydrate epitope. In 1990, when we began this study, we could find only one reference in the literature that gave some support to this possibility [41], although subsequently two further reports provided stronger evidence that the epitope might be a glycoprotein [42] or glycolipid [43].

(There is, however, one major difference between the problems of ABO incompatibility in allografting and those of discordant xenografting. In the latter situation, the transplanted organ expresses complement-inhibiting proteins that are heterologous and therefore believed to be less able to protect the organ from the effects of host complement. This may prove a significant difference, but experimental studies have not yet progressed to the stage where this can be determined.)

Human plasma was infused through pig hearts or kidneys and the anti-pig antibodies were eluted out [12, 13, 16, 44–47]. Human preformed antibodies reacting with porcine heart endothelium were found to belong to three immunoglobulin classes (IgG, IgA, and IgM), all of which bound to the surface of cultured pig kidney cells. Anti-pig immunoglobulins also competed for the pig cell surface epitopes with the *Griffonia simplicifolia* iso-lectin GS1-B4 which is specific for oligosaccharides with a terminal α-galactose.

These anti-pig antibodies were then tested against a panel of synthetic carbohydrate hapten-BSA conjugates, and the specificity of the antibodies was determined. By far the strongest binding was to oligosaccharides with an α-galactosyl (αGal) terminal residue (Fig. 2); these included (a) αGal-R (α-galactose), (b) αGal1–3βGal-R (αGal disaccharide), (c) α1–3βGal1–4GlcNAc-R (αGal type 2 trisaccharide), and (d) αGal1–3βGal1–4βGlc-R (αGal type 6 trisaccharide), where R is $(CH_2)_8COOCH_3$ [12, 13, 16, 44, 45]. Both IgG and IgM anti-αGal components were identified [44, 45], and later IgA anti-αGal antibodies were also recognized [48, 49].

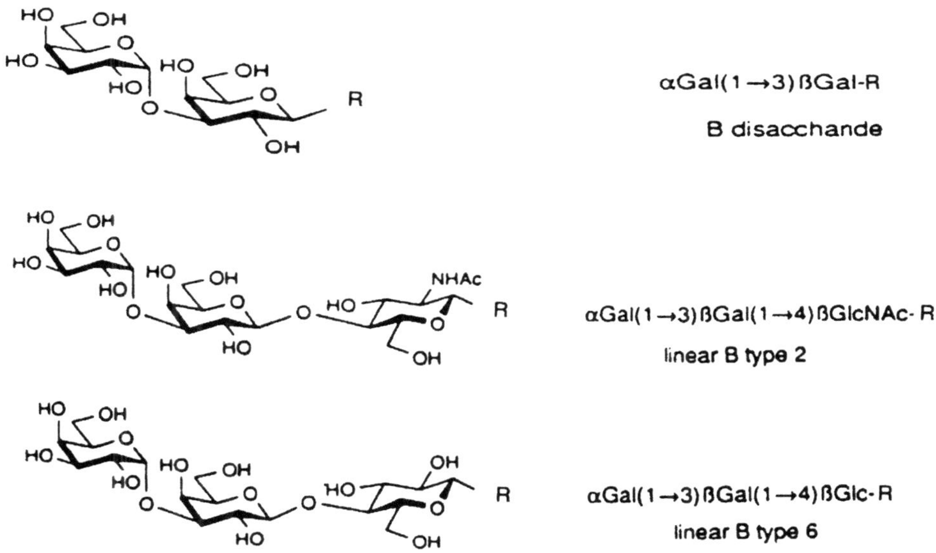

Fig. 2. Three of the major carbohydrate structures that bind human antibodies eluted from pig heart, kidney, and red blood cell stroma: αGal disaccharide (*top*), αGal trisaccharide type 2 (*middle*), and αGal trisaccharide type 6 (*bottom*). R=$(CH_2)_8COOCH_3$

Some of the individual eluted antibody preparations also bound to other carbohydrate antigens (Table 1), including A or A-like carbohydrates, Forssman disaccharide and trisaccharide, α-L-rhamnose and rhamnose-containing structures, and *N*-acetyl-β-D-glucosaminide (βGlcNac)-containing structures. However, none of these antigens was bound by significant levels of antibody in all preparations, whereas antibodies reacting with the αGal type 2 and type 6 trisaccharides and the αGal disaccharide were present in every preparation tested. Based on enzyme-linked immunosorbent assay (ELISA), the anti-αGal1-3Gal antibody specificity appeared to represent by far the most significant human anti-pig carbohydrate antibodies. The important role of anti-αGal antibodies in the HAR of pig organs by human (and baboon) serum, documented originally by Good et al. in 1991 [44], has subsequently been confirmed by several other groups [50–55], although other antibodies may possibly play a role in xenograft rejection in some subjects [56].

More recent studies by our group, in collaboration with Michler and his colleagues in New York, have included an investigation of the presence of anti-αGal antibody in newborn humans and baboons. Anti-αGal antibody has been identified in one of four newborn baboons [57] and two of five newborn humans (unpublished data). They were of the IgG class and presumably were of maternal origin, having crossed the placenta antenatally. The absence of antibody in several neonates of both species lends support to the concept that these antibodies, like the anti-ABH antibodies, develop in neonates in response to the presence of certain microorganisms in the gastrointestinal tract [58], and therefore probably play a role in the body's defense mechanism against infection. Avila and collea-

Table 1. Carbohydrate structures that bind to human anti-pig kidney and/or anti-pig heart antibodies (from [44])

Antigen group	Trivial name	Chemical structure	Anti-pig samples with strong binding (OD ⩾ 0.5)			
			Anti-pig kidney (n=4)		Anti-pig heart (n=2)	
			Human O plasma	Human AB plasma	Human O plasma	Human AB plasma
B-like	Linear B type 2	αGal(1→3)βGal (1→4)βGlcNAc-R	4	4	1	2
	Linear B type 6	αGal(1→3)βGal (1→4)βGlc-R	4	4	1	2
	B disaccharide	αGal(1→3)βGal-R	4	4	1	2
	α-D-Galactoside	αGal-R	3	4	ND	ND
B	B type 4	αGal(1→3)βGal (1→3)βGalNAc-R (1→2)αFuc	3	0	0	0
	B type 5	αGal(1→3)βGal (1→3)βGal-R (1→2)αFuc	3	0	1	0
A-like	A disaccharide	αGalNAc(1→3) βGal-R	2	0	1	2
	Linear A type 6	αGalNAc(1→3)βGal (1→4)βGlc-R	2	0	0	1
	Forssman disaccharide	αGalNAc(1→3)βGal NAc-R	2	0	1	2
	Forssman trisaccharide	αGalNAc(1→3) βGalNAc(1→3) αGal-R	3	0	1	2
A	A trisaccharide	αGalNAc(1→3) βGal-R(1→2)αFuc	3	0	0	0
	A type 4	αGalNAc(1→3)βGal (1→3)βGalNAc-R (1→2)αFuc	2	0	1	0
	A type 5	αGalNAc(1→3)βGal (1→3)βGal-R (1→2)αFuc	2	0	1	0
	A type 6	αGalNAc(1→3)βGal (1→4)βGlc-R (1→2)αFuc	2	0	1	0
P	P1	αGal(1→4)βGal-R	3	0	1	2
	Paragloboside	βGal(1→4)βGlcNAc (1→3)βGal (1→4)βGlc-R	0	0	1	0
βGlcNAc-containing	*N*-Acetyl-β-D-glucosaminide	βGlcNAc-R	2	3	1	2
		βGlcNAc(1→4) βGlcNAc-R	0	1	1	2
Rhamnose-containing	α-L-Rhamnose	α-L-Rha-R	0	2	1	2
		α-L-Rha(1→3) βGlcNAc(1→2) α-L-Rha-R	2	2	1	2

Table 1. (Continued)

Antigen group	Trivial name	Chemical structure	Anti-pig samples with strong binding (OD ⩾ 0.5)			
			Anti-pig kidney (n=4)		Anti-pig heart (n=2)	
			Human O plasma	Human AB plasma	Human O plasma	Human AB plasma
Other		αGalNAc(1→2)βGal-R	1	1	1	2
		αGalNAc(1→4)βGal-R	1	0	1	1
		βGalNAc(1→2)βGal-R	0	2	1	2
		βGal(1→3)βGalNAc-R	0	1	1	0
		αGlc(1→2)βGal-R	1	0	1	1
		βGlc(1→2)βGal-R	1	0	1	1
		βGlc(1→2)αMan-R	1	1	1	1
		αMan(1→6)αMan-R	0	1	1	2

Modified from [45]).
R, O-$(CH_2)_8$-CO-NH-bovine serum albumin; Gal, galactose, Fuc, fucose, Rha, rhamnose, GlcNAc, *N*-acetylglucosamine, GalNAc, *N*-acetylgalactosamine, Man, mannose, ND, not done.

gues, however, demonstrated an absence of anti-αGal antibody in only 10 % of newborn infants (J.L., Avila, personal communication).

Considerable variation in the degree of cytotoxicity in individual human sera towards cultured pig (PK15) cells has been demonstrated [48]. Samples of human serum from 75 individuals of histo-blood group AB (to exclude any possible cytotoxic effect of anti-A or anti-B antibodies) showed widely differing cytotoxicity to pig cells in vitro, with PK15 cell death ranging from 1 % to 100 % (although 67 % of sera killed at least 50 % of the cells). The degree of cytotoxicity correlated with the titer of anti-αGal antibody, which also varied considerably among human sera. This finding is in contradistinction to previously reported data that suggested that all human sera showed a similar degree of cytotoxicity towards pig tissues [59]. Furthermore, we have found it easier to adsorb out or inhibit anti-αGal antibodies in some individuals than in others.

Anti-αGal antibodies were first identified in 1984 by Galili and his colleagues, who subsequently reported that these antibodies could only be detected in humans, apes and Old World monkeys and are not present in the lower nonhuman primates or other mammals [60–62]. The αGal antigen, however, is present in lower mammals. The gene encoding for α1,3-galactosyltransferase, which is essential for the production of α-galactose, is present in humans as a processed pseudogene [63] or has undergone a frameshift mutation and is no longer functional [64]. Galili et al. [65] initially focused their studies on autoimmune disorders, but in 1993 presented evidence supporting the concept that anti-αGal antibodies play a significant role in the hyperacute rejection of transplanted pig organs [51].

Identification of the Carbohydrate Epitopes on Pig Vascular Endothelium

Pig tissues were screened by immunofluorescence with lectins, monoclonal antibodies and human natural antibodies for the presence of carbohydrate antigens on the vascular endothelium which may be potential targets for HAR in pig-to-human xenotransplantation. The results, reviewed elsewhere in this volume (Chap. 4), demonstrated the presence of αGal epitopes on the vascular endothelium of all organs examined [66,67]. Samuelsson et al. [68, 69] in Goteborg confirmed the structure of the epitope and determined the complete pentasaccharide structure of the major pig kidney αGal neutral glycosphingolipid to be αGal1–3βGal1–4βGlcNAc1–3βGal1–4βGlc1–1 ceramide.

Inhibition of Serum Cytotoxicity by αGal Oligosaccharides In Vitro

Initial studies using the chromium (^{52}Cr) release assay with labeled target cells of pig kidney cell line LLC PK1, pig erythrocytes, and pig lymphocytes demonstrated that cytotoxicity of human serum of any ABO group could be signifi-

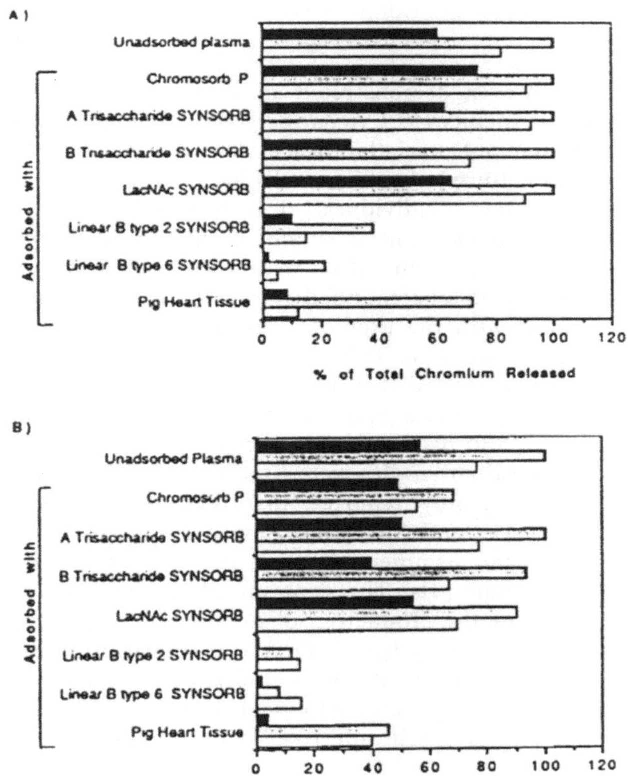

Fig. 3. A Human O plasma and **B** human AB plasma were incubated alone, with uncoated Chromosorb P, or with various carbohydrate structures attached to the Chromosorb P (SYNSORB). These plasmas were also perfused through pig heart tissue and then collected. Samples were used to measure antibody-mediated lysis using chromium release from labeled target cells of pig kidney cell line LLCPK1 (total release, 17300 cpm), pig erythrocytes (total release, 9100 cpm), and pig lymphocytes (total release, 11300 cpm). *LacNAc SYNSORB*, βGal1–4βGlcNAc bound to Synsorb. (From [44]) Solid bars-pig kidney cells. Shaded bars-pig RBC. Open bars-pig lymphocytes

cantly reduced after passage through an immunoaffinity column of an αGal trisaccharide or disaccharide [44] (Fig. 3). Antibody-mediated lysis of sheep and bovine erythrocytes was also reduced by preadsorption of human plasma with immobilized αGal1–3Gal oligosaccharides, suggesting that human anti-αGal antibodies were directed against the same αGal epitopes in several nonprimate mammals. Lysis of pig kidney cells was also virtually abolished when human plasma was incubated with any one of the three soluble αGal oligosaccharides. Haptens of unrelated structure did not inhibit these cytotoxic antibodies.

These initial experiments demonstrated some heterogeneity in the population (later confirmed independently by Cairns et al. [70]), since the cytotoxic antibodies found in some plasma apparently required adsorption by the αGal trisaccharide structure while the αGal disaccharide was sufficient in other plasma. Similarly, the cytotoxicity of some sera was more markedly reduced by immunoadsorption with the type 2 trisaccharide than the type 6, and vice versa.

In 1992, Koren et al. [71] developed a simple in vitro test to measure human and baboon serum cytotoxicity to pig cells. Pig kidney (PK15) cells, which were demonstrated to express abundant αGal epitopes, are grown in cell culture, and live cells are differentiated from dead using a two-color fluorescence technique. Unmodified human or baboon plasma, when incubated with these cells for 60 min, leads to death of a percentage of cells (the percentage varying between individuals [48]). Extensive studies utilizing this test have confirmed that cytotoxicity of both human and baboon sera can only be significantly reduced or abolished by αGal structures with an α1–3 linkage, and not by a large selection of other carbohydrates [49, 72] (Table 2). Inhibition of cytotoxicity is dependent on the concentration of αGal oligosaccharide (Fig. 4). Importantly, we (F.A. Neethling et al., unpublished) and others [73] have demonstrated that cell death can be prevented by prior treatment of the cells with α-galactosidase,

Table 2. Concentration of oligosaccharides needed to obtain 50 % inhibition of cytotoxicity of unmodified human or baboon serum on PK15 cells

Oligosaccharide	Concentration (in μM) in serum	
	Human	Baboon
1. Fucα1–2Galβ1-R	>10 000	>10 000
2. Galβ1-R	>10 000	>10 000
3. Galα1–2Galβ1-R'	7000	>10 000
4. Galα1–3Gal	386(±149)[a]	301(±44)[e]
5. Galα1–3Galβ1–4Gal	163(±73)[b]	141(±60)[f]
6. Galα1–3Galβ1–4Galα1–3Gal	54(±31)[c]	119(±30)[g]
7. Galα1–3Galβ1–4GlcNAc	27(±11)[d]	31(±4)[h]

From [74].
Bold type indicates structural differences of the oligosaccharide from the major pig vascular endothelium glycolipid Galα1–3Galβ1–4GlcNAcβ1–3Galβ1–4Glcβ1-Cer. R represents one to three or one to four linkages to Gal or to GlcNAc; R' is -$O(CH_2)_3NHCOCF_3$. The results of the strong inhibitors[a–h] are expressed as mean ± SD (n=3). Statistical significance: a vs. c (t, 3.1); a vs. d (t, 3.9); b vs. d (t, 3.1); e vs. h (t, 9.7); f vs. h (t, 3.1); g vs. h (t, 5.4), all with p<0.02. The other comparisons did not reach the p=0.05 level of significance.

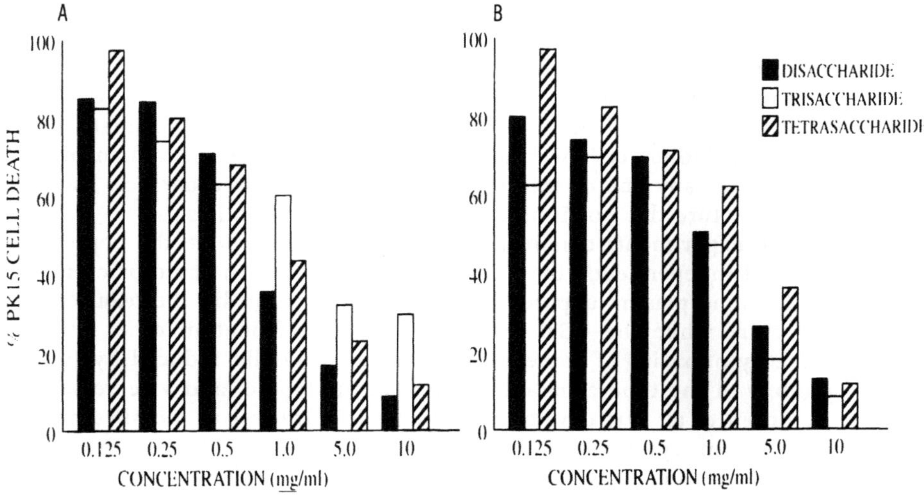

Fig. 4A,B. Reduction in cytotoxicity of (A) human and (B) baboon serum on PK15 cells after incubation of serum with increasing concentrations of α-galactosyl oligosaccharides (Dextra, Reading, UK). B disaccharide is αGal1–3Gal; B trisaccharide is αGal1–3βGal1–4Gal; B tetrasaccharide is αGal1–3βGal1–4αGal1–3Gal. (From [72])

which removes the terminal αGal molecule, thus confirming the importance of anti-αGal antibody-antigen binding to the cytotoxicity of the serum.

Recent observations suggest that, although anti-αGal antibodies recognize the epitope from its non-reducing end, substitutions at the reducing terminus can also modify the antibody-binding capacity [74]. The addition of methyl-α-Gal to human serum gives weak inhibition of cytotoxicity (Fig. 4), whereas the Galα1–3Gal disaccharide substantially inhibits the reaction, and the Galα1–3Galβ1–4GlcNAc trisaccharide is ten times more efficient. The modification from α to β anomeric configuration of the non-reducing end results in a complete loss of activity, while substitutions at the reducing end induce only a partial loss of activity. Modified tri- and tetrasaccharides are better inhibitors than the disaccharide, but not as good as the trisaccharide Galα1–3Galβ1–4GlcNAc. The reducing terminus therefore contributes some energy to the reaction, indicating that certain oligosaccharides will be of more potential clinical use than others. Furthermore, data from Rieben et al. [49] suggest that the stereochemical presentation of the αGal oligosaccharide plays an important role and must be considered in designing oligosaccharides intended for neutralization of anti-pig antibodies.

In Vivo Studies of "Oligosaccharide Therapy" in Baboons

Having shown in vitro that the antibody could be readily adsorbed from human or baboon plasma by an immunoaffinity column of αGal trisaccharide and, furthermore, that the adsorbed plasma was not cytotoxic to pig PK15 cells (but that the anti-αGal antibodies eluted from the column were highly cytotoxic [72], in vivo studies were undertaken [75, 76].

Initially, none of the αGal1-3Gal oligosaccharides was available to us in the large quantities required for extracorporeal immunoadsorption (EIA) or continuous i.v. infusion in baboons. As our in vitro studies had demonstrated that melibiose (αGal1-6Glc) and arabinogalactan (an impure polysaccharide of plant origin with an αGal terminal residue) had some protective effect on the cytotoxic activity of both human and baboon sera [72], we chose to infuse these, even though they were effective only at 50–100 times the concentration of the αGal disaccharide.

The i.v. infusion of melibiose and/or arabinogalactan at extremely high concentrations (<50 g/h) completely eliminated the cytotoxicity of the serum to PK15 cells in four of 15 baboons, and greatly reduced it in all others. (The i.v. infusion of carbohydrates devoid of terminal αGal, such as dextrose, dextran, or mannitol, even in high concentrations, i.e., <40 g/h, had no effect). However, if continued for more than a few hours or days, these infusions were toxic, manifested by hemorrhage in the kidneys and lungs and, although pig heart survival in one baboon was extended (from a control of 10 min) to more than 12 h, were clearly not suitable for the long-term infusion necessary to allow accommodation to develop.

The efficacy of EIA was also demonstrated in these studies. Utilizing an immunoaffinity column of melibiose, the EIA of baboon plasma on four consecutive days reduced serum cytotoxicity to PK15 cells to less than 20 %. After the fourth immunoadsorption, the addition of an i.v. infusion of arabinogalactan or melibiose reduced serum cytotoxicity further to 2 %–12 %.

More recently, we have been able to obtain sufficient αGal disaccharide to make up an immunoaffinity column for the EIA of anti-αGal antibodies in three baboons [77, 78]. In all three cases, EIA was effective in significantly reducing serum cytotoxicity and the level of anti-αGal antibody in the baboon serum. When pharmacologic immunosuppression was added and prior splenectomy carried out, anti-αGal antibody levels and cytotoxicity were both negligible after a course of EIA. This state persisted in one baboon for a period of almost 3 weeks (Fig. 5). Although no pig organ transplants were performed in this initial study, the protocol clearly reduced serum cytotoxicity to the point that it would seem likely that HAR would not occur and that accommodation might develop. Studies are progressing to confirm this conclusion.

Porcine Stomach Mucin as a Source of αGal Oligosaccharide

Chemically synthesized oligosaccharides are expensive and difficult to produce in large quantities (although these disadvantages are likely to be overcome by the use of enzymatic techniques of production). We therefore searched for another cheaper and more plentiful source of αGal oligosaccharide. After studies by Zhao et al. [79] had demonstrated that porcine stomach mucin (PSM) at various concentrations reduced the cytotoxic activity of human serum on pig endothelial cells, we undertook an extensive study of PSM both in vitro and in vivo [80–82]. (Chemical analysis indicates that PSM comprises of (w/w): 37 % hexosamine, 27 % total hexose, 10 % fucose, 20 % protein, and 6 % neuraminic (sialic) acid [83].

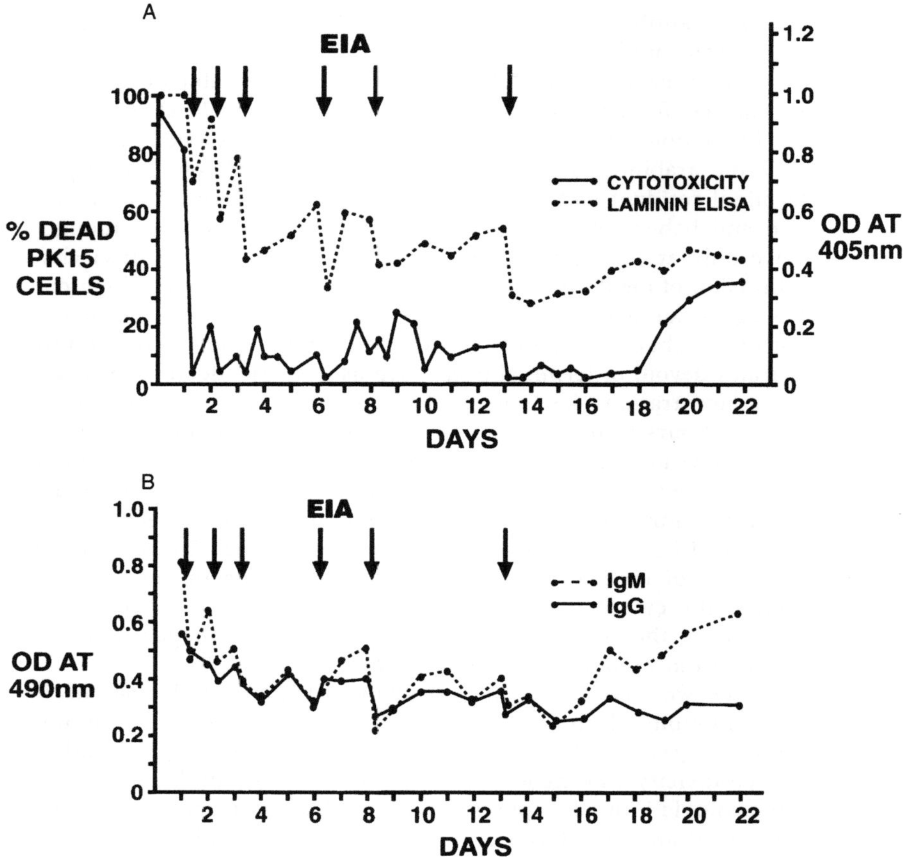

Fig. 5A,B. Changes in (A) serum cytotoxicity to PK15 cells and anti-αGal antibody level (measured by mouse laminin enzyme-linked immunosorbent assay, *ELISA*) and (B) anti-pig IgM and IgG levels (measured by pig PK15 cell ELISA). *EIA*, extracorporeal immunoadsorption; *OD*, optical density. (From [77])

Carbohydrate compositional analysis of PSM shows that it contains primarily four monosaccharides – fucose, galactose, *N*-acetyl-galactosamine (GalNAc), and *N*-acetyl-glucosamine (GlcNAc) (S.F. Li, unpublished).

A crude preparation of PSM inhibited the cytotoxicity of both baboon and human sera to PK15 cells in vitro, reducing pig cell death to 7% and 30%, respectively, at 2.5 mg/ml. Passage of human serum over an immunoaffinity column of crude PSM also resulted in a reduction in cytotoxicity to 24%–44% (depending on the solid matrix used). The i.v. administration of crude PSM to a baboon led to significant, but incomplete, inhibition of serum cytotoxicity to PK15 cells.

Due to the size and composition of the PSM molecules, PSM is almost certainly immunogenic. Crude PSM was therefore purified by β-elimination (to remove the protein fraction) and immunoaffinity chromatography on a column

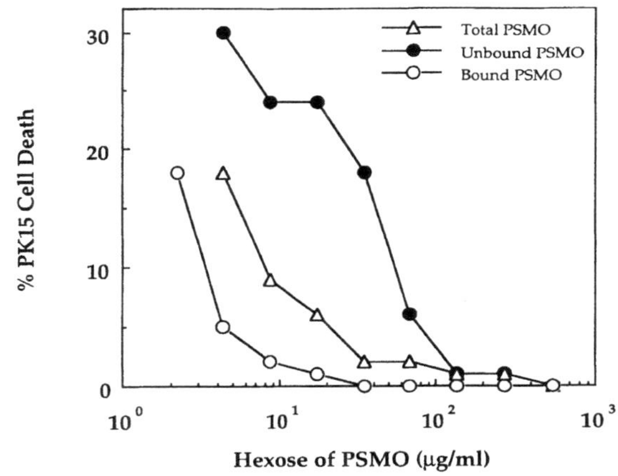

Fig. 6. Reduction of cytotoxicity of baboon serum to cultured PK15 cells by porcine stomach mucin oligosaccharides (*PSMO*). The initial cytotoxicity of the serum was low. The antibody column-bound PSMO was approximately 15 times more efficient than the antibody column-unbound PSMO, and four times more efficient than the total (β-eliminated) PSMO in reducing cytotoxicity of baboon serum to PK15 cells

of anti-αGal antibody to give rise to three different PSM oligosaccharide fractions (PSMO): (1) β-eliminated (total), (2) antibody (Ab) column-bound, and (3) Ab column-unbound. These PSMO were also tested both in vitro and in vivo. The most potent inhibitor of the cytotoxicity of baboon serum to PK15 cells in vitro was the anti-αGal Ab column-bound PSMO (i.e., predominantly αGal oligosaccharides), followed by the β-eliminated PSMO, with the Ab column-unbound PSMO being the least effective (Fig. 6). In vivo studies demonstrated that both β-eliminated and, particularly, Ab column-bound PSMO significantly inhibited (a) baboon serum cytotoxicity and (b) binding of baboon anti-αGal antibodies to mouse laminin for 72 h after i.v. infusion (Fig. 7).

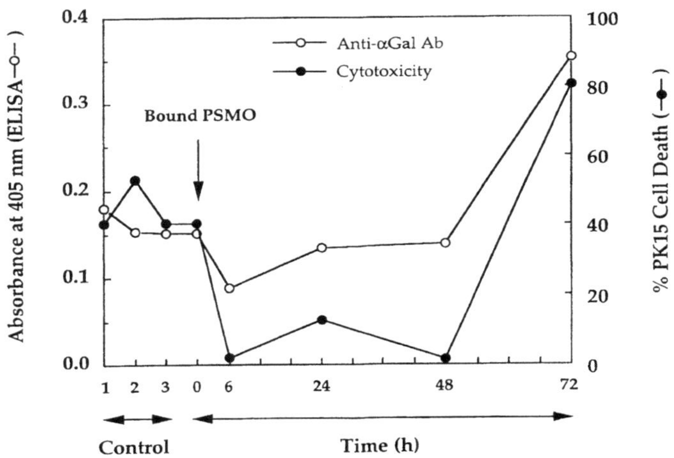

Fig. 7. Inhibition of baboon serum cytotoxicity to PK15 cells and of anti-αGal antibody binding to mouse laminin by the intravenous infusion of 6.8 mg antibody column-bound porcine stomach mucin oligosaccharides (*PSMO*) administered over 10 min. Both cytotoxicity and antibody binding were markedly reduced for 48 h, at which time a rebound of both cytotoxicity and antibody binding is seen. The *arrow* indicates the time of infusion of antibody column-bound PSMO

Comment

In summary, therefore, we have documented that HAR is primarily initiated by preformed anti-αGal antibodies present in human (and nonhuman primate) serum directed against αGal epitopes on the surface of the vascular endothelium of the pig. Present evidence is that no other antibodies play a major role, although this cannot be totally excluded in all cases. Activation of the complement system follows, leading to rapid destruction of the transplanted organ. When HAR is avoided by some form of immune manipulation, other mechanisms (possibly also related to the presence of anti-αGal antibody) lead to early graft destruction by what has been termed "delayed xenograft (vascular) rejection" [27, 84, 85], which is discussed elsewhere in this volume. For example, when complement activity is completely negated by the administration of cobra venom factor to the host, features suggestive of vascular or mixed vascular/cellular rejection, (although not hyperacute), still develop within a few days [27, 85].

We have therefore suggested the development of immunoaffinity columns of an αGal oligosaccharide capable of being used in an EIA system to deplete anti-αGal antibodies from the host, during which period the pig organ would be transplanted into the human recipient. Alternatively, or in addition, the continuous i.v. infusion of an oligosaccharide into the host to "neutralize" antibody would also be beneficial until the organ is accommodated. Whether prior splenectomy will increase the likelihood of accommodation occurring (by reducing the rebound of anti-αGal antibody) remains uncertain. Observations in this regard from the related field of organ allotransplantation in the presence of ABO incompatibility are conflicting, with Alexandre et al. observing improved results in splenectomized patients [9, 10], although splenectomy was not essential in our own studies in baboons [14, 15]. As it has been well-documented that splenectomy results in less rebound of antibody after antibody depletion [86], this procedure may well be beneficial.

Concomitant pharmacologic immunosuppressive therapy will clearly be required to prevent the subsequent development of cellular rejection and perhaps also to reduce the production of new antibody by B lymphocytes, particularly during the early post-transplant period while accommodation is taking place. If accommodation proves not to be a mechanism by which discordant xenotransplantation can be achieved, then acceptance of a discordant xenograft might still be possible if, following removal of the human anti-pig antibodies, their titer could be maintained at very low levels by one or a combination of immunosuppressive drugs.

Three groups independently suggested that the ultimate solution to the problem of discordant xenotransplantation might be to genetically engineer a pig that does not express αGal epitopes on its vascular endothelium [51, 87, 88]. To prevent expression of the enzyme α1,3-galactosyltransferase (α1,3GT), the encoding gene would need to be deleted, interrupted, or replaced, either within the coding region or within the regulatory sequences, so that enzyme is not produced.

Genes encoding α1,3GT from various species have been identified [89–91], including a pig genomic DNA clone [88]. Although techniques to inactivate or "knockout" the expression of the galactosyltransferase gene in pigs have not yet been demonstrated, such techniques are established in the mouse and, with the current rate of advancement in the field of genetic engineering, it is likely that they will prove feasible in swine in the future. However, McKenzie's group in Australia have reported that knockout of the αGal leads to expression of other oligosaccharides (that are normally cryptic) against which there are also antibodies in human serum (I.F.C. McKenzie, personal communication) and does not result in complete protection from the cytotoxicity of human serum.

Alternative methodologies to produce animals with altered expression of α1,3GT have been suggested and have been discussed previously [87]. For example, the DNA encoding for another enzyme (such as a fucosyltransferase or sialyltransferase) that would modify the sugar structures could be inserted into the embryo where it would be incorporated into the chromosomes and expressed to modify or mask the immunoreactivity of the αGal structure of the cell surfaces (Fig. 4). Progress in this respect is being made by Sandrin et al. [92] (Chap. 50), who transfected COS cells simultaneously with cDNA clones encoding α1,2-fucosyltransferase (α1,2FT) and α1,3GT and demonstrated preferential expression of the H histo-blood group oligosaccharide (αFuc1–2βGal1–4βGlcNAc) rather than αGal. Furthermore, in a pig kidney cell line that expressed (natural) αGal and H (by transfection) epitopes, the increased expression of H resulted in a major decrease in expression of αGal. Coexpression of two enzymes (α1,2FT and α1,3GT) in both the COS and pig cells resulted in a major decrease in human antibody binding and in complement-mediated cell lysis.

As a knockout pig cannot as yet be bred, and as expression of the H antigen does not completely obscure expression of αGal, we suggested a further possible approach [77], namely a genetically engineered pig that expresses a cDNA encoding α-galactosidase [93–95] together with a cDNA encoding α1,2-fucosyltransferase. Such a combined approach might well result in pigs that are αGal-negative.

Recent developments in gene therapy techniques suggest another possible future direction in depleting or masking the αGal epitope that may prove an alternative to the genetic engineering techniques discussed above. Techniques of introducing a gene directly into the endothelium of an organ, either in vivo [96] or ex vivo [97] by organ perfusion of the arterial system (e.g., of the heart by the coronary circulation) have recently been described. The selected gene could therefore be introduced into the pig organ's arterial system by the use of a balloon catheter either before or immediately after excision. Such gene function in the vascular endothelium would be anticipated to persist at least for some weeks, which may be sufficient time to allow accommodation to develop.

In summary, numerous studies since 1991 have clearly confirmed the important role of anti-αGal antibodies in the HAR (and possibly in the delayed vascular rejection) of pig organs by humans and nonhuman primates. A satisfactory method of preventing this antibody-antigen binding might well resolve the major problems of discordant xenotransplantation. Approaches to achieve this include (a) anti-αGal antibody depletion or inhibition in the recipient and (b) modification of oligosaccharide epitope expression in the donor pig.

References

1. ROSENBERG, J.C., BROERSMA, R.J., BULLEMER, G., et al. Relationship of platelets, blood coagulation, and fibrinolysis to hyperacute rejection of renal xenografts. Transplantation. 1969, 8, 152
2. ROSENBERG, J.C., HAWKINS, E., RECTOR,F. Mechanisms of immunological injury during antibody-mediated hyperacute rejection of renal heterografts. Transplantation. 1971, 11, 151
3. HAMMER, C., CHAUSSEY, C.H., BRENDEL, W. Preformed natural antibodies in animals and man. Outlook on xenotransplantation. Eur. Surg. Res. 1973, 5, 162
4. HAMMER, C. Isohemagglutinins and preformed natural antibodies in xenogeneic organ transplantation. Transplant. Proc. 1987, 19, 4443
5. WIENER, A.S. Origin of naturally-occurring hemagglutinins and hemolysins: a review. J. Immunol. 1951, 66, 287
6. SPRINGER, G.F., HORTON, R.F. Blood group isoantibody stimulation in man by feeding blood group-active bacteria. J. Clin. Invest. 1969, 48, 1280
7. PLATT, J.L., BACH, F.H. Mechanism of tissue injury in hyperacute xenograft rejection. In: Xenotransplantation. (Cooper, D.K.C. et al., eds) Springer, Heidelberg, 1991, p. 69
8. ROSE, A.G., COOPER, D.K.C., HUMAN, P.A., REICHENSPURNER, H., REICHART, B. Histopathology of hyperacute rejection of the heart- experimental and clinial observations in allografts and xenografts. J. Heart Lung Transplant. 1991, 10, 223
9. ALEXANDRE, G.P., SQUIFFLET, J.P., DE BRUYERE, M., et al. Splenectomy as a prerequisite for successful human ABO-incompatible renal transplantation. Transplant. Proc. 1985, 17, 138
10. ALEXANDRE, G.P.J., SQUIFFLET, J.P., DE BRUYERE, E.M., et al. Present experiences in a series of 26 ABO-incompatible living donor renal allografts. Transplant. Proc. 1987, 19, 4538
11. BANNETT, A.D., McALACK, R.F., RAJA, R., BAQUERO, A., MORRIS, M. Experiences with known ABO-mismatched renal transplants. Transplant. Proc. 1987, 19, 4543
12. COOPER, D.K.C. Depletion of natural antibodies in non-human primates – a step towards successful discordant xenografting in humans. Clin. Transplantation. 1992, 6, 178
13. COOPER, D.K.C. Is xenotransplantation a realistic clinical option? Transplant. Proc. 1992, 24, 2393
14. COOPER, D.K.C., YE, Y., KEHOE, M., et al. A novel approach to "neutralization" of preformed antibodies: cardiac allotransplantation across the ABO-blood group barrier as a paradigm of discordant xenotransplantation. Transplant. Proc. 1992, 24, 566
15. COOPER, D.K.C., YE, Y., NIEKRASZ, M., et al. Specific intravenous carbohydrate therapy – a new concept in inhibiting antibody-mediated rejection: experience with ABO-incompatible cardiac allografting in the baboon. Transplantation. 1993, 56, 769
16. COOPER, D.K.C., GOOD, A.H., MALCOLM, A.J., et al. Specific intravenous carbohydrate therapy – a new approach to the inhibition of antibody-mediated rejection following ABO-incompatible allografting and discordant xenografting. Transplant. Proc. 1993, 25, 377
17. BACH, F.H., TURMAN, M.A., VERCELLOTTI, G.M., PLATT, J.L., DALMASSO, A.P. Accommodation: a working paradigm for progressing toward clinical discordant xenografting. Transplant. Proc. 1991, 23, 205

18. COOPER, D.K.C. Clinical survey of heart transplantation between ABO-blood group incompatible recipients and donors. J. Heart Transplant. 1990, 9, 376
19. COOK, D.J., GRAVER, B., TERASAKI, P.I. ABO-incompatibility in cadaver donor kidney allografts. Transplant. Proc. 1987, 19, 4549
20. OPELZ, G. Collaborative Kidney Transplant Study Newsletter 2, 1988
21. GORDON, R.D., IWATSUKI, S., ESQUIVEL, C.O., et al. Experience with primary liver transplantation across ABO blood groups. Transplant. Proc. 1987, 19, 4575
22. COOPER, D.K.C., LEXER, G., ROSE, A.G., et al. Cardiac allotransplantation across major blood group barriers in the baboon. J. Med. Primatol. 1988, 17, 333
23. COOPER, D.K.C., HUMAN, P.A., LEXER, G., et al. Effects of cyclosporine and antibody adsorption on pig cardiac xenograft survival in the baboon. J. Heart Transplant. 1988, 7, 238
24. ALEXANDRE, G.P.J., GIANELLO, P., LATINNE, D., et al. Plasmapheresis and splenectomy in experimental renal xenotransplantation. In: Xenograft 25. (Hardy, M.A., ed) New York, Elsevier, 1989, p. 259
25. FISCHEL, R.J., PLATT, J.L., MATAS, A.J., et al. Prolonged survival of a discordant cardiac xenograft in a rhesus monkey. Transplant. Proc. 1991, 23, 589
26. ROSLIN M.S., ZISBROD, Z., BURACK, J.H., et al. 15-day survival in pig-to-baboon heterotpic cardiac xenotransplantation. Transplant. Proc. 1992, 24, 572
27. KOBAYASHI, T., TANIGUCHI, S., YE, Y., et al. Delayed xenograft rejection in C3-depleted discordant (pig-to-baboon) cardiac xenografts treated with cobra venom factor. Transplant. Proc. In press
28. WHITE, D.J.G., BRAIDLEY, P., DUNNING, J., et al. Hearts from pigs transgenic for human DAF are not hyperacutely rejected when xenografted to primates. Presented to the Third International Congress for Xenotransplantation. Boston, 1995.
29. LIOYD, K.O., KABAT, E.A., LICERIO, E. Immunochemical studies on blood groups. 38: Structures and activities of oligosaccharides produced by alkaline degradation of blood-group Lewis-a substance. Proposed structure of the carbohydrate chains of human blood-group A, B, H, Le^a, and Le^b substances. Biochemistry. 1968, 7, 2976
30. WATKINS, W.M. Genetic regulation of the structure of blood-group-specific glycoproteins. Biochem. Soc. Symp. 1974, 40, 125
31. WATKINS, W.M. Biochemistry and genetics of the ABO, Lewis, and P blood group systems. In: Advances in Human Genetics, Vol. 10. Harris, H., Hirschhorn, K. (eds) Plenum, New York, 1980, p. 1
32. WATKINS, W.M. Biosynthesis. Molecular basis of antigenic specificity in the ABO, H and Lewis blood group systems. In: Glycoproteins, Montreuil, J., Schachter, H., Vligenhart, J.F.G. (eds) Elsevier, Amsterdam, 1995, p. 313
33. LEMIEUX, R.U. Human blood groups and carbohydrate structures. Chem. Soc. Rev. 1978, 7, 423
34. PINTO, B.M., BUNDLE, D.R. Preparation of glycoconjugates for use as artificial antigens: a simplified procedure. Carbohydrate Res. 1983, 124, 313
35. BENSINGER, W.I., BAKER, D.A., BUCKNER, C.D., CLIFT, R.A., THOMAS, E.D. Immunoadsorption for removal of A and B blood group antibodies. N. Engl. J. Med. 1981, 304, 1360
36. BENSINGER, W.I., BAKER, D.A., BUCKNER, C.D., CLIFT, R.A., THOMAS, E.D. In vitro and in vivo removal of anti-A erythrocyte antibody by adsorption to a synthetic immunoadsorbent. Transfusion. 1981, 21, 335

37. BENSINGER, W.I., BUCKNER, C.D., CLIFT, R.A. Whole blood immunoadsoption of anti-A or anti-B antibodies. Vox. Sang. 1985, 48, 357
38. ROMANO, E.L., BHARDWAJ, J., KELLY, S., et al. Interaction of IgG and IgM anti-A with synthetic oligosaccharides. Transplant. Proc. 1987, 19, 4479
39. ROMANO, E.L., SOYANO, A., LINARES, J. Preliminary human study of synthetic trisaccharide representing blood substance A. Transplant. Proc. 1987, 19, 4475
40. ROMANO, E.L., SOYANO, A., LINARES, J., LAUZON, G.J. Neutralization of ABO blood group antibodies by specific oligosaccharides. Transplant. Proc. 1987, 19, 4426
41. LAUS, R., ULRICHS, K., MULLER-RUCHHOLTZ, W. Carbohydrate-specific human heterophile antibodies in normal human sera that react with xenogeneic cells. Arch. Allergy Appl. Immun. 1988, 85, 201
42. PLATT, J.L., LINDMAN, B.J., CHEN, H., SPITALNIK, S.L., BACH, F.H. Endothelial cell antigens recognized by xenoreactive human natural antibodies. Transplantation. 1990, 50, 817
43. HOLGERSSON, J., CAIRNS, T.D.H., BREIMER, M.E., et al. Carbohydrate antigen specificity of pig lymphocytotoxic IgM antibodies produced by 2 EBV transformed human B cell lines. Glycoconjugate J. 1991, 8, 172
44. GOOD, A.H., COOPER, D.K.C., MALCOLM, A.J., et al. Identification of carbohydrate structures which bind human anti-porcine antibodies: implications for discordant xenografting in man. Transplant. Proc. 1992, 24, 559
45. COOPER, D.K.C., GOOD, A.H., KOREN, E., et al. Identification of α-galactosyl and other carbohydrates that are bound by human anti-pig antibodies: relevance to discordant xenografting in man. Transpl. Immunol. 1993, 1, 198
46. KOREN, E., NEETHLING, F.A., YE, Y., et al. Heterogeneity of preformed human anti-pig xenogeneic antibodies. Transplant. Proc. 1992, 24, 598
47. KOREN, E., NEETHLING, F.A., RICHARDS, S., et al. Binding and specificity of major immunoglobulin classes of preformed human anti-pig heart antibodies. Transplant. Int. 1993, 6, 351
48. KUJUNDZIC, M., KOREN, E., NEETHLING, F.A., et al. Variability of anti-Gal antibodies in human serum and their relation to serum cytotoxicity against pig cells. Xenotransplantation. 1994, 1, 58
49. RIEBEN, R., VON ALLMEN, E., KORCHAGINA, E.Y., et al. Detection, immunoadsorption, and inhibition of cytotoxic activity of anti-αGal antibodies using newly developed substances with synthetic Galα1–3Gal disaccharide epitopes. Xenotransplantation. 1995, 2, 98
50. SANDRIN, M.S., VAUGHAN, H.A., DABKOWSKI, P.L., McKENZIE, I.F.C. Anti-pig IgM antibodies in human serum react predominantly with Gal(α1–3)Gal epitopes. Proc. Natl. Acad. Sci. USA 1993, 90, 11391
51. GALILI, U. Interaction of the natural anti-Gal antibody with α-galactosyl epitopes: a major obstacle for xenotransplantation in humans. Immunology Today. 1993, 14, 480
52. CAIRNS, T., KARLSSON, E., HOLGERSSON, J., et al. Confirmation of a major target epitope of human natural IgG and IgM anti-pig antibodies: terminal galactose α1,3galactose. Transplant. Proc. 1994, 26, 1384
53. CAIRNS, T., HAMMELMANN, W., GRAY, D., WELSH, K., LARSEN, G. Enzymatic removal from various tissues of the galactose α1,3galactose target antigens of human antispecies antibodies. Transplant. Proc. 1994, 26, 1279

54. FOURNIER, A.M., BIRCHALL, I.E., KYRIAZIS, A.G., PEARSE, M.J., d'APICE, A.J.F. A human naturally-occurring antibody, anti-Gal, recognizes epitopes in pig kidney, heart and liver and is cytotoxic to endothelial cells in the presence of rabbit complement. Second International Congress on Xenotransplantation, Cambridge, U.K., 1993 (abstract 113), p. 142
55. KARLSSON, E., CAIRNS, T., HOLGERSSON, J., WELSH, K., SAMUELSSON, B.E. Pig-to-human xenotransplantation. Confirmation of a major target epitope of preformed human natural IgG and IgM anti-pig-terminal galactose α1,3galactose. Glycoconjugate J. 1993, 10, 297
56. WIESLANDER, J., MANSSON, O., KALLIN, E., et al. Specificity of human antibodies against Galα1-3Gal carbohydrate epitope and distinction from natural antibodies reacting with Galα1-2Gal or Galα1-4Gal. Glycoconjugate J. 1990, 7, 85
57. MINANOV, O., ITESCU, S., KWIATKOWSKI, P., et al. Preformed and induced anti-Gal cytotoxic antibodies in newborn humans and baboons. (Abstract) J. Heart Lung Transplant., 1996, 15, 101
58. GALILI, U., MANDRELL, R.E., HAMADEH, R.M., SHOHET, S.B., GRIFFISS, J.M. Interaction between the human natural anti-α-galactosyl Immunoglobulin G and bacteria of the human flora. Infect. Immun. 1988, 57, 1730
59. WELSH, K.I., TAUBE, D.H., THICK, M., et al. Human antibodies to pig determinants and their association with hyperacute rejection of xenografts. In: Xenotransplantation. (Cooper, D.K.C., et al., eds) Heidelberg, Springer, 1991, p. 501
60. GALILI, U., RACHMILEWITZ, E.A., PELEG, A., FLECHNER, I. A unique natural human IgG antibody with anti-α-galactosyl specificity. J. Exp. Med. 1984, 160, 1519
61. GALILI, U., CLARK, M.R., SHOHET, S.B., BUEHLER, J., MACHER, B.A. Evolutionary relationship between the natural anti-Gal antibody and the Galα1-3Gal epitope in primates. Proc. Natl. Acad. Sci. USA. 1987, 84, 1369
62. GALILI, U., SHOHET, S.B., KOBRIN, E., STULTS, C.L.M., MACHER, B.A. Man, apes and Old World monkeys differ from other mammals in the expression of α-galactosyl epitopes on nucleated cells. J. Biol. Chem. 1988, 263, 17755
63. JOZIASSE, D.H., SHAPER, J.H., JABS, E.W., SHAPER, N.L. Characterization of an αGal1-3-galactosyltransferase homologue on human chromosome 12 that is organized as a processed psdeudogene. J. Biol. Chem. 1991, 266, 6991
64. LARSEN, R.D., RIVERA-MARRERO, C.A., ERNST, L.K., CUMMINGS, R.D., LOWE, J.B. Frameshift and nonsense mutations in a human genomic sequence homologous to a murine UDP-Gal:β-D-Gal(1-4)-D-GlcNAcα(1-3)-galactosyl transferase cDNA. J. Biol. Chem. 1990, 265, 7055
65. GALILI, U. The natural anti-Gal antibody: evolution and autoimmunity in man. Immunol. Series. 1991, 55, 355
66. ORIOL, R., YE, Y., KOREN, E., COOPER, D.K.C. Carbohydrate antigens of pig tissues reacting with human natural antibodies as potential targets for hyperacute vascular rejection in pig-to-man organ xenotransplantation. Transplantation. 1993, 56, 1433
67. ORIOL, R., BARTHOD, F., BERGEMER, A-M, et al. Monomorphic and polymorphic carbohydrate antigens on pig tissues: implications for organ xenotransplantation in the pig-to-man model. Transplant. Int. 1994, 7, 405

68. BACKER, A.E., HOLGERSSON, J., KARLSSON, H., BINNS, R.M., SAMUELSSON, B.E. (1993) Structural characterization of glycosphingolipids in different organs of a semi-inbred pig strain using GC/MS of ceramide glycanase-released oligosaccharides. Second International Congress on Xenotransplantation. Cambridge, U.K. (abstract 24) p. 52
69. RYDBERG, I., CAIRNS, T.D.H., GROTH, C.G., et al. Specificities of human IgM and IgG anticarbohydrate xenoantibodies found in the sera of diabetic patients grafted with fetal pig islets. Xenotransplantation. 1994, 1, 69
70. CAIRNS, T., LEE, J., GOLDBERG, L., et al. Polymorphism within the human IgG anti-pig repertoire. (Abstract) Presented to the British Transplantation Society. Manchester, U.K., 1995
71. KOREN, E., NEETHLING, F.A., KOSCEC, M., et al. In vitro model for hyperacute rejection of xenogeneic cells. Transplant. Proc. 1994, 26, 1166
72. NEETHLING, F.A., KOREN, E., YE, Y., et al. Protection of pig kidney (PK15) cells from the cytotoxic effect of anti-pig antibodies by α-galactosyl oligosaccharides. Transplantation. 1994, 57, 959
73. LA VECCHIO, J.A., DUNNE, A.D., EDGE, A.S.B. Enzymatic removal of alpha-galactosyl epitopes from porcine endothelial cells diminishes the cytotoxic effect of natural antibodies. Transplantation. 1995, 68, 841
74. NEETHLING, F., JOZIASSE, D., BOVIN, N., et al. The reducing end of αGal oligosaccharides contributes to their efficiency in blocking natural antibodies of human and baboon sera. Transplant. Int. 1996, 9, 98
75. YE, Y., NEETHLING, F.A., NIEKRASZ, M., et al. Intravenous administration of α-galactosyl carbohydrates reduces in vivo baboon serum cytotoxicity to pig kidney cells and transplanted pig hearts. Transplant. Proc. 1994, 26, 1399
76. YE, Y., NEETHLING, F.A., NIEKRASZ, M., et al. Evidence that intravenously administered α-galactosyl carbohydrates reduce baboon serum cytotoxicity to pig kidney cells (PK15) and transplanted pig hearts. Transplantation. 1994, 58, 330
77. TANIGUCHI, S., NEETHLING, F.A., BOVIN, N., et al. In vivo immunoadsorption of anti-pig antibodies in baboons using a specific αGal1–3Gal column. Transplantation. In press
78. COOPER, D.K.C., KOREN, E., ORIOL, R. Manipulation of the anti-αGal antibody-αGal epitope system in experimental discordant xenotransplantation. Xenotransplantation. 1996, 3, 102
79. ZHAO, Z., MICHALSKI, J.C., CHEREAU, C., et al. An approach to the structure of carbohydrate epitopes recognized by human natural antibodies on porcine endothelial cells. Transplant. Proc. 1994, 26, 1390
80. LI, S.F., YEH, J-C, COOPER, D.K.C., CUMMINGS, R.D. Inhibition of human anti-αGal IgG by oligosaccharides derived from porcine stomach mucin. Xenotransplantation. 1995, 2, 279
81. LI, S.F., NEETHLING, F.A., YEH, J-C, COOPER, D.K.C. Potent inhibition of human and baboon anti-αGal antibodies by a subfraction of oligosaccharides derived from porcine stomach mucin. Transplant. Proc. 1996, 28, 558
82. LI, S.F., NEETHLING, F.A., TANIGUCHI, S., et al. Glycans derived from porcine stomach mucin are effective inhibitors of natural anti-αGal antibodies in vitro and in vivo. Transplantation. In press

83. GLENISTER, D.A., SALAMON, K.E., SMITH, K., BEIGHTON, D., KEEVIL, C.W. Enhanced growth of complex communities of dental plaque bacteria in mucin-limited continuous culture. Microbiol. Ecol. in Health and Dis. 1988, 1, 31
84. INVERARDI, L., SAMAJA, M., MARELLI, F., BENDER, J.R., PARDI, R. Cellular immune recognition of xenogeneic vascular endothelium. Transplant. Proc. 1992, 24, 459
85. LEVENTHAL, J.R., DALMASSO, A.P., CROMWELL, J.W., et al., Prolongation of cardiac xenograft survival by depletion of complement. Transplantation. 1993, 55, 857
86. REDING, R., WHITE, D.J.G., DAVIES, H.ff.S., et al. Effect of splenectomy on antibody rebound after plasma exchange. Transplantation. 1989, 48, 145
87. COOPER, D.K.C., KOREN, E., ORIOL, R. Genetically engineered pigs. Lancet. 1993, 342, 682
88. DABKOWSKI, P.L., VAUGHAN, H.A., McKENZIE, I.F.C., SANDRIN, M.S. Characterization of a cDNA clone encoding the pig α1,3galactosyltransferase: implications for xenotransplantation. Transplant. Proc. 1993, 25, 2921
89. LARSEN, R.D., RAJAN, V.P., RUFF, M., et al. Isolation of a cDNA encoding murine UDP galactose: β-D-galactosyl-1,4-N-acetyl-D-glucosaminide α-1,3-galactosyltransferase: Expression cloning by gene transfer. Proc. Natl. Acad. Sci. USA. 1989, 86, 8227
90. LOWE, J.B., LARSEN, R.D., RUFF, M.M., CUMMINGS, R.D. Isolation of cloned cDNAs that direct expression of oligosaccharides recognized by Griffonia simplicifolia isolectin B_4. J. Cell. Biochem. 1989, 13A, 129
91. JOZIASSE, D.H., SHAPER, J.H., VAN DEN EIJNDEN, D.H., et al. Bovine α1–3 galactosyltransferase: isolation and characterization of a cDNA clone. Identification of homologous sequences in human genomic DNA. J. Biol. Chem. 1989, 264, 14290
92. SANDRIN, M.S., FODOR, W.L., MOUHTOURIS, E., et al. Enzymatic remodeling of the carbohydrate surface of a xenogeneic cell substantially reduces human antibody binding and complement-mediated cytolysis. Nature Med. 1995, 1, 1248
93. BISHOP, D.F., CALHOUN, D.H., BERNSTEIN, H.S., et al. Human α-galactosidase A: nucleotide sequence of a cDNA clone encoding the mature enzyme. Proc. Natl. Acad. Sci. USA. 1986, 83, 4859
94. DEN HERDER, I.F., MATEO ROSELL, A.M., VAN ZUILEN, C.M., PUNT, P.J., VEN DEN HONDEL, C.A.M.J.J. Cloning and expression of a member of the Aspergillus niger gene family encoding αgalactosidase. Mol. Gen. Genet. 1992, 233, 404
95. ZHU, A., GOLDSTEIN, J. Cloning and functional expression of a cDNA encoding coffee bean α-galactosidase. Gene. 1994, 140, 227
96. LIM, C.S., CHAPMAN, G.D., GAMMON, R.S., et al. Direct in vivo gene transfer into the coronary and peripheral vasculatures of the intact dog. Circulation. 1991, 83, 2007
97. ARDEHALI, A., FYFE, A., LAKS, H., et al. (1995) Direct gene transfer into donor hearts at the time of harvest. J. Thorac. Cardiovasc. Surg. 1995, 109, 716

26 Removal of Natural Antibodies by Immunoadsorption: Results of Experimental Studies

J.R. Leventhal

Introduction

The clinical application of xenotransplantation from swine into humans will likely require the use of effective and well-tolerated techniques for antibody removal. This assumption is based upon the growing body of scientific evidence which implicates xenoreactive antibody binding and activation of the complement cascade as central events in the process of hyperacute xenograft rejection [1, 2]. Although transgenic approaches are presently being employed to engineer porcine organs which are inherently resistant to human antibody-dependent, complement-mediated damage (i.e., expression of human regulators of complement activation; αGal1–3Gal "knockout" swine), it is more than likely that removal of pre-existing xenoreactive antibodies will be necessary in the pretransplant period. In addition, it may be necessary to remove antibodies from the xenograft recipient after transplantation on a regular basis until a process of graft adaptation or accomodation takes place.

This chapter will first briefly review a number of strategies for antibody removal and/or blockade which have been used in xenotransplantation. Secondly, it will present in detail work from our laboratories using adsorptive columns for removal of human and baboon anti-pig antibodies. Finally, the utility of immunoadsorption using column technologies for prevention of porcine xenograft rejection in humans will be discussed.

Techniques for Removal of Preformed Natural Antibodies

As reviewed by Bach et al. [3], a number of methods have been used for the removal or neutralization of circulating preformed natural antibodies. These include: (a) plasma exchange or plasmapheresis, (b) nonspecific antibody sorbents, such as protein A columns, (c) specific antibody sorbents, such as xenogeneic organs or cell stroma, (d) injectable antigen, (e) nonspecific reducing agents, such as penicillamine, which disrupt the activity of IgM, and (f) blockade of antibody binding (i.e., Fab fragment administration). To date, removal of xenoreactive antibodies has been achieved in experimental models predominantly by either plasmapheresis or organ perfusion.

Plasmapheresis is a nonselective technique for antibody removal in which whole blood is removed from the circulation, followed by the separation and return of the erythrocyte fraction to the subject in an appropriate crystalloid or colloid solution. Plasmapheresis has been employed clinically for a number of immunologic conditions, including systemic lupus erythematosus, myasthenia gravis, and thrombotic thrombocytopenic purpura. This technique has been applied to xenotransplantation with some success. Early experience with plasmapheresis for xenotransplantation involving nonprimate species during the 1960s and 1970s found antibody depletion using this method extended xenograft survival (4). In pig-to-primate xenotransplantation, Alexandre et al. used preoperative plasmapheresis and immunosuppression in splenectomized baboons to extend porcine renal xenograft survival, with one organ surviving for 22 days [5].

However, plasmapheresis has several limitations. The effectiveness of plasmapheresis is a function of the starting concentration of antibody component; thus the efficiency of the procedure for antibody removal decreases with each successive passage of plasma volume. Furthermore, plasmapheresis removes all circulating plasma proteins, including clotting factors, and may therefore result in a deleterious effect upon the coagulation system. This effect is likely to restrict the use of plasmapheresis in the peritransplant period, since bleeding complications may result. Replacement of clotting factors with fresh frozen plasma would be hazardous, since this blood product contains high levels of xenoreactive antibodies. Alternatively, it has been suggested that the stress of plasmapheresis might lead to the increased synthesis of acute phase reactants, which include coagulation factors, thus promoting the development of a hypercoaguable state in the post-pheresis period [6].

Another, more selective, approach to removal of xenoreactive antibodies is organ perfusion, where the recipient antibodies are removed through binding to an extracorporeal source of target xenoantigens. Antibody depletion by organ perfusion can delay hyperacute xenograft rejection [7–9]. In addition, the combination of organ perfusion with immunosuppression has extended pig-to-nonhuman primate xenograft survival for many days [8, 9]. Cooper et al. [7] used organ perfusion to deplete xenoreactive natural antibodies from baboons. Reduction in antibody titers to undetectable levels was associated with extension of heterotopic porcine cardiac xenograft survival to 60–120 h (mean, 52 h). Fischel et al. [9] used organ perfusion to remove xenoreactive antibodies from rhesus monkeys receiving porcine cardiac xenografts. Organ perfusion was well tolerated, resulted in significant removal of anti-pig antibodies and allowed for prolonged survival of cardiac xenografts. Organ perfusion, although effective, also has several disadvantages. Organ perfusion with whole blood leads to depletion of complement and clotting factors and a loss of intravascular blood volume. Although some of these effects may be mitigated by selective passage of recipient plasma without cellular elements through the target organ, organ perfusion would still be cumbersome to perform, requirng sacrifice of suitable donor animals. This logistic problem is magnified if one considers the potential need for repeated antibody depletions in the post-xenotransplant period.

An attractive alternative to plasmapheresis and organ perfusion is the application of immunoapheresis using affinity columns to specifically bind and remove antibodies. This approach avoids the consequences of wholesale plasma protein removal and costly replacement fluids seen with plasmapheresis, and is technically easier than organ perfusion. Columns containing immobilized staphylococcal proteins A and G have been used successfully for antibody removal in a number of autoimmune diseases and for renal transplant recipients with anti-HLA antibodies [10–12]. Shapiro et al. [13] have used a staphylococcal protein A column for antibody removal in a pig-to-dog renal transplant model. They achieved 84% and 71% reductions in total canine IgG and IgM, respectively. However, only a two- to fourfold reduction in dog anti-pig crossmatch titer was observed. Although time to onset of hyperacute rejection was prolonged in dogs treated with protein A column adsorption, significant morbidity and mortality in the treatment group occurred. Furthermore, clinical application of staphylococcal protein A and G columns for antibody removal in humans may be limited by the poor binding affinity of these immunosorbents for human IgM antibodies, the isotype closely associated with hyperacute xenograft rejection [1].

Columns using antibody conjugates as immunosorbents represent a novel approach for the selective removal of plasma components. Contrary to plasmapheresis or organ perfusion, antibody-based immunoadsorption (immunoapheresis) provides a highly specific depletion technique, using immobilized antibodies generated against one or several predetermined plasma components [14]. In fact, columns containing an immobilized antibody against human low-density lipoproteins (LDL-Therasorb) are in successful clinical use [15–17]. In an effort to develop an improved method for xenoreactive antibody removal, we have studied the utility of extracorporeal columns containing polyclonal antibodies directed against human immunoglobulins to selectively bind and remove antibodies from human and baboon plasma. These columns have been extensively tested using in vitro, ex vivo, and in vivo systems. As discussed below, our results indicate that columns containing anti-human IgG or IgM are extremely effective for removing baboon and human anti-porcine IgG and IgM natural antibodies from plasma. Removal of antibody was not associated with a significant reduction in coagulation factors. In addition, employment of both columns in vivo resulted in significant reductions in anti-pig antibodies in baboons. Furthermore, application of these columns in an ex vivo perfusion model has been shown to prevent hyperacute rejection. Finally, the combination of antibody removal pre- and post-transplant by immunoapheresis with immunosuppression prevented the hyperacute rejection of pig-to-baboon renal transplants. Reviews of these experimental observations have recently been reported [18, 19].

Methodology

Columns

Removal of antibodies was accomplished with two sterile and pyrogen-free columns containing polyclonal anti-human antibodies conjugated to cyanogen-bromide activated Sepharose beads. The first column (Ig-Therasorb column, Baxter Corp.) contained polyclonal sheep anti-human IgG (heavy and light chain specific) with a total column volume of 300 cc. The second column contained polyclonal sheep antihuman IgM (μ-chain specific) with a total column volume of 150 cc. Columns were kept filled with storage buffer (1X phosphate-buffered saline, 0.01% sodium azide, pH 7.2) at a temperature of 4 °C until use.

In Vitro Column Testing for Antibody Removal

Anti-human Ig columns were initially tested with recently outdated fresh frozen human plasma (500 cc per experiment) obtained from the University of Minnesota blood bank, or fresh baboon plasma (300–500 cc per experiment) obtained from baboon blood collected onto anticoagulant citrated dextrose. Columns were flushed with 4 l of 0.9N saline to remove their storage buffer prior to the application of plasma. Plasma was then run over the column for a total of two plasma volumes. Plasma retained in the column was removed by flushing the columns with one column volume of normal saline. Pre- and post-column plasma samples were obtained for measurement of total IgG and IgM, anti-pig IgG and IgM, transferrin, fibrinogen, factor 5, factor 8, and complement (CH50). The columns were regenerated at the end of each experiment by antibody desorption using three column volumes of 0.2 *M* glycine, pH 2.8. Column pH was then readjusted by passage of three column volumes of 1X phosphate-buffered saline. The regenerated columns were then either reused, or filled with one column volume of storage buffer and kept at 4 °C until further use.

Ex Vivo Testing of Anti-IgG and Anti-IgM Columns

Experiments were conducted using an ex vivo cardiac perfusion system that we have previously described [19]. Briefly, heart-lung blocks were harvested from from 20–25 kg outbred donor swine after topical cold-induced cardiac arrest. The heart was then instrumented and perfused with oxygenated blood via a Biomedicus centrifugal blood pump (Medtronic, Eden Prarie MN). For control studies, porcine blood was obtained from heart donors prior to organ harvest. Fresh human blood was obtained from normal donors. Blood was anticoagulated with 1.2 units heparin/ml and used within 3 h. All human blood was separated into plasma and cellular components by centrifugation (4200 rpm for 6 min). Plasma was either unmodified and recombined with cells at the time of priming of the perfusion circuit or passed through the Therasorb columns and then recombined with cellular components at perfusion circuit priming. An operational circuit volume of 600 ml was used in all experiments; perfusion circuits were primed and circulated for approximately 15 min prior to initiaiting cardiac reperfusion. During cardiac reperfusion, free water, glucose, insulin, and calcium were supplied to maintain stable serum osmolarity, electrolyte concentrations, and to provide a source of energy for cardiac metabolism. Functional parameters, including heart rate, ECG R wave voltage, oxygen consumption, and coronary artery resistance were measured. Blood samples were obtained at defined intervals for measurement of antibody,complement, and complete blood cell counts.

In Vivo Column Testing for Antibody Removal

Anti-human Ig columns were used to remove antibodies from naive baboons (10–15 kg) as shown in Fig. 1. Baboons were placed under general anesthesia and underwent placement of a double-lumen dialysis catheter in the internal jugular vein, under standard sterile operating room conditions. On line plasma separation with a Baxter Autopheresis C plasmapheresis machine was then instituted. Separated plasma was passed into an anti-human Ig column which had been flushed with 4 l of 0.9N saline. The column effluent was then recombined with the separated baboon blood cells and returned to the subject through the central venous line. A total of two plasma volumes were passed through the column during each procedure. In several experiments, the column was regenerated between the first and second plasma volume.

Measurement of Antibody. Human and baboon anti-porcine antibodies were measured by a previously described endothelial cell-targeted enzyme-linked immunosorbent assay (ELISA) with slight modifications [20]. Total IgG and IgM levels were determined by nephelometry using a polyclonal fluoresceinated anti-human IgG or IgM antibody.

Preparation and Staining of Tissue Sections. The immunohistochemical reagents used and section preparation for porcine tissues have been described in detail [21]. Briefly, frozen sections from porcine hearts and kidneys were stained with fluorescein isothiocyanate (FITC)-conjugated goat antibodies specific for human IgG, IgM, C1q, and C3. FITC-conjugated rabbit antibodies specific for properdin and fibrinogen were also used. In some experiments, a murine

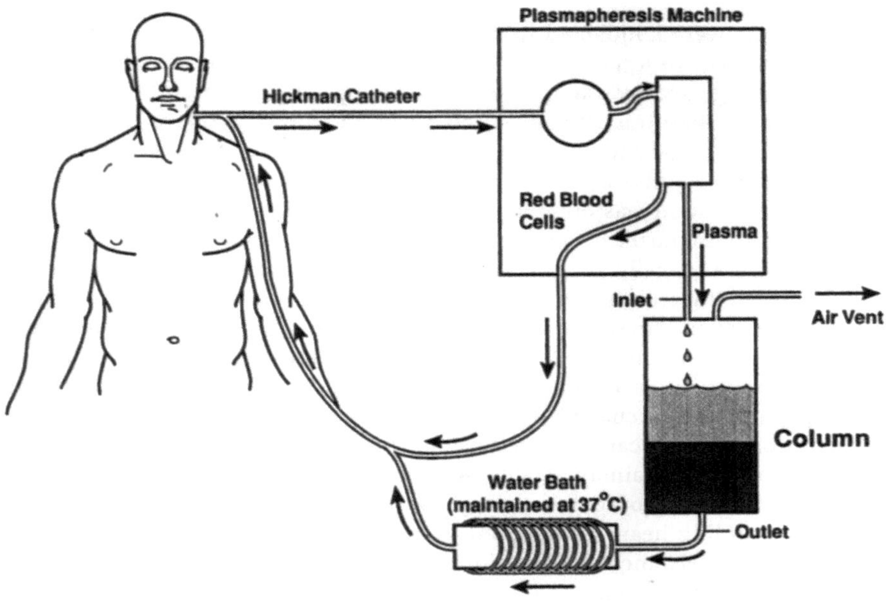

Fig. 1. Online immunoadsorption used for in vivo studies

monoclonal antibody (mAb) specific for human C9 neoantigen was also used. Xenograft biopsies were also analyzed by hematoxylin and eosin (H&E) staining.

Measurement of Complement Activity. Hemolytic C activity of the classical pathway (CH50) was determined using a modification of the technique of Kabat and Mayer [22]. In some experiments, complement deposition on porcine endothelial cells by column-treated serum was studied by C3bi neoantigen determination [23].

Measurement of Other Nonimmunoglobulin Serum Proteins. Serum transferrin, fibrinogen, factor 5, and factor 8 levels were determined using standard laboratory techniques in the clinical laboratory facility at the University of Minnesota.

Anesthesia. Baboons were sedated with ketamine hydrochloride (10 mg/kg i.m.) for all blood draws and injections. Primates undergoing transplantation were sedated with ketamine (as above) and thiamylal sodium (0.75–1.0 mg/kg i.v.). An endotracheal tube was inserted, and ventilation maintained with a Siemens C 900 ventilator with a closed circuit providing oxygen at 4l/min, nitrous oxide at 2–3 l/min, and halothane at 0.5%–1.5%. Muscle relaxation in baboons was achieved with 2 mg succinylcholine chloride/kg i.v. During primate surgeries, blood gases and acid base balance were maintained within normal limits. Continuous blood pressure readings and electrocardiographic monitoring of baboons were done. Pigs used as donors for transplant and harvesting aortae were sedated with a combination of ketamine and xylazine, then intubated and managed anesthetically in a fashion similar to baboons.

Transplant Procedure and Post-transplant Monitoring. Animals receiving porcine xenografts underwent splenectomy and placement of a 13.5 French double-lumen dialysis catheter 7 days pretransplant. Subsequently these animals received antibiotics (50 mg cefuroxime/kg i.v. twice daily) and nystatin popsicles (1 million units per popsicle twice daily). Four days before transplant, the animals began an immunosuppressive protocol based upon one which we have previously described [24], receiving a single dose of cyclophosphamide (20 mg/kg i.v.) and were begun on daily 15-deoxyspergualin (DSG, 4 mg/kg i.v.). DSG dosage was reduced if a decrease in absolute neutrophil count to less than 1500 cells/mm^3 occurred. Three days before transplant, a dose of horse anti-baboon anti-lymphocyte globulin was adminstered (20 mg/kg i.v.). Two days before transplant, subjects underwent plasmapheresis with and Autopheresis C device (Baxter Corp.) for two plasma volumes; plasma was replaced 1:1 with 5% human albumin. One day before transplant, subjects underwent column absorption with the Ig-Therasorb column as described above for two plasma volumes, with a regeneration step between each plasma volume. On the day of transplant, baboon subjects again underwent a two plasma volume column absorption with the Ig-Therasorb immediately before surgery. Porcine kidneys were harvested from 15–25 kg outbred swine using standard techniques and flush preservation with Euro-Collins solution. Baboons then underwent laparotomy, bilateral nephrectomy, and renal xenotransplantation with a single porcine kidney. Furosemide and mannitol were given prior to unclamping of the renal vessels to ensure a brisk diuresis.

Baboons were begun on a continuous infusion of cyclosporine A (3–4 mg/kg per day) to achieve whole blood chromatographic levels of 200–300. Intravenous steroids (methylprednisolone) were also instituted with a single bolus dose of 500 mg, followed by a daily taper to 1 mg/kg per day. Daily monitoring of subject complete blood cell count, serum electrolytes, transferrin, and total IgG and IgM was performed. Serum was also collected to measure hemolytic complement activity and anti-porcine antibodies as described above. Baboons underwent column absorption in the post-transplant period if a rise of total IgG and/or IgM antibodies to more than 25 % of pretreatment levels was observed. An open kidney biopsy was also obtained at these timepoints.

Results

Effect of Ig-Therasorb Column on Antibody Levels in Human and Baboon Plasma

In eight experiments the passage of human plasma through the Ig-Therasorb column was associated with a 97.5 % and 78.4 % mean reduction in total IgG and IgM, respectively ($n=6$). Similar results were achieved with baboon plasma (97.2 % and 81.5 % mean reductions of IgG and IgM, $n=3$). The majority of antibody removal occurred during the first passage of plasma through the column, suggesting that the potential absorptive capacity of the column was being reached at this time. The pronounced reduction in IgM antibodies by the Ig-Therasorb has been shown to be attributable to the anti-light chain specificity of the immobilized antibodies (J. Mueller-Derlich, unpublished data). Based

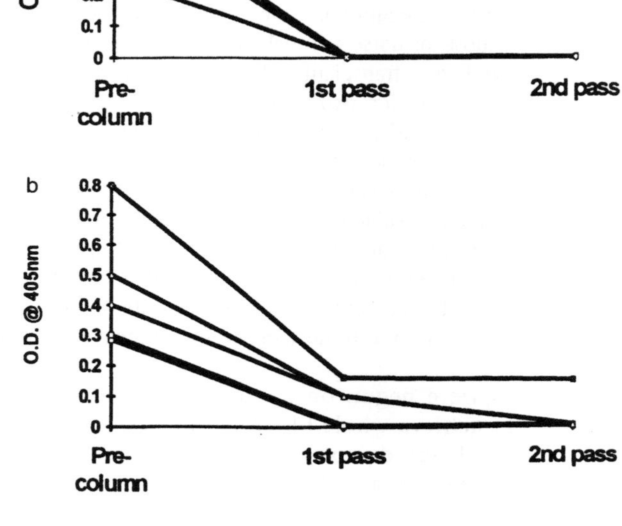

Fig. 2A,B. Effect of immunoadsorption upon levels of **A** anti-pig IgG and **B** anti-pig IgM antibodies in human plasma. Each line represents an individual experiment in which plasma samples at a 1:2 dilution from different time points during immunoadsorption were tested for reactivity against pig endothelial cells by enzyme-linked immunosorbent assay (ELISA; see "Methodology"). Data displayed following subtraction of background absorbance (0.12)

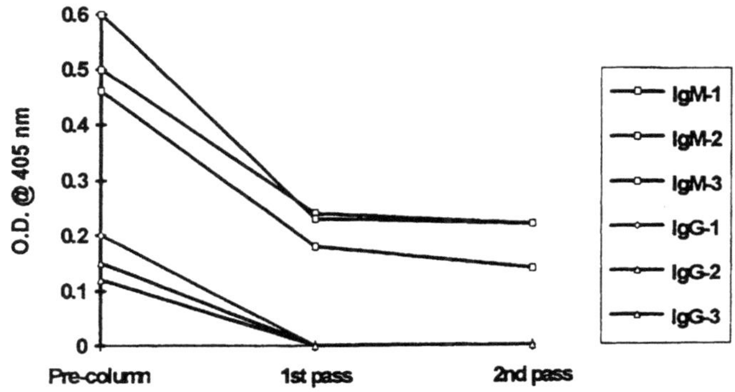

Fig. 3. Effect of immunoadsorption upon levels of anti-pig IgG and IgM antibodies in baboon plasma. Each line represents an individual experiment in which plasma samples at a 1:2 dilution from different time points during immunoadsorption were tested for reactivity against pig endothelial cells by enzyme-linked immunosorbent assay (ELISA; see "Methodology"). Data displayed following subtraction of background absorbance (0.13)

upon starting concentrations of Ig in plasma used for our experiments, the Ig-Therasorb column appeared capable of removing approximately 3100 mg IgG and 200 mg IgM.

We also examined the impact of antibody removal with the Ig-Therasorb column upon anti-pig antibody levels in human and baboon plasma. As shown in Fig. 2, passage of human plasma through this column was associated with marked reductions in levels of anti-pig IgG and IgM antibodies. Anti-pig IgG was reduced 54- to 486-fold, while anti-pig IgM was lowered by nine- to 54-fold. The effect of Ig-Therasorb absorption upon baboon anti-pig antibody levels is shown in Fig. 3. As for human plasma, marked reductions in both antipig IgG and IgM levels is observed.

Effect of IgM Column on Antibody Levels in Human and Baboon Plasma

Using the IgM column, a mean reduction in total IgM for both human (83.9 %, n=4) and baboon (82.6 %, n=2) plasma occurred, primarily during the the first pass through the column. Only a 13 %–18 % reduction in total IgG was seen. These experiments indicated the IgM column possessed a binding capacity of approximately 300 mg Ig. The marked reduction in total IgM by this column correlated with a 27 %–54 % reduction in anti-pig IgM antibodies from human and baboon plasma (data not shown); no signficant reduction in human or baboon anti-pig IgG levels was observed.

Effect of Colunn Absorption on Nonimmunoglobulin Serum Proteins

A potential advantage of immunoapheresis is the specific removal of immunoglobulins, with minimal impact upon other important plasma proteins, such as clotting factors. The passage of human or baboon plasma through our columns in this experimental setting was associated with 30 % mean reduction in transferrin levels; this reduction correlated with the reduction in plasma proteins expected from the amount of saline introduced during the column adsorption procedure in order to recover all experimental plasma from the columns. Similar reductions in plasma fibrinogen (26 %), factor 5 (25 %), and factor 8 (31 %) were observed. However, complement activity in plasma passaged over the Ig-Therasorb was reduced by 70 %, indicating that complement protein binding and/or activation by the column was taking place. As noted below, little or no reduction in CH50 activity was associated with passage over the IgM column.

Effect of Ig-Therasorb Column on Hyperacute Rejection: Ex Vivo Studies

Using our ex vivo model, swine hearts perfused with autologous blood (n=5) consistently demonstrated stable heart rate and rhythm for greater than 360 min, at which time point each study was electively terminated. Hearts perfused with unmodified human blood (n=5) underwent cessation of of normal cardiac activity at a mean time of 25.2±5.6 min. The hearts perfused with human blood depleted of antibodies with the Ig-Therasorb column (n=5) demonstrated a marked prolongation of normal heart rate and rhythm for and average of 252±48.1 min (p<0.01 vs. unmodified human blood). Column adsorption of plasma followed by recombination of plasma and cell fractions in the perfusion system produced a 90.5 % and 86 % reduction in total IgG and IgM, respectively. A 47 % reduction in anti-pig IgG and a 69.4 % reduction in anti-pig IgM antibodies was also noted. Total and anti-porcine Ig levels in immunoadsorbed plasma was lower prior to recombination with cellular components in the perfusion system, suggesting that unabsorbed plasma was retained in the cell fraction.

Unmodified human blood perfused through porcine hearts showed a significant drop in xenoreactive antibodies , with a 64.6 % and 73.3 % mean reduction in human anti-porcine IgG and IgM, respectively, by the end of the reperfusion period. This reduction in circulating levels of anti-pig IgG and IgM was associated with antibody deposition within porcine cardiac xenografts. In contrast, column adsorbed blood had stable levels of antibody during the reperfusion period.

Hearts perfused with non-depleted human blood demonstrated characteristic changes of hyperacute rejection, with marked tissue edema, interstitial hemorrhage, microvascular thrombosis, and endothelial detachment. Immunopathology demonstrated marked deposition of IgM, IgG, C1q, C3, and C4. In contrast, sequential endomyocardial biopsies obtained from hearts perfused with Ig-Therasorb-adsorbed human blood showed no evidence of hyperacute rejection; only minimal deposits of IgG and essentially no IgM, C1q, C3, or C4 was identified.

Effect of IgM Column on Hyperacute Rejection: Ex Vivo Studies

In these perfusion system experiments, passage of human plasma over the IgM column resulted in approximately 90 % reduction in total and swine-specific

IgM antibodies. No significant reduction in total or anti-porcine IgG antibodies occurred. The reduction in IgM levels was associated with prolonged survival of porcine hearts on the perfusion circuit (228.5±45.2 min, $p<0.01$ vs. unmodified controls). The passage of human plasma over the IgM column did not significantly reduce CH50 levels. However, we observed a reduction in the complement activating capacity of IgM-depleted human blood. It has been demonstrated that human IgM xenoreactive antibodies, but not IgG, are capable of activating complement (i.e., through C3bi generation) when bound to the surface of porcine endothelial cells [25]. The reduced IgM levels in our column-adsorbed plasma was associated with an approximate 80% decrease in C3bi binding to porcine endothelial cells in vitro (Kroshus et al., unpublished observations).

Histologic analysis of control swine hearts perfused with unmodified human blood showed typical widespread features of hyperacute rejection. Diffuse deposits of IgG, IgM, C1q, C3, C4, and C9 neoantigen were seen. Hearts perfused with IgM-reduced human blood showed similar deposition of IgG, but only minimal IgM binding. Marked reduction in deposits of C1q, C3, and C4 was also observed. This association between human IgM and complement protein binding therefore suggests that IgM, and not IgG, is responsible for vascular deposition of complement in the perfused porcine xenografts.

Effect of Ig-Therasorb and IgM Columns on Circulating Levels of Antibodies in Baboons

We next examined the ability of our anti-human Ig columns to remove Ig from baboon plasma in vivo. Our in vitro studies indicated that the adsorptive capacity of our columns was limited, and would be exceeded by the Ig load in the plasma volume of our baboon subjects. In order to avoid prolonged anesthetic time during repeated column passage and regeneration required to deplete all plasma antibodies, we elected to reduce the antibody load of each animal by performing plasmapheresis the day before column absorption. As shown in Fig. 4, column adsorption with the Ig-Therasorb following plasmapheresis achieved marked reductions in total IgG and IgM levels; cessation of column adsorption was followed by a rapid rise in Ig levels. These reductions in total IgG and IgM correlated with similar reductions in antipig IgG and IgM levels (Fig. 5A). In vivo antibody removal with the IgM column following plasmapheresis resulted in sustained reduction in total IgM, while total IgG was not markedly reduced and indeed rose slightly over this period (Fig. 4). A selective reduction in baboon antipig IgM levels was also observed (Fig. 5B).

Impact of Pre- and Post-Transplant Antibody Removal With Ig-Therasorb Column Combined with Immunosuppression on Pig-to-Baboon Xenograft Survival

Based upon the safety and efficacy of column adsorption in naive baboons, we postulated that columns used immediately pretransplant would achieve extremely low levels of xenoreactive antibodies and prevent hyperacute xenograft rejection.

Fig. 4. Effect of immunoadsorption with either the Ig-Therasorb (*left*) or IgM columns (*right*) upon total IgG and IgM levels in baboons. Data displayed are from representative experiments involving single animals. *P*, plasmapheresis; *C*, column adsorption

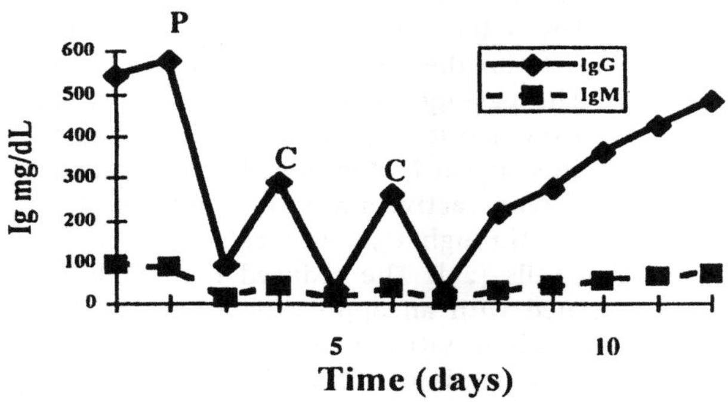

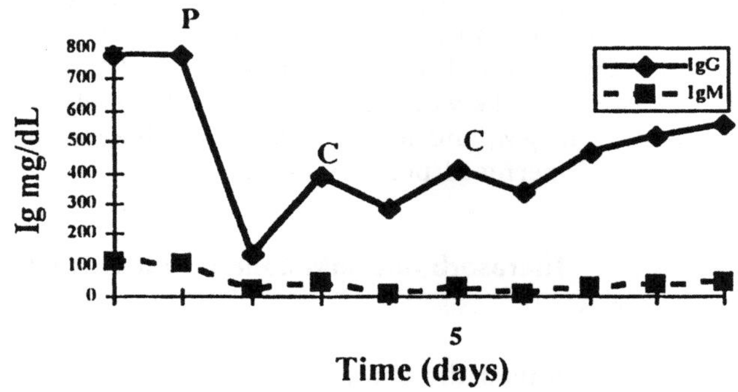

a

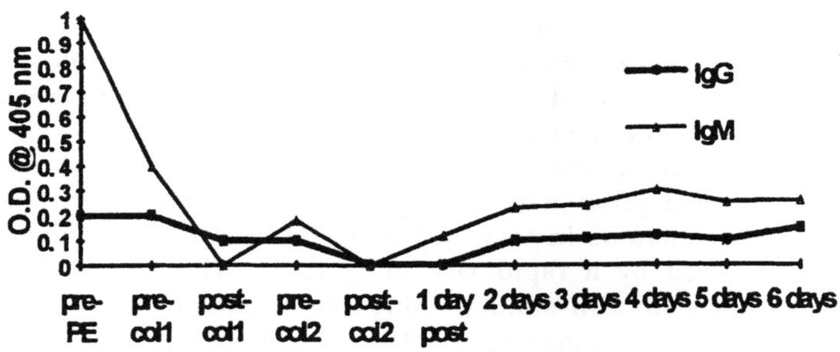

b

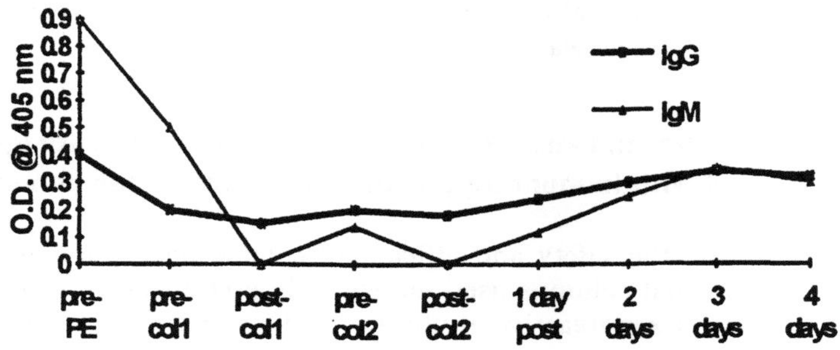

Furthermore, we posited these lowered levels could be maintained by immunosuppression and repeated immunoapheresis post-transplant. Two baboon subjects underwent a protocol of immunosuppression and antibody removal using the Ig-Therasorb column prior to bilateral nephrectomy and placement of a porcine renal xenograft (see "Methodology"). Marked reductions in total Ig and anti-pig antibodies were achieved in both xenograft recipients (Fig. 6). These reductions in IgG and IgM levels were associated with prevention of hyperacute xenograft rejection. Both baboons exhibited persistent graft function up until the time of subject sacrifice after 11 and 13 days. The first baboon was euthanized for a pulmonary infection, while the second succumbed following an episode of hypotension during a kidney biopsy. All post-transplant kidney biopsies did not show evidence of vascular xenograft rejection. Glomeruli were undamaged, while varying degrees of acute tubular necrosis was observed. No significant cellular infiltration was noted. Immunohistochemical staining of renal xenograft biopsies failed to reveal vascular deposits of IgG, IgM, C3, properdin, or fibrinogen (Table 1).

Table 1. Immunopathologic findings in renal biopsies from baboons undergoing immunoadsorption, immunosuppression, and pig-to-baboon kidney transplantation

	IgM	IgG	C3	Fibrin
Pre-transplant	–[a]	–[a]	–	–
Post-transplant				
3 h	–[a]	–[a]	–	–
Day 2	–	–	–	–
Day 5	–[a]	–[a]	–[a]	1+[b]
Day 9	–[a]	–[a]	–[a]	–
Days 11/13	–[a]	–[a]	–[a]	–

[a]Denotes trace mesangial deposition.
[b]Focal intravascular thrombi in less than 10 % of glomeruli.

Comment

Hyperacute rejection of porcine xenografts by humans and nonhuman primates is thought to be initiated by the binding of xenoreactive antibodies to antigens expressed on the surface of xenogeneic endothelium [1]. Efforts to prevent hyperacute rejection of porcine xenografts have therefore concentrated in part upon developing techniques for the reduction or removal of xenoreactive antibodies.

Fig. 5A,B. Effect of immunoadsorption with either the A Ig-Therasorb or B IgM column upon anti-pig IgG and IgM levels in baboons. Data displayed are from representative experiments involving single animals. Measurements performed with serum samples at 1:2 dilutions at the time points indicated using porcine endothelial cell enzyme-linked immunosorbent assay (ELISA). Data displayed following subtraction of background absorbance (0.12)

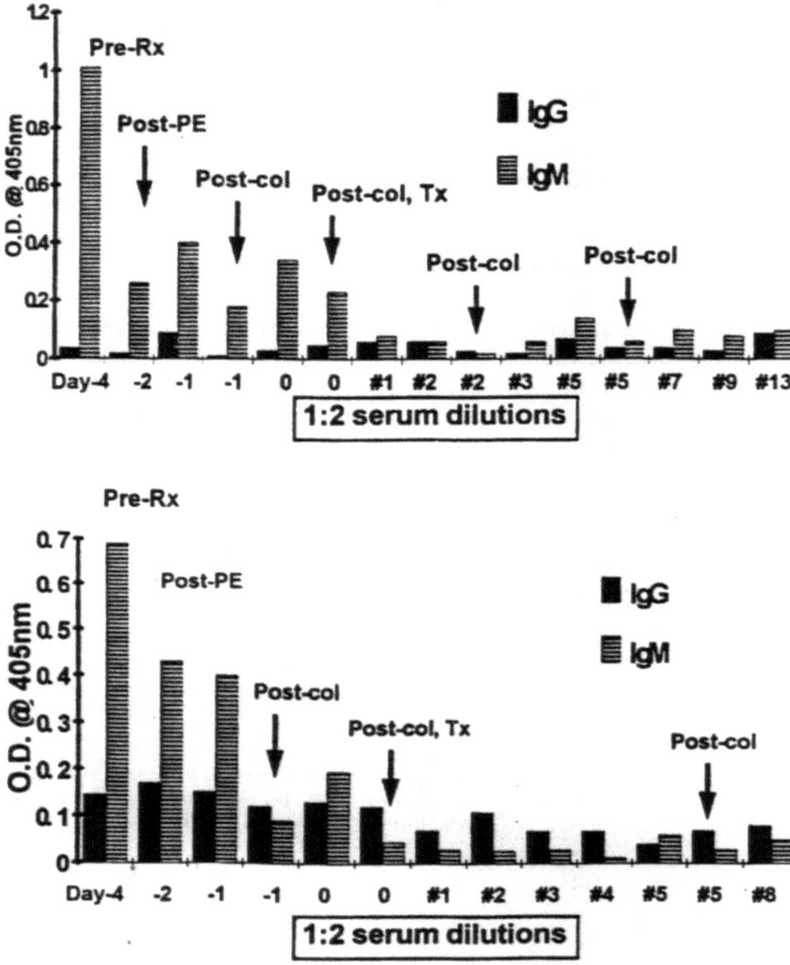

Fig. 6. Antipig antibody levels in two baboons undergoing immunoadsorption, immunosuppression, and pig-to-baboon renal transplantation. Antibody measurement performed by pig endothelial cell enzyme-linked immunosorbent assay (ELISA). Data displayed following subtraction of background absorbance (0.12)

The problem of xenoreactive natural antibodies has been approached using a variety of selective and non-selective techniques. Plasmapheresis and organ perfusion represent two of the most commonly used methods for antibody removal in xenotransplantation. Although both approaches have demonstrated some effectiveness [5, 7–9], they also possess distinct disadvantages. Plasmapheresis is hampered by the removal of non-immunoglobulin plasma proteins – such as clotting factors – which may make its use dangerous in the peritransplant period. Organ perfusion suffers from sequestration and loss of blood volume, as well as activation of the complement and coagulation cascades, as the perfused organ is rejected. Organ perfusion is also cumbersome to perform, requiring sacrifice of a donor animal to obtain target organs.

In an effort to develop an improved method for xenoreactive antibody removal, we have studied the utility of extracorporeal columns to selectively bind and remove antibodies from human and baboon plasma. Contrary to plasmapheresis or organ perfusion, antibody-based immunoadsorption (immunoapheresis) provides a highly specific depletion technique, using immobilized antibodies generated against one or several predetermined plasma components [14]. In our studies, columns containing polyclonal antibodies directed against human immunoglobulins were evaluated. Our results suggest that immunoapheresis with columns containing polyclonal anti-human Igs as the immunosorbent are a safe and effective means for antibody removal with advantages over other methods of antibody depletion. Antibody removal by either anti-human Ig column was not associated with any immunoapheresis-related morbidity and mortality in our study. These columns exerted minimal effects upon the coagulation system, indicating they would be safe to use in the perioperative period. Indeed, we observed no bleeding complications in our baboons during the short periods of heparinization required by the column absorption procedures. Column adsorption was not associated with loss of intravascular blood volume, and could be performed over several hours. Thus, this method of antibody depletion would appear to be superior to plasmapheresis or organ absorption.

Ex vivo perfusion studies were conducted to expand upon our in vitro and in vivo studies. Although isolated heart preparations have been used as a basic model for the study of cardiac metabolism and function for many years, they have been utilized in a more limited fashion for the study of mechanisms of hyperacute rejection in different species combinations. Ex vivo preparations using other organs such as kidneys and livers have been used to study the role of antibody, complement, and cellular blood elements in the process of hyperacute rejection, as well as to assess the impact of certain therapeutic interventions on xenograft survival [26–28]. Cardiac perfusion models have an advantage compared to other solid organ perfusion models due to the number of functional parameters that can be analyzed. Although there are limitations to such perfusion models, results obtained may help establish the effectiveness of different interventions, and serve as the foundation for subsequent in vivo studies.

Although immunoadsorption with either the Ig-Therasorb or IgM column resulted in prolongation of porcine xenograft survival ex vivo, these columns differ markedly in their effects upon the complement sytem. Perfusion of human plasma over the Ig-Therasorb resulted in a significant reduction in complement activity; this effect is likely due to the binding of C1 to Fc regions of Igs adsorbed to the Sepharose column, with subsequent reduction in total complement hemolytic activity. In contrast, the IgM column did not cause significant depletion of complement activity. This suggests that immunoadsorbed IgM exists in conformation which hinders the binding of C1q to the Fc region of antibodies. Moreover, that selective removal of IgM achieves extension of ex vivo perfused xenograft survival comparable to that seen with the less selective and complement-depleting Ig-Therasorb column underscores the importance of xenoreactive IgM in the pig-to-primate species combination.

In our studies the Ig-Therasorb column and not the anti-IgM column was used for antibody removal in baboons receiving porcine renal xenografts. We felt it would be necessary to remove both IgG and IgM antibodies in the peri-transplant period, since we have observed rising titers of both anti-pig IgG and IgM following xenografting in this model [21, 24]. Thus, the question of whether selective depletion of IgM anti-pig antibodies prevents hyperacute rejection has not been directly addressed in vivo. This issue is important, since anti-pig IgM antibodies have been implicated as critical to the inititation of hyperacute porcine xenograft rejection. Based upon our results in the ex vivo perfusion model with the IgM column, we are presently instituting in vivo pig to baboon transplant studies using selective removal of IgM.

Antibody depletion by our Ig-Therasorb column was associated with prevention of hyperacute rejection and extension of xenograft survival in baboons. Although it is possible that depletion of complement activity during immunoapheresis may have contributed to these effects, both transplanted baboons exhibited return of complement activity to more than 90 % of normal levels in the post-transplant period (data not shown), while antibody titers remained low. Furthermore, experiments conducted in our ex vivo system with the IgM column support the notion that antibody removal, and not complement depletion, is responsible for extension of xenograft survival. Therefore, the combination of immunoadsorption and immunosuppression – and not complement depletion – appear to be critical for continuing xenograft survival in this study. These results appear to differ from our previous study in which both antibody removal by plasmapheresis and complement depletion were required to achieve prolonged survival of pig xenografts in baboons [10]. However, comparision of xenoreactive antibody levels in transplanted baboons from each study has shown immunoapheresis to result in a two- to fourfold greater reduction of anti-pig antibodies than pre-transplant plasmapheresis alone (J. Leventhal, unpublished observations). Thus, intervention with the complement system may not be necessary under conditions where extremely low antibody titers exist.

Removal of antibodies with both anti-human Ig columns did not result in consumption of clotting factors. These columns could therefore be used to prepare antibody-free blood products for use in xenotransplantation. The recent experience with pig-to-human liver xenografting indicates that antibody-free blood products would be desirable, if not an absolute necessity for the safe clinical application of xenografting [29].

Ongoing trials in humans have shown the Ig-Therasorb column to be both safe and effective for repeated antibody removal in patients with autoimmune diseases and anti-HLA antibodies [30, 31]. Unlike baboons, these or similar columns could be used repeatedly at the bedside in patients to achieve marked antibody depletion, thus avoiding the need for adjunctive pretransplant plasmapheresis. Moreover, implementation of an automated column regeneration process presently in clinical use for the LDL-Therasorb would minimize plasma dilution to less than 10 %, thus reducing the chance of volume overload [14]. Furthermore, with the identification of terminal galactose residues in the αGal1–3Gal linkage as the major porcine endothelial cell epitopes recognized by human xenoreactive antibodies, it may be possible to generate highly selective columns with bound carbohydrates, or mimetic compounds with high binding affinity for xenoreactive antibodies. We therefore propose that column adsorption represents an effective and clinically applicable method for antibody removal in xenotransplantation.

Acknowledgments. The authors would like to thank Man Qiu Yang and Pamela Simone, for excellent technical assistance, Barbara Burke for reviewing all xenograft biopsies, Franz Bieber for early work in development of anti-IgM sepharose, and the laboratory of A.P. Dalmasso for running of complement assays.

References

1. Platt JL, Vercellotti GM, Dalmasso AP, et al. Transplantation of discordant xenografts: A review of progress. Immunology Today 1990; 11:450
2. Platt JL, Bach FH. The barrier to xenotransplantation. Transplantation 1991; 52:1037
3. Bach FH, Platt JL, Cooper DKC. Accomodation-the role of natural antibody and complement in discordant xenograft rejection. In: Cooper DKC, et al., eds. Xenotransplantation.Heidelberg, Springer 1991; p. 81
4. Auchincloss H. Xenogeneic Transplantation. Transplantation 1988; 46:1
5. Alexandre G, Gianello P, Latinne D, et al. Plasmapheresis and splenectomy in experimental renal xenotransplantation. In: Hardy MA, ed. Xenograft 25. New York, Elsevier 1989; p. 259
6. Platt JL Therapeutic strategies for hyperacute xenograft rejection. In: Platt JL Hyperacute Xenograft Rejection.Austin: RJ Landes Co. 1995; p. 165
7. Cooper DKC, Human PA, Lexer G,et al. Effects of cyclosporine and antibody absorption on pig cardiac xenograft survival in the baboon. J Heart Transplant 1988; 7:238
8. Roslin MS, Zisbrod Z, Tranbaugh RF, et al. 15-Day survival in pig to baboon heterotopic cardiac xenotransplantation. Presented to the First International Congress on Xenotransplantation, Minneapolis, 1991
9. Fischel RJ, Platt JL, Matas AJ, et al. Prolonged survival of a discordant cardiac xenograft in a rhesus monkey. Transplant Proc 1991; 23:589
10. Barocci S, Nocera A In vitro removal of anti-HLA IgG antibodies from highly sensitized transplant recipients by immunoadsorption wit protein A and protein G sepharose columns: a comparision. Tranplant Int 1993;6:29
11. Palmer A, Welsh K, Gjorstrup P, et al. Removal of anti-HLA antibodies by extracorporeal immunoadsorption to enable renal transplantation. Lancet 1989; 1:10
12. Palmer A, Gjorstrup P, Severn A, et al. Treatment of systemic lupus erythematosus by extracorporeal immunoadsorption Lancet 1988; 2:272
13. Shapiro R, Tzakis AG, Scantlebury V, et al. Immunodepletion in xenotransplantation. J Invest Surg 1990;3:39
14. du Moulin A, Mueller-Derlich J, Bieber F, et al. Antibody-based immunoadsorption as a therapeutic means. Blood Purif 1993;11:145
15. du Moulin A: LDL immunoaphereis technique: In Gotto AM Jr, et al. (eds): Treatment of Severe Hypercholesterolemia in the Prevention of Coronary Heart Disease.Basel, Karger, 1990:170

16. Stoffel W, Borberg H, Greve V. Application of specific extracorporeal removal of low density lipoprotein in familial hypercholesterolemia. Lancet 1981; 1:1005
17. Richter WO, Suehler K, Schwandt P: Extracorporeal elimination by immunoadsorption: side effects and influences on other serum lipoproteins and serum parameters; In Gotto AM Jr, et al. (eds): Treatment of Severe Hypercholesterolemia in the Prevention of Coronary Heart Disease. Basel, Karger, 1990:183
18. Leventhal JR, John R, Fryer JP, et. al. Removal of baboon and human antiporcine IgG and IgM natural antibodies by immunoadsorption. Results of in vitro and in vivo studies. Transplantation 1995; 59:294
19. Kroshus TJ, Dalmasso AP, Leventhal JR, et al. Antibody removal by column immunoabsorption prevents tissue injury in an ex vivo model of pig-to-human xenograft hyperacute rejection. J Surg Res 1995; 59:43
20. Platt JL, Turman MA, Noreen H, et al. An ELISA assay for xenoreactive natural antibodies. Transplantation 1990; 49:1000
21. Leventhal JR, Dalmasso AP, Cromwell JW, et al. Prolongation of cardiac xenograft survival by depletion of complement. Transplantation 1993; 55:857
22. Kabat EA, Mayer MM, eds. Experimental Immunochemistry. 1961 (2nd ed.) Charles C Thomas: 149
23. Kroshus TJ, Dalmasso AP. . Selective IgM removal by column immunoabsorption prevents tissue injury and delays hyperacute rejection in an ex vivo model of pig-to-human xenografting. (Manuscript in preparation.)
24. Leventhal JR, Sakiyalak P, Witson J, et al. Synergistic effect of combined antibody and complement depletion upon discordant cardiac xenograft survival in non-human primates. Transplantation 1994; 57:974
25. Vercellotti GM, Platt JL, Bach FH, Dalmasso AP. Neutrophil adhesion to xenogeneic endothelium via iC3b. J Immunol 1991;146:730
26. Tuso PJ, Cramer DV, Yasunaga C, et al. Removal of natural human xenoantibodies to pig vascular endothelium by perfusion of blood through pig kidneys and livers. Transplantation 1993; 55:1375
27. Citterio F, Maggiano N, Tartaglione R et al. Detection of targets of human performed natural antibodies. Transplant Proc 1992; 24:437
28. Collins BH, Chari R, Magee J, et al. Mechanisms of injury in porcine livers perfused with blood of patients with fulminant hepatic failure. Transplantation 1994; 58:1162
29. Makowka L, Wu GD, Hoffman A, et al. Immunohistopathologic lesions associated with the rejection of a pig-to-human liver xenograft. Presented at the Second International Congress on Xenotransplantation, Cambridge, 1993
30. Mueller-Derlich J, du Moulin A, Spaethe R. Removal of human immunoglobulins with Ig-Therasorb. Transfusion Med 1993;3:31
31. Mueller-Derlich J, du Moulin A, Spaethe R. Removal of human immunoglobulins with Ig-Therasorb. Artif Organs 1993;17:546

27 Neutralization of the Cytotoxic Effect of Anti-αGal Antibodies with Monoclonal Anti-idiotypic Antibodies

E.Koren, F. Milotic, F.A. Neethling, and D.K.C. Cooper

Introduction

The use of the pig (or other widely divergent species) as a donor of organs for humans is dependent upon the development of a successful method of overcoming the hyperacute rejection (as well as any subsequent immune response) that is mounted in humans against grafted pig organs. The initiating factor in this hyperacute rejection is believed to be the presence of preformed antibodies in the recipient's serum [1–4]. Recipient xenoreactive antibodies bind target molecules on the vascular endothelial cell surface of the xenografted organ and activate complement, leading to endothelial cell destruction and resulting in interstitial hemorrhage and edema.

Good et al. [5, 6] were the first to demonstrate clearly that the human preformed anti-pig antibodies that initiate hyperacute vascular rejection are directed against carbohydrate structures expressed on the cell surface, particularly those that have terminal αGal1–3Gal (αGal) residues (Chap. 25). Although these antibodies may prove not to be the only antibodies binding to pig cells [5, 6], their abundance makes them of great importance in the initiation of hyperacute rejection.

Successful transplantation of pig organs into humans will require the development of methods for the removal and/or neutralization of preformed "anti-pig" (i.e., anti-αGal) antibodies. There are several possible approaches, many of which are described in this volume. This chapter will discuss the potential application of anti-idiotypic antibodies (AIAs) specifically directed against idiotypes expressed on anti-αGal antibodies. AIAs recognize specific idiotypes that are antigenic determinants localized within the variable regions of immunoglobulins [7]. Furthermore, AIAs are also directed against the B lymphocyte subpopulations that bear the same idiotypes on their surface. AIAs could, therefore, neutralize circulating anti-pig antibodies *and* inhibit production of these antibodies, thus inducing a specific and long-lasting immunosuppression resulting in prolonged survival of the xenograft.

The aim of our investigations was to produce and characterize murine monoclonal AIAs that specifically bind human anti-αGal antibodies and identify those that neutralize the cytotoxic activity of anti-αGal antibodies on pig cells [8].

Production of Mouse Monoclonal Anti-idiotypic Antibodies

In order to produce AIAs, BALB/c mice were injected with purified human anti-pig antibodies (eluted from pig hearts after perfusion with human serum) biweekly for a period of 6 months. Each animal was bled from the tail vein before immunization in order to collect pre-immune sera for use as negative controls. Every 4 weeks from the day of the first injection, samples of blood were drawn in order to determine anti-idiotypic activity and optimal time for fusion.

The serum samples were analyzed in an enzyme-linked immunosorbent assay (ELISA) as follows. Cell culture 96-well plates were seeded with pig kidney (PK15) cells, which were grown until confluent, and fixed. Mixtures of human serum and immunized mouse sera were prepared, consisting of increasing quantities of mouse serum and a constant concentration of human serum. These mixtures were incubated on plates followed by washing and incubation with peroxidase-labeled antibody to human immunoglobulins. Peroxidase substrate was added and the optical density of the developed color was measured. As AIAs in the mouse sera inhibited the binding of human anti-pig antibodies to the pig cells attached to the plate, the color was diminished proportionally to the concentration of AIA. Preimmune mouse sera were used as respective negative controls in each case.

Two out of ten immunized mice that developed the highest anti-idiotypic titer were sacrificed and splenectomized. Isolated splenocytes of each mouse were separately fused with mouse myeloma cells using the conventional polyethylene-glycol method [9]. Supernates from macroscopically visible hybridomas were screened for the presence of mouse immunoglobulins. Hybridomas producing detectable quantities of antibodies were cloned and further tested for binding to human anti-αGal IgG as well as to total human IgG. The human anti-αGal IgG was isolated by immunoaffinity chromatography of human AB serum over an immobilized αGal(1–3)Gal column (Chembiomed, Edmonton, Alberta, Canada) as described previously [10].

Hybridoma antibodies that reacted at least five times as highly with anti-αGal IgG, compared to total IgG, were considered specific for variable regions of the anti-αGal IgG and potentially anti-idiotypic. Their specificity for variable regions was corroborated by high reactivity with purified anti-αGal Fab_2 fragments. Antibodies that reacted equally with anti-αGal IgG and total IgG were considered specific for the constant regions of the IgG molecule and, therefore, non anti-idiotypic. The described screening was also carried out with baboon anti-αGal IgG and baboon total IgG in order to find AIAs that cross-reacted with human and baboon anti-αGal antibodies.

Twenty-nine out of 312 clones (9 %) produced antibodies that showed at least five times higher reactivity in regard to anti-αGal IgG than to total human IgG. The same monoclonal antibodies that specifically bound to idiotypes on human anti-αGal were also tested against baboon anti-αGal IgG and baboon total IgG. These experiments showed that 15 of the 29 monoclonal AIAs cross-reacted with human and baboon anti-αGal antibodies. Eleven out of 29 AIAs showed relatively high affinity for human anti-αGal IgG and Fab_2 fragments based on

Table 1. Characteristics of monoclonal anti-idiotypic antibodies directed against human and baboon anti-αGal antibodies

Antibody code	Immuno-globulin class	Relative affinity[a] for: Human anti-αGal IgG	Human anti-αGal Fab_2	Baboon anti-αGal IgG	Cytotoxicity[b] (% dead cells): Human serum	Baboon serum
cD_6	IgG_3	1.21[a]	1.11[a]	1.32[a]	58 (±7.6)[b]	2 (±1.5)[b]
dA_8	IgM	2.53	2.25	0.25	7 (±2.5)	5 (±1.8)
dC_4	IgG_1	1.36	1.28	0.71	27 (±6.7)	3 (±1.5)
dD_4	IgG_2A	0.87	0.93	0.68	15 (±6.0)	3 (±1.8)
dE_2A_2	IgM	2.21	2.08	0.98	8 (±7.5)	12 (±5.5)
dE_2C_3	IgM	2.43	2.38	0.76	3 (±1.1)	1 (±0.7)
dF_4	IgG_2B	1.27	1.34	1.23	6 (±3.5)	3 (±2.0)
eB_8D_3	IgG_1	2.09	1.89	0.81	45 (±7.2)	ND
eC_7C_1	IgM	1.83	1.97	0.65	3 (±1.2)	4 (±1.9)
eF_1D_6	IgM	2.12	1.96	1.13	38 (±5.9)	ND
gD_7A_3	IgM	2.09	2.16	0.64	2 (±0.6)	2 (±1.4)
jB_3 (control)	IgG_1	NA	NA	NA	100 (±0.3)	98 (±4.6)

NA, not applicable; ND, not done.
[a] Relative affinity is expressed as the slope of the binding curve.
[b] Cytotoxicity of sera is expressed as a percentage of dead PK15 cells (mean of four tests ± standard deviation).

the slopes of binding curves (Table 1). Furthermore, four of these high affinity antibodies (cD_6, dE_2A_2, dF_4, and dF_1D_6) also reacted with baboon anti-αGal IgG with relatively high affinity (Table 1).

In Vitro Neutralization of Serum Cytotoxic Activity

In six examined unmodified *human* AB sera, the average cytotoxic activity (expressed as the percentage of killed PK15 cells) was more than 80 %. However, after preincubation with ascites fluid containing high affinity AIAs, the cytotoxic activity of all human sera decreased significantly (Table 1). Some of the antibodies (such as gD_7A_3 and dE_2C_3) reduced the average cytotoxicity to less than 5 % of the starting serum activity. Others (eB_8D_3, cD_6, dC_4, and dF_1D_6) were less effective, reducing the cytotoxicity to 45 %, 58 %, 26 %, and 38 %, respectively. The protective effect of all examined AIAs was concentration dependent and reached the saturation point at a 1:4 dilution of ascites.

Some combinations of two AIAs were more effective than any of the single antibodies (Table 2). For example, mixtures of dA_8 + dF_4, dE_2C_3 + dF_4, or gD_7A_3 + dF_4, completely inhibited the cyotoxicity of human serum towards PK15 cells.

The protective activity of single AIAs against the cytotoxicity of *baboon* sera was generally higher (Table 1). In eight cases, the cytotoxicity of baboon serum was reduced to less 5 % of the starting activity using quantities of ascites that

Table 2. Protective activity of two combined anti-idiotypic antibodies against the cytotoxicity of human serum to pig (PK15) cells

Antibody codes	Cytotoxicity[a] (% dead cells)
$dA_8 + dE_2C_3$	1 (±0.8)
$dA_8 + dF_4$	0
$dE_2C_3 + dF_4$	0
$gD_7A_3 + dF_4$	0
$gD_7A_3 + dA_8$	2 (±1.1)
$gD_7A_3 + dE_2C_3$	2 (±0.8)
$eB_8D_3 + dF_4$	11 (±4.1)
$dC_4 + dF_4$	5 (±3.1)

[a] Cytotoxicity of sera is expressed as a percentage of dead PK15 cells (mean of three tests ± SD).

were ten times lower than those necessary to accomplish similar protection against human serum. Again, mixtures of AIAs were more effective than the single antibodies (data not shown). As with human sera, the protective effect of AIAs against baboon sera was concentration-dependent and saturable.

In Vivo Inhibition of Serum Cytotoxicity

In vitro analyses revealed certain mixtures of AIAs as particularly effective in the neutralization of baboon serum cytotoxicity. For example, both $dE_2C_3 + dA_8$ and $dE_2A_2 + cD_6$ reduced the number of dead cells to 2%. On the basis of these in vitro data, a mixture of $dE_2C_3 + A_8$ was infused i.v. twice into a female baboon (Fig. 1A). Serum samples drawn after the first infusion showed a slight decrease in cytotoxic activity during the first 8 h. However, a second infusion of AIAs 48 h later decreased serum cytotoxicity by 50% from its initial value.

In a second experiment, a mixture of the AIAs $dE_2A_2 + cD_6$ was administered in two i.v. injections given within 1 h to a male baboon (Fig. 1B). The inhibitory effect of the AIAs was evident immediately, the cytotoxic activity of the serum being reduced to less than 20% or the initial level within 1 h. Cytotoxicity rose to 38% 8 h after the second injection, at which level it remained for 24 h.

In a further two in vivo experiments, other combinations of two AIAs were injected i.v. into each of two baboons. By 1 hour postinjection, a drop in cytotoxicity was evident in both cases by 59% and 90%, respectively (Fig. 1C,D). This protective effect continued for 24 hours postinjection.

Binding of Anti-idiotypic Antibodies to Peripheral Blood B Lymphocytes

B cells express on their surface the same idiotypes as the antibodies they produce. Therefore, if one were to attach ricin, or some other toxin, to the AIAs specific for anti-αGal antibodies, B-cells producing anti-αGal antibodies could be eliminated for several weeks.

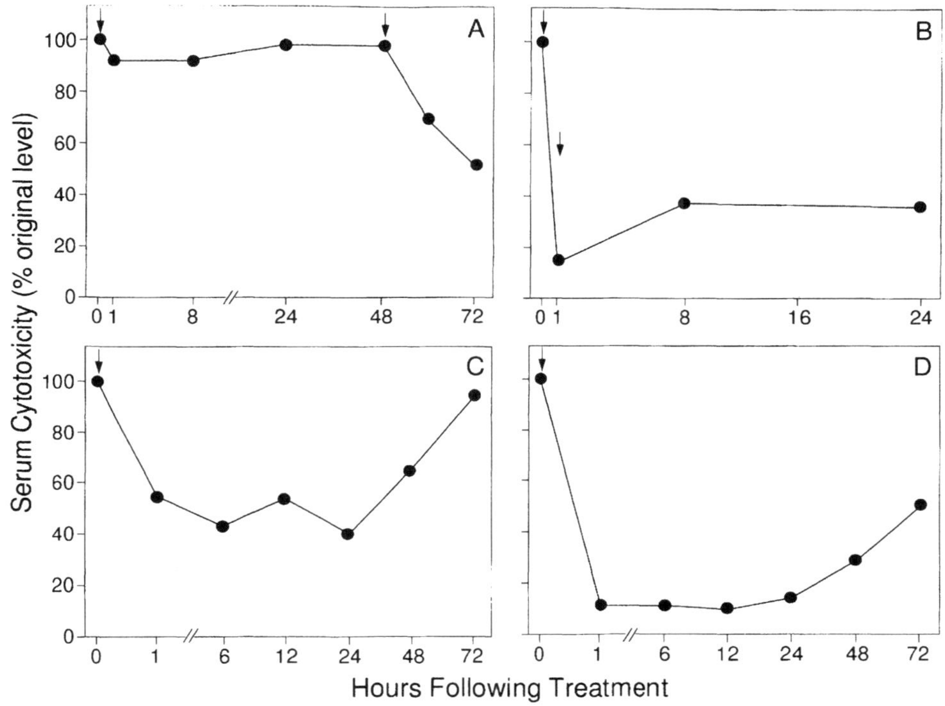

Fig. 1. A Effect of the intravenous injection (*arrows*) of monoclonal anti-idiotypic antibodies (AIAs) on the cytotoxicity of baboon serum. A mixture of dE_2C_3 and dA_8 AIAs caused a slight decrease (8 %) in cytotoxicity during the initial 8 h after the first injection. This was followed by restoration of cytotoxicity to the preinjection level at the 24- and 48-hour time intervals. However, a second injection, given 48 h after the first, had a more pronounced effect, causing a 45 % decrease in cytotoxicity over the subsequent 48 h. **B** Effects of the intravenous injection of monoclonal AIAs dE_2A_2 and cD_6 on the cytotoxicity of baboon serum. Two bolus injections (*arrows*) were given within 1 h, causing an initial 87 % decrease in cytotoxicity that was largely maintained (at approximately 38 % of the original level) for at least 24 h. **C** Effect of treatment with AIAs dE_2C_3 and dA_8. After one bolus injection of higher concentration (twice as high as shown in **A**) of these antibodies into a new baboon, the serum cytotoxicity dropped by approximately 50 % and remained at that level for 24 h. **D** Effects of AIAs dE_2C_3 + gD_7A_3 after a single bolus injection. The serum cytotoxicity abruptly decreased by 90 % within 1 h and stayed at that level for 24 h

In an attempt to explore the expression and accessibility of anti-αGal idiotypes on the surface of human B lymphocytes, peripheral blood lymphocytes were stained with each of the above 11 AIAs combined with an antibody specific for B cells (anti-CD-20). An example of the flow cytometry analysis (Fig. 2) demonstrates the binding of one of the AIAs (cD_6) to a subpopulation of B lymphocytes. Only seven of the described 11 AIAs were capable of staining B lymphocytes. The results of flow cytometry analyses of five normal human donors are shown in Table 3. The expression of most idiotypes is quite variable and relatively low (<5 % of B cells), which is in accordance with the variability [11] and concentration [12] of anti-αGal antibodies in human sera.

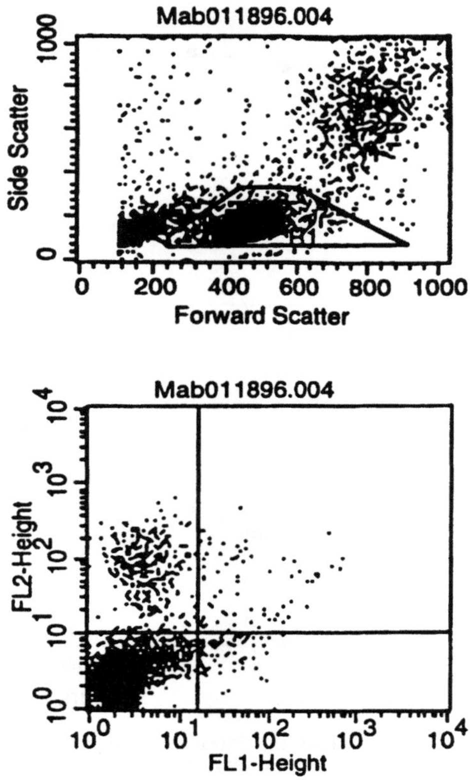

Fig. 2. Results of flow cytometry analysis of human peripheral blood lymphocytes fluorescently stained with anti-idiotypic antibody cD_6 (FL1) and with antibody to CD20 (FL2). *Top*, lymphocytes were gated based on Side/Forward Scatter pattern (*R1*) in order to eliminate contaminating platelets and monocytes. *Bottom*, fluorescence of gated lymphocytes. Nonfluorescent cells are shown in the *lower left quadrant*, representing 90.16 % of all gated lymphocytes. Cells in the *upper left quadrant* are stained only with anti-CD20 and represent 6.87 % of the gated population, corresponding to B lymphocytes that do not express the cD_6 idiotype. Cells in the *upper right quadrant* are stained with both anti-CD20 and anti-idiotypic antibody cD_6, and represent 1.31 % of gated cells. These doubly labeled cells belong to the subpopulation of B lymphocytes expressing cD_6 idiotype on their surface. Interestingly, there is a population of gated cells that appear to express cD_6 idiotype (*lower right quadrant*, 1.66 %) but are not B lymphocytes. These might be T lymphocytes bearing the cD_6 idiotype

Table 3. Reactivity of anti-idiotypic antibodies (AIA) with human peripheral B lymphocytes

Antibody	Normal human donors (initials/gender)					
	KM/f	KR/m	NB/f	TO/m	BY/f	MS/f
cD_6	0[a]	0	0.76	16.01	1.15	0.99
dC_4	2.2	0	0	0.46	0.2	0.99
dD_4	0	0.65	0	2.6	0	0.14
dE_2A_2	0	0.17	0	4.16	1.14	0
dE_2C_3	0	0.13	0	4.11	1.27	0
dF_4	0	0.55	0	3.65	0.81	0.51
gD_7A_3	0	0	0	3.67	3.39	0

[a] Each number represents the percentage of B lymphocytes (CD20 positive) bearing the corresponding idiotype.

Comment

Beneficial effects from the presence of naturally occurring AIAs have been demonstrated in kidney allograft recipients [13–16]. Survival time of allografts has been reported to be significantly longer in some cases when the patient had received donor-specific blood transfusions pretransplant. Stimulated by the transfused blood cells, the immune system responded by producing antibodies against incompatible HLA antigens. After a certain period, these anti-HLA antibodies elicited the production of specific AIAs capable of binding to idiotypes on the anti-HLA immunoglobulins and thus neutralizing their activity in regard to humoral rejection of the allograft. In these examples, naturally occurring AIAs helped to maintain long-term allograft function.

By analogy, arteficially generated AIAs directed against anti-αGal immunoglobulins could play a similar role in xenotransplantation. Indeed, this role would be more important than in the case of allografts as humoral mechanisms play a much greater role in the rejection of xenografts than of allografts.

Our data clearly demonstrate the feasibility of such an approach. Many of the monoclonal antibodies produced in this study reacted equally with total human IgG and anti-αGal IgG, but some showed specificity for anti-αGal IgG. High reactivity with anti-αGal IgG demonstrated the specificity of 29 monoclonals for epitopes expressed only on anti-αGal molecules. These epitopes were most likely localized in the variable regions of anti-αGal immunoglobulins since the monoclonal antibodies also bound with high affinity to purified anti-αGal Fab_2 fragments.

Some of the monoclonal AIAs strongly cross-reacted with baboon anti-αGal antibodies, but showed minimal reactivity with total baboon IgG, suggesting that some anti-αGal idiotypes may be shared between humans and non-human primates. Consequently, the same AIAs could protect pig organs transplanted into either species. This is of considerable practical importance because pig-to-baboon engraftment is considered one of the closest experimental models to pig-to-human xenotransplantation.

More than one third of the AIAs were capable of inhibiting the cytotoxic activity of human sera in vitro, the average levels of inhibition ranging from 42 % to more than 95 %. However, none of the AIAs could alone completely protect cultured pig kidney cells. Furthermore, considerable variability was observed among the levels of inhibition accomplished in different human and baboon sera. These two observations indicate that several idiotypes may exist on anti-αGal immunoglobulins and the expression thereof may be variable in populations.

Two different combinations of antibodies (dE_2C_3 + dF_4 and dA_8 + dF_4) completely abolished the cytotoxic activity of human sera. which suggests that at least three major epitopes (i.e., dE_2C_3, dA_8 and dF_4) were represented within the examined human population. Although none these three AIAs alone could completely inhibit the serum cytotoxicity, it took only two of them to achieve complete inhibition, suggesting that the three epitopes (idiotopes) belong to two separate idiotypes. For example, dE_2C_3 and dA_8 could be confined within one idiotype, whereas dF_4 could be a part of the second. The identification as well as distribution of idiotypes of anti-αGal antibodies remain to be further explored.

Anti-idiotypes of the IgM class were generally more effective when compared to those of the IgG class [8]. This could be explained by larger size and higher number of binding sites on IgM molecules, both of which would contribute towards the more efficient inhibition of binding of anti-αGal antibodies to the surface of pig cells.

The results of the four in vivo experiments in baboons carried out in this study suggest that the i.v. administration of AIAs could be effective in protecting transplanted pig organs from hyperacute rejection, providing that the appropriate AIA combination and dose are selected. The protective effect of the injected AIAs was demonstrated by the cell culture method instead of by survival of a xenograft in a live animal. However, work in our laboratory has demonstrated a close correlation between the results using the above in vitro technique with those of actual xenograft survival [17, 18]. Further experiments with purified AIAs are necessary to determine their optimal combinations and dosage.

AIAs could be administered into a recipient intravenously or could be a constituent part of an immunoaffinity column to be used extracorporeally; both of these methods have been used to overcome ABO incompatibility of transplanted organs [19, 20]. Intravenously infused AIAs could specifically neutralize anti-pig antibodies without interfering with other non-anti-pig immunoglobulins. Immunoaffinity columns could be used as an extracorporeal device capable of the selective removal of anti-pig antibodies. Furthermore, both modalities could be applied even more efficiently in the same recipient, with primary extracorporeal immunoadsorption (to deplete the subject of anti-αGal antibodies) followed by subsequent intravenous infusion (to neutralize any remaining or newly produced anti-αGal antibodies).

Intravenously administered mouse monoclonal AIAs would obviously be immunogenic to human recipients, which could result in only a limited period of efficacy. The use of "humanized" murine antibodies could greatly, if not completely, reduce this immunogenicity [21–23].

Anti-idiotypic antibody or antibodies recognizing B-lymphocytes that produce anti-αGal antibodies could be coupled with toxins, such as ricin, and used to eliminate these cells [24–26]. It appears, however, that various combinations of AIAs would be necessary to accomplish a specific and long-lasting immunosuppression.

In conclusion, AIAs directed against human anti-αGal antibodies may prove valuable in therapy to prevent the antibody-mediated rejection of pig organs in humans.

References

1. Rosenberg, J.C., Hawkins, E., Rector, F. Mechanisms of immunological injury during antibody-mediated hyperacute rejection of renal heterografts. Transplantation, 1971; 11:151
2. Hammer, C., Chaussey, C.H., Brendel, W. Preformed natural antibodies in animals and man. Outlook on xenotransplantation. Eur. Surg. Res., 1973; 5:162
3. Paul, L.C. Mechanism of humoral xenograft rejection. In: Cooper, D.K.C., et al., (eds) Xenotransplantation. Springer, Heidelberg, 1991, p. 47

4. Platt, J.L. Bach, F.H. Mechanism of tissue injury in hyperacute xenograft rejection. In: Cooper, D.K.C., et al., (eds) Xenotransplantation. Springer, Heidelberg, 1991, p. 69
5. Good, A.H., Cooper, D.K.C., Malcolm, A.J., et al. Identification of carbohydrate structures that bind human antiporcine antibodies: implications for discordant xengrafting in humans. Transplant. Proc., 1992; 24:559
6. Cooper, D.K.C., Good, A.H., Koren, E., et al. Identification of α-galactosyl and other carbohydrates that are bound by human anti-pig antibodies: relevance to discordant xenografting in man. Transplant. Immunol., 1993; 1:198
7. Cooke, A. Regulation of the immune response. In: Roitt, I., et al. (eds) Immunology. Mosby-Year Book, Europe, Ltd., London, 1993, p. 94
8. Koren E, Milotic F, Neethling FA, Koscec M, Fei D, Kobayashi T, Taniguchi S, Cooper DKC. Murine monoclonal anti-idiotypic antibodies directed against human anti-αGal antibodies reduce in vitro and in vivo cytotoxicity of human and baboon sera to pig cells in culture: implications for pig-to-human organ xenotransplantation. Transplantation, 1996; 62:837
9. Goding, J.W. Production of monoclonal antibodies. In: Goding, J.W. Monoclonal Antibodies: Principles and Practice. Academic Press, London, 1986, p.71
10. Koren, E., Kujundzic, M., Koscec, M., et al. Cytotoxic effects of human preformed anti-Gal IgG and complement on cultured pig cells. Transplant. Proc., 1994; 26:1336
11. Kujundzic, M., Koren, E., Neethling, F.A., et al. Variability of anti-αGal antibodies in human serum and their relation to serum cytotoxicity against pig cells. Xenotransplantation, 1994; 1:58
12. Galili, U., Macher, B.A., Buehler, J., Shohet, S.B. Human natural anti-α-galactosyl IgG. II. The specific recognition of α(1-3)-linked galactose residues. J.Exp.Med., 1985; 162:573
13. Miyajima, T., Higuchi, R., Kashiwabara, H., Yokoyama, T., Fujimoto, S. Anti-idiotypic antibodies in a patient with a functioning renal graft. Nature, 1980; 283:306
14. Pohanka, E., Manfro, R.C., Oto, C., et al. Anti-idiotypic antibodies to HLA after donor-specific blood transfusion (DST). Transplant. Proc., 1989; 21:1806
15. Reed, E., Hardy, M., Benvenisty, A., et al. Effect of anti-idiotypic antibodies to HLA on graft survival in renal allograft recipients. New Engl. J. Med., 1987; 316:1450
16. Rodey, G.A., Phelan, D.L. Association of anti-idiotypic antibody with successful second transplant of a kidney sharing HLA antigens with the previous hyperacutely rejected first kidney. Transplantation, 1989; 48:54
17. Ye Y., Neethling, F.A., Niekrasz, M., et al. Intravenous administration of α-galactosyl carbohydrates reduces in vivo baboon serum cytotoxicity to pig kidney cells and transplanted pig hearts. Transplant. Proc., 1994; 26:1399
18. Kobayashi, T., Taniguchi, S., Ye, Y., et al. Prolongation of graft survival following pig-to-baboon heart transplantation by cobra venom factor (CVF) without natural antibody depletion. Submitted for publication
19. Cooper, D.K.C., Ye, Y., Niekrasz., et al. Specific intravenous carbohydrate therapy – a new concept in inhibiting antibody-mediated rejection: experfience with ABO-incompatible cardiac allografting in the baboon. Transplantation, 1993; 56:769
20. Bannett, A.D., McAlack, R.F., Raja, R., et al. Experiences with known ABO-mismatched renal transplants. Transplant. Proc., 1987; 19:4543
21. Adair, J.R. Engineering antibodies for therapy. Immunol Rev., 1992; 130:5
22. Jolliffe, L.K. Humanized antibodies: enhancing therapeutic utility through antibody engineering. Int. Rev. Immunol., 1993; 10:241

23. Woodle, E.S., Thistlewaite, J.R., Jolliffe, L.K., et al. Humanized antibodies: successful transfer of immune modulating properties and idiotype expression. J. Immunol., 1992; 148:2756
24. Ghetie, V., Swindell, E., Uhr, J.W., Vitetta, E.S. Purification and properties of immunotoxins containing one vs two deglycosylated ricin A chains. J. Immunol. Methods., 1993; 166:117
25. Amlot, P.L., Stone, M.J., Cunningham, D., et al. A phase I study of an anti-CD22-deglycosylated ricin A chain immunotoxin in the treatment of B-cell lymphomas resistant to conventional therapy. Blood, 1993; 82:2624
26. Grossbard, M.L., Gribben, J.G., Freedman, A.S., et al. Adjuvant immunotoxin therapy with anti-B4-blocked ricin after autologous bone marrow transplantation for patients with B-cell non-Hodgkin's lymphoma. Blood, 1993; 81:2263

28 Designer Tissues and Organs: Mouse to Man

D. Faustman

Introduction

A long-standing goal of the transplant community has been to overcome immunological rejection of transplanted tissues and organs. While much of the research has been devoted to identifying new immunosuppressive agents and new combinations of existing agents for allotransplantation, immunosuppression still carries significant short-term and long-term side effects, especially enhanced susceptibility to infection. For xenografts, even stronger immunosuppressive regimens are expected to be necessary. One solution to xenograft acceptance may reside in novel therapeutic strategies that strive to prevent the need for immunosuppression.

Several years ago, our laboratory attempted to avert transplant rejection by immunologically intervening at a new attack point in the rejection cascade. Tissues and cells were treated before transplantation to conceal or eliminate the antigens that summon immune rejection. This technology is sometimes referred to as "donor antigen modification" or, more stylistically, "designer tissue and organs." Our intention was to modify the graft at the molecular level in order to avoid immunosuppression of the host. Earlier efforts at modifying the graft at the cellular level by elimination of donor lymphoid cell populations were successful in mice in the allograft setting, but ineffective for whole organ survival in even lower species or in cellular transplants in higher species. Designer tissues and organs modified at the molecular level offered greater selectivity and latitude in tailoring the graft to escape immune detection. Donor antigen modification contrasts with bone marrow chimerism (i.e., a bone marrow transplant and a solid organ transplant from the same donor to ensure acceptance of the organ) where host immune manipulations are employed.

Without the risks of systemic immunosuppression, designer tissues and organs could be therapeutic for a broad range of chronic conditions that are not life-threatening. They also could be offered to conventional organ transplant patients at earlier stages of their disease when patients are healthier and better able to withstand surgical intervention. The main risk with designer tissues and organs is that the modified donor tissue could be rejected, a risk commonly encountered with any transplant. Because designer tissue can be potentially rendered safer and may ultimately avoid host intervention, a broader spectrum of diseases could be treated.

The purpose of this chapter is to describe the research evolution of designer tissues and to trace its contribution to a growing body of transplant research.

Research in murine hosts demonstrated the successful transplantation of xenogeneic cells and tissues modified at the molecular level without immunosuppression. Transplant success of cells across species by donor antigen modification allowed the extension of these concepts to the genetic level. The ability to modify antigens either at the DNA, RNA, or protein level offers tremendous latitude in the development of new biological therapies. Variations on the designer tissue concept are being probed in animal models of diabetes, solid organ failure, and neurological diseases. A concept launched in the laboratory in the early 1990s has already culminated in landmark human clinical trials for Parkinson's disease using donor-modified pig neurons into humans.

The wide range of applications of designer tissues and organs for allo- and xenotransplantation is readily apparent; modified donor cells, tissues, and organs can be considered potential therapies for an almost limitless number of conditions as long as the dominant antigens are identified and then effectively shielded or eliminated prior to implantation.

Origin of the Designer Tissue Concept

Our idea of targeting donor antigens instead of modification of the host immune system was stimulated by research on the molecular events surrounding the killing of target cells by cytotoxic T lymphocytes (CTLs, hereinafter referred to as T cells). In an elegant study, Spits and coworkers [1] identified the sequential stages of T cell destruction of the target cell. In contrast to earlier research, which focused primarily on the T cell, they examined the roles of cell surface markers on both the T cell and the target cell. By using antibodies against different cell surface markers to block distinct stages, they were able to tease apart in vitro the interactions between molecules on the T cell and the target cell. They were among the first to identify three stages in T cell cytotoxicity: (1) adhesion between T cell and target cell, (2) T cell receptor activation, and (3) T cell lysis of the target cell (Fig. 1).

A critical finding was that one of the major classes of histocompatibility antigens on the surface of the target cell – the major histocompatibility complex (MHC) class I molecules – were involved in both adhesion to, and activation of, the T cell. Class I antigens and other classes of antigens encoded by the MHC complex serve to distinguish "self" from "non-self" because they differ across species and between members of the same species. Class I antigens have long been implicated in eliciting T cell cytotoxicity, but this study offered more detailed insight into their pivotal role. What this study also demonstrated was that antibodies to class I antigens could prevent T cell adhesion and activation, thereby interfering with lysis.

Spits and coworkers crystallized the importance of class I antigens in immune rejection of tumors. With this study's goal centering on enhancing tumor rejection, we departed upon the idea of a central role of target class I antigens as pivotal in tumor escape, and perhaps similarly pivotal in an opposing role for manipulation in transplantation. As a test antigen, we chose to mask class I on donor cells with antibody fragments, and then transplant the donor antigen-modified cells into non-immunosuppressed hosts.

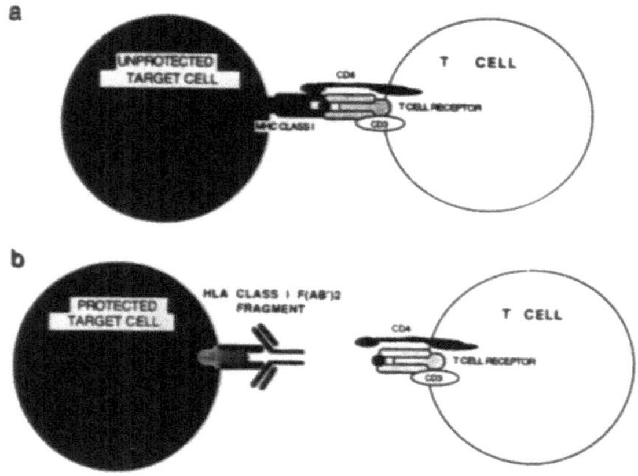

Fig. 1a,b. Adhesion, activation, and lysis by cytotoxic T lymphocytes (CTLs). *MHC*, major histocompatibility complex

First Demonstration of the Concept

Using a xenogeneic model, the first successful demonstration of the designer tissue concept was demonstrated [2]. We found that when we coated the graft with antibody fragments to conceal class I antigens, the graft eluded the host immune system indefinitely and functioned normally. The host developed tolerance to the treated graft because secondary transplants of untreated tissue were later accepted. The mechanism of donor specific tolerance is still not fully defined, but may involve induction of T cell anergy through altered donor class I density. Altered class I density may be pivotal in T cell shaping in both the periphery as well as the thymus [3–5].

The graft consisted of purified human cadaveric islets that had been incubated with antibody fragments before being implanted into non-immunosuppressed mice. We decided to produce very pure antibody fragments because they lacked the portion of the antibody molecule that binds complement, the Fc fragment. When the Fc fragment is enzymatically cleaved from the $F(ab')_2$ fragment (Fig. 2), the purified $F(ab')_2$ fragment binds to the graft for several days without fixing complement which would have destroyed the graft. Grafts survived for 200 days and functioned appropriately, as determined by assays for human C peptide, a proinsulin processing product. Finally, human liver cells similarly treated with antibody fragments also survived for an extended period.

Treatment with *whole* antibodies to class I antigens failed to prolong graft survival, as did treatment with whole antibodies and antibody fragments to CD29. CD29 is an antigen uniquely expressed on the passenger lymphocytes which accompany the graft because they cannot be entirely eliminated during the purification process. Finally, treatment of the graft with polyclonal antibody fragments to all antigenic determinants on human islets prolonged graft survival until the point when class I antibody fragments were removed from the mixture. Graft rejection ensued at a slowed rate, attesting to the critical role of class I antigens as pivotal for this transplantation barrier, although recognizing the possible importance of other antigens in additional immune responses.

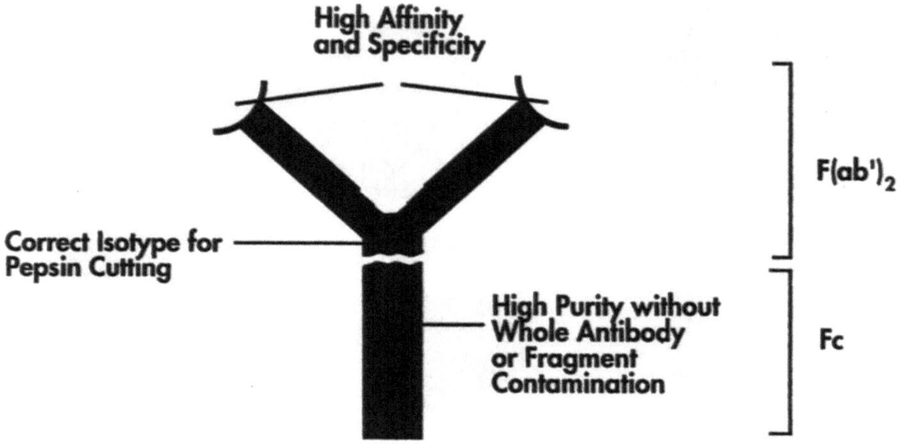

Fig. 2. Fab fragment cleaved from Fc fragment. Requirements for a masking antibody

For the sake of rigor, we selected a xenogeneic instead of an allogenic model to test the designer tissue concept. If designer tissues could succeed in the demanding case across a species barrier, then they could be considered for simpler allogeneic models. In other respects, however, our xenogeneic model represented the height of simplicity. First, the tissue contained only one dominant antigen that needed to be masked. We found that human islet tissue highly expressed class I antigens, while displaying only minimal expression of adhesion molecules intercellular adhesion molecule (ICAM)-1 and lymphocyte function-associated antigen (LFA)-3 (which in other tissues are thought to stabilize binding and to contribute to T cell activation). Second, the vasculature could be separated from the tissue to avoid hyperacute rejection, the earliest and most formidable barrier to discordant xenograft acceptance. Third, our model targeted antigens at the protein level rather than at the genetic level. Our goal was to conceal protein antigens that already appeared on the surface of graft cells. Other approaches, discussed later in this chapter, target antigens not at the protein level, but at the DNA and RNA level. The use of more sophisticated transgenic and antisense technology, respectively, can similarly prevent antigen expression and validated the donor antigens as a target for the immune response.

In summary, this tough xenogeneic model confirmed the paramount role of class I antigens in islet cell rejection. By providing a challenging test of the designer tissue concept, it also helped to launch a novel therapeutic strategy.

Expansion of Research on Designer Tissues

After our first study was published, our laboratory and others began to probe the potential of designer tissues, using a variety of donor antigen modification techniques as well as masking antigens with protein fragments in varying transplan-

Table 1. Designer donor tissues

Tissues	Allo/xeno	Donor/recipient	Target	Reference
Masking antibody				
Islets	Xeno	Human/mouse	Class I	[2]
Islets	Xeno	Human/mouse	All surface antigens	[2]
Islets	Allo/xeno	Human or monkey/monkey	Class I	[7]
Islets	Allo	Mouse/mouse	Class I	[6]
Neurons	Xeno	Pig/rat	Class I	[8]
Neurons	Xeno	Pig/monkey	Class I	[9]
Liver cells	Xeno	Human/mouse	Class I	[2]
Gene ablation				
Islets	Allo	Mouse/mouse	Class I	[11]
Islets	Allo	Mouse/mouse	Class I	[12]
Islets	Allo	Mouse/mouse	Class I	[6]
Liver cells	Allo/xeno	Mouse/mouse or guinea pig or frog	Class I	[13]
Kidneys	Allo	Mouse/mouse	Class I	[10]
Gene addition				
White blood cells	Xeno	Mouse or pig/human[a]	CD59	[15]
Endothelial cells	Xeno	Pig/human[a]	CD46, CD55, CD46/CD55 hybrid	[16]
Endothelial cells	Xeno	Pig/human[a]	CD46, CD55, CD59	[17]
Hearts	Xeno	Pig/baboon	CD55, CD59	[18]
Hearts, kidneys, lungs	Xeno	Pig/monkey	CD59	[19]
COS cells	Xeno	Pig/human[a]	H transferase	[20]

[a]Human serum in vitro.

tation settings. The body of research, summarized in Table 1, can be classified into four distinct groups based on the technique used to modify the donor tissue. The techniques currently employed for donor antigen modification are the following: (a) antibody masking, (b) gene ablation, (c) gene addition, and (d) RNA ablation.

Antibody Masking

Antibody masking of xenogeneic tissue is the first of the donor antigen modification techniques to progress to primate and human trials. Pancreatic islet cells and neurons are the most common types of donor cells to be camouflaged with antibody masking, although any type of tissue can theoretically be treated once the dominant antigens have been identified. All of the studies cited below targeted class I antigens using antibody fragments.

Islet cell masking for the treatment of diabetes has been pursued with mixed results. Osorio and colleagues [6] targeted class I antigens in a mouse allograft model. To approximate a diabetic state, the mice first were treated with a drug that chemically induced hyperglycemia. Then they received islet allografts which had been pretreated with antibody fragments. Graft survival was prolonged relative to controls, but within 1 month the grafts were eventually rejected. Investigators attributed eventual allograft rejection to a variety of possibilities, including the absence of sufficient quantities of $F(ab')_2$ fragments, anti-idiotypic antibodies against the $F(ab')_2$ fragment, and an immune pathway independent of class I activation of T cells.

Steele and colleagues [7] investigated islet cell transplants in a primate model. Cynomolgus monkeys received either allogeneic or xenogeneic (human) islets. The grafts were pretreated with antibody fragments to class I antigens. Histologic evidence of donor islets were present months after transplantation into non-immunosuppressed monkeys.

Neuronal xenografts with antibody masking have been investigated for Huntington's disease [8] and Parkinson's disease [9]. In the first study, fetal pig striatal cells were implanted into rats whose striatum had been lesioned one week earlier with injections of quinolinic acid. These injections destroy striatal neurons in an attempt to simulate the dysfunction present in Huntington's disease. Rats received either untreated tissue or tissue pretreated with $F(ab')_2$ fragments against porcine class I antigens. Of the control rats receiving untreated tissue, some were immunosuppressed with cyclosporine (CsA) while others were not. Three to four months later, graft survival was found to be prolonged in animals given $F(ab')_2$-treated grafts and in the CsA treated animals given unaltered grafts. Grafts did not survive in non-immunosuppressed controls. Graft volume, determined histologically with the aid of computer image analysis, was significantly larger in the CsA group compared with the $F(ab')_2$ group. Yet in both of these groups, immunohistochemistry revealed graft cytoarchitecture to be well organized and graft axons to have correctly grown in the direction of their target nuclei. It was encouraging that pig neurons appeared to be capable of locating their target.

In a similar study design, Burns and coworkers [9] applied antibody masking to a primate model of Parkinson's disease. Porcine mesencephalic neuroblasts were implanted into monkeys with 1-methyl-4-phenyl-1,2,3,6-tetrahydropyridine (MPTP)-induced Parkinsonism. Measures of locomotor activity and dopamine fiber density in the host striatum confirmed that pretreatment of donor tissue with $F(ab')_2$ fragments succeeded at restoring motor function and replenishing dopamine fibers at the site of implantation. A control animal, maintained on CsA after receiving untreated cells, showed similar improvement. A non-immunosuppressed control showed no improvement after transplantation, suggesting graft rejection. These and other findings from the same laboratory have led to the inauguration of a clinical trial for Parkinson's disease. In this trial, porcine neuroblasts are treated with antibody fragments to class I before implantation into patient's striatum (O. Isacson, personal communication).

The studies described in this section highlight the range of potential applications of antibody masking to both allo- and xenotransplants. Islet cell masking has encountered unexpected hurdles in the application to type I diabetes, a topic discussed in the next section. However, neuronal cell masking has been sufficiently effective to usher in human clinical trials.

Gene Ablation

Gene ablation, or gene "knockout" technology, offers another vehicle to modify donor tissue and organs. With gene ablation, the gene or genes encoding protein antigens can be permanently deleted, thereby eliminating antigen expression in all cells. In one common method of gene ablation, the target gene is inactivated in cultured embryonic stem cells via homologous recombination; a target vector containing an inactive version of the gene recombines with, and thereby replaces, the wild type gene. Through reintroduction of the embryonic cells into a foster mother and through selective breeding, progeny can be produced that are homozygous for the mutation. Rejection by the host immune system is expected to be avoided when the targeted gene encodes a protein antigen slated for expression on the surface of donor cells.

The major advantage of gene ablation over protein modification of donor tissue is that the antigen is permanently eliminated in all cells, tissues, and organs in which it is expressed. The major limitation is that it is only available in mice, which are too phylogenetically distant from humans to be considered as suitable donors. The permanent nature of the modification also can sometimes be a limitation, especially when the protein encoded by the gene has additional functions. Inactivation of the gene might lead to physiological changes that compromise the utility of the donor tissue. Gene ablation can also target genes that encode proteins essential for the target protein expression.

Several transplantation laboratories have exploited the availability of knockout mice deficient in β_2-microglobulin. β_2-Microglobulin is a peptide that forms part of the class I molecule and is necessary for its assembly and expression. Mice homozygous for the β_2-microglobulin mutation fail to display class I antigens on the cell surface, a feature that makes them highly desirable for transplantation studies. While much of the research described below has focused on islet cell and liver cell xenotransplants, one project examined whole organ allografts. Coffman and coworkers [10] found that kidneys from β_2-microglobulin-deficient mice functioned significantly better in allogeneic recipients than did kidneys from normal mice.

The fate of pancreatic islet transplants from β_2-microglobulin-deficient mice has been explored in several studies. The islets showed prolonged survival when implanted into a normal mouse strain [11, 12]. Most grafts survived indefinitely and were capable of reversing hyperglycemia that had been chemically induced prior to transplantation. Investigators attributed the few instances of graft rejection to three possibilities. First, some surface expression of class I antigens can occur in the absence of β_2-microglobulin. The presence of even a fraction of the total number of class I antigens may be sufficient for T cell recognition and lysis. Second, β_2-microglobulin circulating in the serum of the recipient can be used to reconstitute class I antigens on the donor tissue (since β_2-microglobulin is a highly conserved protein not encoded by genes at the MHC locus.)

Third, rejection of the tissue from β_2-microglobulin-deficient donors may be mediated by other immune pathways, such as by natural killer cells. Support for the second and third possibilities was presented by Li and Faustman [13] in their study of liver cell allo- and xenografts.

Graft rejection almost invariably occurs, however, when the recipients are nonobese diabetic (NOD) mice [11, 14]. Islet allografts from β_2-microglobulin-deficient mice are rejected by NOD mice at a slightly delayed rate but still soon after implantation. This is in contrast to the success with recipients whose diabetes is chemically induced. NOD mice, unlike those with chemically induced diabetes, spontaneously develop an autoimmune form of diabetes that destroys the graft because it displays a variety of antigens identical to autoantigens. In this respect, NOD mice more closely resemble humans with type I diabetes. These findings suggest that elimination of class I antigens alone will not be sufficient for the treatment of humans with type I diabetes. One of the many directions for future research is to pinpoint the autoantigens on the graft which induce autoimmune rejection.

Elimination of class I antigens also may be insufficient for selected tissues and selected combinations of donor and host species. Liver cells from β_2-microglobulin-deficient donors were implanted into allogeneic recipients and two separate species of xenogeneic recipients [13]. The allotransplants and the xenotransplants into guinea pigs were not that effective, in contrast to xenotransplant effectiveness in frog recipients. When liver cells were transplanted from humans to mice in antibody masking experiments, they were accepted [2]. These studies show the results of class I antigen removal to vary according to the species combination of donor and host.

Gene ablation experiments have demonstrated the advantages and limitations of eliminating class I antigens. They are clearly a dominant antigen on islet cells and neurons in some allogeneic and xenogeneic combinations. However, class I antigens may play a secondary role depending on the type of donor tissue, the species combination, and/or the disease state of the recipient. In these cases, other dominant antigens need to be identified and targeted.

Gene Addition

Gene addition is a technique especially promising for transplantation of solid organs, the most challenging type of transplant, and represents another form of donor antigen modification. What makes solid organs particularly troublesome from the point of view of transplantation is that they are subject to hyperacute rejection. Hyperacute rejection, the first wave of assault against discordant xenografts, results in rapid rejection within minutes to hours. The vascular endothelium, which cannot be removed prior to transplant, expresses the αGal1–3Gal (αGal) epitope, the target of hyperacute rejection [15]. Preformed antibodies that bind to αGal activate complement, resulting in loss of vascular integrity, hemorrhage, ischemia, and necrosis.

Gene addition involves the insertion of a foreign gene (or transgene) early in development. The desired gene is microinjected into the nucleus of a fertilized egg, thereby giving rise to a mature animal with the transgene incorporated into the genome of each cell. The desired gene or genes used thus far in xenograft research encode proteins designed to inhibit hyperacute rejection. Gene addition is advantageous because it can be readily undertaken in many kinds of donor animals, particularly swine. Swine are among favored donor animals for solid organ transplants because of their ease of breeding, domestication, low maintenance costs, similarities to humans in organ size and physiology, and fewer ethical objections. The other advantages of gene addition, like those for gene ablation, are permanence and versatility.

The body of research described below employs gene addition mostly with porcine donors. In all but one study, the transgenes encode human complement regulatory proteins, cell surface molecules that are species specific and act to control the complement cascade. Complement regulatory proteins protect host endothelial cells from activated complement. Were it not for complement regulatory proteins, autologous cells would be killed by hundreds of their own complement molecules which readily diffuse from their targets. Investigators are modifying donor organs with *human* complement inhibitors, because the organs are eventually to be transplanted into humans. However, before human trials can be undertaken, the efficacy of transgenic organs in withstanding complement-mediated cell lysis must be tested in animal models and in vitro.

Most studies have created transgenic cell lines or transgenic animals expressing human CD46 (membrane cofactor protein), CD55 (decay-accelerating factor, DAF), and/or CD59. The first two are complement regulatory proteins that block distinct reactions in the early stages of the complement cascade, whereas, CD59 inhibits the final reaction, the formation of the membrane attack complex which lyses cells.

Fodor and colleagues [16] produced transgenic animals expressing human CD59. To enhance expression of the transgene in selected cell types, the transfected DNA also contained a promoter sequence. Using immunohistochemistry, they verified the presence of human CD59 on the surface of endothelial cells and a variety of cell types taken from the transgenic animals. Then they harvested peripheral blood mononuclear cells (PMBCs) and exposed them in vitro to human sera. PMBCs from transgenic swine were superior to controls in resisting complement attack.

Extending this concept to other complement regulatory proteins, Miyagawa and coworkers [17, 18] engineered swine endothelial cells to express human CD46, CD55, and/or CD59. These studies had the advantage of examining the protective effects of complement regulatory proteins in the same cells that trigger hyperacute rejection. They also had the advantage of examining the joint expression of more than one complement regulatory protein. They found that transfection of CD55 and a hybrid CD46/CD55 suppressed complement cytotoxicity by 50 %–80 %. Both were more effective than transfection with CD46 alone, which suppressed activity by 15 %–50 %. In a follow-up study, they compared the efficacy of CD46, CD55, and CD59. CD59 was the only protein of the three which offered minimal protection, in contrast to the findings of Fodor and coworkers, who studied the effects of CD59 in a different cell line.

These in vitro studies set the stage for whole organ transplants from transgenic pigs into nonhuman primates. Transgenic organs expressing human CD55 and CD59 [19] and human CD59 alone (T. Kroshus et al., unpublished) were implanted into baboons and Old World monkeys, respectively. Hearts, lungs, and kidneys survived up to 48 h, a significant improvement over control organs which survived for only 60–90 min. Hyperacute rejection still took place, suggesting that human complement regulatory proteins were capable of providing some, but not enough, protection to surmount hyperacute rejection.

With the realization that complement regulatory proteins may not prove sufficiently effective in combating hyperacute rejection, Sandrin and coworkers [20] have devised another transgenic strategy: to reduce the expression of the epitope eliciting hyperacute rejection (αGal) through competitive inhibition. These investigators created transgenic cell lines and animals expressing the human enzyme, H transferase. Known also as α1,2-fucosyltransferase, this enzyme was selected because it shares a common acceptor substrate with α1,3-galactosyltransferase, the enzyme that normally generates αGal by placing a terminal galactose moiety onto a cell surface glycoprotein. Investigators demonstrated that H transferase out-competes α1,3-galactosyltransferase and places a fucosyl residue on the substrate. Instead of forming αGal, a fucosylated *N*-acetyllactosamine is generated. This is the universally tolerated human blood group O antigen. Without the expression of αGal, porcine cells transfected with H transferase exhibited enhanced survival in vitro when incubated with human serum. The major advantage of this strategy is its prevention of the first stage of hyperacute rejection, i.e., the binding of preformed antibodies, which may also cause direct damage to the endothelial surface [15]. The binding of preformed antibodies was previously believed to be benign as long as complement fixation was avoided.

RNA Ablation

RNA ablation is another promising strategy that strives to prevent antigen expression at the RNA level by blocking transcription or translation. RNA ablation can be achieved through the creation of oligodeoxynucleotides that are complementary to, and hybridize with, DNA or RNA sequences to inhibit transcription or translation, respectively.

The only studies of RNA ablation in the transplant field to-date are those by Ramanathan and coworkers [21, 22]. They identified an oligodeoxynucleotide that inhibited induction of class I and ICAM expression by interferon-gamma. The studies were performed in vitro in a cell line, K562, that normally has low level expression of class I antigens. They first postulated that the oligodeoxynucleotide acted in the early stages of interferon-γ induction rather than post-translationally. In their follow-up study, they showed the oligodeoxynucleotide to act even earlier via a novel mechanism – it inhibited binding of interferon-γ to the cell surface [21, 22]. This may be an unusual mechanism for an oligodeoxynucleotide, but it only enhances the possibilities for xenotransplant research. What these studies provide is yet another means of blocking expression of class I antigens.

Comment

Designer tissues and organs through donor antigen modification hold tremendous promise for xenotransplantation. Research in animal models has already demonstrated that long-term xenograft survival can be achieved without immunosuppression. This achievement has galvanized the transplantation community, for it shows that an overwhelming obstacle to xenograft acceptance can be alleviated. Immune rejection need not occur if graft antigens can be immunologically masked or genetically eliminated. Researchers now have at their disposal a battery of techniques which operate at the DNA, RNA, or protein level to remove or conceal antigens. Xenotransplantation is within reach, not just for patients with life-threatening conditions, but also for patients with chronic conditions. As testimony to the widespread applications for chronic conditions, the first clinical trial of designer tissues is for patients with Parkinson's disease.

The successes with cellular and tissue xenografts bode well for the far more difficult task of whole organ xenotransplantation. Solid organs have a multiplicity of antigens, particularly those which elicit hyperacute rejection. Once all of the dominant antigens are identified, the therapeutic strategy for whole organs and tissues is conceptually identical - modify the donor, not the host.

References

1. SPITS, H., VAN SCHOOTEN, W., KEIZER, H., et al. Alloantigen recognition is preceded by nonspecific adhesion of cytotoxic T cells and target cells. Science. 232:403, 1986
2. FAUSTMAN, D., COE, C. Prevention of xenograft rejection by masking donor HLA class I antigens. Science. 252:1700, 1991
3. HOGQUIST, K.A., JAMESON, S.C., HEATH, W.R., et al. T cell receptor antagonist peptides induce positive selection. Cell. 76:17, 1994
4. ASHTON-RICKARDT, P.G., BANDEIRA, A., DELANEY, J.R., et al. Evidence for a differential avidity model of T cell selection in the thymus. Cell. 76:651, 1994
5. SEBZDA, E., WALLACE, V.A., MAYER, J., et al. Positive and negative thymocyte selection induced by different concentrations of a single peptide. Science. 263:1615, 1994
6. OSORIO, R.W., ASCHER, N.L., STOCK, P.G. Prolongation of in vivo mouse islet allograft survival by modulation of MHC class I antigen. Transplantation. 57:783, 1994
7. STEELE, D.J.R., HERTEL-WULFF, B., CHAPPELL, S., et al. Long-term survival of pancreatic islets in diabetic monkeys. Cell Transplant. 3:216, 1994
8. PAKZABAN, P., DEACON, T.W., BURNS, L.H., et al. Enhanced survival of neural xenografts after masking of donor major histocompatibility complex class I. Soc. Neurosci. 16:1708, 1995
9. BURNS, L.H., PAKZABAN, P., DEACON, T.W., et al. Xenotransplantation of porcine ventral mesencephalic neuroblasts restores function in primates with chronic MPTP-induced Parkinsonism. Soc. Neurosci. 19:1330, 1994
10. COFFMAN, T., GEIER, S., IBRAHIM, S., et al. Improved renal function in mouse kidney allografts lacking MHC class I antigens. J. Immunol. 151:425, 1993

11. MARKMANN, J.F., BASSIRI, H., DESAI, N.M., et al. Indefinite survival of MHC class I-deficient murine pancreatic islet allografts. Transplantation. 54:1085, 1992
12. OSORIO, R.W., ASCHER, N.L., JAENISCH, R., et al. Major histocompatibility complex class I deficiency prolongs islet allograft survival. Diabetes. 42:1520, 1993
13. LI, H., FAUSTMAN, D. Use of donor β2-microglobulin-deficient transgenic mouse liver cells for isografts, allografts, and xenografts. Transplantation. 55:940, 1993
14. OSORIO, R.W., ASCHER, N.L., MELZER, J.S., et al. Beta-2-microglobulin gene disruption prolongs murine islet allograft survival in NOD mice. Transplant. Proc. 26:752, 1994
15. PLATT, J.L. A perspective on xenograft rejection and accommodation. Immunol. Rev. 141:127, 1994
16. FODOR, W.L., WILLIAMS, B.L., MATIS, L.A. Expression of a functional human complement inhibitor in a transgenic pig as a model for the prevention of xenogeneic hyperacute organ rejection. Proc. Natl. Acad. Sci. USA. 91:11153, 1994
17. MIYAGAWA, S., SHIRAKURA, A., IWATA, K., et al. Effects of transfected complement regulatory proteins, MCP, DAF, and MCP/DAF hybrid, on complement-mediated swine endothelial cell lysis. Transplantation. 58:834, 1994
18. MIYAGAWA, S., SHIRAKURA, R., NAKATA, S., et al. Effect of transfected MACIF (CD59) on complement-mediated swine endothelial cell lysis, compared with those of membrane cofactor protein (CD46) and decay-accelerating factor (CD55). Transplant. Proc. 27:328, 1995
19. McCURREY, K.R., KOOYMAN, D.L., ALVARADO, C.G., et al. Human complement regulatory proteins protect swine-to-primate cardiac xenografts from humoral injury. Nature Med. 1:423, 1995
20. SANDRIN, M.S., FODOR, W.L., MOUHTOURIS, E., et al. Enzymatic remodeling of the carbohydrate surface of a xenogeneic cell substantially reduces human antibody binding and complement-mediated cytolysis. Nature Med. 1:1261, 1995
21. RAMANATHAN, M., LANTZ, M., MACGREGOR, R.D., et al. Characterization of the oligodeoxynucleotide-mediated inhibition of interferon-gamma-induced major histocompatibility complex class I and intercellular adhesion molecule-1. J. Biol. Chem. 269:24564, 1994
22. RAMANATHAN, M., LANTZ, M., MACGREGOR, R.D., et al. Inhibition of interferon-gamma-induced major histocompatibility complex class I expression by certain oligodeoxynucleotides. Transplantation. 57:612, 1994

29 Use of Anti-μ Monoclonal Antibodies in Xenotransplantation: A Potential Approach To Overcome Vascular Rejection

M. Soares, X. Havaux, F. Cormont, F. Nisol, T. Besse, P. Gianello, D. Latinne, and H. Bazin

Introduction

In 1982, Alexandre and colleagues demonstrated that hyperacute rejection (HAR) of ABO-incompatible kidney allografts could be overcome if the recipient's circulating preformed natural antibodies were depleted prior to transplantation. Although anti-ABO natural antibodies regain normal serum levels in the few days following transplantation, HAR usually does not occur [1, 3, 4, 36]. As first hypothesized by F.H. Bach [8], the acceptance of an ABO-incompatible allograft could result from modification of endothelial cells (EC) physiological response, characteristics leading to "accommodation," i.e., allowing the survival of the transplant in the presence of high levels of circulating IgM natural antibodies and complement, after a period of depletion.

These pioneering studies suggested that HAR of immediately vascularized discordant xenografts might also be bypassed if the recipient's circulating xenoreactive natural antibodies (XNA) could be removed prior to xenotransplantation [6, 7, 55]. Using similar treatments to those previously shown to inhibit the HAR of ABO-incompatible kidney allografts, Alexandre and colleagues obtained a significant prolongation of the survival time of pig-to-baboon kidney xenografts, but these xenografts were still rejected after 2–3 weeks following transplantation [2, 30].

As is the case with ABO-incompatible allografts, transplantation of immediately vascularized xenografts across phylogenetically distant species, such as pigs and primates, results in the loss of the xenograft due to a rapid and violent humoral immunological phenomenon termed as hyperacute rejection (HAR). The pathology of the HAR of pig-to-primate discordant xenografts is similar to that observed in ABO-incompatible allografts and is characterized by the rapid and irreversible occurrence of interstitial hemorrhage, edema, diffuse intravascular platelet and fibrin thrombi, together with marked EC injury [11, 49]. Discordant xenografts undergoing HAR show extensive intraluminal vascular depositions of recipient's XNA (of the IgM and, to a lesser extent, the IgG isotypes) along with complement C1q, C4, C3, and C5b-9 (membrane attack complex) proteins [49].

Circulating XNA recognize on the surface of porcine EC several glycoproteins expressing the oligosaccharide Gal-α(1,3)-Gal-β(1,4)-GlcNAc-R epitope [27, 31, 56]. It is know clear that XNA recognize a restricted number of EC glycoproteins (gp115/135) which have been demonstrated to be the porcine equivalents of human integrins α_1, α_v, α_3/α_5, β_1, β_3, and von Willebrand factor [51].

Together with XNA, complement activation plays a central role on the pathogenesis of HAR of discordant xenografts [50]. Therefore, a great deal of effort has recently been aimed towards suppressing complement activation in xenograft recipients. Probably one of the most promising approaches consists of using transgenic pigs, overexpressing one or several human complement inhibitory proteins (CD55, CD46, or CD59) on the surface of EC [22]. The use of CD55 transgenic pigs seems to be particularly interesting for xenotransplatation in primates since, in the absence of further immunosuppressive treatment, these transgenic organs are no longer hyperacutely rejected (White et al., oral communication, Third International Meeting of Xenotransplantation, Boston, 1995). However, 4–6 days after transplantation cardiac xenografts from CD55 transgenic pigs stop functioning, probably due to delayed xenograft rejection, a process mediated mainly by recipient elicited XNA as well as by monocyte and NK cell infiltration [11]. Since in the pig-to-primate combination complement activation is thought to take place primarily through the classical pathway, HAR may be overcome using therapeutic protocols resulting in the sustained depletion of circulating XNA.

Following the demonstration that successful ABO-incompatible kidney allografting could be achieved after preoperative depletion of circulating natural antibodies by plasma exchange and splenectomy, similar protocols have been used to deplete circulating XNA (and other factors) and prolong survival time of discordant xenografts [2–4, 24, 37, 38, 40, 53, 54,58, 66]. Although splenectomy and plasma exchange have proven to be useful in depleting circulating XNA (to 80%–85% of pretreatment levels) and prolonging the survival of discordant xenografts, rejection always occurs upon the return of circulating XNA (and other factors).

The high efficiency of splenectomy in decreasing the levels of circulating IgM XNA (50%–60% depletion as compared to pretreatment levels) in adult rats may be related to our recent finding that IgM XNA-secreting cells (SC) are exclusively located in the spleen where they account for approximately 0.1% of the total number of IgM SC [54, 60].

The combination of splenectomy and B cell immunosuppressive drugs, such as 15-deoxyspergualin (DSG), brequinar sodium, or mycophenolate mofetil (RS61443), in protocols involving complement inactivation by cobra venom factor (CVF) has been shown to prolong guinea pig-to-rat cardiac xenograft rejection from a few minutes to 6–7 days [15, 33, 35, 39]. Similar protocols using CVF, splenectomy, plasma exchange, cylophosphamide and DSG have also been shown to significantly prolong the survival time of porcine-to-primate cardiac xenografts from a few hours to 17 days [40].

An alternative approach which has been shown to be successful in achieving profound depletion of circulating IgM XNA in both humans and nonhuman primates consists of the extracorporeal perfusion of the recipient's blood through one or several porcine vascularized organs prior to the xenotransplant [26, 44, 65]. In addition, the extracorporeal perfusion of recipient serum using immunoabsorbent columns containing the oligosaccharide epitopes recognized by circulating XNA, such as the Gal-α(1,3)-Gal-β(1,4)-GlcNAc-R epitope, or by anti-human IgM and IgG antibodies has also been reported to be useful in depleting circulating XNA [17, 41]. However, it should be noted that these ex vivo perfusion techniques do not act on XNA production and thus will only deplete circulating

XNA for a relative short period of time, which may be inadequate for EC "accommodation" to take place. As recently demonstrated, the continuous intravenous infusion of synthetic A or B tissue antigens in baboons leads to the inhibition of circulating natural antibodies and to the prolongation of survival of ABO-incompatible allografts, which would suggest that the continuous infusion of synthetic oligosaccharides containing the Gal-α(1,3)-Gal-β(1,4)-GlcNAc-R epitope may be able to inhibit circulating XNA in primates and probably suppress the HAR of porcine-to-primate discordant xenografts [19, 20].

It is our belief, however, that, in order to achieve "accommodation" of discordant xenografts, total depletion of circulating XNA for a relative long period of time may have to be achieved by removing not only the circulating "pool" of XNA, but probably more importantly by inhibiting the production of XNA by B cells.

Previous work from our and other laboratories has demonstrated that, in rodents, treatment from birth with polyclonal anti-μ antibodies (a model which mimics the antigen recognition by surface IgM) arrests B cell development and migration of newly formed immature B cells from the bone marrow to the spleen [12, 13, 18, 45]. Several studies have also demonstrated the crucial role of cross-linking and internalization of membrane IgM (mIgM) or IgD (mIgD) on the surface of immature B cells in the induction of B cell tolerance [16, 25, 32]. This inhibition B cell of B cell maturation by signaling through the B cell antigen receptor (mIgM or mIgD) may result from a lack of appropriate costimulating signals through other surface receptors, such as the CD40 molecule [25, 46, 64]. The ability of mIgM cross-linking to arrest immature B cell maturation and differentiation has led us to propose a new model of B cell suppression based on the administration of anti-μ monoclonal antibody (mAb) in adult animals.

Guinea Pig-to-Rat Model

The role of circulating XNA in the pathogenesis of the HAR of discordant xenografts has been difficult to assess, mainly because the methods used to deplete circulating XNA in vivo are often not totally specific and probably insufficiently performed [24, 38]. To address this question we have depleted circulating IgM XNA to undetectable levels by administrating high doses of an anti-μ mAb in adult rats (30 mg/kg at day −3 and 15 mg/kg at day −1 before xenotransplantation) and subsequently analyzed the outcome of guinea pig cardiac discordant xenografts.

The survival time of guinea pig cardiac xenografts was significantly prolonged in IgM-depleted animals (62 min, $p<0.01$) as compared to controls treated with PBS (18 min survival time) or isotype-matched anti-IgA mAb (12 min survival time) [59]. Prolongation of the xenograft survival time in the anti-μ-treated group correlated with an undetectable serum level of IgM and IgM XNA and with the absence of detectable IgM XNA deposits on the rejected xenograft vascular endothelium. Furthermore, the prolongation of the survival time of guinea pig xenografts in anti-μ-treated rats was not due to a decrease in complement activity since at the time of rejection no significant decrease in C1q, C4, C3, B factor, and C5-dependent complement hemolytic activity was observed between controls and anti-μ-treated animals [59]. At the time of rejection both IgM-depleted and control animals showed intense C3 deposition on the rejected xenograft vascular endothelium and myocardium, clearly indicating that complement activation occurs in absence of IgM XNA [59]. Although HAR of guinea pig cardiac xenografts was not bypassed by the depletion of circulating IgM XNA, our data clearly indicate that IgM XNA are directly implicated in the pathogenesis of HAR and that the anti-μ approach is a potential therapeutic treatment for discordant xenografts.

It is also clear from these experiments that IgM-independent activation of complement through the alternative pathway is one of the main mechanisms responsible for the pathogenesis of HAR in the guinea pig-to-rat xenograft model [58].

In order to achieve the long-term depletion of circulating XNA which may allow the induction of EC "accommodation" we have developed an approach based on the injection into adult animals of repeated high doses (15–30 mg/kg) of an anti-μ mAb [58]. The first version of this protocol consisted of the injection into adult rats of an anti-rat IgM mAb (MARM-7) after splenectomy, plasma exchange, and the administration of the anti-B cell immunosuppressive drug, RS61443 [58]. This procedure was able to deplete circulating IgM and IgM XNA to undetectable levels for a period of 2.5–4 weeks. Depletion time was dose-dependent; the higher the dose of injected anti-μ, the longer the period for which circulating IgM and IgM XNA remained at undetectable levels [58]. Moreover, depletion of circulating IgM was correlated with the detection of free circulating anti-μ mAb (i.e., noncomplexed to circulating IgM). Finally, anti-μ administration was significantly more efficient in rats that had decreased levels of circulating IgM after splenectomy, plasma exchange and administration of the RS61443 immunossuppresive drug [58]. These experiments suggested that the anti-μ approach may allow the depletion of IgM XNA for a sufficiently long period of time to test the hypothesis of "accommodation" in other xenograft models such as the porcine-to-primate xenograft or even in ABO incompatible allografts.

Administration of an anti-μ mAb certainly generates large amounts of anti-μ/IgM immune complexes in the circulation which, however, have never been detected by immunolocalization in the kidneys or lungs of anti-μ-treated rats. Interestingly, we recently found that as early as 1–4 h after the first anti-μ administration (30 mg/kg) both IgM and anti-μ mAb colocalize within sinusoidal spaces in the liver and, in particular, a strong granular staining was observed in Kupffer cells. The processing of these complexes must be extremely rapid since at 24 h they were no longer detected in the liver [34].

Although in adult rats we have not been able to detect any pathological signs related to the formation of these immune complexes, the possibility of decreasing the doses of anti-μ should certainly be taken into consideration if one is to attempt to use this approach clinically. Our data (as well as data from Bach and colleagues) demonstrate that the combination of anti-μ with anti-B and T cell immunosuppressive drugs (such as brequinar sodium, cyclosporine, or rapamycin) permits a reduction by at least tenfold in the dose of anti-μ mAb required to achieve complete depletion of circulating IgM XNA in adult rats [11, 58].

In order to explain the sustained effect of the anti-μ treatment we have hypothesized that the long-term depletion of the serum levels of circulating IgM results not only from the direct binding of the anti-μ mAb to circulating IgM molecules, followed by rapid removal of the resulting complexes by Kupffer cells in the liver, but more importantly from the effect of the anti-μ mAb on B cell maturation and certainly on the differentiation of these B cells into IgM-secreting cells (SC) [37].

To test this hypothesis we have analyzed in vivo the effect of anti-μ administration on B cells and, in particular, on the differentiation of B cells into the stage of Ig SC. When administered without further treatment, anti-μ induced specific and intense cross-linking and internalization of mIgM but not of mIgD, CD45RB and MHCII, which were all still expressed at normal levels on the surface of mature B cells [63]. Furthermore, anti-μ administration led to the rapid depletion in spleen and bone marrow of immature and short-lived Thy-1^+CD45RB^+ B cells and to the rearrangement of the morphological localization of mature and long-lived Thy-1^-CD45RB^+ B cells in the periphery. In particular, the marginal zone B cell population (CD45$RB^{low}$$MHCII^{low}$$IgD^{low}$$IgM^{high)}$ usually detected in the spleen was particularly affected [63]. In addition, anti-μ mAb administration resulted in the specific depletion of the number of IgM SC, but not of IgA, IgG1, IgG2a, IgG2b SC, in the spleen, which paralleled the depletion of circulating IgM but not IgA, IgG1, IgG2a, IgG2b. In contrast to the other IgG subclasses, IgG2c SC, as well as circulating IgG2c, were increased by tenfold in anti-μ-treated rats as compared to controls. Finally, anti-μ-treated rats showed a significant inhibition in the generation of primary thymus-dependent as well as thymus-independent antibody responses. Taken together these data suggest that upon anti-μ administration B cell differentiation in adult rats is strongly modulated, resulting in the early arrest of B cell differentiation in the bone marrow at the stage of Thy-1^+CD45$RB^+$$IgM^+$, which causes the downregulation of IgM production. Furthermore, anti-μ mAb administration directly or indirectly activates a particular subset of mature B cells which differentiate into IgG2c SC in the spleen [63].

Contrary to previous reports where the administration of anti-μ or anti-δ mAbs to adult mice generated a strong specific antibody response, in anti-μ-treated rats antibodies directed against the anti-μ mAb remained at undetectable levels during the time period of our experiments (i.e., 14 days). This may be explained by the fact that the large majority of mature B cells "activated" upon mIgM cross-linking by anti-μ mAb (mouse IgG1) may not receive the necessary rescuing co-signals from the restricted number of anti-mouse IgG1 T helper cell clones available. Furthermore, our data are in keeping with the recent finding that the recognition of soluble thymus-dependent antigens by activated B cells undergoing clonal affinity maturation in the germinal centers results in massive B cell apoptosis [52, 57]. Given the continuous administration of the anti-μ mAb to adult rats, one may predict that the few B cells "activated" upon cross-linking of mIgM and receiving rescuing T cell help may still be deleted in the presence of circulating anti-μ. This is certainly an interesting feature of the anti-μ approach since the sustained administration of this mAb would inhibit per se the generation of a specific immune response that would potentially result in the formation of immune complexes and the subsequent elimination of circulating anti-μ.

Taken together, the data from these experiments support the idea that, by suppressing B cell differentiation towards the stage of IgM SC, anti-μ administration achieves a profound and sustained depletion of circulating IgM as well as IgM-XNA in adult animals. Furthermore, this treatment may not result in the generation of a "neutralizing" antibody response directed against the anti-μ mAb. Given the above, we propose that the administration of an anti-μ mAb in combination with other immunosuppressive agents, including complement inhibitory drugs, may provide a potential approach to overcome the HAR of discordant xenografts.

To determine the mechanism of B cell inhibition resulting from the administration of an anti-μ mAb to adult animals is of both theoretical and practical importance. If B cell differentiation could be suppressed at an early stage of B cell maturation, one would be able to inhibit the overall differentiation of immature B cells into the stage of Ig SC, resulting in the depletion of circulating XNA of the IgM isotype but also those of the IgG isotype. Because XNA of the IgG isotype are probably involved in the pathogenesis of the delayed rejection of discordant xenografts, the administration of an anti-μ mAb would be a potential approach to bypass both the hyperacute and delayed rejection of discordant xenografts.

In anti-μ-treated rats, cross-linking of mIgM may arrest B cell differentiation either by acting (a) at an early stage of B cell differentiation, probably on immature B cells in the bone marrow, inhibiting their maturation into all Ig isotypes SC, or (b) at a later stage of B cell differentiation, once mature B cell are already committed to produce IgM, and specifically inhibit the maturation of these immunocompetent B cells into IgM SC.

In order to detect at which stage of B cell development an anti-μ mAb may inhibit B cell differentiation, adult rats expressing the Ig κ-1b light chain allotype were treated for 7 days with the anti-μ mAb, and bone marrow nucleated cells were transferred into nonlethally irradiated congeneic rats expressing the Ig κ-1a light chain allotype. Upon bone marrow transplantation, recipients were further treated with anti-μ mAb for the following 30 days, and bone marrow-driven B cells and Ig SC were analyzed [62].

The results from this experiment showed that, in contrast to control animals treated with isotype-matched control mAb, there were virtually no mature $CD45RB^{+}MHCII^{+}IgM^{+}IgD^{+}$ B cells and IgA, IgM and IgG SC driven from the maturation of donor bone marrow Ig κ-1b^{+} in the spleen of chimera Ig κ-1a/Ig κ-1b anti-μ-treated rats. These data strongly support the early hypothesis that the administration of an anti-μ mAb to adult rats blocks B cell differentiation at an early stage of B cell maturation in the bone marrow (M. Soares et al., submitted).

Moreover, using this experimental protocol we have compared the effect of the administration of an anti-μ mAb with that of an anti-δ mAb in order to analyze in which measure mIgM or mIgD cross-linking on the surface of immature B cells may inhibit their development and differentiation. We found that cross-linking of both mIgM or mIgD suppressed the maturation of rat immature B cells early during B cell development in the bone marrow. However, in anti-δ treated rats a subset of immature B cells in the bone marrow may not express sufficient levels of mIgD, and thus "escapes" deletion upon cross-linking of mIgD (M. Soares et al., submitted). Furthermore, the results from these experiments suggest that the B cells that "escape" deletion in anti-δ- treated rats belong to a distinct B cell lineage that may be responsible for the generation of thymus-independent antibodies, including XNA (M. Soares et al., submitted). Taken together, our data support the mechanism of inhibition of B cell differentiation illustrated in Fig. 1.

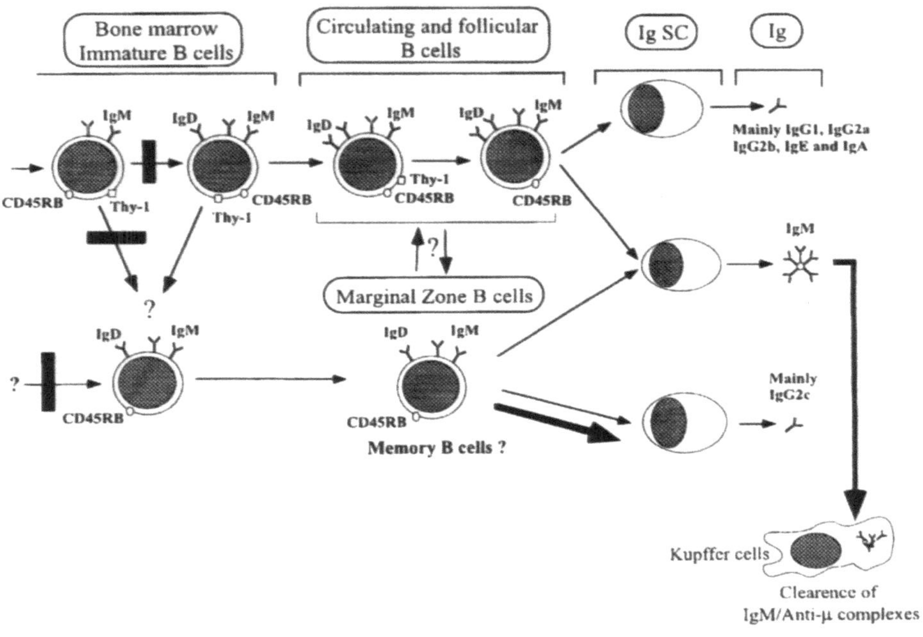

Fig. 1. The effect of anti-μ administration on B cell differentiation and IgM production. In adult rats, newly formed $CD45RB^+IgM^+IgD^+Thy\text{-}1^+$ B cells are continuously generated in the bone marrow and migrate to the spleen, where they account for up to 10%–15% of B cells [21, 63]. Mature B cells in the spleen and other secondary lymphoid organs do not express the Thy-1 marker [21]. At least two major populations of mature B cells have been identified in the spleen of adult rats: (1) follicular $CD45RB^{high}IgM^{low}IgD^{high}$ $MHCII^{high}$ B cells and (2) marginal zone $CD45RB^{low}IgM\text{-}^{highIgDlow}MHCII^{high}$ B cells [37, 43]. In contrast to follicular B cells, which are involved in thymus-dependent antibody responses (IgM, IgG1, IgG2a, IgG2b), marginal zone B cells are thought to generate mainly thymus-independent responses (IgM, IgG2c, IgA) [43]. Interestingly, a significant percentage of B cells in the marginal zone are thought to be memory B cells [23, 42]. A single high dose (30 mg/kg) of anti-μ results in the rapid depletion of circulating IgM through the generation and subsequent clearance of circulating IgM–anti-μ immune complexes by Kupffer cells in the liver (represented by a *thick arrow*) [34, 58, 63]. The sustained administration of lower doses of anti-μ (15 mg/kg) induces intensive cross-linking of mIgM on the surface of B cells, resulting in the total arrest of newly formed $Thy\text{-}1^+CD45RB^+IgM^+IgD^+$ B cell differentiation in the bone marrow (represented by *black bars*). The arrest of B cell differentiation in the bone marrow results in the depletion of IgM and IgG secreting cells (*SC*), which leads to the depletion of circulating IgM and IgG, including XNA of the IgM and IgG isotypes [63] (M. Soares et al., submitted). When used without further treatment, anti-μ administration also results in the activation of a particular subset of mature B cells, probably in the marginal zone of the spleen, which differentiates specifically into the secretion of IgG2c (represented by a *thick arrow*)

Pig-to-Primate Xenograft Model

In order to analyze the effect of splenectomy and/or plasmapheresis on the serum level of XNA, Papio anubis baboons were treated with splenectomy alone, plasma exchange alone, or both (splenectomy at day 0 and plasma exchanges on days 0, 1, and 2). Two baboons were included in each group. Circulating IgM and IgG were measured by enzyme-linked immunosorbent assay (ELISA), and IgM and IgG XNA by flow cytometry using pig lymphocytes as targets. In contrast to the significant circulating IgM depletion described in rats , in baboons no more than 30%–40% reduction of the IgM serum levels was observed following splenectomy. These data might result from a different distribution of peripheral mature B cells in primates when compared to rats. Plasma exchange resulted in a transient decrease of circulating IgM at day 2 (approximately 60% reduction as compared to pre-plasma exchange level), immediately followed by a "rebound" to approximately 170% of pre-plasma exchange level by the following week. The combination of splenectomy and plasma exchange decreased serum IgM by 75% as compared to the presplenectomized level. As described in the rat model [54], the combination of splenectomy with plasma exchange totally suppressed the rebound of circulating IgM. However, neither splenectomy nor plasma exchange were sufficient to decrease IgM to undetectable levels, as measured by ELISA. Plasma exchange, but not splenectomy, allowed a reduction in the IgG serum level, and the combination of splenectomy with plasma exchange does not suppress the rebound observed after plasma exchange alone.

Two mAb (LO-BM-1 and LO-BM-2) produced in our laboratory [14] have been selected for their specificity and high avidity for baboon IgM. LO-BM-1 is a rat IgG2b Ig κ-1a light chain mAb which binds to baboon IgM with an avidity of 1×10^{-9} *M*. LO-BM-2 is a rat IgG2a Ig κ-1a light chain mAb which binds to baboon IgM with an avidity of 2.4×10^{-9} *M*. These two mAb recognize human IgM but do not cross-react with baboon or human IgA, IgD, or IgG isotypes. Interestingly, LO-BM-2, but not LO-BM-1, cross-links and internalizes mIgM on cultured splenic baboon and human B cells. Given the ability of anti-rat IgM mAb (MARM-4) to suppress B-cell maturation following internalization of mIgM in adult rats, we have hypothesized that LO-BM-2 mAb might have similar effects on baboon B cells.

We tested the ability of these two mAb to deplete circulating IgM XNA, either in association with splenectomy and plasmapheresis or with splenectomy alone. One baboon was treated with LO-BM-1 mAb (i.v. injection of 2.5 mg/kg per day for 10 days) after splenectomy and plasma exchange. A second baboon was given LO-BM-2 mAb (i.v. injection of 10 mg/kg per day for 4 days) after splenectomy and plasma exchange, and a third baboon received LO-BM-2 mAb (i.v. injection of 18 mg/kg per day for 4 days) after splenectomy alone. No significant decrease of IgM or IgG serum concentration was observed following administration of LO-BM-1 mAb, the lowest dose of anti-μ used. In the second treated baboon, IgM and IgM XNA serum levels were very significantly decreased (98% decrease as compared to the pre-splenectomy serum level) following LO-BM-2 mAb administration. Serum levels of IgG were reduced (around 70%) after plasma exchanges, but very high values (up to 500 % of the pre-level) were reached after the end of the mAb treatment. IgG XNA were depleted by plasma exchanges (80 % of the initial value) but returned progressively to 60 % of the pre-levels within 1 week. However, over the time of maximal depletion, between day 2 and day 7, 100 μg/ml circulating IgM were still detectable by ELISA. Finally, in the third baboon, IgM and IgM XNA serum levels were very significantly depleted (96 % decrease as compared to the pre-splenectomy level) following splenectomy and LO-BM-2 mAb administration, the highest dose of anti-μ used. Residual 200 μg/ml of IgM serum concentration was still detectable by ELISA after this last injection of anti-μ. IgG serum levels did not change significantly.

Although in this study formation of IgM/anti-μ complexes is believed to be the main mechanism accounting for depletion of circulating IgM, immunohistological analyses of kidney from the anti-μ-treated baboons did not reveal pathological features of immune complex deposition. All baboons treated with high doses of anti-μ developed anti-rat antibodies between day 13 and day 20. In these experiments the doses of' anti-μ administered were probably not sufficient to act at the B cell level, as observed in rats. However, if the anti-μ mAb is administered at a dose sufficient to act on B cell maturation, then this approach might be able to block the humoral immune response against the mAb. We believe that the use of approximately 18–20 mg/kg per day doses of LO-BM-2 anti-μ mAb, following splenectomy and plasma exchange, should be able to act on IgM^+ B cells and totally deplete circulating IgM XNA for a longer period of time. The use of immunosuppressive drugs, such as DSG or leflunomide, in combination with this protocol might be able to still further reduce the doses of anti-μ required to cause a long-term depletion of circulating IgM XNA. Such protocols have been started and the experiments are in progress.

References

1. Alexandre, G.P.J., Squifflet, J.P., De Bruyère, M., et al. (1987) Present experiences in a series of 26 ABO-incompatible living donor renal allografts. Transplant. Proc. 19, 4538
2. Alexandre, G.P.J., Gianello, P., Latinne, D., et al. (1989) Plasmapheresis and splenectomy in experimental renal xenotransplantation. In: Xenograft 25. Hardy, M. (ed), p. 259
3. Alexandre, G.P.J., Latinne, D., Carlier, M., et al. (1991a) ABO-incompatibility and organ transplantation. Transplant. Rev. 5, 230
4. Alexandre, G.P.J., Latinne, D., Gianello, P., Squifflet, J.P. (1991b) Preformed cytotoxic antibodies and ABO-incompatible grafts. Clin. Transplantation. 5, 583
5. Auchincloss, J.H. (1988) Xenogeneic transplantation. A review. Transplantation. 46, 1
6. Bach, F.H. (1991a) Revisiting a challenge in transplantation: discordant xenografting. Hum. Immunol. 30, 262
7. Bach, F.H. (1991b) Xenotransplantation: problems for consideration. Clin. Transplantation. 5, 595
8. Bach, F.H., Turman, M.A., Vercellotti, G.M., Platt, J.L., Dalmasso, A.P. (1991) Accommodation: A working paradigm for progressing toward clinical discordant xenografting. Transplant. Proc. 23, 205

9. Bach, F.H., Blakely, M.L., van der Werf, W., et al. (1993) Discordant xenografting: a working model of problems and issues. Xeno. 1, 8
10. Bach, F.H. (1994) Discordant xenografts: problems beyond antibodies and complement. Xeno. 2, 57
11. Bach, F.H., Robson, S.C., Ferran, C., et al. (1994) Endothelial cell activation and thromboregulation during xenograft rejection. Immunol. Rev. 141, 5
12. Bazin, H., Platteau, B., Beckers, A., Pauwels, R. (1978) Differential effect of neonatal injections of anti-μ or anti-δ antibodies on the synthesis of IgM, IgD, IgE, IgA, IgG1, IgG2a, IgG2b and IgG2c immunoglobulin classes. J. Immunol. 121, 2083
13. Bazin, H., Platteau, B., MacLennan, I.C.M., Johnson, G.D. (1985) B-cell production and differentiation in adult rats. Immunology. 54, 79
14. Bazin, H. (1990) Rat Hybridomas and Rat Monoclonal Antibodies. Bazin H. (ed.) CRC Press, Boca Raton
15. Blakely, M.L., Van der Werf, W.J., Hancock, W.W., Bach, F.H. (1993) Rejection of guiena pig cardiac xenografts post-cobra venom factor therapy is associated with endothelial cell activation and mononuclear cell infiltration. Surg. Forum. 44, 399
16. Brink, R., Goodnow, C.C., Crosbie, J., et al. (1992) Immunoglobulin M and D antigen receptors are both capable of mediating B lymphocyte activation, deletion, or anergy after interaction with specific antigen. J. Exp. Med. 176, 991
17. Cairns, T., Karlsson, I., Holgersson, J., Welsh, K., Samuelsson, B. (1993) Confirmation of a major target epitope of human natural IgG and IgM anti-pig antibodies: terminal galactose α1,3 galactose. 2nd Int. Congress in Xenotransplantation 56 (Abstract) Transplant. Proc
18. Cerny, A., Heusser, C., Sutter, S., et al. (1986) Generation of agammaglobulinaemic mice by prenatal and postnatal exposure to polyclonal or monoclonal anti-IgM antibodies. Scand. J. Immunol. 24, 437
19. Cooper, D.K.C., Ye, Y., Niekrasz, M., et al. (1993) Specific intravenous carbohydrate therapy. Transplantation. 56, 769
20. Cooper, D.K.C., Koren, E., Oriol, R. (1994) Oligosaccharides and discordant xenotransplantation. Immunol. Rev. 141, 31
21. Deenen, G. J., F. G. Kroese. (1993). Kinetics of B cell subpopulations in peripheral lymphoid tissues: evidence for the presence of phenotypically distinct short-lived and long-lived B cell subsets. Int. Immunol. 5, 735
22. Dalmasso A. P., Vercellotti J. L., Platt J. L., F. H. Bach (1991) Inhibition of complement-mediated endothelial cell cytotoxicity by decay-acclerating factor. Transplantation. 52, 530
23. Dunn, W. D., P. G. Isaacson, J. Spencer. (1995) Analysis of mutations in immunoglobulin heavy chain variable region genes of microdissected marginal zone (MGZ) B cells suggests that the MGZ of human spleen is a reservoir of memory B cells. J. Exp. Med. 182, 559
24. Figueroa, J., Fuad, S.A., Kunjummen, B.D., Platt, J.L., Bach, F.H. (1993) Suppression of synthesis of natural antibodies by mycophenolate mofetil (RS-61443). its potential use in discordant xenografting. Transplantation. 55, 1371
25. Finkelman, F. D., J. M. Holmes, O. I. Dukhanina, S. C. Morris. (1995) Cross-linking of membrane immunoglobulin D, in the absence of T cell help, kills mature B cells in vivo. J. Exp. Med. 181, 515
26. Fischel, R.J., Bolman III, R.M., Platt, J.L., et al. (1990) Removal of IgM anti-endothelial antibodies results in prolonged cardiac xenograft survival. Transplant. Proc. 22, 1077

27. Galili, U., Rachmilewitz, E.A., Peleg, A., Flechner, I. (1984) A unique natural human IgG antibody with anti-α-galactosyl specificity. J. Exp. Med. 160, 1519
28. Galili, U., Buehler, J., Shohet, S.B., Macher, B.A. (1987) The human natural anti-Gal IgG. III. The subtlety of immune tolerance in man as demonstrated by crossreactivity between natural anti-Gal and anti-B antibodies. J. Exp. Med. 165, 693
29. Galili, U. (1993) Interaction of the natural anti-Gal antibody with α-galactosyl epitopes: a major obstacle for xenotransplantation in humans. Immunol. Today. 14, 480
30. Gianello, P., Latinne, D., Alexandre, P.G.J. (1995) Pig to baboon renal xenograft. Xeno. 3, 26
31. Good, A.H., Cooper, D.K.C., Malcolm, A.J., et al. (1992) Identification of carbohydrate structures that bind human antiporcine antibodies: implications for discordant xenografting humans. Transplant. Proc. 24, 559
32. Goodnow, C.C. (1992) Transgenic mice and analysis of B-cell tolerance. Annu. Rev. Immunol. 10, 489
33. Hancock, W.W., Bach, F.H. (1994) The immunopathology of discordant xenograft rejection. Xeno. 2, 68
34. Havaux, X.B., Seiji Hori, Soares M. Processing of IgM/anti-IgM immune complexes by the liver of rats treated with anti-IgM monoclonal antibodies. Transplant. Proc. 1996, 29, 345–347
35. Hayashi, S., Ito, M., Yokoyama, I., Takagi, H. (1994) Evidence that combination therapy using cobra venom factor, splenectomy, and deoxyspergualin is effective in guinea pig to rat cardiac xenotransplantation. Transplantation. 57, 777
36. Latinne, D., Squifflet, J.P., De Bruyère, M., et al. (1989) Subclasses of ABO isoagglutinins in ABO-incompatible kidney transplantation. Transplant. Proc. 21, 641
37. Latinne, D., Soares, M., Havaux, X., et al. (1994) Depletion of IgM xenoreactive natural antibodies by injection of anti-μ monoclonal antibodies. Immunol. Rev. 141, 94
38. Leventhal, J.R., Flores, H.C., Gruber, S.A., et al. (1992) Evidence that 15-deoxyspergualin inhibits natural antibody production but fails to prevent hyperacute rejection in a discordant xenograft model. Transplantation. 54, 26
39. Leventhal, J.R., Matas, A.J., Sun, L.H., et al. (1993) The immunopathology of cardiac xenograft rejection in the guinea pig-to-rat model. Transplantation. 56, 1
40. Leventhal, J.R., Sakiyalak, P., Witson, J., et al. (1994) The synergistic effect of combined antibody and complement depletion on discordant cardiac xenograft survival in non-human primates. Transplantation. 57, 974
41. Leventhal, J.R., John, R., Fryer, J.P., et al. (1995) Removal of baboon and human anti-porcine IgG and IgM natural antibodies by immunoadsorption. Results of in vitro and in vivo studies. Transplantation. 59, 294
42. Liu, Y. J., S. Oldfield, I. C. MacLennan. (1988) Memory B cells in T cell-dependent antibody responses colonize the splenic marginal zones. Eur. J. Immunol. 18:355
43. MacLennan, I.C.M., Gray, D., Kumararatne, D.S., Bazin, H. (1982) The lymphocytes of splenic marginal zones: A distinct B cell lineage. Immunol. Today. 3, 305
44. Makowka, L., Cramer, D.V., Hoffman, A., Sher, L., Podesta, L. (1993) Pig liver xenografts as a temporary bridge for human allografting. Xeno. 1, 27
45. Manning, D.D., Jutila, J.W. (1976) Immunosuppression in mice injected with heterologous anti-immunoglobulin antisera. J. Immunol. 144, 288
46. Noelle, R.J., Ledbetter, J.A., Aruffo, A. (1992) CD40 and its ligand, an essential ligand-receptor pair of thymus-dependent B-cell activation. Immunol. Today. 13, 431

47. Platt, J.L., Lindman B. J., Chen H., Spitalnik S. L., Bach, F.H. (1990) Endothelial cell antigens recognized by xenoreactive human natural antibodies. Transplantation. 44, 712
48. Platt, J.L., Vercellotti, G.M., Dalmasso, A.P., et al. (1990) Transplantation of discordant xenografts: a review of progress. Immunol. Today. 11, 450
49. Platt, J.L., Fishel, R.J., Matas, A.J., et al. (1991) Immunopathology of hyperacute xenograft rejection in a swine-to-primate model. Transplantation. 52, 214
50. Platt, J.L., Bach, F.H. (1991) The barrier to xenotransplantation. Transplantation. 52, 937
51. Platt, J.L., Holzknecht, Z.E. (1994) Porcine platelet antigens recognized by human xenoreactive natural antibodies. Transplantation. 57, 327
52. Puledran B., Kannourakis S., Smith K., Nossal J. V. (1995) Soluble antigens can cause enhanced apoptosis of germinal center B cells. Nature. 375, 331
53. Reding, R., White, D.J.G., Wright, L.J., et al. (1989) Qualitative analysis of antibody rebound after plasma exchange in the rat. Transplant. Proc. 21, 777
54. Reding, R., Soares, M., Baranski, A., et al. (1994) Preformed antibody and complement rebound after plasma exchange. Analysis of immunoglobulin isotypes and effect of splenectomy. Transplant. Immunol. 2, 231
55. Sachs, D.H., Bach, F.H. (1990) Immunology of xenograft rejection. Hum. Immunol. 28, 245
56. Sandrin, M.S., Vaughan, H.A., Dabkowski, P.L., McKenzie, I.F.C. (1993) Anti-pig IgM antibodies in human serum react predominantly with Gal(a1–3)Gal epitopes. Proc. Natl. Acad. Sci. USA. 90, 11391
57. Shokat, K. M., C. C. Goodnow. (1995) Antigen-induced B-cell death and elimination during germinal-centre immune responses. Nature. 375, 334
58. Soares, M., Latinne, D., Elsen, M., et al. (1993) In vivo depletion of xenoreactive natural antibodies with an anti-μ monoclonal antibody. Transplantation. 56, 1427
59. Soares, M., Lu, X., Havaux, X., et al. (1994a) In vivo IgM depletion by anti-μ monoclonal antibody therapy: the role of IgM in hyperacute vascular rejection of discordant xenograft. Transplantation. 57, 1003
60. Soares, M., Van Beneden R., Havaux, X., et al. (1994b) Characterization of xenoreactive natural antibodies secreting cells in rats. Xenotransplantation. 1, 118
61. Soares, M., Nisol, F., Bach, F.H., Latinne, D. (1994c) Use of anti-μ monoclonal antibody as a therapeutic approach to achieve depletion of xenoreactive natural antibodies. Transplant. Proc. 26, 1357
62. Soares, M., Havaux, X., Latinne, D., Bazin, H. (1994d) Depletion of xenoreactive natural antibodies by anti-μ monoclonal antibodies. Xeno. 2
63. Soares, M., Havaux, X., Nisol, F., Bazin, H., Latinne, D. Modulation of rat B cell differentiation in vivo by the administration of a anti-μ monoclonal antibody. J. Immunol. (1996) 158, 108–118
64. Tsubata, T., Wu, J., Honjo, T. (1993) B-cell apoptosis induced by antigen receptor crosslinking is blocked by a T-cell signal through CD40. Nature. 364, 645
65. Tuso, P.J., Cramer, D.V., Yasunaga, C., et al. (1993) Removal of natural human xenoantibodies to pig vascular endothelium by perfusion of blood through pig kidneys and livers. Transplantation. 55, 1375
66. Van De Stadt, J., Vendeville, B., Weill, B., et al. (1988) Discordant heart xenografts in the rat. Transplantation. 45, 514

30 Use of Intravenous Immunoglobulin as a Therapeutic Approach To Prevent Rejection Between Widely Disparate Species

C. Gautreau, J. Cardoso, and D. Houssin

Introduction

Among non-primate mammals, the pig may be an ideal donor for human transplantation [1]. Unfortunately, xenotransplantation of pig organs into untreated humans will probably result in immediate xenogeneic hyperacute rejection (HAR) involving human anti-pig natural antibodies and complement [2]. Such rejection, occurring between disparate species, cannot be controlled with currently used immunosuppressive agents.

In 1992, our group began a series of experiments to test the possibility of using intravenous immunoglobulin to prevent HAR. In this short chapter we review our own work [3, 4] and that of others [5–7] concerning this topic.

Intravenous Immunoglobulin

Intravenous immunoglobulin G (IVIG) is from human origin, prepared from a plasma pool of more than one thousand donors. IVIG is used for the treatment of primary or secondary immunodeficiencies, chronic inflammatory diseases, bacterial and viral infections, and several autoimmune disorders [8–12]. Amelioration of acute graft-versus-host-disease in bone marrow transplantation [13] and HLA alloantibody suppression in heart and renal transplantation have also been observed after IVIG administration [14, 15].

The intravenous infusion of large amounts of immunoglobulin G (400–2000 mg/kg body weight over 2–5 days) can modify immunological reactions. Several mechanisms of the beneficial effect of IVIG in immune-related disorders are possible [10, 16]: (a) IVIG acts as an anti-inflammatory agent [17], (B) it induces Fcγ receptor blockade on reticuloendothelial cells [18], or (c) it contains public anti-idiotypes that downregulate autoimmune phenomena [19, 20].

Experimentation showed that supraphysiological levels of IVIG were efficient in attenuating or preventing the develoment of acute complement-mediated tissue damage in a guinea pig model. The infusion of anti-Forssman antibody in guinea pigs leads to the occurence of irreversible shock and death. The previous administration of high doses of IVIG increased survival time and prevented death of guinea pigs injected with anti-Forssman antiserum [21]. It thus appears that IVIG may act as a complement activation modulator, probably by preventing active C3 fragments from binding to target cells. Several studies have demonstrated that C3b might be covalently linked to IgG [22, 23]. Thus high amounts of IgG might divert C3b from target cells and suppress complement-mediated damage.

When we initiated this work, we began with the hypothesis that IVIG might prevent the complement-dependent tissue damage observed in HAR.

Use of Intravenous Immunoglobulin G in the Prevention of Guinea Pig-to-Rat Cardiac Xenograft Rejection

This study [4] was carried out to investigate the delaying action of IVIG administration on the HAR of a guinea pig heart grafted into a rat.

Male outbred guinea pigs were used as heart donors and male inbred Lewis rats as recipients. Rats were heparinized, then slowly infused through the portal vein with a single dose of IVIG at a concentration of 1500 mg/kg or with an equivalent volume of 9 g/l NaCl. Guinea pig-to-rat heterotopic cardiac xenotransplantation was performed, and rejection defined as the cessation of visible cardiac contractions. Heart graft survival time was calculated from the time of graft reperfusion.

The mean guinea pig cardiac survival time in rats treated with IVIG prior to xenoengraftment was significantly longer (167.8±29.8 min, $p<0.005$) than the mean survival time measured in rats treated with NaCl (12.4±1.2 min). Macroscopically, congestion of the graft with cyanosis was observed in all cases (with or without IVIG) and was rapidly followed by cessation of beating. No such event occurred to the native heart of the recipient. Our results are consistent with those of another group [5] who demonstrated prolongation of the heart survival up to 97 min following IVIG treatment.

In the guinea pig-to-rat combination, complement activation is critical for hyperacute rejection which can proceed without the involvement of rat xenoreactive natural antibodies directed against the guinea pig heart [24]. An increase of guinea pig heart survival (to 25 min) in rats depleted of xenoreactive antibodies by previous plasma exchange has been reported [24], whereas the survival time can be prolonged up to 112 [25], or 189 min [26] when rats are complement-depleted by soluble complement receptor, and to 88 h when they are complement-depleted by cobra venom factor [24]. Our own results, therefore, suggest that, in this model, IVIG probably interferes with the alternative pathway of complement activation, and possibly also with the classical pathway.

In our guinea pig-to-rat model, high doses of IVIG (1500 mg/kg) were infused into the rat prior to engraftment. A similar dose was used in the study that demonstrated IVIG-related prevention of lethal Forssman shock in guinea pigs injected with anti-Forssman antiserum [21]. Several studies have shown that C3b generated during complement activation by the alternative [22] and the classical pathway [23] binds readily to IgG. In our model, high-dose IVIG may thus act as a complement modulator by diverting the attachment of the activated C3 to the endothelial target cells on the grafted heart.

We have also found that human serum and IVIG are able to agglutinate rat red blood cells, suggesting the existence of human anti-rat natural xenoantibodies.

The xenoantibodies contained in IVIG may induce activation of the complement system of the rat; the subsequent depletion of rat complement contributes to the beneficial effect of IVIG in the guinea pig-to-rat xenograft model.

Use of Intravenous Immunoglobulin G in the Pig-to-Human Combination

Inhibitory effect on Complement-Dependent Cytotoxicity Assays

Cytotoxicity of human sera, with or without addition of IVIG, have been assessed in vitro by complement-dependent cytotoxicity assays using three different pig target cells: endothelial cells (EC), lymphocytes, and red blood cells (RBC) [3, 4].

The level of human natural anti-pig antibodies varies widely from one serum to another. Some sera (especially of blood group A or O) may contain up to 500 times more anti-pig xenoantibodies than others (especially of blood group AB) [27]. To assess in vitro the inhibitory effect of IVIG on the lysis of pig cells, we have thus used human sera diluted to the last dilution giving 100 % cells lysis in the presence of rabbit complement. Cytotoxic activity of human serum to pig EC was determined by a colorimetric MTT assay and the results were expressed in percentage of cytotoxicity (cell death,%C). The addition of IVIG to human serum inhibited in a dose-dependent manner the cytotoxicity to pig EC. The%C decreased from 34 % without IVIG to 14 % with 12.5 g/l IVIG (p=0.03).

The cytotoxic activity of human serum to pig lymphocytes in the presence of rabbit complement was determined using a modified standard protocol of the complement-mediated cytotoxicity test in Terasaki plates. Cell death was visualized by a trypan blue coloration. Results were expressed in cytotoxicity score by a microscopic evaluation of the percentage of cells lysed. When 16 g/l IVIG was added to human serum, an inhibitory effect of 100 % was observed.

The most precise inhibition curves were obtained by using pig RBC as targets. Hemolysis assays performed on microtitration plates were easy to standardize and allowed simultaneous comparisons between numerous assays. Assays were performed by adding diluted decomplemented human serum to a suspension of pig RBC in the presence of rabbit complement. Hemolysis was measured in supernatants by optical density determination of free hemoglobin, and percent hemolysis was calculated. Incubation lasted 150 min at 37 °C. When increasing concentrations of IVIG (0.5–20 g/l final concentration) were added, a dose-dependent inhibitory effect of IVIG on pig RBC lysis by human serum was observed. The inhibitory effect was 80 % with 10 g/l IVIG and 90 % with 20 g/l IVIG.

In a recent study, Magee et al. [6, 7] found that the addition of human IgG to human serum inhibited in a dose-dependent manner (a) the deposition of iC3b, (b) cytotoxicity, and (c) the release of heparan sulfate from the pig cellular targets mediated by that serum.

IVIG exerts a dose-dependent inhibitory effect on the complement-dependent lysis of pig cells induced by human serum. Though the mechanism of the in vitro action of IVIG remains to be determined, several hypotheses can be put forward: (a) inhibition of complement activation, (b) neutralization of the xenoantibodies directed to pig antigens via the antiidiotypic antibodies which may be present in IVIG, and (c) IVIG may contain IgG anti-pig xenoantibodies that may mask the recognition of pig xenoantigens by IgM anti-pig xenoantibodies.

Intravenous Immunoglobulin G Contains Anti-pig Xenoantibodies

IVIG is a product of human origin and may thus contain human anti-pig natural xenoantibodies of IgG isotype. Numerous data strongly suggest that in the pig-to-human combination IgM, and not IgG, xenoantibodies are primarily involved in initiating HAR [2, 28]. However, IgG xenoantibodies may also contribute to porcine xenograft rejection, as suggested by reports showing that human IgG are cytotoxic to cultured pig cells [29] and mediate antibody-dependent cell cytotoxicity [30, 31]. We have revealed the presence of anti-pig xenoantibodies in IVIG by using pig RBC [32]. Although the in vivo target of HAR is pig EC, several previous reports have shown that human xenoantibodies recognize cross-reactive epitopes on pig EC and pig RBC [33, 34].

Hemagglutination of pig RBC by IVIG was performed by using microtyping cards (Diamed). IVIG contained hemagglutinating anti-pig xenoantibodies. A 30% direct hemolysing activity of IVIG on pig RBC was also found when the incubation lasted overnight. On the contrary, after depletion of anti-pig xenoantibodies from IVIG by incubation of IVIG with washed pig RBC, IVIG no longer agglutinated or hemolysed pig RBC. After incubation of IVIG with pig RBC, anti-pig xenoantibodies were eluted from pig RBC by thermal extraction, then detected by hemagglutination. These results are consistent with others showing that IVIG contain IgG antibodies that bind to pig EC [6]. However, in this last study, IVIG did not initiate the activation of complement [6].

The anti-pig xenoantibodies contained in IVIG may impair its inhibitory effect on pig cell cytotoxicity induced by human serum. In fact, when IVIG were depleted of anti-pig xenoantibodies, its in vitro inhibitory effect on pig RBC lysis was markedly enhanced.

Pig Livers Perfused with Human Blood

The objective of the experiments reported here was to evaluate the inhibitory effect of IVIG on the xenogeneic hyperacute rejection occurring on pig livers perfused with human blood [3].

Pig livers were surgically excised and connected to a closed oxygenated and heated recirculating system. Perfusions were performed through the portal vein and the hepatic artery. The perfusate was heparinized and composed of Krebs buffer, prewashed human RBC, and compatible extemporaneously defrozen fresh frozen plasma as a source of human anti-pig xenoantibodies and complement. Control experiments were performed with homologous whole pig blood.

Sequential biopsies of the pig liver were performed to assess the time-related occurence of histological lesions as well as the deposition of immunoglobulins (IgG, IgM) and complement factors (C1q, C3). Liver viability was evaluated by measurement of bile production and release of liver enzymes (ALT, AST).

Three experimental groups were studied: pig livers perfused with human blood (G1), pig livers perfused with human blood and IVIG (G2), and pig livers perfused with pig blood (G3). Perfusion lasted at least 4 h.

Histological lesions observed were sinusoidal dilatation and congestion, endothelial disruption of the sinusoidal border with intralobular hemorrhage (peliosis), hepatocytal atrophy and necrosis, and portal hemorrhage. Sinusoidal dilatation and congestion were constantly observed in G1 and G2 from the first 30 min. Other histological lesions were heterogeneous, involving some lobules or part of a lobule, and varying from one lobe to another. In an attempt to determine the time-related appearance of the lesions, we considered only obvious lesions involving more than 5 %–10 % of the tissue.

Sinusoidal dilatation and congestion were scarcely observed in G3. In G1, most of the histological lesions appeared during the first hour of perfusion, then increased and were almost constant at 4 h perfusion. In contrast, no lesion was observed in G3 at 4 h perfusion, though lobular hemorrhages appeared after 5 h. In G2, hepatocytal atrophy and necrosis and portal hemorrhage were never observed, but peliosis appeared at 1 h in two experiments. We consider lobular hemorrhage to be an early parameter of rejection in this ex vivo model [35]. The delay before occurence of lobular hemorrhage was significantly longer in the group with IVIG (G2) than in the group without (G1) (262 min vs. 48 min).

Sequential deposition of IgG, IgM, C1q, and C3, were investigated in two experiments in each group. No deposition of any components was observed in G3. In G1, 10 min after the beginning of the perfusion, intense and linear IgG deposits were observed along the sinusoidal border. Deposits of IgM were focal and positive along the sinusoidal border or the portal vein at various time (5 min in the first experiment and 100 min in the second). In both experiments, C1q and C3 were found positive as faint focal deposits between 5 min and 30 min of perfusion, then became intense after 30–60 min perfusion.

In G2, IgG deposits were intensely positive and linear 5 min after the introduction of human blood and IVIG into the circuit. IgM was faint and focal along the sinusoidal border at 30 min perfusion. Focal deposits of C1q and C3 became positive between 1 h and 3 h of perfusion. After 3 h of perfusion, liver enzyme release was lower in G2 than in G1. The volume of bile secreted was not different between the groups.

In this model, the effect of IVIG on HAR may be summarized as a delaying effect on complement activation, on the occurence of histological lesions usually described in pig livers perfused with human blood [35–37], and on liver enzyme release.

Use of Intravenous Immunoglobulin G in the Prevention of Pig-to-Primate Cardiac Xenograft Rejection

Magee et al. [6, 7] described successful prevention of HAR in pig-to-cynomolgus monkey and the pig-to-baboon combinations by using IVIG. Heterotopic porcine cardiac xenografts were placed in primates that were treated with IVIG. In four of six experiments, HAR of the pig heart was prevented and the xenografts functioned 18 h, 7.5, 7.5, and 10 days, respectively. Immunohistological analysis of the functioning xenografts revealed deposits of IgG and IgM along blood vessels, but little or no C4, C3, C5b, or membrane attack complex (MAC) deposits. The mechanism by which IgG protects against complement-mediated injury in this model appears to involve complement deposition rather than inhibition of IgM binding.

Comment

In this chapter, we have briefly summarized the experiments performed by us and others to assess the inhibitory effect of IVIG on the HAR that occurs between disparate species. In vitro experiments demonstrated that IVIG inhibits in a dose-dependent manner the cytotoxicity and activation of pig cells in the presence of human serum. By using an ex vivo model of pig liver perfused with human blood, we have shown a delaying effect of IVIG on both complement activation and the development of the histological lesions usually found in HAR. Xenotransplantation experiments performed in vivo in the guinea pig-to-rat and the pig-to-primate combinations showed that a delay in (and even prevention of) HAR can be obtained after infusion of IVIG into the recipient. Though its mechanism of action remains to be clarified, these results suggest that IVIG may interefere with HAR by complement modulation. Among the multiple strategies being explored with the aim of preventing xenograft rejection between widely disparate species, immunoglobulin infusion may represent a simple therapeutic approach. This product is already widely used in humans in a variety of diseases.

Acknowledgements. This work was supported by an INSERM Grant CRI-950301. Thanks are due to Dr. Monique Fabre (Laboratoire d'Anatomo-pathologie, Faculte de Medecine Le Kremlin Bicetre, Paris, France) for histological and immunohistological analysis.

References

1. Ye Y, Niekrasz M, Kosanke S, et al. The pig as a potential organ donor for man. Transplantation 1994; 57:694
2. Platt JL, Vercellotti GM, Dalmasso AP, et al. Transplantation of discordant xenografts: a review of progress. Immunol Today 1990; 11:450
3. Gautreau C, Cardoso J, Woimant G, et al. Prevention of hyperacute xenograft rejection by intravenous immunoglobulin in the pig-to-human combination. Transplant Proc 1994; 26:1281
4. Gautreau C, Kojima T, Woimant G, et al. Use of intravenous immunoglobulin to delay xenogeneic hyperacute rejection. An in vivo and in vitro evaluation. Transplantation 1995; 60:903
5. Latremouille C, Haeffner-Cavaillon N, Goussef N, et al. Normal human polyclonal immunoglobulins for intravenous use significantly delay hyperacute xenograft rejection. Transplant Proc 1994; 26:1285

6. Magee JC, Collins BH, Harland RC, et al. Prevention of hyperacute xenograft rejection by intravenous immunoglobulin. Transplant Proc 1995; 27:271
7. Magee JC, Collins BH, Harland RC, et al. Immunoglobulin prevents complement-mediated hyperacute rejection in swine-to-primate xenotransplantation. J. Clin. Invest. 1995; 96:2404
8. Buckley RH, Schiff RI. The use of intravenous immune globulin in immunodeficiency diseases. N Engl J Med 1991; 325:110
9. Kaveri SV, Dietrich G, Hurez V, Kazatchkine MD. Intravenous immunoglobulins (IVIG) in the treatment of autoimmune diseases. Clin Exp Immunol 1991; 86:192
10. Dwyer JM. Manipulating the immune system with immune globulin. N Engl J Med 1992; 326:107
11. Nydegger UE. Intravenous immunoglobulin in combination with other prophylactic and therapeutic measures. Transfusion 1992; 32:72
12. Dalakas MC, Illa I, Dambrosia JM, et al. A controlled trial of high-dose intravenous immune globulin infusions as treatment for dermatomyositis. N Engl J Med 1993; 329:1993
13. Sullivan KM, Kopecky KJ, Jocom J, et al. Immunomodulatory and antimicrobial efficacy of intravenous immunoglobulin in bone marrow transplantation. N Engl J Med 1990; 323:705
14. Glotz D, Haymann JP, Sansonetti N, et al. Supression of HLA-specific alloantibodies by high-dose intravenous immunoglobulins (IVIg). A potential tool for transplantation of immunized patients. Transplantation 1993; 56:335
15. Tyan DB, Li VA, Czer L, Trento A, Jordan SC. Intravenous immunoglobulin suppression of HLA alloantibodies in highly sensitized transplant candidates and transplantation with a histoincompatible organ. Transplantation 1994; 57:553
16. Rosen FS. Putative mechanisms of the effect of intravenous γ-globulin. Clin Immunol Immunopathol 1993; 67:S41
17. Newburger JW, Takahashi M, Beiser AS, et al. The treatment of Kawasaki syndrome with intravenous gamma-globulin. N Engl J Med 1991; 324:1633
18. Debre M, Bonnet MC, Fridman WH, et al. Infusion of Fcγ fragments for treatment of children with acute immune thrombocytopenic purpura. Lancet 1993; 342:945
19. Sultan Y, Kazatchkine MD, Maisonneuve P, Nydegger UE. Anti-idiotypic suppression of autoantibodies to factor VIII (antihaemophilic factor) by high-dose intravenous gammaglobulin. Lancet 1984; 2:765
20. Fremeaux Bacchi V, Maillet F, Berlan L, Kazatchkine MD. Neutralising antibodies against C3NeF in intravenous immunoglobulin. Lancet 1992; 340:63
21. Basta M, Kirshbom P, Frank MM, Fries LF. Mechanism of therapeutic effect of high-dose intravenous immunoglobulin. Attenuation of acute complement-dependent immune damage in a guinea pig model. J Clin Invest 1989; 84:1974
22. Gadd KJ, Reid KBM. The binding of complement component C3 to antibody-antigen aggregates after activation of the alternative pathway in human serum. Biochem J 1981; 195:471
23. Brown EJ, Berger M, Joiner KA, Frank MM. Classical complement pathway activation by antipneunoccocal antibodies leads to covalent binding of C3b to antibody molecules. Infect Immun 1983; 42:594
24. Leventhal JR, Dalmasso AP, Cromwell JW, et al. Prolongation of cardiac xenograft survival by depletion of complement. Transplantation 1993; 55:857

25. Pruitt SK, Baldwin WM, Marsh HC Jr, et al. The effect of soluble complement receptor type 1 on hyperacute xenograft rejection. Transplantation 1991; 52:868
26. Zehr KJ, Herskowitz A, Lee PC, et al. Neutrophil adhesion and complement inhibition prolongs survival of cardiac xenografts in discordant species. Transplantation 1994; 57:900
27. Gautreau C, Cardoso J, Jeyaraj P, Houssin D, Weill B. Relationship between human natural anti-A, anti-B alloantibodies and anti-pig xenoantibodies. Transplant Proc 1993; 25:389
28. Sandrin MS, Vaughan HA, Dabkowski PL, McKenzie IFC. Anti pig IgM antibodies in human serum react predominantly with Galα(1,3) gal epitopes. Proc Natl Acad Sci USA 1993; 90:11391
29. Koren E, Kujundzic M, Koscec M, et al. Cytotoxic effect of human preformed anti-Gal IgG and complement on cultured pig cells. Transplant Proc 1994; 26:1336
30. Galili U. Interaction of the natural anti-Gal antibody with a-galactosyl epitopes: a major obstacle for xenotransplantation in humans. Immunol Today 1993; 14:480
31. Schaapherder AFM, Daha MR, Telbute MTJW, Van der Wonde FJ, Gooszen HG. Antibody-dependent cell-mediated cytotoxicity against porcine endothelium induced by a majority of human sera. Transplantation 1994; 57:1376
32. Gautreau C, Cardoso J, Zhao Z, et al. Human natural cytotoxic antibodies recognize cross-reactive antigens on pig endothelial cells and pig red blood cells. Transplant Proc. 1994; 26:
33. Platt JL, Lindman BJ, Chen H, Spitalnik SL, Bach FH. Endothelial cell antigens recognized by xenoreactive human natural antibodies. Transplantation 1990; 50:817
34. Vaughan HA, Loveland BE, Sandrin MS. Galα(1,3) gal is the major xenoepitope expressed on pig endothelial cells recognized by naturally occuring cytotoxic human antibodies. Transplantation 1994; 58:879
35. Cardoso J, Gautreau C, Wroblewski T, et al. Lobular hemorrhage: an early parameter of rejection in isolated pig livers perfused with heparinized human blood. Transplant Proc. 1994; 26:1308
36. Collins BH, Chari RS, Magee JC et al. Mechanisms of injury in porcine livers perfused with blood of patients with fulminant hepatic failure. Transplantation 1994; 58:1162
37. Makowka L, Wu GD, Hoffman A, et al. Immunohistopathologic lesions associated with the rejection of a pig-to-human liver xenograft. Transplant Proc. 1994; 26:1074

31 Control of Complement-Mediated Tissue Damage by γ-Globulin: Application in Xenotransplantation

J.L. Platt and M.M. Frank

Introduction

The complement system is regulated by a series of glycoproteins circulating in the plasma and expressed on cell surfaces. Among the plasma proteins which do so are factor H and I which control initiation of the alternative complement pathway C3 convertase, C1 inhibitor which regulates the function of C1qrs and C4 binding protein which controls activation of the classical complement pathway C3 convertase. Immunoglobulin is generally thought to be an activator of the complement system, particularly of the classical complement pathway. However, it was recently discovered that immunoglobulin also regulates the activation of the complement system [1] and that this function of immunoglobulin may be used advantageously in xenotransplantation [2].

The involvement of antibody in the activation of the complement system has been known for over a century. After incubation of a target with an heat inactivated immune serum, cytotoxicity is shown to be initiated in part by binding of heat-stable and heat-labile components of the serum to the target. The heat stable molecules are, of course, immunoglobulins; the heat-labile molecules are in general components of the complement system. Antibody may also activate complement through the alternative pathway on some cell surfaces. It is believed that by attaching to and blocking acidic sugars such as sialic acid or heparan sulfate, antibody impairs the interaction between C3b and factor H and I. Antibody also augments the alternative pathway by serving as an acceptor to which C3b attaches and having done so is partially protected from factors H and I [3].

We have developed the concept that immunoglobulin also controls the activation of complement by acting as an alternative acceptor for reactive complement proteins. This concept was based on the observation that high plasma levels of IgG prevent complement deposition on antibody coated target cells [1] suggesting that the immunoglobulin might serve as a regulator of the complement cascade and modulate the effect of complement activators in the formation of C3 convertases. The concept was first tested in the guinea pig. Administration of IgG anti-Forssman antibodies to unmanipulated guinea pigs leads invariably to cataclysmic shock and death. However, guinea pigs treated with purified immunoglobulin are protected from the Forssman reaction in nearly 50 % of cases. Guinea pig IgG was as effective as human IgG in preventing tissue injury.

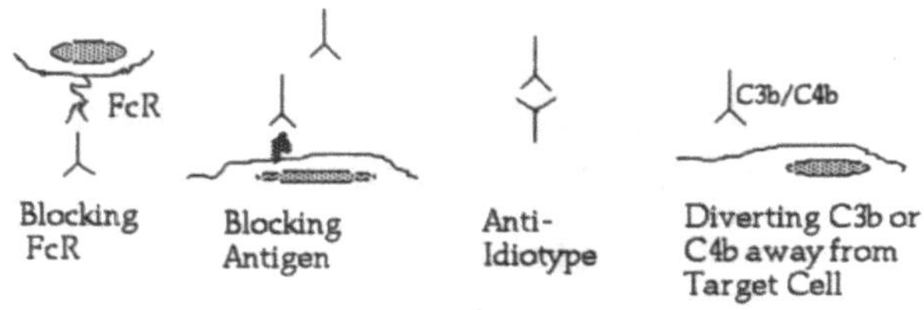

Fig. 1. Mechanisms of humoral regulation by γ-globulin. Among the mechanisms underlying the therapeutic efficacy of γ-globulin, four are shown. γ-globulin may block Fc receptors (*FcR*) and thus impair the ability of pathogenic antibodies, attached to target cells, to interact with leukocytes or reticuloendothelial cells bearing Fc receptors. γ-Globulin may also bind to antigens blocking interaction of those antigens with pathogenic antibodies or antigen specific receptors. It may inhibit some immune responses through anti-idiotype–idiotype interactions. It may form covalent complexes with C3b or C4b, diverting these components away from target cell surfaces. It is through the diversion of active complement components away from xenograft endothelium that γ-globulin is thought to prevent complement-mediated tissue injury in pig-to-primate models

Mechanisms of Action of γ-Globulin

γ-Globulin might interfere with humoral immune reactions at one or more of a number of steps (Fig. 1). γ-Globulin might influence the binding of a specific antibody to a target antigen. One mechanism may involve idiotype-anti idiotype interaction, a mechanism proposed to account for the ability of γ-globulin to decrease levels of circulating anti-HLA and anti-platelet antibodies [4–6]. γ-Globulin preparations might contain soluble contaminants which could block antibody binding. γ-Globulin might block Fc receptors, impairing interaction of phagocytic or cytolytic cells with target cells.

γ-Globulin might also control the binding of activated complement proteins to target antigens and such control is the best explanation for the effects of γ-globulin in the Forssman reaction. One mechanism for such control might involve the consumption of complement proteins through the action of immune aggregates. This mechanism does not appear to contribute to the protection of guinea pigs from the Forssman reaction as complement levels remain unchanged following administration of γ-globulin to unmanipulated guinea pigs. Nor does γ-globulin prevent the action of anti-Forssman antibodies in this model. Because the blood of the treated animals with high levels of IgG was defective in depositing complement on target cells, it was hypothesized that the high IgG levels prevented complement binding to endothelium.

Effects of γ-Globulin in a Porcine-to-Primate Xenograft Model

We reasoned that analysis of the effects of γ-globulin on the reactions involved in the rejection of porcine organ xenografts by primates might yield insights into the mechanism or mechanisms of action of γ-globulin. Human γ-globulin, which is known to contain immunoglobulins which can control complement function, also should contain IgG directed against Galα1–3Gal the major target of human xenoreactive antibodies [7–9]. Infusing human γ-globulin into the recipient of a porcine xenograft might thus allow the weighing of the various pathogenic and protective effects of immunoglobulins. Our initial studies analyzed of the immune and regulatory properties of human immunoglobulin in in vitro systems [2, 10]. Using endothelial cells as a target, we found that commercial preparations of γ-globulin indeed contain significant amounts of IgG, but very little or no IgM that bound to porcine cells. The IgG in commercial γ-globulin bound to porcine endothelial cells in part by recognizing Galα1–3Gal, digestion of porcine endothelial cells with α-galactosidase abrogating the binding of IgG by 20 %–50 %. Although IgG bound to the porcine cells, it did not induce complement binding when the cells with human IgG attached were incubated with human complement [2, 11]. This result is consistent with our prior observations that it is IgM and not IgG in human serum which activates complement when a human serum is exposed to porcine cells [12]. We also showed that although human γ-globulin contains IgG directed against Galα1–3Gal, the same epitope as xenoreactive IgM [9], the binding of that IgG to porcine endothelial cells did not prevent the binding of xenoreactive IgM from a human serum or the ability of that IgM to activate complement on washed cells. These results suggest that within the limits of the system used whatever anti-idiotypic or "blocking" effects γ-globulin might have on the antibodies in a normal human serum, those effects do not materially influence the interaction of xenoreactive antibodies with a target cell.

The next question was whether γ-globulin would control complement in this system as in the other systems previously analyzed. When γ-globulin was added to a human serum, it prevented, in a dose dependent manner, the binding of human complement to porcine cells as measured by the lysis of the cells and the release of heparan sulfate from the cells, a reaction we previously showed to depend on the activation of complement leading to formation of C5a [13].

To gain further insight into the mechanisms through which γ-globulin might regulate a humoral immune reaction, we tested how the administration of γ-globulin might modify the course of complement-mediated tissue injury in xenotransplantation The initial experiments were conducted in a model system in which the blood of cynomolgus monkeys was circulated through porcine kidneys using an ex vivo circuit. When the circuit was established and perfusion begun, the porcine kidneys maintained a normal color for a few minutes, but its color soon changed, taking on a mottled appearance and blood flow to the organ rapidly decreased. These external changes were associated with histologic lesions consisting of hemorrhage, glomerular microthrombi, etc., characteristic of hyperacute rejection of the kidney. However, when the cynomolgus monkey was treated with human γ-globulin (2 g per kg) prior to establishing the circuit, the porcine kidneys maintained a normal appearance and blood flow. Histologic studies revealed very little evidence of anatomic abnormality in the kidneys perfused by the treated animals, there being only a few focal hemorrhages and few microthrombi. The porcine kidneys perfused by untreated cynomolgus monkeys contained substantial deposits of IgM, some IgG, and the complement components C3, C5b, C4, and the membrane attack complex along glomerular and interstitial capillaries. Kidneys from the treated preparations contained deposits of IgM and especially prominent deposits of IgG along endothelial surfaces, but practically no deposits of C4, C3, C5b, or the membrane attack complex.

The results observed in the ex vivo perfusion model were confirmed in pig-to-cynomolgus monkey and pig-to-baboon cardiac xenograft models [2]. Administration of γ-globulin to primates prevented the development of hyperacute rejection of porcine hearts transplanted in most treated animals. The immunopathology of the xenografts in these treated recipients revealed host immunoglobulins and C1q along endothelial surfaces. However, although plasma C4 and CH50 levels progressively decreased there was little or no evidence of complement components other than C1q in the grafts suggesting that the complement reactions had indeed been diverted. The histology of the xenografts was consistent with the idea that the γ-globulin had conferred substantial protection against complement-mediated injury. In the several cases in which hyperacute acute rejection did occur, the alternative pathway of complement had been activated and there was no evidence of classical pathway components. This finding provides evidence that γ-globulin may be especially effective in controlling the classical complement pathway.

Our studies using nonhuman primates supported other evidence summarized above concerning the mechanism of action of γ-globulin. The presence of human γ-globulin in the blood of non-human primates did not impair the binding of xenoreactive antibodies, particularly IgM, in the serum of the nonhuman primates to porcine endothelial cells. Although complement levels in the primates decreased after administration of γ-globulin, the CH50 and the levels of C3 and C4 remained appreciable, suggesting that the complement system remained intact. After the xenografts were reperfused, the level of complement in the plasma of the recipients declined rapidly, consistent with the idea that consumption was initiated in the graft and then diverted away. Also consistent with this view was the presence of C1q and the near absence of C4 and C3 in the grafts suggesting that following reperfusion, the very rapid and profound decrease in complement components in the recipient's blood reflected consumption initiated in the graft with the reactive molecules of C4 and/or C3 diverted away.

Comment

Our findings have several implications for the field of xenotransplantation. Of interest from a theoretical perspective is the nature of the interactions between xenoreactive antibodies and the graft. Although the pathogenesis of rejection in pig-to-primate xenografts clearly involves binding of xenoreactive antibodies to the graft leading to activation of the complement system [14, 15], and although xenoreactive antibodies may also mediate injury by directly altering the physiology of the endothelial cells to which they attach [9, 16], we must now consider that immunoglobulins also may serve a protective role. Immunoglobulins may cause endothelial cells to adopt a posture of resistance to complement-mediated injury and immunoglobulins may help to divert reactive complement molecules away from the target. Whether xenoreactive antibodies offer more or less benefit in these functions compared to the other 98 % of immunoglobulins in plasma we do not yet know.

From a practical perspective, our findings show that there is, in γ-globulin, a readily available and presumably safe agent which can be used to prevent complement-mediated injury to xenografts. One potential advantage of this agent over some others that have been reported is what appears to be selectively greater effects on the classical complement pathway, with the alternative complement pathway remaining functionally intact. Since the alternative complement pathway confers protection against invasive microorganisms, the administration of γ-globulin would likely have less tendency than other approaches to compromise host defense.

There is yet another implication of our findings. As the effects of γ-globulin appear to be manifest at all concentrations tested it may be that physiologic concentrations of immunoglobulin in the blood contribute to the regulation of the complement system. In this case, manipulation of total serum immunoglobulin levels by immunosuppression or by immunoabsorption might make vascularized xenografts more susceptible than they would otherwise be to complement and might thus be found to have some paradoxically detrimental effects on the well-being of a xenograft.

Acknowledgments. Some of the work reviewed here was supported by grants from the National Institutes of Health (HL509585, HL52297 and AI35033).

References

1. Basta, M., Kirshbom, P., Frank, M.M., Fries, L.F. Mechanism of therapeutic effect on high-dose intravenous immunoglobulin–attenuation of acute, complement-dependent immune damage in a guinea pig model. J.Clin.Invest. 84, 1974, 1989
2. Magee, J.C., Collins, B.H., Harland, R.C., et al. Immunoglobulin prevents complement mediated hyperacute rejection in swine-to-primate xenotransplantation. J.Clin.Invest. 96, 2404, 1995
3. Fries, L.F., Gaither, T.A., Hammer, C.H.Frank, M.M. C3b covalently bound to IgG demonstrates a reduced rate of inactivation by factors H and I. J.Exp.Med. 160, 1640, 1984
4. Glotz, D., Haymann, J-P., Sansonetti, N., et al. Suppression of HLA-specific alloantibodies by high-dose intravenous immunoglobulins (IVIg). Transplantation 56, 335, 1994
5. Dwyer, John M. Manipulating the immune system with immune globulin. N.Engl.J.Med. 326, 107, 1994
6. Ronda, N., Hurez, V.Kazatchkine, M.D. Intraveneous immunologbulin therapy of autoimmune and systemic inflammatory diseases. Vox Sang. 64, 65, 1993
7. Good, A.H., Cooper, D.K.C., Malcolm, A.J., et al. Identification of carbohydrate structures that bind human antiporcine antibodies: implications for discordant xenografting in humans. Transplant. Proc. 24, 559, 1992
8. Sandrin, M.S., Vaughan, H.A., Dabkowski, P.L., McKenzie, I.F.C. Anti-pig IgM antibodies in human serum react predominantly with Galα(1,3)Gal epitopes. Proc.Natl.Acad.Sci.USA 90, 11391, 1993
9. Holzknecht, Z.E.Platt, J.L. Identification of porcine endothelial cell membrane antigens recognized by human xenoreactive antibodies. J.Immunol. 154, 4565, 1995

10. Magee, J.C., Collins, B.H., Harland, R.C., et al. Prevention of hyperacute xenograft rejection by intravenous immunoglobulin. Transplant. Proc. 27, 271, 1995
11. Platt, J.L., Lindman, B.J., Geller, R.L., et al. The role of natural antibodies in the activation of xenogenic endothelial cells. Transplantation 52, 1037, 1991
12. Platt, J.L., Vercellotti, G.M., Lindman, B.J., et al. Release of heparan sulfate from endothelial cells: Implications for pathogenesis of hyperacute rejection. J.Exp.Med. 171, 1363, 1990
13. Platt, J.L., Dalmasso, A.P., Lindman, B.J., Ihrcke, N.S.Bach, F.H. The role of C5a and antibody in the release of heparan sulfate from endothelial cells. Eur.J.Immunol. 21, 2887, 1991
14. Perper, R.J.Najarian, J.S. Experimental renal heterotransplantation. I. In widely divergent species. Transplantation 4, 377, 1966
15. Platt, J.L., Fischel, R.J., Matas, A.J., et al. Immunopathology of hyperacute xenograft rejection in a swine-to-primate model. Transplantation 52, 214, 1991
16. Platt, J.L.Holzknecht, Z.E. Porcine platelet antigens recognized by human xenoreactive natural antibodies. Transplantation 57, 327, 1994

32 Prolongation of Xenograft Survival by Cobra Venom Factor

T. Kobayashi, E. Kemp, and D.K.C. Cooper

Introduction

In the 1960s, the very important role of complement in hyperacute xenograft rejection was detected and investigated, particularly by two groups headed by Gewurz and Nelson, respectively [1–4]. Complement activation was demonstrated to be an important event in hyperacute rejection. Two circumstances had delayed the clear understanding of this conclusion. The first was that, as early as 1953, Simonsen [5] found no alterations in serum complement concentrations during rejection of allografts (in dogs), and neither did Hume et al. [6] in transplanted patients undergoing acute allograft rejection. Today, we know the great differences between allograft rejection and xenograft rejection, but it was natural at that time to link these two phenomena together. The second factor was the absence of knowledge (or denial of the existence) of the alternative pathway. The existence and very important role of this pathway was only fully acknowledged 10 years after the basic experiments by Gewurz et al. and Nelson.

While it had hitherto been thought that the classical pathway was the only one operating in discordant xenograft rejection, in the 1970s it became evident that both the classical and alternative pathways could be activated and lead to graft destruction. In a book on xenotransplantation written in 1978 by Kemp [7], the following statement was made: "It is probable that the complement system in hyperacute xenograft rejection can be activated by both the classical and alternative pathways – if one is blocked it is possible that the other is activated more strongly" (Fig. 1). Important experimental evidence was documented by Schilling et al. [8], who, using organ perfusion experiments, proposed that xenograft rejection took place in some animal models even after depletion of natural antibodies.

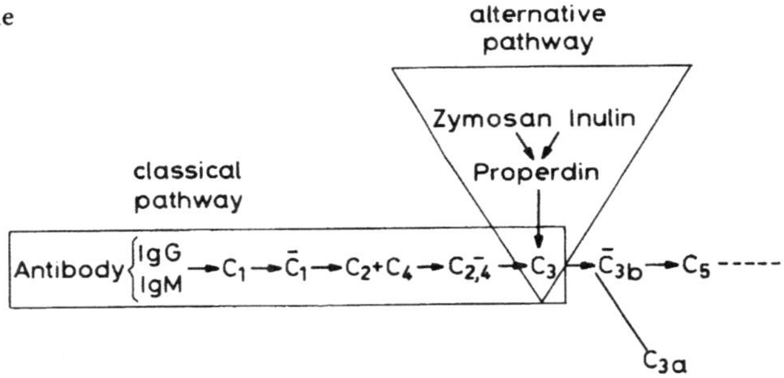

Fig. 1. The two pathways of the complement system [7]

During the 1980s, several investigations confirmed that both pathways can be activated and lead to destruction of a discordant xenograft. Kissmeyer-Nielsen, Olsen, Petersen, and Fjeldborg [9] as early as 1966 demonstrated the importance of antibodies in allotransplantation. In some experimental models the classical pathway has major influence, but if this pathway is not functioning, the alternative pathway may come into play. Nonsuckling pigs, which do not yet harbor immunoglobulins, exhibit delayed rejection of transplanted rabbit kidneys [10]. Experiments in Kemp's laboratory showed that no transplanted kidney was rejected by a non-suckling pig, while 3-week-old pigs rejected rabbit kidneys within 15–45 min.

Much longer survival was seen in the newborn pig-to-newborn baboon cardiac xenograft model by Kaplon et al. [11]. Eventually, however, the grafts transplanted into newborn animals without immunoglobulins in the serum are rejected. Thus it seems that the immunological system has several defense barriers against xenotransplantation. In addition to the classical and alternative pathways of complement, and the acute cellular response, probably other factors may also be activated in order to combat foreign tissue [12]. Today, in the 1990s, investigations have clarified some of the mechanisms of discordant xenograft rejection (Chap. 2).

Thirty years ago, Gewurz et al. and Nelson detected the profound effect of cobra venom factor (CVF) upon hyperacute xenograft rejection [1–4]. By ingenious methods they developed preparations of CVF that were tolerated

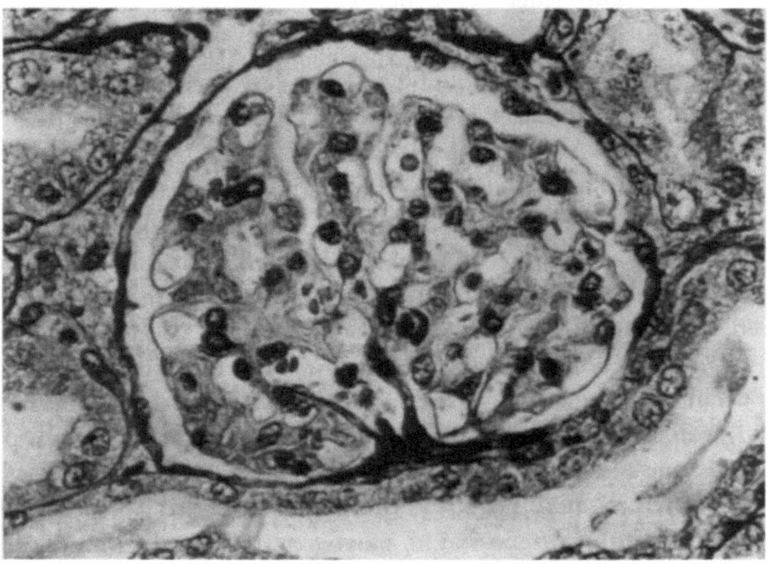

Fig. 2. Histopathology of a rabbit kidney transplanted into a bilaterally nephrectomized cat that received treatment with cobra venom factor. Seven days after transplantation, the serum creatinine was 630 µmol/l. The kidney functioned, as judged by creatinine and good diuresis. The glomeruli, the arterioles, and the interstitial tissue were normal, but a focal tubular degeneration was seen in the cortex. (Courtesy of Prof. Svend Larsen)

Table 1. Graft survival and histology of rabbit renal xenografts in cats

Group	Drug	Xeno-grafts (n)	Graft survival (mins)			Glome-rular platelet aggre-gation	Vascular endo-thelial damage	Immuno-fluores-cence (rabbit anti-cat)
			Mean	Range	p			
Control		8	12	5–20		8	0	2
ACE inhibitors	Captopril	5	56	45–60	0.001	5	0	0
	Enalapril	5	34	20–50	0.002	5	0	0
Vaso-dilators	Nifedipine	3	15	15–15	NS	3	0	0
	Prostacyclin	3	42	22–54	0.02	3	0	0
Immuno-suppres-sants	Corticosteroids + azathioprine	19	8	1–30	NS	19	0	2[a]
	Cyclosporine A	4	11	10–13	NS	4	0	1
	Lomudal (sodium chromoglycate)	3	22	22–22	0.01	3	0	0
	Cobra venom factor	13	2700	180–10 000	0.001	0	0	4[b]

From [13].
NS, not significant.
[a]Out of 12 xenografts.
[b]Out of 11 xenografts.

by the recipient animal and that could delay rejection from minutes to several hours. In our own (Kemp's) laboratory, we demonstrated even longer prolongation of discordant xenograft function by using CVF [13] (Fig. 2, Table 1). Unfortunately, the CVF used was toxic. CVF-treated animals lost appetite and did not thrive. Furthermore, the preparation used had nephrotoxic properties, resulting in some tubular necrosis in transplanted kidneys which, however, functioned for several days. The toxicity of CVF is related to the purity of the preparation (now greatly improved) and also to the experimental model used. For example, rats are more vulnerable to CVF toxicity than cats, and special purification procedures are necessary before CVF can be used in rat experiments.

Inherited deficiency in one of the complement factors can also result in prolonged survival of discordant xenografts in certain experimental animals, the best known of which is the C6-deficient rabbit [14]. Prolongation of survival of discordant xenografts was also demonstrated following treatment with monoclonal antibodies directed against complement factors. Thus we found prolongation (but also side effects) using a preparation of anti-C3 [15].

Cobra Venom Factor

CVF is a glycoprotein isolated from cobra venom which depletes complement activity through consumption of the C3 component. Crude cobra venoms have long been known to have various toxic actions, most notably the peripheral respiratory paralysis that is the primary cause of death following cobra venom poisoning [16, 17]. Various pharmacologically active toxins and enzymes, such as neurotoxins, cardiotoxins and phospholipase A2, have been separated from cobra venoms, and their functions have been determined [18, 19].

Toxicity

The clinical symptoms of systemic intoxication develop within 1–12 h and include drowsiness, apathy, a feeling of "alcoholic intoxication" or of receding consciousness, diplopia, blurred vision, headache, and heaviness of the eyelids (ptosis). Paralysis of the extrinsic ocular muscles, palate, tongue, and neck muscles is common. The intercostal muscles, diaphragm, and limbs may also be affected. Coma, and twitching movements or convulsion, may be seen as terminal events [18].

Purification

Purification of CVF, therefore, is essential for in vivo administration. Ion exchange chromatography and gel filtration are used for the isolation of CVF from the cobra venom [20]. Briefly, cobra venom is dissolved in 0.01 *M* phosphate buffer (pH7.5) and passed down a diethylaminoethanol (DEAE) cellulose column. After the major proteins, including the neurotoxins, have passed through the column, CVF is eluted with a 0.5 *M* NaCl gradient. The CVF fraction is then concentrated and purified further by gel filtration using Sephadex G-200. However, since this two-step purified CVF still contains phospholipase A2, further sequential chromatography or isoelectric focusing is necessary to yield a product that is free of phospholipase A2 [21–23].

It has been shown that purified CVF retains the capacity to cause lung damage [24], since CVF activates the alternative pathway of complement, thereby generating vasoactive and chemotactic complement fragments, C3a and C5a, which are known to induce aggregation of platelets and leukocytes [25, 26]. However, C3a and C5a are rapidly converted to C3a des Arg and C5a des Arg by carboxypeptidase N (SCPN), and therefore infusion of purified CVF is nonlethal and, indeed, is no longer associated with significant morbidity [27].

Mechanism of Action

CVF, which is a structural and functional analogue of C3 [28], is a complement-activating protein (Fig. 1). CVF binds factor B to form the complex CVFB [29], which is also cleaved by factor D into CVFBb and Ba [30]. The biomolecular complex CVFBb is a C3/C5 convertase that activates C3 and C5 analogously to the C3/C5 convertase formed with C3b. Although the two C3/C5 convertases, C3bBb and CVFBb, share molecular architecture, the active site-bearing Bb subunits, and substrate specificity, the two enzymes exhibit significant functional differences. The CVFBb enzyme is physicochemically far more stable than

C3bBb. The half-life of decay dissociation at 37 °C is 1.5 min for C3bBb [31] but is 7 h for CVFBb [30]. C3bBb is disassembled by Factor H [32], and C3b is inactivated by the combined action of factors H and I [33], whereas CVFBb is resistant to these regulatory complement proteins [34, 35]. C3bBb requires additional C3b for C5 cleavage, while CVFBb can cleave C5 directly [36].

Experience in Experimental Xenotransplantation

Therefore, CVF provides the opportunity for the in vitro and in vivo experimental study of complement depletion. The administration of CVF has been used in many experiments relating to the hyperacute rejection of xenotransplants in which complement is believed to play a major role (Tables 2, 3). In the early experiments using CVF, the role of complement in the development of hyperacute rejection after discordant xenotransplantation was examined. Since CVF was demonstrated to inhibit hyperacute rejection, more recently CVF has been used to help elucidate the mechanisms of delayed xenograft rejection [37–40]. In concordant xenotransplantation, the complement-mediated rejection that occurs after the initial increase in antibody production has also been investigated using CVF.

Although CVF is the most commonly known and well characterized complement-reactive factor, the existence of at least two other anticomplementary factors from cobra venoms has been reported [41, 42]: (1) high molecular weight factor (H-CoF; *MW*, $0.8–1.0 \times 10^6$), which is known to inhibit early reactions of the classical pathway of complement and (2) complement inhibitor (CI; *MW*, 26 000), which interferes at various steps of the complement cascade, including reactions of both the classical and the alternative pathways.

Two CVFs – one from *Naja naja* and the other from *N. haje* cobra venom – have been purified and compared regarding their function and pharmacokinetics [36, 43]. The differences reported include the following: (a) CVF from *N. naja* has C3- and C5-depleting effects, while CVF from *N. haje* has a selectively C3-deplet-

Table 2. Xenotransplantation experiments involving the use of cobra venom factor (CVF) in nonrodents

Donor/recipient species	Transplant	Longest graft survival	Reference
Rabbit/dog	Kidney	150 min	[4]
Pig/dog	Kidney	26 h	[56]
Pig/dog	Kidney	21 h	[3]
Pig/dog	Kidney	60 min	[57]
Dog/rabbit	Kidney	75 min	[58]
Rabbit/cat	Kidney	3 days	[59]
Rabbit/cat	Kidney	7 days	[13]
Rabbit/pig	Heart	18 h	[60]
Pig/baboon	Heart	17.5 days	[37]
Pig/baboon	Heart	25 days	[38]

Table 3. Xenotransplantation experiments involving the use of cobra venom factor (CVF) in rodents

Donor/recipient species	Graft survival		Reference
	Mean	Longest	
Rat/rabbit	4.4 h	–	[61]
Hamster/rat (sensitized)	1.8 days	–	[61]
Guinea pig/rat	2.9 days	–	[62]
Guinea pig/rat	–	3 days	[63]
Hamster/rat	49.1 days	105 days	[64]
Hamster/rat	3.2 days	4 days	[65]
Guinea pig/rat	3.7 days	–	[66]
Guinea pig/rat	2.3 days	–	[67]
Hamster/rat	4.0 days	5 days	[68]
Guinea pig/rat	6.6 days	7 days	[69]
Guinea pig/rat	3.2 days	–	[39]
Guinea pig/rat	–	–	[40]
Hamster/rat	–	19 days	[70]
Mouse/rat (sensitized)	–	4 days	[71]
Guinea pig/rat	6.0 days	8 days	[72]

Heart transplantation was performed in all cases.

ing effect in humans and mice, (b) approximately tenfold higher dosages of *N. haje* CVF than of *N. naja* CVF are necessary to obtain similar effectiveness in mice, and (c) the functional half-life of *N. naja* CVF is 11.5 h, while that of *N. haje* CVF is 4.5 h in mice. According to other papers, however, the half-life of *N. naja* CVF in rabbits [44] and in mice [45] is reported to be 32 h and 24 h, respectively. Therefore, *N. naja* CVF appears to be more efficient for the depletion of complement activity than *N. haje* CVF.

A major obstacle in performing CVF experiments is that the elimination of CVF in vivo is accelerated by the production of neutralizing antibody. Since CVF is a foreign protein and is highly immunogenic, anti-CVF antibody is generally produced after CVF administration, reducing its efficacy [38, 44–46]. Repeated CVF injection after approximately 1 week led to a reduced effect on complement depletion in rabbits [44] and in mice [45]. When CVF was injected in guinea pigs every 3 days, complement activity was suppressed for only 8 days after initial administration [46]. In xenotransplantation experiments, we need to consider the possibility that it is the reduced efficacy of repeated administration of CVF caused by anti-CVF antibody production that leads to complement-mediated rejection, rather than other factors.

In studies at one of our own centers [38], we documented greatly decreased efficiency of CVF when readministered to a baboon 2 weeks after an initial injection. Anti-CVF antibody was detected as early as 6 days after the initial CVF administration in a baboon that had also undergone splenectomy and pig heart transplantation. Frequent CVF injections were required to maintain complement activity at a low level. However, when given in a combination with pharmacologic immunosuppressive therapy (consisting of cyclosporine, methylprednisolone, cyclophosphamide, ±methotrexate) the administration of CVF (0.25 mg/kg) every 3 days proved sufficient to suppress complement activity for at least 25 days with no anti-CVF antibody being detected. Therefore, the concomitant administration of pharmacologic immunosuppressive therapy appeared to be beneficial in suppressing the production of anti-CVF antibody and in maintaining the efficacy of CVF.

Cobra Venom Factor and Anti-αGal Antibodies

Recent work from other centers has demonstrated that the structure of CVF includes N-linked complex-type oligosaccharides which contain terminal α-galactosyl (αGal) residues. Therefore, the naturally occurring anti-αGal antibody present in human serum [47–49] can cross-react with CVF [50]. Although anti-αGal antibody does not affect the complement-activating activity of CVF in humans in vivo (because the oligosaccharide chains of CVF are not required for its complement-activating function), it has been suggested that anti-αGal antibody will modulate the effect of complement activation by CVF by forming immune complexes, which presumably result in a more rapid removal of CVF from the circulation [50].

Pig-to-baboon heart transplantation experiments at our center [38] confirmed previous reports demonstrating that purified CVF is nontoxic and highly effective in depleting complement activity [43–46, 50]. However, in combination with heavy pharmacologic immunosuppression, a high incidence of infection was observed in the recipient baboons. If CVF is used clinically together with pharmacologic immunosuppressive therapy to prevent complement-mediated vascular rejection, it seems likely that this combined therapy will put the patient at a significant risk of developing infection.

Comment

Other agents are also being explored in an effort to inhibit complement-mediated rejection. The effects of (a) soluble complement receptor type I (sCR1) [51], (b) anti-C5 monoclonal antibody [52], (c) FUT-175 (a synthetic serine protease inhibitor) [53], and (d) K76COOH (a monocarboxylic acid derivative of a fungal product) [53] have all been reported. Since these agents, unlike CVF, do not release the potent proinflammatory mediator C5a (which activates endothelial cells and attracts leukocytes, resulting in graft damage by fibrin deposition and platelet aggregation) they may prove preferable to CVF in the prevention of hyperacute rejection.

CVF delays hyperacute xenograft rejection but delayed vascular rejection is not avoided. At the present time, one of the great unanswered questions concerns the causes and mechanisms of rejection in the presence of complement inactivation.

Other means of inactivation of the complement system have been developed, but CVF is still as effective as newer agents, such as SCR1 [54] and C1-inhibitors [55]. One of the most exciting developments today is the breeding of transgenic animals with human complement regulator genes (Chap. 49). This is a most promising method of obtaining successful xenografting, and was, in fact, developed to some considerable extent on the basis of results from the early experiments with CVF.

References

1. GEWURZ, H., CLARK, D.S. Participation of complement and complement-fixing antibody in the rejection of vascularized grafts. J. Lab. Clin. Med. 1964; 64:861
2. GEWURZ, H., CLARK, D.S., VARCO, R.L., et al. Serum complement: an indicator of accelerated homograft rejection in man. J. Peds. 1965; 67:1031
3. NELSON, R.A. Jr. A new concept of immunosuppression in hypersensitivity reactions and in transplantation immunity. Survey Ophthal. 1966; 11:498
4. GEWURZ, H., CLARK, D.S., FINSTAD, J., et al. Role of the complement system in graft rejection in experimental animals and man. Ann. N.Y. Acad. Sci. 1966; 129:673
5. SIMONSEN, M. Biological incompatibility in kidney transplantation in dogs: serological investigations. Acta. Path. Microb. Scand. 1953; 32:36
6. HUME, D.M., MERRILL, J.P., MILLER, B.F., et al. Experiences with renal homotransplantation in the human: report of nine cases. J. Clin. Invest. 1955; 34:327
7. KEMP, E. Xenografting. The Future of Organ Transplantation. Odense University Press, Denmark, 1978
8. SCHILLING, A., LAND, W., PRATSCHKE, E., et al. Dominant role of complement in the hyperacute xenograft rejection reaction. Surg. Gynecol. Obstet. 1976; 142:29
9. KISSMEYER-NIELSEN, F., OLSEN, S., PETERSEN, F.P., FJELDBORG, O. Hyperacute rejection of kidney allografts associated with preexisting humoral antibodies against donor cells. Lancet. 1966; 2:662
10. KEMP, E., WHITE, D., DIEPERINK, H., et al. Delayed rejection of rabbit kidneys transplanted into baby pigs. Transplant. Proc. 1987; 19:1143
11. KAPLON, R.J., MICHLER, R.E., XU, H., et al. Absence of hyperacute rejection in newborn pig-to-baboon cardiac xenografts. Transplantation. 1995; 59:1
12. KEMP, E. Experimental xenotransplantation between distantly related nonprimate species. In: Cooper, D.K.C., Kemp, E., Reemtsma, K., White, D.J.G. (eds). Xenotransplantation. (First edition) Heidelberg, 1991, p. 377
13. KEMP, E., STEINBRUCHEL, D., STARKLINT, H., et al. Renal xenograft rejection: prolonging effect of captopril. ACE-inhibitors, prostacyclin, and cobra venom factor. Transplant. Proc. 1987; 19:4471
14. MEJIA-LAGUNA, J.E., GARCIA-CORNEJO, M., LOPEZ-SORIANO, F., et al. The role of the sixth component of complement in the rejection of kidney xenografts. Immunol. 1970; 19:767
15. KEMP, E., DIEPERINK, H., LETH, P., et al. Monoclonal antibodies to complement C3 prolong survival of discordant xenografts: guinea pig heart to rat transplantation. Transplant. Proc. 1994; 26:1011

16. SARKAR, B.B., MAITRA, S.R., GHOSH, B.N. The effect of neurotoxin, haemolysin and choline esterase isolated from cobra venom on heart, blood pressure and respiration. Ind. J. Med. Res. 1942; 30:453
17. LEE, C.Y., PENG, M.T. An analysis of the respiratory failure produced by the Formosan elapid venoms. Arch. Int. Pharmacodyn. 1961; 133:180
18. MELDRUM, B.S. The actions of snake venom on nerve and muscle. The pharmacology of phospholipase A and of polypeptide toxins. Pharmacol. Rev. 1965; 17:393
19. LEE, C.Y., CHEN, Y.M. Central neurotoxicity of cobra neurotoxin, cardiotoxin and phospholipase A2. Toxicon. 1977; 15:395
20. HARRISON, R.A., LACHMANN, P.J. Complement technology. In: Handbook of Experimental Immunology, 4th Edition. Weir, D.M., Herzenberg, L.A., Blackwell, C., Herzenberg, L.A. (eds). Oxford, Blackwell, 1986
21. VOGEL, C.W., MULLER-EBERHARD, H.J. Cobra venom factor: improved method for purification and biochemical characterization. J. Immunol. Methods. 1984; 73:203
22. LACHMANN, P.J., HALBWACHS, L., GEWURZ, A., GEWURZ, H. Purification of cobra venom factor from phopholipase A contaminant. Immunology. 1976; 31:961
23. PEPYS, M.B., TOMKINS, C., SMITH, A.D. An improved method for the isolation from Naja Naja venom of cobra venom factor (CoF) free of phospholipase A. J. Immunol. Meth. 1979; 30:105
24. TILL, G.O., JOHNSON, K.J., KUNKEL, R., WARD, P.A. Intravascular activation of complement and acute lung injury, dependency on neutrophils and toxic oxygen metabolites. J. Clin. Invest. 1982; 69:1126
25. GROSSKLAUS, C., DAMERAU, B., LEMGO, E., VOGT, W. Induction of platelet aggregation by the complement-derived peptides C3a and C5a. Naunyn-Schmiedeberg's Arch. Pharmacol. 1976; 295:71
26. HAMMERSCHMIDT, D.E., HARRIS, P.D., WAYLAND, J.H., CRADDOCK, P.R., JACOB, H.S. Complement-induced granulocyte aggregation in vivo. Am. J. Pathol. 1981; 102:146
27. HUEY, R., BLOOR, C.M., KAWAHARA, M.S., HUGLI, T.E. Potentiation of the anaphylatoxins in vivo using an inhibitor of serum carboxypeptidase N (SCPN). Am. J. Pathol. 1983; 112:48
28. VOGEL, C-W., SMITH, C.A., MULLER-EBERHARD, H.J. Cobra venom factor: structural homology with the third component of human complement. J. Immunol. 1984; 133:3235
29. HENSLEY, P., O'KEEFE, M.C., SPANGLER, C.J., OSBORNE, J.C. JR, VOGEL, C-W. The effect of metal ions and temperature on the interaction of cobra venom factor and human complement factor B. J. Biol. Chem. 1986; 261:11038
30. VOGEL, C-W., MULLER-EBERHARD, H.J. The cobra venom factor-dependent C3 convertase of human complement. A kinetic and thermodynamic analysis of a protease acting on its natural high molecular weight substrate. J. Biol. Chem. 1982; 257:8292
31. MEDICUS, R.G., GOTZE, O., MULLER-EBERHARD, H.J. Alternative pathway of complement: recruitment of precursor properdin by the labile C3/C5 convertase and the potentiation of the pathway. J. Exp. Med. 1976; 144:1076
32. WHALEY, L., RUDDY, S. Modulation of the alternative complement pathway by β1H globulin. J. Exp. Med. 1976; 144:1147
33. PANGBURN, M.K., SCHREIBER, R.D., MULLER-EBERHARD, J.H. Human complement C3b inactivator: isolation, characterization and demonstration of an absolute requirement for the serum protein β1H for cleavage of C3b and C4b in solution. J. Exp. Med. 1977; 146:257

34. LACHMAN, P.J., HALBWACHS, L. The influence of C3b inactivator (KAF) concentration on the ability of serum to support complement activation. Clin. Exp. Immunol. 1975; 21:109
35. NAGAKI, K., IIDA, K., OKUBO, M., INAI, S. Reaction mechanisms of β1H globulin. Int. Archs. Allergy Appl. Immunol. 1978; 57:221
36. VON ZABERN, I., HINSCH, B., PRZYKLENK, H., SCHMIDT, G., VOGT, W. Comparison of Naja n. naja and Naja h. haje cobra venom factors: correlation between binding affinity for the fifth component of complement and mediation of its cleavage. Immunobiol. 1980; 157:499
37. LEVENTHAL, J.R., SAKIYALAK, P., WITSON, J., et al. The synergistic effect of combined antibody and complement depletion on discordant cardiac xenograft survival in nonhuman primates. Transplantation. 1994; 57:974
38. KOBAYASHI, T., TANIGUCHI, S., YE, Y., et al. Delayed xenograft rejection in C3-depleted discordant (pig-to-baboon) cardiac xenografts treated with cobra venom factor. Transplant. Proc. 1996; 28:560
39. BRAKELY, M.L., VAN DEL WERF, W.J., BERNDT, M.C., et al. Activation of intragraft endothelial and mononuclear cells during discordant xenograft rejection. Transplantation. 1994; 58:1059
40. FRYER, J.P., LEVENTHAL, J.R., DALMASSO, A.P., et al. Cellular rejection in discordant xenografts when hyperacute rejection is prevented: analysis using adoptive and passive transfer. Transplant. Immunol. 1994; 2:87
41. BALLOW, M., COCHRANE, C.G. Two anticomplementary factors in cobra venom: hemolysis of guinea pig erythrocytes by one of them. J. Immunol. 1969; 103:944
42. VON ZABERN, PRZYKLENK, H., DAMERAU, B., ZIMMERMAN, B. Isolation and properties of a complement inhibitor from Naja haje venom, distinct from known anticomplementary factors in cobra venom. Scand. J. Immunol. 1981; 14:109
43. VAN DEN BERG, C.W., AERTS, P.C., VAN DIJK, H. In vivo anti-complementary activities of the cobra venom factors from Naja naja and Naja haje. J. Immunol. Methods. 1991; 136:287
44. COCHRANE, C.G., MULLER-EBERHARD, J.H., AIKIN, B.S. Depletion of plasma complement in vivo by a protein of cobra venom: its effect on various immunologic reactions. J. Immunol. 1970; 105:55
45. PEPYS, M.B. Studies in vivo of cobra factor and murine C3. Immunol. 1975; 28:369
46. PLEYER, U., MONDINO, B.J., SUMNER, H.L. The effect of systemic decomplementation with cobra venom factor on corneal complement levels in guinea pigs. Invest. Ophthalmol. Vis. Sci. 1992; 33:2212
47. GALILI, U., RACHMILEWITZ, E.A., PELEG, A., et al. A unique natural human IgG antibody with anti-α-galactosyl specificity. J. Exp. Med. 1984; 260:1519
48. GOOD, A.H., COOPER, D.K.C., MALCOLM, A.J., et al. Identification of carbohydrate structures that bind human anti-porcine antibodies: implications for discordant xenografting in humans. Transplant. Proc. 1992; 24:559
49. COOPER, D.K.C., GOOD, A.H., KOREN, E., et al. Identification of α-galactosyl and other carbohydrates that are bound by human anti-pig antibodies: relevance to discordant xenografting in man. Transpl. Immunol. 1993; 1:198
50. GOWDA, D.C., PETRELLA, E.C., RAJ, T.T., BREDEHORST, R., VOGEL, C-W. Immunoreactivity and function of oligosaccharides in cobra venom factor. J. Immunol. 1994; 152:2977

51. PRUITT, S.K., KIRK, A.D., BOLLINGER, R.R., et al. The effect of soluble complement receptor type 1 on hyperacute rejection of porcine xenografts. Transplantation. 1994; 57:363
52. KROSHUS, T.J., ROLLINS, S.A., DALMASSO, A.P., et al. Complement inhibition with an anti-C5 monoclonal antibody prevents acute cardiac tissue injury in an ex vivo model of pig-to-human xenotransplantation. Transplantation. 1995; 60:1194
53. KOBAYASHI, T., NEETHLING, F., TANIGUCHI, S., et al. Investigation of the anticomplement agents, FUT-175 and K76COOH, in discordant xenotransplantation. Xenotransplantation. In press
54. CRUPCALA, M., POMER, P., STAEHLER, G., WALDHERR, R., KIRSCHFINK, M. Prolongation of discordant renal xenograft survival by depletion of complement. Comparative effects of systemically administered cobra venom factor and soluble complement receptor type 1 in a guinea pig-to-rat model. Transplant. Int. 1994; 7:650
55. DALMASSO, A.P., PLATT, J.L. Potentiation of C1 inhibitor plus heparin in prevention of complement-mediated activation of endothelial cells in a model of xenograft hyperacute rejection. Transplant. Proc. 1994; 28:1246
56. SNYDER, G.B., BALLESTEROS, E., ZARCO, R.M., LINN, B.S. Prolongation of renal xenografts by complement suppression. Surg. Forum. 1966; 14:478
57. MOBERG, A.W., SHONS, A.R., GEWURZ, H., MOZES, M., NAJARIAN, J.S. Prolongation of renal xenografts by the simultaneous suquestration of preformed antibody, inhibition of complement, coagulation and antibody synthesis. Transplant. Proc. 1971; 3:538
58. MEJIA-LAGUNA, J.E., MARTINEZ-PALOMO, A., BIRO, C.E., et al. Morphologic study of the participation of the complement system in hyperacute rejection of renal xenotransplants. Am. J. Pathol. 1972; 69:71
59. KEMP, E., KEMP, G., LARSEN, S. Survival of discordant renal xenografts up to 3 days: assessment of function, light and immunofluorescent microscopy. Scand. J. Urol. Nephrol. 1980; suppl 54:150
60. JOHNSTON, P.S., WANG, M., LIM, S.M.L., WRIGHT, L.J., WHITE, D.J.G. Discordant xenograft rejection in an antibody-free model. Transplantation. 1992; 54:573
61. ROSENGARD, B.R., HALL, T.S., IMAGAWA, D.K., et al. Hyperacute rejection of cardiac xenografts: two new models showing differences in pathogenesis. Surg. Forum. 1985; 36:361
62. ADACHI, H., ROSENGARD, B.R., HUTCHINS, G.M., et al. Effects of cyclosporine, aspirin, and cobra venom factor on discordant cardiac xenograft survival in rats. Transplant. Proc. 1987; 19:1145
63. MIYAGAWA, S., HIROSE, H., SHIRAKURA, R., et al. The mechanism of discordant xenograft rejection. Transplantation. 1988; 46:825
64. VAN DEN BOGAERDE, J., ASPINALL, R., WANG, M-W., et al. Induction of long-term survival of hamster heart xenografts in rats. Transplantation. 1991; 52:15
65. CHEN, H., ,XU, D., WU, J., DALOZE, P. Prolongation of hamster to rat xenograft survival by rapamycin. Transplant. Proc. 1992; 24:715
66. LEVENTHAL, J.R., MATAS, A.J., SUN, L.H., et al. The immunopathology of cardiac xenograft rejection in the guinea pig-to-rat model. Transplantation. 1993; 56:1
67. TAVAKOLI, R., MICHEL, A., CARDOSO, J., et al. Prolonged survival of guinea pig-to-rat heart xenografts using repeated low doses of cobra venom factor. Transplant. Proc. 1993; 25:407

68. MOHIUDDIN, M., KLINE, G., SHEN, Z., et al. Experiments in cardiac xenotransplantation. J. Thorac. Cardiovasc. Surg. 1993; 106:632
69. HAYASHI, S., ITO, M., YOKOYAMA, I., TAKAGI, H. Evidence that combination therapy using cobra venom factor, splenectomy, and deoxyspergualin is effective in guinea pig to rat cardiac xenotransplantation. Transplantation. 1994; 57:777
70. SCHUURMAN, H-J., JOERGENSEN, J., KUIPERS, H., et al. Vascular transplantation of Syrian hamster heart into Lewis rat: effect of brequinar, cyclosporine, cobra venom factor, and splenectomy. Transplant. Proc. 1994; 26:1217
71. GANNEDAHL, G., KARLSSON-PARRA, A., WALLGREN, A.C., et al. Role of antibody synthesis and complement activation in concordant xenograft retransplantation. Transplantation. 1994; 58:337
72. SCHERINGA, M., BLANKER, R., BEMELMAN, M., et al. Prolonged survival of guinea pig hearts in rats after combined antibody and complement depletion. Transplant. Proc. 1995; 27:303

33 Therapeutic Effect of Soluble Complement Receptor Type 1 in Xenotransplantation

H.C. Marsh and U.S. Ryan

Introduction

The immediate and devastating effects of hyperacute rejection in xenotransplantation have tended to focus research and therapeutic strategies on this major hurdle, and there is no question that without such strategies the problems facing xenotransplantation cannot even be studied experimentally [1]. Nevertheless, if xenotransplantation is to become a clinical alternative, it will be necessary to confront the full spectrum of pathophysiological mechanisms at play. Many of these are well known clinically in the context of allotransplantation [2]. In xenotransplantation, the most critical steps are the immediate deposition of xenoreactive natural antibodies on graft endothelium causing complement activation, the activation of coagulation and thrombotic mechanisms, the intermediate inflammatory and immune cellular responses, and the anticipated longer-term processes of tissue hyperplasia and remodeling. Many of the cellular and molecular culprits driving or amplifying these pathways are known and inextricably linked: others yet to be discovered or fully understood will have to be woven into the existing tapestry. Despite the individual and collective complexities of the pathways involved, some points emerge clearly:

1. Complement activation is central to the initiation, progression and amplification of the destructive processes of hyperacute rejection.
2. It will be hard to overestimate the amplifying role of the endothelium as a target and source of activation responses.
3. In order to alleviate early or late responses to xenotransplantation, therapeutic regimens that limit the amplification cascades are likely to be more effective than those that block individual molecular effectors of damage.

Before considering the effects of soluble complement receptor type 1 (sCR1) in xenotransplantation, it may be useful to outline the mechanisms of complement activation and its consequences on the cell types most critically involved in the progression of responses to xenografting.

Complement Activation

Upon reperfusion of the xenograft, pre-existing, xenospecific natural antibodies bind to the graft endothelium thus activating complement through the classical pathway, leading to hyperacute rejection. Interventions which deplete natural antibodies or complement are both effective in delaying hyperacute reaction in models of xenotransplantation. For Old World monkey recipients receiving non-Old World monkey grafts, the predominant xenoreactive antigen appears to be the carbohydrate epitope Galα1–3Gal [3], which appears to play an important role in hyperacute rejection [4]. Natural antibodies are also present in non-primate recipients although the specificity of these xenoreactive antibodies is not as well defined. Nonprimate recipients also appear to activate complement through antibody-independent mechanisms, possibly involving the alternative pathway [5, 6]. Alternative pathway activation as reflected by the capacity to lyse erythrocytes is clearly species dependent. For example, rat complement efficiently lyses guinea pig erythrocytes by the alternative pathway and is an order of magnitude more efficient than the alternative pathway lysis of pig erythrocytes by human complement [7]. Alternative pathway activation may result from species incompatibilities between donor complement regulatory molecules and the complement components of the recipient – a lack of homologous restriction [8]. Antibody-dependent alternative pathway activation has also been reported [9, 10]. Complement activation by either pathway in discordant combinations such as guinea pig-to-rat or pig-to-primate leads to rapid hyperacute rejection, which appears strongly dependent on the terminal complement components.

The relative contribution of late versus early components of the complement cascade has been examined using C6-deficient rats in a model of guinea pig to rat discordant cardiac xenografting [11]. The C6-deficient rats were compared with similar strains of complement-sufficient rats. All rats with adequate complement activity rejected the cardiac xenografts between 15 and 80 min, whereas C6-deficient rats rejected the cardiac xenografts in 1–2 days despite the fact that they had high preexisting IgM natural antibody titers. These results confirmed earlier studies of cat kidneys transplanted into C6-deficient rabbits [12]. Transfer of serum from complement-sufficient rats caused hyperacute rejection within 116 min. Transfer of heat-inactivated or C6-deficient serum did not induce hyperacute rejection. The hyperacute rejection process was characterized by intravascular platelet aggregation and interstitial hemorrhage. Organs transplanted into the C6-deficient animals had patent vessels at 30 min, but at 2 days were heavily infiltrated by granulocytes and monocytes. This study [11] clearly illustrates that a deficiency in C6 prevents C5b-9-driven cellular damage and procoagulant activity, but that it allows an accelerated acute rejection, presumably mediated by C3a and C5a, with vasoactive and inflammatory consequences.

In addition to factors which are peculiar to xenotransplantation, such as xenospecific antibodies and the lack of homologous restriction, more common mechanisms of complement activation are also likely to be involved, especially when therapeutic intervention delays hyperacute rejection. Such mechanisms include ischemia and reperfusion injury which likely activates both complement pathways as demonstrated in a rat model of myocardial infarction [13] and which may result from the exposure of subcellular activators [14–16]. Complement activation by ischemic and injured tissues is clearly not responsible for hyperacute rejection but may contribute to the overall inflammatory process. Finally, complement, and in particular fragments of C3, facilitate primary and secondary antibody responses, especially to low-dose antigen challenges [17, 18]. Any mature xenospecific antibody response that might possibly be generated under conditions of extended xenograft survival, would in turn activate complement and other antibody-dependent inflammatory mechanisms including those mediated by receptors such as FcR [19] and C1qR [20–23].

Complement Effects on Endothelial Cells and Platelets

In the resting situation, normal endothelial cells maintain a barrier between cells and molecules of the vascular lumen and those of the organ parenchyma. Resting endothelial cells actively resist thrombosis via molecules such as thrombomodulin, antithrombin III, tissue factor pathway inhibitor and ADPase. Heparan sulfate on the endothelial surface binds endothelial cell superoxide dismutase, thus promoting antioxidant activities of the endothelium. Immediately upon xenotransplantation, the situation is transformed (see Fig. 1). Xenoreactive natural antibodies bind to graft endothelium activating complement which in turn activates the endothelium causing disruption of endothelial junctions leading to edema and hemorrhage. This process also exposes subendothelial procoagulant surfaces to platelets which adhere by the interaction of platelet receptor gpIb and von Willebrand factor (vWF). Platelet binding to C1q or vWF associated with the exposed subendothelial matrix could result in the activation of the platelet receptor gpIIbIIIa with expression of P selectin and procoagulant activity by the platelets [24]. Surface expression of the adhesion molecule P selectin promotes the interaction of platelets and leukocytes [25] resulting in tissue factor expression on monocytes following direct adhesive contact [26]. Production of superoxide anion and other reactive oxygen species could be enhanced through the interaction of P selectin and sialyl-Lewis^x (sLeX) carbohydrate antigen as has been demonstrated in vitro [27]. In turn these events would result in further endothelial activation and consequent thrombosis [28]. Thus the immediate effects of antibody-driven complement activity on the endothelial surface result in loss of barrier function and an upregulation of procoagulant and prothrombotic mechanisms as well as the initiation of downstream inflammatory amplification loops.

Activation of the complement cascade by either the classical or alternative pathways, leads to cleavage first of C3 and then of C5 into biologically active products. The smaller cleavage products (anaphylatoxins C3a and C5a) are extremely potent proinflammatory mediators. Both C3a and C5a dramatically increase vascular permeability, trigger release of histamine from mast cells and basophils, and stimulate smooth muscle contraction. C5a activates endothelial cells [29, 30], although C5a receptors on endothelial cells are expressed at low density [31]. Endothelial activation results in release of heparan sulfate [29], synthesis of tissue factor [32], secretion of vWF from Weibel-Palade bodies and transient expression of P selectin [31]. The acute consequences of endothelial cell activation, in the context of xenotransplantation, are dire. Fibrin deposition, augmented thrombin-mediated platelet aggregation, and vascular leak and hemorrhage all serve to limit xenograft survival.

The terminal effector phase of complement activation results in the formation and deposition of the membrane attack complex (MAC, C5b-9), a pore-forming

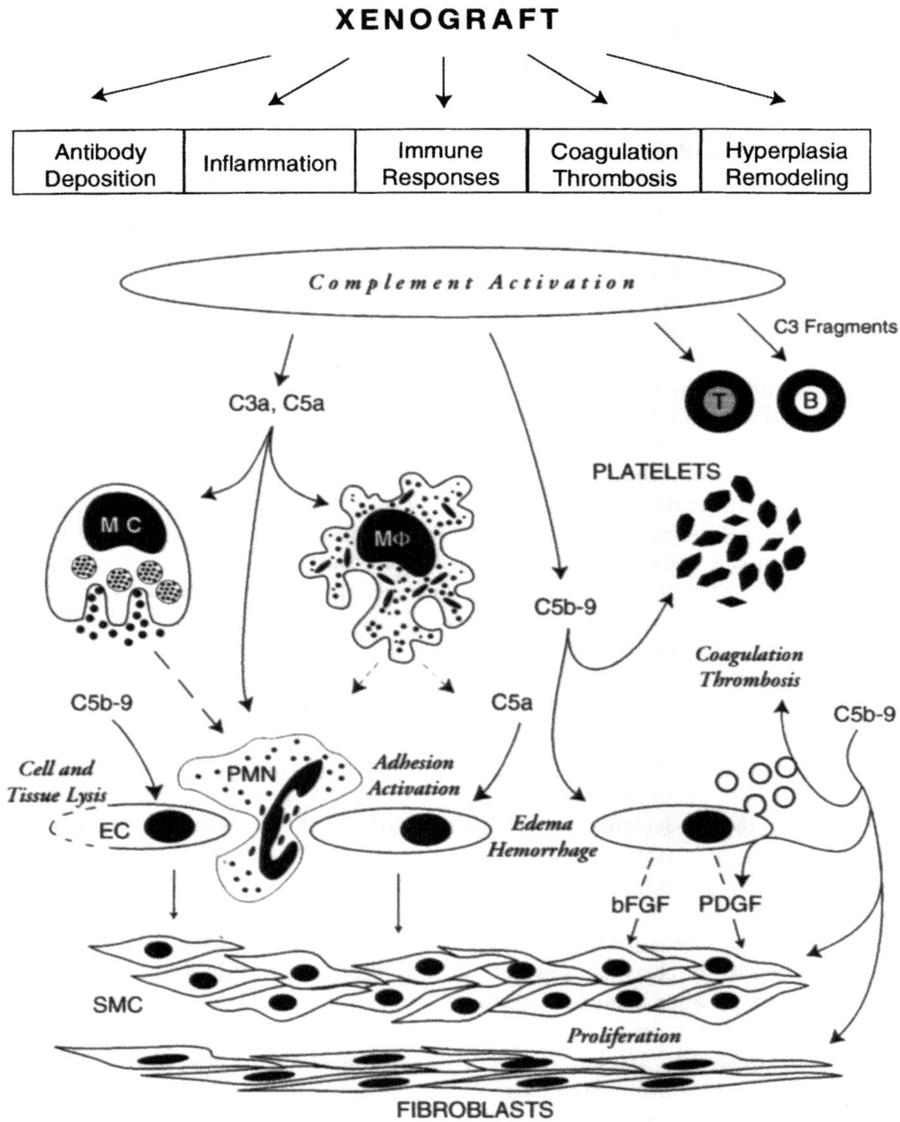

Fig. 1. Introduction of a xenograft immediately sets in motion events that culminate in hyperacute rejection. Xenoreactive natural antibodies are deposited on the graft endothelium and complement activation ensues. Early split products of complement activation, such as the anaphylatoxins C3a and C5a and the terminal complement complex C5b-9, activate a wide variety of cells to cause activation, adhesive interactions, and release of a host of mediators, cytokines, chemokines, and growth factors. The cellular and molecular interactions result in coagulation and thrombosis, edema and hemorrhage, inflammatory reactions, and cell and tissue destruction and may lead to proliferation of underlying cells and tissues. *FGF*, fibroblast growth factor; *PDGF*, platelet-derived growth factor; *EC*, endothelial cell; *SMC*, smooth muscle cell; *PMN*, polymorphonuclear neutrophil; *MΦ*, macrophage

complex of multiple complement components (C5b, C6, C7, C8, and C9). C5b-9 assembly on cell membranes causes ion and water fluxes that ultimately lead to cell death by lysis. Sublytic deposition of C5b-9 and consequent cytosolic ionic changes may initiate signaling cascades that activate a variety of proinflammatory responses [33] including the release of reactive oxygen metabolites, production of prostaglandins and leukotrienes and secretion of cytokines including interleukin (IL)-1. Insertion of C5b-9 into endothelial cells leads to the release of platelet derived growth factor (PDGF) and basic fibroblast growth factor (bFGF) [34]. These potent mitogens for smooth muscle cells may contribute to chronic proliferative changes similar to those observed in vessels with transplant arteriosclerosis associated with chronic allograft rejection. Insertion of C5b-9 causes a rapid fusion of cytoplasmic granules with the endothelial cell membrane exposing P selectin leading to interact ions among platelets, neutrophils and monocytes [35]. In addition, the vesiculation of the plasma membrane exposes a catalytic surface on vascular endothelial cells for assembly of the prothrombinase enzyme complex that can contribute to fibrin-deposition associated with acute immune endothelial injury [36]. Platelet aggregation and activation can be augmented by C5b-9 deposition on platelets [37]. C5b-9 activated platelets also increase thromboxane synthesis, secrete storage granule contents, and express procoagulant activity. The involvement of platelets in hyperacute rejection has been demonstrated and the contribution of platelets to accelerated arteriosclerosis and chronic rejection is widely accepted. Through the action of C5b-9, complement activates a wide-range of cell types, circumventing any requirement for a specific receptor–ligand interaction. Thus the formation of the terminal complement complex can lead both to endothelial cell destruction and to sublytic triggering mechanisms which mimic the effects of endothelial cell and platelet agonists.

Complement Effects on Leukocytes

C5a is a powerful chemoattractant for granulocytes (eosinophils and basophils as well as neutrophils) and monocytes. C5a activates these cells and causes enzyme release by granulocytes [38, 39], cytokine (IL-1, IL-6, IL-8, and tumor necrosis factor-α, TNF-α) production by monocytes [40–42] and up-regulation of the complement receptor type 1 (CR1) and type 3 (CR3) [43, 44]. C3a activates basophils [45] and eosinophils which may in turn activate neutrophils [46]. The release of proinflammatory cytokines amplifies downstream adhesion and activation events, augments the proliferative responses of T lymphocytes, and enhances antibody production by B lymphocytes. C3b and its inactive product, iC3b, can serve as accessory adhesion molecules strengthening the contact between target and effector cells expressing CR1 and CR3 [47]. CR3 (CD11b/CD18) is a member of the leukocyte integrin family and binds to fibrinogen, factor X, β-glucan, as well as iC3b [48, 49]. C5a activation of neutrophils and monocytes not only enhances CR1 and CR3 attachment to fixed C3b and iC3b, but also exposes a binding site in CR3 for intercellular adhesion molecule (ICAM)-1 [50]; the latter is known to be upregulated in allografts during rejection [51–56]. C5a also upregulates the leukocyte adhesion molecules CR4 (CD11c/CD18) and LFA-1 (CD11a/CD18) that bind to iC3b and ICAM-1, -2, and -3. Thus C5a promotes adherence to endothelial cells and extravasation of monocytes and neutrophils.

It is interesting that Fc receptors (FcR) are coexpressed with receptors for iC3b, C3b, and C1q on monocytes, macrophages, neutrophils, platelets and some lymphocytes. C5a upregulates monocyte expression of both CR1 and FcR [57] further increasing their potential contribution to target cell destruction. Engagement of FcR on macrophages increases their secretion of C3 at the site of inflammation [58]. Thus activation of complement augments inflammatory injury in the presence of even low levels of antibody. Allograft infiltrates containing large numbers of macrophages expressing both FcR and complement receptors have been correlated with severe rejection episodes in clinical biopsies [59] and animal models [60] and these mechanisms probably play a role in accelerated acute or delayed xenograft rejection.

Possible Long-Term Effects of Complement Activation

When allowed to proceed to completion, activation of the complement system can inflict severe damage to endothelial cells and graft tissues via insertion of C5b-9. At sublytic levels of C5b-9, the effects of complement activation can target a wide range of cells without the need for specific receptor ligand interactions. Taken together, components of the complement system trigger or amplify numerous inflammatory processes largely mediated via the actions of the anaphylatoxins, C3a and C5a, in adherence and activation reactions. Similar recruitment and activation of key cellular components of the hyperacute reaction to xenografts are mediated by C1q, C3b, and C5b-9. The activation of platelets and the coagulation cascade are constant features of the irreversible failure of the xenografts. Ongoing complement activation would tend to perpetuate these responses. Whether acute problems predict chronic outcome is still unknown in the allograft situation and no clear extrapolation can be made to the xenograft situation. However, complement activation, in particular effects of sublytic C5b-9 on endothelial cells, leads to proliferation of smooth muscle cells and fibroblasts in ways that could cause or contribute to the accelerated arteriosclerosis and obliterative bronchiolitis seen in successful heart and lung transplants, respectively. In view of the multiplicity of the effects of complement activation and the downstream amplification of these effects, an inhibitor of complement activation likely to be useful in the clinical arena should be able to block the tissue damaging and procoagulant effects of complement, largely driven by C5b-9, as well as the proinflammatory consequences of complement activation driven by the anaphylatoxins C3a and C5a.

Complement Inhibition

Human CR1 (C3b/C4b receptor; CD35) is a single-chain, cell surface glycoprotein found on erythrocytes, some T lymphocytes, all mature B lymphocytes, neutrophils, eosinophils, basophils, monocytes/macrophages, glomerular podocytes and follicular dendritic cells [61]. CR1 is also found circulating as a soluble form in plasma at low concentrations [62]. Most CR1 is found at low levels on erythrocytes where it binds to immune complexes bearing C3b and C4b, thereby clearing them from the circulation in a process known as immune adherence [63]. CR1 on neutrophils and macrophages mediates phagocytosis of opsonized immune complexes, particles, or cells [64]. CR1 on lymphocytes and follicular dendritic cells appears to facilitate antibody responses and antigen presentation [65]. In some cases, the interaction of the C3b or C4b with CR1 may be involved in cellular activation [66, 67].

The interaction of CR1 with C3b and C4b also serves to regulate complement activation through its convertase decay accelerating activity and its factor I cofactor activity [68–70]. Thus CR1 binds to C3b and C4b, components of the multisubunit C3 and C5 convertases, promoting the irreversible dissociation of the catalytic subunit C2a in the classical pathway and of the subunit Bb in the alternative pathway, and resulting in convertase inhibition. In addition, CR1 serves as a necessary cofactor for the proteolytic degradation by factor I of C3b to iC3b and subsequently to C3dg and of C4b to iC4b and on to C4d, again resulting in downregulation of the complement cascade. CR1 is therefore unique among the regulators of complement activation (RCA) protein family – which includes decay-accelerating factor (DAF, CD55), membrane cofactor protein (MCP, CD46), CR2 (CD21), factor H and C4-binding protein – because it possesses both convertase decay-accelerating factor activity and factor I cofactor activity in both the classical and alternative complement pathways.

CR1 also differs from other cell-surface RCA proteins in that it functions extrinsically to the cell on which it resides [71]. The structural basis for this extrinsic activity was suggested by the cDNA sequence of CR1 [72, 73] in which multiple binding sites for C4b and C3b are arranged in a tandem linear array on a single polypeptide chain. The multiple binding sites make possible high-affinity interactions of independent CR1 molecules with polymeric ligands which include the covalent C3b dimer of the alternative C5 convertase [74], the properdin-stabilized C3b dimer of the alternative C3 convertase [75], the covalent C4b-C3b dimer of the classical C5 convertase [76, 77], and the localized clustering of C3b which covalently attaches to surfaces near an active C3 convertase [78].

Recognizing the potential for high-affinity, multivalent binding by single CR1 molecules as well as the capacity to inhibit both complement pathways by two separate mechanisms, Fearon and colleagues constructed from the most common allotype of CR1, a soluble form which lacked the transmembrane and cytoplasmic protein domains [79]. The resulting soluble complement receptor type 1 (sCR1) was expressed by Chinese hamster ovary cells and shown to retain all the known activities of the native, cell surface receptor. sCR1 was demonstrated in vitro to be a potent and selective inhibitor of both the classical and alternative complement pathways and to block proinflammatory consequences of complement activation, namely, the generation of C3a, C5a, and C5b-9. Furthermore, by serving as a cofactor for factor I, sCR1 facilitates the degradation of C3b and C4b to inactive forms which no longer bind sCR1, releasing it to recycle in the inhibitory process [79].

The cofactor activity of sCR1, like the soluble regulatory protein factor H, makes possible the factor I cleavage of C3b to iC3b and of C4b to iC4b. Unlike factor H, however, sCR1 can also serve as a cofactor for the further cleavage by factor I of iC3b to C3dg and iC4b to C4d. sCR1 is thus capable of degrading the ligands for CR1 and CR3 expressed on macrophages and neutrophils which may mitigate cellular inflammatory responses. The consequences of generating C3dg, a ligand for CR2 on B cells, using sCR1 as a cofactor remain unclear. It is likely that this conversion is normally effected by CR1 which is found complexed with CR2 on the surface of B cells [80].

Because the sequence homology of the complement proteins has been generally well conserved through evolution, sCR1 – which is derived from a human gene product – retains significant, albeit not total, regulatory activity for many non-human complement systems. This has made possible the evaluation of complement inhibition by sCR1 in a wide variety of animal models in several species including rats, guinea pigs, mice, pigs and monkeys.

Models of Xenograft Rejection

Hyperacute rejection has been long considered a primary barrier to successful xenotransplantation. However, sCR1 was first demonstrated to delay hyperacute rejection in an ACI-to-sensitized Lewis rat cardiac allograft model. In this model, repeated skin grafting from ACI rat donors to Lewis rat recipients was used to generate an allo-specific antibody titer followed by heterotopic cardiac transplantation. Complement depletion using cobra venom factor (CVF), a potent activator of complement, had previously shown the model to be complement dependent [81] which was confirmed using a single dose of sCR1 (3 mg/kg) which prolonged graft survival to 32 h compared to 3 h for vehicle-treated controls [82]. These results suggested the potential for sCR1 to control hyperacute rejection in recipients presensitized by alloantigen exposure such as from a prior transplant or transfusion. These results also demonstrated that complement-mediated hyperacute rejection can occur in the context of normal expression levels of the endogenous complement regulatory proteins including DAF, MCP and CD59 – in the context of homologous restriction.

Encouraged by the results in the sensitized allograft model, Pruitt and colleagues examined the effects of sCR1 in the complement-dependent [5, 83] Hartley guinea pig-to-Lewis rat cardiac xenograft model. They found that a single dose of sCR1 at reperfusion prolonged graft survival from a mean of 17 min in vehicle-treated controls to over 12 h for the highest (60 mg/kg) dose tested [84]. As shown in Fig. 2, the dose-dependence of graft survival time which they observed has been subsequently confirmed by other investigators in related studies. Histologic assessment of rejected grafts from buffer-treated recipients revealed intravascular platelet aggregation, interstitial hemorrhage and myocardial necrosis – all characteristic of hyperacute rejection. In grafts harvested at early times (21 min) from sCR1-treated recipients, platelet aggregation, hemorrhage and necrosis were only minimally present. In grafts harvested at rejection from recipients in the high dose (60 mg/kg) group, marked PMN infiltration in addition to

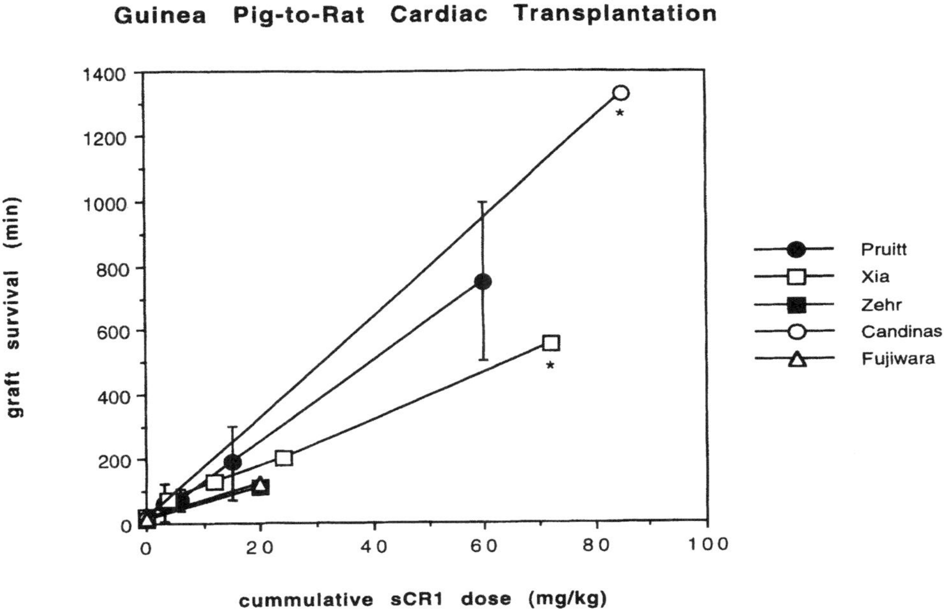

Fig. 2. Mean xenograft survival times are a function of sCR1 dose in the guinea pig-to-rat cardiac xenotransplantation model performed in different laboratories. The *error bars* shown represent the standard deviations observed in the first such study by Pruitt and colleagues [84] (*filled circles*). Additional agents were combined with sCR1 in some of the related studies, but the data presented here represent groups of rats treated with sCR1 alone. The other studies represented are from Xia [88, 89] (*open squares*), Zehr [97] (*filled squares*), Candinas [90] (*open circles*), Fujiwara [96] (*open triangles*), and their respective colleagues. The *asterisks* indicate a repetitive sCR1 dosing regimen, whereas all other data are from single bolus sCR1 groups

myocardial necrosis, interstitial hemorrhage and occasional platelet aggregation was observed. This cellular infiltrate is typical of the rejection of xenografts at longer survival times in the presence of complement depletion or inhibition recently referred to as "accelerated acute rejection" [11] or "delayed xenograft rejection" [85]. As expected, a single bolus of sCR1 (60 mg/kg) had no marked effect on xenospecific IgM natural antibody titers at early times during rejection [86].

The capacity of sCR1 to delay hyperacute rejection likely involves suppression of cellular-independent mechanisms and possibly cellular-dependent mechanisms as well. In an ex vivo model in which rabbit hearts were perfused with 6% human plasma, inclusion of sCR1 at 4.8 μg/ml in the perfusate protected against the increase in diastolic pressure, the decrease in developed pressure, the increase in coronary perfusion pressure, and the increase in cardiac muscle lymphatic fluid flow rate observed in untreated controls [87]. Thus complement inhibition by sCR1 was protective under cellular-independent conditions where neither circulating cells or thrombin-dependent coagulation could contribute to the injury.

The effects of single doses of sCR1 in the guinea pig-to-rat cardiac xenograft model were confirmed [88] and extended to a repetitive dosing regimen (approximately 24 mg/kg at times of -1, 60, and 150 min) which prolonged graft survival beyond that obtained with a single 24 mg/kg dose [89]. Repetitive higher doses of sCR1 (25 mg/kg prereperfusion followed by 20 mg/kg at 5 min, 4 h, and every 12 h subsequent to reperfusion) extended graft survival to a median of 23 h relative to 14 min for controls. Continuous infusion of sCR1 (25 mg/kg prereperfusion followed by 20 mg/kg at 5 min, followed by infusion at 40 mg/kg per 24 h) yielded a similar median graft survival time of 30 h. These high doses of sCR1 were well tolerated by the rat recipients [90].

In an albino guinea pig-to-Wistar rat renal discordant xenograft model, a single 50 mg/kg dose of sCR1 prolonged graft survival to 18.8 h compared to 10.5 min in saline-treated control rats [91]. Renal graft function reflected by the duration of diuresis was 2.3 h compared to no measured function after graft reperfusion in the saline-treated control group.

Having demonstrated the capacity of sCR1 alone to delay hyperacute rejection in discordant rat recipients, studies were carried out in more clinically relevant porcine-to-primate cardiac transplantation models. In an ex vivo model in which porcine hearts were perfused with whole human blood, inclusion of sCR1 at 300 μg/ml in the perfusate maintained cardiac function (heart rate and developed pressure) for up to 4 h compared to a loss of function within 34 min for controls [92]. In a pig-to-cynomolgus monkey heterotopic cardiac xenotransplantation model, a single dose of sCR1 at 15 mg/kg prolonged xenograft survival to between 48 and 90 h compared with untreated controls which rejected in less than 1 h [92].

Analogous to the results obtained using extended dosing regimens in the guinea pig-to-rat model, continuous infusion of sCR1 (25 mg/kg bolus followed by 40 mg/kg per day infusion) in the pig-to-cynomolgus monkey cardiac xenotransplantation model prolonged xenograft survival to 5 days (120 h) in one recipient (for which the infusion catheter was inadvertently occluded and restarted on day 3) and to 7 days (>168 h) in a second recipient [93]. It should be emphasized that this 5- to 7-day xenograft survival time – compared to less than 1 h for untreated controls – was obtained from complement inhibition by sCR1 alone and utilized no other immunosuppressive agents.

Combination Therapies

A large body of evidence – including complement depletion with CVF, inhibition with sCR1, and the use of complement-deficient recipients – clearly establishes the important role of complement activation in hyperacute rejection associated with xenotransplantation. It is clear, however, that other important mechanisms of rejection will also have to be controlled in order to achieve successful xenotransplantation. As previously described, these other mechanisms include B and T lymphocyte responses, vascular endothelial cell activation, responses of natural killer (NK) cells, macrophages and neutrophils, cytokine release, platelet activation, and coagulation. To address these responses efficiently, it is important to focus on those elements of the immune response which, like complement activation, are capable of discriminating self from non-self and thus able to initiate the complete array of defensive responses. Foremost among these are the T and B cell responses to antigen and the responses of a variety of cell types to reactive antibodies mediated by receptors such as FcR and C1qR. Thus successful xenotransplantation will likely require at least some sort of intervention in the complement cascade as well as some form of cellular immunosuppression or, alternatively, the induction of T cell tolerance.

In the pig-to-cynomolgus monkey cardiac xenotransplantation model, continuous infusion of sCR1 (25 mg/kg bolus followed by 40 mg/kg per day infusion) combined with a triple therapy protocol of cyclosporine, cyclophosphamide, and high-dose steroids yielded graft survival times of 11, 21, and 32 days in three recipients (in the latter two, grafts were not rejected but the recipients died of infectious complications) [94]. These very encouraging results point to unanswered questions regarding the best regimen for cellular immunosuppression, the inclusion of additional agents, and the duration of complement inhibition which may be required. Initially, many of these questions can be posed in small animal models such as the guinea pig-to-rat combination.

Complement depletion using CVF has proven effective in prolonging graft survival in the guinea pig-to-rat cardiac xenograft model [83, 95]. It was questioned whether the addition of sCR1 to CVF therapy might further prolong graft survival or otherwise attenuate inflammatory responses caused by the intense complement activation by CVF, either by (a) inhibiting newly synthesized complement components, especially those synthesized within the xenograft by endothelial cells and infiltrating mononuclear cells, or by (b) promoting the factor I degradation of C3b to iC3b and on to C3dg, thus mitigating interactions with the adhesion receptor CR3 (CD11b/CD18) on macrophages and neutrophils. Repetitive doses of sCR1 (25 mg/kg prereperfusion followed by 20 mg/kg at 5 min, 4 h, and every 12 h subsequent to reperfusion) in combination with complement depletion using CVF did not prolong graft survival beyond that obtained using CVF alone, but did result in decreased macrophage activation and reduced levels of cytokines (TNF-α and IL-1β) within xenografts compared to the CVF alone group [90].

In the first study of sCR1 in a discordant xenotransplantation model, a reduction in intravascular platelet aggregation was observed in the grafts of the sCR1-treated rat recipients [84]. The exact mechanisms which result in platelet aggregation during hyperacute rejection and which of these mechanisms are complement-dependent remain to be defined. As described earlier, complement activation of endothelial cells leads to a wide range of responses including the release of heparan sulfate and the increased expression of tissue factor. On the other hand, interspecies incompatibilities of the various factors regulating thrombosis and coagulation could result in platelet aggregation by mechanisms totally independent of complement action. It is not known whether human antithrombin III interacts effectively with rat thrombin, but it is thought to inhibit platelet aggregation in rats by stimulating endothelial cell production of prostacyclin (PGI_2) through binding to heparin-like glycosaminoglycans. In the guinea pig-to-rat cardiac xenotransplantation model, a single 20 mg/kg dose of sCR1 prolonged graft survival to a mean of 2.0 h compared to 18.6 min for the control group, corroborating earlier studies. Treatment with antithrombin III alone did not significantly prolong graft survival (mean of 32.3 min) but did prolong survival to 4.2 h when combined with 20 mg/kg sCR1 [96]. These results suggest the possible combinations of sCR1 with antithrombin III as well as a wide range of anti-platelet agents, including prostacyclin and platelet-activating factor (PAF) antagonists.

When xenograft survival was extended by complement inhibition with sCR1, cellular infiltrates in the grafts were eventually observed by 6.7 h in the guinea pig-to-rat model [84] and by 2–3 days in the pig-to-monkey model [92]. Recently, a variety of agents targeting cellular adhesion receptors has been developed to interrupt the process of rolling, adherence and extravasation of leukocytes at sites of injury and inflammation. The leumedins are one such group of agents and are thought to inhibit neutrophil adhesion by blocking the upregulation of the adhesion receptor CR3 (CD11b/CD18). In the guinea pig-to-rat cardiac xenotransplantation model, a single 20 mg/kg dose of sCR1 again prolonged graft survival to a mean of 1.9 h compared to 8.7 min for the control group. Treatment with the leumedin NPC 15669 alone did not significantly prolong graft survival (mean of 9.9 min) but did prolong survival to 6.2 h when combined with 20 mg/kg sCR1 [97]. As in the above examples, the combination of sCR1 with an agent which alone does not prolong xenograft survival, led to further prolonged survival times.

In light of the synergy obtained from sCR1 used in combination with other agents, we have chosen to incorporate additional functional activities directly into a second generation form of sCR1. Specifically, we have chosen to produce sCR1 under conditions which allow for the incorporation of the sLeX oligosaccharide during the post-translational glycosylation of the protein. sCR1 appears especially well-suited for such sLeX decoration because of its elongated, flexible structure bearing 25 potential asparagine-linked glycosylation sites [79]. The sLeX oligosaccharide is the common carbohydrate ligand for the P, E, and L selectin adhesion receptors which mediate early intercellular contacts, in particular, the rolling of leukocytes on the vascular endothelium. Thus sCR1 expressing sLeX (sCR1sLeX) has the potential not only to inhibit complement activation and selectin-mediated cellular interactions, but also may localize these activities at sites of inflammation where activated endothelium has up-regulated the expression of P and E selectin. Cell lines expressing sCR1sLeX have been developed and the purified protein will be examined in xenotransplantation and other animal model studies.

Potential in Clinical Xenotransplantation

The importance of complement in the hyperacute rejection following xenotransplantation has been recognized using recipient animals depleted of complement with CVF. However, as yet no agents in clinical practice can prevent the hyperacute rejection process. Administration of sCR1 has now been shown to prevent hyperacute rejection in rodent and primate recipients following discordant xenografting and provides a clinically relevant therapeutic option. Continuous administration of sCR1 coupled with standard immunosuppression leads to xenograft survival in the pig-to-primate model of up to a month. Such graft survival times would potentially allow bridging until a suitable human donor organ became available and provides a viable clinical window. Other approaches to limiting complement-mediated hyperacute rejection involve breeding donor animals made transgenic for human membrane-bound complement regulatory molecules, such as MCP, DAF and CD59 [98–100]. This approach has the advantage of localizing complement regulatory molecules at the sites where they are most needed (the vessels of potential donor organs) and, assuming expression levels are maintained, could provide complement inhibition for extended periods. If complement inhibition is required throughout the life of the xenograft, this approach clearly has merit. However, if complement inhibition is required predominantly to stave off the initial onslaught of xenoreactive antibodies on donor endothelium, later to be subdued by accommodation or modulation responses [101–103], it is clearly preferable to use a drug which can be administered subject to physician judgment regarding the dosing and safety needs of the transplant patient [104]. sCR1 provides this opportunity.

References

1. Ryan, U. S. Complement inhibition: the sine qua non of xenotransplantation. Xeno 1994, 2, 19
2. Thomas, L. J.; Ryan, U. S. Immunological consequences of organ transplantation: Implications for therapeutic development. J. of Heart and Lung Transplantation 1995, 14, 938
3. Good, A.H.; Cooper, D.K.C.; Malcolm, A.J.; et al. Identification of carbohydrate structures that bind human anti-porcine antibodies: implications for discordant xenografting in humans. Transplant. Proc. 1992, 24, 559
4. Collins, B. H.; Cotterell, A. H.; McCurry, K. R.; et al. Cardiac xenografts between primate species provide evidence for the importance of the alpha-galactosyl determinant in hyperacute rejection. J. Immunol. 1995, 154, 5500
5. Migagawa, S.; Hirose, H.; Shirakura, R.; et al. The mechanism of discordant xenograft rejection. Transplantation 1988, 46, 825
6. Pruitt, S. K.; Baldwin, W. M.; Barth, R. N.; Sanfilippo, F. The effect of xenoreactive antibody and B cell depletion on hyperacute rejection of guinea pig-to-rat cardiac xenografts. Transplantation 1993, 56, 1318
7. Ish, C.; Ong, G. L.; Desai, N.; Mattew, M. J. The specificity of alternative complement pathway-mediated lysis of erythrocytes: a survey of complement and target cells from 25 species. Scand. J. Immunol. 1993, 38, 113
8. Hansch, G.; Hammer, C. H.; Vanguri, P.; Shin, M. L. Homologous species restriction in lysis of erythrocytes by terminal complement proteins. Proc. Natl. Acad. Sci. USA 1981, 78, 5118
9. Lachmann, P. J.; Hughes-Jones, N. C. Initiation of complement activation. Springer Semin. Immunopathol. 1984, 7, 143
10. Farries, T. C.; Knutzen Steuer, K. L.; Atkinson, J. P. The mechanism of activation of the alternative pathway of complement by cell-bound C4b. Mol. Immunol. 1990, 27, 1155

11. Brauer, R. B.; Baldwin, W. M.; Daha, M. R.; Pruitt, S. K.; Sanfilippo, F. Use of C6-deficient rats to evaluate the mechanism of hyperacute rejection of discordant cardiac xenografts. J. Immunol. 1993, 151, 7240
12. Zhow, X. J.; Niesen, N.; Pawlowski, I.; et al. Prolongation of survival of discordant kidney xenografts by C6 deficiency. Transplantation 1990, 50, 896
13. Murohara, T.; Guo, J. P.; Delyani, J. A.; Lefer, A. M. Cardioprotective effects of selective inhibition of the two complement activation pathways in myocardial ischemia and reperfusion injury. Meth. Find. Exp. Clin. Pharmacol. 1995, 17, 499
14. Giclas, P. C.; Pinckard, R. N.; Olson, M. S. In vitro activation of complement by isolated human heart subcellular membranes. J. Immunol. 1979, 122, 146
15. Pinckard, R. N.; Olson, M. S.; Giclas, P. C.; Boyer, J. R.; O'Rourke, R. A. Consumption of classical complement components by heart subcellular membranes in vitro and in patients after actue myocardial infarction. J. Clin. Invest. 1975, 56, 740
16. Storrs, S. B.; Kolb, W. P.; Pinckard, R. N.; Olson, M. S. Characterization of the binding of purified C1q to heart mitochondrial membranes. J. Biol. Chem. 1981, 256, 10924
17. Hebell, T.; Ahearn, J. M.; Fearon, D. T. Suppression of the immune response by a soluble complement receptor of B lymphocytes. Science 1991, 254, 102
18. Pepys, M. B. Role of complement in induction of antibody production in vivo: effect of cobra venom factor and other C3-reactive agents on thymus-dependent and thymus-independent antibody responses. J. Exp. Med. 1974, 140, 126
19. Sylvestre, D. L.; Ravetch, J. V. Fc receptors initiate the Arthus reaction: redefining the inflammatory cascade. Science 1994, 265, 1095
20. Daha, M. R.; Miltenburg, A. M. M.; Hiemstra, P. S.; et al. The complement subcomponent C1q mediates binding of immune complexes and aggregates to endothelial cells in vitro. Eur. J. Immunol. 1988, 18, 783
21. Bobak, D. A.; Gaither, T. A.; Frank, M. M.; Tenner, A. J. Modulation of FcR function by complement: subcomponent C1q enhances the phagocytosis of IgG-opsonized targets by human monocytes and culture-derived macrophages. J. Immunol. 1987, 138, 1150
22. Ghebrehiwet, B.; Lim, B. L.; Peerschke, E. I.; Willis, A. C.; Reid, K. B. Isolation, cDNA cloning, and overexpression of a 33-kD cell surface glycoprotein that binds to the globular "heads" of C1q. J. Exp. Med. 1994, 179, 1809
23. Zhang, S. C.; Schultz, D. R.; Ryan, U. S. Receptor-mediated binding of C1q on pulmonary endothelial cells. Tissue & Cell 1986, 18, 13
24. Peerschke, E.; Reid, K.; Ghebrehiwet, B. Platelet activation by C1q results in the induction of alpha IIb/beta 3 integrins (GPIIb-IIIa) and the expression of P-selectin and procoagulant activity. J. Exp. Med. 1993, 178, 579
25. Ryan, U. S.; Worthington, R. E. Cell-cell contact mechanisms. Curr. Opinion Immunology 1992, 4, 33
26. Celi, A. P-selectin induces the expression of tissue factor on monocytes. Proc. Natl. Acad. Sci. USA 1994, 91, 8767
27. Tsuji, T.; Nagata, K.; Koike, J.; Todoroki, N.; Irimura, T. Induction of superoxide anion production from monocytes and neutrophils by activated platelets through the P-selectin-sialyl Lewis X interaction. J. Leukoc. Biol. 1994, 56, 583
28. Esmon, C. T. Cell mediated events that control blood coagulation and vascular injury. Annu. Rev. Cell Biol. 1993, 9, 1

29. Platt, J. L.; Dalmasso, A. P.; Lindman, B. J.; Ihrcke, N. S.; Bach, F. H. The role of C5a and antibody in the release of heparan sulfate from endothelial cells. Eur. J. Immunol. 1991, 21, 2887
30. Murphy, H. S.; Shayman, J. A.; Till, G. O.; et al. Superoxide responses of endothelial cells to C5a and TNF-alpha: divergent signal transduction pathways. Am. J. Physiol. 1992, 263, L51
31. Foreman, K. E.; Vaporciyan, A. A.; Bonish, B. K.; et al. C5a-induced expression of P-selectin in endothelial cells. J. Clin. Invest. 1994, 94, 1147
32. Carson, S. D.; Johnson, D. R. Consecutive enzyme cascades: complement activation at the cell surface triggers increased tissue factor activity. Blood 1990, 76, 361
33. Morgan, B. P. Complement membrane attack on nucleated cells: resistance, recovery and non-lethal effects. Biochem. J. 1989, 264, 1
34. Benzaquen, L. R.; Nicholson-Weller, A.; Halperin, J. A. Terminal complement proteins C5b-9 release basic fibroblast growth factor and platelet-derived growth factor from endothelial cells. J. Exp. Med. 1994, 179, 985
35. Hattori, R.; Hamilton, K. K.; McEver, R. P.; Sims, P. J. Complement proteins C5b-9 induce secretion of high molecular weight multimers of endothelial von Willebrand factor and translocation of granule membrane potein GMP-140 to the cell surface. J. Biol. Chem.. 1989, 264, 9053
36. Hamilton, K. K.; Hattori, R.; Esmon, C. T.; Sims, P. J. Complement proteins C5b-9 induce vesiculation of the endothelial plasma membrane and expose catalytic surface for assembly of the prothrombinase enzyme complex. J. Biol. Chem. 1990, 265, 3809
37. Sims, P. J.; Wiedmer, T. The response of human platelets to activated components of the complement system. Immunol. Today 1991, 12, 338
38. Konteatis, Z. D.; Siciliano, S. J.; Vanriper, G.; et al. Development of C5a receptor antagonists - differential loss of functional responses. J. Immunol. 1994, 153, 4200
39. Gulbins, E.; Schlottmann, K.; Rauterberg, E. W.; Steinhausen, M. Effects of rC5a on the circulation of normal and split hydronephrotic rat kidneys. Am. J. Physiol. 1993, 265, F96
40. Ember, J. A.; Sanderson, S. D.; Hugli, T. E.; Morgan, E. L. Induction of interleukin-8 synthesis from monocytes by human C5a anaphylatoxin. Am. J. Pathol. 1994, 144, 393
41. Morgan, E. L.; Ember, J. A.; Sanderson, S. D.; et al. Anti-C5a receptor antibodies -characterization of neutralizing antibodies specific for a peptide, C5aR-(9–29), derived from the predicted amino-terminal sequence of the human C5a receptor. J. Immunol. 1993, 151, 377
42. Barton, P. A.; Warren, J. S. Complement component C5 modulates the systemic tumor necrosis factor response in murine endotoxic shock. Infect. Immunol. 1993, 61, 1474
43. Fearon, D. T.; Collins, L. A. Increased expression of C3b receptors on polymorphonuclear leukocytes induced by chemotactic factors and by purification procedures. J. Immunol. 1983, 130, 370
44. Arnaout, M. A.; Spits, H.; Terhorst, C.; Pitt, J.; Todd, R. F. Deficiency of a leukocyte surface glycoprotein (LFA-1) in two patients with Mo1 deficiency: effects of cell activation on Mo1/LFA-1 surface expression in normal and deficient leukocytes. J. Clin. Invest. 1984, 74, 1291
45. Glovsky, M. M.; Hugli, T. E.; Ishizaka, T.; Lichtenstein, L. M.; Erickson, B. W. Anaphylatoxin-induced histamine release with human leukocytes. Studies of C3a leukocyte binding and histamine release. J. Clin. Invest. 1979, 64, 804

46. Daffern, P. J.; Pfeifer, P. H.; Ember, J. A.; Hugli, T. E. C3a is a chemotaxin for human eosinophils but not for neutrophils. 1. C3a stimulation of neutrophils is secondary to eosinophil activation. J. Exp. Med. 1995, 181, 2119
47. Wahlin, B.; Perlmann, H.; Perlmann, P.; Schreiber, R. D.; Muller-Eberhard, H. J. C3 receptors on human lymphocyte subsets and recruitment of ADCC effector cells by C3 fragments. J. Immunol. 1983, 130, 2831
48. Diamond, M. S.; Garcia-Aguilar, J.; Bickford, J. K.; Corbi, A. L.; Springer, T. A. The I domain is a major recognition site on the leukocyte integrin Mac-1 (CD11b/CD18) for four distinct adhesion ligands. J. Cell Biol. 1993, 120, 1031
49. Rosen, H.; Law, S. K. The leukocyte cell surface receptor(s) for the iC3b product of complement. Curr. Top. Microbiol. Immunol. 1990, 153, 99
50. Diamond, M. S.; Staunton, D. E.; Marlin, S. D.; Springer, T. A. Binding of the integrin Mac-I (CD11b/CD18) to the third immunoglobulin-like domain of ICAM-1 (CD54) and its regulation by glycosylation. Cell 1991, 65, 961
51. Bechtel, U.; Scheuer, R.; Landgraf, R.; Konig, A.; Feucht, H. E. Assessment of soluble adhesion molecules (sICAM-1, sVCAM-1, sELAM-1) and complement cleavage products (sC4d, sC5b-9) in urine – clinical monitoring of renal allograft recipients. Transplantation 1994, 58, 905
52. Bishop, G. A.; Hall, B. M. Expression of leucocyte and lymphocyte adhesion molecules in the human kidney. Kidney Int. 1989, 36, 1078
53. Taylor, P. M.; Rose, M. L.; Yacoub, M. H.; Pigott, R. Induction of vascular adhesion molecules during rejection of human cardiac allografts. Transplantation 1992, 54, 451
54. Brockmeyer, C.; Ulbrecht, M.; Schendel, D. J.; et al. Distribution of cell adhesion molecules (ICAM-1, VCAM-1 ELAM-1) in renal tissue during allograft rejection. Transplantation 1993, 55, 610
55. Fuggle, S. V.; Sanderson, J. B.; Gray, D. W.; Richardson, A.; Morris, P. J. Variation in expression of endothelial adhesion molecules in pretransplant and transplanted kidneys –correlation with intragraft events. Transplantation 1993, 55, 117
56. Hancock, W. W.; Whitley, W. D.; Tullius, S. G.; et al. Cytokines, adhesion molecules, and the pathogenesis of chronic rejection of rat renal allografts. Transplantation 1993, 56, 643
57. Yancey, K. B.; O'Shea, J.; Chused, T.; et al. Human C5a modulates monocyte Fc and C3 receptor expression. J. Immunol. 1985, 135, 465
58. Bajtay, Z.; Falus, A.; Erdei, A.; Gergely, J. Fc gamma R-dependent regulation of the biosynthesis of complement C3 by murine macrophages: the modulatory effect of IL-6. Scand. J. Immunol. 1992, 35, 195
59. Svalander, C.; Nyberg, G.; Blohme, I.; et al. Acute early allograft failure and the C3/macrophage phenomenon. Transplant. Proc. 1993, 25, 903
60. Hayry, P.; von Willebrand, E.; Parthenais, E.; et al. The inflammatory mechanisms of allograft rejection. Immunol. Rev. 1984, 77, 85
61. Ahearn, J. M.; Fearon, D. T. Structure and function of the complement receptors, CR1 (CD35) and CR2 (CD21). Adv. Immunol. 1989, 46, 183
62. Yoon, S. H.; Fearon, D. T. Characterization of a soluble form of the C3b/C4b receptor (CR1) in human plasma. J. Immunol. 1985, 134, 3332
63. Nelson, R. A. The immune-adherence phenomenon. Science 1953, 118, 733
64. Gigli, I.; Nelson, R. A. Complement dependent immune phagocytosis. I. Requirements for C'1, C'4, C'2, C'3. Exp. Cell Res. 1968, 51, 45

65. Thornton, B. P.; Vetvicka, V.; Ross, G. D. Natural antibody and complement-mediated antigen processing and presentation by B lymphocytes. J. Immunol. 1994, 152, 1727
66. Fallman, M.; Andersson, R.; Andersson, T. Signaling properties of CR3 (CD11b/CD18) and CR1 (CD35) in relation to phagocytosis of complement-opsonized particles. J. Immunol. 1993, 151, 330
67. Bacle, F.; Haeffner-Cavaillon, N.; Laude, M.; Couturier, C.; Kazatchkine, M. D. Induction of IL-1 release through stimulation of the C3b/C4b complement receptor type one (CR1, CD35) on human monocytes. J. Immunol. 1990, 144, 147
68. Fearon, D. T. Regulation of the amplification C3 convertase of human complement by an inhibitory protein isolated from human erythrocyte membrane. Proc. Natl. Acad. Sci. USA 1979, 76, 5867
69. Gigli, I.; Fearon, D. T. Regulation of the classical pathway convertase of human complement by the C3b receptor from human erythrocytes. Fed. Proc. 1981, 40, 1172 (abstr)
70. Iida, K.; Nussenzweig, V. Complement receptor is an inhibitor of the complement cascade. J. Exp. Med. 1981, 153, 1138
71. Medof, M. E.; Iida, K.; Mold, C.; Nussenzweig, V. Unique role of the complement receptor CR1 in the degradation of C3b associated with immune complexes. J. Exp. Med. 1982, 156, 1739
72. Klickstein, L. L.; Bartow, T. J.; Miletic, V.; et al. Identification of distinct C3b and C4b recognition sites in the human C3b/C4b receptor (CR1, CD35) by deletion mutagenesis. J. Exp. Med. 1988, 168, 1699
73. Klickstein, L. B.; Wong, W. W.; Smith, J. A.; et al. Human C3b/C4b receptor (CR1). Demonstration of long homologous repeating domains that are composed of the short consensus repeats characteristic of C3/C4 binding proteins. J. Exp. Med. 1987, 165, 1095
74. Kinoshita, T.; Takata, Y.; Kozono, H.; et al. C5 convertase of the alternative complement pathway: covalent linkage between two C3b molecules within the trimolecular complex enzyme. J. Immunol. 1988, 141, 3895
75. Fearon, D. T.; Austen, K. F. Properdin: binding to C3b and stabilization of the C3b-dependent C3 convertase. J. Exp. Med. 1975, 142, 856
76. Takata, Y.; Kinoshita, T.; Kozono, H.; et al. Covalent association of C3b with C4b within C5 convertase of the classical complement pathway. J. Exp. Med. 1987, 165, 1494
77. Kozono, H.; Kinoshita, T.; Kim, Y. U.; et al. Localization of the covalent C3b-binding site on C4b within the complement classical pathway C5 convertase, C4b2a3b. J. Biol. Chem. 1990, 265, 14444
78. Mardiney, M. R.; Muller-Eberhard, H. J.; Feldman, J. D. Ultrastructural localization of the third and fourth components of complement on complement-cell complexes. Am. J. Pathol. 1968, 53, 253
79. Weisman, H. F.; Bartow, T.; Leppo, M. K.; et al. Soluble human complement receptor type 1: in vivo inhibitor of complement suppressing post-ischemic myocardial inflammation and necrosis. Science 1990, 249, 146
80. Tuveson, D. A.; Ahearn, J. M.; Matsumoto, A. K.; Fearon, D. T. Molecular interactions of compalement receptors on B lymphocytes: a CR1/CR2 complex distinct from the CR2/CD19 complex. J. Exp. Med. 1991, 173, 1083
81. Knechtle, S. J.; Halperin, E. C.; Murphy, C. E.; et al. The effect of cyclosporine, total lymphoid irradiation, and cobra venom factor on hyperacute rejection. J. of Heart Transplantation 1985, 4, 541

82. Pruitt, S. K.; Bollinger, R. R. The effect of soluble complement receptor type 1 on hyperacute allograft rejection. J. Surg. Res. 1991, 50, 350
83. Adachi, H.; Rosengard, B. R.; Hutchins, G. M.; et al. Effects of cyclosporine, asprin, and cobra venom factor, on discordant cardiac xenograft survival in rats. Transplant. Proc. 1987, 19, 1145
84. Pruitt, S. K.; Baldwin, W. M.; Marsh, H. C.; et al. The effect of soluble complement receptor type 1 on hyperacute xenograft rejection. Transplantation 1991, 52, 868
85. Blakely, M. L.; Van der Werf, W. J.; Berndt, M. C.; et al. Activation of intragraft endothelial and mononuclear cells during discordant xenograft rejection. Transplantation 1994, 58, 1059
86. Pruitt, S. K.; Baldwin, W. M.; Marsh, H. C.; et al. Effect of soluble complement receptor type 1 on natural antibody levels during xenograft rejection. Transplant. Proc. 1992, 24, 477
87. Homeister, J. W.; Satoh, P. S.; Kilgore, K. S.; Lucchesi, B. R. Soluble complement receptor type 1 prevents human complement-mediated damage of the rabbit isolated heart. J. Immunol. 1993, 150, 1055
88. Xia, W.; Fearon, D. T.; Moore, F. D.; et al. Prolongation of guinea pig cardiac xenograft survival in rats by soluble human complement receptor type 1. Transplant. Proc. 1992, 24, 479
89. Xia, W.; Fearon, D. T.; Kirkman, R. L. Effect of repetitive doses of soluble human complement receptor type 1 on survival of discordant cardiac xenografts. Transplant. Proc. 1993, 25, 410
90. Candinas, D.; Lesnikoski, B. A.; Robson, S. C.; et al. Soluble complement receptor type 1 and cobra venom factor in discordant xenotransplantation. Transplant. Proc., 1996, 28, 581
91. Chrupcala, M.; Pomer, S.; Staehler, G.; Waldherr, R.; Kirschfink, C. Prolongation of discordant renal xenograft survival by depletion of complement. Comparative effects of systemically administered cobra venom factor and soluble complement receptor type 1 in a guinea-pig to rat model. Transpl. Int. 1994, 7, S650
92. Pruitt, S. K.; Kirk, A. D.; Bollinger, R. R.; et al. The effect of soluble complement receptor type 1 on hyperacute rejection of porcine xenografts. Transplantation 1994, 57, 363
93. Pruitt, S. K.; Bollinger, R. R.; Collins, B. H.; et al. Continuous complement inhibition using soluble complement receptor type 1: Effect on hyperacute rejection of pig-to-primate cardiac xenografts. 1995. Third International Congress for Xenotransplantation, Boston MA (abstr. #215)
94. Sanfilippo, F. Effects of complement inhibitors on discordant rodent and pig-to-primate cardiac xenograft rejection. 1995. Third International Congress for Xenotransplantation, Boston MA (abstr. pl-26)
95. Leventhal, J. R.; Dalmasso, A. P.; Cromwell, J. W.; et al. Prolongation of cardiac xenograft survival by depletion of complement. Transplantation 1993, 55, 857
96. Fujiwara, I.; Arakawa, K.; Akami, T.; et al. Prolongation of xenograft survival by soluble complement receptor type 1 (sCR1) and antithrombin-III (AT-III) combination therapy. Transplant. Proc., 1996, 28, 685
97. Zehr, K. J.; Herskowitz, A.; Lee, P. C.; et al. Neutrophil adhesion and complement inhibition prolongs survival of cardiac xenografts in discordant species. Transplantation 1994, 57, 900

98. McCurry, K. R.; Kooyman, D. L.; Alvarado, C. G.; et al. Human complement regulatory proteins protect swine-to-primate cardiac xenografts from humoral injury. Nature Med. 1995, 1, 423
99. Fodor, W. L.; Squinto, S. P. Engineering of transgenic pigs for xenogeneic organ transplantation. Xeno 1995, 3, 23
100. Bach, F. H.; Robson, S. C.; Winkler, H.; et al. Barriers to xenotransplantation. Nature Med. 1995, 1, 869
101. Bach, F. H.; Turman, M. A.; Vercellotti, G. M.; Platt, J. L.; Dalmasso, A. P. Accomodation: a working paradigm for progressing toward discordant xenografting. Transplant. Proc. 1991, 23, 205
102. Bannett, A. D.; McAlack, R. F.; Raja, R.; Baquer, A.; Morris, M. Experiences with known ABO-mismatched renal transplants. Transplant. Proc. 1987, XIX, 4543
103. Alexandre, G. P. J.; Squifflet, J. P.; De Bruyere, M.; et al. Present experiences in a series of 26 ABO-incompatible living donor renal allografts. Transplant. Proc. 1987, XIX, 4538
104. Ryan, U. S. Complement inhibitory therapeutics and xenotransplantation. Nature Med. 1995, 1, 967

34 Immunobiology of Pig-to-Baboon Lung Xenotransplantation

A.S. Shah, S. Itescu, and R.E. Michler

Introduction

Pulmonary allotransplantation is now recognized as the best therapeutic option for patients with end-stage pulmonary disease. One-year survival for persons receiving pulmonary allografts for emphysematous lung disease currently exceeds 80 % and rivals survival for heart allotransplantation [1]. However, despite these impressive figures, expansive growth within the field has been limited by a scarcity of donor organs adequate for transplantation. The donor organ shortage for lungs is more pronounced than for any other solid organ, with only 5 %–10 % of donors of heart, liver, kidneys, and pancreas of acceptable quality having lungs of similar suitability [2, 3].

Two alternatives have emerged in the search for viable solutions to the problem of the donor lung shortage – cross-species transplants and mechanical devices. While each is theoretically valuable as a temporary solution (i.e., as a bridge to eventual allograft replacement), the benefit of either as a temporary or permanent alternative to allotransplantation remains to be proven.

The purpose of this chapter is to discuss the emerging field of cross-species lung transplantation in disparate (discordant) species combinations. The field will be discussed in the light of (a) advances made for other solid-organ xenografts and (b) recent results in new experimental pulmonary xenotransplant models. The histopathologic features of discordant pulmonary xenograft rejection in primate recipients will be described and potential mechanisms of graft rejection discussed. Clinically relevant donor sources will also be reviewed, as will the future of pulmonary xenotransplantation and its potential for clinical reality.

Cross-Species Transplantation

Clinical xenotransplantation itself dates to the early twentieth century, at which time kidney xenotransplants were performed from rabbit, pig, goat, nonhuman primate, and lamb donors. Following these early failures, the scientific literature was devoid of reports documenting clinical xenotransplantation for over 40 years. In 1963, the field of clinical xenotransplantation was pioneered by Reemtsma and colleagues, who transplanted chimpanzee kidneys into humans and achieved functional graft survival of up to 9 months using azathioprine and steroid immunosuppression [4]. During the past decade, advances in experimental cardiac xenotransplantation have confirmed the feasibility and potential benefit of cross-species heart transplantation from concordant species donors. However, parallel advances have not occurred in the field of lung xenotransplantation, and lung xenotransplants in humans have not been attempted to date.

Relevant Donor Sources

Concordant species such as nonhuman primates have been considered as a potential source of donor organs for clinical xenotransplantation. Unlike the fields of cardiac and renal transplantation, very few studies have investigated this option with regards to pulmonary xenotransplantation. However, nonhuman primate xenotransplantation as a clinical therapeutic option is limited, since it cannot adequately address the donor organ shortage. Limitations in the size of these donor animals, the infrequency of universal donor blood group O, and the possibility of transmitting epizootic disease may, at least in the short term, limit widespread clinical application of this option.

Therefore, the retrieval of organs from disparate species must be pursued in order to adequately address the donor organ shortage. Large animals such as the pig, which has remarkably similar cardiopulmonary physiology and anatomy to humans and can be bred in a specific pathogen-free environment, may represent the most likely source of donor organs which could potentially alleviate the organ shortage.

Discordant Pulmonary Xenotransplantation

Experience with experimental lung xenotransplantation between disparate species has been quite limited in comparison to other large organs [5], and the pathogenesis of discordant pulmonary xenograft rejection has not yet been clearly defined. Studies from our laboratory have suggested that, following transplantation into unmodified baboons, pig lungs undergo a form of hyperacute rejection which differs from that seen in other large vascularized organs such as the heart and kidneys [5, 6]. Hyperacute rejection of pig lung xenografts may result from antibody-mediated mechanisms of rejection that are primarily directed against xenoantigens expressed proximally in the pulmonary macrovasculature. The proximal nature of this vascular attack may lead to intense vasoconstriction, elevated pulmonary vascular resistance, poor peripheral lung perfusion, and a paucity of immunoglobulin and complement deposition on the microvasculature. This is in contrast to classical antibody and complement-mediated hyperacute rejection, which is directed against xenoantigens expressed peripherally on microvascular endothelium.

In our preliminary studies, orthotopic single lung xenotransplants (n=10) performed from pigs-to-unmodified primate recipients were engrafted for periods of up to 72 h and demonstrated no significant microvascular endothelial cell (EC) deposition of xenoreactive natural antibody or complement proteins [6]. However, significant graft injury did occur as evidenced by intra-alveolar hemorrhage

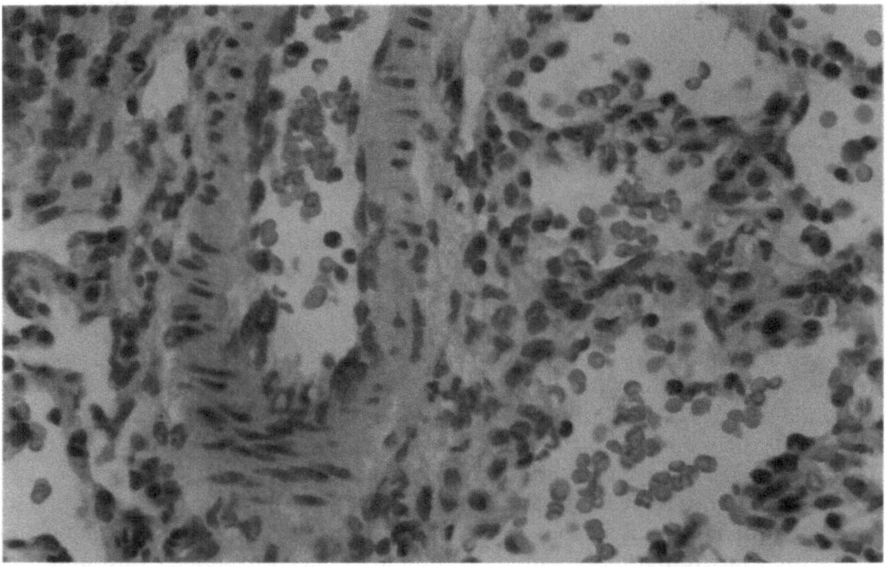

Fig. 1. Intra-alveolar hemorrhage and edema in lung xenograft 15 min after reperfusion

and edema, and examination of large vessels revealed binding of IgM and complement components to endothelial cell surfaces (Fig. 1).

In order to further investigate the roles of natural antibody and complement in mediating discordant pulmonary xenograft rejection in primates, we recently performed orthotopic pig-to-baboon double lung xenotransplants. This procedure necessitated recipient survival to be dependent upon graft function, and allowed us to obtain survival data in non-immunosuppressed animals. All double lung xenografts performed (n=5) underwent rejection within 3.5 h of implantation.

Pulmonary vascular resistance (PVR) was normal in all recipients prior to transplantation, but increased at least twofold within 15 min of graft reperfusion and tenfold within 3 h of graft implantation. Histopathology of the rejected tissue revealed interstitial hemorrhage with endothelial cell denudation and an influx of neutrophils within 15 min of implantation, which was followed by progressive mononuclear cell infiltration. At 2 h following graft reperfusion there was evidence of endothelial cell denudation with increasing interstitial edema and hemorrhage and focal intravascular fibrin and platelet thrombi.

Immunofluorescence of lung xenograft biopsies performed serially revealed focal deposition of IgM and complement on arteriolar endothelium at 1 and 2 h after xenograft reperfusion (Fig. 2). Circulating levels of IgM anti-pig natural antibodies decreased by a mean of 48 % within 2 h of graft reperfusion, presumably reflecting binding to the pulmonary vasculature. Unlike IgM, there were only trace deposits of IgG detected on the arteriolar endothelial surfaces at these time points. Similarly, in the microvascular endothelium only trace deposits of IgG,

IgM, C3, C4, properdin, or MAC were detected. These findings are similar to those observed in a rodent model of discordant lung xenograft rejection [7]. Tavakoli and colleagues performed orthotopic single lung transplants from guinea pigs to Lewis rats and reported the presence of IgM, IgG, and C3 deposits on the arteriolar endothelium of the rejected xenografts by immunofluorescence staining. These observations suggest that hyperacute rejection of pig-to-primate lung xenografts occurs by antibody and complement-mediated mechanisms preferentially targeted against the lung endothelial macrovasculature.

This proximal pattern of antibody binding to macrovascular endothelium in pig lung tissues differs strikingly from the diffuse microvascular endothelial deposition of IgM, C3, C4, and MAC observed in hyperacute rejection of pig-to-baboon cardiac xenografts [5]. In all xenografts studied, there was a progressive influx of $OKM1^{+}$ cells detected as early as 15 min following graft reperfusion, consistent with the presence of neutrophils, macrophages and natural killer cells.

The results of these experiments demonstrate that unmodified transplanted porcine double lung xenografts cannot support the survival of untreated baboon recipients. In all instances graft dysfunction and right ventricular failure occurred as a result of a severe increase in PVR to levels tenfold greater than those pretransplantation.

The significant increase in PVR observed in both our single and double lung xenotransplant studies, as well those from other investigators, suggests that an increase in PVR may be the earliest and most specific indicator of lung xenograft

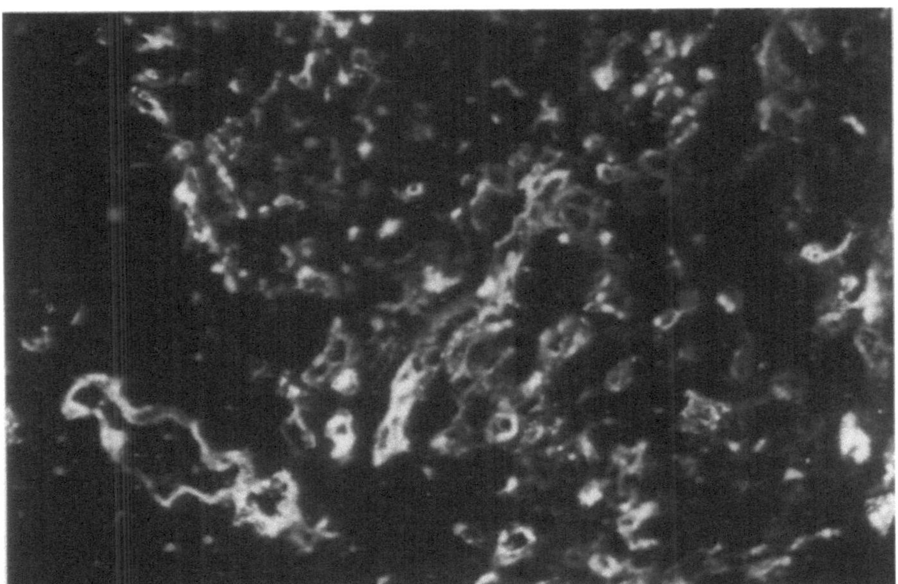

Fig. 2. Immunofluorescence of lung xenograft biopsy revealed focal deposition of IgM on arteriolar endothelium at 2 h after reperfusion

rejection. In the report of Tavakoli and colleagues involving orthotopic single lung transplants from guinea pigs to Lewis rats, there was a delay of 2–15 min before there was visible evidence of graft reperfusion following the restoration of flow to the xenografts. The authors attributed this observation to a sudden increase in pulmonary arteriolar resistance. Similarly, in a model in which pig heart-lung blocs were perfused ex vivo with human blood, an increase in PVR was found to be the earliest indicator of lung injury [8]. We propose that deposition of immunoglobulin and complement on the surface of pulmonary arteriolar endothelium initiates an inflammatory and vascular response that leads to arteriolar damage, vasoconstriction, rise in PVR, and reduced peripheral lung perfusion.

Complement activation occurred in our orthotopic double lung transplant model following the institution of cardiopulmonary bypass and as a result of natural antibody deposition on the large vessels, leading to the recruitment and local deposition of complement proteins. Activation of the complement pathway causes the formation of anaphylatoxins C3A and C5a, which can induce leukocyte aggregation and activation [9, 10]. Activated neutrophils can adhere to and migrate across endothelial cell surfaces, causing local lung injury by the release of free radicals, peroxidase, and proteolytic enzymes, resulting in noncardiogenic pulmonary edema [11]. In this regard, intravenous infusion of complement-activated plasma has been shown to cause pulmonary vascular sequestration of neutrophils, increased PVR, and interstitial pulmonary edema in large animals [10]. The physiologic response by arteriolar endothelium to this damage is to vasoconstrict, thus preventing further damage from occurring to the pulmonary parenchyma. This response may explain the lack of immunoglobulin and complement deposition detected in the distal microvasculature of the pig lung in our orthotopic lung transplant model.

The most potent vasoconstricting polypeptide identified to date is endothelin-1 (ET-1) [12]. Endothelins have been identified in large concentrations in pulmonary tissues, where they are primarily located in vascular endothelial cells as well as in epithelial cells in the trachea and bronchus [13]. Vascular endothelial cells are induced to produce ET-1 following activation of cell surface receptors by physiologic stimuli such as binding of complement [13]. Another source of ET-1 are activated neutrophils, which can convert the precursor of ET-1 to its activated form by proteolytic cleavage [12]. Endothelins have also been shown to induce the release of eicosanoids such as thromboxane A_2 [12], which has been reported to be an important hemodynamic mediator of renal allograft rejection [14]. Suspensions of activated mononuclear cells isolated from rejecting lung allotransplants in dogs have been shown to cause vasoconstriction of pulmonary arteries, and these effects were mediated in part by endothelins and prostanoids [15]. Finally, it is possible that the release of ET-1 or other vasoactive mediators may also be directly induced by the binding of IgM natural antibody to endothelial cells. In this regard, IgM anti-endothelial cell antibodies in humans with systemic lupus erythematosus have been reported to induce ET-1 release from endothelial cells [16]. We are currently evaluating ET-1 expression in pig lung xenografts rejected by baboons.

Various physiologic responses unrelated to immunologic mechanisms may have also contributed, in part, to the increased PVR following xenograft reperfusion. The "reimplantation" response is a unique complication of lung transplantation manifest by pulmonary edema, reduced lung compliance, increased pulmonary vascular resistance, and impaired gas exchange [17]. This is thought to be due primarily to ischemic reperfusion injury, but other factors, including surgical trauma, lymphatic interruption, and denervation, may also play a role. Alterations in pulmonary arterial reactivity resulting from denervation have also been reported following lung allotransplantation in animal studies [18].

In summary, our findings suggest that lung xenografts transplanted across disparate species barriers in primates may not undergo classic antibody-mediated hyperacute rejection targeted against microvascular endothelial cells. Instead, the rejection response in this model appears to be initiated by humoral mechanisms directed against xenoantigens on more proximal levels of the graft vasculature, resulting in endothelial damage, arteriolar vasoconstriction, and severe elevations in PVR. Investigations are currently ongoing to further delineate the nature of this vascular injury.

Pulmonary Xenotransplantation – Future Prospects

Pulmonary xenotransplantation primarily remains an experimental procedure. The field will benefit from lessons learned in the discordant xenotransplantation of other solid organ grafts. At present, major areas of consideration for future investigation exist. First, the roles of natural antibody and complement in mediating rejection of discordant lung xenografts must be more clearly defined and strategies to inhibit these responses, such as through the production of transgenic organs expressing human complement-inhibitory proteins, need to be developed in order to prolong xenograft survival. Additionally, future inquiries must also address in detail host cellular immune responses directed against the lung xenograft. These investigations are likely to lead to a more complete understanding of the mechanisms of lung xenograft rejection and to the development of strategies for modifying these responses which could eventually be applied to humans.

References

1. Hosenpud JD, Novick RJ, Breen TJ, Daily OP. The Registry of the International Society for Heart and Lung Transplantation: Eleventh Official Report-1994. J Heart Lung Transplant 1994; 13: 561
2. Evans RW, Orians CE, Asher NL. The potential supply of organ donors: an assessment of the efficiency of organ procurement efforts in the United States. JAMA 1992; 267: 239
3. Kaiser LR, Cooper JD. The current status of lung transplantation. Adv Surg 1992; 25: 259
4. Reemtsma K, McCraken BH, Schlegel JU, et al. Renal heterotransplantation in man. Ann Surg 1964; 160: 384
5. Platt JL, Fischel RJ, Matas AJ, et al. Immunopathology of hyperacute xenograft rejection in a swine-to-primate model. Transplantation 1991; 52: 214

6. Kaplon RJ, Platt JL, Kwiatkowski PA, et al. Absence of hyperacute rejection in pig-to-primate orthotopic pulmonary xenografts. Transplantation 1995; 59: 410
7. Tavakoli R, Devaux JY, Nonnenmacher L, et al. Discordant lung xenograft rejection in the rat. Transplantation 1992; 53: 235
8. Pierson RN, Tew DN, Konig WK, et al. Pig lungs are susceptible to hyperacute rejection by human blood in a working ex vivo heart-lung model. Transplant Proc 1994;26: 1318
9. Butler J, Rocker GM, Westaby S. Inflammatory response to cardiopulmonary bypass. Ann Thorac Surg 1993; 55: 552
10. Moat NE, Shore DF, Evans TW. Organ dysfunction and cardiopulmonary bypass: the role of complement and complement regulatory proteins. Eur J Cardiothorac Surg 1993; 7: 563
11. Grace PA. Ischaemia-reperfusion injury. Brit J Surg 1994; 81: 637
12. Sessa WC, Kaw S, Hecker M, Vane JR. The biosynthesis of endothelin-1 by human polymorphonuclear leukocytes. Biochem Biophys Res Comm 1991; 174: 613
13. Felip JG. Endothelin peptides: biological actions and pathophysiological significance in the lung. Life Sciences 1992; 52: 119
14. Tonshoff B, Busch C, Schweer H, Scharer K, Seyberth HW. In vivo prostanoid formation during acute renal allograft rejection. Nephrol Dial Transplant 1993; 8: 631
15. Cale ARJ, Ricagna F, Wiklund L, McGregor CGA, Miller VM. Mononuclear cells from dogs with acute lung allograft rejection cause contraction of pulmonary arteries. Circulation 1994: 90: 952
16. Yoshio T, Masuyama J, Mimori A, et al. Endothelin release from cultured endothelial cells induced by sera from patients with systemic lupus erythematosus. Ann Rheum Dis 1995; 54: 361
17. Reitz BA. Heart-lung transplantation: a review. Heart Transplant 1982; 1: 291
18. Nilsson FN, McGregor CGA, Miller VM. Pulmonary arterial reactivity after transplantation. J Thorac Cardiovasc Surg 1992; 103: 751

35 Experimental Lung Xenografting

R.N. Pierson III and G. Pino-Chavez

Introduction

Lung and heart–lung transplantation are now established as therapeutic interventions for many terminal conditions affecting the pulmonary system. Unfortunately, the growth in supply of donor lungs has lagged behind demand. Paradoxically, our increasing clinical success exacerbates the donor organ shortage by broadening indications for transplantation and increasing referrals of appropriate patients at an earlier stage in their disease. As a consequence, appropriate organs are often not available in time, and many of those accepted for transplant die waiting. One third of cystic fibrosis patients (181 of 544) listed between 1990 and 1994 died before transplantation; similar mortality occurs for patients with other underlying pathology [1]. The most acute need is among patients with congenital heart disease and those with cystic fibrosis, for both of whom a heart–lung bloc or double lung graft represents their best or only viable option, and patients with idiopathic pulmonary fibrosis, whose unpredictable, often fulminant course frequently results in mortality shortly after listing. Patients with these and other end-stage pulmonary disorders might benefit if xenogeneic lungs were available.

In choosing a xenogeneic lung donor for human recipients, one would intuitively choose a species phylogenetically closely related to man. But while relative physiologic, biochemical, and immunologic similarity might favor concordant primates, there are important ethical, infectious, and logistical factors mitigating against this option. The transplant community has therefore focused its investigative efforts on an improved understanding of the processes contributing to hyperacute rejection (HAR), in order to devise strategies which might allow eventual clinical application of discordant xenografts.

Concordant Lung Xenotransplantation

We are aware of only three studies describing lung xenografting between concordant species. Veith et al. performed fox-to-dog orthotopic lung xenografts without immunosuppression [2]. Xenografts exhibited radiographic, physiologic, and histologic patterns of rejection similar to those observed with dog allografts. Onset of rejection occurred within 3 days and progressed to complete graft necrosis by 6–12 days. In a subset of animals the contralateral pulmonary artery was ligated shortly after completing the lung implant in order to render the recipient entirely dependent upon the graft. Four of 16 animals succumbed intraoperatively due to high pulmonary vascular resistance. The remaining animals lived between 1 and 5 days. Despite only mild-to-moderate rejection on light microscopy, all lungs exhibited moderate to extensive parenchymal edema, and the recipients died of respiratory failure. The authors report no evidence of HAR on histological examination, but immunohistologic studies of antibody binding and complement activation were not done.

Takeda et al. performed 15 left single lung transplants from Macaque monkeys to baboons using FK506 and splenectomy [3]. Without immunosuppression, grafts were rejected by 4 days. Cellular infiltrates observed at 4 days in treated animals stabilized or resolved with methotrexate, yielding a median survival of 12 days. However, the contralateral pulmonary artery was not occluded; thus the capacity of the xenograft to support the recipient was not assessed.

Using cyclosporine and steroid-based immunosuppression, 12 of 15 baboons receiving cynomolgus monkey heart-lung transplants by Sadeghi et al. survived for 3–90 days [4]. Addition of total lymphoid irradiation (6 Gy) with antithymocyte globulin doubled mean survival time for operative survivors, from 8 to 16 days, but was associated with important infectious morbidity.

These experiences indicate that concordant lung xenografts are capable of providing total pulmonary support acutely. The etiology of the elevated vascular resistance and immediate lung dysfunction in Veith's study [2], which together accounted for early failure in 44 % of cases, is not clear; a similar phenomenon was observed in 20 % of Sadeghi's experiments [4]. It is possible that concordant lung xenografts are particularly susceptible to intravascular thrombosis, inflammation, or other ischemia/reperfusion phenomena. That intensive conventional immunosuppression can permit clinically meaningful graft function is evident from the work of both Takeda et al. and Sadeghi et al., but it was accompanied by evidence of significant toxicity. Extrapolation from a variety of other concordant xenograft models implicates both B and T cell-mediated immune processes in what appears to be an accelerated acute rejection response in control animals [5]. Whether an immunosuppressive regimen for concordant lung xenografting can be developed which has a reasonable therapeutic index is unknown. The potential clinical impact of these moderately encouraging experimental results is limited by the absence of a readily available concordant donor species for human recipients.

Discordant Lung Xenotransplantation

Lack of a biocompatible blood oxygenator for use in conjunction with extracorporeal circulatory support spurred early experiments in which animal lungs were perfused with human blood. Campbell et al. used dog lungs as an oxygenator for seven patients; high pulmonary vascular resistance (PVR) limited flow to 4–800 ml/min over the 15- to 49-min duration of extracorporeal perfusion [6]. Lung injury was apparent, developing more rapidly when high pulmonary artery perfusion pressures were required.

Waldhausen et al. perfused human blood through dog lungs in an ex vivo experimental model [7]. When the calcium chelator ACD was used as an anticoagulant, transpulmonary blood flows of 7–1500 ml/min were observed; importantly, calcium is critical to activation of complement. When heparin was used, a high PVR limited flow to 200 ml/min. Pulmonary edema usually occurred within 10 min with either anticoagulant.

Together, these studies demonstrate that duration of function of the dog lung in a human blood environment is brief and compares unfavorably with function of an allograft. While the mechanisms contributing to acute lung xenograft injury were not rigorously evaluated by these investigators, their findings are consistent with the hypothesis that both complement-dependent and complement-independent processes may contribute.

Bryant et al. perfused pig lungs with human blood using an ex vivo perfusion system [8]. Initial flow rates were typically less than 300 ml/min (10 % of normal human transpulmonary blood flow), attributable to a rapid rise in PVR. PVR elevation was the most important factor limiting oxygen transfer. Intraparenchymal hemorrhage and pulmonary edema uniformly evolved within 3 h (and often within one hour) despite a variety of interventions which blunted vasoconstriction. The pulmonary vasodilator isoproterenol decreased PVR and was associated with a modest delay in lung injury relative to other vasodilators (cyproheptadine, methysergide, and promethazine). Thus rapid elevation of PVR and subsequent parenchymal damage usually occur promptly when pig lungs are perfused with human blood. Indeed, rapid elevation of PVR and acute lung injury have been observed in every experimental model of lung xenotransplantation between species known to be discordant for other organs [9–17].

Whether the pig lung is privileged with respect to HAR by primates is the focus of ongoing controversy. Recently, Kaplon et al. reported short-term (1–3 day) survival of single pig lungs orthotopically transplanted into baboons [18]. Relative blood flow measured in the main pulmonary artery and in the transplanted lung's pulmonary artery indicated that PVR elevation did not prohibit perfusion of the transplant, with 10 %–40 % of the cardiac output perfusing the xenograft. Blood gas measurements from the pulmonary vein of the transplant had a high pO_2, consistent with efficient gas transfer in the xenograft. However, the orthotopic single lung grafts were unable to support the recipient when the contralateral native pulmonary artery was transiently occluded; very high PVR in the graft resulted in right heart failure and circulatory collapse.

Two subsequent double-lung recipients could not be weaned from bypass due to right heart failure [19]. A modest decline in anti-pig endothelial antibody, coupled with patchy deposition of IgM and complement pathway components (relative to that seen in hyperacutely rejected pig hearts) were interpreted as consistent with an absence of activation of the classical mediators of HAR. However, these histologic findings might also be explained by hypoperfusion of some pulmonary capillary beds due to intravascular thrombosis or vasoconstriction. Anti-endothelial antibody levels did decline, implying some sequestration in the transplanted lung. High pulmonary venous pO_2 and pulmonary artery flow probe measurements did not predict the capacity of unilateral or bilateral grafts to support the recipient, suggesting that these parameters are insensitive to hemodynamically important phenomena, and that single lung transplantation without contralateral pulmonary artery occlusion may not be an appropriate model for detecting clinically relevant lung dysfunction.

The pig lung is rapidly damaged by human blood when perfused ex vivo using a working heart–lung model [16]. The injury is characterized by a profound rise in PVR within 5 min despite high-dose vasodilator therapy (with the prostacyclin analogue Prostin VR). Oxygen transport function is lost within 30 min with rare exceptions, in association with massive intraparenchymal hemorrhage and pulmonary edema. Immunohistochemical staining clearly demonstrates immunoglobulin deposition (IgM>IgG) as well as deposition of complement components from both classical and alternative pathways [20]. Prevention of antibody binding and complement activation (by antibody absorption combined with heat treatment) results in significantly prolonged graft function (>4 h), similar to that seen with heterologous pig blood perfusion [17]. While this model has a number of important drawbacks (anticoagulation, exposure of blood to artificial surfaces), these findings suggest that the pig lung, like other pig organs, is susceptible to HAR by antibody- and complement-mediated processes. Further, while the experimental design and the specific interventions employed may also influence other pathways important to acute lung injury, they suggest that antibody binding and complement activation contribute to both the vasoconstrictive and cytotoxic facets of pulmonary damage in this species combination.

In our estimation, Kaplon's physiologic and histologic observations are in large measure consistent with our own; elevated PVR occurs with single or bilateral lung grafts, and, although perhaps less prominent than in hearts, antibody and complement deposition are clearly present [18]. We believe that, in aggregate, the available data support the conclusion that primate anti-pig antibody and complement trigger injury to the lung, including a rapid rise in PVR and subsequent capillary leak. If complement-mediated HAR of the lung does not occur in the pig-to-primate combination, and pig lung is privileged with regard to HAR in baboons, this exceptional finding apparently does not obtain for the pig-to-human combination. A central role for complement has been shown conclusively for the hyperacute (minutes to hours) dysfunction of vascularized organs transplanted between discordant species; its importance has been confirmed for the pig-to-primate combination [21, 22]. Prevention of complement activation alone permits prolonged survival of heart grafts for days [21–24], and survival is extended to weeks if additional immunosuppression is used [23, 24]. The importance of complement in the HAR of the pig lung is demonstrated by our ex vivo heart-lung experiments, reviewed above. However, these heart-lung experiments used blood stored overnight at 4 °C and were consequently depleted of formed blood elements. In addition, high-dose prostacyclin analog, which has potent vasodilatory, cytoprotective, and anti-inflammatory effects, was used to blunt the rise in PVR. With antibody depletion and heat treatment of fresh blood, without prostacyclin, only occasional survivals over 30 min are obtained (unpublished data). This result suggests that complement-independent processes also contribute to the dysfunction observed. If so, inhibition of complement activation may prove insufficient to achieve clinically important function of discordant pulmonary xenografts.

Two groups have recently achieved significant prolongation of pig heart survival in primates using hearts from pigs transgenic for human complement regulatory proteins [24, 25]. Parallel experiments used lungs from animals transgenic for human decay-accelerating factor (hDAF), testing for protection from HAR by ex vivo perfusion with fresh human blood [26] (Figs. 1, 2). Despite high-dose prostacyclin, none of these transgenic lungs was protected from evolution of high PVR. Only two of nine lungs expressed levels of hDAF on the pulmonary endothelium comparable to those seen in man; in one of these two cases the rise in PVR resolved spontaneously, and graft function (as measured by oxygen transport) persisted for 90 min (versus <20 min for controls and other transgenics with low endothelial hDAF expression).

Norin et al. observed that pig lung transgenic for CD59 did not exhibit the extensive inflammatory infiltrates and hemorrhage seen in CD59 lungs within one hour of revascularization in baboons; however injury was evident by 3 h,

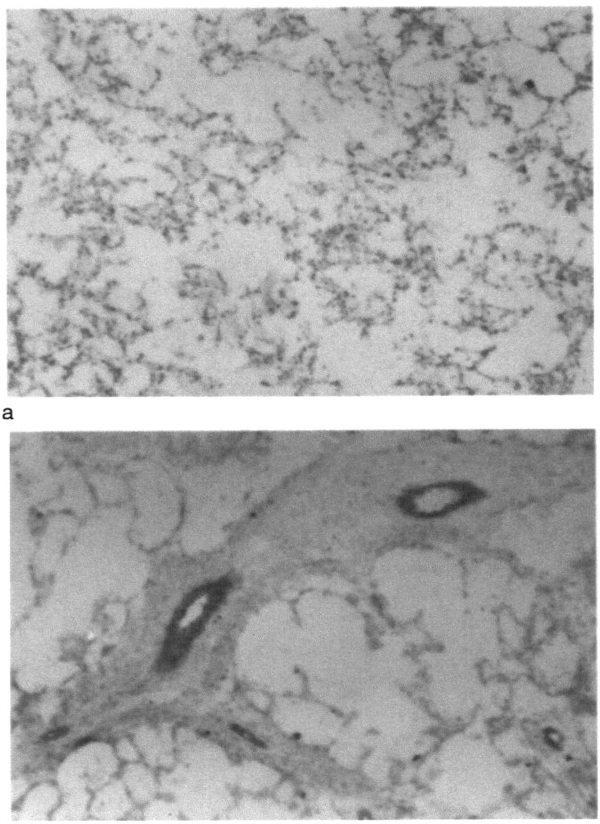

a

b

Fig. 1a–h. Expression of human decay-accelerating factor (hDAF) is assessed by immunohistochemical staining of preperfusion biopsies. Biopsies obtained after 5 min of perfusion with human blood were processed in formalin for routine histology (H&E) or frozen for immunohistochemical evaluation of antibody binding, complement component deposition, and P selection expression [37]. Dark reaction product indicates primary antibody binding, visualized by avidin/biotin-mediated deposition (via secondary antibodies) of peroxidase reaction product; nuclear counterstaining is with hemytoxylin. **a** In a control (non-transgenic) pig lung, hDAF is absent, in contrast to **b** strong expression, particularly in arterioles but also in alveolar interstitium and on epithelial structures (not shown), in a heterozygous (+/–) high hDAF-expressing transgenic lung. Intra-alveolar hemorrhage, perivascular and subepithelial edema, and interstitial congestion are reduced in **d** transgenic compared to **c** control biopsies performed after 5 min. **e,f** IgM binding is not affected by hDAF expression, but **g,h** P selectin expression on arterioles is less prominent

Fig. 1 (continued)

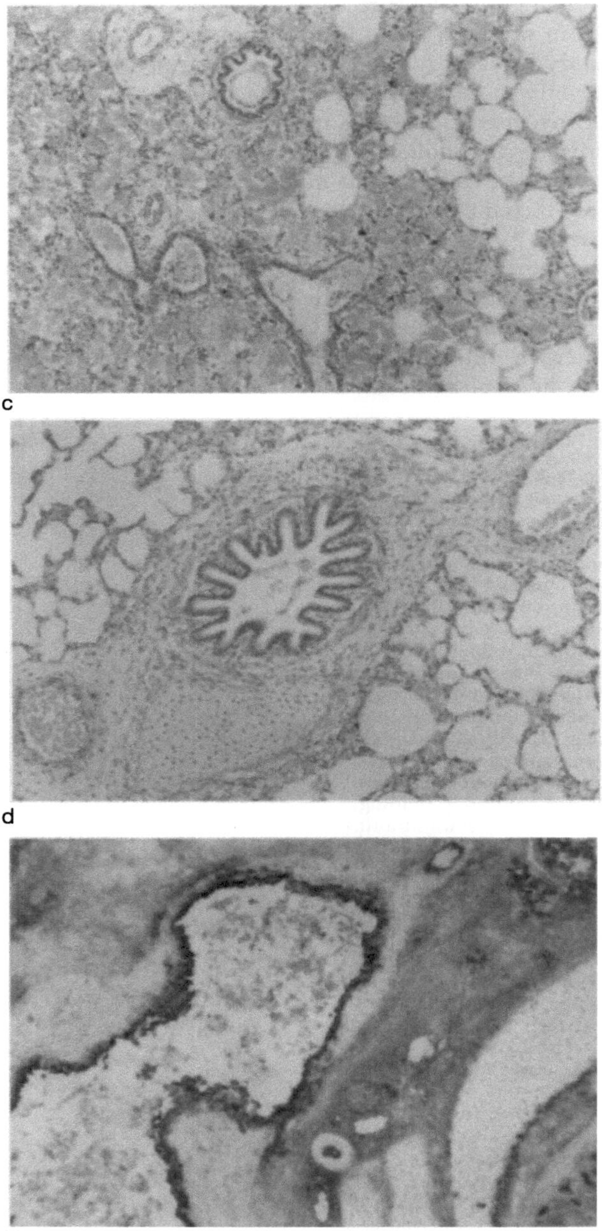

Fig. 1 (continued)

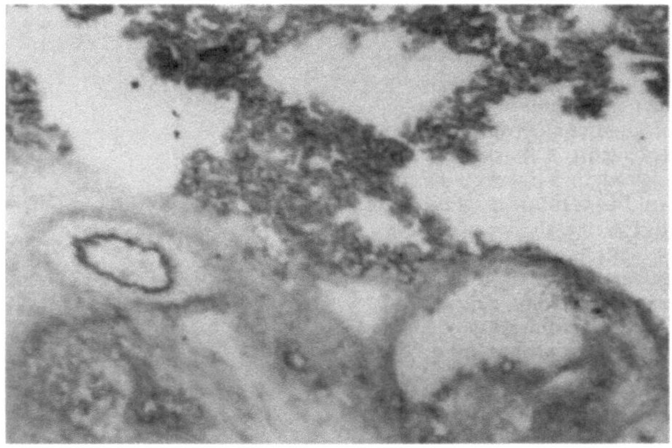

f

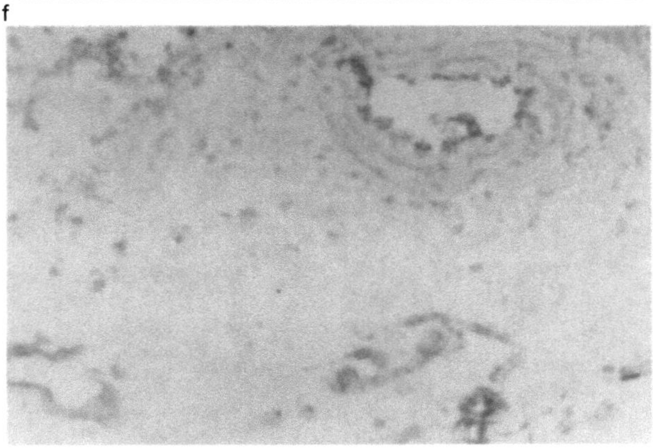

g

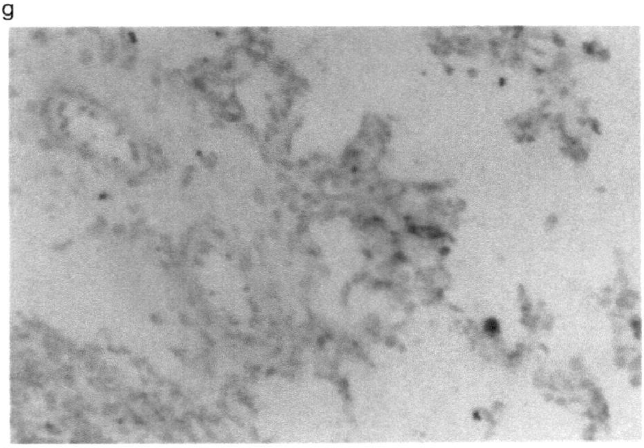

h

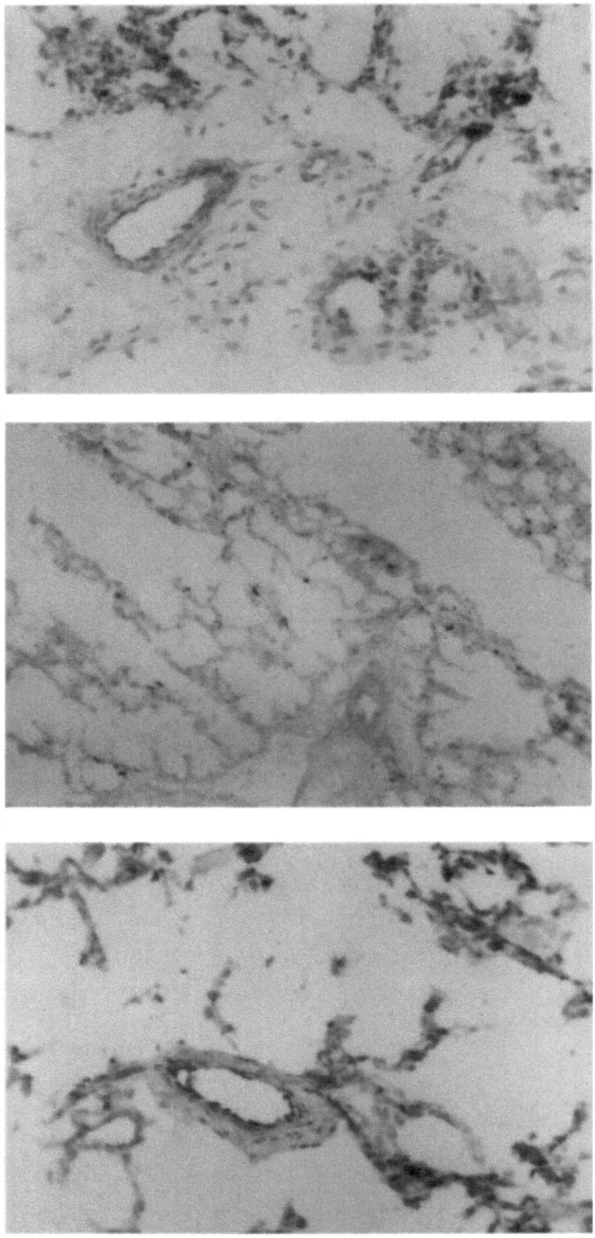

a

b

c

Fig. 2a–h. Biopsies obtained after 5 min of perfusion of pig lung with human blood, frozen, and processed as in Fig. 1. Alternative pathway complement (Properdin) deposition is markedly reduced in **b** transgenic compared to **a** nontransgenic lung. **c,d** The classical pathway is less completely blocked, as indicated by strong binding of C4 on arteriolar epithelium; **d** alveolar interstitial deposition is less prominent in the transgenic lung. C3b (common pathway) and C9 (membrane attack complex) are both significantly reduced on arterioles and in the interstitium of **f,h** transgenic lung compared to **e,g** nontransgenic lung

Fig. 2 (continued)

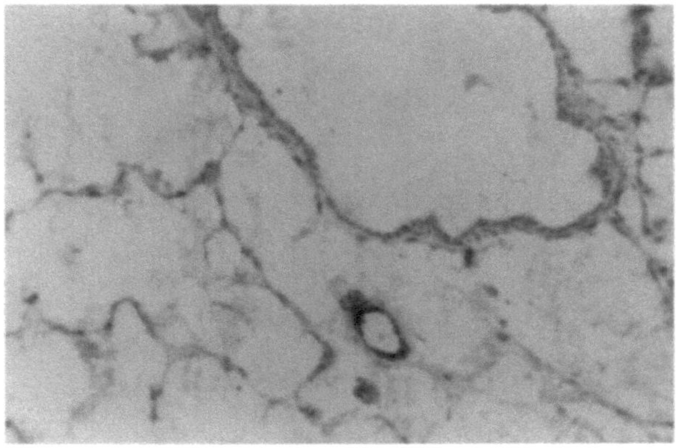

d

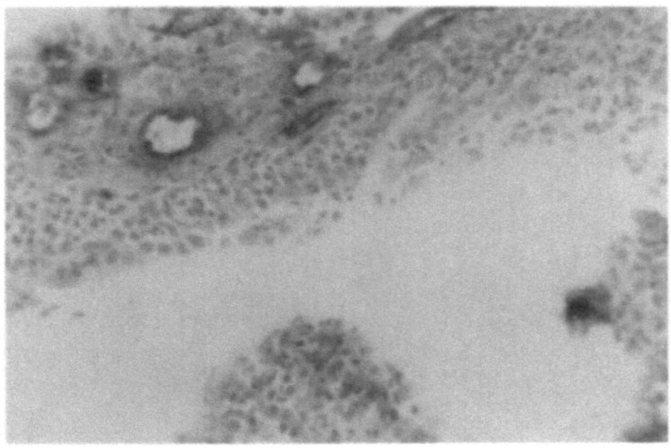

e

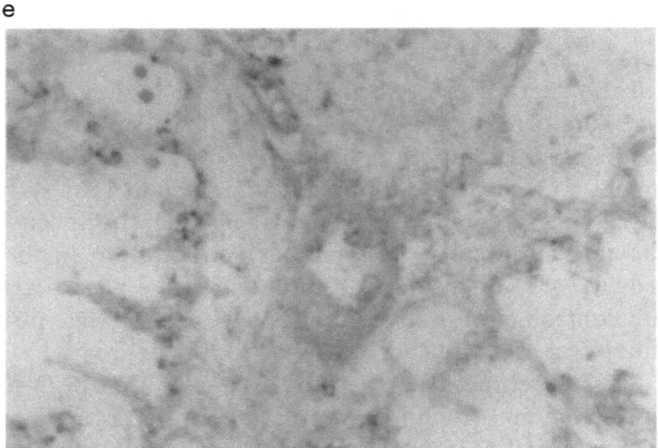

f

Fig. 2 (continued)

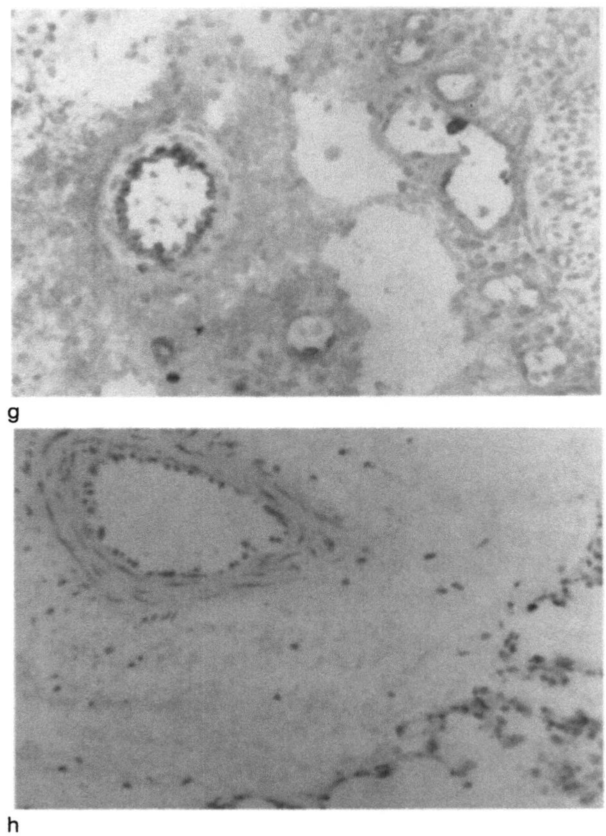

and the grafts were rejected within 12 h [27]. Whether the transgenic lung could have supported the recipient was not tested. Davis et al. found substantial prolongation of graft function in lungs expressing hDAF and CD59 at levels approximately 20 % of those found in human lung [28]. When transplanted to baboons which had previously rejected a pig heart, one of four transgenic single lungs was able to support the recipient's circulation; in three others elevated PVR limited flow to 500 ml/min despite aggressive vasodilator therapy, and occlusion of the contralateral native pulmonary artery was poorly tolerated. Parenchymal injury was delayed, but did evolve over 12–72 h.

These preliminary experiences suggest that high levels of expression of one or more human complment regulatory proteins may contribute to prolongation of survival of discordant lung xenografts, but that higher expression levels than those achieved to date and control of other cellular and humoral mechanisms may be crucial to eventual clinical success.

We have attempted to further define the role of factors other than complement in discordant lung transplant dysfunction using a traditional model, namely depletion of recipient complement with cobra venom factor (CVF) [29]. CVF acts as a C3 convertase, consuming C3 and thus depleting the complement component common to both the classical and alternative pathways (Chap. 32). Pig lungs were perfused with human blood depleted of complement by pretreatment of plasma with CVF. Neither elevation of PVR nor capillary leak was prevented [29]. Even when antibody absorption was added to CVF treatment, hyperacute lung injury and vasoconstriction occurred (unpublished data). This result might be taken as evidence for complement-independent mechanisms governing HAR of the lung. However, while CVF depletes C3, in the process it generates high levels of the neutrophil attractant and anaphylatoxin C3a; in other models, CVF causes neutrophil-mediated, P selectin-dependent pulmonary capillary leak [30]. When Davis et al. administered CVF on the day of a pig-to-baboon single lung transplant, profound vasoconstriction and rapid lung injury occurred [28]. When animals were instead treated for the 2 days prior to transplant, PVR elevation prohibited contralateral pulmonary artery occlusion, and progressive lung injury occurred within 4 h.

We suspect that C3a is at least in part responsible for the vasoconstriction and pulmonary injury observed in these experiments, thus simulating inflammatory facets of complement-mediated HAR, and obscuring the role of complement-independent mechanisms to discordant lung xenograft dysfunction.

Several lines of evidence suggest that the lung may be particularly vulnerable to injury by mechanisms independent of anti-species antibody and complement. The lung appears to be more sensitive than the heart or other organs to a variety of systemic insults, as manifested by the pulmonary capillary leak and acute respiratory distress syndromes (ARDS) which sporadically occur during sepsis and shock or following cardiopulmonary bypass. These insults have in common not only complement activation but the activation and intrapulmonary sequestration of neutrophils, platelets and macrophages. Neutrophil depletion, adhesion molecule blockade, and anti-tumor necrosis factor (anti-TNF) antibody each has a salutary effect on lung injury in these nontransplant models, suggesting that cytokines and formed blood elements may contribute to pulmonary dysfunction by mechanisms perhaps distinct from (but not necessarily independent of) those mediating classic complement-driven HAR [30–34]. In our estimation, it is unlikely that a xenogeneic lung would be privileged with regard to such processes, which one might expect to be triggered by surgical manipulations inherent in clinical and experimental lung xenotransplantation.

Formed blood elements may contribute to the pace of hyperacute discordant xenogeneic lung injury. In two HAR models, the anti-inflammatory agent methylprednisolone, which among its actions inhibits neutrophil binding and degranulation, attenuates the pace of hyperacute pulmonary injury [13, 15]. Neutrophils and platelets are rapidly sequestered in pig lungs perfused by fresh or stored human blood, accompanied by evidence of free radical-mediated membrane lipid injury (unpublished data).

Bryant et al. found that human blood retrieved from the cardiopulmonary bypass machine and stored for 48–96 h gave better results than fresh blood, suggesting that formed blood elements, which are depleted and defunctionalized by storage, contribute to the pace of the rejection response. However, unlike hearts perfused ex vivo [35], no prolongation of lung function is conferred by depletion of formed blood elements by Pall filtration (unpublished observations), confirming Bryant's similar findings using glass or Dacron wool filters to remove formed blood elements from the perfusate. Thus formed blood elements by themselves are not necessary for acute xenograft lung dysfunction to occur, although they may be sufficient to damage the graft under some circumstances (e.g., after CVF treatment).

In light of these observations and the results obtained with transgenic lungs expressing human complement regulatory proteins, it is likely that complement-independent mechanisms, driven either by xenospecific antibody or by other effectors of the immune response such as neutrophils and platelets, may render protection of the lung incomplete even with effective control of complement activation. Prevention of both neutrophil-mediated inflammation and platelet and macrophage activation may thus prove important adjuncts to complement regulation for clinical lung xenografting.

Although the pathogenesis of elevated PVR in lung xenografts remains uncertain, one important specific mediator has been identified. Thromboxane A_2 contributes to elevated PVR associated with infusion of mismatched heterologous blood or human blood in sheep [10]. Similarly, our work identifies thromboxane as the central mediator of pulmonary vasoconstriction, and a contributor to complement activation and capillary leak, in pig lungs perfused with human blood [36]. Addition of antibody absorption (without heat treatment) to thromboxane blockade yields impressive protection of lung function, beyond 4 h in one preliminary experiment. Platelets and pulmonary interstitial macrophages are two known sources of thromboxane. We postulate that activation of one or both cell populations triggers thromboxane production; whether this occurs consequent to or independent of complement activation is an unresolved question of major importance to programs hoping to use transgenic lungs for clinical discordant lung xenotransplantation.

Comment

Concordant pulmonary xenografting is unlikely to be clinically important for a variety of ethical, infectious disease, and logistical reasons. Discordant lung xenotransplantation is currently prevented by acute lung injury, which we believe represents HAR. Prevention of complement activation is likely to result in improved survival, but whether the protection afforded by expression of human complement regulatory proteins will prove sufficient for clinical application is unknown. Vasodilators, steroids, and thromboxane antagonists confer only modest protection, but offer important clues as to mechanisms underlying the acute vasoconstriction and subsequent capillary leak. It is possible that complement-independent mechanisms, driven either by xenospecific antibody or by other effectors of the immune response such as neutrophils and platelets, will render protection of the lung by complement-directed strategies incomplete. Thus, pig-to-human lung transplantation may prove more difficult than the heart or kidney due to susceptibility of the lung to non-xenospecific or complement-independent insults.

Resolution of the relative importance of complement-dependent and complement-independent mechanisms to dysfunction of discordant lung xenografts awaits results of experiments using pharmacologic blockade of complement activation, or study of pigs with higher pulmonary endothelial expression of human complement regulatory proteins. Notwithstanding the discouraging experimental results to date, donor modifications to prevent complement injury, coupled with anticipated advances in our understanding of HAR of the lung, may facilitate clinical application in the foreseeable future.

References

1. UNOS Registry statistics
2. VEITH, F.J., RICHARDS, K.U., HAGSTROM, J.W.C, MONTEFUSCO, C.M. Intrafamilial lung xenografts from fox to dog. J. Thorac. Cardiovasc. Surg. 81:546, 1981
3. TAKEDA, M., KAWAUCHI, M., NAKAJIMA, J., FURUSE, A. Methotrexate in rescue therapy for xenotransplanted lung in primates. (Abstract po-46) Third International Congress for Xenotransplantation, Boston, 1995
4. SADEGHI, A.M., LAKS, H., DRINKWATER, D.C., et al. Heart-lung xenotransplantation in primates. J. Heart Lung Transplant. 10:442, 1991
5. MARKMAN, J.F., BARKER, C.F. Basic and clinical considerations in the use of xenografts. Curr. Probl. Surg. 31:385, 1994
6. CAMPBELL, G.S., CRIPS, N.W., BROWN, E.B. Total cardiac bypass in humans utilizing a pump and heterologous lung oxygenator (dog lungs). Surgery. 40:364, 1956
7. WALDHAUSEN, J.A., WEBB, R.C. SPENCER, F.C., BAHNSON, H.T. Study of the canine lung as an oxygenator of human and canine blood in extracorporeal circulation. Surgery. 42:726, 1957
8. BRYANT, L.R., EISEMAN, B., AVERY, M. Studies of the porcine lung as an oxygenator for human blood. J. Thorac. Cardiovasc. Surg. 55:255, 1968
9. HALMAGYI, D.F.J., STARZECKI, B., McRAE, J., HORNER, G.J. The lung as the main target organ in the acute phase of transfusion reaction in sheep. J. Surg. Res. 3:418, 1963
10. MORAL, D.R., GYSIN, I., PITTET, J.F., COSTABELLA, P.M.M. Role of thromboxane A2 during incompatible homologous and heterologous blood transfusion in sheep. Anesthesiology. 69:A122, 1988
11. COOK, W.A., KLAUSNER, S.K., SINHA, S., KIKKAWA, Y., VEITH, F.J. A new look at hyperacute rejection. Ann. Thorac. Surg. 13:388, 1972
12. TAVAKOLI, R., DEVAUX, J.Y., NONNENMACHER, L., et al. Discordant lung xenograft rejection in the rat. Transplantation. 53:235, 1992
13. KUSAJIMA, K., WAX, S.D., WEBB, W.R., AUST, J.C. Cinemicroscopy of hyperacute pulmonary rejection. Ann. Thorac. Surg. 21:341, 1976
14. KUSAJIMA, K., AUST, J.C., WAX, S.D., WEBB, W.R. Hemodynamic and functional changes in xenogeneic, perfused, isolated lungs. J. Thorac. Cardiovasc. Surg. 72:115, 1976
15. SPEILLER, P.B., KIKKAWA, Y., VEITH, F.J., COOK, W.A. Steroid protection of a pulmonary xenograft model. Surg. Forum. 23:272, 1972

16. PIERSON, R.N. III, TEW, D.N., KONIG, W.K., et al. Pig lungs are susceptible to hyperacute rejection by human blood in a working ex vivo heart-lung model. Transplant. Proc. 26:1318, 1994
17. PIERSON, R.N. III, DUNNING, J.J., KONIG, W.K., et al. Mechanisms governing the pace and character of pig heart and lung rejection by human blood. Transplant. Proc. 26:2337, 1994
18. KAPLON, R.J., PLATT, J.L., KWIATKOWSKI, P.A., et al. Absence of hyperacute rejection in pig-to-primate orthotopic pulmonary xenografts. Transplantation. 59:410, 1995
19. SHAH, A.S., O'HAIR, D.P., KAPLON, R.J., et al. Absence of hyperacute rejection in pig-to-primate double lung xenografts. (Abstract 188) J. Heart Lung Transplant. 14:S83, 1995
20. PIERSON, R.N. III, KASPAR-KONIG, W., TEW, D.N., et al. Hyperacute rejection in a pig-to-human lung transplant model. 1: The role of antipig antibody and complement. TRANSPLANTATION, in the press.
21. FISCHEL, R.J., DALMASSO, A.P., VERCELLOTTI, G.M., et al. Mechanism of complement activation in the hyperacute rejection of porcine organs transplanted into primate recipients. Am. J. Pathol. 140:1157, 1992
22. PRUITT, S.K., KIRK, A.D., BOLLINGER, R.R., et al. The effect of soluble complement receptor type 1 on hyperacute rejection of porcine xenografts. Transplantation. 57:363, 1994
23. FUKUSHIMA, N., BOUCHART, F., GUNDRY, S.R., et al. The role of anti-pig antibody in pig-to-baboon cardiac xenotransplant rejection. Transplantation. 57:923, 1994
24. WHITE, D.J.G., BRAIDLEY, P., DUNNING, J., et al. Hearts from pigs transgenic for human DAF are not hyperacutely rejected when xenografted to primates. (Abstract pl-28) Third International Congress for Xenotransplantation, Boston, 1995
25. McCURRY, K.R., KOOYMAN, D., DIAMOND, L., et al. Human complement regulatory proteins in transgenic animals regulate complement activation in xenoperfused organs. (Abstract 288) Fifteenth International Congress of the Transplantation Society, Kyoto, 1994
26. PIERSON, R.N. III, YOUNG, V.K., KASPAR-KONIG, W., WHITE, D.J.G., WALLWORK, J. Expression of human complement regulatory protein may protect pig lung against hyperacute rejection by human blood. (Abstract 233) J. Heart Lung Transplant. 14:S94, 1995
7. NORIN, A.J., BREWER, R.J., FODOR, W.L., et al. Enhanced survival of porcine endothelialized PTFE vascular grafts and porcine lung xenografts in primates expressing human CD59. (Abstract po-39) Third International Congress for Xenotransplantation, Boston, 1995
28. DAVIS, D. Personal communication
29. PIERSON, R.N. III, TEW, D.F., KONIG, W.K., WHITE, D.J.G., WALLWORK, J. Profound pulmonary hypertension, characteristic of pig lung rejection by human blood, is mediated by xenoreactive antibody independent of complement. Transplant. Proc. 27:274, 1995
30. MULLIGAN, M.S., PAULSON, J.C., DE FREES, S., et al. Protective effects of oligosaccharides in P-selectin-dependent lung injury. Nature. 364:149, 1993
31. COLLETTI, L.M., BURTCH, G.D., REMICK, D.G., et al. The production of tumor necrosis factor alpha and the development of a pulmonary capillary injury following hepatic ischemia/reperfusion. Transplantation. 49:268, 1990

32. WHEELER, A.P., JESMOK, G., BRIGHAM, K.L. Tumor necrosis factor's effects on lung mechanics, gas exchange, and airway reactivity in sheep. Am. J. Physiol. 161:2542, 1990
33. BANDO, K., PILLAI, R., CAMERON, D.E., et al. Leukocyte depletion ameliorates free radical-mediated lung injury after cardiopulmonary bypass. J. Thorac. Cardiovasc. Surg. 99:873, 1990
34. DUKE, S.S., GUERRY-FORCE, M.L., FORBES, J.T., et al. Acute endotoxin-induced lymphocyte subset sequestration in sheep lungs. Lab. Invest. 62:355, 1990
35. YOUNG, V.K., PIERSON, R.N. III, KASPAR-KONIG, W., et al. White blood cells and platelets are integral to the hyperacute rejection of the pig heart by human blood. Transplant. Proc. 27:272, 1995
36. PIERSON, R.N. III, PARKER, R.E. Thromboxane mediates pulmonary vasoconstriction and contributes to cytotoxicity in pig lungs perfused with fresh human blood. Transplant. Proc. 28:635, 1996
37. ROSENGARD, A.M., CARY, N.R., LANGFORD, G.A., TUCKER, A.W., WALLWORK, J., WHITE, D.J.G. Tissue expression of human complement inhibitor, decay-accelerating factor, in transgenic pigs. A potential approach for preventing xenograft rejection. Transplantation 59(9):1325–33, 1995

36 Newborn Pig-to-Baboon Cardiac Xenotransplantation: A Model of Delayed Xenograft Rejection

S. Itescu, O.P. Minanov, and R.E. Michler

Introduction

Cardiac transplantation is currently the best therapeutic option available to patients with end-stage heart disease. However, the supply of human donor hearts remains inadequate to meet the ever-increasing demand. Approximately 17 000 people per year under the age of 55 could benefit from cardiac allotransplantation in the United States alone. Unfortunately, no more than 2200 donor hearts per year are currently available [1]. As a result of this shortage, 30 % of adult patients awaiting cardiac transplantation die before a donor is found [2]. The need for grafts is particularly desperate among newborn infants with congenital malformations, for whom the wait for an available organ results in death even more frequently than in adults.

The severe shortage of organs has led to intensive efforts to develop alternative strategies for organ replacement. "Bridge" therapy with mechanical left ventricular assist devices has recently witnessed relative success in carefully selected adult patients with left ventricular failure [3]. However, use of these devices is not possible for patients with severe biventricular failure or for those patients with a total body surface area of less than $1.5\,m^2$ (due to the large size of such devices). Thus virtually all children, and many adults, are not candidates for mechanical left ventricular assistance. Another approach which obviates these limitations is the use of xenografts.

The preferred source of the xenograft would be a concordant species, such as a nonhuman primate. In concordant xenotransplantation, humans do not have preformed anti-donor cytotoxic antibodies and the graft is not at risk of hyperacute rejection. Widespread use of nonhuman primates, however, is not feasible. The use of chimpanzees is limited by ethical concerns, and the use of baboons is limited by their small size and by their potential for epizootic disease transmission. For these reasons, much interest has focused recently on the use of discordant xenografts, such as those from pig donors. Pigs represent a reasonable alternative donor source based on their similar physiology and size to humans. Moreover, they can be easily bred in large numbers and appear to be relatively free of pathogens capable of causing infection in the human recipient.

However, in common with other discordant donor–recipient pairs, pig xenografts transplanted into primates undergo hyperacute rejection within minutes to hours. The histological hallmarks of this process are rapid thrombotic occlusion of the graft vasculature, platelet aggregation, and infiltration with polymorphonuclear leukocytes. High levels of preformed natural xenoreactive antibodies of IgM isotype are present in all adult primates and appear to be primarily responsible for initiating this process [4]. Immediately following perfusion of a pig xenograft implanted into a primate, binding of xenoreactive IgM antibodies to endothelial cells of the xenograft activates complement, leading to endothelial cell activation, followed by cell injury, thrombosis, and ischemia of the graft [5]. Endothelial cell activation leads to the development of a procoagulant state due to loss of thrombomodulin and heparan sulfate/antithrombin III, thus initiating the extrinsic pathway of coagulation, and increased production of plasminogen activator inhibitor, an inhibitor of fibrinolysis. Together, these conditions lead to fibrin clot formation, platelet activation, and vascular thrombosis. Additionally, activated endothelial cells have increased expression of surface adhesion molecules which enhance the ability of inflammatory cells, such as macrophages and neutrophils, to migrate into the xenograft, further amplifying the inflammatory response.

Humoral Immunity in Discordant Xenotransplantation

The major antigenic determinant on pig endothelium recognized by primate xenoreactive antibodies is the oligosaccharide residue, galactose α1–3 galactose (αGal1–3Gal; αGal). This residue is incorporated in many structures expressed by the endothelium of species that are widely disparate from humans. Evidence that naturally occurring xenoantibodies are directed against αGal are derived from experiments demonstrating prolongation of xenograft survival following depletion of circulating anti-αGal antibodies, infusion of αGal oligosaccharides, or cleavage of αGal residues from pig endothelium [6–8]. Expression of the αGal residue on proteins and lipids depends on the presence of a functional galactosyltransferase gene, encoding a glycosidation enzyme. The phylogenetically related group of primates, which includes humans, apes, and Old World monkeys (the platyrrhines), contains an inactivated α1,3-galactosyltransferase gene [9, 10]. This presumably explains the lack of expression of αGal, as well as the presence of antibodies directed against this epitope, in human adults. In contrast, all other mammalian species contain an intact α1,3-galactosyltransferase gene, and αGal is expressed on their endothelium.

Newborn Pig-to-Baboon Discordant Xenotransplantation: A Model of Natural Antibody Depletion

Since anti-αGal antibodies are hypothesized to develop in humans early in life after exposure to gut microorganisms expressing the αGal epitope, we addressed the possibility that there may be a "window" period during which newborn primates may not yet have developed cytotoxic IgM anti-αGal antibodies. We reasoned that transplacental transfer from the maternal circulation could lead to detectable levels of anti-αGal IgG antibodies, but not of IgM antibodies, which are too large to cross into the fetal circulation. Sera were collected from infant baboons, and pooled adult baboon sera were used as controls. A whole cell

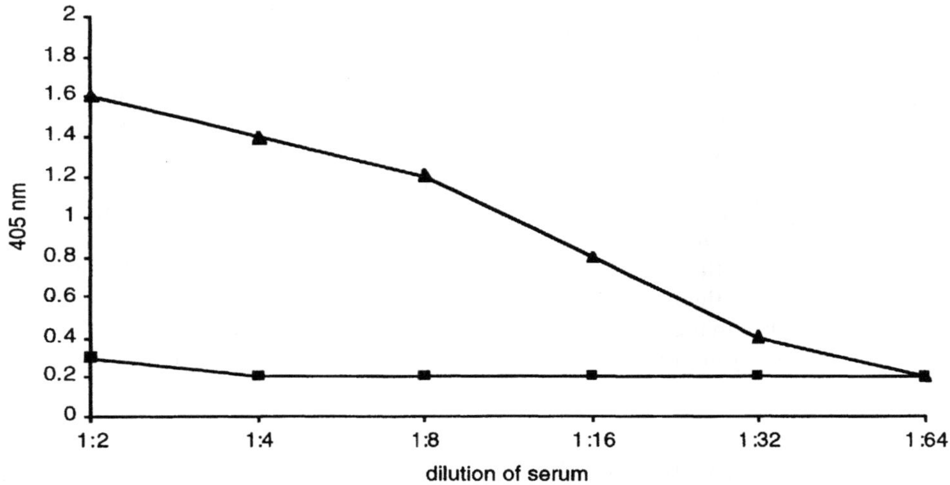

Fig. 1. Binding of baboon natural IgM xenoantibody to cultured pig aortic endothelial cells, measured by enzyme-linked immunosorbent assay (ELISA). *Triangles*, adult; *squares*, newborn

enzyme-linked immunosorbent assay (ELISA) was performed to determine the binding of xenoantibodies to pig aortic endothelial cells and lymphocytes. We found that sera from newborn baboons younger than 7 weeks contained minimally detectable levels of natural IgM xenoantibodies to either cultured pig aortic endothelial cells or lymphocytes [11] (Fig. 1). Pooled adult baboon sera demonstrated high binding levels of natural IgM xenoantibodies to both cell cultures. In contrast to IgM, newborn baboon sera were found to contain IgG antibodies with activity against pig aortic endothelial cells and pig lymphocytes, but at less than 50 % of the binding levels detected in adult baboons (Fig. 2). Adult baboon

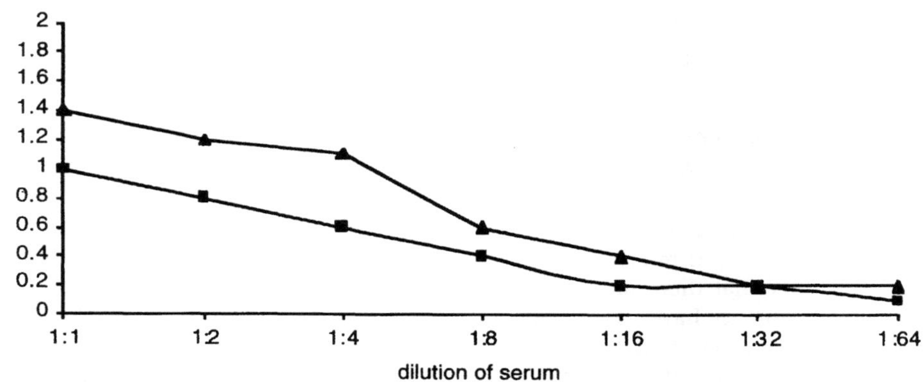

Fig. 2. Binding of baboon natural IgG xenoantibody to cultured pig aortic endothelial cells, measured by enzyme-linked immunosorbent assay (ELISA)

sera demonstrated high levels of cytotoxicity to pig endothelial cells, as measured by an MTT (3-(4,5-dimethyl-thiazoyl-2-y) 2,5 diphenyl-tetrazolium bromide) assay. Newborn baboon sera had very low levels of cytotoxicity, confirming IgM to be the primary xenoreactive antibody for hyperacute rejection. These results were subsequently confirmed, and extended, in an ELISA using bovine serum albumin (BSA)-conjugated αGal residues as specific antigenic targets.

These studies suggested that discordant pig-to-primate xenotransplantation might be feasible in the newborn primate, since the newborn could be viewed as being a natural model of cytotoxic IgM antibody depletion. On the basis of these observations, we performed seven successful procedures of heterotopic cervical cardiac xenotransplantation from newborn pigs to baboons [12, 13]. All xenografts survived beyond the "hyperacute period", with a median survival time of 3.4 days (range, 0.7–6 days). Histologic examination of the explanted xenografts did not demonstrate typical findings of severe hyperacute rejection in any of the tissues studied; however, a mild-to-moderate degree of microscopic hemorrhage and thrombosis was observed in the longest-surviving grafts (Fig. 3). By immunofluorescence, there was only minimal evidence of IgM or IgG binding to pig endothelium, and similarly of complement components, C3, C4, C5b, or membrane attack complex (MAC). These findings were more prominent in the longest-surviving grafts (4 and 6 days).

Using both a whole pig endothelial cell ELISA and purified αGal conjugated to BSA, we observed in two of two newborn baboons that the anti-αGal IgG antibody levels dropped significantly at the time of xenograft rejection, consistent with their binding to the xenoantigens on the pig graft. Moreover, in both ani-

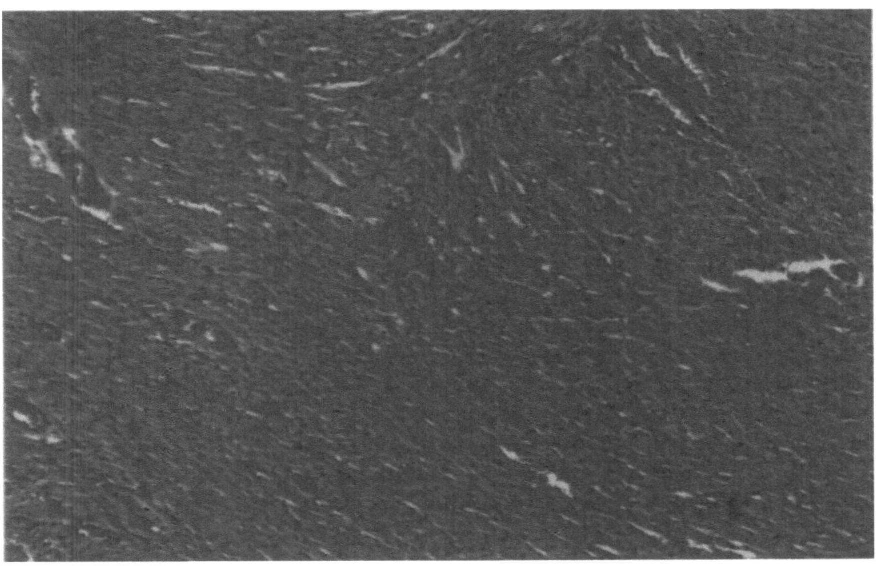

Fig. 3. Histopathology of a heterotopic porcine graft that failed 4 days after xenotransplantation. There is a mild-to-moderate degree of hemorrhage and intravascular thrombosis

mals there was an induction of anti-αGal antibodies post-transplant, an IgM response which peaked by day 14, and an IgG response which progressively increased over time. These results confirm that the absence of preformed IgM antibodies in newborn primates allows them to accept a pig organ for periods well beyond those associated with hyperacute rejection. Unfortunately, the introduction of the heavy antigenic load of αGal present in the transplanted xenograft induces a "delayed" antibody response, which may subsequently contribute to the rejection process.

Cellular Immunity in Discordant Xenotransplantation

In addition to humoral immunity, discordant xenografts induce prominent cellular responses in recipients. A number of studies have addressed the role of T cell immunity in discordant xenograft rejection. In widely disparate species combinations, such as mouse-to-human, direct recognition of xenoantigens appears to be diminished in comparison to alloantigens [14]. This perhaps reflects structural incompatibilities between human CD4 molecules, T cell receptors, adhesion molecules, and their respective ligands on mouse endothelium. In contrast, pig endothelium induces vigorous direct proliferative T cell responses in humans [15–17]. This appears to involve recognition of swine leukocyte antigen (SLA) class II molecules and to involve binding of human CD4 T cells to pig endothelium via lympocyte function-associated antigen (LFA)-1 and CD2.

In addition to direct stimulation, pig xenoantigens activate human T cells by the indirect recognition pathway. To examine the relative contribution of indirect xenoantigen recognition, we performed various experiments designed to study the interactions between recipient macrophages and CD4 T cells [18]. In these studies, we observed high levels of T cell proliferation and IL-2 production following exposure of human mononuclear cells to porcine endothelium, and inhibition of these proliferative responses by 25%–75% in the presence of Monoclonal antibodies directed against either human HLA-DR or CD4. These results suggest that the indirect pathway of antigen recognition might play a more prominent role in xenotransplantation than in allotransplantation. We and others have demonstrated reactivity of human natural killer (NK) cells to porcine endothelium by mechanisms that are both dependent and independent of antibody-dependent cellular cytotoxicity (ADCC) [19, 20]. We investigated whether macrophage-derived cytokines had an effect on human NK cell lysis of pig endothelium. Pretreatment of pig endothelium with IL-1-alpha or tumor necrosis factor (TNF)-alpha was associated with decreased endothelial cell lysis by human NK cells. The mechanism of this endothelial cell protection from lysis is currently being investigated in our laboratory. Together, these studies emphasize the central role of macrophage activation on both the afferent and efferent arms of the human cellular immune response against pig xenoantigens.

Cellular Elements Involved in the Rejection of Newborn Pig-to-Baboon Cardiac Xenografts

In guinea pig-to-rat cardiac xenotransplantation, treatment of recipients with cobra venom factor to deplete serum complement prevented hyperacute rejection and prolonged xenograft survival [21]. However, a delayed form of xenograft rejection occurred, which was accompanied by tissue infiltration with macrophages and NK cells. Since the in vitro primate response to pig xenoantigens appears to depend in great part on macrophage activation, we studied pig hearts rejected by newborn baboons to determine whether a cellular immune response resembling that observed in lower species might also occur in rejection of discordant xenografts in primates [13]. Histologic examination of four pig hearts demonstrated dense mononuclear infiltrates extending from the subepicardial regions into the myocardium (Fig. 4). Immunophenotypic analysis revealed the mononuclear cell infiltrate to consist primarily of 40%–45% macrophages ($CD68^{+}CD14^{+}DR^{+}$) and 30%–35% NK cells ($CD16^{+}$). In addition, 15%–20% of the cells were B cells ($CD20^{+}$), while less than 10% were $CD3^{+}$ T cells. These in vivo studies suggest that the delayed rejection of newborn pig-to-baboon cardiac xenografts occurs in large part due to cellular immune mechanisms involving macrophages and NK cells. Moreover, it is likely that the preexisting and induced anti-αGal IgG response in the recipients amplified the cellular reactivity by binding to Fc receptors on the effector cells.

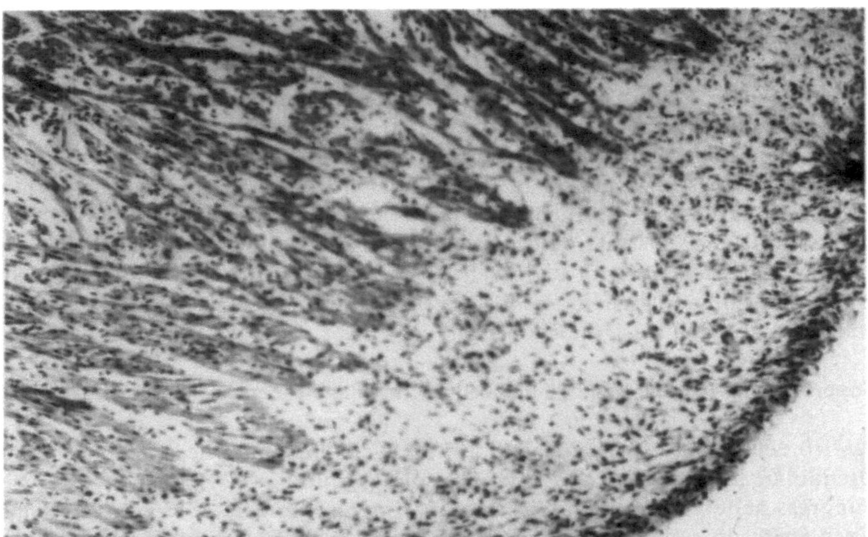

Fig. 4. Histopathology of subepicardial region of a heterotopic porcine graft that failed 4 days after xenotransplantation, demonstrating a dense mononuclear cell infiltrate. Note that there is only a scattering of polymorphonuclear neutrophils

Strategies To Prevent Xenograft Rejection in Newborn Primate Recipients

Modification of Xenograft Endothelium

A great deal of effort has been devoted recently to genetically modifying pig organs such that endothelial cells express membrane-bound human complement regulatory proteins which protect native cells from damage by endogenous human complement. Three of these regulatory proteins - decay accelerating factor (DAF; CD55), homologous restriction factor (HRF; CD59), and membrane cofactor protein (MCP; CD46) - have been expressed in transgenic pigs or mice and appear promising in conferring protection against complement-mediated hyperacute rejection of the xenograft [22]. In several recent studies, pig organs expressing human CD59 or DAF were reported to be protected from complement-mediated injury in pig-to-primate heterotopic cardiac transplantation. In untreated recipient monkeys, these organs survived for 5 days, and for up to 60 days when the recipients were immunosuppressed [23, 24]. Our goal is for the next group of newborn recipients to receive transgenic pig organs. However, transgenic organs expressing complement inhibiting proteins will not affect the induced production of anti-αGal IgG antibodies and their binding to pig endothelium. If these antibodies augment the primate anti-pig cellular response, for example by increasing tissue accumulation of macrophages and NK cells via Fc-CD16 interactions, delayed xenograft rejection will proceed unabated despite transgene expression.

An alternative approach is to modify pig endothelium so that αGal epitopes are either not expressed, or are significantly reduced. Although αGal expression has been successfully eliminated in mice by genetically "knocking out" the enzyme necessary for its manufacture, the technology necessary to similarly manipulate higher mammals is not yet available [25]. Reduction in the number of αGal epitopes may be possible through alteration in its biochemical synthesis. Increased expression of fucosyltransferase in mice is associated with elevated competition for substrate with galactosyltransferase, ultimately leading to significantly decreased levels of endothelial αGal expression [26]. However, it remains to be determined whether the low levels of xenoantigen expressed in such animals can still induce IgG production.

Suppression of Induced Humoral and Cellular Immune Responses Against the Xenograft

Anti-B cell agents, such as azathioprine, cyclophosphamide, 15-deoxyspergualin, brequinar, leflunomide, and mycophenolate mofetil (MMF), have been used to suppress xenoreactve antibodies in experimental models of xenotransplantation. Each agent, in combination with steroids and the anti-T cell agents, cyclosporine or tacrolimus, has extended graft function in various rodent xenotransplantation models from days to weeks [27–32]. We treated one newborn baboon recipient with cyclosporine, cyclophosphamide, and corticosteroids prior to xenotransplantation. The xenograft in this animal survived approximately 6 days, a period over 50 % greater than in untreated recipients. Of particular interest was the observation that post-transplant induced anti-αGal antibody levels were eightfold lower than in untreated recipients. These results are encouraging and suggest that use of these agents is rational. The particular form of cellular rejection which we have described in newborn pig-to-baboon cardiac transplantation appears to be unique to xenogeneic models of transplantation and will require treatment modalities that may differ from those currently used in allotransplantation. These modalities will likely specifically target macrophages and NK cells.

Comment

The severe shortage of human donor hearts, and the limited application of left heart mechanical assist devices (excluding smaller individuals and those with biventricular heart failure), underscore the need for investigative efforts directed toward the clinical application of cardiac xenotransplantation. To date, the major barrier to the use of discordant xenografts in primates has been hyperacute rejection. As a result of the recent success in experimental trials using pig organs transgenically modified to resist lysis by human complement, there is optimism that pig-to-human xenotransplantation may witness formal clinical trials in the next 3–5 years. These trials will likely be patterned after "bridge" trials of mechanical heart assistance and directed toward patients in imminent danger of death for whom a mechanical heart is not an option.

However, our studies of pig cardiac xenotransplantation in newborn baboons, a model of natural antibody depletion, suggest that, before human trials can be contemplated, there are significant barriers of cellular immunity that must be additionally overcome. Of particular concern is a delayed form of rejection that appears to be unique to discordant donor-recipient pairs. This is mediated primarily by recipient macrophages and NK cells, and may be amplified by induced xenoreactive IgG antibodies. Future investigations will need to address the molecular interactions and activation pathways by which these cellular elements initiate the rejection process, and the antigenic determinants against which the response is directed. Detailed understanding of these processes will enable the development of additional rational anti-rejection strategies, enabling xenotransplantation to become a clinical reality.

References

1. Evans RW, Orians CE, Ascher NL: The potential supply of organ donors: An assessment of the efficiency of organ procurement efforts in the United States. JAMA 1993, 267:239
2. Michler RE, Chen JM: Cardiac xenotransplantation: experimental advances, ethical issues, and clinical potential. In Handbook of Cardiac Transplantation.Emery RW, Miller LW (eds). Philadelphia: Hanley and Belfus, 1996:231
3. Levin HR, OZ MC, Chen JM, et al. Reversal of chronic ventricular dilation in patients with end-stage cardiomyopathy by prolonged mechanical unloading. Circulation 1995, 91:2717

4. Xu H, Edwards NM, Dong X, et al. Age-related development of human preformed anti-porcine endothelial cell xenoantibody. J. Thorac. Cardiovasc. Surg. 1995, 110:1023
5. Blakely ML, van der Werf WJ, Berndt MC, et al. Activation of intragraft endothelial and mononuclear cells during discordant xenograft rejection. Transplantation 1994, 10:1059
6. Good, AH, Cooper, DKC, Malcolm, AJ, et al. Identification of carbohydrate structures which bind human anti-porcine antibodies: implications for discordant xenografting in man. Transplant. Proc. 1992, 24:559
7. Ye Y, Neethling FA, Niekrasz M, et al. Evidence that intravenously administered alpha-galactosyl carbohydrates reduce baboon serum cytotoxicity to pig kidney cells (PK15) and transplanted pig hearts. Transplantation 1994, 58:330
8. Collins BH, Cotterell AH, McCurry KR, et al. Cardiac xenografts between primate species provide evidence for the importance of the alpha galactosyl determinant in hyperacute rejection. J. Immunol. 1995, 154:5500
9. Galili U. Evolution and pathophysiology of the human natural anti-alpha-galactosyl IgG (anti-Gal) antibody. Springer Seminars in Immunopathology 1993, 15:155
10. Galili U., Swanson K. Gene sequences suggest in activation of alpha-1,3-galactosyltransferase in catarrhines after the divergence of apes from monkeys. Proc. Natl. Acad. Sci. USA. 1991, 88:7401
11. Xu H, Edwards NM, Chen JM, et al. Newborn baboon serum lacks natural anti-pig xenoantibody. Transplantation 1995, 59:1189
12. Kaplon RJ, Michler RE, Xu H, et al. Absence of hyperacute rejection in newborn pig-to-baboon cardiac xenografts. Transplantation 1995, 59:1
13. Michler RE, Xu H, O'Hair DP, et al. Pig to newborn baboon cardiac xenotransplantation: a model of natural antibody depletion. Transplant Proc. 1996, In press
14. Markmann JF, Barker CF. Basic and clinical considerations in the use of xenografts. Curr. Prob. Surg. 1994, 31:387
15. Rollins SA, Kennedy SP, Chodera AJ, et al. Evidence that activation of human T cells by porcine endothelium involves direct recognition for LFA-1, and CD2. Transplantation 1994, 57:1709
16. Murray AG, Khodadoust MM, Pober JS, Bothwell AL. Porcine aortic endothelial cells activate human T cells: direct presentation of MHC antigens and costimulation by ligands for human CD2 and CD28. Immunity 1994, 1:57
17. Bravery CA, Rose ML, Yacoub MH. Proliferative responses of highly purified human CD4+ T cells to porcine endothelial cells. Transplant. Proc. 1994, 26:1157
18. Itescu S, Wang SF, Minanov O, Xu H, Michler RE. Cellular immunity against pig xenoantigens in humans and baboons. (Abstract) Presented to the International Society for Heart and Lung Transplantation, 1996
19. Inverardi L, Pardi R. Early events in cell-mediated recognition of vascularized xenografts: cooperative interactions between selected lymphocyte subsets and natural antibodies. Immunol. Rev. 1994, 141:71
20. Itescu S, Wang SF, Kwiatkowski P, Minanov O, Michler. Human NK cells are activated by IL-2 to lyse pig endothelial cells, and are inhibited by anti-CD2 Mabs. (Abstract) Presented to the American Society for Transplant Physicians, 1996
21. Hancock WW, Blakely ML, Van der Werf W, Bach FH: Rejection of guinea pig cardiac xenografts post-cobra venom factor therapy is associated with infiltration by mononuclear cells secreting interferon-gamma and diffuse endothelial activation. Transplant. Proc. 1993, 25:2932

22. Thorley BR, McInnes B, Chrisiansen D, McKenzie IFC, Loveland BE: Construction of CD46 minigenes for the production of transgenic mice. Transplant. Proc. 1995, 27: 2177
23. Byrne G, McCurry K, Martin M, Platt J, Logan J. Development and analysis of transgenic pigs expressing the human complement regulatory proteins CD59 and DAF. (Abstract oral 47) Presented at the Third International Congress for Xenotransplantation, Boston. 1995
24. White DJG, Braidley P, J. Dunning, et al. Hearts from pigs transgenic for human DAF are not hyperacutely rejected when xenografted to primates. (Abstract plenary 28) Presented at the Third International Congress on Xenotransplantation, Boston, 1995
25. Tange MJ, Katerelos, Crawford RJ, et al. Analysis of alpha 1,3 galactosyltransferase knockout mice. (Abstract oral 90) Presented at the Third International Congress on Xenotransplantation, Boston, 1995
26. Sandrin MS, Fodor WL, Cohney S, et al. Reduction of the major porcine xenoantigen gal alpha 1,3-Gal by expression of alpha 1,2 fucosyltransferase. (Abstract oral 23) Presented at the Third International Congress for Xenotransplantation, Boston, 1995
27. Schuurman HJ, Joergensen J, Kuipers H, et al. Vascular transplantation of syrian hamster heart into Lewis rat: effect of brequinar, cyclosporin, cobra venom factor, and splenectomy. Transplant. Proc. 1994, 26:1217
28. Xiao F. Chong A, Foster P, et al. Effect of leflunomide in control of acute rejection in hamster-to-rat cardiac xenografts. Transplant. Proc. 1994, 26:1263
29. Lin Y, Sobis H, Vandeputte, M., Waer M: Induction therapy of leflunomide and cyclosporin allows for long-term xenograft survival under cyclosporin alone. Transplant. Proc. 1994, 26:3052
30. Lin Y,Sobis H, Vandeputte M, Waer M: Mechanism of leflunomide-induced prevention of xenoantibody formation and xenograft rejection in the hamster to rat heart transplantation model. Transplant. Proc. 1995, 27:305
31. Cosenza CA, Cramer DV, Tuso PJ, et al. Combination therapy with brequinar sodium and cyclosporine synergistically prolongs hamster-to-rat cardiac xenograft survival. J. Heart Lung Transplant. 1994, 13:489
32. Thomas F, Araneda D, Quarantillo P: Long-term survival of disparate cardiac xenografts: induction of tolerance and humoral accommodation. Transplant. Proc. 1994, 26:1220

37 Total Lymphoid Irradiation – Immunosuppressive Therapy for Xenotransplantation

A.J. Norin

Introduction

A major obstacle to successful xenotransplantation has been the lack of reliable therapeutic methods to inhibit the induction of antibody directed against determinants on macromolecules that differ between species (xenoantibodies, XNA). In this article we summarize our studies utilizing total lymphoid irradiation (TLI) for immunosuppression of xenograft rejection mediated by induced XNA. For purposes of clarity, we define the term " induced XNA" as antibodies that are synthesized as a direct result of interspecies organ, tissue or cell transplantation. "Natural preformed XNA" are distinct from induced XNA in that the former are induced prior to transplantation by exposure to environmental immunogens that have reactive determinants in common with those of the xenograft. In our initial studies with TLI, we employed a concordant xenograft model rather than a discordant model to avoid the difficulty of evaluating an induced XNA response in the presence of preformed XNA [1].

Immunosuppression with fractionated-dose TLI has been utilized for several decades in experimental and clinical settings. Slavin et al. [2] first utilized TLI as pretransplant immunosuppressive therapy, in which long-term survival of murine skin allografts was observed after administration of allogeneic bone marrow from the skin donor. It is presumed that successful skin allograft acceptance was due to the chimeric state of the hematopoetic compartment of the recipients since TLI without bone marrow from the skin donor strain was relatively ineffective. Many investigators have subsequently examined the effect of TLI either alone or in combination with chemical immunosuppressants in experimental and clinical allo- and xeno-transplantation. Excellent results using TLI treatment have been obtained with low-total dose, wide-field irradiation as utilized in our studies. Myburgh and colleagues [3] (Chap. 22) have reported greater than 1-year survival of kidney and liver allografts in baboons treated with TLI alone. Human kidney allograft survival in TLI and cyclosporin A (CsA)-treated patients was 80% at 5 years for all recipients whose panel reactive activity (PRA) was less than 30% [4]. Renal allograft survival was less than 30% at 5 years for patients with a PRA greater than 30%, suggesting the deleterious effect of preformed antibody. Ryanasiewcz et al. [5] observed a synergistic effect of TLI and low-dose CSA in a rabbit cardiac allograft model, and Knechtle et al. [6] observed a similiar effect in a rodent model. Pennock et al. [7], however, failed to detect such an effect in a primate xenograft model, perhaps due to over-immunosuppression.

Synergism of TLI and pharmacologic agents in xenotransplantation is likely morc apparent than in allotransplantation due to poor survival of the former type of grafts with conventional therapy (i.e., therapy that is not effective in suppressing antibody responses) [6, 8–10]. More recently, however, perioperative or postoperative TLI has been used successfully in the treatment of early resistant rejection or recurrent rejection in clinical heart allotransplantation [11, 12] and in experimental heart-lung transplantation [13].

Concordant Xenotransplantation

We studied four groups of baboons that received heterotopic cervical heart xenografts from cynomolgous monkeys *(Macaca fasicularis)* [14, 15]. Group 1 was untreated, group 2 was treated with CsA and methylpredinsolone (MP), group 3 received 8 Gy TLI (1 Gy twice a week for 4 weeks), and group 4 was treated with TLI, CsA, and MP. Mean survival of the concordant cardiac xenografts was 6, 25, 29, and 255 days, respectively, for groups 1–4. Hearts in group 4 survived >77, >108, >142, 184, >480, and 540 days. Two of the latter recipients rejected their grafts, while the other four baboons expired with functioning grafts that had minimal evidence of rejection. Two of these four recipients died of sepsis, one died from a perforated duodenal ulcer, and the other died of unknown causes. Addition of the TLI treatment to CsA + MP immunosuppression, therefore, had a synergistic effect in this preclinical concordant primate model.

Immunohistochemical studies revealed alternate mechanisms of cardiac rejection in CsA + MP-treated versus TLI-treated recipients (i.e., group 2 vs. group 3). In the CsA + MP-treated baboons microscopic evidence of humoral rejection was detected, including mixed cellular infiltrates, edema, hemorrage, thrombosis, and myocyte necrosis. Additionally, IgM and complement (C3 and C4) were detected on frozen sections of the monkey heart xenografts. In contrast, sections of cardiac tissue from TLI only-treated recipients (group 3) demonstrated evidence of cell-mediated rejection, i.e., infiltrates of mononuclear cells without hemorrage and thrombosis. IgM, C3, and C4 were not detected on cardiac tissue of TLI only-treated baboons. Further evidence of humoral cardiac rejection in CsA + MP-treated baboons was demonstrated by the detection of high levels of anti-monkey XNA (1>1:256). TLI only-treated recipients had low levels of anti-monkey XNA (titer, <1:8). Recipients treated with TLI only or with TLI + CsA + MP that experienced rejection had high levels of intragraft cytolytic lymphocytes (20 % and 40 % cytotoxicity, respectively) at necroscopy providing additional evidence for a predominately cell-mediated rather than a humorally mediated mechanism of rejection. TLI + CsA + MP-treated recipients had no histologic evidence of rejection on biopsies obtained up to 100 days after transplantation and no evidence of anti-monkey XNA at that time. The two animals that rejected their monkey xenografts at 184 and 540 days had evidence of cell-mediated rejection on microscopic examination of heart specimens, while the other recipients had little evidence of rejection at their deaths.

Previous studies of the mechanism of concordant xenograft rejection had been contradictory, some suggesting a cell-mediated mechanism ([13–15], while others suggesting that humoral mechanisms predominate [6]. Our studies and those of other investigators have clarified this matter. Firstly, rodent skin grafts are only susceptible to antibody-mediated rejection after vascularization, and therefore may be rejected by a cellular mechanism before induction of XNA [16, 17]. Secondly, we demonstrated in a vascularized concordant primate model that antibody-mediated rejection phenomena predominate in recipients that receive potent anti-T cell therapy but ineffective anti-B cell therapy [14, 15].

Prior to our studies [14, 15, 21] it had not been possible with standard pharmacologic immunosuppression to prolong concordant xenograft survival in primates to a duration that would be useful in human organ transplantation. These reports suggested that the early destruction of concordant primate heart xenografts in recipients treated with pharmacologic agents only (e.g., CsA) is likely due to inability of this therapy to adequately suppress the high levels of XNA produced after transplantation. The addition of TLI to the chemical immunosuppressive regimen had a synergistic effect in that cardiac xenograft survival was increased 20-fold compared with either treatment alone. The prolongation of xenograft survival was associated with significantly lower levels of serum XNA. The decreased level of serum XNA was not merely due to its adsorption by the transplanted organ, since monkey-specific antibodies could not be detected on cardiac tissue of TLI or TLI + CsA + MP-treated recipients. Furthermore, low serum XNA titers were not the result of the presence of noncomplement-fixing antimonkey antibodies as only low levels of serum IgM and IgG were detected in monkey lymphocyte-binding assays utilizing fluorescence-activated flow cytometry [14]. Finally, the TLI + CsA + MP-treated recipients did not exhibit clinical signs of generalized B cell immunodeficiency and had normal Ig levels [15]. These latter findings are in agreement with previous studies showing relatively intact humoral immunity in transplant recipients given low cumulative doses of TLI (8 Gy) [22]. Animals and humans receiving higher cumulative doses (20–34 Gy) have exhibited reduced humoral immune responses [23, 24]. While the above results in the recipients of low-dose TLI + CsA + MP are consistent with an inability to mount a specific anti-monkey XNA response, further studies on the response to third-party antigens would provide confirmation of this hypothesis.

The mechanism(s) by which TLI prevented a XNA response is not clear. The reduced level of XNA may occur by a direct effect of the immunosuppressive therapy on B cells, particularly IgM-secreting cells, to produce a specific state of nonresponsiveness [14]. Another possibility is that TLI may indirectly induce nonreactivity of B cells through its effects on T cells which regulate humoral responses. Previous reports have demonstrated reduced B cell responses to nominal antigens in animals and humans following TLI, although a period of unresponsiveness to these antigens has not been reported [23–25]. In rheumatoid arthritis patients and in mice treated with TLI, reduced T cell-dependent B cell responses with normal or elevated T-independent B cell reactivity were observed [23]. Other investigators have reported a reduction in in vitro B cell responses to T-independent antigens in TLI-treated mice [25]. In the latter study, antibodies to diphtheria and tetanus toxoids decreased twofold after TLI therapy, and did not rise significantly after booster innoculation. The hyporeactive period lasted for approximately 20 days after the last dose of irradiation and may have been due to unresponsiveness in immature $IgM^{(+)}$, $IgD^{(-)}$ cell populations that repopulate the spleen of TLI-treated recipients. In addition, adherent suppressor cells were described that may contribute to B cell hyporesponsiveness in TLI-treated recipients [25]. It is possible that the presence of a large sustained source of xenoantigen (i.e., the cardiac graft) immediately following TLI is important in promoting a nonreactive state in the B cell and/or T helper cell compartments [26–29]. It is clear, however, that substantial T cell reactivity develops against the monkey xenograft in the fourth week after low-dose TLI, since CsA therapy is essential in preventing the cytolytic lymphocyte (CTL and activated NK)-mediated rejection that occurs during this period [15]. Furthermore, relatively normal in vitro cytolytic responses to xenoantigens in mixed lymphocyte culture (MLC) were generated in lymphocytes from TLI-treated recipient lymphocytes 1 month following xenotransplantation. TLI combined with bone marrow transplantation, as has been demonstrated in murine allotransplantation models [2], has not as yet been studied for induction of tolerence in concordant primate xenograft models.

Discordant (Swine-to-Primate) Xenotransplantation

Because of the encouraging results obtained in preventing the early loss of concordant monkey hearts in the baboon from induced XNA, we investigated the effect of TLI in a discordant swine-to-baboon cardiac xenograft model. Baboons were treated with TLI and CsA + MP, as described above. Specific absorption of XNA was performed just prior to surgery by either (a) continous hemoperfusion (HP) through a porcine spleen or (b) continous membrane plasmaphoresis and perfusion through a porcine spleen/liver (MPP) [30, 31]. Xenografts survived 6, 8, and 15 days in the HP group and 1, 7, and 8 days in the MP group, both groups significantly longer than untreated controls (less than 2 h) [32, 33]. Serial analysis of the level of serum XNA (a) before transplantation, (b) after absorption by donor species organ perfusion, and (c) at various times after transplantation, was performed. Pretransplant XNA titers generally were in the 1:128 to 1:256 range. XNA titers as assessed by CDC in the hemoperfused recipients were reduced following the latter procedure and remained below the level of the pretransplant titer even on the day of rejection. XNA levels as assessed by flow cytometry were initially lowered by the MP technique, but frequently increased by the following day [30, 33]. The initial rise in titer after donor organ perfusion is likely due to equilibration with XNA from the extravascular space [30].

The effect of the timing of donor organ perfusion relative to the time of transplantation on elevation of XNA (IgG) was studied. Recipients that received MPP 1–7 days before transplantation had a more than eightfold increase in peak IgG XNA more than 6 days after transplantation. Recipients that received MPP on the day of transplantation had a zero to twofold increase in IgG XNA. MPP treatment without organ transplantation was a sensitizing event with XNA titers increasing 30- to 100-fold. TLI had no effect on preexisting anti-porcine XNA titers, but clearly prevented the induction of exceedingly high levels(>1:2000) of XNA in the presence of a cardiac xenograft. In contrast, porcine antigen shed from perfused organs without transplantation or perfusion 1 day before transplantation induced a high XNA titer, even though TLI had been administered. These results suggest an interaction between the altered immune response (due to TLI) and the presence of a vascularized xenograft, resulting in inhibition of the humoral response. This effect is apparently negated by exposure of the recipient to porcine antigens as little as 24 h before xenotransplantation.

Comment

In summary, TLI-treated baboons receiving heterotopic monkey heart xenotransplants have demonstrated a lack of an induced XNA response as long as a well-functioning vascularized graft is present. At first it may be somewhat surprising to observe a similar effect of TLI in the discordant swine-to-baboon model as in the concordant monkey-to-baboon model, i.e., inhibition of induced XNA. The humoral immune response of a baboon to a porcine graft is nevertheless likely to be a primary response rather than a secondary one. Though the antigenic determinants on porcine proteins (Galα1–3Gal residues) that react with natural XNA [34, 35] are the same as on the putative immunogen of bacterial origin, the carrier molecules are dissimilar. The baboon's immune system is therefore naive to the Galα1–3 galactosylated porcine proteins, and thus a primary response is induced as a result of an organ transplant. The results of our studies [15, 30–33] support the above hypothesis, suggesting that appropriately timed TLI may prevent the induced XNA response following discordant transplants between swine and primate species.

Three major obstacles to successful transplantation of discordant swine organs into humans are presently known: (1) hyperacute rejection mediated by anti-Gal α1–3Gal antibodies and complement, (2) acute rejection mediated by induced XNA and complement, and (3) rejection mediated by activated NK cells and T lymphocytes, in particular CTL [36, 37]. In future studies we will determine whether TLI in combination with anti-T cell pharmacologic agents, such as CsA or FK506, will prevent an induced XNA response to swine organs that express human transgenes (which inhibit hyperacute rejection) [38–41].

Acknowledgments. The author gratefully acknowledges the participation of past and present members of the SUNY-Health Science Center at Brooklyn Xenotransplant Research Program: R. Brewer, M. Del Rio, M. Roslin, A. Panza, R. Tranbaugh, M. Coons, Y.D. Kim, T. Chang, J. Cunningham, M. Vaynblatt T. Brown, Q. Liu, D. Hochman, R. Mushnitsky, S. Kamholz, Z. Zisbrod, J. Burack I. Alexandropoulos, M. Sadeghian, C. Chen, A. Strashun, G. Grijalva, and N. Lawson. We appreciate the support of the Foundation for Surgical Education and Research, Maimonides Research and Development Foundation, The Brooklyn Medical Foundation, and USPHS Grant CA47548 and our enjoyable collaboration with colleagues at Alexion Pharmaceuticals, Inc., New Haven, CT.

References

1. Calne RY, Organ transplantation between widely disparate species. Transplant Proc 1970; 2:550
2. Slavin S. Strober S, Fuks S, et al. Induction of specific transplantation tolerance using fractionated total lymphoid irradiation in adult mice: long term survival of allogeneic bone marrow and skin grafts. J. Exp Med 1977; 146:34
3. Myburgh JA, Smit JA, Stark JH, Browde S. Total lymphoid irradiation in kidney and liver transplantation in the baboon: prolonged graft survival and alterations in T cell subsets with low cumulative dose regimens. J. Immunol 1984; 132: 1019
4. Myburgh JA, Meyers AM, Margolies L, et al. Total lymphoid irradiation in clinical renal transplantation: results in 73 patients. Transplant Proc 1991; 23: 2033
5. Ryanasiewicz JJ, Sutherland DET, Kawahara K, Kim T, Najarian JS. Total lymphoid irradiation in rat heart allografts: dose fractionization and combination with cyclosporine A. Transplant Proc 1981; 13:452
6. Knechtle SJ, Halperin WC, Bollinger RR. Xenograft survival in two species combinations using total lymphoid irradiation and cyclosporine. Transplantation 1987; 43:173
7. Pennock JJ, Reitz BA, Bieber CP, et al. Survival of primates following orthotopic cardiac transplantation treated with total lymphoid irradiation and chemical immune suppression. Transplantation 1981; 32: 467
8. Reichenspurner H, Human PA, Boehm DH, et al. Optimalization of immunosuppression after xenogeneic heart transplantation in primates. J Heart Transplant 1989; 8: 200
9. Sachs DH, Bach FH. Immunology of xenograft rejection. Hum Immunol 1990; 28: 245
10. Platt J, Vercellotti GM, Dalmasso AP, et al. Transplantation of discordant xenografts: a review of progress. (Commentary by Auchincloss H Jr.) Immunol Today 1990; 11: 450
11. Evans MA, Schomberg PJ, Rodeheffer RH, et al. Total lymphoid irradiation: a novel and successful therapy for resistant cardiac allograft rejection. Mayo Clin. Proc 67: 785. 1992
12. Salter SP, Salter MM, Kirklin JK, Bourge RC. Total lymphoid irradiation in the treatment of early or recurrent heart transplant rejection. Int J. Radiat Oncol Biol Phys 33:83 1995
13. Sadeghi AM, Laks H, Drinkwater DC, Pearl JM et al. Heart-lung xenotransplantation in primates. J. Heart Lung Transplant 10:442, 1991
14. Norin AJ, Roslin MS, Panza A, et al. TLI induces specific B cell unresponsiveness and long-term monkey heart xenograft survival in cyclosporine treated baboons. Transplant Proc 1992; 24:508
15. Roslin MS, Tranbaugh RE, Panza A, et al. One year monkey heart xenograft survival in cyclosporine treated baboons. Transplantation 54: 949, 1992
16. Manning DD, Reed ND, Shaffer CF, et al. Maintenance of skin xenografts of widely divergent phylogenetic origin on congenitally athymic (nude) mice. J. Exp Med 1973; 138: 488
17. Steinbruchel D, Kemp E, Starklint H, et al. Synergistic effect of cyclosporine A, cyclophosphamide and steroids in rabbit-to-rat skin xenotransplantation. Transplant Proc 1987; 19: 1168
18. Thomas FT, Marchman W, Carrobi A, et al. Immunobiology of the xenograft response: xenograft rejection in immunodeficient animals. Transplant Proc 1991; 23: 208

19. Baldamus CA, McKenzie IFC, Winn HJ, et al. Acute destruction by humoral antibody of rat skin grafted to mice. J Immunol 1973; 110: 1532
20. Bogman MJJT, Berden JHM, Hageman JFHM, et al. Patterns of vascular damage in the antibody mediated rejection of skin xenografts in the mouse. Am J Pathol 1980; 100: 727
21. Panza, A, Roslin M, Coons M, et al. Successful cardiac xenogeneic transplantation in primates using total lymphoid irradiation. Eur J. Cardio Thorac Surg 1991; 5:161
22. Myburg JA, Smit JA, Meyers AM, et al. Total lymphoid irradiation in renal transplantation. World J Surg 1986; 10:369
23. Tanay A, Strober S, Logue GL, Schiffman G. Use of total lymphoid irradiation (TLI) in studies of the T cell-dependence of autoantibody production in rheumatioid arthritis. J Immunol 1984; 132:1036
24. Tanay A, Strober S. Opposite effects of total lymphoid irradiation. J Immunol 1984; 132: 979
25. May RD, Slavin S, Vitetta ES. The partial characterization of suppressor cells in the spleens of mice conditioned with fractionated total lymphoid irradiation (TLI). J Immunol 1983; 131: 1108
26. Katz DH, Benacerraf B. Reversible and irreversible B cell tolerance: distinguishing properties and mechanisms. In: Katz DH, Benacerraf C. eds. Immunological Tolerance: Mechanisms and Potential Therapeutic Applications.New York: Academic, 1974: p. 249
27. Teale JM, Klinman NR. Induction of self-tolerance in mature peripheral B lymphocytes. Nature 1980; 288:385
28. Goodnow CC, Crosbie J, Jorgenson H, et al. Induction of self -tolerance in mature peripheral B lymphocytes. Nature 1989; 342: 385
29. Smith CA, Williams GT, Kingston R, et al. Antibodies to CD3/T cell receptor complex induce death by apoptosis in immature T cells in thymic. Nature 1989; 337: 181
30. Brewer RJ, Del Rio MJ, Roslin MS, et al. Depletion of preformed antibody in primates for discordant xenotransplantation by continuous donor organ plasma perfusion. Transplant Proc 1993; 385:386
31. Brewer RJ, Del Rio, MJ, Vaynblat M, et al. Adsorption of xenoantibodies for cardiac xenotransplantation in total lymphoid irradiation – treated baboons. Transplant Proc 1994; 1355:1356
32. Brewer RJ, Roslin MS, Del Rio MJ, et al. Prevention of induced antibody response in discordant cardiac xenotransplantation: role of the graft in total lymphoid irradiation-treated recipients. Transplant Proc 1994; 1351:1352
33. Roslin MS, Zisbrod Z, Burack JH, et al. 15-day survival in pig-to-baboon heterotopic cardiac xenotransplantation. Transplant Proc 1992; 572:573
34. Good AH, Cooper DKC, Malcolm AJ, et al. Identification of carbohydrate structures which bind human anti-porcine antibodies: implications for discordant xenografting in man. Transplant Proc 1992; 24:559
35. Sandrin MS, Vaughan HA, Dabkowski PL, McKenzie IFC. Anti-pig antibodies in serum react predominantly with Galα1–3Gal epitopes . Proc Natl Acad Sci USA 1993; 90: 11391
36. Norin AJ, Kamholz SL, Pinsker KL, et al. Cyclosporine-induced tolerance in experimental organ transplantation: evidence of diminished donor-specific cytotoxicity relative to donor-specific proliferative response. J Immunol 1987; 139:332
37. Norin AJ, Kamholz SL. Evidence of intragraft interleukin-2 activated killer cells and allospecific cytolytic T lymphocytes in rejecting lung allografts. Transplantation 1989; 48: 856

38. McCurry KR, Kooyman DL, Alvarado CG, et al. Human complement regulatory proteins protect swine – to- primate cardiac xenografts from humoral injury. Nature Med 1995; 1: 403
39. Carrington CA, Richards AC, Cozzi E, et al. Expression of DAF and MCP on pig endothelial cells protects from human complement. Transplant Proc 27; 319, 1995
40. Fodor WL, Williams BL, Matis LA, et al. Expression of a functional human complement inhibitor in a transgenic pig as a model for the prevention of xenogeneic hyperacute organ rejection . Proc Natl Acad Sci USA 1994; 91: 11153
41. Norin AJ, Brewer RJ, Lawson N, et al. Enhanced survival of porcine endothelialized PTFE vascular grafts and porcine lung xenografts in primates expressing human CD 59. Transplant Proc. In press

38 Xenogeneic Tolerance Through Hematopoietic Cell and Thymic Transplantation

M. Sykes and D.H. Sachs

Introduction

Induction of donor-specific tolerance would be desirable and might even be essential to the success of clinical xenotransplantation for several reasons:

1. It would eliminate the risk of acute or chronic rejection. Chronic rejection currently leads to eventual graft loss in a high percentage of allograft recipients, despite recent improvements in immunosuppressive therapy. In view of the frequently greater difficulty that is encountered in attenuating xenoresponses than alloresponses [1], it seems likely that both acute and chronic rejection might be a major limitation to xenogeneic organ transplantation, even if the initial natural antibody-induced hyperacute rejection problem could be overcome.
2. A state of tolerance would obviate the need for chronic imunosuppressive therapy with its attendant risks of opportunistic infection, malignancy and organ toxicity.

The tolerance approach might be most readily applied to xenotransplantation, since the use of xenogeneic donors provides the opportunity for obtaining tolerance-inducing cell populations (e.g., bone marrow) from the donor, then waiting for the recipient to recover from the procedure with a tolerant immune system, followed by grafting with a solid organ from the same donor. In addition, the potential for generating fully inbred xenograft donors (e.g., miniature swine) provides the possibility of using an unlimited source of genetically homogeneous tissue whenever required for maintenance of the tolerant state. Furthermore, xenogeneic donors could potentially be modified using gene therapy to facilitate the ability to induce tolerance to xenoantigens.

In this review, we shall discuss two approaches to inducing central tolerance to xenogeneic donors. The first involves the use of xenogeneic hematopoietic cell transplantation to induce a state of mixed chimerism. The second involves host thymectomy followed by replacement with a xenogeneic donor thymus after depletion of the pre-existing peripheral T cell repertoire.

Non-myeloablative Conditioning Regimen Allowing Induction of Mixed Xenogeneic Chimerism

Rationale for the Mixed Chimerism Approach

The use of xenogeneic bone marrow transplantation (BMT) may provide an approach to the induction of specific tolerance toward a xenogeneic organ donor, while preserving otherwise normal immune function. Numerous studies in allogeneic animal models have demonstrated that specific transplantation tolerance can be produced by transplanting hematopoietic cells across full major histocompatibility (MHC) barriers [2–8]. However, it has not yet been possible to use this approach to the induction of transplantation tolerance in humans, largely due to the unacceptable nonhematopoietic toxicity associated with myeloablative conditioning regimens, the excessive risk of graft-versus-host disease (GVHD) in HLA-mismatched transplantation [9], and the difficulty in achieving bone marrow engraftment across major histocompatibility barriers. The latter difficulties have presented major limitations to the use of clinical bone marrow allotransplantation [10,11], and, as illustrated below, resistance to reconstitution by xenogeneic hematopoietic cells may be even greater than that observed for allogeneic hematopoietic cells.

The use of lethal whole body irradiation (WBI) and BMT has also been shown to permit induction of transplantation tolerance across concordant xenogeneic barriers in rodent models [3, 12–15]. The clinical applicability of this approach is also limited by the toxicity of preparative regimens [16, 17], by GVHD [9, 18, 19], and by difficulties in achieving marrow engraftment [11, 20, 21]. Therefore, if BMT is to be a useful method of inducing transplantation tolerance in the clinical setting, it will be essential to develop conditioning regimens which specifically target those host elements which resist marrow engraftment, rather than to use regimens which nonspecifically destroy proliferating cells such as hematopoietic stem cells and gut epithelium. Furthermore, it will be important to develop means of achieving xenoengraftment without GVHD. Elimination of GVHD-producing T cells in bone marrow has been associated with an increased incidence of failure of engraftment of allogeneic marrow in both clinical [20, 22, 23] and experimental [24, 25] studies.

An additional obstacle must be addressed when considering bone marrow transplantation across complete histocompatibility barriers (allogeneic or xenogeneic). Since MHC restriction specificity is determined by host thymic epithelial cells during the time when T cells are regenerating post-BMT [26], a source of antigen-presenting cells (APC) bearing the same host MHC phenotype is required to present antigen effectively in the periphery. Since such peripheral APC are bone marrow-derived, they will eventually consist only of donor-type cells in fully allogeneic or fully xenogeneic chimeras. Thus, a state of immunoincompetence would exist, since the restricting elements required to present antigen to host-restricted T cells would be absent from the periphery [27]. One way of circumventing this difficulty would be to provide a source of host-type BMC and thus produce a mixed chimera, so that a continuous source of host-type APC is provided. Indeed, superior immunocompetence has been demonstrated in mixed allogeneic chimeras compared to fully allogeneic chimeras prepared across complete MHC barriers [26–30]. Thus preparation of mixed xenogeneic chimeras might be an optimal approach to the use of BMT for the induction of transplantation tolerance across species barriers.

Non-myeloablative Regimen Permitting Induction of Mixed Xenogeneic Chimerism

Recent studies have demonstrated that mixed chimerism and transplantation tolerance can be induced across complete allogeneic MHC barriers in mice using a relatively nontoxic, non-myeloablative preparative regimen. This regimen involves elimination of host T lymphocytes by in vivo administration of monoclonal antibodies (mAbs) specific for $CD4^+$ and $CD8^+$ T cells, followed by a low dose (3 Gy) of WBI and a higher dose (7 Gy) of local irradiation to the thymus [31]. We have extended this approach to a xenogeneic rat→mouse species combination using the modified conditioning regimen shown in Fig. 1 [32]. This regimen was similar to that used for allogeneic mixed chimerism, except that mAbs against host Thy1-positive cells and against the natural killer (NK) cell marker NK1.1 were added to the preparative regimen. When T cell-depleted (TCD) rat

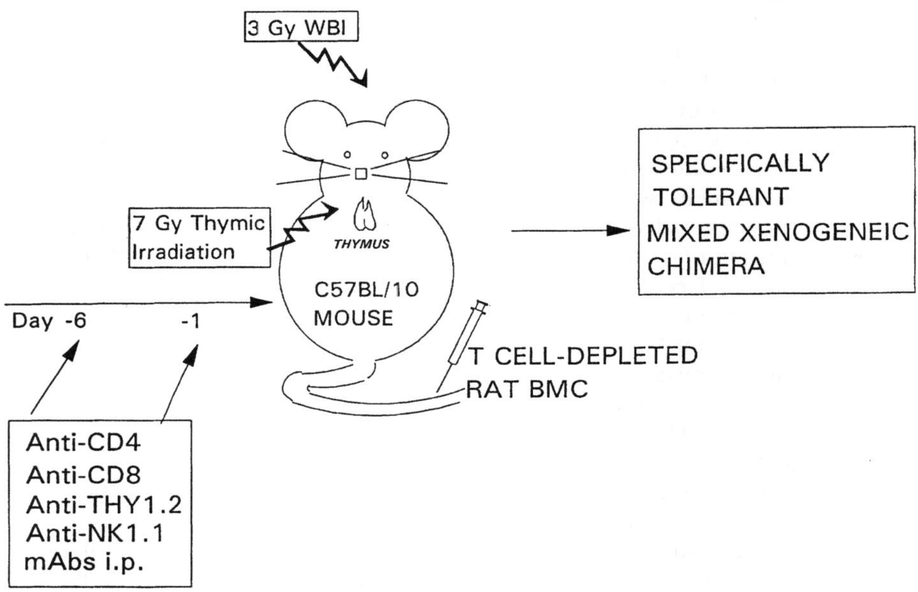

Fig. 1. Method for producing mixed xenogeneic (rat→mouse) chimeras using a non-myeloablative conditioning regimen. Each mouse received 6×10^7 rat bone marrow cells that were T cell depleted as described [32]. *WBI*, whole body irradiation; *BMC*, bone marrow cell; *NK*, natural killer; *mAbs*, monoclonal antibodies

marrow was administered to mice conditioned as shown in Fig. 1, mixed chimerism and specific transplantation tolerance were successfully induced [32]. T cell depletion of rat marrow was essential in order to avoid the development of GVHD in this model. Thus our regimen achieves the goal of allowing the engraftment of TCD rat marrow without GVHD.

A comparison of the host conditioning required to achieve allogeneic versus xenogeneic marrow engraftment suggests that NK cells may play a more important role in resisting rat marrow engraftment than in resisting allogeneic marrow engraftment in mice. Recent studies suggest that a major mechanism by which NK cells are prevented from killing "self" targets is the transmission of inhibitory signals through NK cell surface molecules that recognize specific class I MHC determinants [33, 34]. Since recognition of some, even fully allogeneic, class I molecules appears to lead to reduced NK activity compared to that observed for cells deficient in class I expression [34, 35], it seems possible that the greater disparity of xenogeneic MHC molecules than allogeneic MHC molecules could lead to a greater role for NK cells in rejecting xenografts than allografts.

The reason that anti-Thy1.2 mAb treatment is so important to the achievement of rat marrow engraftment in mice is unclear. It is possible that $CD4^-CD8^-$ $\alpha\beta$ T cell receptor $(TCR)^+$ or $\gamma\delta$T cells may play a role in resisting rat marrow engraftment. $CD4^-CD8^-$ $\alpha\beta TCR^+$ T cells expressing the NK cell-associated molecule NK1.1 may resist allogeneic marrow engraftment in a specificity pattern that resembles that of NK cell-mediated resistance [36–38]. Murine $\gamma\delta$T cells have recently been shown to be capable of mediating cytotoxicity against normal rat target cells [39]. We are currently evaluating the role of both of these cell types in resisting rat marrow engraftment in mice.

Recent studies in the allogeneic model have demonstrated that lasting multilineage chimerism and donor-specific tolerance can be achieved when thymic irradiation is omitted from the conditioning regimen if additional injections of anti-T cell mAbs are given prior to BMT (i.e., mAbs are administered on days -6 and -1 with respect to BMT) [40]. Similarly, we have observed no difference in the level of chimerism in mice receiving rat BMT after treatment with a similar regimen to that shown in Fig. 1, except that thymic irradiation is omitted [41]. These results suggest that, if this approach were to be applied clinically, toxicity of the conditioning regimen might be further reduced by the omission of thymic irradiation.

Donor-Specific T Cell Tolerance in Mixed Xenogeneic Chimeras

Mixed xenogeneic rat→mouse chimeras show markedly prolonged donor-specific rat skin graft survival. Non-donor type rat skin grafts are rapidly rejected, indicating that the chimeras are immunocompetent, and are specifically tolerant to the bone marrow donor [32] (Fig. 2). In vitro studies demonstrating long-term donor-specific mixed lymphocyte reaction (MLR) and cell-mediated lympholysis (CML) tolerance for at least 1 year following BMT confirm the existence of a state of donor-specific tolerance in these mice. However, donor-specific skin grafts are often eventually chronically rejected in these animals. This rejection probably

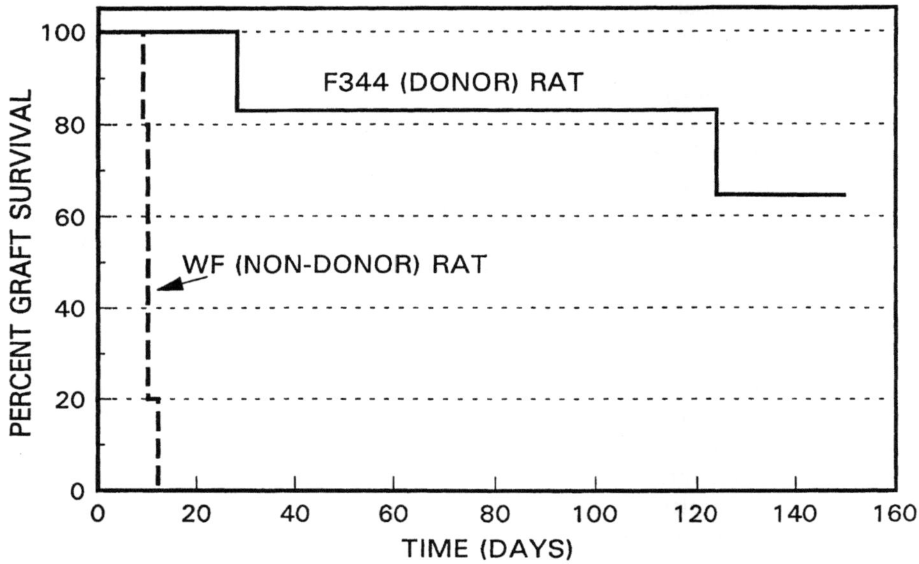

Fig. 2. Survival of donor-type (*solid line*, F344) and non-donor type (*dashed line*, WF) rat skin grafts placed 4 months after bone marrow transplant in rat→mouse chimeras prepared with the regimen shown in Fig. 1

reflects recognition of skin-specific antigens, since, even after this rejection has occurred, specific unresponsiveness to donor antigens expressed on lymphohematopoietic cells is still observed in vitro (B. Nikolic et al., unpublished data).

The capacity of hematopoietic tissue to induce tolerance results in large part from the ability of bone marrow-derived cells in the thymus to induce clonal deletion of developing thymocytes with T cell receptors that recognize their antigens [5, 42–45], resulting in the generation of a T cell repertoire that is tolerant of the hematopoietic cell donor. Several marrow-derived cell types, including dendritic cells [46], B cells [47], and thymocytes [44], have been shown to have the capacity to induce intrathymic deletional tolerance. Tolerance induction in the allogeneic BMT model upon which the xenogeneic regimen is based has been shown to be due primarily to an intrathymic deletional mechanism following depletion of the majority of preexisting peripheral T cells [45]. Active suppression or anergy does not appear to play a significant role in the maintenance of tolerance in these animals. Maintenance of this state is dependent upon the continued presence of donor antigen in the thymus, which continues to generate new T cells for most of the life of the chimera [74]. Clonal deletion of donor-reactive host thymocytes is apparent at the time when thymic regeneration first occurs post-BMT, and is associated with the early intrathymic appearance of donor class II MHC-bearing cells with dendritic morphology [45, 48]. In addition, a small population of residual host T cells that escapes antibody-mediated depletion in the periphery may be tolerized by an anergy mechanism when donor marrow is transplanted [45].

Similar to the allogeneic model, tolerance in our rat→mouse chimeras probably results primarily from initial ablation of the existing T cell repertoire with mAbs, followed by intrathymic generation of a new T cell repertoire that is tolerized by a clonal deletion mechanism. Studies of recipient T cell families using particular Vβ genes (Vβ5 and Vβ11) provide evidence for clonal deletion as a major mechanism of tolerance induction and maintenance in these rat-mouse chimeras [41]. Concomitant with the observed deletion of these Vβ families, rat class II$^+$ cells with dendritic morphology are detectable in the thymi of chimeric, tolerant mice (H. Lei et al., unpublished data). These results suggest that rat marrow-derived cells participate in negative selection in the thymus. Since rats are not known to encode endogenous superantigens in their genomes that could account for the observed deletion of Vβ families in chimeras, and the murine recipients were unable to express the class II MHC antigens required to present superantigens that would lead to deletion of these Vβ, we believe that deletion is due to the presentation of endogenous superantigens encoded in the mouse genome by rat class II molecules on rat APC that enter the host thymus. However, as chimerism disappears from the thymi of these animals, recipient T cells expressing Vβ5 and Vβ11 eventually appear in the thymus and periphery of the mice. In spite of this failure of deletional tolerance after the eventual loss of intrathymic chimerism in long-term chimeras, CML tolerance and skin graft prolongation persist (B. Nikolic et al., unpublished data).

Humoral Tolerance in Mixed Xenogeneic Chimeras

Mixed chimeras do not show a significant IgG antibody response to the donor, even after eventual rejection of a donor-specific skin graft [49]. Anti-rat antibodies were not detected even at late time points when chimerism had completely or almost completely disappeared from peripheral blood [32, 49]. In contrast, rat skin grafting led to immunization and development of a marked IgG response in control mice receiving conditioning without BMT [49]. Since IgG responses are largely T cell-dependent, these observations provide further evidence for T cell tolerance in mixed xenogeneic chimeras, even as the level of xenogeneic donor repopulation declines.

We have recently demonstrated that sera of normal, untreated mice contain natural IgM antibodies that are cytotoxic for rat BMC but not for rat spleen cells [50]. Using adoptive transfer of normal serum to SCID mice, we obtained evidence that natural antibodies (NAb) can significantly impede rat marrow engraftment [51]. Since initial chimerism and transplantation tolerance can be induced in the rat→mouse species combination using BMT, the type of natural antibodies we have detected clearly do not prevent marrow engraftment. However, this does not imply that NAb do not reduce the level of engraftment of rat BMC, and, indeed, their presence might explain the large numbers of rat BMC which are required in order to achieve engraftment in mice [3, 12, 31, 32].

In view of our observation that normal mouse serum contained "rat BMC-specific" NAb, we considered the possibility that these NAb were responsible for the gradual loss of chimerism in mixed xenogeneic chimeras. However, the results of our studies argue against this possibility, and actually suggest that xenogeneic chimerism may be associated with a state of tolerance among natural antibody-forming B cells. The level of donor bone marrow-reactive IgM antibodies was markedly lower in mixed xenogeneic chimeras than in similarly conditioned non-BMT controls [49, 52]. This reduction was not likely due to absorption by rat hematopoietic cells, as it persisted even as the level of chimerism declined [52]. Furthermore, donor cells that were not coated with NAb could be detected in the blood of long-term chimeras, in which the reduction in NAb levels persisted. The observation that induction of mixed xenogeneic chimerism appear to tolerize NAb-forming B cells suggests a novel approach to overcoming the NAb problem which presents a major obstacle to vascularized discordant xenografts. If mixed chimerism could be established well before the time of solid organ grafting, a state of NAb tolerance might obviate the requirement for absorption procedures, and most importantly, would assure life-long freedom from antibody-mediated rejection.

Since swine are excellent potential xenogeneic organ donors for humans (see below), we recently evaluated the potential of swine marrow to induce NAb tolerance for determinants expressed on swine endothelial cells. Absorption studies indicated that most human NAb target antigens expressed on swine endothelial cells are also shared by swine BMC and their progeny [53]. Thus, induction of mixed swine → human chimerism might not only induce cellular tolerance, but could also induce tolerance among NAb-forming B cells and eliminate the risk of hyperacute rejection when solid organ transplantation from swine donors was subsequently performed.

NAb-producing B cell tolerance may be due to cross-linking of Ig receptors on these B cells by donor antigens, resulting in apoptosis, as has been shown in a model in which $CD5^+$ B cells of Ig receptor-transgenic mice make autoantibody against their red blood cells [54]. Furthermore, it is possible that the 3 Gy WBI used in our conditioning regimen depletes a significant fraction of NAb-producing B cells. Since substantial levels of rat-reactive NAb recover in animals receiving conditioning without rat BMT, it is clear that, if these B cells are depleted by irradiation, progenitor cells capable of replacing them are present in the adult recipients. If mature NAb-producing B cells are in fact depleted by the conditioning regimen in BMT recipients, recovering donor-reactive B cells may be deleted at an early developmental stage due to the presence of membrane-bound antigen on rat marrow-derived cells.

In summary, these results demonstrate a lack of humoral immunity against donor antigens during the period when chimerism declines and following skin grafting in mice preconditioned with the complete tolerizing mAb regimen. Thus it is unlikely that antibody mediates either bone marrow graft failure or skin graft rejection in these mice. Together, our results suggest a persistence of specific cellular tolerance in these mice to antigens expressed on bone marrow-derived cells, despite the gradual loss of chimerism. Importantly, they also suggest that a state of mixed xenogeneic chimerism could lead to a state of NAb tolerance toward the donor, thus providing a new approach to avoiding hyperacute rejection.

Competitive Advantage for Host Hematopoiesis in Xenogeneic Bone Marrow Transplant Recipients

Despite the evidence for lasting T cell and B cell tolerance described above, the level of rat hematopoietic reconstitution gradually declines in chimeras prepared with the non-myeloablative regimen shown in Fig. 1, and rat cells are sometimes undetectable by flow cytometry by 6–12 months following BMT [32] (Fig. 3). However, donor-specific cellular and humoral tolerance are still observed in studies performed as late as 1–1.5 years post-BMT (B. Nikolic, unpublished data). In addition, a second injection of donor-type rat bone marrow cells to chimeras receiving 3 Gy WBI 5 months after the initial BMT resulted in a significant boost in the level of rat hematopoietic repopulation (Fig. 3) and did not induce a significant anti-donor antibody [55] or CML response (B. Nikolic, unpublished data). This boost in chimerism prolongs the period during which deletion of $V\beta5^+$ and $V\beta11^+$ cells is observed [55]. We therefore believe that donor-specific T cell tolerance is maintained during the period when donor-type reconstitution declines.

To address the possibility that the gradual loss of donor repopulation was due to rejection by recipient NK cells, we compared long-term chimerism in control chimeras and animals receiving chronic murine NK cell depletion with anti-NK1.1 mAb. The two groups showed no discernable difference in the rate of

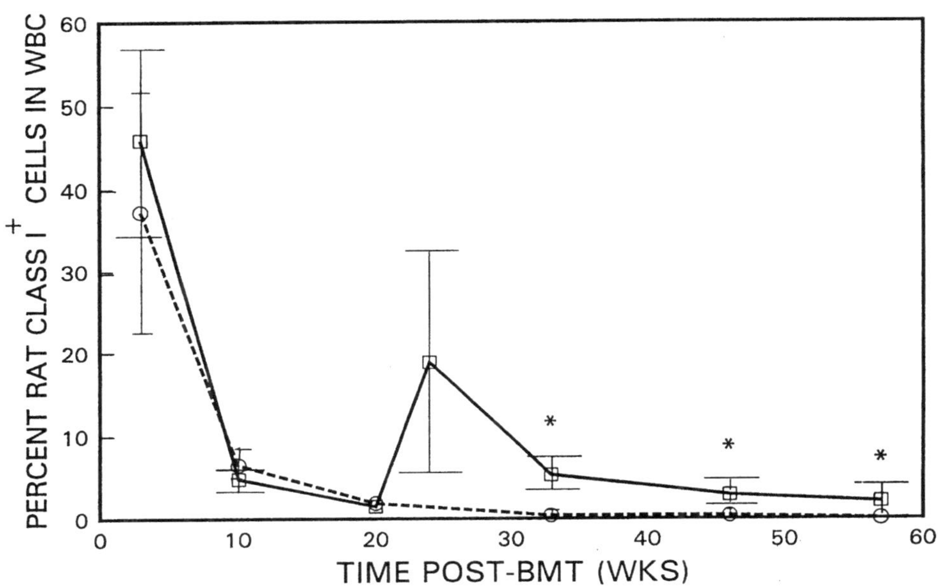

Fig. 3. Enhanced rat white blood cell (*WBC*) repopulation in recipients of 3 Gy whole body irradiation (WBI) and repeat marrow infusion (6×10^7 T cell-depleted bone marrow cells) 22 weeks following conditioning with the complete non-myeloablative regimen and TCD rat bone marrow transplantation (*BMT*). The mean (±SD) percentage of rat class I$^+$ cells in WBC as determined by two-color flow cytometry (FCM) is shown for control animals (*dashed line, circles*) and for those receiving 3 Gy WBI and an additional rat BMT at 22 weeks following the initial BMT (*solid line, squares*). $^*p<0.05$

decline of chimerism [55], suggesting that a failure of NK cell "tolerance" was not responsible for this decline. Although further studies will be needed to clarify the state of host NK cell "tolerance" to the donor in these mice, our studies suggest that the gradual loss of donor-type repopulation is most likely due to a competitive advantage enjoyed by host hematopoietic cells over xenogeneic ones. Mixed rat/mouse marrow reconstitution studies in SCID mice have confirmed the importance of this "competition factor" in determining rat cell reconstitution of specific lineages in mice [55a]. This advantage could be due to species differences in cytokines, adhesion molecules and their ligands, and other components of the marrow stromal environment. Thus it is not surprising that host hematopoiesis would gradually supersede donor rat hematopoiesis after recipient stem cells have recovered from the initial myelosuppressive irradiation.

Attempts To Achieve Bone Marrow Engraftment in Discordant Species Combinations

Choice of the Pig as a Xenograft Donor

Because donor organ availability has become a major limitation to the field of transplantation, there has been a resurgence of interest in xenografting over the past few years. Although nonhuman primates would provide the closest potential donors for man phylogenetically, there are a variety of reasons, including availability and ethical considerations, which mitigate against wide-scale use of primates as xenograft donors. Furthermore, recent evidence indicating that potentially lethal retroviruses and other viruses can be transmitted from nonhuman primates to humans has raised questions about the safety of using such closely related species as xenograft donors [56]. We and others have therefore turned our attention to more discordant species as a potential xenograft donor source. The miniature swine which we have inbred over the past 20 years as a large animal model for transplantation [57, 58] have a variety of advantages over other potential xenograft donors:

1. Size
2. Immunologic Characterization
3. Breeding characteristics
4. Reproducibility of genetics
   a) For cellular and organ transplant
   b) For retransplantation
5. Genetic engineering
   a) One set of vectors for all potential recipients
   b) Breeding of transgenics

The chief advantage of pigs is their breeding characteristics, which make it possible to manipulate the genetics of these animals in a relatively short time. These characteristics include large litter size (three to ten piglets), short gestation time (15 weeks), frequent estrus cycles (every 3 weeks), and sexual maturity at the early age of 4–6 months. Thus, the generation time of these animals is approximately 1 year, with the potential for selection of breeders at every generation. These characteristics have enabled us to establish three herds of MHC homozygous pigs as well as several intra-MHC recombinant strains. Another advantage of these animals is their size, which is very similar to that of human beings, with maximal weights of approximately 250 lb. Thus one might choose an appropriate donor for any potential human recipient.

Pig-to-Mouse Bone Marrow Transplantation

In view of the competitive advantage of host marrow over marrow from the closely related rat species in mice, even greater physiologic barriers may inhibit reconstitution by hematopoietic cells from more widely disparate species. Consistent with this hypothesis, when porcine bone marrow cells were administered to sublethally irradiated severe combined immunodeficient (SCID) mice, which lack T and B cell-mediated immunity [59], only a low level of swine myeloid cell repopulation of recipient hematopoietic tissues was observed. Swine Ig was initially detected in the serum of these mice, but became undetectable by about 5 months following BMT. However, swine hematopoietic progenitors were detected long term in the marrow of some mice, suggesting that a low level of pluripotent hematopoietic stem cell engraftment may have been achieved [60].

NK cells did not appear to limit porcine marrow engraftment in SCID mice [60], which lack other forms of immunity. This inability to demonstrate a role for NK cells in xenoresistance in this species combination may reflect a failure of cellular interactions that are critical for cytolytic function, e.g., lymphocyte function-associated antigen (LFA)-1/intercellular adhesion molecule (ICAM), to function between the pig and the mouse. We believe that the species specificity of environmental factors such as cytokines and adhesion molecules may present the major limitation to engraftment and reconstitution of mice by swine marrow. Consistent with this possibility, in vitro mixing studies demonstrated a competitive advantage for growth of human hematopoietic progenitors over xenogeneic porcine ones on pre-established human stromal layers [61]. In an attempt to improve the ability of swine marrow cells to compete for hematopoietic repopulation in a xenogeneic environment, we have begun to evaluate exogenously administered swine-specific cytokines. Administration of recombinant porcine IL-3, the most species-specific of the hematopoietic growth factors, has resulted in a marked increase in the level of swine hematopoietic repopulation and in the number of swine progenitor cells in marrow of SCID mouse recipients. The addition of donor cytokines and/or genetic engineering to make swine marrow more "human-like" in its responsiveness to human environmental stimuli might be necessary for the successful application of BMT to the induction of xenotolerance in human recipients [62].

As discussed above, absorption studies have indicated that most human NAb target antigens expressed on swine endothelial cells are also shared by swine BMC and their progeny [53]. Thus induction of mixed swine → human chimerism might not only induce cellular tolerance, but could also induce tolerance among

NAb-forming B cells and eliminate the risk of hyperacute rejection when solid organ transplantation from swine donors was subsequently performed.

Pig-to-Primate Bone Marrow Transplantation

Tolerance Induction in an Allogeneic Primate Bone Marrow Transplant Model

Because the non-myeloablative preparative regimen used in mice as described above was far less toxic than the lethal preparative regimen utilized in previous studies, we have considered it for potential clinical applicability. We have therefore recently developed a similar protocol in cynomolgus monkeys as a pre-clinical large animal model [63]. Pairs of animals were selected following serologic and MLR testing to assure that they were MHC mismatched at class I and class II/oci. Animals were chosen such that at least one mAb was available which reacted with the donor MHC and not with the recipient, for detection of chimerism by flow cytometry (FCM) post-transplant. As illustrated in Fig. 4, animals received 3.0 Gy WBI, 7.0 Gy thymic irradiation, and horse anti-human ATG preoperatively. Bilateral nephrectomy, splenectomy, orthotopic kidney transplantation and donor bone marrow administration were all performed on day 0 (see below for further details on the preparative regimen). In order to supplement suppression of mature T cells by ATG, treatment with cyclosporin A i.m. was begun on day 1 and continued for 4 weeks. No further immunosuppression was administered after this time. This protocol was thus highly analogous to that utilized in our previous murine studies [31].

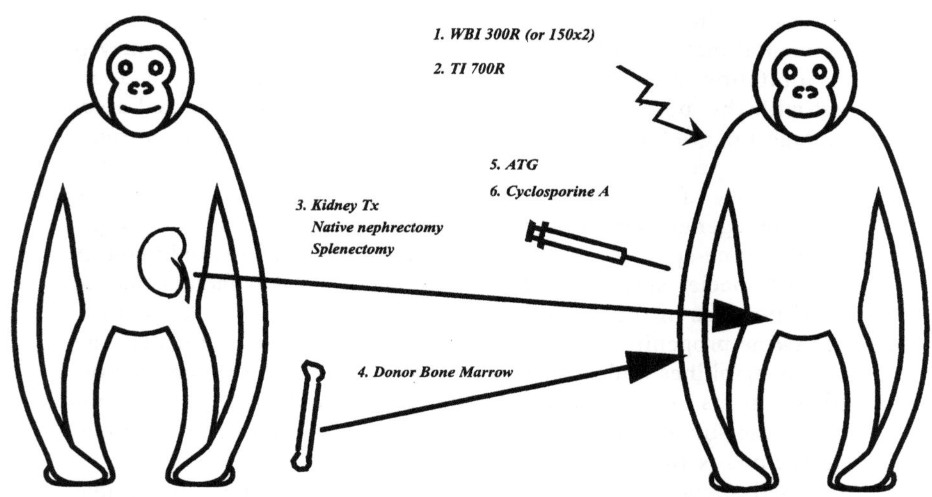

Fig. 4. Protocol for non-myeloablative preparative regimen to induce tolerance between full major histocompatibility complex (MHC) haplotype-mismatched cynomolgus monkeys. *WBI*, whole body irradiation; *ATG*, antithrombocyte globulin

Monkeys treated by this regimen became pancytopenic on day 8, but recovered thereafter, becoming essentially normal hematologically by day 30. Sequential FCM analyses showed clear evidence for chimerism among lymphoid, myeloid and monocytic subpopulations, generally detected first on about day 8, and persisting until day 30. Thereafter, the levels of detectable chimerism decreased progressively, becoming difficult to distinguish from background staining with isotype control antibodies (i.e., less than 1%–2%) by FCM. In all six animals treated by this protocol, transplantation tolerance was induced, as assessed by MLR assays, by monitoring of kidney transplant function, and in one case by acceptance of a full thickness graft of frozen skin from the kidney donor [63]. In none of these animals was any additional exogenous immunosuppression administered after day 30. We have therefore concluded that specific transplantation tolerance can be induced in primates by this procedure [63].

Mixed Chimerism in a Pig-to-Primate Discordant Xenograft Combination

Non-myeloablative Protocol. We have recently begun studies attempting to extend the nonmyeloablative regimen for production of mixed chimerism to this discordant pig ⟶ primate combination [64]. The protocol we have used is illustrated schematically in Fig. 5. This protocol parallels very closely that which we have previously demonstrated to be effective for inducing long-term graft acceptance in allogeneic mouse combinations [31], concordant rat to mouse xenogeneic combinations [32], and fully MHC mismatched cynomolgus monkeys [63]. The one main difference from previous protocols involves the need to remove natural antibodies from the recipient's circulation in order to avoid hyperacute rejection. As illustrated in Fig. 5, this has been accomplished in our model by intraoperative perfusion of the monkey's blood either through an isolated pig liver or through specific antigen-bearing columns via silastic catheters inserted into the aorta and vena cava on day 0, immediately prior to renal transplantation [64]. It is interesting to note that a similar procedure utilizing ex vivo pig liver perfusion has been used clinically to treat hepatic coma [65,66]. Our use of solid matrix columns bearing appropriate α1,3-galactose sugar linkages is based on reports suggesting that the majority of primate anti-swine natural antibodies are directed to this epitope [67, 68], which has been confirmed in our laboratory. Our early results with such columns are encouraging (Lorf et al., manuscript in preparation).

The preparative regimen we have used is very similar to that utilized in our monkey allotransplantation model, as described above. Sublethal irradiation consisting of three fractions of WBI, 1.0 Gy each, were administered on days −6 and −5, and 7.0 Gy of thymic irradiation was administered on day −1. While it is not clear in either of these large animal models whether or not thymic irradiation is required, we have retained it in the protocols, and are presently testing its necessity in the allogeneic model. Similarly, splenectomy on day 0, although not yet proven to be a necessary part of the preparative regimen, has been included in the protocol because of its apparent usefulness in other transplant models involving preformed antibodies [69, 70]. Because no monoclonal antibodies to remove mature T cells from monkeys in vivo are yet available, we have utilized ATG (Upjohn) for this purpose. This reagent was administered on days −2, −1, and 0 (50 mg/kg, i.v.). As described for our allogeneic primate model [63], examina-

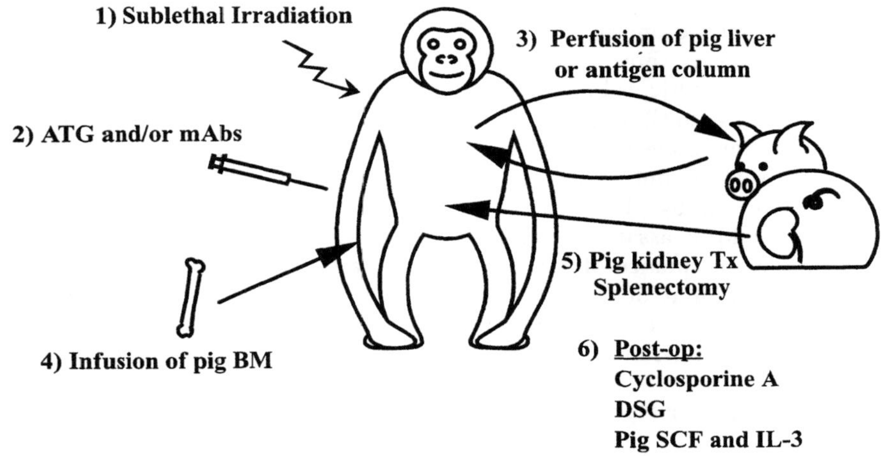

Fig. 5. Non-myeloablative protocol for attempts to induce transplantation tolerance across the discordant xenogeneic barrier pig → cynomolgus monkey through establishment of mixed chimerism. *ATG*, antithrombocyte globulin; *mAbs*, monoclonal antibodies; *BM*, bone marrow; *DSG*, 15-deoxyspergualin; *IL*, interleukin

tion of lymph nodes indicated that this T cell depletion was not complete, so we have also included a postoperative course of immunosuppression with cyclosporin A (15 mg/kg per day, i.v.) to further suppress T cell function in the immediate post-transplant period. Recently, 2 weeks of treatment with 15-deoxyspergualin was also added to the protocol because of its ability to suppress antibody responses [71]. On day 0, a pig kidney was transplanted into the same large vessels utilized for the perfusion procedure. Pig bone marrow was harvested and prepared from the same donor, and was infused at approximately 5×10^8 cells/kg perioperatively.

Removal of Natural Antibodies. Removal of NAbs in this combination has been successful in avoiding hyperacute rejection in more than 15 pig to monkey xenotransplants performed to date [72]. A summary of kidney survivals in this series of animals is shown in Fig. 6. Following the full preparative regimen, kidney grafts have functioned normally for up to 15 days, achieving normal blood urea nitrogen (BUN) and creatinine levels. Open biopsies during this time have revealed normal kidneys grossly and have shown normal kidney histology. However, in all of these animals the kidney subsequently succumbed to a vascular form of rejection, and no long-term kidney survivals were achieved. In addition, with the exception of recent animals in which pig recombinant growth factors were used (see below), there has only been transient evidence for pig cell chimerism, with a low level of pig cells (1 %–5 %) in the peripheral blood [72].

The absorption procedure led to an almost complete removal of IgM and IgG anti-pig antibodies, and these antibodies remained at very low levels until shortly before rejection. In those animals which rejected the xenografts, IgG antibodies were observed in the serum at the time of rejection and were found by immunofluorescence in large vessels [72]. Preliminary data indicate that this IgG antibody detected additional determinants to those detected by natural antibodies, suggesting that the production of monkey anti-pig IgG represents a T cell dependent immune response to the transplant, and that this phenomenon, return of natural antibodies, in addition to the contributed to loss of grafts by vascular rejection during the second week.

Current Status. Our studies in allogeneic systems have demonstrated that chimerism is a requirement for achieving lasting transplantation tolerance [31, 73, 74]. Our current efforts have therefore focused on means for increasing the reconstitution by pig bone marrow cells in monkey recipients. One of the methods being tested involves the use of pig recombinant cytokines (SCF and IL-3) in the postoperative period. Recent results suggest that administration of these cytokines to a monkey receiving the full preparative regimen prolonged survival of pig bone marrow progeny in the monkey's bone marrow for over 6 months (T. Sablinski et al., manuscript in preparation). In addition, pig cytokines were used postoperatively in the animal with the longest kidney survival in Fig. 6 (#1094, 15-day survival). Unfortunately, this cynomolgus monkey died from a complication of thrombocytopenia with a functioning kidney transplant (T. Sablinski et al., manuscript in preparation). We consider these results to be preliminary, but very encouraging. We are also planning to test the use of fetal pig thymic tissue, which, in the mouse model described above, leads to discordant xenograft tolerance [75]. It is our hope that, by combining approaches being pursued in other laboratories toward avoiding hyperacute rejection with our own approach to inducing cellular tolerance, long-term acceptance of discordant xenografts will be achieved in the pig to primate combination.

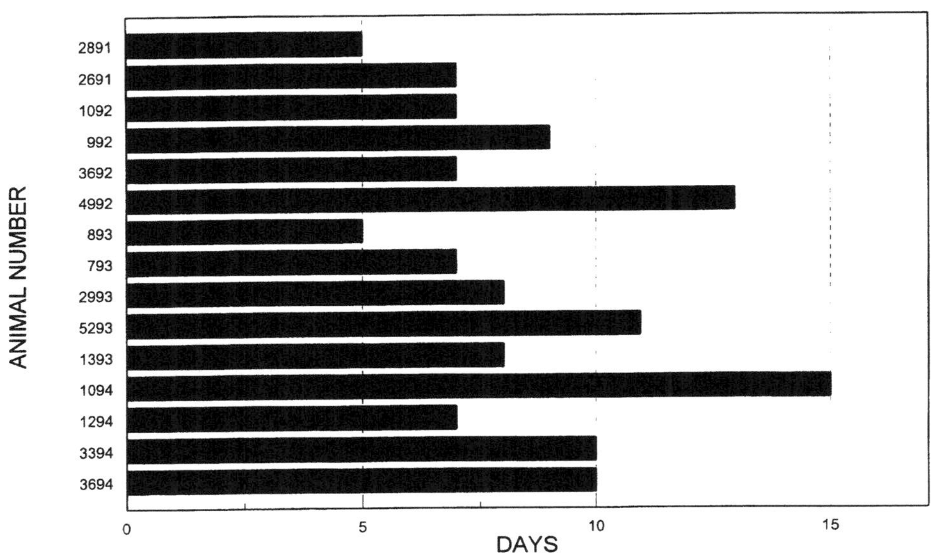

Fig. 6. Survival of technically successful pig kidney xenografts in our series of cynomolgus monkeys

Xenogeneic Thymic Transplantation as an Approach to Inducing Tolerance

Xenogeneic Thymic Tissue Replaces the Host Thymus in Immunocompetent Thymectomized and T Cell Depleted Mice

In the pig to mouse transplantation studies performed thus far, we have not succeeded in inducing porcine hematopoietic cells to mature and home to the recipient thymus and induce deletional tolerance there. Since thymic tissue itself can induce T cell tolerance by a variety of mechanisms [76–80], an alternative approach to inducing central tolerance would be to replace the host thymus with a xenogeneic donor thymus. We therefore evaluated the potential of swine fetal thymus/liver grafts to induce tolerance in immunocompetent mice. The fetal liver was added as a source of porcine hematopoietic cells that could potentially induce deletional tolerance in the porcine thymus graft. Results of these studies demonstrated that, in adult thymectomized (ATX), otherwise immunocompetent mice receiving a modification of the conditioning regimen shown in Fig. 1 prior to implantation of fetal pig thymus/liver grafts, murine $CD4^{+}$ T cells that are specifically tolerant of the swine donors develop in the grafts and migrate to the periphery (Fig. 7).

Murine T cells developing in fetal pig thymic grafts are capable of responding to alloantigens in vitro [75] (Fig. 8) and in vivo [75a]. Our results therefore demonstrate a method for inducing specific tolerance across discordant species barriers [75, 75a]. However, as is discussed above, MHC restriction is generally believed to be determined by the MHC of the thymus [81–84]. It would therefore be expected that murine T cells that differentiated in a pig thymus would not be able to respond to peptide antigens presented by host MHC. Immunoincompetence would occur due to a mismatch between the class II MHC restriction imposed by the pig thymus and the MHC of host-type APC present in the periphery. However, preliminary studies indicate that the predicted immunoincompetence may not be a problem in these mice, as their T cells appear to be capable of recognizing peptide antigens in the context of host MHC (Y. Zhao et al., unpublished data). These results are consistent with studies showing reconstitution of functional murine T cells in thymi from another xenogeneic species (human) grafted into immunodeficient beige-nude-xid mice [85]. The apparent discrepancy between these results and those involving T cell selection in a thymus graft from the same species [86] suggest that marrow-derived or other host cell types may be capable of mediating positive selection only in xenogeneic thymic grafts. Further definition of the cell types responsible for positive selection of mouse thymocytes in pig thymus/liver grafts will be essential to a full understanding of immunocompetence in these mice.

The human thymus is known to involute at puberty, and recent studies have suggested that the capacity of the adult human thymus to repopulate CD4 T cells following destruction of the existing T cell pool by irradiation or chemotherapy may be limited [87,88]. Thus, a xenogeneic thymus graft may prove to be important to the achievement of T cell recovery and immunocompetence

Fig. 7a,b. Growth of fetal pig thymus/liver grafts in the presence of mature mouse T cells in the periphery. **a** An increase in fetal pig thymus/liver graft size was observed upon exploratory laparotomy performed at 5 and 19 weeks post-transplant, despite **b** the presence of mature $CD4^+/\alpha,\beta$-T cell receptor (*TCR*)$^+$ T cells in the peripheral white blood cells (WBC; shown 16 weeks after monoclonal antibodies were discontinued). Control adult thymectomized mice which received fetal swine liver grafts without a thymus fragment did not maintain their grafts and developed <5% $\alpha\beta$-TCR^+ T cells in the periphery

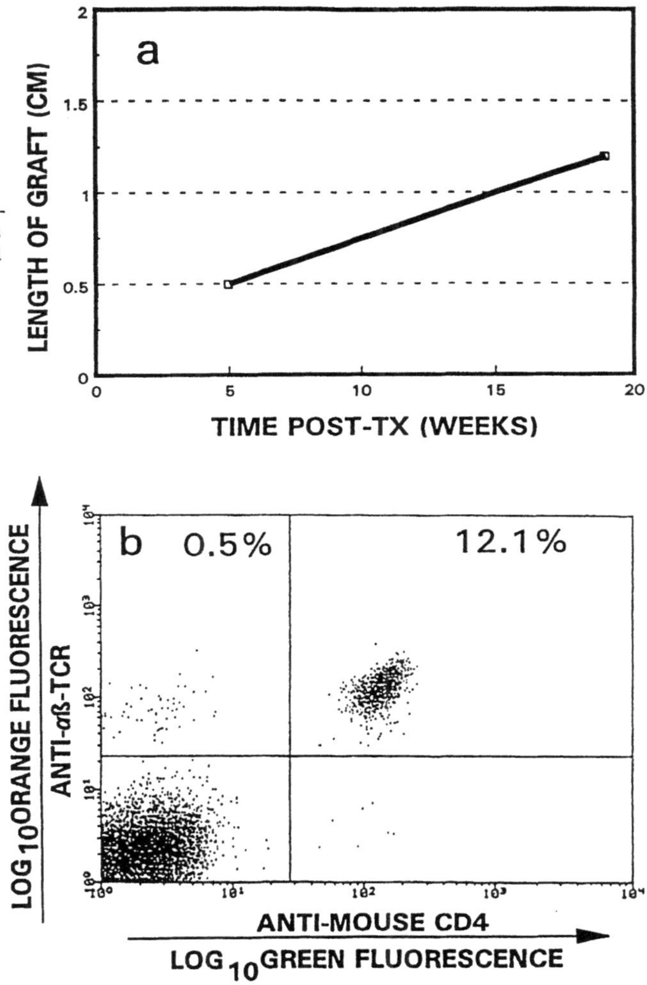

when regimens that involve depletion of preexisting peripheral T cells are used to condition recipients.

In addition to its potential to induce donor-specific tolerance for xenografting, the xenogeneic thymus grafting approach may also have potential to contribute to the treatment of patients infected with human immunodeficiency virus (HIV). The thymus appears to be a significant target of HIV infection [89–92], and its destruction would likely preclude the recovery of $CD4^+$ T cells even if effective antiretroviral therapy were given. Thus the provision of a xenogeneic thymic graft might provide an important adjunct to pharmacotherapy or other approaches in patients with acquired immunodeficiency syndrome (AIDS).

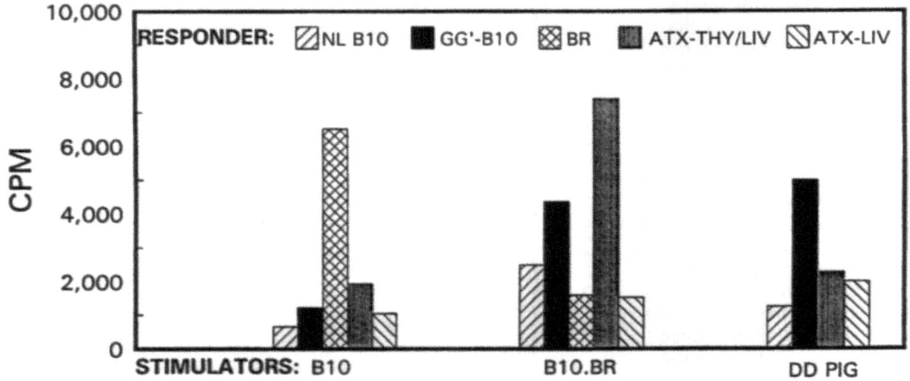

Fig. 8. Specific unresponsiveness of B10 mice transplanted with fetal pig thymus/liver (*THY/LIV*) grafts to pig antigens in mixed lymphocyte reaction (*MLR*). Adult thymectomized (*ATX*)-THY/LIV B10 (H-2b) mice demonstrated specific unresponsiveness to pig antigens, despite the presence of normal allo-responsiveness to a fully major histocompatibility complex (MHC)-mismatched B10.BR (H-2k) stimulator. Control ATX-B10 mice which received a swine liver graft without a thymus fragment (*ATX-LIV*) mounted no responses to any stimulator, demonstrating the importance of the pig thymus graft in the development of functional mouse T cells. Responses are shown for spleen cells from representative normal B10 mice (*NL B10*), a normal B10 mouse grafted with GG (SLA-Ic/SLA-IId) pig skin 12 weeks earlier (*GG'-B10*), normal B10.BR (*BR*), or thymectomized B10 mice conditioned with the non-myeloablative regimen described above and transplanted with either a fetal pig THY/LIV graft (*ATX-THY/LIV*) or a fetal pig liver graft only (*ATX-LIV*). Indicated 30 Gy-irradiated stimulator cell populations were used

Tolerance to the Discordant Xenogeneic Donor and the Host in Adult Thymectomized Recipients of Thymus Tissue

Tolerance to the discordant porcine donor in the above studies has been illustrated by the growth of the thymic xenografts as murine CD4 T cells repopulate the periphery (Fig. 7), the long-term coexistence of murine and porcine thymocytes in these grafts, and by unresponsiveness to pig antigens in MLR reactions (Fig. 8). Furthermore, partial deletion of Vβ families (Vβ5 and Vβ11) recognizing endogenous superantigens that could only be presented by donor (pig) class II molecules and not by recipient ($I\text{-}E^- H\text{-}2^b$) MHC is observed [75]. This result suggests that pig antigens participate in negative selection of murine thymocytes developing in swine thymic grafts. Immunohistochemical stains have demonstrated the presence in the grafts of cells with dendritic morphology that express high levels of porcine MHC class II, and these cells may be involved in negative selection of pig-reactive murine T cells [75a]. The most striking illustration of the tolerant state in these animals is provided by recent studies demonstrating the long-term survival of donor-type pig porcine skin grafts while murine skin allografts are rejected in ATX mice reconstituted with a pig thymus [75a]. This result provides the first demonstration of donor-specific skin graft tolerance across a discordant xenogeneic barrier.

As shown in Fig. 8, these animals also show MLR tolerance to host antigens. The presence of host class II$^+$ cells with dendritic morphology in the grafts, concomitant with complete deletion of Vβ families that recognize host superantigen/host MHC complexes [75] suggest that this tolerance also occurs by an intrathymic deletional mechanism.

Comment

Xenogeneic hematopoietic cell and thymic transplantation provide promising approaches to the induction of both humoral and cellular tolerance across species barriers, and might potentially make pig to human xenotransplantation a clinical reality. The development of specific and nontoxic methods of overcoming the immunologic and physiologic barriers to xenogeneic marrow engraftment is a major challenge that must be met before this goal can be achieved. A greater understanding of the species specificity of molecular interactions important for hematopoiesis and cell homing will be a first step toward transcending these physiologic barriers. Perhaps most promising is the potential application of genetic engineering technologies to make porcine donor tissues more readily capable of surviving and, in the case of hematopoietic cells, competing with host tissues for survival in a human environment.

Acknowledgements. We thank Dr. Hugh Auchincloss, Jr. and Dr. Boris Nikolic for helpful review of the manuscript and Ms. Diane Plemenos for expert assistance with the manuscript. This work was supported in part by NIH Grants #RO1-AI37692 and RO1-HL49915 and through a sponsored research agreement between the Massachusetts General Hospital and BioTransplant, Inc. Dr. Sykes and Dr. Sachs serve as consultants to BioTransplant, Inc.

References

1. Auchincloss HA. Why is cell-mediated xenograft rejection so strong? Xeno 1995, 3: 19
2. Billingham RE, Brent L, Medawar PB. "Actively acquired tolerance" of foreign cells. Nature 1953, 172: 603
3. Ildstad ST, Sachs DH. Reconstitution with syngeneic plus allogeneic or xenogeneic bone marrow leads to specific acceptance of allografts or xenografts. Nature 1984, 307(5947): 168
4. Sykes M, Sheard M, Sachs DH. Effects of T cell depletion in radiation bone marrow chimeras. I Evidence for a donor cell population which increases allogeneic chimerism but which lacks the potential to produce GVHD. J Immunol 1988, 141: 2282
5. Marrack P, Lo D, Brinster R, et al. The effect of thymus environment on T cell development and tolerance. Cell 1988, 53: 627
6. Slavin S. Total lymphoid irradiation. Immunol Today 1987, 3: 88
7. Pierce GE. Allogeneic versus semiallogeneic F1 bone marrow transplantation into sublethally irradiated MHC-disparate hosts. Effects on mixed lymphoid chimerism, skin graft tolerance, host survival, and alloreactivity. Transplantation 1990, 49: 138

8. Mayumi H, Good RA. Long-lasting skin allograft tolerance in adult mice induced across fully allogeneic (multimajor H-2 plus multiminor histocompatibility) antigen barriers by a tolerance-inducing method using cyclophosphamide. J Exp Med 1989, 169: 213
9. Clift RA, Storb R. Histoincompatible bone marrow transplants in humans. Ann Rev Immunol 1987, 5: 43
10. O'Reilly RJ, Collins NH, Kernan N, et al. Transplantation of marrow depleted of T cells by soybean lectin agglutination and E-rosette depletion: major histocompatibility complex-related graft resistance in leukemic transplant recipients. Transplant Proc 1985, 17: 455
11. Anasetti C, Amos D, Beatty PG, et al. Effect of HLA compatibility on engraftment of bone marrow transplants in patients with leukemia or lymphoma. N Engl J Med 1989, 320: 197
12. Ildstad ST, Wren SM, Sharrow SO, Stephany D, Sachs DH. In vivo and in vitro characterization of specific hyporeactivity to skin xenografts in mixed xenogeneically reconstituted mice (B10 + F344 rat→B10). J Exp Med 1984, 160: 1820
13. Santos GW, Cole LJ. Effects of donor and host lymphoid and myeloid tissue injections in lethally X-irradiated mice treated with rat bone marrow. J Natl Cancer Inst 1958, 21: 279
14. Bau J, Thierfelder S. Antilymphocytic antibodies and marrow transplantation. Transplantation 1973, 15: 564
15. Muller-Rucholtz W, Muller-Hermelink HK, Wottge HU. Induction of lasting hematopoietic chimerism in a xenogeneic (rat→mouse) model. Transplant Proc 1979, 11: 517
16. Deeg HJ, Storb R, Thomas ED. Bone marrow transplantation: a review of delayed complications. Br J Haematol 1984, 57: 185
17. Freirich EJ, Gehan EA, Rall DP, Schmidt LH, Skipper HE. Quantitative comparison of toxicity of anti-cancer agents in mouse, rat, hamster, dog, monkey, and man. Cancer Chemotherapy Rep 1966, 50: 219
18. Sullivan K M, Witherspoon R P, Storb R, et al. Chronic graft-versus-host disease: recent advances in diagnosis and treatment. In: Gale R P, Champlin R, eds. Alan R. Liss, Inc., New York, 1989: 511
19. Makinodan T. Circulating rat cells in lethally irradiated mice protected with rat bone marrow. Proc Soc Exp Biol Med 1956, 92: 174
20. Gale RP, Reisner Y. Graft rejection and graft-versus-host disease: mirror images. Lancet 1986, i: 1468
21. Poynton CH. T cell depletion in bone marrow transplantation. Bone Marrow Transplant 1988, 3: 265
22. Martin PJ, Hansen JA, Buckner CD, et al. Effects of in vitro depletion of T cells in HLA-identical allogeneic marrow grafts. Blood 1985, 66: 664
23. Kernan NA, Flomenberg N, Dupont B, O'Reilly RJ. Graft rejection in recipients of T-cell-depleted HLA-nonidentical marrow transplants for leukemia. Transplantation 1987, 43: 842
24. Soderling CCB, Song CW, Blazar BR, Vallera DA. A correlation between conditioning and engraftment in recipients of MHC-mismatched T cell-depleted murine bone marrow transplants. J Immunol 1985, 135: 941

25. Ferrara JLM, Lipton J, Hellman S, Burakoff S, Mauch P. Engraftment following T-cell-depleted marrow transplantation. Transplantation 1987, 43: 461
26. Zinkernagel RM, Callahan GN, Althage A, Cooper S, Klein PA, Klein J. On the thymus in the differentiation of "H-2 self-recognition" by T cells: evidence for dual recognition? J Exp Med 1978, 147: 882
27. Singer A, Hathcock KS, Hodes RJ. Self recognition in allogeneic radiation chimeras. A radiation resistant host element dictates the self specificity and immune response gene phenotype of T-helper cells. J Exp Med 1981, 153: 1286
28. Ildstad ST, Wren SM, Bluestone JA, Barbieri SA, Sachs DH. Characterization of mixed allogeneic chimeras. Immunocompetence, in vitro reactivity, and genetic specificity of tolerance. J Exp Med 1985, 162: 231
29. Zinkernagel RM, Althage A, Callahan G, Welsh Jr RM. On the immunocompetence of H-2 incompatible irradiation bone marrow chimeras. J Immunol 1980, 124: 2356
30. Ruedi E, Sykes M, Ildstad ST, et al. Antiviral T cell competence and restriction specificty of mixed allogeneic (P1+P2 → P1) irradiation chimeras. Cell Immuol 1989, 121: 185
31. Sharabi Y, Sachs DH. Mixed chimerism and permanent specific transplantation tolerance induced by a non-lethal preparative regimen. J Exp Med 1989, 169: 493
32. Sharabi Y, Aksentijevich I, Sundt III TM, Sachs DH, Sykes M. Specific tolerance induction across a xenogeneic barrier: production of mixed rat/mouse lymphohematopoietic chimeras using a nonlethal preparative regimen. J Exp Med 1990, 172: 195
33. Moretta L, Ciccone E, Moretta A, Hoglund P, Ohlen C, Karre K. Allorecognition by NK cells: nonself or no self? Immunol Today 1992, 13: 300
34. Bix M, Liao N-S, Zijlstra M, Loring J, Jaenisch R, Raulet D. Rejection of class I MHC-deficient haemopoietic cells by irradiated MHC-matched mice. Nature 1991, 349: 329
35. Salcedo M, Hoglund P, Ljunggren H-G. Natural killer cell interaction with murine allogeneic MHC class I molecules. Transplantation 1995, 60: 281
36. Yankelevich B, Knobloch C, Nowicki M, Dennert G. A novel cell type responsible for marrow graft rejection in mice. T cells with NK phenotype cause acute rejection of marrow grafts. J Immunol 1989, 142: 3423
37. Kikly K, Dennert G. Evidence for a role for T cell receptors (TCR) in the effector phase of acute bone marrow graft rejection. TCR Vb5 transgenic mice lack effector cells able to cause graft rejection. J Immunol 1992, 149: 3489
38. Takeda K, Moore MW, Dennert G. Acute rejection of marrow grafts in mice. Dependence on and independence of functional TCR in the rejection process. J Immunol 1994, 152: 4407
39. Okumura C, Suto R, Furukawa K, et al. Induction of murine gamma-delta T cells cytotoxic for xenogeneic rat cells. J Immunol 1995, 154: 1114
40. Tomita Y, Sachs DH, Khan A, Sykes M. Additional mAb injections can replace thymic irradiation to allow induction of mixed chimerism and tolerance in mice receiving bone marrow transplantation after conditioning with anti-T cell mAbs and 3 Gy whole body irradiation. Transplantation 1996, 61: 469
41. Tomita Y, Lee LA, Sykes M. Engraftment of rat bone marrow and its role in negative selection of murine T cells in mice conditioned with a modified non-myeloablative regimen. Xenotransplantation 1994, 1: 109
42. van Ewijk W, Ron Y, Monaco J, et al. Compartmentalization of MHC class II gene expression in transgenic mice. Cell 1988, 53: 357

43. Ramsdell F, Fowlkes BJ. Clonal deletion versus clonal anergy: the role of the thymus in inducing self tolerance. Science 1990, 248: 1342
44. Schonrich G, Strauss G, Muller K-P, et al. Distinct requirements of positive and negative selection for selecting cell type and CD8 interaction. J Immunol 1993, 151: 4098
45. Tomita Y, Khan A, Sykes M. Role of intrathymic clonal deletion and peripheral anergy in transplantation tolerance induced by bone marrow transplantion in mice conditioned with a non-myeloablative regimen. J Immunol 1994, 153: 1087
46. Matzinger P, Guerder S. Does T cell tolerance require a dedicated antigen-presenting cell? Nature 1989, 338: 74
47. Inaba M, Inaba K, Hosono M, et al. Distinct mechanisms of neonatal tolerance induced by dendritic cells and thymic B cells. J Exp Med 1991, 173: 549
48. Tomita Y, Khan A, Sykes M. Mechanism by which additional monoclonal antibody injections overcome the requirement for thymic irradiation to achieve mixed chimerism in mice receiving bone marrow transplantation after conditioning with anti-T cell mAbs and 3 Gy whole body irradiation. Transplantation 1996, 61: 477
49. Aksentijevich I, Sachs DH, Sykes M. Humoral tolerance in xenogeneic BMT recipients conditioned with a non-myeloablative regimen. Transplantation 1992, 53: 1108
50. Aksentijevich I, Sachs DH, Sykes M. Normal mouse serum contains natural antibody against bone marrow cells of a concordant xenogeneic species. J Immunol 1991, 147: 79
51. Aksentijevich I, Sachs DH, Sykes M. Natural antibodies can inhibit bone marrow engraftment in the rat → mouse species combination. J Immunol 1991, 147: 4140
52. Lee LA, Sergio JJ, Sachs DH, Sykes M. Mechanism of tolerance in mixed xenogeneic chimeras prepared with a non-myeloablative conditioning regimen. Transplant Proc 1994, 26: 1197
53. Latinne D, Vitiello D, Sachs DH, Sykes M. Tolerance to discordant xenografts: I. Human natural antibody determinants are shared on miniature swine bone marrow cells and endothelial cells. Transplantation 1994, 57: 238
54. Murakami M, Tsubata T, Okamoto M, et al. Antigen-induced apoptotic death of Ly-1 B cells responsible for autoimmune disease in transgenic mice. Nature 1992, 357: 77
55. Lee LA, Sergio JJ, Sykes M. Evidence for non-immune mechanisms in the loss of hematopoietic chimerism in rat → mouse mixed xenogeneic chimeras. Xenotransplantation 1995, 2: 57
55a. Gritsch, H.A. and Sykes, M. Host morrow for a competitive advantage which limits donor hematopoietic repopulation in mixed xenogeneic chimeras. In press, Xenotransplantation
56. Taylor R. A pig in a poke? Xenotransplants and infectious disease. Nature Med 1995, 1: 728
57. Sachs D H. MHC-Homozygous miniature swine. In: Swindle M M, Moody D C, Phillips L D, eds. Iowa State University Press, Ames,IA, 1992: 3
58. Sachs DH, Leight G, Cone J, Schwarz S, Stuart L, Rosenberg S. Transplantation in miniature swine. I. Fixation of the major histocompatibility complex. Transplantation 1976, 22: 559
59. Schuler W, Weiler IJ, Schuler A, et al. Rearrangement of antigen receptor genes is defective in mice with severe combined immunodeficiency. Cell 1986, 46: 963
60. Gritsch HA, Glaser RM, Emery DW, et al. The importance of non-immune factors in reconstitution by discordant xenogeneic hematopoietic cells. Transplantation 1994, 57: 906

61. Emery DW, Sykes M, Sachs DH, LeGuern C. Mixed swine/human long-term bone marrow cultures. Transplant Proc 1994, 26: 1313
62. Yang Y-G, Sergio JJ, Swenson K, Glaser RM, Monroy R, Sykes M. Donor-specific growth factors promote swine hematopoiesis in SCID mice. Xenotransplantation 1996, 3: 92
63. Kawai T, Cosimi AB, Colvin RB, et al. Mixed allogeneic chimerism and renal allograft tolerance in cynomologous monkeys. Transplantation 1995, 59: 256
64. Latinne D, Gianello P, Smith CV, et al. Xenotransplantation from pig to cynomolgus monkey: An approach toward tolerance induction. Transplant Proc 1993, 250: 336
65. McDermott WV, Norman JC. Extracorporeal pig liver perfusion in the treatment of hepatic coma. Epatologia 1972, 18: 265
66. Collins BH, Chari RS, Magee JC, et al. Mechanisms of injury in porcine livers perfused with blood of patients with fulminant hepatic failure. Transplantation 1994, 58: 1162
67. Oriol R, Ye Y, Koren E, Cooper DKC. Carbohydrate antigens of pig tissues reacting with human natural antibodies as potential targets for hyperacute vascular rejection in pig-to-man organ xenotransplantation. Transplantation 1993, 56: 1433
68. Sandrin MS, McKenzie IF. Gal alpha (1,3)Gal, the major xenoantigen(s) recognised in pigs by human natural antibodies. Immunol Rev 1994, 141: 169
69. Alexandre G P J, Gianello P, Latinne D, et al. Plasmapheresis and splenectomy in experimental renal xenotransplantation. In: Hardy M A, ed. Excerpta Medica, New York, 1989: 259
70. Alexandre GP, Squifflet JP, De Bruyere M, et al. Present experiences in a series of 26 ABO-incompatible living donor renal allografts. Transplant Proc 1987, 19: 4538
71. Thomas FT, Tepper MA, Thomas JM, Haisch CE. 15-Deoxyspergualin: a novel immunosuppressive drug with clinical potential. Ann NY Acad Sci 1993, 685: 175
72. Tanaka M, Latinne D, Gianello P, et al. Xenotransplantation from pig to cynomolgus monkey: the potential for overcoming xenograft rejection through induction of chimerism. Transplant Proc 1994, 26: 1326
73. Sharabi Y, Abraham VS, Sykes M, Sachs DH. Mixed allogeneic chimeras prepared by a non-myeloablative regimen: requirement for chimerism to maintain tolerance. Bone Marrow Transplant 1992, 9: 191
74. Khan A, Tomita Y, Sykes M. Thymic dependence of loss of tolerance in mixed allogeneic bone marrow chimeras after depletion of donor antigen. Peripheral mechanisms do not contribute to maintenance of tolerance. Transplantation 1996, 62: 380
75. Lee LA, Gritsch HA, Sergio JJ, et al. Specific tolerance across a discordant xenogeneic transplantation barrier. Proc Natl Acad Sci USA 1994, 91: 10864
75a Zhao Y., Swenson K, Sergio JJ, Arn JS, Sachs DH, Syker M. Skin graft tolerance across a discordant xenogeneic barrier. Nature Med 1996, 2: 1211
76. Speiser DE, Pircher H, Ohashi PS, Kyburz D, Hengartner H, Zinkernagel RM. Clonal deletion induced by either radioresistant thymic host cells or lymphohemopoietic donor cells at different stages of class I-restricted T cell ontogeny. J Exp Med 1992, 175: 1277
77. Salaun J, Bandeira A, Khazaal I, et al. Thymic epithelium tolerizes for histocompatibility antigens. Science 1990, 247: 1471
78. Gao E-K, Lo D, Sprent J. Strong T cell tolerance in parent→F1 bone marrow chimeras prepared with supralethal irradiation. J Exp Med 1990, 171: 1101

79. Bonomo A, Matzinger P. Thymus epithelium induces tissue-specific tolerance. J Exp Med 1993, 177: 1153
80. Ramsdell F, Lantz T, Fowlkes BJ. A nondeletional mechanism of thymic self tolerance. Science 1989, 246: 1038
81. Bradley SM, Kruisbeek AM, Singer A. Cytotoxic T lymphocyte response in allogeneic radiation bone marrow chimeras. The chimeric host strictly dictates the self-repertoire of Ia-restricted T cells but not K/D-restricted T cells. J Exp Med 1982, 156: 1650
82. Geha RS, Rosen FS. The evolution of MHC restrictions in antigen recognition by T cells in a haploidentical bone marrow transplant recipient. J Immunol 1989, 143: 84
83. Chu E, Umetsu D, Rosen F, Geha RS. Major histocompatibility restriction of antigen recognition by T cells in a recipient of haplotype mismatched human bone marrow transplantation. J Clin Invest 1983, 72: 1124
84. Roncarolo MG, Yssel H, Touraine J-L, et al. Antigen recognition by MHC-incompatible cells of a human mismatched chimera. J Exp Med 1988, 168: 2139
85. Kollman TR, Goldstein MM, Goldstein H. The concurrent maturation of mouse and human thymocytes in human fetal thymus implanted in NIH-biege-nude-xid mice is associated with reconstitution of the murine immune system. J Exp Med 1993, 177: 821
86. Bevan MJ, Fink PJ. The influence of thymus H-2 antigens on the specificity of maturing killer and helper cells. Immunol Rev 1978, 42: 3
87. Mackall CL, Fleisher TA, Brown MR, et al. Age, thymopoiesis, and CD4+ T-lymphocyte regeneration after intensive chemotherapy. N Engl J Med 1995, 332: 143
88. Annett G, Weinberg K, Kashyap A, et al. Post-transplantation thymic function predicts immunocompetence. Blood 1994, 84: 250a.(Abstract)
89. Stanley SK, McCune JM, Kaneshima H, et al. Human immunodeficiency virus infection of the human thymus and disruption of the thymic microenvironment in the SCID-hu mouse. J Exp Med 1993, 178: 1151
90. Grody WW, Fligiel S, Naeim F. Thymus involution in the acquired immunodeficiency syndrome. Am J Clin Pathol 1985, 84: 85
91. Kollman TR, Kim A, Pettoello-Mantovani M, et al. Divergent effects of chronic HIV-1 infection on human thymocyte maturation in SCID-hu mice. J Immunol 1995, 154: 907
92. Schuurman H-J, Krone WJA, Broekhuizen R, et al. The thymus in acquired immune deficiency syndrome. Comoparison with other types of immunodeficiency diseases, and presence of components of human immunodeficiency virus type 1. Am J Pathol 1989, 134: 1329

39 Chimerism and Tolerance as an Approach to Xenotransplantation

J.S. Gammie and S.T. Ildstad

Introduction

The modern era of clinical transplantation has made solid organ transplantation a viable therapeutic option for patients with organ failure. Despite reasonable success (3-year survival rates for heart, kidney, and lung transplantation of 75 %, 69 %, and 58 %, respectively) [1], clinical transplantation is limited by problems in three key areas: (1) an insufficient supply of organs, (2) complications associated with nonspecific immunosuppression (infection and malignancy), and (3) the failure of current immunosuppressive regimens to prevent the development of rejection. At the present time, chronic rejection remains the primary cause of late graft loss and, as such, contributes to the shortage of donor organs available for transplantation.

As of 1994, 37 000 people were on the waiting list for a solid organ transplant, while 2900 died while awaiting an organ in the previous year [2]. Despite aggressive educational and organizational initiatives, the supply of solid organs has remained constant at around 4000 per year between 1987 and 1991.

Xenotransplantation could provide a solution to the scarcity of human organs. The formidable immunologic barriers to successful interspecies transplantation are highlighted by the aggregate clinical experience to date. Development by Carrel of the techniques of vascular anastomosis permitted several early attempts at xenografting [3]. Jaboulay in 1906 performed two renal xenotransplants to recipients suffering from renal failure, one using a pig and the other a goat donor [4]. In both cases the grafts failed to function and at explantation were found to have vascular thrombosis. Several other early failures precipitated a long hiatus in clinical xenotransplantation.

Advances in immunology and the development of nonspecific immunosuppressants in the 1960s led to early success in renal allografting and a renewed interest in xenografting. Reemtsma performed a series of chimpanzee to human renal transplants in 1963 and 1964 at Tulane University utilizing an immunosuppressive regiment consisting of azathioprine, steroids, actinomycin C and graft irradiation [5]. Most grafts were rejected within 2 months, although a single kidney survived and functioned well for 9 months. Additional renal xenografts were carried out by Hitchcock [6] and Starzl [7] with similar results. In 1964 Hardy and colleagues performed the first heart xenotransplant, using a chimpanzee donor [8]. An undersized graft and perhaps hyperacute rejection contributed to cardiac failure and recipient death in the operating room. Starzl performed three chimpanzee to human liver xenografts in the late 1960s, the longest of which survived only 14 days [9]. These disappointing results and the wider availability of human donors as a result of a newly accepted definition of brain death again led to a cessation of clinical xenotransplants.

The development of new T cell directed immunosuppressive agents (cyclosporine in 1978 and subsequently tacrolimus) stimulated a 1984 baboon heart transplant to an infant with hypoplastic left heart syndrome [10]. While the graft functioned well for 2 weeks, cardiac failure supervened and the infant died 20 days postoperatively. Autopsy showed evidence of antibody-mediated rejection, but importantly only minimal cellular infiltrates, suggesting that cyclosporine had been effective in abrogating the cellular arm of the xenoimmune response. More recently, Starzl performed two liver transplants using baboon livers and immunosuppression with tacrolimus (FK506), steroids, cyclophosphamide, and prostaglandin E_1 (PGE_1) [11]. The first recipient survived 70 days before succumbing to infection. In this case early liver biopsies showed both humoral damage and lymphocytic infiltration, but these changes were mild and had resolved by the time of death. A second recipient died of peritonitis after 25 days. Despite these bold clinical efforts, long-term xenograft acceptance to date has not been achieved.

The principle that transplantation between distantly related species results in hyperacute rejection, while transplantation between more closely related species does not, was established by Perper and Najarian in the mid-1960s [12]. Calne later introduced the terms *discordant* and *concordant* to refer to the degree of transplantation disparity between two species [13]. This was an operational definition: transplants between discordant species experienced hyperacute rejection, whereas those between concordant species did not.

A promising approach to xenotransplantation that might reduce or eliminate the need for nonspecific immunosuppression and avoid rejection is the induction of donor-specific transplantation tolerance through bone marrow chimerism. Donor-specific transplantation tolerance is a state in which the recipient permanently accepts an allograft or xenograft without the need for immunosuppressive drugs, yet retains the ability to respond to nondonor foreign antigens such that immunocompetence and resistance to infection are preserved. This chapter will explore the history, present status, and future directions of tolerance induction through bone marrow transplantation.

What We Know About Mechanisms for Xenoreactivity

Humoral Response

There are fundamental differences between the allogeneic and xenogeneic immune response. In xenotransplantation, the humoral response is predominant. Xenoreactive antibodies are termed "natural" or "preformed" and are analogous to the antibodies that exist for blood group antigens. Natural antibodies exist in the absence of prior immunization and are believed to function as a first line of defense against microbes. They are primarily of the IgM isotype (in contrast to allosensitization, where the predominant antibodies are of the IgG isotype) and function by binding to endothelium and initiating the classical complement pathway [14]. The ensuing reaction is qualitatively similar to hyperacute allograft rejection and is characterized by endothelial activation with a change from an anti- to a procoagulant environment and loss of vascular integrity [15]. These changes are responsible for the pathologic findings of interstitial edema, cellular necrosis, hemorrhage and a sparse cellular infiltrate. Destruction of the graft occurs within minutes, rather than the 7–10 days required for cell-mediated rejection to occur. Natural antibodies derive exclusively from that subpopulation of B cells which express CD5, which comprise 50 % of fetal B cells, but only 2 %–3 % of B cells in adults [16]. Platt et al. have developed an assay for the detection of natural antibodies which utilizes donor endothelial cells in vitro [17]. They have identified a triad of glycoproteins termed GP113/135 which represent the primary target of natural antibodies on the endothelial surface. Glycosidase treatment halted natural antibody binding, suggesting that the epitope(s) of importance are the oligosaccharide portions of the glycoprotein.

The important role of antibody-mediated rejection in the xenograft response has been confirmed by experiments in which recipient serum is depleted of antibody prior to xenograft placement. In one experiment, perfusion of rhesus serum through a porcine kidney before transplantation of a porcine heart increased graft survival from 2 to 80 h [18]. In some species combinations, hyperacute xenograft rejection is less dependent on the presence of natural antibody and activation of the classical complement pathway, but is rather mediated by direct activation of the *alternative* complement pathway by interaction of complement components with the xenogeneic endothelial cell surface. Experimental manipulations to deplete the xenograft recipient of natural antibodies as well as attempts to inactivate the complement system have achieved only modest success in prolonging xenograft survival [19], and none appears clinically feasible at present.

Cellular Response

In addition to the first barrier presented by the humoral immune response, xenograft rejection is also mediated by the cellular arm of the immune system. Cellular responses to xenoantigens are dependent upon recognition of foreign antigen in the context of the major histocompatibility complex (MHC) molecule [20]. Because the MHC is highly conserved, such interactions are possible and do function across a wide phylogenetic range. It has been difficult to study the cellular immune response in xenotransplantation, because the explosive nature of the humoral response leads to such rapid destruction of the graft that the cellular response is masked [21]. Clearly a vigorous cellular response to xenografts does exist in vivo. Even in concordant interspecies transplants (which have minimal or no preformed antibodies) a vigorous cellular response occurs and destroys the graft at a somewhat more attenuated pace than hyperacute rejection. Combinations of powerful immunosuppressive agents in these models have been unsuccessful in controlling the cellular response, suggesting a powerful and perhaps fundamentally different type of response.

$CD4^+$ T cells seem to have an enhanced role in the xenogeneic cellular immune response: antibody depletion of CD4 cells only minimally prolongs skin allograft survival, whereas similar depletion markedly extends xenograft survival [22]. Depletion of CD4 cells in a xenogeneic mixed lymphocyte reaction completely eliminated proliferation, whereas the allogeneic response was only partially diminished [23]. $CD4^+$ cells have been classified into two subgroups based on the characteristic cytokines they produce: the T-helper 1 (TH1) subset makes interleukin (IL)-2 and interferon (IFN)-γ and predominates in cell-mediated responses whereas the TH2 subset produces IL-4 and IL-10 and predominates in the humoral response [24]. Wren et. al. examined the mRNA cytokine profile of normal mouse lymphocytes in response to allo- and xenogeneic stimulation in MLR assays and found that TH1 responses were predominant in the allogeneic response (i.e., increased production of IL-2 and IFN-γ), while TH2 responses were predominant in the xenogeneic response (increased production of IL-4 and IL-10) [25]. Such differential cellular responses for allo-versus xenoreactivity may explain the failure of conventional immunosuppressive agents in xenotransplantation and might be exploited to develop new targeted immunosuppressive agents to control xenoreactivity.

Donor-Specific Tolerance Through Bone Marrow Chimerism

One approach to overcome the problem of vigorous xenoreactivity is the induction of donor-specific tolerance through bone marrow chimerism. The association between bone marrow chimerism and donor specific tolerance for transplanted grafts was first reported in the late 1940s and early 1950s [26]. Ray Owen first described red blood cell chimerism in Freemartin cattle. Freemartin cattle are dizygotic twins that share a common placenta during intrauterine life. Owen observed that exchange of blood between the twins' circulation in utero led to the development of stable, life-long red blood cell chimerism in both of the animals: a portion of each twin's red cells were phenotypically identical to its twin's. He hypothesized that the "...critical interchange is of embryonal cells ancestral to the erythrocytes of the adult animal."

Shortly thereafter, Sir Peter Medawar, who had developed a technique of histocompatibility typing based on skin grafting and had been commissioned by the British Agricultural Society to use this technique to determine which cattle twins were Freemartin, noted that skin grafts from one dizygotic twin to its Freemartin sibling were permanently accepted [27]. Aware of Owen's report, Medawar and his team hypothesized that the red blood cell chimerism in some way permitted donor-specific graft acceptance. This state of tolerance was believed to result from the clonal deletion of antigen-specific T cells [28]. Attempts to duplicate this experiment of nature in unconditioned adult mice were unsuccessful.

Subsequently, Billingham, Brent and Medawar [29] successfully injected hematopoietic cells into neonatal mice and demonstrated donor specific tolerance to skin grafts. During a privileged time period (which in mice lasts until about 72 h after birth and in humans is present only until the 14th to 16th week of gestation), marrow engrafted without cytoreductive conditioning. These experiments established the foundation for bone marrow transplantation with engraftment of the pluripotent stem cell as a means of rendering a recipient specifically tolerant to solid organ, tissue, and cellular grafts from a specific donor.

Bone marrow is unique in that it is the only tissue that, once transplanted, does not require immunosuppression to maintain graft acceptance. Moreover, acceptance of bone marrow also confers acceptance of donor derived organs and cellular grafts. In order to achieve engraftment of marrow, however, an adult recipient must undergo cytoreductive conditioning to create a "niche" for the transplanted cells, and in addition must receive standard immunosuppression to prevent residual host cells from rejecting the graft. Immunosuppressive agents used to prevent solid organ allograft rejection do not alone provide the necessary conditions for bone marrow engraftment. Experience has shown that specific cytoreductive agents such as radiation or busulfan (commonly employed in clinical bone marrow transplantation) are necessary for the pluripotent stem cell to engraft, even in autologous recipients [30].

Since Medawar's initial demonstration of lymphohematopoietic chimerism and donor-specific tolerance, several models have been developed in which engraftment of bone marrow has been achieved across species barriers. Congdon and Lorenz in 1954 demonstrated rescue of lethally irradiated mice with unmodified rat bone marrow [31]. Donor-specific tolerance to rat skin grafts after lethal irradiation of recipient mice and reconstitution with rat bone marrow was first demonstrated in 1957 [32]. These and other studies were limited by poor survival of recipients, as well as limited technology for demonstrating species-specific origin of myeloid and erythroid cells (i.e., chromosomal morphology at metaphase) [33].

Mixed Xenogeneic Chimeras

The preparation of mixed xenogeneic chimerism with donor-specific tolerance and excellent survival of recipients was first reported by Ildstad and Sachs in 1984 [34]. In that model, lethally irradiated mice were reconstituted with a combination of 5×10^6 T cell-depleted syngeneic (mouse) and 4×10^7 T cell-depleted xenogeneic (rat) bone marrow cells. These mixed xenogeneic chimeras (mouse + rat $\rightarrow$ mouse, Fig. 1) exhibited excellent survival and some exhibited detectable low-level chimerism (0 %–2.6 % rat). Survival of subsequent donor-specific (rat) skin grafts was prolonged. Systemic donor-specific tolerance was also evident in vitro, as recipient lymphocytes were specifically unreactive to donor alloantigens yet remained responsive to MHC-disparate third-party alloantigens in MLR and CML assays. Mixed allogeneic chimeras similarly had excellent survival and donor-specific tolerance to skin grafts. Chimerism in these animals occurred at a higher level (5 %–92 %) than in xenogeneic chimeras. The tolerance which developed in both groups of chimeras was an all-or-none phenomenon. Animals with 0.5 % donor cells were as tolerant as those with greater than 90 % donor cells.

In contrast to mixed chimerism, fully allo- or xenogeneic chimeras are prepared by lethally irradiating the host and reconstituting only with donor allo- or xenogeneic marrow (A $\rightarrow$ B). While fully allogeneic chimerism also leads to

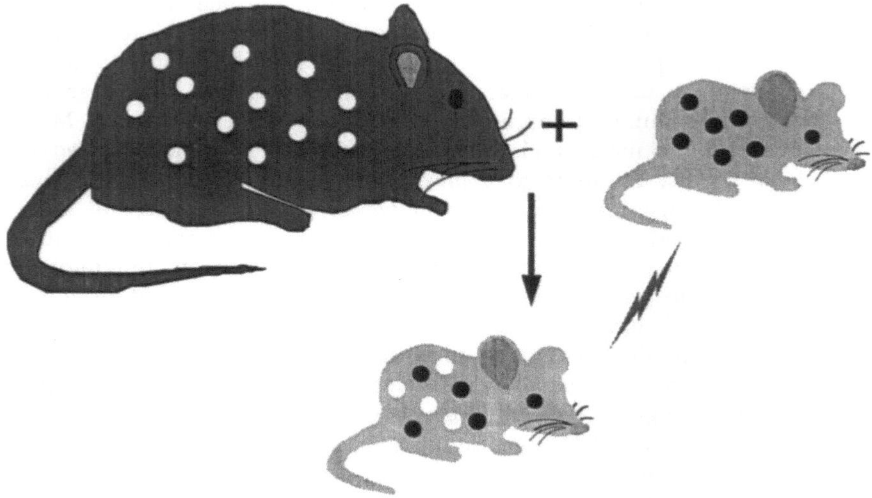

Fig. 1. Mixed xenogeneic chimerism (rat + mouse → rat)

donor-specific tolerance, complete replacement of the recipient's immune system is associated with a state of relative immunoincompetence [35–37], and recipients are prone to graft-versus-host disease (GVHD) [38]. A clear advantage of mixed allogeneic chimerism is improved immunocompetence and lack of susceptibility to GVHD relative to fully allogeneic chimeras. An explanation for this difference is found by considering T cell development in a foreign host. In fully allogeneic chimeras, nascent T cells undergo education and development in a foreign (host) thymic environment and emerge restricted to recognizing antigen in the context of host MHC on antigen-presenting cells (APCs). Since the recipient has been ablated, the only APCs available express foreign MHC, so T cells must see antigen in the context of foreign MHC. Defects in T cell recognition and activation result in a state of immunoincompetence for all primary immune responses (antibody production, antiviral reactivity) and therefore decreased survival.

Mixed chimerism is associated with engraftment of both host and donor pluripotent hematopoietic stem cells, with production of multilineage progeny by each of the stem cells. This provides both donor and host APCs with which T cells restricted to host APC can interact. Immunocompetence for primary immune responses (antibody production, antiviral responses) is thereby preserved. The presence of the syngeneic bone marrow provides the host-type APCs essential for full immunocompetence while the allogeneic marrow provides a persistent source of antigen for induction and maintenance of donor-specific tolerance.

Mixed xenogeneic chimeras (rat + mouse → mouse) prepared without T cell depletion of the xenogeneic (rat) bone marrow (preserving components essential for stem cell engraftment) demonstrate excellent survival, freedom from GVHD, and donor-specific tolerance to skin and islet grafts [39, 40]. Levels of chimerism range from 1%–48% rat. Xenogeneic T lymphocytes in this model undergo phenotypically normal maturation in the xenogeneic stromal environment: rat T lymphocytes with an immature staining pattern are present in the thymus while those with a mature phenotype are found in the periphery of a mixed xenogeneic chimera [41].

The model of mixed allogeneic chimerism has been applied to determine the influence of syngeneic and allogeneic components on engraftment, as well as to define the role of various cell types in failure of engraftment. The initial mixed allogeneic chimerism model ($A + B \rightarrow A$) incorporated T cell depletion of both syngeneic (A) and allogeneic (B) components of bone marrow. When the syngeneic component was not T cell depleted (irrespective of whether the allogeneic component was T cell depleted), recipients repopulated exclusively with host-type cells [35]. This suggested the existence of an alloreactive component in the syngeneic marrow that prevented allogeneic marrow engraftment and which was functionally removed with T cell depletion.

T cell depletion of the syngeneic component of the mixed marrow inocula permitted engraftment of the allogeneic component, whether or not it had been T cell-depleted. In combination with untreated allogeneic marrow, recipients repopulated exclusively with donor-type cells, whereas when both syngeneic and allogeneic bone marrow were T cell depleted, the recipients repopulated as mixed donor/host chimeras with variable percentages of donor and host-type lymphoid elements. In all cases the engraftment of allogeneic bone marrow was associated with specific tolerance to allogeneic skin grafts.

The fact that T cell depletion of donor marrow in both allogeneic and xenogeneic systems somehow impaired subsequent engraftment suggested the existence of cells in bone marrow which express T cell markers and exert a facilitatory effect on engraftment. Such observations are in accord with the experience in clinical bone marrow transplantation. Realization that T cells were the primary effector of GVHD stimulated clinical trials aimed at preventing GVHD by T cell depletion of the bone marrow. While the incidence of GVHD was decreased, the benefit was offset by a substantial increase in failure of engraftment [42, 43]. GVH activity and facilitation of engraftment were deemed inseparable, and further efforts to perform T cell depletion of donor marrow were abandoned.

The model of mixed allogeneic chimerism is an ideal one to study because the endpoint measured is the level of chimerism, rather than death. In studies of the engraftment "facilitating" effect, a model of allogeneic chimerism was established in which the majority of lethally irradiated recipients repopulated with low levels of donor cells (a ratio of 1:1 T cell-depleted syngeneic to T cell-depleted allogeneic cells resulted in a mean 17% level of allogeneic chimerism) [44]. Rare events multiparameter live sterile cell sorting was utilized to isolate specific, highly purified subpopulations of bone marrow cells which could then be added back to the above system to determine if this population enabled engraftment of stem cells in allogeneic recipients. A "facilitating cell" population characterized by the presence of specific cell-surface markers, including $CD3^+$, $CD8^+$, $CD45^+$, $CD45R^+$, class II dim/intermediate, but T cell receptor $(TCR)^-$ was identified. Ten thousand allogeneic stem cells alone will not rescue a lethally irra-

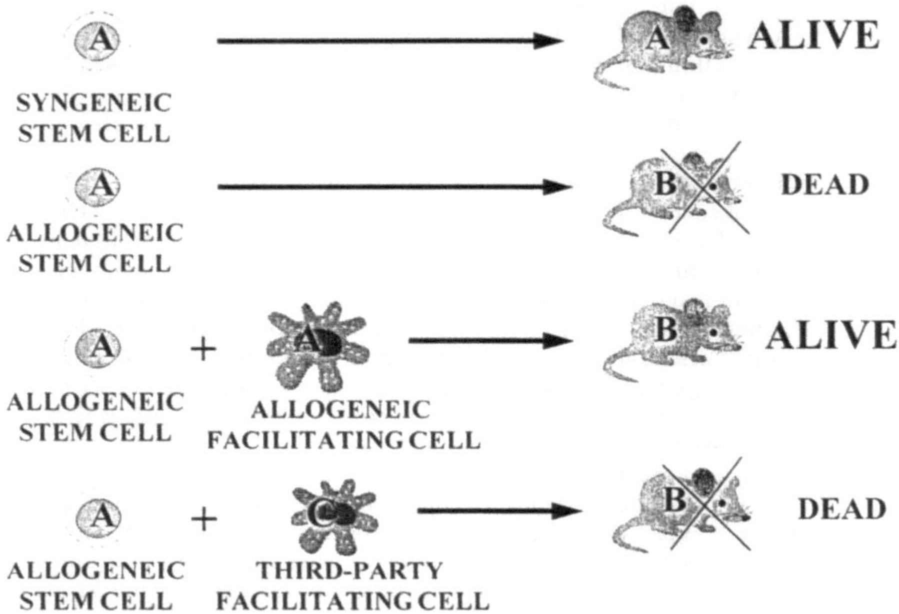

Fig. 2. Major histocompatibility complex (MHC)-matched facilitating cells permit the engraftment of allogeneic stem cells

diated recipient; however the addition of as few as 30 000 purified facilitating cells permits reliable engraftment. Importantly, the facilitating cell and the stem cell must be MHC matched for this effect to occur (Fig. 2).

Recipients of the facilitating and stem cell inoculum demonstrated durable multilineage allogeneic engraftment, confirming that the pluripotent hematopoeietic stem cell had indeed engrafted without GVHD. The identification of a facilitating cell population may allow selective graft engineering in bone marrow transplantation, such that cells mediating GVHD can be selectively removed while stem cells, progenitors, and those cells mediating the facilitating effect preserved. The scope of bone marrow transplantation may be widened to include induction of donor-specific transplantation tolerance for xeno- and allotransplantation as well as its application to nonmalignant disease states including various enzyme deficiency states, hemoglobinopathies, and autoimmune disorders.

Nonlethal Conditioning

While bone marrow transplantation and the development of donor-specific tolerance is an attractive strategy to permit xenotransplantation, the requirement for lethal irradiation of the recipient has its significant toxicity and limits clinical applicability. This has stimulated efforts to achieve bone marrow chimerism with nonlethal conditioning of the recipient. A number of nonlethal methods for producing mixed chimerism and donor-specific tolerance have been described.

Monaco and Wood were the first to demonstrate that infusion of large numbers of lymphoid cells during a state of immunosuppression induced by adult thymectomy and anti-lymphocyte serum produced specific tolerance and long-lasting lymphohematopoietic cell chimerism [45]. Tolerance was achieved in a single-MHC-mismatched parent → F1 model, but similar efforts in fully mismatched models were hampered by GVHD and were unsuccessful. A radiation-free model has been described by Muyami and Good, in which tolerance to MHC-disparate skin grafts was achieved with in vivo recipient depletion with anti-Thy1.2 monoclonal antibodies followed by infusion of spleen and bone marrow cells as well as cyclophosphamide. Levels of chimerism were low (1 %–3 %), and the requirement for large numbers of allogeneic spleen cells and thus a high risk of GVHD would make such a model impractical for clinical application [46]. Cobbold et al. were able to achieve tolerance across MHC barriers using depleting anti-CD4 and anti-CD8 monoclonal antibodies, but required sublethal doses of radiation (600 cGy) to reliably achieve this effect [47].

Sharabi and Sachs lessened the requirement for total body irradiation to 300 cGy in a similar model using 700 cGy thymic irradiation in combination with anti-CD4 and anti-CD8 monoclonal antibodies [48]. Extension of this technique to a xenogeneic (rat → mouse) model required the addition of anti-NK1.1 and anti-Thy1.2 antibodies in order to achieve reliable engraftment [49]. Although significant xenogeneic chimerism was initially achieved, levels declined and by 6 months were undetectable. Donor-specific tolerance for skin grafts was present. Further observations showed a significant attenuation of the humoral response against rat bone marrow cells, suggesting that a degree of humoral tolerance in addition to cellular tolerance had been achieved [50].

In our own hands, a total body irradiation (TBI)-based model for incomplete recipient myeloablation was first established in an allogeneic model [51]. The incidence and level of chimerism in a mixed allogeneic model were determined at various levels of TBI. Durable engraftment of MHC-disparate bone marrow occured in 100 % of recipients at 700 cGy, 51 % at 600 cGy, 13 % at 500 cGy, and none at 400 cGy TBI. When cyclophosphamide, an alkylating agent widely used for cytoreduction in preparation for bone marrow transplantation, was administered in combination with radiation, substantially lower doses of radiation (500 cGy) were sufficient to permit reliable engraftment. Finally, addition of antilymphocyte globulin (ALG) to the above model reduced the radiation requirement further to 300 cGy [52]. This regimen was non-myeloablative and nonlethal, as 100 % of animals so treated and not given bone marrow repopulated with syngeneic cells and survived. The chimerism produced in this model was stable, multilineage, and conferred donor-specific tolerance to skin and cardiac allografts. A similar, nonlethal conditioning regimen has recently been applied to the xenogeneic model. Mice conditioned with 700 cGy TBI and transplanted with untreated rat bone marrow developed permanent (stable) multilineage chimerism and demonstrated donor-specific tolerance to simultaneous islet xenografts [53].

Human->Baboon Mixed Xenogeneic Chimeras

Recent efforts in our laboratory have been directed at preparation of human->baboon mixed xenogeneic chimeras. The establishment of a human immune system in a large primate model would provide an experimental model for a number of disease states, including human immunodeficiency virus (HIV) infection. Human marrow enriched for both stem and facilitating cell phenotypes is given to a nonlethally conditioned baboon. Dose-escalation studies are currently in progress. We have established that baboons tolerate the infusion of large doses of human marrow without toxicity. Preliminary results suggest that human chimerism at levels as high as 20% is achievable in this model [54]. Conversely, transplantation of baboon marrow (which is resistant to infection with HIV-1) into a human with late-stage acquired immunodeficiency syndrome (AIDS) might restore the recipient's immunocompetence. This therapeutic strategy is being explored in pilot clinical studies.

Comment

The benefits of xenotransplantation include a large supply of organs, the opportunity to modify organs prior to transplant, and the resistance of certain species to common human pathogens, such as hepatitis and HIV. In order for these benefits to be realized, the xenogeneic immune response must be harnessed. Donor-specific transplantation tolerance following successful engraftment of xenogeneic hematopoietic stem cells offers a unique solution to the daunting problem of vigorous xenoreactivity.

References

1. 1994 Annual Report of the U.S. Scientific Registry for Transplant Recipients and the Organ Procurement and Transplantation Network – Transplant Data: 1988–1993. UNOS, Richmond, VA, and the Division of Organ Transplantation, Bureau of Health Resources and Development, Health Resources and Services Administration, U.S. Department of Health and Human Services, Bethesda, MD, p. E-21
2. Guo TJ, Daily OP, Davies DB: The UNOS OPTN Waiting List: 1988 to 1994. In: Clinical Transplants 1994, Terasaki, P.I., Cecka, J.M., eds. UCLA Tissue Typing Laboratory
3. Carrell A. La technique operatoire des anasomoses vasculaires et la transplantation des visceres. Lyon Med. 1902; 98:859–64
4. Jaboulay M. Greffe de reins au pli du coude par soudures arterielles et veineuses. Lyon Med. 1906; 107:575
5. Reemtsma R. Xenotransplantation – a brief history of clinical experiences: 1900–1965. In: Xenotransplantation, Cooper DKC, et al., eds. Springer, Heidelberg, 1991
6. Hitchcock CR, Kiser JC, Telander RL, et al. Baboon renal grafts. JAMA 1964; 189:934
7. Starzl TE, Marchioro T, Peters GN, et al. Renal heterotransplantation from baboon to man: experience with six cases. Transplantation, 1964; 2:752

8. Hardy JD, Kurrus FE, Chavez CM, et al. Heart transplantation in man: developmental studies and report of a case. JAMA, 1964; 188:1132
9. Starzl TE. Experience in Hepatic Transplantation. Saunders, Philadelphia, 1969, p. 408
10. Bailey LL, Nehlsen-Cannarella SL, Concepcion W, et al. Baboon to human cardiac xenotransplantation in a neonate. JAMA, 1985; 254:3321
11. Starzl TE, Fung J, Tzakis A, et al. Baboon to human liver transplantation. Lancet, 1993; 341:65
12. Perper RJ, Najarian JS. Experimental renal heterotransplantation: I. In widely divergent species. Transplantation, 1966; 4:377
13. Calne RY. Organ transplantation between widely disparate species. Transplant Proc, 1970; 2:550
14. Markmann JF, Barker CF. Basic and clinical considerations in the use of xenografts. Curr Probl Surg, 1994; 5:385
15. Kaufman CL, Gaines BA, Ildstad ST. Xenotransplantation. Annu Rev Immunol, 1995; 13:339
16. Platt JL, Vercellotti GM, Dalmasso AP, et al. Transplantation of discordant xenografts: a review of progress. Immunol Today, 1990; 11:450
17. Platt JL, Lindaman BJ, Chen H, et al. Endothelial cell antigens recognized by xenoreactive human natural antibodies. Transplantation, 1990; 50:817
18. Fischel RJ, Matas AJ, Perry E, et al. Plasma exchange, organ perfusion, and immunosuppression reduce "natural" antibody levels as measured by binding to xenogeneic endothelial cells and prolong discordant xenograft survival. Transplant Proc, 1992; 24:574
19. Leventhal JR, Dalmasso AP, Cromwell JW, et al. Prolongation of cardiac xenograft survival by depletion of complement. Transplantation, 1993; 55:857
20. Swain SL, Dutton RW, Schwab R, et al. Xenogeneic human anti-mouse T cell responses are due to the activity of the same functional T cell subsets responsible for allospecific and major histocompatibility complex restricted responses. J Exp Med, 1983; 157:720
21. Auchincloss H. Xenogeneic transplantation. Transplantation, 1988; 45:1
22. Pierson RN III, Winn HJ, Russell PS, Auchincloss H Jr. Xenogeneic skin graft rejection is especially dependent on CD4+ T cells. J Exp Med, 1989; 170:991
23. Moses RD, Pierson RN, Winn JH, et al. Xenogeneic proliferation and lymphokine production are dependent on CD4+ helper T cells and self antigen-presenting cells in the mouse. J Exp Med, 1990; 172:567
24. Mossman TR, Schumacher JH, Street NF, et al. Diversity of cytokine synthesis and function of mouse CD4+ T cells. Immunol Rev, 1991; 123:209
25. Wren SM, Wang SC, Thai NL, et al. Evidence for early Th2 T cell predominance in xenoreactivity. Transplantation, 1993; 56:905
26. Owen RD. Immunogenetic consequences of vascular anastomoses between bovine twins. Science, 1945; 102:400
27. Billingham RE, Lamphin HG, Medawar PB, et al. Tolerance of homografts, twin diagnosis and the freemartin conditions in cattle. Heredity, 1952; 6:201
28. Burnet FM. The Clonal Selection Theory of Acquired Immunity. Cambridge: Cambridge University Press, 1959
29. Billingham RE, Brent L, Medawar PB. Actively acquired tolerance to foreign cells. Nature, 1953; 172:606

30. Down JD, Tarbell NJ, Thames HD, Mauch PM. Syngeneic and allogeneic bone marrow engraftment after total body irradiation: dependence on dose, dose rate, and fractionation. Blood, 1991; 77:661
31. Congdon CG, Lorenz E. Humoral factor in irradiation protection: modification of lethal irradiation injury in mice by injection of rat bone marrow. Am J Physiol, 1954; 176:297
32. Zaalberg O, Vos O, Van Bekkum D. Surviving rat skin grafts in mice. Nature, 1957; 180:238
33. Ford CE, Hamerton JL, Barnes DW, Loutit JF. Cytological identification of radiation chimeras. Nature, 1956; 177:452
34. Ildstad ST, Sachs DH. Reconstitution with syngeneic plus allogeneic or xenogeneic bone marrow leads to specific acceptance of allografts or xenografts. Nature, 1984; 307:168
35. Ildstad ST, Wren SM, Bluestone JA, et al. Effect of selective T cell depletion of host and/or donor bone marrow on lymphopoietic repopulation, tolerance, and graft-vs-host disease in mixed allogeneic chimeras (B10 + B10.D2 → B10). J Immunol, 1986; 136:28
36. Zinkernagel RM, Althage A, Callahan G, Welsh RM. On the immunoincompetence of H-2 incompatible irradiated bone marrow chimeras. J Immunol, 1980; 124:2356
37. Rayfield LS, Brent L. Tolerance, immunocompetence, and secondary disease in fully allogeneic radiation chimeras. Transplantation, 1983; 36:183
38. Korngold R, Sprent J. Lethal GvHD after bone marrow transplantation across minor histocompatibility barriers in mice: prevention by removing mature T cells from marrow. J Exp Med, 1978; 148:1687
39. Ildstad ST, Boggs SS, Vecchini F, et al. Mixed xenogeneic chimeras (rat + mouse to mouse): evidence of rat stem cell engraftment, strain-specific transplantation tolerance, and skin-specific antigens. Transplantation, 1992; 53:815
40. Li H, Ricordi C, Demetris AJ, et al. Mixed xenogeneic chimerism (mouse + rat → mouse) to induce donor-specific tolerance to sequential or simultaneous islet xenografts. Transplantation, 1994; 57:592
41. Ildstad ST, Vacchio MS, Markus PM, et al. Cross-species transplantation tolerance: rat bone marrow-derived cells can contribute to the ligand for negative selection of mouse T cell receptor Vbeta in chimeras tolerant to xenogeneic antigens (mouse + rat → mouse). J Exp Med, 1992; 175:147
42. Soderling CCB, Song CW, Blazar BR, Vallera DA. A correlation between conditioning and engraftment in recipients of MHC-mismatched T cell-depleted murine bone marrow transplants. J Immunol, 1985; 125:941
43. Kernan NA, Bordignon C, Heller G, et al. Graft failure after T cell-depleted human leukocyte antigen identical marrow transplant for leukemia: I. Analysis of risk factors and results of secondary transplants. Blood, 1989; 74:2227
44. Kaufman C, Colson Y, Wren S, et al. Characterization of a novel cell that facilitates engraftment of purified stem cells in an allogeneic MHC-disparate environment. Blood, 1994; 84:2436
45. Monaco AP, Wood ML, Russell PS. Induction of immunological tolerance and chimerism across the H-2 locus in mice following adult thymectomy and antilymphocyte serum (ALS). Transplantation, 1966; 4:543

46. Muyami H, Good RA. Long-lasting skin allograft tolerance in adult mice induced across fully allogeneic (multimajor H-2 plus multiminor histocompatibility) antigen barriers by a tolerance-inducing method using cyclophosphamide. J Exp Med, 1989; 169:213
47. Cobbold SP, Martin G, Waldmann H. Monoclonal antibodies to promote marrow engraftment and tissue graft tolerance. Nature, 1986; 323:164
48. Sharabi Y, Sachs DH. Mixed chimerism and permanent specific transplantation tolerance induced by a nonlethal preparative regimen. J Exp Med, 1989; 169:493
49. Sharabi Y, Aksentijevich I, Sundt TM, et al. Specific tolerance induction across a xenogeneic barrier: production of mixed rat/mouse lymphohematopoietic chimeras using a nonlethal preparative regimen. J Exp Med, 1990; 172:195
50. Aksentijevich I, Sachs DH, Sykes M. Humoral tolerance in xenogeneic BMT recipients conditioned by a non-myeloablative regimen. Transplantation, 1992; 53:1108
51. Colson YL, Wren SM, Schuchert MJ, et al. A nonlethal conditioning approach to achieve durable multilineage mixed chimerism and tolerance across major, minor and hematopoietic histocompatibility barriers. J Immunol, 1995; 155:4179–4188
52. Colson YL, Li H, Boggs SS, et al. Durable mixed allogeneic chimerism and tolerance by a nonlethal radiation based cytoreductive approach. J Immunol, 1996; 157:2820–2829
53. Li H, Abou El-Ezz AY, Cambrell BE, Ildstad ST. Mixed xenogeneic chimerism and tolerance. III. A nonlethal approach to induce donor-specific transplantation tolerance to simultaneous islet xenografts. Transplantation, 1995; 60:59
54. Michaels M, Kaufman C, Huneke R, et al. Multilineage mixed chimerism in nonhuman primates using a nonlethal conditioning approach. Presented at the Symposium on Tolerance Induction, Breckenridge, 1995

VI Experimental Pancreatic Islet Cell Xenotransplantation

40 Introduction

R.P. Lanza and W.L. Chick

Xenotransplantation of pancreatic islets offers the possibility of a cure for diabetes mellitus. There are over 100 million people with diabetes in the world, and the incidence levels continue to increase by approximately 2% per year. In patients with insulin-dependent diabetes mellitus (IDDM), there is a marked decrease in the number of insulin-producing beta cells in the pancreas. In the past, animal or recombinant human sources of insulin have provided the replacement therapy required by these patients. Unfortunately, injected insulin cannot precisely mimic the ability of the normal pancreas to regulate blood glucose concentrations. The concentration of insulin in the blood is normally linked to the blood glucose concentration by moment-to-moment fluctuations in insulin secretion by the beta cells of the pancreatic islets. These fluctuations in insulin secretion, which serve to control blood glucose concentrations, are dependent upon a complex series of biochemical pathways in the living beta cell, and are extremely difficult or impossible to simulate by insulin injection. The results of the Diabetes Control and Complications Trial (DCCT) suggest that failure to achieve physiologic glucose control with injected insulin is responsible for the serious complications of this disease including diabetic nephropathy, retinopathy and neuropathy [1].

There is hope that the transplantation of islets of Langerhans will not only eliminate the need for daily insulin injections, but will prove effective in preventing or retarding the development of complications associated with the disease. Unfortunately, like other human organs, donor pancreases are in very short supply. In the United States, it is estimated that only approximately 1000 pancreases are recovered each year. Even with improved procurement of human organs, the supply of donor tissue would remain quite inadequate if pancreatic islet transplantation were to be developed as an effective therapy. For the immediate future, the logical alternative is to use nonhuman donor islets. For example, methods have been developed to isolate pancreatic islets from porcine and bovine glands; insulins from these animals are fully active in man and have been used to treat diabetics for over 70 years. Pig and cow islets are an attractive option because they are readily available and the amino acid sequences of these insulins are similar to human insulin. Furthermore, herds of specific pathogen-free (SPF) animals are already available as a potential safeguard against the transfer of infectious organisms to human islet recipients.

Although fundamental advances in our understanding of the human immune system and the immune rejection process may eventually lead to means for developing therapies which will overcome the vigorous humoral and cellular immune responses associated with the transplantation of xenogeneic tissues, many of these solutions are likely to be decades in the future. Immunoisolation [2] and immunomodulation [3] techniques offer great promise for solving this problem in a reasonable time frame, and may, in the next several decades, prove the only way to establish prolonged survival of islet xenografts. Islets offer an advantage in this respect; the tissue can be maintained and manipulated more easily than whole organ grafts and may allow several approaches for the induction of tolerance to be linked together resulting in a more effective therapy [4]. Moreover, the opportunity for encapsulation of islet tissue to isolate it from the immune system of the host by a selectively permeable membrane may allow the xenotransplantation of islets to be achieved without generalized immunosuppression [5].

Much experimental work is currently in progress exploring these approaches for transplanting islet xenografts. For the most part, these studies involve transplantation of concordant islets into rodents, although work exploring immunoisolation strategies for transplanting discordant islets is also underway in both rodents and dogs. In this brief introduction, we will simply touch on some of the broader strategies that have been explored in experimental models of islet xenotransplantation. More detailed discussions of some of these approaches will be furnished by the other chapters in this book.

Immunomodulation

A number of strategies have been developed to reduce the immunogenicity of isolated islet tissue prior to transplantation (Fig. 1). These include culturing the islets under different conditions [6–8], exposing the islets to ultraviolet B (UV-B) irradiation [9], and pretreatment with antibodies to either eliminate passenger

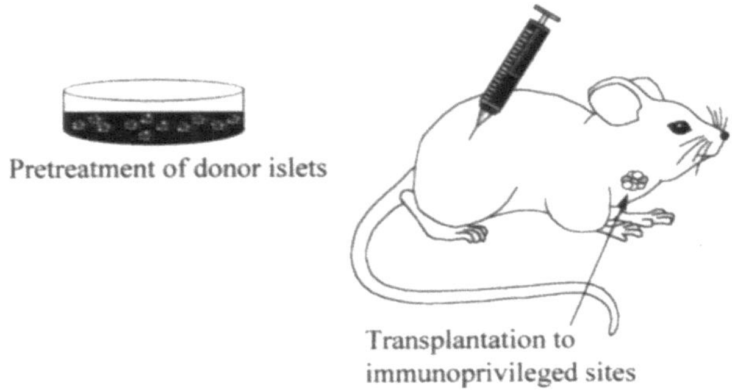

Fig. 1. Immunomodulation. A number of pretreatment strategies have been developed to reduce the immunogenicity of islets prior to transplantation. These include culturing the islets under different conditions, exposing the islets to ultraviolet B irradiation, and treatment with antibodies to either eliminate passenger lymphocytes or to camouflage or mask donor transplant antigens before transplantation. Other approaches aim to transplant islets to immunologically privileged sites such as the thymus, testis, or brain. Alternative techniques involve modulating the immune system of the host with either drugs, antibodies, or other agents

lymphocytes [10] or to camouflage or mask donor transplant antigens [11] before transplantation. Other approaches aim to transplant islets intrathymically [12] or to immunologically privileged sites such as the testis or brain [13]. Alternative techniques involve modulating the immune system of the host with either antibodies, drugs or oral antigens [14–16].

Immunomodulation of Islets by Culture

Culturing islets in hyperbaric oxygen (95%) or at low temperatures (22°–24°C) has been shown to reduce islet immunogenicity in a number of different rodent models [8]. The first attempts to use culture at high oxygen concentrations to reduce the immunogenicity of donor tissue were reported in the mid-1970s, when it was demonstrated that this technique could prolong survival of both thyroid allografts [17] and thyroid xenografts [18]. Subsequent experiments using islet xenografts cultured in high O_2 or at low temperature were also successful [6]. To date, however, the utilization of this procedure has been limited to studies in rodents. The reason for the beneficial effects of these various culture procedures is unclear. One well accepted theory, initially proposed by Snell [19] and later strengthened by Lafferty et al. [20], suggests that these approaches act on major histocompatibility complex (MHC) class II-positive antigen-presenting cells (APCs) carried in the islet tissue. Both high oxygen tension and low temperature are known to exert a deleterious effect on the resident leukocytes, most commonly referred to as passenger leukocytes; the passenger leukocyte-depleted islet graft is then unable to initiate a rejection response, although rejection will occur if the immune system of the recipient is deliberately activated by challenge with donor leukocytes or a skin graft [21, 22].

Immunomodulation of Islets by Ultraviolet B Irradiation

The effects of ultraviolet B irradiation (290–320 nm) on donor/host immunogenicity and on the downregulation of host immune responses has also been studied by several groups [23, 24]. Hardy et al. [25] have shown that the state of hyporesponsiveness or anergy induced by exposing islet allografts to UV-B irradiation is also beneficial in reducing xenograft immunogenicity. UV-B irradiated rat islets were successfully xenotransplanted into streptozotocin-induced diabetic mice. The islets were accepted by B10/BR recipients (low responder), while high-responder Balb/C mice showed only modest prolongation of islet xenograft survival. Although the underlying mechanism(s) of the UV-B effect on APC function is poorly defined, recent studies suggest that impairment of accessory cell function is due to defect(s) at the molecular level [9].

Antibodies Directed to Major Histocompatibility Complex Determinants

Antibodies are another mode of therapy that have been used to prevent graft rejection of both islet allografts and xenografts [11]. There are three contrasting immunological targets for immune interference using antibodies: (1) the administration of antibodies to the host to inactivate or destroy the host's T cells, (2) the use of antibodies to eliminate specifically passenger lymphocytes from the donor tissue prior to transplantation, and (3) the use of nonlytic antibodies to camouflage or mask donor transplant antigens prior to transplantation. Using the latter approach, Faustman et al. [26] prevented human islet xenograft rejection in murine recipients without immunosuppression by masking donor HLA class I antigens. Although masking all donor surface molecules with nonlytic polyclonal serum similarly allowed long-term survival, other less dense surface proteins such as lymphocyte function-associated antigen (LFA)-3 and intercellular adhesion molecule (ICAM)-1 played a less important role and allowed less extended survival when masked prior to xenotransplantation.

Intrathymic Islet Transplants and Systemic Tolerance

The use of the thymus as a site of pancreatic islet transplantation is based on several morphologic and functional attributes [12]. Anatomic data suggest that the thymic parenchyma is relatively sequestered from peripheral immune surveillance [27, 28]. Furthermore, the thymus is known to play a central role in the acquisition of T cell tolerance to self-MHC and non-MHC antigens [29]. The ability of the thymus to promote indefinite survival of rat islet allografts and render recipients unresponsive to donor alloantigens led Mayo et al. [30] and others [31] to evaluate the capability of the thymus to promote survival of concordant islet xenografts (rat-to-mouse). In these experiments, it was demonstrated that the thymus provided a similar degree of protection to the xenografts, and that long-term residence of intrathymic islet xenografts promoted the development of a donor-specific unresponsive state. The mechanism of the induction of this unresponsive state to xenogeneic antigens remains uncertain, although it may be due to deletion or functional inactivation of xenoantigen-reactive T cell clones [30].

Islet Xenotransplantation to Other Immunoprivileged Sites

In addition to the thymus, there are a number of other immunologically privileged sites that have been explored for purposes of experimental islet transplantation. These include the anterior chamber of the eye, the cheek pouch of the hamster, the brain and cerebrospinal fluid (CSF) space, and the testis [13]. Of course, only the latter two sites have direct clinical potential. Tzu et al. [31] have shown prolonged survival of rat islet xenografts in the brain and in the intrathecal/subarachnoid space of monkeys, and Selawry et al. [32] have demonstrated the long-term survival of hamster islets in the testes of rats treated with cyclosporine. More recently, the latter group has demonstrated extended survival of discordant islet xenografts (pig to rat) without sustained immunosuppression using a composite of islets and Sertoli cells [33]. The authors believe this immunoprotection was provided by a substance or substances secreted by the Sertoli cells.

Modulation of the Immune System with Antibodies and/or Drugs

Islet xenograft survival has been prolonged in various animal models using a wide range of immunosuppressive agents, including cyclosporine [34–36], 15-deoxyspergualin [37, 38], FK506 (tacrolimus) [39], leflunomide [40, 41], antilymphocyte/antithymocyte serum [42, 43], CTLA4Ig [44, 45], and monoclonal antibodies directed against CD4 and CD8 epitopes [35, 46, 47] among others [14]. Unfortunately, use of these agents is associated with a variety of problems [48, 49], and some of them, including cyclosporine [50–53] and FK506 [54, 55], have dose-dependent deleterious effects on glucose homeostasis and beta cell function.

Immunoisolation

A number of immunoisolation systems have been developed and refined during the past several decades which have set the stage for a quantum advance in cell and tissue transplantation. These systems, may, during the next several decades, prove the best way to establish prolonged survival of cell and tissue xenotransplants in patients with diseases caused by the loss of specific vital metabolic functions. In addition to diabetes, they have broad application to treating major diseases such as cancer and acquired immunodeficiency syndrome (AIDS) and a wide range of other disorders resulting from functional defects of native cell systems [5]. These include the use of (a) hepatocytes in the treatment of liver failure and enzymatic defects [56–62], (b) adrenal cells in Parkinson's disease [63–65], (c) cells which produce nerve growth factors in Alzheimer's disease [66–68], epilepsy, Lou Gehrig's disease, Huntington's disease [69–71], spinal cord injuries [72], and strokes, (d) cells which produce clotting factors VIII and IX in hemophilia [73, 74], and (e) endocrine cells in other disorders resulting from hormone deficiency [75, 76]. Moreover, by using recombinant DNA and cell engineering technologies in conjunction with encapsulation technologies, it should also prove possible to treat patients suffering from chronic pain [65], Kaposi's sarcoma, and various hematologic disorders.

To date, most of the research in the area of encapsulated cell transplantation has been carried out with pancreatic islets. There are several reasons for this: (a) diabetes is a leading cause of morbidity and mortality in the world, at a cost of approximately $94 billion in the United States alone, (b) pancreatic islets, which comprise only 1%–2% of the human adult pancreatic volume, can be isolated from animal sources, and (c) the quantity of differentiated islet tissue to be transplanted is within a reasonable range (less than 1 g).

Three major types of encapsulation system have been studied by our own and other groups (Fig. 2). These include devices anastomosed to the vascular system as arteriovenous (AV) shunts, hollow fibers and wider-bore membrane diffusion chambers, macroporous membrane devices, and microcapsules and reactors. Islet xenotransplantation studies in diabetic rodents and dogs indicate that these systems can function for periods of several months to more than 1 year [2, 77]. However, clinical application of these devices is hindered in many cases by problems such as fragility, limited surface area, and, in the case of perfused vascular devices, the surgery required for implantation and shunt connection with risks of hemorrhage, thrombosis, embolism and infection, and the relatively high diffusion resistance inherent in the plastic membranes. We have recently developed a microencapsulation technology that bypasses these problems and provides more options for the method and site of implantation. These biodegradable microreactors can simply be injected under the skin, or placed intraperitoneally or in other extravascular sites using a needle and syringe. These studies will be discussed in greater detail in the proceeding section (see Chap. 43).

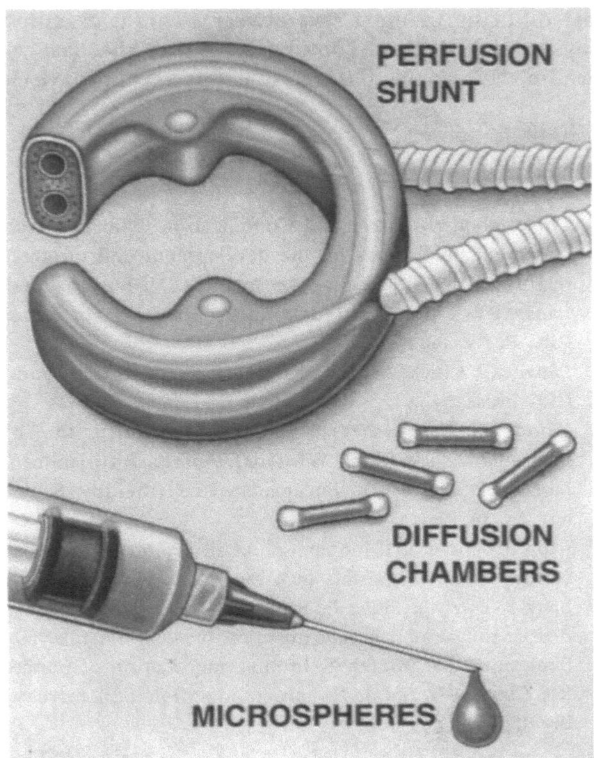

Fig. 2. Immunoisolation. In the form of a vascular implant, islets can be distributed in a chamber surrounding a permselective membrane, and the device implanted as a shunt in the vascular system. Alternatively, islets can be immunoisolated within membrane diffusion chambers or microcapsules and placed intraperitoneally, intramuscularly, subcutaneously, or in other sites. The islets within these devices are generally immobilized in hydrogels such as alginate or agar. One of the important functions of these gels is to provide more uniform islet distribution by preventing settling and subsequent aggregation of the tissue into larger, necrotic masses. (Reprinted with permission from [5])

Comment

Studies involving transplantation of human islets in type I diabetics have been of significant value both in documenting the potential importance of islet transplantation as a therapeutic modality, and in defining some of the problems which must be overcome before this approach can be used in large numbers of patients. The currently limited supply of adult human pancreatic glands, and the fact that multiple glands may be required to isolate sufficient numbers of islets to treat a single patient, indicate that techniques must be further developed and refined for xenografting of isolated islets from animal sources to diabetic patients. Development of methods for propagating islets in culture, although still at an early stage, are likely to resolve the problem of islet procurement in the more distant future.

Techniques for transplanting islets must overcome both classical immune rejection of transplanted cells and tissues, and autoimmune destruction of beta cells known to occur in type I diabetics. Islet transplantation should be simple and practical, and should be associated with minimal side effects. Finally, the approaches developed must not produce islet damage or dysfunction.

An increasing body of evidence involving islet transplantation in animals using immune isolation and immune modulation strongly suggests that methods for successful xenografting of islets in diabetic patients will be developed and tested during the next several years. This is certain to revolutionize current therapy for this disease. Looking back over the past 75 years since the discovery of insulin, few would disagree that this revolution is long overdue.

References

1. The Diabetes Control and Complication Trial Research Group. The effect of intensive treatment of diabetes on the development and progression of long-term complications in insulin-dependent diabetes mellitus. N. Engl. J. Med. 329, 977, 1993
2. Lanza RP, Chick WL (eds), Immunoisolation of Pancreatic Islets.Austin, R.G.Landes/CRC Press, 1994
3. Lanza RP, Chick WL (eds), Immunomodulation of Pancreatic Islets.Austin, R.G.Landes/CRC Press, 1994
4. Wood KJ. Approaches to achieving tolerance. In: Immunomodulation of Pancreatic Islets. Lanza RP, Chick WL (eds). Austin, R.G.Landes/CRC Press, 1994. p.1–16
5. Lanza RP, Chick WL. Encapsulated cell therapy. Scientific American Science & Medicine. 2, 16, 1995
6. Lacy PE, Finke EH, Janney CG, et al. Prolongation of islet xenograft survival by in vitro culture of rat megaislets in 95% O2. Transplantation. 33, 588, 1982
7. Lacy P, Davie J, Finke E. Prolongation of islet allograft survival following in vitro culture (240C) and a single injection of ALS. Science. 204, 312, 1979
8. Benhamou PY, Mullen Y. Immunomodulation of pancreatic islets by culture. In: Lanza RP, Chick WL (eds), Immunomodulation of Pancreatic Islets.Austin, R.G.Landes/CRC Press, 1994. p99–109

9. Hardy MA, Goodman ER, Athan ES, et al. Immunomodulation by ultra-violet B irradiation. In: Lanza RP, Chick WL (eds), Immunomodulation of Pancreatic Islets. Austin, R.G.Landes/CRC Press, 1994. p111–127
10. Faustman DL, Steinman RM, Gebel HM, et al. Prevention of rejection of murine islet allografts by pretreatment with anti-dendritic cell antibody. Proc. Natl. Acad. Sci. USA 81, 3864, 1984
11. Faustman D. Antibodies directed to MHC determinants for transplantation. In: Lanza RP, Chick WL (eds), Immunomodulation of Pancreatic Islets.Austin, R.G.Landes/CRC Press, 1994. p111–127
12. Mayo GL, Posselt AM, Campos L, et al. Intrathymic islet transplants and systemic tolerance. In: Lanza RP, Chick WL (eds), Immunomodulation of Pancreatic Islets. Austin, R.G.Landes/CRC Press, 1994. p87–98
13. Selawry HP. Islet transplantation to immunoprivileged sites. In: Lanza RP, Chick WL (eds), Immunomodulation of Pancreatic Islets.Austin, R.G.Landes/CRC Press, 1994. p75–86
14. Thomas FT. Immunomodulation of islet transplantation: Future prospects. In: Lanza RP, Chick WL (eds), Immunomodulation of Pancreatic Islets.Austin, R.G.Landes/CRC Press, 1994. p161–172
15. Gores PE, Sutherland DER. Immunosuppression for islet transplantation. In: Lanza RP, Chick WL (eds), Immunomodulation of Pancreatic Islets.Austin, R.G.Landes/CRC Press, 1994. p63–74
16. Sayegh MH, Weiner HL, Carpenter CB. Oral tolerence. In: Lanza RP, Chick WL (eds), Immunomodulation of Pancreatic Islets.Austin, R.G.Landes/CRC Press, 1994, p153–160
17. Lafferty KJ, Cooley M, Woolnough J, Walker KZ. Thyroid allograft immunogenicity is reduced after organ culture. Science. 188, 259, 1975
18. Sollinger HW, Burkenholder PM, Rasmus WR, Bach FH. Prolonged survival of xenografts after organ culture. Surgery.81, 74, 1977
19. Snell G. The homograft reaction. Ann. Rev. Microbiol. 11,439, 1957
20. Lafferty K, Prowse S, Simeonovic C, et al. Immunology of tissue transplantation: a return to the passenger leukocyte concept. Annu. Rev. Microbiol. 1, 143, 1983
21. Bowen K, Prowse S, Lafferty K. Reversal of diabetes by islet transplantation: vulnerability of the established allograft. Science. 213, 1261, 1981
22. Morrow C, Sutherland D, Steffes M, et al. Lack of donor specific tolerance in mice with established anti-IA treated islet allografts. Transplantation. 36, 691, 1983
23. Pamphilon DH, Alnaqdy AA, Wallington TB. Immunomodulation by ultraviolet light: Clinical studies and biological effects. Immunol. Today. 2, 119, 1991
24. Hardy MA, Oluwole SF. Effect of ultraviolet radiation on immunogenicity of tissues and organ allografts. Transplant. Rev. 5, 46, 1991
25. Hardy MA, Lau H, Weber C, Reemtsma K. Pancreatic islet transplantation: Induction of graft acceptance by ultraviolet irradiation of donor tissue. Ann. Surg. 200, 441, 1984
26. Faustman D, Coe C. Prevention of xenograft rejection by masking donor HLA class I antigens. Science. 252, 1700, 1991
27. Raviola E, Karnovsky MJ. Evidence for a blood-thymus barrier using electron-opaque tracers. J. Exp. Med. 136,466, 1972
28. Weiss L (ed), The Blood Cells and Hematopoietic Tissues.McGraw-Hill, 1977. p503–522
29. Schwartz RH. Acquisition of immunological self-tolerance. Cell. 57, 1973, 1989

30. Mayo GL, Posselt AM, Campos L, et al. Intrathymic transplantation promotes survival of iselt xenografts (rat to mouse). Transplant. Proc. 26, 758, 1994
31. Tzu WJ, Tai J. Xenotransplantation of rat pancreatic endocrine cells in spontaneously and streptozotocin-induced diabetic monkeys. Transplant. Proc. 21, 2736, 1989
32. Selawry HP, Whittington K, Bellgrau D. Abdominal, intratesticular islet-xenograft survival in rats. Diabetes. 38 (Suppl 1), 220, 1989
33. Selawry H, Cameron D, Wang X, Ghawji M, Alloush L. Extended survival of discordant islet xenografts (pig to rat) without sustained immunosuppression. Proceedings of the 5th International Congress on Pancreas and Islet Transplantation (Miami Beach, Florida, June 18–22, 1995) p 3.5
34. Terasaka R, Lacy PE, Bucy RP, Davie JM. Effect of cyclosporine and low temperature culture on rejection of islet xenografts (rat-to-mouse). Transplantation. 41, 661, 1986
35. Hering BJ. Islet xenotransplantation. In: C Ricordi(ed), Pancreatic Islets Transplantation. Austin, R.G.Landes, 1992. p313–335.
36. Stegall M, Chabot J, Weber C, Reemtsma K, Hardy MA. Pancreatic islet transplantation in cynomolgus monkeys. Transplantation. 48, 944, 1989
37. Nakajima Y, Yabuuchi H, Kanehiro H. Prolongation of pancreatic islet xenograft survival and thymus alteration by 15-deoxyspergualin. Transplantation. 48, 351, 1989
38. Thomas F. Comparative immunosuppression for xenografting. In: Xenograft 25.MA Hardy (ed) Elsevier; Amsterdam, New York, Oxford, 1989, p55
39. Yabuuchi H, Nakajima Y, Segawa M, Kanehiro H. Prominent prolongation of islet xenograft survival in combination therapy with FK506 and 15-deoxyspergualin. Transplant. Proc. 23, 859, 1991
40. Wennberg L, Wallgren AC, Rafael E, et al. Treatment with cyclosporin A in combination with Leflunomide and RS-61443 prevents rejection of pig islets transplanted into rats. Presented at the Third International Congress for Xenotransplantation, Boston, 1995. Transplant. Proc. In press
41. Lakey J, Yatscoff R, Koshal A, Rajotte R. Prolongation of concordant islet xenografts with Leflunomide. Presented at the Third International Congress for Xenotransplantation, Boston, 1995. Transplant. Proc. In press
42. Lacy PE, Davie J, Finke EH. Prolongation of islet xenograft survival (rat to mouse). Diabetes. 30, 285, 1981
43. Gotoh M, Porter J, Monaco AP, Maki T. Prolongation of islet xenograft survival by islet irradiation and antilymphocyte serum treatment of recipients. Transplant. Proc. 20, 997, 1988
44. Harlan DM, June CH. Tolerance and the costimulatory pathway. In: Lanza RP, Chick WL (eds), Immunomodulation of Pancreatic Islets.Austin, R.G.Landes/CRC Press, 1994. p141–152
45. Weber CJ, Hagler MK, Chryssochoos J, et al. CTLA4Ig prolongs survival of microencapsualted rabbit islet xenografts in spontaneously diabetic NOD mice. Presented at the Third International Congress for Xenotransplantation, Boston, 1995. Transplant. Proc. In press
46. Lacy PE, Ricordi C, Finke E. Effect of transplant site and L3T3 treatment on survival of rat, hamster and rabbit islet xenografts in mice. Transplantation. 47, 761, 1989
47. Ricordi C, Lacy PE, Sterbenz K, Davie JM. Low temperature culture of human islets or in vivo treatment with L3T4 antibody produces a marked prolongation of human-to-mouse islet xenograft survival. Proc. Natl. Acad. Sci. USA 84, 8080, 1987

48. Kahan BD: Cyclosporine. N. Engl. J. Med. 321, 1725, 1989
49. Fung JJ, Alessiani M, Abu-Elmagd K, et al. Adverse effects associated with the use of FK 506. Transplant. Proc. 23, 3105, 1992
50. Gunnarsson R, Klintmalm G, Lundgren G, et al. Deterioration in glucose metabolism in pancreatic transplant recipients given cyclosporin. Lancet. 2, 571, 1983
51. Alejandro R, Feldman EC, Bloom AD, Kenyon NS: Effects of cyclosporin on insulin and C-peptide secretion in healthy beagles. Diabetes. 38, 698, 1989
52. Schlumpf R, Largiader F, Uhlschmid GK, Baumgartner D: Is cyclosporine toxic for transplanted pancreatic islets? Transplant. Proc. 28, 1169, 1986
53. Van Schilfgaarde R, van der Burg MPM, van Suylichem HG, Goosen HG, Frolich M Does cyclosporin influence beta cell function? Transplant. Proc. 28, 1175, 1986
54. Tze WJ, Tai J, Cheung S: In vitro effects of FK-506 on human and rat islets. Transplantation. 49, 1172, 1990
55. Engfeldt P, Tyden G, Gunnarsson R, Ostman J, Groth CG: Impaired glucose tolerance with cyclosporine. Transplant. Proc. 18, 65, 1986
56. Mito M, Sawa M. Hepatocyte transplantation. In: Lanza RP, Chick WL (eds): 1996/97 Yearbook of Cell and Tissue Transplantation. Dordrecht, The Netherlands, Kluwer Academic Press, 1996
57. Makowka L, Falk RE, Rostein LE, et al. Cellular transplantation in the treatment of experimental hepatic failure. Science. 210, 901, 1980
58. Cai Z, Shi Z, Sherman M, et al. Development and evaluation of a system of microencapsulation of primary rat hepatocytes. Hepatology. 10, 855, 1989
59. Sun AM, Cai Z, Shi Z, et al. Microencapsulated hepatocytes: an in vitro and in vivo study. Biomat. Art Cells Art Org. 15, 1483, 1987
60. Sun AM, Cai Z, Shi Z, et al. Microencapsulated hepatocytes as a bioartificial liver. Trans. Am. Soc. Artif. Intern. Organs.32, 39, 1986
61. Hori M. Will artificial liver therapy ever become a reality? Artif. Organs. 12, 293, 1988
62. Eguchi S, Chen S, Rozga J, Demetriou AA. Tissue Engineering/Hybrid Tissues:Liver, In: Lanza RP, Chick WL (eds): 1996/97. Yearbook of Cell and Tissue Transplantation. Dordrecht, The Netherlands, Kluwer Academic Press, 1996
63. Freed WJ. Neural transplantation: Brain, In: Lanza RP, Chick WL (eds): 1996/97. Yearbook of Cell and Tissue Transplantation. Dordrecht, The Netherlands, Kluwer Academic Press, 1996
64. Widner H, Brundin J, Rehncroma S, et al. Transplanted allogeneic fetal dopamine neurons survive and improve motor function in idiopathic Parkinson's Disease. Transplant. Proc. 23, 793, 1991
65. Sagen J. Chromaffin cell transplantation. In: Lanza RP, Chick WL (eds): 1996/97. Yearbook of Cell and Tissue Transplantation. Dordrecht, The Netherlands, Kluwer Academic Press, 1996
66. Phelps CH, Gage FH, Growdon JH, et al. Potential use of nerve growth factor to treat Alzheimer's disease. Science. (Letter) 243, 11, 1989
67. Phelps CH, Gage FH, Growdon JH, et al. Potential use of nerve growth factor to treat Alzheimer's disease. Neurobiol of Aging. 10, 205, 1989
68. Hefti F, Knusel B. Chronic administration of nerve growth factor and other neurotropic factors to the brain. Neurobiol of Aging. 9, 689, 1988

69. Frim DM, Short MP, Rosenberg WS et al. Local protective effects of nerve growth factor-secreting fibroblasts against excitotoxic lesions in the rat striatum. J. Neurosurg. 78, 267, 1993
70. Schumacher JM, Short MP, Hyman BT et al. Intracerebral implantation of nerve growth factor-producing fibroblasts protects striatum against neurotoxic levels of excitatory amino acids. Neuroscience. 45, 561, 1991
71. Winn SR, Hammang JP, Emerich DF et al. Polymer-encapsulated cells genetically modified to secrete human growth factor promote the survival of axotomized septal cholinergic neurons. Proc. Natl. Acad. Sci. USA 91, 23, 1994
72. Tessler A. Neural transplantation: Spinal cord. In: Lanza RP, Chick WL (eds): 1996/97. Yearbook of Cell and Tissue Transplantation. Dordrecht, The Netherlands, Kluwer Academic Press, 1996
73. Roberts HR. The treatment of hemophilia: past tragedy and future promise. N. Engl. J. Med. 321, 1188, 1989
74. Hellman L, Smedsrod B, Sandberg H, et al. Secretion of coagulant factor VIII activity and antigen by in vitro cultivated rat liver sinusoidial endothelial cells. Br. J. Hematol. 73, 348, 1989
75. Fu XW, Sun AM. Microencapsulated parathyroid cells as a bioartificial parathyroid: in vivo studies. Transplantation. 47, 432, 1989
76. Darquy S, Sun AM. Microencapsulated parathyroid cells as a bioartificial parathyroid: in vitro studies. Trans. Am. Soc. Artif. Intern. Organs. 33, 356, 1987
77. Lanza RP, Sullivan SJ, Chick WL. Islet transplantation with immunoisolation. Diabetes. 41, 1503, 1992

41 Isolated Pancreatic Islet Xenografting

F.T. Thomas

Introduction

At present, short-term success has been obtained with isolated pancreas islet allografts [1, 2]. Clinical success has not been obtained with islet xenografts, although at least one study suggests that the human immune response to islet xenografts may be no stronger than that to allografts in some instances [3]. Recent advances in both islet isolation techniques and suppression of xenogeneic immune reactivity have provided a measure of optimism regarding the future of islet xenografting which was not previously appropriate.

Isolated islet xenografts have a multitude of advantages over islet allografts. At present, islet xenografting is the only realistic hope for the widespread application of pancreas islet replacement therapy. The limited application of whole-organ pancreas allografting to type I diabetes is starkly evident when one considers that there are currently a million or more diabetics in this country who could potentially benefit from islet replacement therapy and that only 500 or so whole-organ pancreas allografts were performed in 1995. Human organ donor shortage severely limits all areas of human organ transplantation but is a particular problem with islet transplants since the shortage of human pancreases is especially acute. In addition, problems with efficiency in islet isolation will probably result in a need for a minimum of two human donors per recipient.

Islet xenografting using discordant donor species, preferably animals which are freely slaughtered for food, provides an immense potential for application of islet replacement therapy to the problem of human type I diabetes. It seems probable that virtually unlimited donor islets could be made available and, at the same time, the many thorny ethical and cost-effective issues involving use of human donors would be obviated. Islet xenografting has recently been demonstrated to represent a unique paradigm for xenografting in that isolated islets from discordant species do not apparently suffer a high rate of hyperacute or accelerated rejection if effective immunosuppression is given. This important matter will be discussed in more detail later using discordant pig donor islet models as examples.

Historically, clinical islet xenografting is now nearly 100 years old, since the first recorded clinical islet xenotransplant of a minced sheep pancreas was performed in 1893 [5]. Modern progress in islet xenografting, however, has only occurred within the last 20 years. In 1975, Weber et al. reported a unique xenograft, placing piscine (fish) islets into rats, with short-term function in irradiated hosts [6]. Eloy et al. in 1979 reversed diabetes in rats on a short-term basis with chicken embryo free pancreas grafts [7]. The first successful islet xenografts surviving for more than 50 days with good function were reported in 1980, and this is essentially the beginning of the modern era in islet xenografting [8].

To our knowledge, there are no published articles devoted entirely to pancreas islet xenografting, so this review, hopefully, will provide a more complete overview of this developing field.

Pancreas Islet Isolation For Xenografting

Effective and efficient techniques for the isolation of islets are essential to both allografting and xenografting. The two major parameters against which islet isolation techniques are measured are the purity and quantity of well-functioning isolated islets obtained. In human allografting, the quantity or efficiency of isolation can be critical because of donor shortfalls. Efficiency is often less critical in xenograft donors lacking ethical or cost-effective restrictions. Purity in isolation would appear to be a virtue in both allotransplantation and xenotransplantation since the vigor of the rejection response, as well as problems of primary nonfunction, appear at least partially related to islet contamination by exocrine tissue and the resulting inflammation response, insulitis, and islet injury [9, 10]. Thus, this discussion is pertinent to allografting or xenografting, but it will be focused on isolation factors most germane to xenografting.

In 1965, Moskalewski reported the isolation of guinea pig pancreatic islets by collagenase digestion. In 1967, Lacy and Kostianovsky reported on the use of collagenase and a Ficoll density gradient to isolate intact islets from the rat pancreas [11]. Lacy was the first investigator to report short-term success in islet xenotransplantation. He reported that low-temperature (24 °C) islet culture (and later culture at 37 °C) prolonged survival of xenografts to 50 days when used in combination with short-course antilymphocyte serum (ALS) therapy [8]. Previous attempts at xenografting of islets were only successful on a short-term basis [12].

In 1984, Grey et al. introduced an important variant into islet isolation procedure involving the initial distention of the pancreatic duct with a warm (37°–39 °C) collagenase solution together with an initial incubation period under these conditions [13]. Although these techniques were described for the human pancreas, they were quickly adapted to islet isolation from the nonhuman pancreas.

In 1988, Ricordi described an "automated" (semiautomated) method for pancreatic islet isolation [14]. The basic features of this procedure are the use of an isolation-perfusion chamber into which collagenase at 37 °C is circulated until free islets are seen on microscopy. The isolation machine is then switched to filtration–dilution–cooling phase to protect the islets from overdigestion. In 1990, Ricordi published the best description of a reproducible high-yield isolation technique for pig islets incorporating a gentle shaking motion of the digestion chamber to avoid disruption of the fragile pig islets [15]. Using this technique, he showed a yield of 5000–10 000 islets/g tissue – by far the best results recorded to date – in a large series of digestion of pig islets. Calafiore has reported similar yields of pig islets using a somewhat different technique with a multienzyme digestion and variants in techniques of islet purification [16].

There have been few descriptions of techniques for isolation of the other non-human species islets. Lacy described a technique for bovine pancreas islet isolation using velcro strips which has been improved upon recently by Hering et al. [17]. The utility of bovine islets is questionable because of their peculiar insulin secretory parameters. The major stimuli for insulin secretion from bovine islets are fatty acids, and glucose stimulates insulin release poorly [18]. Thus, it is doubtful that these islets would closely replicate human insulin secretion patterns, although a recent description of two separate populations of bovine islets responding to different physiological stimuli suggests the need to reexamine this matter [19].

A number of workers have developed efficient techniques for isolating dog pancreas islets. Alejandro has reported a large and excellent experience with the dog pancreas [20]. Rajotte et al. have developed techniques for consistent isolation of large volumes of dog islets (2000–5000 islets/g pancreatic tissue) [21]. This group has also developed techniques for reliable cryopreservation of islets permitting the retained viability of the islets after thawing [22].

Immunoisolation of Islet Xenografts in the Recipient

Immunoisolation is applied here to denote the separation of the donor tissue from recipient tissue compartments in which recipient responder cells have full access and are fully operational.

Immunologically Privileged Sites

One type of immunoisolation has been traditionally termed the "immunologically privileged site" (Chap. 15). In the case of xenografts, at least two sites have been shown to confer some degree of immunoisolation upon islet xenografts – the brain and/or intrathecal space, and the testes. Tzu showed prolonged survival of xenografts in the intrathecal space, the subarachnoid space, and in the brain [23]. Selawry et al. demonstrated the long-term survival of xenograft islets in the tests [24]. Naji has recently demonstrated that the intrathymic space is immunologically privileged for islet allografts, and preliminary studies in his laboratory have suggested that xenografts may also be immunoisolated in the intrathymic space [25].

All of these sites pose practical problems for future xenograft application. Intracerebral injection poses many potential problems of a complex nature. The intrathecal space is perhaps more attractive but also has potential for morbidity, as does the subarachnoid space. The use of the intrathymic space is complicated by the involution of the adult human thymus and the associated questions concerning its immunological activities in adulthood, any of which could be involved in active mechanisms of generating immune tolerance in privileged sites. Nevertheless, these privileged sites could well serve as an excellent repository for the small-volume islet xenograft and, therefore, deserve careful study.

Bioencapsulation

The second concept of immunoisolation that has shown promise for xenografting of islets is the use of so-called bioencapsulation techniques [26] (Chap. 43). While a number of techniques of bioencapsulation or mechanical isolation of islets have been demonstrated, the most attractive and promising technique would appear to be the use of the bilayered polylysine-alginate membrane. This technique, devised primarily by Sun and Lim, places a capsule of polylysine-alginate around pancreatic islets [27]. As few as one and as many as eight to ten islets can be enclosed in the capsules, which are usually 300–800 μm in diameter. Nutrients diffuse nicely into the capsule and are available to the islet from which insulin (and presumably the other β-cell hormones) diffuses out. Immune cells, γ-globulin, and even middle molecules such as interleukin-1 (IL-1) can be shown to be blocked from entering the capsule [28]. Rather remarkable survivals of discordant islets have been recorded with bioencapsulation, and the function of the islets has also been clearly demonstrated [29].

There are a host of potential problems involving these encapsulation membranes, including their ability to avoid rupture, proteinaceous collections, and attachment of immune cells, especially macrophages, on their surface [30]. Nevertheless, they are an attractive and novel device for blocking islet xenograft rejection. If bioencapsulation has any place in transplantation, it may well be in xenografting, where there is a clear and present need for immunoisolation because of the hyper-reactive xenogeneic immune responses operative in this situation.

Donor Islet Immunoalteration for Xenografting

Islet Cell Culture

Pioneering work by Lafferty et al. in 1975 demonstrated that cultured endocrine tissue enjoyed prolonged survival when allografted [31]. He suggested that this immunoalteration culture was related to a loss of the so-called passenger leukocytes, leading to a decrease in what Lafferty has termed "the second signal to immune reactivity." His culture technique was also shown to prolong survival of thyroid xenografts [32].

In 1979, Lacy et al. reported prolongation of islet allografts by culturing for 7 days at 24 °C, together with a single injection of rabbit ALS [33]. Without the ALS, prolonged survival was not produced, but with the ALS prolongation of more than 100 days was achieved. Lacy reported in 1980 a marked prolongation, with over 70 % of islet xenografts surviving over 60 days if islets were cultured for 7 days at 24 °C, together with a single injection of rabbit ALS [8]. Lacy's group later expanded this work to demonstrate that culture at both 24 °C and 37 °C was able to produce prolongation of xenografts as well as allografts in a number of different models.

The precise mechanism by which this immunoalteration occurs is not clear, and more recent work has suggested that it may be related to either loss of class II surface antigen cells or, in fact, loss of class I donor antigens, which could be expected to directly stimulate the CD8 cell [34]. There is much evidence that xenograft rejection occurs via indirect presentation of antigens and that, therefore, the direct stimulation of the CD8 cell by a class I antigen would not be a major factor in xenograft immunogenicity [35].

Despite these uncertainties, it is clear culturing cells does reduce immunogenicity. It should be mentioned that the explanation for this could clearly range from the simple to the complex, and that the known reduction in exocrine contamination of the cultured islets that occurs within 1–2 weeks after initiation of culture could well be responsible for the decreased immunogenicity seen. Certainly, the cultured cells show none of the hyperimmunogenicity seen with fresh islets which results in early rejection (1–3 days) of grafts. Our group has recently shown prolonged graft survival with culture for 7–10 days at 37 °C, and this is our preference for graft culture prior to xenotransplantation at the present time [36].

Cryopreservation

Rajotte's group has shown that cryopreservation of islets results in immunoalteration of the donor cells [37]. Again, the precise mechanism by which this occurs is not evident. It has been postulated that cryopreservation results in a loss of class II antigen cells during the process of freezing and thawing. Because of this, cryopreservation could be utilized in future xenogeneic efforts to provide extra donor tissue or donor tissue from multiple sources for elective use, and further study of this technique for immunoalteration is clearly desirable. Rajotte's work strongly suggests that the cryopreservation technique needs to be precise in terms both of the rapidity of freezing and thawing and of the techniques utilized (such as rapid-thaw procedures) in order to provide optimal viability and function of the islets.

Depletion of Antigen-Bearing Cells

A number of techniques have been used to deplete the class II antigen-bearing cells from the islets prior to transplantation [38]. Faustman et al. were able to demonstrate significant prolongation of islets with depletion of dendritic cells using monoclonal antibodies [39]. Antidendritic cell antibodies and anti-Ia antibodies are clearly also useful in depletion of these cells. Recently, this matter has become clouded by demonstrations that dendritic cells in fact proliferate locally within the tissue and that initial removal of the dendritic cells may be followed by a prompt reaccumulation of the cells. Dendritic cells are known to be marrow-derived which is a likely source of the repopulation.

In a novel series of studies, Morris' group recently demonstrated that dendritic cells actually migrate out of the allograft and into the spleen and other extra graft lymph node depots [40]. These studies suggest that previous attempts to deplete class II cells with antibodies may not have been done in an optimal manner. Nevertheless, the results justify optimism in this area, and future studies designed to remove class II antigen-bearing cells and/or dendritic cells from islet xenografts may yield valuable donor immunoalteration techniques.

Exposure to Ultraviolet Light

Hardy's group demonstrated that ultraviolet (UV) light is capable of decreasing the immunogenicity of islets in culture [41]. They demonstrated a marked prolongation of islet xenografts following treatment with UV light. The UV light treatment is quite simple and, if effective, it could be easily applied to islet therapy. This is another example of the great potential for application of immunoalteration techniques in xenograft islets, which can be programmed into precise protocols of immunoalteration due to the elective nature of the donor islet procurement and the lack of limits on donor pretreatment.

In summary, immunoalteration of xenograft islets is a technique with great potential for xenogeneic islet transplantation. This is especially so because of all of the islet grafts, xenografting lends itself to the widest variety of immunoalteration since it is the most elective of the islet transplant procedures. In contrast, islet allografting, involving as it does the emergent procurement of human islet tissue, creates constraints in the ability to electively pretreat islets to produce immunoalteration. In addition, the procurement of the pancreas is often compromised by the need to use techniques for optimal procurement of other organs which may not complement the pancreas procurement. Thus immunoalteration of islets is most applicable to xenotransplantation, and it is likely that it will receive its greatest use in this area.

Immunology and Immunosuppression in Islet Xenografting

Islet Graft Survival

Early studies of rodent allografting of islets indicated that the isolated islets evoked a strong, early immunological response [6, 9]. This response was manifested primarily as early nonfunction of the islets or as a pattern of early function followed by rapid rejection [10]. Both of these phenomena are quite relevant and pertinent to the matter of islet xenografting since heightened immune reactivity seen in disparate species can be expected to result in a high incidence of primary nonfunction and a high rate and tempo of early graft rejection.

Most early studies in this area were quite discouraging with prolongation of grafts beyond 30 days representing, in general, a distinct exception [4]. Recent results have provided more optimism concerning the potential for isolated islet xenografting between concordant species combinations [8]. Equally encouraging have been the reports, such as those of Ricordi et al., in which certain islet treatments are able to prolong disparate xenografts [43]. The greatest hope is that tolerance to islet xenografts could be induced in a manner similar to reported induction of tolerance to islet allografts [44].

Results at the present time have improved, perhaps because of better knowledge of islet isolation techniques as well as the availability of better immunosuppressive drugs [13]. Recently, rather striking successes with achievement of long-term graft survival in the range of more than 200 days without immunoisolation have been obtained. Of immense interest also is the recent description of functional tolerance of islets whereby islets retain function over 200 days after discontinuance of all immunosuppression.

Importance of Experimental Methodology

Many studies of islet xenografting are compromised by experimental techniques and reporting peculiarities. A number of studies have looked at islet xenografting but have not serially measured the blood glucose levels following xenotransplantation. This is regarded by many investigators as an inappropriate omission, especially since it is such an easy thing to do. In many of these xenograft models, reversal of hyperglycemia with proven lack of function of native islets previously treated with streptozotocin (STZ) has not been demonstrated clearly. It is sincerely hoped that future studies in this area will all include a clear demonstration of islet function by serial monitoring of blood glucose.

The matter of the possible return of islet function following STZ treatment is a highly problematic one [4, 46–48]. There seems to be no question that many of the animals do have return of their native islets and, therefore, it is necessary to demonstrate that the euglycemia is related to function of the islet transplant and not the native islets. In some studies it has been clearly shown that this is precisely what has happened to maintain hypoglycemia in the late posttransplant period [48]. Often, islet function returns at about 100–120 days after transplantation following STZ treatment. The demonstration of clear-cut rejection of pancreas islet transplants by the development of hyperglycemia for a period of time, which may later revert to euglycemia, is strong evidence that the native islets have resumed functioning. Thus euglycemia in the late posttransplant period does not rule out the possibility of late return of function of native islets later after STZ treatment [49].

Reach's group has recently demonstrated a nice technique using high-performance liquid chromatography (HPLC) to separate pig insulin from rat insulin, and to demonstrate that late insulin secretion is related to the transplanted islets (pig insulin) and not due to the native rat islets (rat insulin) [50]. Our group has accomplished similar studies using rat C peptide which has less than 1% cross-reactivity with pig C peptide. Together with the pig and rat insulin levels, the rat C peptide studies can be combined to establish from what source the insulin is being secreted.

Immunosuppression

Immunosuppression for pancreas islet xenografts is a poorly developed area. A number of studies have shown that cyclosporine (CsA) only poorly prolongs xenograft islet survival [51, 52]. Nakajima et al. showed that total lymphoid irradiation (TLI) would prolong pancreatic xenografts to the range of 30 days [53]. Lacy's group has demonstrated prolongation of concordant xenografts with the use of an LT34 monoclonal antibody [54]. FK506 prolongs islet grafts but, like CsA, has inherent islet cell toxicity [56].

Thomas et al. recently reported prolongation of survival of pig islet xenografts to over 200 days in strong-responder Lewis rats [57]. In addition, pig xenografts have been prolonged in nonobese diabetic (NOD) mice and functional tolerance of these discordant xenografts has been reported using rabbit antithymocyte globulin (RATG) and 15-deoxyspergualin (DSG) [58]. Islet cell function was observed for 12–14 weeks in these recipients which were given a combination of RATG and DSG, with or without splenectomy. This combination looks to be the most promising one for current treatment of islet xenografts. DSG has been previously shown by our group and others to be a quite effective suppressive agent for xenografts [58].

Lack of knowledge of the immune mechanisms of islet xenograft rejection is a major impediment to development of better immunosuppression. The role of humoral antibody in islet destruction has not been well-established. Naji, Barker, and coworkers have shown that islets appear to be more sensitive to antibody destruction than, for example, comparable grafts of skin [59]. Delmonico's findings, however, do not support this concept [60]. Our own results, showing a low rate (<40 %) of primary nonfunction and also a low rate (<10 %) of early graft rejection of pig islets grafted to Lewis rats which have high levels of anti-donor preformed antibodies, support Delmonico's findings, but this area requires further, more detailed, study.

A number of studies have suggested that the macrophage may be important in islet xenograft rejection. This would explain the effectiveness of DSG in preventing islet rejection since this agent is known to have anti-macrophage activity [58]. Studies have also shown that $CD4^+$ cells are prominent in islet allograft, as well as islet xenograft, rejection [55]. Studies of nonislet xenografts have suggested a possible role for antibody-dependent cellular cytotoxicity (ADCC), natural killer (NK), killer (K), or lymphocyte-activated killer (LAK) effector cells in xenograft rejection, but little is known of the role of these cells in islet xenograft rejection. Other studies using skin and heart xenografts have not accorded the NK cell a central role in xenograft rejection.

Islet cells, both allografts and xenografts, are apparently injured and destroyed by inflammatory reactions consequent to contamination of the islet preparation by pancreatic exocrine cells, leading to a severe inflammatory response [10]. Hence, the importance of purity in islet preparations is paramount. The ability of depletion of class II antigens to prolong islet xenografts is in keeping with the suggestion by Auchincloss that indirect antigen presentation is a major mechanism in xenograft rejection [35]. Hopefully, future studies will develop better conceptual schemes of islet xenograft rejection.

Practical Considerations in Islet Xenografting

Site of Placement of Islet Xenografts

Currently, there is a preference for the intraportal placement of islet xenografts, but the intrasplenic placement, as well as the renal subcapsular placement, have also received a great amount of attention. The renal subcapsular placement, despite its unphysiological nature (drainage into the systemic venous circulation), has produced consistently good results in xenografting and, in fact, in some authors' studies, the results are superior to those seen with intraportal placement. Intrapancreatic placement is a novel concept, recently tested.

Intraportal placement has much to recommend it, including the physiological nature of the placement, with drainage of secreted insulin into the portal bed and, hence, to the liver, to where it would normally be secreted [62]. By adding a small laparotomy incision in which the omentum is brought up into the wound, the islets can be placed intraportally by injection into an omental vein or a mesenteric vein through the same incision used for a kidney transplant. The intraportal placement can also be accomplished by cannulation of the obliterated umbilical vein, which drains into the left portal vein, or the percutaneous placement of islets into the portal system under fluoroscopic or ultrasonic guidance.

The intrasplenic placement is a procedure midway between portal placement and a more distal splanchnic placement. There is evidence that many of the islets placed into the spleen, especially if placed into a clamped arterial pedicle, will reflux into the portal system or later migrate to the liver [63].

Placement of the islets directly under the kidney capsule of the transplanted kidney could potentially permit the biopsy of these islets clinically. This may be an important consideration because little thought has been given at present to the problem of rejection of islets, diagnosis of rejection, and the need to modulate immunosuppression to reverse rejection. It should be remembered that, in allografting where immune reactivity is even less than that in the xenograft, survival of kidney transplants, for example, could be as low as 10% if we did not have the capability to reverse rejection crises after diagnosing them by administering large doses of steroids and other immunosuppressive agents. In short, there are multiple factors which may provide important considerations in the placement of islet xenografts.

Repeated Administration

Another technical consideration which seems destined to come to the forefront in islet xenografting, because of the ease of application to xenografting, is the matter of administration of large numbers of donor islets or repeated injection of donor islets [65]. In a number of clinical cases to date, advantage has been taken of the easy opportunity to simply do another islet injection should the first injection prove to be (a) of borderline adequacy for maintenance or normoglycemia, or (b) simply inadequate, or (c) rejected. In the longest surviving patients in the St. Louis and Miami series, second islet injections were given after prolonged survival after the first islet injection, and these appeared to restore normoglycemia [66, 67].

If one reasons from the parallelism drawn by Teraski's group between the length of function of the first and the second allograft, one could reason that long-surviving first xenografts might well presage a long-surviving second, repeat xenograft [68]. In the case of xenografts, this principle could be easily exploited because of the essentially unlimited availability of donor islets.

Use of Multiple Donors

Another matter which deserves future consideration is the consideration of multiple donors brought forth by Monaco's group [69]. This group has achieved superior results in rodent xenografting, using islets from multiple donors. The theoretical basis for this is not certain [70]. Regardless of the conceptual scheme, the experimental facts indicate this system may be valuable.

This system, again, would have unique application to xenografting, since it would be possible to simultaneously graft islets with antigens of marked antigenic disparity, such as a bovine graft with a pig graft or a sheep graft. This, again, illustrates one of the major advantages of xenografting over allografting in that the amount and variety of donor tissue available for grafting is large and provides many potential options.

Possibility of Ex Vivo Pretreatment

As a clinical surgical procedure, islet xenografting has a number of unique properties. In contrast to a cadaver allograft, an islet xenograft is an elective surgical procedure. The procedure can be scheduled well in advance and, in the usual situation where donor islets are maintained in culture, one would schedule the procedure some 5–10 days in advance, when the availability of islets was anticipated. The entire procedure would be quite leisurely and orderly and would even involve lengthy final testing of the islet preparation over perhaps a 2- or 3-day period before the final decision is made to transplant the islets.

This completely elective nature of the xenograft procedure also makes it possible to engage in novel and unusual ex vivo pretreatment of the donor islets, as well as recipient pretreatment by techniques designed to induce tolerance. Induction of functional tolerance across xenogeneic barriers has currently been achieved. The work of Sachs and others suggest that xenogeneic chimerism and xenogeneic tolerance is indeed possible, at least in relatively concordant species [71].

Choice of Donor Species

The first necessary prerequisite for human xenografting would be the isolation in viable and rather pure form of animal islets which would be suitable for human implantation. Furthermore, these islets should preferably be from a disparate species, nonprimate in type, in which no ethical constraints exist regarding the obtaining of adequate pancreas donor tissue. Animals satisfying these criteria are almost all disparate to the human. The animals which logically come to mind are the pig, the cow, and other species of animals freely used for human food and freely slaughtered. In general, there are few ethical constraints to the use of virtually any of the disparate species, including sheep, goats, horses, or other farm animals. Rodent donors are impractical, since the number of islets obtained is so small that up to thousands of individual rodents might be required for a single human transplantation.

A broad prerequisite for adequacy of a species for human xenotransplantation is that the physiology of the pancreas islets in these species ought to be near that of the human. The physiology of islets varies throughout the animal kingdom, and patterns of maintenance of specific levels of blood sugar, patterns that influence secretion, counter-regulatory mechanisms, etc., do vary between species [72, 73]. There is evidence that quite distant species including fish and chickens will maintain a carbohydrate metabolism relatively close to that of the human. However, Ricordi et al. reported on hamster islets transplanted into mice and found that the hamster islets maintained a fasting blood sugar level of around 66 mg%, which corresponds to blood sugar levels in hamsters, but is considerably different from the average 145 mg% in fasting mice [74]. Thus careful study of comparative xenograft physiology is important.

Practical considerations and outright cost-effectiveness, however, are a salient feature of our current medical environment. Thus it is highly likely that the pig and/or cow might prove to be the most practical animals for xenograft donation if the physiology of these animals islets is appropriate and the difficulty of preventing rejection is not overwhelming. Both pigs and cows grow to large size, and it is not unusual to find pig pancreases in the range of 300 g and cow pancreases in the range of 500–600 g containing millions of islets which could potentially provide adequate donor islets for five to ten human transplants from a single animal.

In addition, insofar as we know, the pig, in particular, and, to a large degree, the cow are free of pathogens that would endanger the human species. Pig and cow products are widely consumed by the human without ill effects, including fresh products such as cow's milk, which are the result of lactation processes and, therefore, might be expected to contain any of the shedding viruses and other pathogens found in such tissues.

In contrast to this situation, for example, the primates represent problematic donors. It is clear that these animals harbor a number of viruses and other pathogens which can be quite dangerous and even fatal to the human, such as the monkey B virus [75]. Some monkey species have a human immunodeficiency virus (HIV), and it is quite possible that monkeys also have viruses which are unknown at the present time [76]. These considerations will most certainly form the basis for future direction in xenografting.

Insulitis and Recurrence of Diabetes

In the case of islet transplantation for diabetes, an interesting and probably important area is the recurrence of the original disease process (diabetes) in the transplanted islets. Recurrence of diabetes in islet transplants has been well-documented by the Minnesota group in human leukocyte antigen (HLA)-identical siblings [77]. The insulitis that precedes type I diabetes is an immune attack upon the islets, which seems, at least to some degree, to be related to the major histocompatibility antigens that lead to the possibility of the recurrence of disease.

In this respect, the xenograft, especially from a disparate species, could be expected to be relatively immune to recurrence of disease, since the membrane antigens which would form the target of an immune insulitis are quite dissimilar to those which were the targets of the original disease process. In fact, there is some experimental evidence for this in the NOD mouse, in which isografts are shown to suffer the heaviest early insulitis after transplant, with allografts in between, and xenografts showing the least amount of early immune damage following transplantation [78].

Modification of Donor Tissue

In this respect, techniques of immunoalteration of donor tissue will be critically important. At the present time, it would seem that the potentially most efficacious techniques for decreasing islet immunogenicity would be focused primarily upon islet cell xenograft culture for a minimum of 5–7 days. Studies to date would suggest that culture at either 24 °C or 37 °C would be useful in reducing immunogenicity.

Xenografting permits the widest use of immunoalteration techniques on donor tissue because of our ability to carefully program the donor procurement and to define its time frame and parameters, and also because there is a lack of ethical constraint on treatment of donors. It is entirely possible that treatment such as total body irradiation of the donor, prohibitive in human donors, could become a well-accepted procedure in xenograft donors.

Modification of the Recipient Immune Response

Second only to immunoalteration of the xenograft donor is the modification of the recipient immune response, which is currently the Achilles heel of xenografting. Approaches to immunosuppression for xenografting could take different avenues. The blockage of humoral antibody and macrophage are clearly desirable goals. Indirect antigen processing has also been shown by Auchincloss to be an important mechanism of xenograft rejection [35], and this was corroborated by islet studies [34].

Development of tolerance to islet xenografts, like allografts, is a very important goal. Xenogeneic tolerance is very difficult to achieve or document by classical criteria. Sublethal irradiation and reconstitution seem a rather drastic solution to xenograft suppression [81]. Finally, one of the most attractive goals for islet xenografting would be the development of immunoisolation techniques either using privileged sites or bioencapsulation. Such systems might permit the elimination of immunosuppression, which must continue to be a goal for all of transplantation, including islet transplantation where suppressive agents are toxic to the islet.

Technical Options

A major potential of pancreas islet xenografting will be to provide for important technical options in the placement of these grafts. These include grafting insequence, the possibility of multiple placement sites, the possibility of utilizing large amounts of tissue from a single donor to induce tolerance over a period of time, as well as many other considerations that will probably come to light with early xenograft experience, e.g., placing islets in immune privileged sites, such as the thymus, or artificial privileged sites, such as bioencapsulation in hollow-fiber membrane systems.

In short, islet xenografting will foster the development of a number of important technical options, both in terms of immunoalteration of donor tissue, timing and technique of transplantation, timing and method of immunosuppression, as well as techniques which would modify the recipients in manners which could favorably alter xenograft survival. Induction of tolerance is yet another example of the large potential for immunomodulation in islet xenografting.

Promising Islet Xenograft Donors

Pig

Because of the large potential for islet xenografting in treating the huge number of diabetics who might require this procedure, our group began investigations to develop techniques for the isolation of pig pancreatic islets approximately 3 years ago. The pig has classically been the source of insulin used for human diabetics. The pig islet has a physiology very much like that of the human [82]. The leading role in the development of techniques for isolation of pig islets has been taken by Camillo Ricordi, working in Lacy's laboratory and, later, in Milan and Pittsburgh [14, 15, 83, 84]. Ricordi's description of isolation of pig islets in April 1990 represents perhaps the first comprehensive demonstration of a consistently successful technique for pig islet isolation using a semiautomated technique [15].

Using Ricordi's techniques, his results have been reproduced by our laboratory recently. We have also had an islet yield of about 8000–10 000 islets per gram prior to Ficoll separation, and 4000–5000 islets per g after Ficoll separation, with a high degree (>90 %) of purity. In addition, recent studies in our laboratory have demonstrated the ability to transplant these pig islets with a low rate

(10 % or less) of primary nonfunction and survival with recipient euglycemia in the difficult pig-to-Lewis rat discordant model for 10–14 weeks using some newer forms of immunosuppression. These results are quite promising since many of the results of islet allografts have been less impressive.

Technique of Pig Islet Isolation

Perhaps the most critical thing about pig islets is their fragility and ease of disruption. It is, therefore, necessary to utilize a gentle technique – far more gentle than that used in islet separation from the human or other animals. The pig pancreas is best digested with a static ductal perfusion after removal of the pancreas with a short warm ischemic time. We have been able to obtain satisfactory pancreases from both old breeding sows, which give large pancreases up to 300 g, as well as market-weight pigs.

The pancreatic duct is perfused with a 2 % collagenase solution at 37 °C to achieve full distention of the gland. The gland is usually cannulated proximally and distally and a catheter sewn in place for perfusion under pressure. We utilize a volume of collagenase which is twice the weight of the pancreas (i.e., 200 ml for a 100-g segment of pancreas). Following a static perfusion for about 5 min, the porcine pancreas is placed in the digestion chamber, described by Ricordi (Fig. 1), consisting of a stainless steel chamber of approximately 350 ml volume. The chamber is capped with a filter 200 μm in diameter and is perfused with a collagenase solution containing 2 % fetal bovine serum at 37 °C. The collagenase solution is heated in a water bath, beginning at a temperature of about 29 °C and gradually warmed to 37 °C. The perfusate enters the chamber and comes into contact with the pancreas; the digested portions of the pancreas pass through the filter exit at the top of the chamber. An inline roller pump maintains a flow of 50 ml per min.

After approximately 10 min of digestion, with sampling of the recirculating fluid, free islets can be seen with a dithizone (DTZ) stain supplemented with a 2 % dimethyl sulfoxide (DMSO) solution. Once free islets are seen, the effluent from the chamber is directed into a beaker in a 4 % water bath. The gland is then perfused at 150 ml per min with a collagenase solution containing 10 % fetal calf serum with usually a 3–4 l volume. The resulting dispersed pancreatic fragments are purified on a Ficoll density gradient to a purity of 80 %–95 % islets. The final preparation is carefully monitored by DTZ staining, concentrated and usually placed in culture prior to transplantation.

Fetal Islets

Hellerstrom et al. [85] recently published data on isolation of fetal pig islets. These islets were obtained from fetal pigs of gestational age 60–70 days. One litter produced about 100 000 islets, and these islets performed well in nude mice. Fetal islets have the advantage of ease of extraction due to a low amount of fibrous tissue in the fetal pancreas, a potential for expansive growth and differentiation, and possibly some degree of hypoimmunogenicity [85]. Fetal xenograft tissue may well be a useful source of donor tissue for islet xenografting.

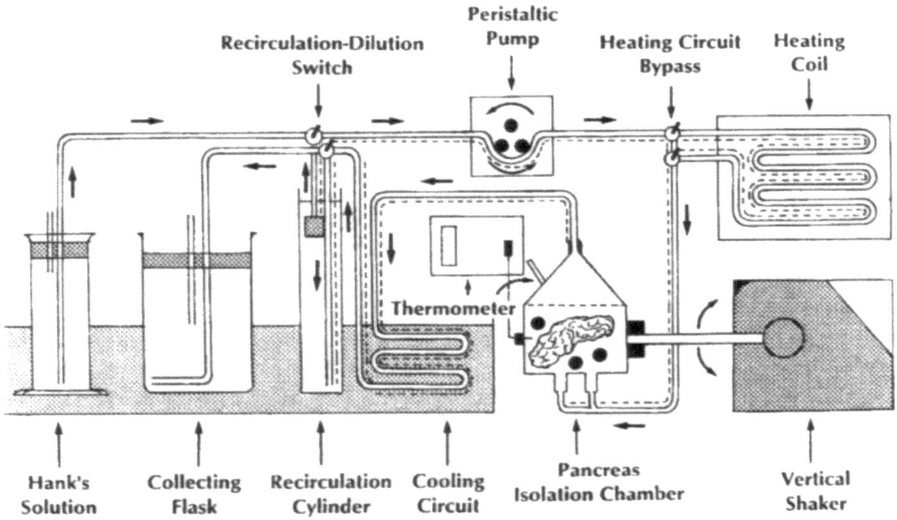

Fig. 1. Automated procedure for isolation of pancreatic islets. (Courtesy of Dr. C. Ricordi [14])

Teleost Fish

In certain teleost fishes, islet tissue is aggregated into visible organs called Brockmann bodies. They are easily identified and have a high purity of islets. Weber performed the original xenografting of piscine islets to rats [6]. Recently, Schrezenmeir et al. identified certain teleost species with blood sugars in the human range (86–89 mg%) [86]. In addition, they showed these islets released insulin and glucagon in a glucose-dependent manner, tolerated mammalian temperatures, and survived encapsulation for weeks. These islets, available from such common fish as flounder and trout, would seem to be an exciting new approach to potential islet donation for xenografting [87].

Dog

Techniques for isolation of islets from dogs have been well established [88, 89]. In general, the dog islet is characterized as easier than the pig to isolate, but harder than the rodent. The size of the dog makes dog islets attractive for human use. There is apparently good physiological compatibility between dog islets and human islets. The major problem with the use of the dog may well be ethical concerns.

Comment

Although this chapter is perhaps the most comprehensive publication solely on islet xenografting to-date, it must necessarily be considered preliminary. The chapter seeks to summarize the state of clinical and, especially, experimental islet xenografting. In addition, it seeks to plan some future strategies for application and expansion of islet xenografting. Hopefully, it more fully outlines the large potential for islet xenografting that has been developed by workers in the pancreas islet isolation field – those who have developed techniques for donor islet immunnoalteration, those publishing on recipient immunoisolation techniques, and those seeking to achieve successful islet xenografting by the traditional manner of immunosuppression of the host response. In the future, these efforts may be complemented by induction of host tolerance to islet xenografts.

Perhaps the highest goal of current work in this area will be to develop the optimal "chimeric" approach to islet xenografting, borrowing the best qualities of these individual areas and molding an elegant composite creature, reflecting the noblest features of them all. Hopefully, the information in this chapter will provide the chimera-creator with strategic information which will aid him or her in this quest.

Acknowledgments. Some of the author's work in relation to this chapter was supported by NIH Grant #R01 A122293, and Diabetes and Education Fund Grant #B39-II89.

References

1. Scharp, D.W., Lacy, P.E., Santiago, J.V., et al. Insulin independence after islet transplantation into type I diabetic patient. Diabetes. 39, 515, 1990
2. Tzakis, A.G., Ricordi, C., Alejandro, R., et al. Pancreatic islet transplantation after upper abdominal exenteration and liver replacement. Lancet. 336, 402, 1990
3. Kondratiev, Y.Y., Sodovnikova, N.V., Petrova, G.N., et al. Islet cell transplantation in type I diabetes mellitus: evaluation of humoral immune response. Exp. Clin. Endocrinol. 93, 147, 1989
4. Weber, C., Zatrigi, A., Weil, R., et al. Pancreatic islet isografts, allografts, and xenografts: comparison of morphology and function. Surgery. 79, 144, 1976
5. Williams, P.W. Notes on diabetes treated with grafts of sheep's pancreas. Br. Med. J. 2, 1303, 1893
6. Weber, C., Weil, R., McIntosh, R., et al. Xenotransplantation of piscine islets into hyperglycemic rats. Surgery. 77, 208, 1975
7. Eloy, R., Haffen, K., Kedinger, M., Grenier, J.F. Chick embryo pancreatic transplants reverse experimental diabetes of rats. J. Clin. Invest. 64, 361, 1979
8. Lacy, P.E., Davie, J.M., Finke, E.H. Prolongation of islet xenograft survival without continuous immunosuppression. Science. 209, 283, 1980
9. Reckard, C.R., Stuart, F., Schulak, J.A. Immunologic comparisons of isolated pancreatic islet and whole-organ allografts. Transplant. Proc. 11, 563, 1979

10. Kaufman, D.B., Rabe, F.L., Platt, J.L., Dunn, D.L., Sutherland, D.E.R. Effect of host immunomodulation on the prevention of islet allograft primary non-function in a murine model. Transplant. Proc. 22, 857, 1990
11. Lacy, P.E., Kostianovsky, M. A method for the isolation of intact islets of Langerhans from the rat pancreas. Diabetes. 16, 35, 1967
12. Sutherland, D.E.R., Matas, A.J., Najarian, J.S. Pancreas islet cell transplantation. Surg. Clin. N. Amer. 58, 365, 1978
13. Morris, P.J., Gray, D.W., Sutton, R. Pancreatic islet transplantation. Br. Med. Bull. 49, 224, 1989
14. Ricordi, C., Lacy, P.E., Finke, E.H., Olack, B.J., Scharp, D.W. Automated method for isolation of human pancreatic islets. Diabetes. 37, 413, 1988
15. Ricordi, C., Socci, C., Davalli, A.M., et al. Isolation of the elusive pig islet. Surgery. 107, 688, 1990
16. Calafiore, R., Basta, G., Callcinaro, F., et al. Islands of Langerhans transplant in the treatment of diabetes mellitus: current status, indications, future perspectives. Recenti. Prog. Med. 81, 94, 1990
17. Hering, B.J., Romann, D., Clarius, A., et al. Bovine islets of Langerhans: potential source for transplantation? Diabetes. 38, 206, 1982
18. Hering, B.J. Romann, D., Clarius, A., et al. Islands of Langerhans of cattle – potential donor tissue for clinical islet transplantation? Z. Exp. Chir. Transplant. Kunstiche Organe, 22, 138, 1989
19. Bonner-Weir, S., Fike, A.A. A dual population of islets of Langerhans in bovine pancreas. Cell Tissue Res. 206, 157, 1980
20. Alejandro, R., Strasser, S., Zucker, P.F., Mintz, D.H. Isolation of pancreatic islets from dogs. Semi-atomated purification on albumin gradients. Transplantation. 50, 207, 1990
21. Finegood, D.L., Warnock, G.L., Kneteman, N.M., Rajotte, R.V. Insulin sensitivity and glucose effectiveness in long-term islet autotransplanted dogs. Diabetes. 38, 189, 1989
22. Rajotte, R.V., Warnock, G.L., Kneteman, N.M., Rajotte, R.V. Optimizing cryopreservation of isolated islets. Transplant. Proc. 21, 2638, 1989
23. Tzu, W.J., Tai, J. Xenotransplantation of rat pancreatic endocrine cells in spontaneous and strepozotocin-induced diabetic monkeys. Transplant. Proc. 21, 2736, 1989
24. Selawry, H.P., Whittington, K.B., Bellgrau, D. Abdominal intratesticular islet-xenograft survival in rats. Diabetes. 38, 220, 1989
25. Mayo, G., Posselt, A., Barker, C., Campos, L., Naji, A. Prolongation of survival of donor strain xenografts by intrathymic innoculation of xenogeneic islets. Transplantation.58, 107, 1994
26. Ricker, A.T., Stockgerger, S.M., Halban, P.A. In: The Immunology of Diabetes Mellitus. Jaworski, M.A. (ed.) Amsterdam, Elsevier, 1986, p. 193
27. O'Shea, G.M., Sun, A.M. Encapsulation of rat islets of Langerhans prolongs xenograft survival in diabetic mice. Diabetes. 35, 943, 1986
28. Siebers, U., Zekorn, T., Bretzel, R.G., et al. Bioartificial pancreas: islet survival and interleukin-1 action. Transplant. Proc. 22, 2035, 1990
29. Wu, Z.G., Shi, Z.Q., Lu, Z.N., et al. In vitro culture and transplantation of encapsulated human fetal islets as an artificial endocrine pancreas. Trans. Am. Soc. Artif. Intern. Organs. 35, 736, 1989

30. Weber, C., Zabinski, S., Koschitzky, T., et al. The role of CD4+ helper T cells in the destruction of microencapsulated islet xenografts in NOD mice. Transplantation. 49, 396, 1990
31. Lafferty, K.J., Cooley, M., Woolnough, J., Walker, K.Z. Thyroid allograft immunogenicity is reduced after organ culture. Science. 188, 259, 1975
32. Sollinger, H.W., Burkenholder, P.M., Rasmus, W.R., Bach, F.H. Prolonged survival of xenografts after organ culture. Surgery. 81, 74, 1977
33. Lacy, P.E., Davie, J.M., Finke, H., Scharp, D.W. Prolongation of islet allograft survival. Transplantation. 27, 171, 1979
34. Stock, P.G., Ascher, N.L., Chen, S., et al. The alloimmune response to murine islets occurs via indirect antigen presentation to LYT2+ and L3T4+ lymphocytes. Transplant. Proc. 22, 841, 1990
35. Auchincloss, H. Xenotransplantation – a review. Transplant. Rev. 46, 1, 1990
36. Thomas, F., Pittman, K. Factors in effective isolation and culture of adult pig islets (API). Submitted for publication
37. Coulombe, M., Warnock, G., Rajotte, R. Prolongation of islet xenograft survival by cryopreservation. Diabetes. 36, 1086, 1987
38. Lafferty, K., Davie, J.M., Finke, E. Prolongation of islet xenograft survival (rat-to-mouse). Diabetes. 36, 1086, 1987
39. Faustman, D.L., Stienman, R.M., Gabel, A.M. Depletion of anti-Ia + dendritic cells. Proc. Natl. Acad. Sci. USA. 81, 3864, 1984
40. Larsen, C., Austyn, J., Morris, P. The role of graft-derived dendritic leukocytes in the rejection of vascularized organ allografts. Ann. Surg. 212, 308, 1990
41. Chabot, J., Weber, C., Hardy, M., et al. Synergy of ALS and UV-B in prolongaton of primate-to-mouse islet xenograft survival. Transplant. Proc. 19, 1160, 1987
42. Walter, P., Lesmeister, F., Leetz, H., et al. Influence of and UVB irradiation on graft survival and function of islets of Langerhans. Diabetes. 38, Suppl. 1, 288, 1989
43. Ricordi, C., Lacy, P.E., Sterbenz, K., Davie, J.M. Low temperature culture of human islets or in vivo treatment with L3T4 antibody produces a marked prolongation of human-to-mouse islet xenograft survival. Proc. Natl. Acad. Sci. USA. 84, 8080, 1987
44. Has, L., Lafferty, K., Allison, A., Eugui, E.M. RS-61443 allows islet allografting and specific tolerance induction in adult mice. Transplant. Proc. 22, 876, 1990
45. Lacy, P.E. Islet transplantation. Clin. Chem. 32/10B, B76, 1986
46. Kruszinska, Y., Hone, D., Morley, A., Alberti, A. Preservation of islet function and morphology in high dose streptozotocin diabetic rats. Diab. Res. 3, 175, 1986
47. Trimble, E., Karakash, C., Malaisse-Lagae, R. Effects of intraportal islet transplantation on the transplanted tissue and recipient pancreas. Diabetes. 29, 341, 1980
48. Richardt, M., Menden, A., Bretzel, R., Federlin, K. Islet transplantation for experimental diabetes of the rat. B cell regeneration following transplant. Horm. Metab. Res. 16, 551, 1984
49. Slipjepcevic, M., Helmke, K., Federlin, K. Islet transplantation in experimental diabetes of the rat. Horm. Metab. Res. 7, 20, 1975
50. Chicheportichi, D., Darquy, S., Lepeintre, J., et al. High-performance liquid chromotography analysis of circulating insulins distinguishes between endogenous insulin production (a potential pitfall with streptozotocin diabetic rats) and islet xenograft function. Diabetologia. 33, 457, 1990

51. Terasaka, R., Lacy, P.E., Bucy, R.P., Davie, J.M. Effect of cyclosporine and low temperature culture on rejection of islet xenografts (rat-to-mouse). Transplantation. 41, 661, 1986
52. Stegall, M., Chabot, J., Weber, C., Reemtsma, K., Hardy, M.A.. Pancreatic islet transplantation in cynomolgus monkeys. Transplantation. 48, 944, 1989
53. Nakajima, Y., Nakano, H., Nakagawa, H., Segawa, M., Shiratori, T. Effect of total lymphoid irradiation on pancreas islet xenograft survival in rats. Transplantation. 34, 98, 1982
54. Lacy, P.E. Present status of islet transplantation. Clin. Inv. Med. 10, 496, 1987
55. Simeonovic, C., Ceredio, R., Wilson, J.D. Effect of GK1.5 antibody dosage on survival of pig proislet xenografts in CD4+ T cell depleted mice. Transplantation. 49, 849, 1990
56. Yosunami, Y., RYU, S. Kamei, T. Characterization of immunosuppressive activity of FK506 in rat islet allografts. Transplant. Proc. 22, 875, 1990
57. Thomas, F., Henretta, J., Pittman, K., Patselas, T., Thomas, J.M. Long-term survival of pig islet xenografts documented by differential species insulin and C-peptide. Transplant. Proc.26, 1138, 1994
58. Thomas, F., Pittman, K., Thomas, J. Induction of functional xenograft tolerance of pig islets in the autommune NOD mouse. Transplant. Proc.27, 3323, 1995
59. Naji, A., Barker, C. Differential susceptibility of endocrine tissues to humoral immunity. Surg. Forum, 29, 349, 1978
60. Delmonico, F., Chase, C.., Russle, P. Transplantation of rat islets of Langerhans into diabetic mice. Transplant. Proc. 9, 367, 1977
61. Sutton, R., Greay, D.W., Burnett, M., et al. Metabolic function of intraportal and intrasplenic islet autografts in cynomolgus monkeys. Diabetes. 38, 182, 1989
62. Alejandro, R., Cutfield, R.G., Steinvold, F., et al. Natural history of intrahepatic canine islet cell autografts. Clin. Invest. 78, 1339, 1986
63. Warnock, G.L. Rajotte, V.R., Procyshyn, A.W. Normoglycemia after reflux of islet-containing pancreas fragments into the spenic vascular bed in dogs. Diabetes. 32, 452, 1983
64. Kaufman, D., Morel, D., Field, M., et al. Canine islet autografts. Functional outcome as influenced by islet number and purity. Transplant. Proc. 22, 771, 1990
65. Kanai, T., Porter, J., Monaco, A.P., Maki, T. Sequential multiple transplantations of multiple-donor pancreatic islet allografts. Diabetes. 38, Suppl. 1, 286, 1989
66. Alejandro, R., Mintz, D.H., Noel, J., et al. Islet cell transplantation in type I diabetes mellitus. Transplant. Proc. 19, 2359, 1987
67. Scharp, D.W., Lacy, P., Ricordi, C., et al. Human islet transplantation in patients with type I diabetes. Transplant. Proc.. 21, 2744, 1989
68. Cicciarelli, J., Cho, R.V. Regraft kidney transplant survival. In: Clinical Transplants. Terasaki, P.I. (ed.) Los Angeles, UCLA Tissue Typing Lab, 1986, p. 285
69. Gotoh, M., Porter, J., Kanai, T., Monaco, A.P., Maki, T. Effect of specific and nonspecific alloantigen stimulation on islet allograft survival. Transplant. Proc. 21, 2746, 1989
70. Kanai, T., Porter, J., Maki, T., Monaco, A.P. Possible mechanisms underlying marked graft survival following multiple donor islet allotransplantation. Transplant. Proc. In press
71. Sachs, D., Bach, F. Immunology of xenograft rejection. Hum. Immunol. 28, 245, 1990

72. Sun, A.M., O'Shea, G.M., Yuan, Z.Y., Ma, F., Cai, Z. Allo- and xenotransplantation of microencapsulated islets of Langerhans (a bioartificial pancreas). In: Advanced Models for Therapy of Insulin Dependent Diabetes. Brunetti, P., Walkausl, W.K. (eds.) New York, Raven Press, Serono Symposia, 37, 303, 1987
73. Manns, J.G., Boda, J.M. Insulin release in lambs and adult sheep. Am. J. Physiol. 212, 747, 1967
74. Lacy, P., Ricordi, C., Finke, E. Effect of transplant site and alpha L3T4 treatment on survival of rat, hamster and rabbit islet xenografts in mice. Transplantation. 47, 761, 1989
75. King, N.W., Chalifoux, L.V., Ringler, D.J., et al. Comparative biology of natural and experimental SIVmac infection in macque monkeys: a review. J. Med. Primatol. 19, 109, 1990
76. Daniel, M.D., Letvin, N.L., Sehgal, P.K., et al. Prevalence of antibodies to 3 retroviruses in a captive colony of macaque monkeys. Int. J. Cancer. 41, 601, 1988
77. Sibley, R.K., Sutherland, D.E.R., Goetz, F., Michael, A.F. Recurrent diabetes in the pancreas iso- and allograft. Lab. Invest. 53, 132, 1985
78. Mandel, T., Koulmanda, M., Loudovaris, T., Bacelj, A. Islet grafts in NOD mice – comparison of iso- allo-and pig xenografts. Transplant. Proc. 21, 3813, 1989
79. Kaufman, D., Platt, J., Rabe, F., et al. Differential roles of Moc 1 + cells and CD4+ and CD8+ T lymphocytes in primary non-function and classic rejection of islet allografts. J. Exp. Med. 172, 291, 1990
80. Moses, R., Pierson, R. III, Winn, H., Auchincloss, H. Xenogeneic proliferation and lymphokine production are dependent upon CD4+ helper T cells and self-antigen presenting cells in the mouse. J. Exp. Med. 172, 567, 1990
81. Ildstad, S., Wren, S., Stephany, D., Sach, D.H. Effect of selective T cell depletions in mixed xenogeneic reconstitution on species hyporeactivity to xenogeneic transplantation. Transplantation. 41, 372, 1986
82. Crowther, N., Gotfreadsen, C., Moody, A.J., Green, I.C. Porcine islet isolation cellular digestion and secretory response. Horm. Met. Res. 21, 590, 1989
83. Ricordi, C., Finke, E., Lacy, P.E. A method for the mass isolation of islets from the adult pig pancreas. Diabetes. 35, 649, 1986
84. Ricordi, C., Soci, A., Dailli, C., et al. Application of the automated method to islet isolation in swine. Transplant. Proc. 22, 784, 1990
85. Hellerstrom, C., Andersson, A., Korsgren, O., Jansson, L., Sandler, S. Aspects of pancreatic islet transplantation in diabetes. Ballieres Clin. Gastroenterol. 3, 851, 1989
86. Schrezenmeir, J., Faust, P., Laue, C., et al. Immunoprotection in biocompatible membranes permits transplantation of piscine islets to rats. Transplant. Proc. 21, 2730, 1989
87. Falkner, S., Ostberg, Y. Comparative morphology of pancreatic islets in animals. In: The Diabetic Pancreas. Volk, B.W., Arquilla, E.R. (eds.) New York, Raven Press, 1977, p. 15
88. Alejandro, R., Cutfield, R., Schienvold, F., et al. Natural history of intrahepatic canine islet cell autografts. J. Clin. Invest. 78, 1339, 1986
89. Warnock, G., Rajotte, R. Critical mass of purified islets that induce normoglycemia after implantation in the dog. Diabetes. 37, 467, 1988

42 Recent Approaches to the Isolation of Adult Porcine Islets of Langerhans

K. Ulrichs and A. Heiser

Introduction

All over the world new strategies for providing alternative organ donors for transplantation have focused on the pig and its capability to provide both vascularized and nonvascularized organs. In this context, the nonvascularized isolated pancreatic islet could serve as a pioneer tissue in xenotransplantation, whereas vascularized organs may be more difficult to transplant due to preformed natural xenogeneic antibodies in human serum that attack the grafted xenogeneic porcine tissue leading to a hyperacute rejection. As long as the onset of type I diabetes cannot be detected and inhibited well in advance of major endocrine tissue destruction and we lack molecular-genetic strategies for treating type I diabetes successfully, one of the major goals in the treatment of this severe autoimmune disease is to graft purified functioning endocrine tissue.

Since 1990, two considerations have forced many laboratories to concentrate on the isolation of islets of Langerhans from the adult pig, in addition to obtaining pancreatic islets from humans: (1) the relative lack of human organ donors and (2) the current concept of treating severe forms of type I diabetes. Based upon the enzymatic digestion method that is successful in rodents and, to a lesser extent, in humans, a number of laboratories have started to develop methods that will work in the pig. Despite undisputed occasional success with one approach or another, the reliability of the techniques and the reproducibility of the results remain questionable. Successful, reproducible technology is, of course, an essential requirement for the continued clinical application of porcine islet xenografting.

The following review concentrates primarily on some major problems that determine the success of porcine islet isolation.

Review of Current Approaches and Results

In 1990, Ricordi published a basic method for the isolation of adult porcine islets of Langerhans [1], based on his original successful method for isolating human islets [2]. It was hardly surprising that other laboratories soon followed in his footsteps [3, 4], since the demand for xenogeneic islets as a source for future clinical transplantation is growing steadily. However, it soon became apparent that the porcine pancreas is a much more difficult tissue to handle than either the rodent or human pancreas. A great variety of factors influence the isolation process and the final results, e.g., the donor material (race, age, weight, sex), the explantation protocol (slaughterhouse vs. operating room, warm and cold ischemia, perfusion solution), the enzymatic digestion procedure (collagenase batch, digestion chamber, mechanical vs. hand shaking, open vs. closed circulation, temperature, pH), the microscopic evaluation (determination of the digestion endpoint, counting of islets or islet equivalents, viability), and the purification protocols (density gradients, centrifugation vs. sedimentation), to name only a few. Hence, it was hardly surprising that the isolation results varied greatly from group to group, ranging from approximately 1500 [5] to 13 000 [6] islets per g organ (IpgO).

In the initial phase, due to good access and limited budgets, many groups favored slaughterhouse pigs as donors [1, 3, 4, 6–10]. This meant using pancreas donors of varying genetic background, approximately 5–36 months old and ready for meat production. A certain amount of warm ischemic time was often considered unavoidable [4, 7–10], particularly in countries of the European Union (EU), where slaughtering is carried out according to strict regulations (anesthesia with CO_2 gas or electroshock, cessation of heart beat after incision of the carotid artery and bleeding, cadaver wash at 60 °C). Visible results of these limitations were the fragmentation of islets [3, 5, 8, 11, 12], poor viability [12] (personal observations) and poor insulin release, particularly from islets from younger individuals [11], which appear to be more vulnerable due to their irregular shape and their loose morphology. Consequently, the basic methods were extended or altered.

The major changes included the following. Instead of young donor pigs (age 10 months), older pigs (2–3 years, "retired breeders") were used. They produced higher islet yields, calculated according to islet volume density and insulin content [6]. Though it would be helpful if more groups could confirm this important finding, the scales presently appear to be tipped in favor of older individuals, as our own observations indicate [see below]. Isolating islets from brain-dead, heart beating donors expectedly improved the yields [1, 3, 6, 13, 14]. This must be interpreted as a clear sign that warm ischemia is a critical factor in the porcine pancreas and should be avoided, as is routinely practiced for other organs, clinically and experimentally. The disappointing results obtained by individual laboratories [13] (personal observations) after cold perfusion and surgical excision of the donor organ cannot be explained at present and need to be further analyzed. However, surgical removal, followed by immediate perfusion by cold collagenase solution that was gradually warmed to 32°C before loading the organ into the digestion chamber, resulted in very good islet yields [15]. Further analyses are needed to clarify this point.

Further modifications included the stainless steel digestion chamber. It was modified by including a window to better control the digestion status [15], or was omitted and mechanical shaking of the organ was replaced by gentle hand-shaking, both yielding better results (P. Marchetti, personal communication). Others developed a one-step, operator-independent isolation system which allows the critical digestion endpoint to be determined independent of the operator [16]. However, these results are still somewhat contradictory. A direct comparison of the automated technique and a simpler manual procedure clearly showed that the automated technique produced better yields [17].

Nearly all investigators use collagenase for the enzymatic digestion of the porcine pancreas, based upon previous experience in rodents and/or humans. However, the quality of the collagenase provided by various suppliers is still poorly defined and concentrations are often indicated as milligrams per milliliter [1, 3, 4, 6, 8–10, 12–14, 17] rather than enzyme activity (units per milliliter), as we prefer to use [7, 18]. Application of purified enzymes [19] should eventually help to detect those collagenase components that are essential to the release of intact islets and those that damage the islet structure. Others use the pancreas' own autodigestive (endogenous) enzymes to disintegrate the tissue, with the side effect of obtaining single beta cells instead of intact islets [20]. Furthermore, a modified University of Wisconsin solution is supposed to be helpful during the digestion step for protecting the fragile porcine islets against oxidative stress [21]. Results obtained after minor technical modifications, e.g., concerning the counting of released islets and their purification, viability and function, are difficult to interpret, since the desired result – a great number of intact, viable and functioning islets of all sizes and profiles – remains the outcome of single isolations but is rarely achieved routinely.

A general observation, and maybe the most striking one, is the fragility of the porcine islet. One can assume that unphysiological explantation of the donor organ, which often includes warm ischemia time, favors the autolytic digestion of the tissue, including the endocrine cells. Furthermore, it is very likely that the reason for the fragility is that the architecture of the porcine pancreatic tissue differs from that of rodent or human tissue. The only informative report on porcine pancreas morphology [22] indicates that there is very little peri-insular capsule present, and that the structural integration of the islet in the exocrine tissue depends almost exclusively on cell-to-cell adhesions [23]. Whether this holds for pigs of different races, ages, and weights, still remains to be elucidated. The lack of information about morphological peculiarities has forced our group to evaluate the porcine tissue histologically in greater detail. In the next section we will briefly summarize the results.

Histology of the Porcine Pancreas

Our contacts with university departments of agricultural science and domestic animal anatomy failed to give us much information on the anatomy and morphology of the porcine pancreas that was useful for the purpose of islet isolation. We investigated seven domestic pig breeds and the wild boar to obtain detailed histological information on islet profiles, numbers and sizes, pancreas mass, volume density of the endocrine tissue, and the collagen content of the capsules surrounding islets.

The main results, which have been published elsewhere in detail [24], can be summarized briefly as follows:

1. Porcine islets are round, oval, dumbbell-shaped and triangular and, as expected, occur in all intermediate profiles. Round and oval islets predominate. These profiles are also detected in crude islet preparations, which indicates that they can withstand the enzymatic and mechanical influences of the digestion process.

2. The total number of islets varies greatly from strain to strain, with, for example, the wild boar showing twice as many islets (approximately 500/cm^2 tissue section) as the experimentally used Goettingen minipig (approximately 250/cm^2).
3. The tail of the pancreas, which is usually used for islet isolation, accounts for about 50 % of the pancreatic mass. Body and head make up the other 50 %.
4. The majority of islets (64.3 %; range, 59.8 %–68.9 %) in the seven domestic breeds are 50–100 μm in diameter. With its 86 %, the wild boar is a remarkable exception. German Landrace pigs show the greatest number (2 %) of large islets (250 to more than 300 μm).
5. German Landrace pigs reveal the greatest islet volume density of all pig breeds (3.4 %; range, 1.2 %–3.4 %).
6. Only 25 % of all islets are surrounded by a collagen capsule that covers more than 75 % of the islet surface.
7. In roughly 33 % of all islets capsules composed of collagen, type I, III, and IV fibers cover less than 25 % of the surface.
8. Theoretical calculation: German Landrace pigs (2–3 years old) have an estimated islet number of 22 000 IpgO and a pancreatic mass of 255 g on average; that makes a total of 5 610 000 theoretically available islets. Presuming a collagenase batch of sufficient activity is at hand and the pancreatic tail (50 % of the total pancreatic mass of approximately 2 805 000 islets) is used as donor tissue, the minimum yield would be approximately 701 250 islets (or 5500 well-digested IpgO, if only the 25 % of all islets with a collagen capsule surrounding >75 % of the islet surface are released from the tissue). These numbers appear to be realistic at present and can be achieved in occasional satisfactory isolations [1, 3, 4, 6, 13, 14, 17].

A histological evaluation of the porcine pancreas, performed prior to islet isolation (as described above) may thus be a great help in predicting the isolation results, especially if pigs of different breeds and ages are used in different parts of the world. The only other report dealing with the morphology of the porcine pancreas, which analyzed six different breeds including the wild boar, appears to have shown comparable results [25]. Unfortunately, these data have not yet been fully reported. Parallel to the histological evaluation our group began to isolate porcine islets and to analyze parameters that have been hitherto insufficiently studied, e.g., the donor pig's breed and age and various enzymes that influence the digestion process.

Isolation of Islets from the "Adult" Porcine Pancreas

Isolation Technique

Pancreata were harvested from brain-dead, non-heart-beating female pigs. Hybrid pigs, which are crossbreeds of three to five races that are commonly used for meat production, were obtained from local slaughterhouses. Purebred pigs, e.g., German Landrace, Piétrain and Munich minipig "Troll," were acquired from commercial breeders. Donor pigs were either young individuals (14 months old) or old ones (2–3 years old, so-called retired breeders). Both age groups are referred to as "adult" pigs, as against newborn or weanling pigs. Because of the hygiene laws in the EU, a warm ischemia time of 25 min was unavoidable.

Only the splenic pancreatic lobe was prepared and removed from the donor organ. Immediately after harvesting, the pancreatic duct was cannulated with a self-made catheter, consisting of a polyethylene tube (inner diameter, 0.58 mm; outer diameter, 0.96 mm; NeoLab, Heidelberg, Germany) and a 23G×1 in. needle. The glands were stored and transported in cool (4 °C) Eurocollins solution (Fresenius, Bad Homburg, Germany). Cold ischemia time ranged from 30 to 240 min. In the initial phase, islets were isolated by Ricordi's semiautomated digestion method [1]. We later modified this basic technique, as we called it, and obtained what we referred to as our standard technique (see below; modifications are indicated by an asterisk). Peripancreatic fat, blood vessels and connective tissue were dissected from the pancreas and discarded. The weight of the organs (part of the pancreatic tail end) ranged from 15.0 to 99.7 g (mean, 45.0±23.4 g).

The collagenase solution, containing Hank's buffered salt solution (HBSS, Gibco/BRL, Eggenstein, Germany), 25 m*M* Hepes* (Boehringer, Mannheim, Germany) and 1.8 U PZ/ml collagenase (cat. no. 17448, Serva, Heidelberg, Germany), was adjusted to pH 7.6*, prewarmed to 28 °C, and then injected into the pancreas via the catheter. After infusion, the organ was loaded into a stainless steel chamber [1] with a Teflon* screen (mesh 420 µm) and five Teflon/steel* beads (diameter, 2 cm). The chamber was connected to a circulation system, including a reservoir, a peristaltic pump, and a heating circuit (45 °C). After the organ was loaded into the chamber, the system was filled with collagenase solution and recirculation (flow rate, 70 ml/min) was started. The chamber was gently shaken by hand* for 10 s every minute. Every other minute, a sample (150 µl) was taken, stained with 50 mg dithizone (DTZ; Sigma, Germany) in 5 ml dimethyl sulfoxide diluted 1:20 with HBSS and supplemented with 5% fetal calf serum (FCS; Conco, Germany) and screened microscopically [26]. During the procedure, the temperature and pH of the solution were constantly recorded.

When a significant number of well-digested intact islets was observed (after 21.5±5.42 min), recirculation was interrupted and elution of the digested tissue was started. Elution was performed with HBSS (supplemented with 25 m*M* Hepes and 5% FCS, precooled to 4 °C*, pH 7.4). Shaking and monitoring were continued during the elution phase. When no more islets were observed (after 17.0±5.68 min), elution was terminated. The eluate was then washed (270×*g*, 4 min, twice) to separate the collagenase from the cells. After sedimentation, the islet yield was quantitated in 150-µl samples. Only well-digested DTZ-stained islets, i.e., intact islets without a detectable exocrine rim, were counted as IpgO or used to calculate islet equivalents (adjusted to an islet of 150 µm in diameter). The viability of the islets was determined by staining them with fluorescein diacetate and propidium iodide (FDA/PI).

Results Obtained with the Basic Technique

Of 103 isolations, 58 were performed to establish the isolation technique according to the original Ricordi method [1]. Sixteen of the 58 were necessary to improve the technical equipment (digestion chamber, heating circuit, pump, cooling device) and islet monitoring (digestion endpoint). Isolation results (IpgO) were not evaluated during this experimental phase. The subsequent 42 isolations with the basic technique [1] were carried out to vary parameters, e.g., warm and cold ischemia time, collagenase batches and concentrations, and isolation media. The results obtained were 475±624 (range, 0–2813) IpgO of varying viability. This experience, with the highly unsatisfactory islet yields, viability and reliability, led us to establish our standard technique (for modifications, see above), which we used for all following isolations.

Influence of the Donor Pig Breed

To analyze the influence of the genetic background of the pig on islet yield and viability, 39 isolations with hybrid pigs (crossbreeds) were compared with results obtained with three purebred breeds, German Landrace (*n*=5), Piétrain (*n*=5), and minipig "Troll" (*n*=5). The results of this study (Fig. 1) can be summarized as follows:

1. The 39 isolations using hybrid pigs as organ donors resulted in a mean islet yield of 1190 IpgO with the large standard deviation of 1440. Testing with FDA/PI staining showed that the islet viability continued to be variable.

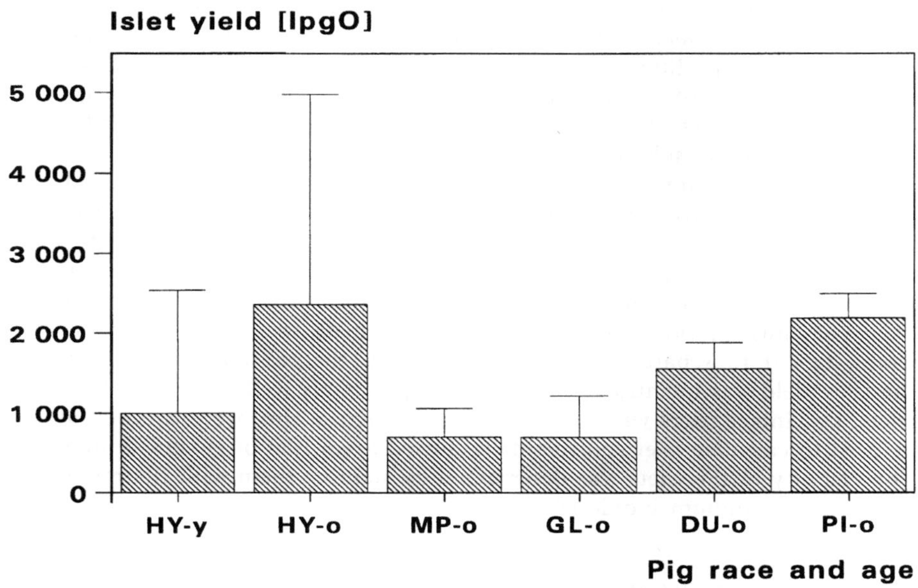

Fig. 1. The influence of donor age and race on islet yields. Results, indicated as islets per g organ (*IpgO*), of isolations performed with young hybrid pigs (*HY-y*, *n*=7) and old hybrid pigs (*HY-o*, *n*=9) and with old individuals of various pig breeds: Munich minipig (*MP-o*, *n*=5), German Landrace (*GL-o*, *n*=5), Duroc (*DU-o*, *n*=5), and Piétrain (*PI-o*, *n*=5)

2. Of the three purebred breeds, Piétrain gave the best results with 2180±317. German Landrace (606±379) and the minipig "Troll" (691±357) resulted in significantly lower islet yields. Thus so far the best and most reproducible islet yields were obtained with purebred Piétrain pigs. Improved yields also resulted in improved islet viability.

We hypothesized that the great variation in yields of islets isolated from hybrid pigs may be caused by genetic differences between these pigs, which are crossbreeds of three to five purebred strains. This was confirmed to some extent by the results obtained with Piétrain pigs. Isolations from these pigs not only produced higher yields, but the yields were more reproducible, as is shown by the smaller standard deviation. In addition, high yields from Piétrain and low yields from minipigs tally quite well with the histological finding that the islet volume density (%) of the total pancreatic mass is much higher in Piétrain pigs (mean, 2.55%, $n=5$) than in minipigs (mean, 1.24%, $n=5$). The observation that German Landrace pigs gave poor islet yields conflicts with the good islet volume density in this breed (mean, 3.38%, $n=3$). Further studies are necessary to clarify this point. As far as the correlation of genetics and islet yield is concerned, it may be necessary to analyze more purebred races or even to breed special pig strains in order to obtain appropriate donor conditions for a satisfying islet isolation.

Influence of Donor Age

To investigate the influence of the donor age on islet yield and viability, isolations were performed in young ($n=7$) and old ($n=9$) hybrid pigs. Unfortunately, Piétrain pigs were not available when this study was started. The islet yield (Fig. 1) was significantly lower in younger pigs (837±326) than in older ones (2930±1450). Additionally, microscopic screening of isolated islets showed larger amounts of fragmented islets in young individuals than in old ones. It is quite obvious from our results that, in addition to genetic aspects, the age of the donor plays an important role, a finding that harmonizes with that of other investigators [6]. However, the increased donor age may cause severe logistic problems due to the greater weight of the animals. Hence, in spite of islet volume limitations [see above], minipigs may provide an answer to this problem.

Influence of Pancreatic Enzymes

To test the influence of four different enzymes, collagenase, clostripain, neutral protease, and trypsin, 12 isolations were performed with the standard technique. Samples of the collagenase solution were collected (a) before injection into the gland and (b) at the end of the recirculation period (21.5±5.4 min) when the first well-digested islets could be identified. The kinetics of the four enzymes are shown in Fig. 2.

Collagenase activity decreased from 1.82±0.22 U PZ: 4-Phenylazobenzyloxycarbonyl-Pro-Leu-Gly-Pro-D-Arg before injection to 1.22±0.19 at the end of the

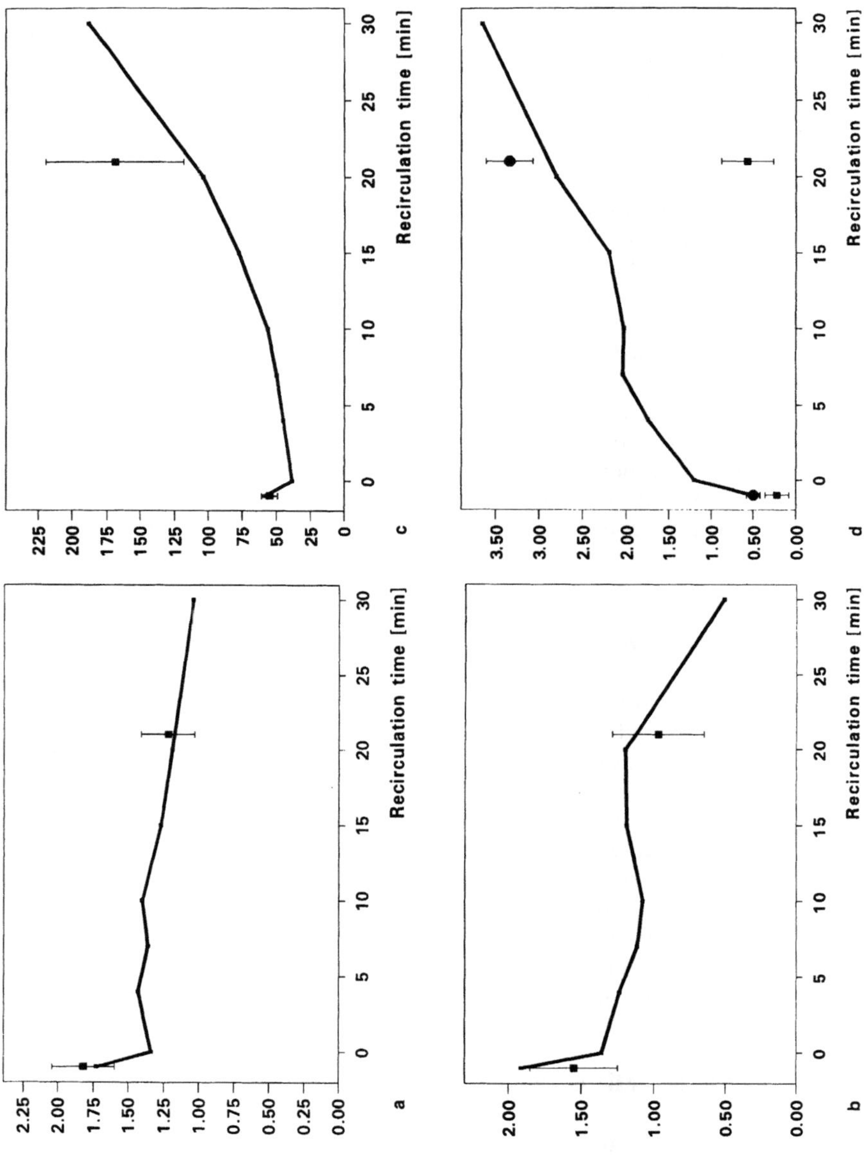

Fig. 2a–d. Enzyme kinetics during the isolation procedure. Results of tests of collagenase **a** with PZ (U/ml) and **b** Falgpa (U/ml) as substrate and of **c** neutral protease (U Azocoll/ml) and **d** trypsin (U BAEE/ml) activity. The *squares* illustrate the results of 12 experiments in which samples of the collagenase solution were taken only before injection into the gland and at the end of recirculation (after 21.5±5.42 min). Each *line* represents the results of a representative experiment, in which samples of the collagenase solution were taken before injection into the gland, immediately after (0 min) and 4, 7, 10, 15, 20, and 30 min after starting the recirculation. Trypsin activity showed two types of kinetics: a strong increase in eight out of 12 (*square*, mean ± SD) or a slight increase in four out of 12 (*circle*, mean ± SD)

recirculation phase, or from 1.55±0.30 U Falgpa/ml to 0.97±0.32. The slight decrease in collagenase may be caused by two effects: (1) binding of collagenase to the donor tissue that was removed by centrifugation before the start of the activity test and (2) proteolytic damage to collagenase molecules. These effects should be considered when determining a suitable collagenase concentration. A concentration of 1.80 U PZ collagenase/ml worked very well in our hands. Clostripain activity was unaffected: 0.48±0.08 U BAEE: N-Benzoyl-L-Arginin-Ethyl-Ester before injection and 0.42±0.07 U BAEE/ml at the end of recirculation. Neutral protease increased from 55.2±6.04 U Azocoll/ml to 169±50.7. Quite unexpectedly, trypsin activity showed two types of kinetics. In eight cases it increased slightly from 0.22±0.14 U BAEE/ml to 0.57±0.31, and in four cases it increased very strongly from 0.50±0.08 U BAEE/ml to 3.34±0.27.

These results can be summarized as follows: during the isolation procedure, collagenase activity decreased slightly, whereas the activity of the pancreatic enzymes neutral protease and trypsin increased; in some cases trypsin activity increased very strongly.

Major variations in the islet yield, ranging from 0 to 12 491 IpgO after the above isolations, forced us to look for a correlation between enzyme activity and islet yield. A close correlation could be found between trypsin activity and islet yield. Poor islet yields (507±739 IpgO) correlated with a strong increase in pancreatic trypsin activity (1.50 U BAEE/ml), whereas low trypsin activity (>1.50 U BAEE/ml) correlated with high islet yields (6795±3697 IpgO). Neutral protease had hardly any effect on islet yield and, if at all, only a mild one.

A major problem faced in isolating islets from the porcine (and the human) pancreas is to achieve reproducibly high yields of good quality islets. That such parameters as the pig breed [7, 24], the donor age [6, 7], and the pH of the isolation medium [7] influence the islet yield has been clearly shown. Using the standard isolation technique and collagenase batches of controlled quality and proteolytic activity, as affirmed by company representatives, we were still unable to achieve satisfactorily reproducible high islet yields. This disappointment forced us to look into the basics, namely the enzymatic digestion process itself. The reasoning behind the enzymatic isolation technique is to specifically disintegrate the collagen-containing connective tissue by means of collagenase. It has been shown that there is an increase in proteolytic activity during the isolation procedure when islets are isolated from various donor species [27].

Our own studies confirmed these findings for porcine islets. Moreover, we determined that, particularly, trypsin was released during the digestion procedure, presumably due to disintegration of the exocrine tissue. Trypsin disintegrates a large number of proteins and thus appears to accelerate this process. The combination of exogenous collagenase and endogenous trypsin may easily initiate an unspecific, fast and uncontrollable tissue disintegration process. Our experiments showed that trypsin activity greater than 1.50 U BAEE/ml damaged the tissue in a way that clearly prevents the release of high islet yields. Furthermore, individual experiments revealed strong variations in trypsin activity. The failure of some islet isolations was apparently caused by the high endogenous trypsin activity of some pancreata (Fig. 3).

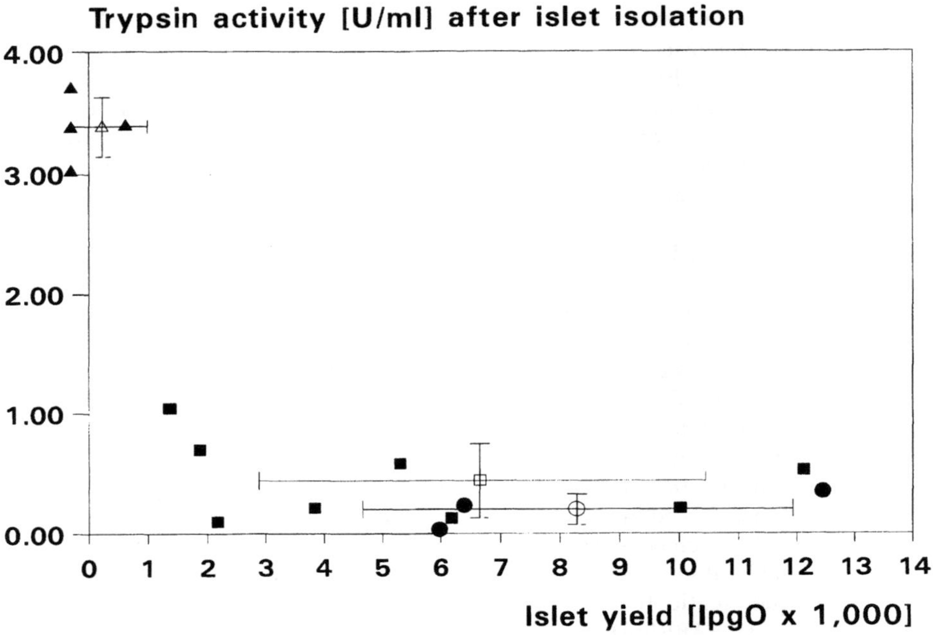

Fig. 3. Correlation of trypsin activity and islet yield. Results of trypsin activity tests and islet yields (islets per g organ, *IpgO*). Three groups of isolations are shown: *triangles*, isolations with trypsin activity >1.5 U BAEE/ml (n=4); *squares*, isolations with trypsin activity <1.5 U BAEE/ml (n=8); *circles*, isolations with trypsin inhibition by Pefabloc (n=3)

We speculate that factors such as the pig breed [7, 24], the donor age [6, 7], perhaps also the nutrition [28] and retrieval procedure [13], may directly influence the trypsin content of the pancreas. This may directly affect the islet yield by altering the trypsin activity during the isolation procedure in an unknown manner. The proteolytic activity of the collagenase preparation may possibly exert an additional effect, because it is known that trypsin activates trypsinogen and other proteolytic enzymes [29].

The negative influence of high trypsin activity on the islet yield induced us to try to inhibit the activity of this particular enzyme. A trypsin inhibitor used in islet isolations had to fulfill at least three requirements: (1) considering the susceptibility of the islets, the inhibitor had to be nontoxic, (2) it should not interfere with the activity tests, and (3) it had to be irreversible. An inhibitor with these properties is Pefabloc (Boehringer, Mannheim, Germany). We performed three isolations with adult pigs using collagenase solutions supplemented with Pefabloc (Fig. 3). There was only a slight increase in neutral protease (from 57.6±3.90 U Azocoll/ml before injection to 62.3±11.4 at the end of recirculation) and trypsin activity (from 0.17±0.09 U BAEE/ml to 0.35±0.15) during these isolations, and the islet yield was satisfactory (8395±3553 IpgO). (Due to logistics and problems with the collagenase suppliers we did not have sufficient time to extend these interesting studies before preparing this manuscript, but they will be continued soon.)

If high trypsin activity causes some isolations to fail, prophylactic inhibition should result in reproducibly high yields. In this context, another laboratory used a collagenase solution supplemented with 10% bovine serum albumin (BSA) as protease inhibitor and described a positive effect (+48%) on rat islet yield [27]. In our opinion, however, BSA has three disadvantages: (1) it interferes with activity tests, (2) it obviously inhibits collagenase activity (data not shown), and (3) it is a competitive inhibitor. Thus Pefabloc appears to be a much more suitable trypsin inhibitor, since it fulfills the above criteria. All isolations performed with Pefabloc resulted in low trypsin activity and a high islet yield.

However, the role of residual trypsin activity needs to be further investigated. To ensure complete and well-timed disintegration of the connective tissue, a small but well controllable degree of proteolytic activity may be necessary. From our experience with trypsin, it cannot be excluded that other pancreatic enzymes, e.g., lipase, elastase, or phospholipase A_2, also interfere with the controlled enzymatic disintegration of the pancreas and thus influence islet yield. Nevertheless, trypsin released by the digested exocrine tissue could function as an indicator or marker enzyme, when one is trying to determine the digestion endpoint, an aspect that needs to be further clarified.

To summarize our experience from 1991 until the present, it is clear (Fig. 4) that a more systematic analysis of the basic porcine islet isolation method has yielded quite a number of important and influential parameters. Undoubtedly, some progress has already been since these parameters were identified and taken into consideration, as far as islet yield and viability, islet fragility, and more reproducible results are concerned.

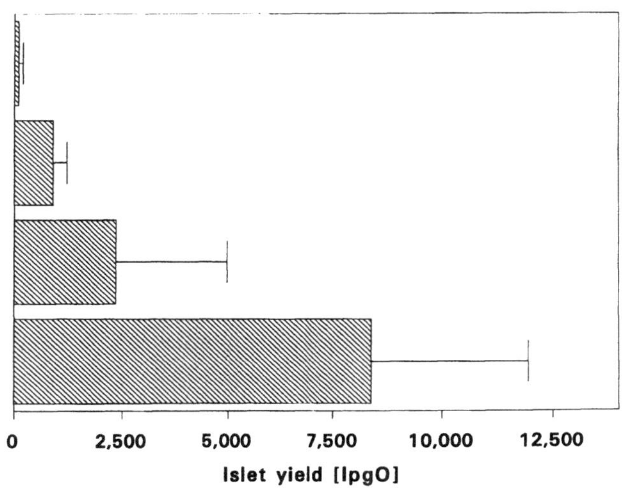

Fig. 4. Modifications of the islet isolation technique and their influence on islet yields. Comparison of the basic method and our standard method, involving various modifications of the islet isolation procedure. The *top row* shows the results obtained in our laboratory with the basic method described by Ricordi [1]. The other rows show islet yields (islets per g organ, *IpgO*) achieved by using an isolation technique with reduced mechanical stress (Teflon mesh, Teflon beads, handshaking; *second row*), purebred old pigs (*third row*), and prophylactic trypsin inhibition (*fourth row*). See text for details

Comment

With due respect to all investigators who claim repeatedly good results, it must be clearly stated that technical devices for isolating islets of Langerhans from the porcine pancreas are not yet sufficiently advanced to provide the clinician reliably with sufficient amounts of viable and functioning islets for future clinical xenotransplantation. Further developmental work will be required in the coming years, and this poses a major challenge to biotechnology and experimental transplantation. However, considering the undeniable achievements by various groups working in this field, a number of factors have surfaced that appear to exert a major influence on the isolation results.

Donor Pig. The transplantation community would be well advised to work closely with university departments of agriculture, commercial breeders, breeding societies, and farmers to find the most suitable purebred (or hybrid) pig breed, preferably of advanced age, to serve as a donor animal that can eventually be bred or bought at a reasonable cost. During this search, a detailed morphological analysis of the porcine pancreas should be performed to provide more essential data than are presently available on islet number and size and islet volume density. The amount of collagen and the collagen types that surround the particularly fragile porcine islets should be analyzed in detail with an eye to developing suitable collagenase preparations.

Logistics and Ischemia. Considering the widely differing and difficult EU regulations for the slaughtering process, as well as the questions of sterility and fragmentation of islets, the donor organ should be explanted with full operating room facilities, to avoid any warm ischemia time and damage before the pancreas is shipped to the laboratory. There have, however, been two reports of disappointing islet yields after surgical excision of the gland [13] (personal observations). Though the cause for this lack of success is presently unknown, we feel there may be a relationship between the organ retrieval procedure and the release and activity of the pancreatic enzymes. Based on all of our experience with an inadequate explantation procedure, it may be predicted that the fragility of islets will then further decrease and islet viability and function will improve considerably, as least as long as the fragility is not determined by poor initial islet architecture.

Collagenase. Researchers and the companies that provide collagenase should cooperate more closely to detect further reactive components of the collagenase enzyme(s), as was successfully achieved in one laboratory isolating rat islets [30]. To-date, eight collagenase subtypes have been described [31]. Their specificity for individual collagen types is still unknown. With increasing research in this field and more information, it should be possible to create a cocktail of various reactive enzymatic fractions that also matches the specific demands of the specific porcine tissue. A combined effort like this would have mutual benefits. The varying quality of poorly defined collagenase batches should hopefully soon become a nightmare of the past. The production of specifically tailored liberase (Boehringer Company) may be a first step in the right direction.

Pancreatic Enzymes. The example of trypsin has directed research into an unexpected new direction, i.e., on enzymes that are released from the tissue during the digestion phase and very likely interfere with the activity of "collagenase." Our preliminary data suggest that other proteolytic pancreatic enzymes, e.g., lipase and/or phospholipase A_2, probably contribute to this problem.

Minor problems involving the digestion chamber, the shaking procedure, purification protocols, and viability and function assays may have to be reevaluated, once a really satisfactory isolation protocol is available, one that reflects all important parameters, including those that have not yet been identified. An effort by all attracted to this field of medical research would not only advance the isolation of porcine islets for future clinical xenotransplantation. It would similarly advance the isolation of human islets for clinical allotransplantation, a field that still suffers from setbacks and awaits a major breakthrough before it is accepted by clinicians and patients alike.

Acknowledgment. The authors gratefully acknowledge the efficient support of Dr. Michael Giesel and Jürgen Pfaff of Biotest Pharma GmbH, Dreieich, Germany and their kind help in screening the current literature.

References

1. Ricordi, C., Socci, C., Davalli, A.M., et al. Isolation of the elusive pig islet. Surgery 107, 688, 1990
2. Ricordi, C., Lacy, P.E., Scharp, D.W. Automated islet isolation from human pancreas. Diabetes 38, 140, 1989
3. Calafiore, R., Calcinaro, F., Basta, G., et al. A method for the massive separation of highly purified, adult porcine islets of Langerhans. Metablolism 39, 175, 1990
4. Marchetti, P., Finke, E.H., Gerasimidi-Vazeou, A., et al. Automated large-scale isolation, in vitro function and xenotransplantation of porcine islets of Langerhans. Transplantation 52, 209, 1991
5. Hesse, U.J., Danis, J., Weyer, J., Meyer, G., Saad, S. In-vitro- und In-vivo-Studien zur Isolierung, Transplantation und Funktion von Langerhans-Inseln am Schwein. Langenbecks Arch Chir 375, 259, 1990
6. Socci, C., Ricordi, C., Davalli, A.M., et al. Selection of donors significantly improves pig islet isolation yield. Horm Metabol Res 25, 32, 1990
7. Heiser, A., Ulrichs, K., Müller-Ruchholtz, W. Influence of porcine race, age, and pH of the isolation medium on porcine pancreatic islet isolation success. Transplant Proc 26, 618, 1994
8. Deng, S., Bühler, L., Andereggen, E., et al. Islet isolation from slaughterhouse pig pancreata: Evidence of in vitro and in vivo function. Transplant Proc 26, 3396, 1994
9. Chadwick, D.R., Robertson, G.S.M., Rose, S., et al. Storage of porcine pancreatic digest prior to islet purification. Transplantation 56, 288, 1993
10. Davalli, A.M., Bertuzzi, F., Socci, C., et al. Paradoxical release of insulin by adult pig islets in vitro. Transplantation 56, 148, 1993
11. Ricordi, C., Finke, E.H., Lacy, P.E. Method for the mass isolation of islets from the adult pig pancreas. Diabetes 35, 649, 1986
12. Bühler, L., Deng, S., Mage, R., et al. Pig islet isolation: New aspects. Transplant Proc 26, 628, 1994

13. Ricordi, C., Socci, C., Davalli, A.M., et al. Effect of pancreas retrieval procedure on islet isolation in the swine. Transplant Proc 22, 442, 1990
14. Kerr-Conte, J., Pattou, F., Hober, C., et al. Induction of cerebral death in slaughterhouse pigs facilitates pancreas harvesting for islet isolation. Transplant Proc 26, 614, 1994
15. Warnock, G.L., Katyal, D., Okamura, J., Lakey, J.R.T., Rajotte, R.V. Studies of the isolation, viability, and preservation of purified islets after surgical pancreatectomy in large pigs. Xenotransplantation 2, 161, 1995
16. Polo, F., Monroy, B., Di Maria, S., et al. Islet isolation from the porcine pancreas, using a continuous digestion method. Xenotransplantation 2, 230, 1995
17. Toomey, P., Chadwick, D.R., Contractor, H., et al. Porcine islet isolation: Prospective comparison of automated and manual methods of pancreatic collagenase digestion. Br J Surg 80, 240, 1993
18. Heiser, A., Ulrichs, K., Müller-Ruchholtz, W. Prophylactic trypsin inhibition during the isolation procedure guarantees reproducible, high porcine islet yields. Xenotransplantation 1, 66, 1994
19. Van Suylichem, P.T.R., Johnson, P.R.V., Vos-Scheperkeuter, G.H., et al. Purified enzymes in pig pancreas dissociation for islet isolation: preliminary observations. Xenotransplantation 2, 172, 1995
20. Ohgawara, H., Kobayashi, A., Chong, S.J., Akaike, T., Hashimoto, Y. Preparation of adult pig pancreatic cells: Comparative study of methods with or without proteolytic enzymes. Cell Transplant 3, 325, 1994
21. Arbet-Engels, C., Darquy, S., Capron, F., Reach, G. Isolation of islets of Langerhans from the rat and pig pancreas using a modified UW solution from organ storage to islet purification. Diab Metabol 19, 590, 1993
22. Van Deijnen, J.H., Hulstaert, C.E., Wolters, G.H., van Schilfgaarde, R. Significance of the peri-insular extracellular matrix for islet isolation from the pancreas of rat, dog, pig, and man. Cell Tiss Res 267, 139, 1992
23. Bonner-Weir, S., Davalli, A.M., Scaglia, L., Hollister, J., Weir, G.C. Myths about the structure and function of porcine islets. Xenotransplantation 2, 207, 1995
24. Ulrichs, K., Bosse, M., Heiser, A., et al. Histomorphological characteristics of the porcine pancreas as a basis for the isolation of islets of Langerhans. Xenotransplantation 2, 176, 1995
25. Kirchhof, N., Hering, B.J., Geiss, V., Federlin, K., Bretzel, R.G. Evidence for breed-dependent differences in porcine islets of Langerhans. Transplant Proc 26, 616, 1994
26. Latif, Z.A., Noel, J., Alejandro, R. A simple staining of fresh and cultured islets. Transplantation 45, 827, 1988
27. Wolters, G.H.J., Suylichem, P.T.R., van Deijnen, J.H.M., van Schilfgaarde, R. Increased islet yield by improved pancreatic tissue dissociation: The effects of bovine serum albumin and calcium. Transplant Proc 21, 2626, 1989
28. Linn, T., Schmitz, P., Kloer, H.U., et al. Experimental islet isolation from donors with different nutrition regimens. Horm Metabol Res 25, 17, 1990
29. McShane, P., Sutton, R., Gray, D.W.R., Morris, P.J. Techniques for islet preparation: Protease activity in pancreas islet isolation by enzymatic digestion. Diabetes 38, 126, 1989

30. Wolters, G.H.J., Vos-Scheperkeuter, G.H., Lin, H.C., van Schilfgaarde, R. Different roles of class I and class II clostridium histolyticum collagenase in rat pancreatic islet isolation. Diabetes 44, 227, 1995
31. Bond, M.D., van Wort, H.E. Characterization of the individual collagenases from clostridium histolyticum. Biochemistry 23, 3085, 1984

43 Xenotransplantation of Encapsulated Pancreatic Islets

R.P. Lanza and W.L. Chick

Introduction

The potential therapeutic applications for cell and tissue transplantation are enormous. Skin, bone, and bone marrow transplantation are already widely used, highly successful clinical procedures [1–3]. Although the transplantation of other cells and tissues is more experimental, these transplants also appear likely to play a major role in medicine in the future [4]. These include the transplantation of pancreatic islets, fetal tissue and cells genetically engineered to produce specific bioactive substances. Diabetes mellitus, for example, afflicts over a 100 million people and is a leading cause of morbidity and mortalitiy in the world. An ideal treatment for this disease would be the transplantation of the islets of Langerhans.

Restoration of normal glucose metabolism has already been achieved in several patients with type I diabetes mellitus by the transplantation of islets of Langerhans [5, 6]. Success, unfortunately, has been sporadic, and the requirement for immunosuppressive drugs exposes these patients to a wide variety of serious complications including cancer, infection, renal failure, and osteoporosis [7, 8].

Ultimately, the goal of islet transplantation is to treat patients without generalized immunosuppression, and early enough in the course of the disease to prevent or retard the development of complications associated with this disease. Encapsulation of islets in biohybrid devices offers a distinct advantage in this respect. Unlike corneal grafts and bone marrow cells, islet tissue can be readily isolated from the immune system of the host by a selectively permeable membrane without interfering with its physiological function. Low molecular weight substances such as nutrients, electrolytes, oxygen, and insulin are exchanged across the membrane while immunocytes, antibodies and other immune rejection effector mechanisms are excluded [9] (Fig. 1). This approach has the potential not only to allow allogeneic transplantation without immunosuppression, but also to allow the use of xenografts.

In the form of a vascular implant, the islets can be distributed in a chamber surrounding the membrane, and the device implanted as a shunt in the vascular system [10–12]. Alternatively, the islets can be encapsulated within diffusion chambers (tubular and planar configurations) [13–16] or spherical micro- or macrocapsules [17–19] and placed intraperitoneally [13–21], subcutaneously [22, 23] or in other sites [24] (Fig. 2). Results in diabetic animals indicate that these systems can function for periods of several months to more than 1 year [25, 26]. Furthermore, results in spontaneously diabetic animals indicate that

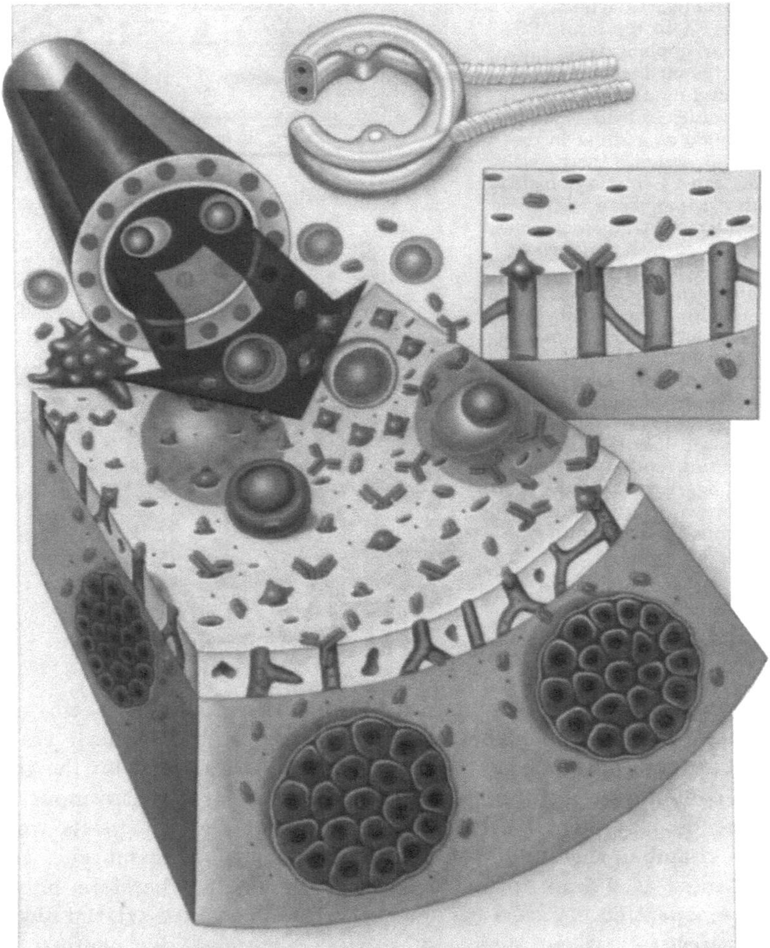

Fig. 1. The principle of immunoisolation is to separate transplanted cells and tissue from the immune system of the host using a selectively permeable membrane (seen in cross-section). Nutrients and oxygen, represented here by *small dots*, and secreted products, in this case proinsulin, are exchanged across the membrane. Complement and immunoglobulins are prevented from reaching the transplanted cells partly because of their size, as shown in this conceptual illustration (Reprinted with permission from [9])

both conventional transplant rejection and autoimmune beta cell destruction can be blocked. However, these data also suggest that because of limitations in functional islet longevity, periodic replenishment of islets will be required in patients. In some designs this may pose significant difficulties. Use of biodegradable materials may well help to solve this potential problem by allowing absorption and excretion of implants when the islet cells which they contain become functionally inactive.

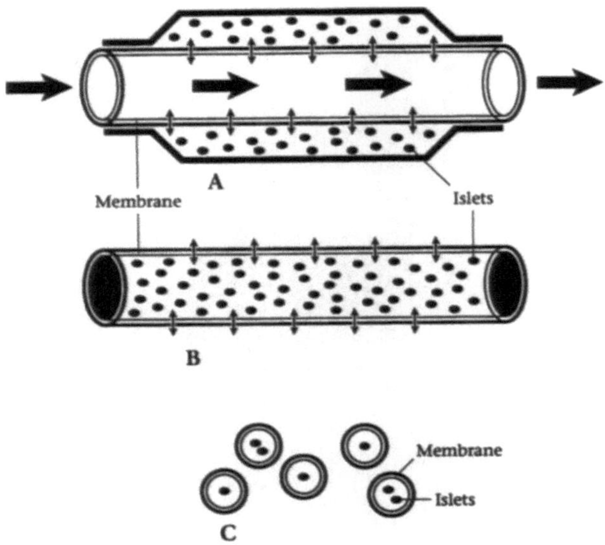

Fig. 2. Biohybrid artificial devices. **A** In the form of a vascular implant, islets can be distributed in a chamber surrounding a perm-selective membrane, and the device implanted as a shunt in the vascular system. Alternatively, islets can be immunoisolated within **B** membrane diffusion chambers or **C** microcapsules and placed intraperitoneally, intramuscularly, subcutaneously, or in other sites. The islets within these biohybrid devices are generally immobilized in hydrogels such as alginate or agar. One of the important functions of these gels is to provide more uniform islet distribution by preventing settling and subsequent aggregation of the islets into larger, necrotic masses. (Reprinted with permission from [25])

Perfusion Devices Implanted as Arteriovenous Shunts

Although much of the immunoisolation work to date has been carried out with tubular diffusion chambers and microcapsules, the modern era of biohybrid device development began approximately 20 years ago with the introduction of islet-containing perfusion devices implanted as arteriovenous (AV) shunts. These devices offered certain obvious advantages. The islets were distributed in a chamber surrounding a selectively permeable membrane, and the device implanted as a shunt in the cardiovascular system. Therefore, only a thin membrane separated the islets from a stream of oxygenated arterial blood with a partial pressure of approximately 100 torr (mmHg). By contrast, extravascular devices implanted intraperitoneally, intramuscularly, or in other tissues must exchange oxygen and nutrients over larger diffusion distances, and with a microvasculature that normally delivers oxygen at a partial pressure of only 40 torr [27, 28]. In this regard, there are data that suggest that islet viability and/or insulin secretory function are detrimentally influenced at low oxygen tensions [29–31]. In addition, it was possible to access the cell chamber of vascular devices for removal and replacement of nonfunctioning islets once the device was implanted. The seeding ports could be designed to be accessible for reseeding using a needle and syringe, and could be positioned just under the surface of the skin.

The original perfusion devices were developed in the early and mid-1970s by Chick et al. [32, 33]. These devices utilized bundles of capillary fibers, seeded on their outside surfaces with isolated islet cells. Tissue culture medium was circulated through the lumen of the fibers, and the islets secreted insulin in response to stimulatory glucose concentrations. However, the use of these small-diameter fibers (ID, <1 mm) as vascular implants was limited to short-term, ex vivo studies because of clotting [32, 34–39]. Experiments in which tubular membranes with an inner diameter of 2.7 mm were used resulted in the first demonstration of extended in vivo patency [40]. These larger diameter fibers remained patent as AV shunts for seven weeks in dogs that did not receive any systemic anticoagulation.

An artificial pancreas device which utilized a single, coiled, tubular membrane with an inner diameter of 5–6 mm was investigated by our group for several years [41–43]. This device design incorporated a poly acrylonitrile-polyvinyl chloride (PAN-PVC) membrane within an acrylic housing. The islet chamber was created by the space between the membrane and the housing. The PAN-PVC membrane could not be sutured so it was connected to standard polytetrafluorethylene graft material of the same diameter which extended beyond the housing and was used for anastomosis to the vascular system.

In vivo studies indicated that this design had excellent biocompatibility with respect to blood clotting. Four dogs which received devices without islet tissue were still ongoing after 3 years. The function of this perfused artificial pancreas was evaluated by implanting devices seeded with canine islet allografts into severely diabetic pancreatectomized dogs using a protocol that had been shown to optimize long-term insulin secretion in devices maintained in vitro [42]. These experiments indicated that the devices significantly improved glucose homeostasis and functioned for more than 1 year [41]. Histologic evaluation of the devices after removal revealed viable islets with granulated alpha cells. No evidence of infiltration of immune cells was observed, suggesting that the membrane was indeed immunoprotective. In two animals in which the devices were removed one year after implantation, the exogenous insulin required to control fasting blood glucose concentrations increased by more than 20 U/day. In addition, approximately 25 % of the islets remained viable after one year in vivo (Fig. 3). One of the devices was perfused with tissue culture medium in vitro following removal, and showed continued release of insulin.

Data from the implantation of devices containing xenogeneic islets were limited but did indicate that discordant xenografts were also feasible [25, 41]. One dog which received devices containing bovine islets demonstrated excellent control of fasting glucose levels for almost 2 months without exogenous insulin. The results using porcine islets were even more preliminary, but in at least one dog a device containing porcine islets substantially decreased the exogenous insulin requirement for more than 6 months.

However, a number of issues remained which appeared to limit the therapeutic potential of this approach. Perhaps most importantly, data suggested that the size and geometry of perfusion devices imposed a critical limitation on the amount of islet tissue that could be transplanted into a patient using a single unit. At present, two perfusion devices would be required to treat a patient with an insulin requirement of approximately 30 units/day. Attempts to lengthen the coiled, tubular membrane, thereby increasing insulin secretion, failed because of clotting. In addition, the glycemic control provided by the perfusion device design clearly was not optimal. Nevertheless, much was learned from these studies. They represent an important step toward developing newer, simpler, more viable strategies for transplanting islets using encapsulation technologies.

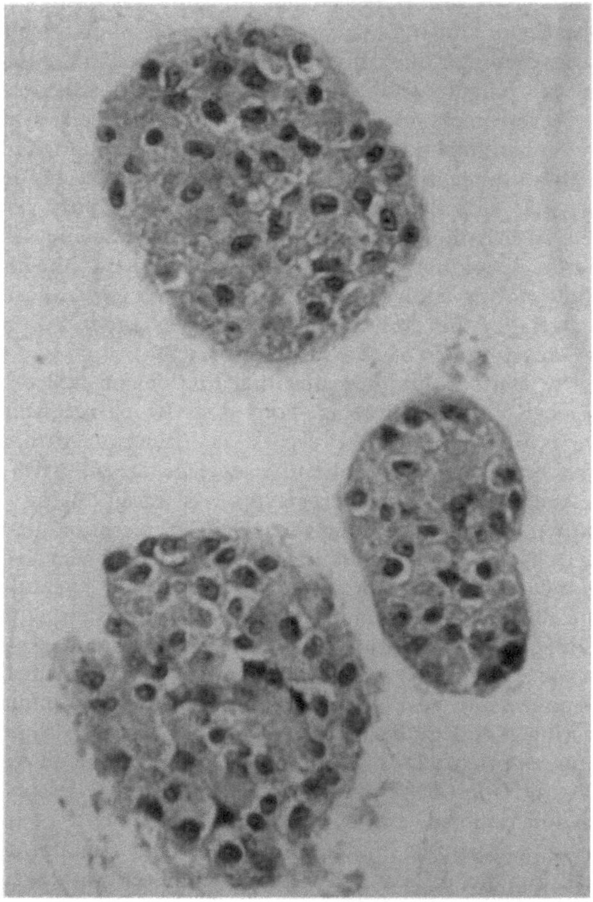

Fig. 3. Canine islets retrieved from a vascular device after more than 1 year in a diabetic dog without any immunosuppression. After device removal, the exogenous insulin requirement of the animal increased more than 20 U/day. (Reprinted with permission from [25])

Diffusion Chambers

Numerous devices of this type have been evaluated by our own and other groups [44]. These are typically tubular or planar designs. Membrane materials used to fabricate these devices include PAN-PVC, polypropylene, polycarbonate, and cellulose nitrate [25, 45]. These studies have been reviewed elsewhere [28, 46–49]; only those systems which have shown significant progress to date will be discussed further.

In 1982, Woodward et al. [50] examined the influence of geometry on the occurrence of fibrosis. He demonstrated that a disc-shaped chamber induced a zone of collagen-rich connective tissue between the implant and the vascular system, whereas a hollow-fiber elicited only a minimal response. A number of investigations have been carried out to assess the potential of tubular chambers as an artificial pancreas. Others found that islet and insulinoma tissue seeded within hollow fibers restored normoglycemia in diabetic rodents when implanted intra-

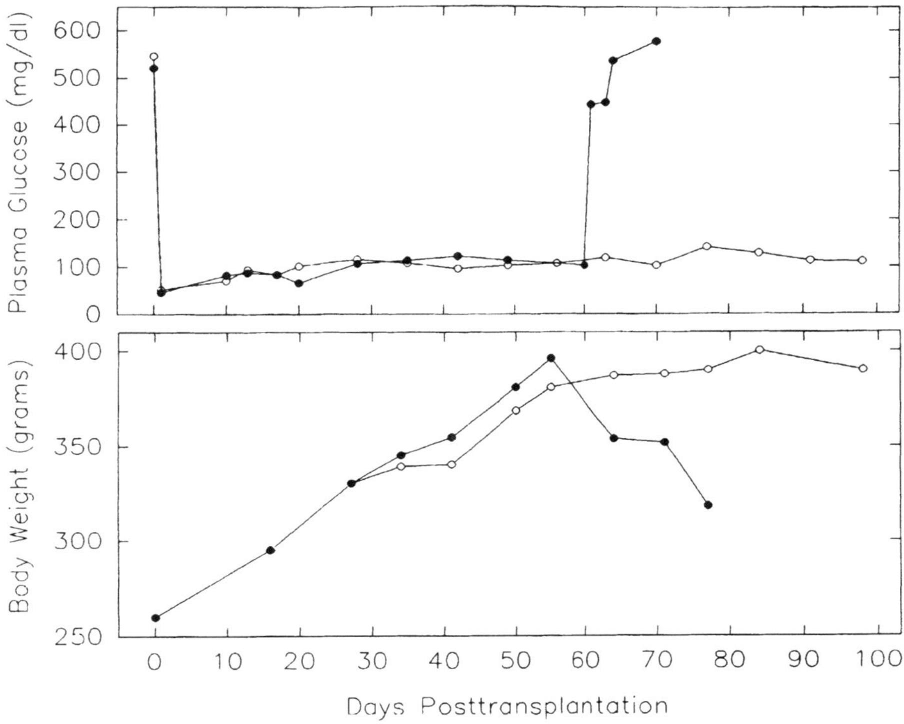

Fig. 4. Fasting plasma glucose concentrations (*top*) and body weight (*bottom*) in two spontaneously diabetic BB/Wor rats that received discordant canine islet xenografts encapsulated in permselective acrylic membranes (i.e, hollow fibers). The membranes were removed from one rat (*filled circles*) at 2 months. The other animal (*open circles*) continued to maintain normoglycemia after more than 8 months. No immunosuppression was used in this study. (Reprinted with permission from [58])

peritoneally [51–53]. Histologic analysis of recovered implants, however, revealed a fibrous tissue layer surrounding the membranes. The same type of fiber was also observed to elicit an inflammatory pericapsular response in the pig [54]. This tissue reaction was generally more intense, though qualitatively similar to that seen in the rat, except for lymphoid clusters with giant and pseudo-epithelioid cells that were observed only in the pigs. The reaction consisted of several layers of fibroblasts and collagen with polymorphonuclear leukocytes, macrophages, histiocytes, and small lymphocytes. The fenestrated outer wall of the tubular membrane was always infiltrated by collagen, fibroblasts, and macrophages.

Reports from our laboratory [55–58] described a series of experiments using wider-bore tubular chambers with a diameter of 1.6–4.8 mm. These studies were carried out with PAN-PVC membranes having a smooth outer skin. Porcine, bovine, and canine islets placed within these chambers restored normoglycemia in streptozotocin (STZ)-induced diabetic rats for more than 1 year without immunosuppression [26]. Only minimal tissue reactivity was observed. The external membrane surfaces were generally free of fibrotic overgrowth and exhibited only occasional host cell adherence. Encapsulated canine xenografts implanted in spontaneously diabetic BB rats also had the same success, resulting in fasting normoglycemia for periods of several weeks to more than eight months [58] (Fig. 4). Intravenous glucose tolerance test (IVGTT) K values (decline in glucose levels, % per min) after implantation in spontaneously diabetic BB and STZ rats were 2.3 %±0.4 % and 2.6 %±0.2 % to 3.5 %±0.3 %, respectively, compared with 3.1 %±0.1 % and 3.3 %±0.1 % for normal control groups. In contrast, the K values for untreated diabetic rats were less than 1. Both light and electron microscopy of long-term functioning grafts revealed well-preserved islets (Fig. 5), with hormone-producing alpha, beta, and delta cells.

While these wider-bore PAN-PVC membranes solved many of the problems associated with diffusion chambers (e.g., fibrosis, abscess formation, adhesions) [45, 59], studies in large animals closer to man will likely be required before clinical trials can be contemplated. Experiments in totally pancreatectomized, severely diabetic dogs have in fact already been performed in our laboratory [57]. They indicated that canine islet implants can provide long-term correction of hyperglycemia without the use of immunosuppressive and/or antiinflamma-

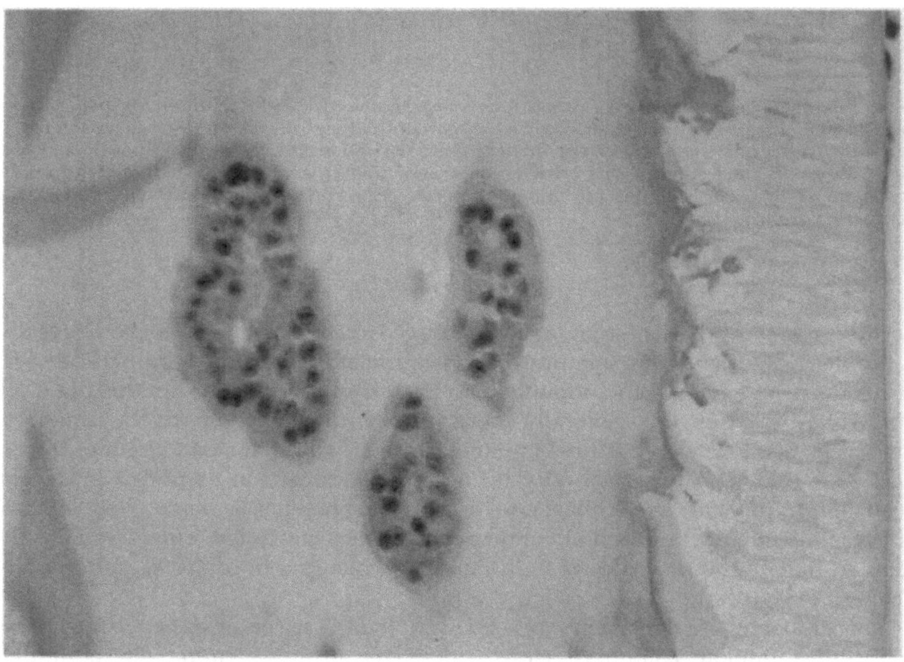

Fig. 5. Encapsulated porcine islets retrieved from the peritoneal cavity of diabetic rats 307 days after xenotransplantation. (Reprinted with permission from [26])

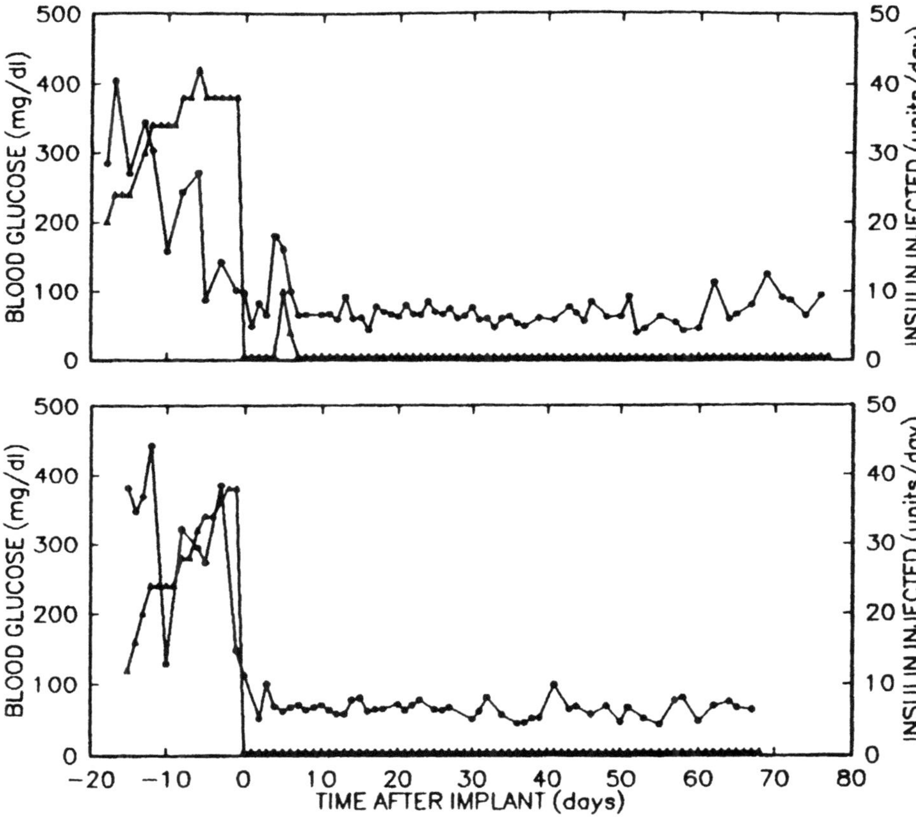

Fig. 6. Successful treatment of experimental diabetes in dogs with encapsulated islets. First description of the ability of an extravascular device to sustain normogyclemia in a large animal model without any immunosuppression. Exogenous insulin requirements (*triangles*) and fasting blood glucose concentrations (*circles*) in two dogs before and after device implantation. (Reprinted with permission from [57])

tory drugs. Insulin independence was achieved for more than 10 weeks in dogs with preimplantation insulin requirements of 30–40 units/ day (a dosage in the range of what many human patients require; Fig. 6). Little or no fibrosis was observed for periods as long as 30 weeks.

In view of these encouraging results, a number of unsolved issues critical to the wide-scale clinical success of these devices must be addressed: (1) long-term biocompatibility (with risk of fibrosis, peritonitis, intestinal adhesions, and abscess formation), (2) membrane breakage, (3) suitability for retrieval (or, alternatively, the use of the peritoneum or other implantation site as a "dumping ground"), (4) further improvements in glycemic control, and (5) potential limitations imposed by the size and geometry of these chambers.

Biocompatibility

Experiments performed in our laboratory have demonstrated the feasibility of long-term immunoisolation of islets by artificial (PAN-PVC) membranes and the long-term biocompatibility of the membrane versus the graft and versus the recipient [26, 55–58]. These data indicate that islet implants can provide correction of hyperglycemia in dogs and rodents for periods of several months to more than 1 year without the use of immunosuppressive drugs. Diffusion chambers fabricated from permselective acrylic membranes showed little or no evidence of an inflammatory response when implanted intraperitoneally in either spontaneously or STZ-induced diabetic rats [26, 58]. Complications such as abscess formation or intestinal adhesions, which have been observed with other technologies [45, 59], were not observed with these implants.

These studies have recently been extended to implantation in the peritoneal cavity of a large animal, the dog, with surgically induced diabetes [57]. Histological examination of the chambers revealed that they were biocompatible. The outer surface showed only scattered foci of macrophages and lymphocytes. Intactness and sterility of the chambers, however, were crucial factors in the success of the implants. In addition to loss of islet viability, damaged or contaminated membranes were often encapsulated by fibrous tissue, which exhibited an interstitial acute and/or chronic inflammatory reaction and development of granulation tissue. Before testing can be undertaken in diabetic patients, it will be important to determine the cause(s) of this peritoneal tissue reaction.

Membrane Breakage

Most of the transplants described above ultimately failed because of membrane breakage. Under stress, the tubular chambers can bend, leading to fracture of the membrane walls and subsequent destruction of the encapsulated islet tissue. By 5–7 months postimplantation, 80 %–90 % of the membrane chambers in dogs had broken. The tubular membranes used in most of these studies had a wall thickness of only 69–105 µm. The chambers fabricated from these membranes were relatively fragile, and susceptible to breakage. An increase in the membrane wall thickness may minimize this problem.

Methods for Removal

Because of limitations imposed by islet longevity and resultant requirements for reseeding, membrane chambers will eventually require localization and removal. If necessary, and depending upon the site of implantation, the devices could be removed by laparoscopy. However, surgical excision would be necessary if diffusion chambers were to become fibroencapsulated and/or vascularized. Open surgery, of course, carries risk of infection and would be a more extensive surgical procedure.

Blood Glucose Control

The motivation for islet transplantation is to provide physiologic control of blood glucose concentration. In vitro and in vivo experiments with tubular chambers have demonstrated only moderately delayed changes (lag time, <10 min) in insulin secretion in response to changes in glucose concentration. Perifusion of encapsulated canine islets with glucose elicited an approximately fourfold average increase from the basal insulin secretion [55]. There was a delay of only 7±1 min before the insulin concentration in the perfusate began to increase. Although this response is well within a time-frame compatible with closed-loop insulin delivery (pharmacokinetic modeling of glucose homeostasis in man suggests that the lag time of the increase in insulin delivery by an artificial pancreas must be less than 15 min to avoid significant overexcursion of postprandial blood glucose) [60], a reduction in the volume of the islet cell compartment would further improve the transmission of the glycemic signal from the blood to the islets, and of insulin from the islets to the recipient.

In a set of experiments [57, 61], wider-bore chambers were implanted into the peritoneum of six totally pancreatectomized dogs, and the animals monitored for glycemic control by fasting and postprandial blood glucose determinations, and by responses to both intravenous and oral glucose. All of the dogs had varying degrees of reduced insulin requirements for control of fasting blood glucose levels. Implantation of the chambers completely supplanted exogenous insulin therapy in three animals for 51 to more than 90 days (each of these implants continued to maintain blood glucose control for more than 20 weeks). The fasting glucose concentrations averaged 81±6 mg/dl for these three animals during the first month. This was lower than the fasting glucose levels prior to pancreatectomy, which averaged 91±3 mg/dl. The precise reason for these slightly lower levels is unclear.

Diffusion Limitations

Immunoisolated islets lack intimate vascular access, and must be supplied with oxygen and nutrients by diffusion from the nearest blood vessels over distances greater than those normally encountered. In wider-bore membrane chambers, the problem of cell death or dysfunction as a result of oxygen supply limitations, or accumulation of wastes or other cellular products is likely to be more severe. Our observations with chambers with an internal diameter of 4–8 mm is consistent with this. Chambers retrieved from the peritoneal cavity of dogs several months after allotransplantation contained a central core of necrotic islets. Only a rim of islets remained viable within approximately 0.5–1 mm of the inner membrane wall. Similar results were obtained with canine islet implants into rats. These findings may also explain the surprisingly large number of islets required to achieve blood glucose control. Clearly, careful attention must be paid to the diffusion distances and transport properties of the membranes. The relatively small volume (and short distances) associated with smaller spherical devices would maximize the transfer of oxygen and nutrients to the islets, and minimize the suppression of function by any islet hormonal or metabolic products which could accumulate in the islet compartment.

Host Sensitization

Although encapsulation systems serve to block uptake of antibodies and complement, the possibility must be considered that antigens released from the cell compartment could stimulate a host humoral response. Such antibodies could be induced by antigens shed from the cell surface, or by proteins secreted by live cells or liberated after cell death. This could lead to an allergic response and/or immune complex disease. Studies have been performed in our laboratory in order to help rule-out the possibility of serious immunologic sequelae in recipients [62, 63]. Although these studies were carried out using islets encapsulated inside tubular membrane chambers, the results may be reflective of other cell encapsulation systems as well, including microcapsules, hollow fibers, devices anastomosed to the vascular system as AV shunts, and other types of implantable diffusion chambers.

In these studies, chambers containing porcine or bovine islets were implanted intraperitoneally into STZ-induced diabetic rats. Sera were collected at various intervals and tested against isolated canine and porcine islets for tissue specificity and interspecies cross-reactivity by fluorescence immunocytochemistry. No immunofluorescence (or only weak background staining) was obtained when islets were exposed to horse sera, or to sera obtained prior to implantation of devices containing xenogeneic islets. Within 2–6 weeks, however, the postimplantation sera showed strong immunoreactivity (Table 1). The antibodies were found to be reactive to multiple tissues, and to possess little or no interspecies cross-reactivity.

The appearance of these xenoantibodies coincided with the appearance of circulating soluble immune complexes. However, none of the respiratory, cutaneous, or gastrointestinal manifestations that are characteristic of an anaphylactic reaction, or of the diseases of immediate-type hypersensitivity were observed, even following the intraperitoneal injection of additional naked islet tissue. Renal glomeruli did not stain for IgG or C3 in islet recipients. These results suggest that

Table 1. Xenogeneic humoral response induced in rats by encapsulated porcine islets (sera tested against porcine islets)

Time (days)	Score (n=15
0 (pre)	±
1–7	±
8–14+	15–21+
22–28	$+^{1}$
29–35	$+^{1}$
36–42	++
43–49	++
76–80	$+++^{1}/_{2}$

Reprinted with permission from [62]

islet cell antigens crossed the membrane and stimulated antibody formation in the host, although they did not appear to cause renal or immune-complex disease during the course of this study.

In theory, the essential feature of immune-complex disease would be the demonstration of immune complexes in tissues and biological fluids. However, the formation, fate, biologic activities, and pathologic potential of immune complexes depend on (a) the nature of the antigens (size, valence, chemical composition, and magnitude and duration of exposure) and antibodies (affinity and reactivity with phlogogenic mediators) involved, (b) the molar ratio and production rate of the two reactants, and (c) the state of the host's phagocytes (both circulating leukocytes and the reticuloendothelial system) [64]. In the experimental serum sickness model, more than 99% of the immune complexes formed are eliminated by phagocytes, predominantly by the liver's Kupffer cells, leaving less than 1% of the complexes capable of producing disease [65]. Overload of this system may be causative in precipitating disease [66–69].

It is important to note that in diseases of immediate-type hypersensitivity (or allergies), genetic factors exert an important influence on many specific immunoglobulin responses [70]. In humans, individual haplotype has been shown to be associated with the magnitude of responsiveness to certain antigens [71–73], and could predispose certain xeno-device-sensitized patients to an anaphylactic reaction following exposure to other xenogeneic proteins in the form of foods (e.g., the ingestion of pork). However, none of the clinical manifestations that are characteristic of the anaphylactic syndrome, or of the diseases of immediate type hypersensitivity, were observed in this study, even after reexposure to a significant quantity of islet material.

Microcapsules

Over the past decade, several methods for microencapsulating islets have been investigated [74]. Microcapsules offer a number of distinct advantages over the use of other biohybrid encapsulation devices, including greater surface to volume ratio, ease of implantation (can simply be injected), and retrievability by lavage and needle aspiration (or alternatively, fabrication from biodegradable materials). However, a variety of problems limit the usefulness of most microcapsules, and only the alginate-poly-L-lysine (PLL) system has resulted in long-term islet function in larger animals. This type of microencapsulation system is also widely used to immobilize microbial cells for industrial applications [75, 76]. The procedure involves extruding a mixture of cells and sodium alginate using a droplet generation device into a $CaCl_2$ solution.

Using this procedure to entrap islets in calcium alginate hydrogels, Lim and Sun [77] then coated these negatively charged gelled droplets with positively charged PLL. However, these capsules were unstable and produced an inflammatory response when implanted into the peritoneal cavity of animals [78, 79]. Modifications in the encapsulation procedure have improved the biocompatibility of the capsules, resulting in a dramatic increase in the duration of islet allograft function in diabetic rodents to more than 1 year [80]. Implanted rat-to-mouse islet xenografts produced blood glucose control for a shorter period of time. Although prolongation of survival of canine islets has also been achieved with the alginate-PLL technique, these studies have been performed in mice, and have usually required adjunctive treatment with immunosuppressive agents [81–83]. Weber et al. [84] found that alginate-PLL microcapsules containing canine islets functioned for less than 2 weeks in diabetic nonobese diabetic (NOD) mice. With anti-CD4 monoclonal antibody treatment, however, long-term functional survival was observed in many of the recipients.

Recently, prolongation of discordant xenograft survival in STZ-induced diabetic mice has been achieved in our laboratory without immunosuppression using alginate microspheres without the synthetic poly (L-lysine) membrane [85]. Uncoated alginate spheres containing porcine and bovine islets routinely reversed hyperglycemia after intraperitoneal injection into diabetic mice. All but one (13 out of 14) of the grafts functioned for at least 1 month, and in 11 animals for at least 10 weeks. In comparison, nonencapsulated islet transplants failed to function, or sustained euglycemia for less than 4 days.

The ability of uncoated microspheres to achieve marked prolongation of discordant xenograft survival is surprising, as the destruction of the grafts might have been expected to occur based on the presence of circulating preformed natural antibodies in the recipients that are reactive to cells of the donor [86]. Our data suggest that proteins of the complement system would also have had access to the encapsulated islet graft. Naturally produced antibody and activation of the complement cascade are generally thought to target the donor endothelium [87, 88]. The cytotoxic antibodies in man against pig xenoantigens are believed to be directed against α-galactosyl epitopes, which are expressed on vascular endothelium but are not expressed on many parenchymal cells [89, 90]. These antibodies appear to trigger the hemorrhagic necrosis that leads to solid organ rejection [91–94]. However, the role of xenoreactive natural antibodies in islet rejection is still uncertain. An explanation for the immunoprotective effect of the alginate spheres also needs to accommodate the fact that cytokines (M_r, 10–30 kDa), nitric oxide and other toxic moieties are small enough to diffuse readily into the gel matrix, yet did not induce obvious dysfunction or destruction of the islet grafts.

Our data suggest that the alginate matrix served as a physical barrier to prevent direct effector cell contact with the donor tissue. However, we cannot rule out the possibility that immunological effector molecules were excluded from the negatively charged alginate gels based on properties other than simply molecular weight. The destruction of discordant islet xenografts may depend upon proteins that carry charges under physiological conditions. For example, one or more of the components of the complement system with its cascading series of plasma enzymes, regulatory proteins, and proteins capable of cell lysis could be affected by the electrostatic interaction between the gel support and protein charges. Other phenomena may also be involved in the mechanism(s) of protection. Zekorn et al. [95] have shown that encapsulated islets are protected from high doses of IL-1 (M_r, 17 kDa) inside hollow-fiber membranes with a molecular weight cutoff of 50 kDa. The authors suggested that a nonspecific coating of the membranes by serum proteins may have caused the protective effect.

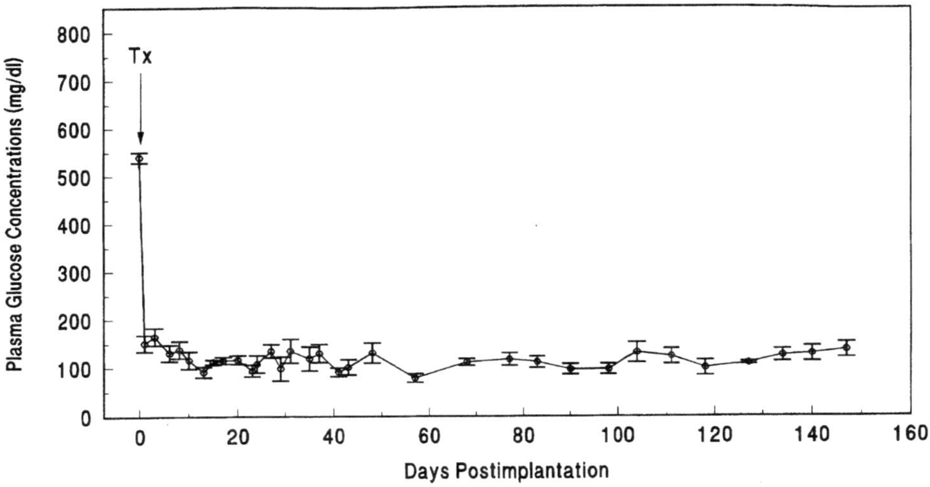

Fig. 7. Mean nonfasting plasma glucose levels in four streptozotocin (STZ)-induced diabetic rats that received intraperitoneal implants of alginate-encapsulated bovine islets. All of the animals received low-dose cyclosporine (CsA, 10–20 mg/kg per day s.c.). Immunohistochemical staining of the grafts (>100–150 days) revealed healthy viable islets (80 %–100 %, comparable to the day 0 control specimens), with well-granulated alpha, beta, and delta cells. This method for transplanting discordant islets into rats is simple and inexpensive and may also be a useful procedure for transplanting other cells and tissues. These spheres can be formed simply by extruding a mixture of cells and sodium alginate with a 16-gauge angiocatheter into a $CaCl_2$ solution. (Reprinted with permission from [96])

Although our results using uncoated alginate microspheres in mice are encouraging, it will be important to study the nature and extent of this immunoprotectivity in other animal models. Preliminary experiments in diabetic rats suggest that uncoated alginate spheres containing porcine and bovine islets can reverse hyperglycemia for periods of up to more than 175 days [96] (Fig. 7). However, these results have been inconsistent and usually have required adjunctive treatment with immunosuppressive agents. Whether this immunosuppression can be eliminated, or the alginate microspheres modified to provide more complete immunoprotection, requires further assessment and study.

Experiments in spontaneously diabetic dogs have also been performed in our laboratory. Results indicate that long-term survival of canine islet allografts can be achieved by encapsulation inside uncoated alginate spheres (Fig. 8). Although low-dose cyclosporine (CsA) was also administered, by 3 weeks postimplantation the whole-blood trough levels of the drug were below detectable limits by high-performance liquid chromatography (HPLC). Implantation of the microspheres completely supplanted exogenous insulin therapy in the dogs for 60 to more than 150 days. These results may have important implications in assessing the potential role for this type of microreactor as therapy for human insulin-dependent diabetes. Moreover, by using recombinant methods and encapsulating other tissues, it may also prove possible to treat patients suffering from a wide variety of other disorders requiring hormone or enzyme replacement therapy.

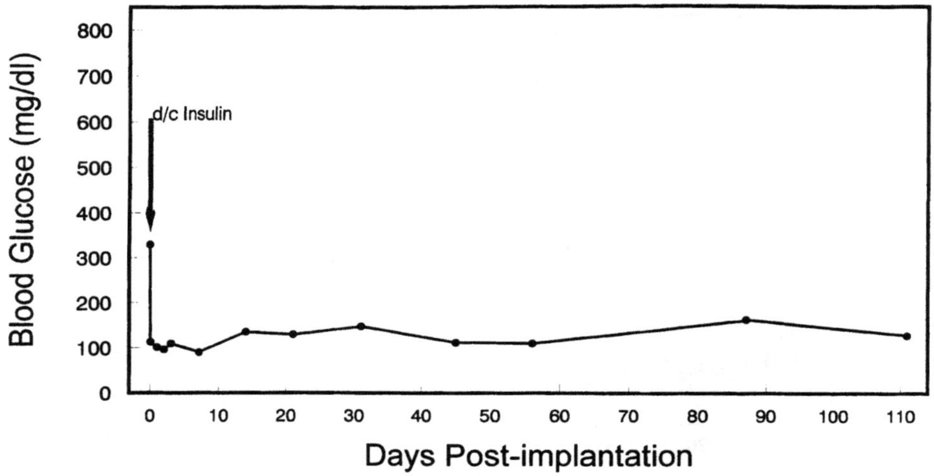

Fig. 8. Fasting blood glucose concentrations in a spontaneously diabetic dog that received an intraperitoneal implant of alginate-encapsulated canine islets. (Reprinted with permission from [13])

Soon-Shiong et al. [97] have also reported successful long-term implantations of microencapsulated allografts in larger animals. They treated spontaneous diabetes in dogs administered low doses of cyclosporine. These PLL-coated microspheres maintained euglycemia for 63–172 days, comparable to the results obtained in our laboratory without the synthetic poly-L-lysine membrane. Using the same technology, Soon-Shiong et al. [98] have also achieved insulin-independence in a patient for approximately 1 month. However, this patient was on a regimen of immunosuppressive drugs, and subsequently required exogenous insulin therapy. Calafiore et al. [99] have also achieved insulin independence in one of three alloxan-induced diabetic dogs and, transiently, in one of two patients without any pharmacologic immunosuppression. However, these microcapsules were coated with PLL and were deposited in artificial prostheses directly anastomosed to blood vessels.

More recently, our laboratory has successfully tested a new type of microreactor in both rodents and normal dogs using discordant islet xenografts [13, 100]. Coated and uncoated islet-containing microreactors were implanted into the peritoneum of normal dogs for periods of four to six weeks. Few or no islets survived in the uncoated microcapsules, even with the use of triple immunosuppressive therapy. However, when bovine islets were immobilized inside the new type of coated microreactor, the tissue remained viable both with and without low-dose immunosuppression (Fig. 9). Immunohistochemical staining revealed well-granulated alpha, beta, and delta cells consistent with functionally active hormone synthesis and secretion. To test further the secretory function of the islets, the explanted microreactors were incubated in solutions containing either basal (50 mg/dl) or stimulatory (300 mg/dl) concentrations of glucose. In both the immunosuppressed and non-immunosuppressed dog experiments, the explanted islets responded with an approximately four- to sixfold average increase above

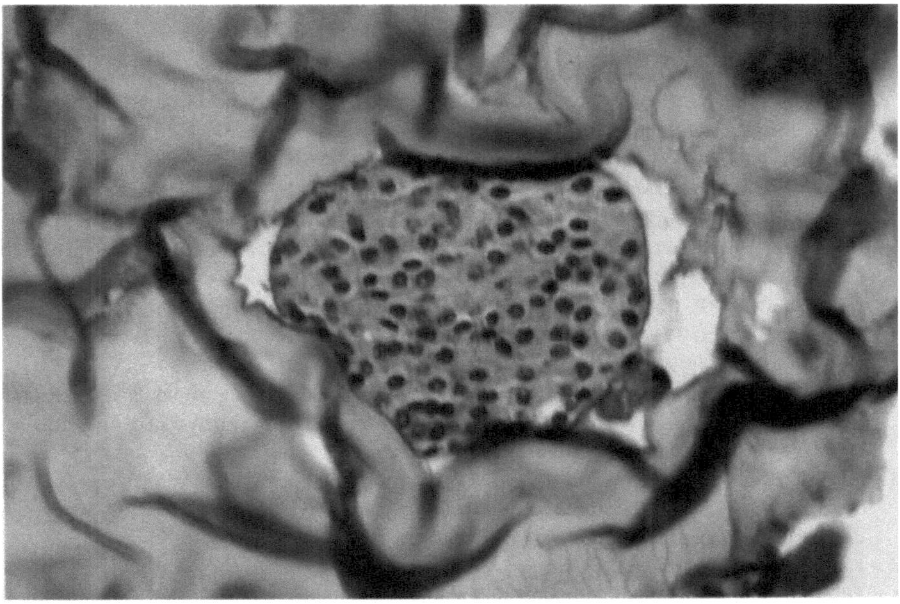

Fig. 9. Encapsulated bovine islet retrieved from the peritoneal cavity of a dog 6 weeks after xenotransplantation. These new biodegradable "microreactors" are injectable and do not appear to require the use of immunosuppressive drugs to prevent rejection

basal insulin secretion. We hope to bring this new approach to xenotransplantation to clinical reality within the next year.

Comment

There is considerable excitement among researchers and clinicians who hope to see the introduction of a hybrid pancreas to replace conventional insulin therapy. The transplantation of encapsulated islets has recently been extended from rodents to larger animals, and is now moving from the laboratory to the patient. Data from our laboratory suggest that this approach has the potential not only to allow the transplantation of islets across a wide species barrier, but that it can be achieved using injectable microreactors fabricated from biodegradable polymers. The next few years should prove to be ones of great challenge and, hopefully, of great excitement and promise to those involved in islet transplantation. It appears likely that by the year 2000 clinical trials utilizing encapsulated islet xenografts to treat diabetic patients will become a reality. This in turn will serve as an important starting point for developing living-drug delivery systems for treating a wide range of additional disorders. For patients with diabetes, as well as those with other diseases such as cancer, hemophilia, liver failure, and Parkinson's, the coming years hold promise for greatly improved therapy using encapsulated cells.

References

1. Hansbrough JF, Williams SK, Lawlor D, Pruitt BA. Section XII: Skin transplantation. In: 1996/1997 Yearbook of Cell and Tissue Transplantation.Lanza RP, Chick WL (eds). Kluwer Academic Press, Dordrecht, 1996. p 205
2. Tomford WW, Mankin HJ. Bone and cartilage transplantation. In: 1996/1997 Yearbook of Cell and Tissue Transplantation.Lanza RP, Chick WL (eds). Kluwer Academic Press, Dordrecht, 1996. p 37
3. Rowlings PA, Passweg JR, Armitage JO, et al. International Bone Marrow Transplant (and ABMTR) Registry Report. In: 1996/1997 Yearbook of Cell and Tissue Transplantation. Lanza RP, Chick WL (eds). Kluwer Academic Press, Dordrecht, 1996
4. Lanza RP, Chick WL (eds). 1996/1997 Yearbook of Cell and Tissue Transplantation. Kluwer Academic Press, Dordrecht, 1996
5. Bretzel RG, Hering BJ, Schultz AO, Geier C, Federlin K: International Islet Transplant Registry report. In: 1996/1997 Yearbook of Cell and Tissue Transplantation.Lanza RP, Chick WL (eds). Kluwer Academic Press, Dordrecht, 1996. p 153
6. Hering BJ, Wahoff DC, Sutherland DER. Clinical islet transplantation. In: 1996/1997 Yearbook of Cell and Tissue Transplantation. Lanza RP, Chick WL (eds). Kluwer Academic Press, Dordrecht, 1996. p 137
7. Kahan BD. Cyclosporine. N. Engl. J. Med. 321, 1725, 1989
8. Fung JJ, Alessiani M, Abu-Elmagd K, et al. Adverse effects associated with the use of FK 506. Transplant. Proc. 23, 3105, 1992
9. Lanza RP, Chick WL. Encapsulated cell therapy. Scientific American Science & Medicine. 2, 16, 1995
10. Sullivan SJ, Maki T, Borland KM, et al. Biohybrid artificial pancreas: Long-term implantation studies in diabetic, pancreatectomized dogs. Science. 252, 718, 1991
11. Lanza RP, Solomon BA, Monaco AP, Chick WL. The hybrid artificial pancreas: diffusion and vascular devices. In: Pancreatic Islet Transplantation. C. Ricordi (ed), R.G. Landes, Austin, 1992, p. 223
12. Monaco AP, Maki T, Ozato H, et al. Transplantation of islet allografts and xenografts in totally pancreatectomized diabetic dogs using the hybrid artificial pancreas. Ann. Surg. 214, 339, 1991
13. Lanza RP, Chick, WL. Encapsulated cell transplantation. Transplant. Rev. 9, 217, 1995
14. Lanza RP, Butler DH, Borland KM, et al. Successful xenotransplantation of a diffusion-based biohybrid artificial pancreas: A study using canine, bovine, and porcine islets. Transplant. Proc. 24, 669, 1992
15. Lanza RP, Borland KM, Lodge P, et al. Treatment of severely diabetic, pancreatectomized dogs using a diffusion-based hybrid pancreas. Diabetes. 41, 886, 1992
16. Race JM, LeGrelle M, Bethoux JP, Cugnenc PH, Altman JJ. Macroencapsulation in small animals. In: Pancreatic Islet Transplantation: Volume III. Immunoisolation of Pancreatic Islets. R.G. Landes, Austin, 1994. p133
17. Lanza RP. Macroencapsulation in large animals. In: Pancreatic Islet Transplantation: Volume III. Immunoisolation of Pancreatic Islets.R.G. Landes, Austin, 1994. p139
18. Lim F, Sun AM. Microencapsulated islets as bioartificial endocrine pancreas. Science. 210, 908, 1980
19. Goosen MFA. Fundamentals of microencapsulation. In: Pancreatic Islet Transplantation: Volume III. Immunoisolation of Pancreatic Islets.R.G. Landes, Austin, 1994. p21

20. Zielinski, BA, Goddard, MB, Lysaght, MJ. Immunoisolation. In: Principles of Tissue Engineering.Lanza, RP, Langer, R, Chick, WL (eds). R.G. Landes/Academic Press, Austin, 1997
21. Soon-Shiong P. Encapsulated islet transplantation: pathway to human clinical trials. In: Pancreatic Islet Transplantation: Volume III. Immunoisolation of Pancreatic Islets.R.G. Landes, Austin, 1994. p81
22. Lacy PE, Hegre OD, Gerasimidi-Vazeou A, et al. Maintenance of normoglycemia in diabetic mice by subcutaneous xenografts of encapsulated islets. Science. 254, 1282, 1991
23. Valente U, Ferro M, Campisi C, et al. Allogeneic pancreatic islet transplantation by means of artificial membrane chambers in 13 diabetic recipients. Transplant. Proc. 12, 223, 1980
24. Icard P, Penfornis F, Gotheil C, et al. Tissue reaction to implanted bioartificial pancreas in pigs. Transplant. Proc. 22, 724, 1990
25. Lanza RP, Sullivan SJ, Chick WL. Islet transplantation with immunoisolation. Diabetes. 41, 1503, 1992
26. Lanza RP, Beyer AM, Staruk JE, Chick WL. Biohybrid artificial pancreas: Long-term function of discordant islet xenografts in streptozotocin diabetic rats. Transplantation. 56, 1067, 1993
27. Spokane RB, Clark LC, Bhargava HK, et al. An implanted peritoneal oxygen tonometer that can be calibrated in situ. Trans. Am. Soc. Artif. Intern. Organs. 1990, 36:M719
28. Colton CK, Avgoustiniatos, ES. Bioengineering in development of the hybrid artificial pancreas. J. Biomed. Eng.1991, 113:152
29. Dionne KE, Colton CK, Yarmush ML. Effect of hypoxia on insulin secretion by isolated rat and canine islets of Langerhans. Diabetes. 1993, 42:12
30. Kuhtreiber WM, Lanza RP, Beyer AM, et al. Relationship between insulin secretion and oxygen tension in hybrid diffusion chambers. ASAIO J. 1993, 39: M247
31. Ohta M, Nelson D, Nelson J, et al. Oxygen and temperature dependence of stimulated insulin secretion in isolated rat islets of Langerhans. J. Biol. Chem. 1990, 265:17525
32. Chick WL, Perna JJ, Lauris V, et al. Artificial pancreas using live β-cells: Effects of glucose homeostasis in diabetic rats. Science. 1977, 197:780
33. Chick WL, Like AA, Lauris V. Beta cell culture on synthetic capillaries: An artificial endocrine pancreas. Science. 1975, 187:847
34. Tze WJ, Wong FC, Chen IM, et al. Implantable artificial endocrine pancreas unit used to restore normoglycemia in the diabetic rat. Nature. 1976, 264:466
35. Whittemore AD, Chick WL, Galletti PM, et al. Effects of the hybrid artificial pancreas in diabetic rats. Trans. Am. Soc. Artif. Intern. Organs. 1977, 13:336
36. Sun AM, Parisius W, Healy GM, et al. The use in diabetic rats and monkeys of artificial capillary units containing cultured islets of Langerhans. Diabetes. 1977, 26:1136
37. Feldman S, Dodi G, Haid K, et al. Artificial hybrid pancreas. Surg. Forum. 1977, 28:439
38. Tze WJ, Wong FC, Chen LM. Implantable artificial capillary unit for pancreatic islet allograft and xenograft. Diabetologia. 1979, 16:247
39. Sun AM, Parisius W, MacMorine HG, et al. An artificial endocrine pancreas containing cultured islets of Langerhans. Artif. Organs. 1980, 4:275
40. Galletti PM, Trudell LA, Panol G, et al. Feasibility of small bore AV shunts for hybrid artificial organs in nonheparinized beagle dogs. Trans. Am. Soc. Artif. Intern. Organs. 1981, 17:185

41. Lanza RP, Solomon BA, Monaco AP, et al. Devices implanted as AV shunts, Lanza RP, Chick WL (eds): Pancreatic Islet Transplantation: Volume III. Immunoisolation of Pancreatic Islets. Austin, Landes/CRC Press, 1994, p154
42. Sullivan SJ, Maki T, Borland KM, et al. Biohybrid artificial pancreas: Long-term implantation studies in diabetic, pancreatectomized dogs. Science. 1991, 252:718
43. Monaco AP, Maki T, Ozato H, et al. Transplantation of islet allografts and xenografts in totally pancreatectomized diabetic dogs using the hybrid artificial pancreas. Ann. Surg. 1991, 214:339
44. Lanza RP, Chick WL. Introduction, Lanza RP, Chick WL (eds): Pancreatic Islet Transplantation: Volume III. Immunoisolation of Pancreatic Islets.Austin, Landes/CRC Press, 1994, p1
45. Theodorou NA, Vrbova H, Tyhurst M et al. An assessment of diffusion chambers for use in pancreatic islet cell transplantation. Transplantation. 1979, 27:350
46. Lanza RP, Soon-Shiong P. Experimental xenotransplantation of encapsulated islets. In: Cooper DKC, et al. (eds): Xenotransplantation.Heidelberg, Springer-Verlag, 1991, 297
47. Colton, CK Implantable biohybrid artificial organs. Cell Transplant. 1995, 4:415
48. Scharp DW, Mason NS, Sparks RE. Islet immuno-isolation: The use of hybrid artificial organs to prevent islet tissue rejection. World J. Surg. 1984, 8:221
49. Scharp DW, Mason NS, Sparks RE, The use of hybrid artificial organs to provide immunoisolation to endocrine grafts in transplantation. In: Slavin S (ed): Bone Marrow and Organ Transplantation. Elsevier Science Publishers, Israel, 1984, p601
50. Woodward CL. How fibroblasts anf giant cells encapsulate implants: considerations in design of glucose sensors. Diabetes Care. 1982, 5:278
51. Altman JJ, Houlbert D, Bruzzo F, et al. Implantation of semipermeable hollow fibers to prevent immune rejection of transplanted pancreatic islets. In: Federlin K, Pfeiffer E, Raptis S (eds): Islet-Pancreas-Transplantation and Artificial Pancreas.New York, Thieme-Stratton, 1982
52. Altman JJ, Houlbert D, Callard P, et al. Long-term plasma glucose normalization in experimental diabetic rats with microencapsulated implants of benign human insulinomas. Diabetes. 1986, 35:625
53. Archer J, Kaye R, Matter G. Control of streptozotocin diabetes in Chinese hamsters by cultured mouse islet cells without immunosuppression. J. Surg. Res. 1980, 28:77
54. Icard P, Penfornis F, Gotheil C, et al. Tissue reaction to implanted bioartificial pancreas in pigs. Transplant. Proc. 1990, 22:724
55. Lanza RP, Butler DH, Borland KM et al. Xenotransplantation of canine, bovine, and porcine islets in diabetic rats without immunosuppression. Proc. Natl. Acad. Sci. 1991, 88;11100
56. Lanza RP, Butler DH, Borland KM, et al. Successful xenotransplantation of a diffusion-based biohybrid artificial pancreas: A study using canine, bovine, and porcine islets. Transplant. Proc. 1992, 24:669
57. Lanza RP, Borland KM, Lodge P, et al. Treatment of severely diabetic, pancreatectomized dogs using a diffusion-based hybrid pancreas. Diabetes. 1992, 41:886
58. Lanza RP, Borland KM, Staruk JE, et al. Transplantation of encapsulated canine islets into spontaneously diabetic BB/Wor rats without immunosuppression. Endocrinology. 1992, 131:637
59. Andersson A. Survival of pancreatic islet allografts. Lancet. 1979, 2:585

60. Kraegen EW, Chisholm DJ, MacNamara ME. Timing of insulin delivery with meals. Horm. Metab. Res. 1981, 13:365
61. Lanza RP, Lodge P, Borland KM et al. Transplantation of islet allografts using a diffusion-based biohybrid artificial pancreas: long-term studies in diabetic, pancreatectomized dogs. Transplant. Proc. 1993, 25:978
62. Lanza RP, Beyer AM, Chick WL. Xenogeneic humoral responses to islets transplanted in biohybrid diffusion chambers. Transplantation. 1994, 57:1371
63. Lanza RP, Kuhtreiber WM, Beyer A et al. Humoral response to encapsulated islets. Transplant. Proc. 1994, 26:3346
64. Theofilopoulos AN, Dixon FJ. The biology and detection of immune complexes. Adv. Immunol. 1979, 28:89
65. Wilson CB, Dixon FJ. Quantitation of acute and chronic serum sickness in the rabbit. J. Exp. Med. 1971, 134:7S
66. Benacerraf B, Sebestyen M, Cooper HS. The clearance of antigen-antibody complexes from the blood by the reticulo-endothethelial system. J. Immunol. 1959, 82:131
67. Cochrane CG, Koffler D. Immune complex disease in experimental animals and man. Adv. Immunol. 1973, 16:185
68. Kijlstra A, Van Der Lelij A, Knutson DW et al. The influence of phagocyte function on glomerular localization of aggregated IgG in rats. Clin. Exp. Immunol. 1978, 32:207
69. Haakenstad AO, Mannik M. Saturation of the reticuloendothelial system with soluble immune complexes. J. Immunol. 1974, 112:1939
70. Austen KF. Diseases of immediate type hypersensitivity. In: JD Wilson, E Braunwald, KJ, Isselbacher, et al (eds): Harrison's Principles of Internal Medicine. (12th edition). New York: McGraw-Hill, 1991, p1422
71. Sasazuki T, Kohno Y, Iwamoto I et al. Association between an HLA haplotype and low responsiveness to tetanus toxiod in man. Nature. 1978, 272:359
72. de Vries RP, Kreeftenberg HG, Loggen HG et al. In vitro immune responsiveness to vaccinea virus and HLA. N. Engl. J. Med. 1977, 297:692
73. Christiansen FT, Hawkins BR, Dawkins RL. Immune function in ankylosing spondylitics and their relatives: influence of disease and HLA B27. Clin. Exp. Immunol. 1978, 33:270
74. Lanza RP, Chick WL (eds). Pancreatic Islet Transplantation. Volume III. Immunoisolation of Pancreatic Islets.Austin, Landes/CRC Press, 1994
75. Hackel V, Klein J, Megret R et al. Immobilization of microbial cells in polymeric matrices. Eur. J. Appl. Microbiol. 1975, 1:291
76. Kierstan M, Bucke C. The immobilization of microbial cells, subcellular organelles and enzymes in calcium alginate gels. Biotechnol. Bioeng. 1977, 9:387
77. Lim F, Sun AM. Microencapsulated islets as bioartificial endocrine pancreas. Science. 1980, 210:908
78. Sun AM, O'Shea G, Van Rooy H et al. Microencapsulation d'ilots de Langerhans et pancreas artificial. J. Ann. Diabetol. (Hotel-Dieu) 1982, 20:161
79. Sun AM, O'Shea GM, Goosen MFA. Injectable microencapsulated islet cells as a bioartificial pancreas. Appl. Biochem. Biotechnol. 1984, 10:87
80. O'Shea GM, Goosen MFA, Sun AM. Prolonged survival of transplanted islets of Langerhans encapsulated in a biocompatible membrane. Biochim. Biophys. Acta. 1984, 804:133

81. Wang Y, Hao L, Gill R et al. Autoimmune diabetes in NOD mouse is L3T4 T-lymphocyte dependent. Diabetes. 1987, 36:535
82. Calafiore R, Janjic D, Koh N et al. Transplantation of microencapsulated canine islets into NOD mice: prolongation of survival with superoxide dismutase and catalase. Clin. Res. 1987, 35:499A
83. Ricker A, Bhatia V, Bonner-Weir S et al. Microencapsulated xenogeneic islet grafts in NOD mouse; dexamethasone and inflammatory response. Cold Spring Harbor Symposium, October 1987:53A
84. Weber CJ, Zabinski S, Koschitzky T et al. The role of CD4+ helper T cells in the destruction of microencapsulated islet xenografts in NOD mice. Transplantation. 1990, 49:396
85. Lanza RP, Kuhtreiber WM, Ecker D et al. Xenotransplantation of porcine and bovine islets without immunosuppression using uncoated alginate microspheres. Transplantation. 1995, 59:1377
86. Platt JL, Bach FH. The barrier to xenotransplantation. Transplantation. 1991, 52:937
87. Platt JL, Vercellotti GM, Dalmasso AP, et al. Transplantation of discordant xenografts: A review of progress. Immunol. Today. 1990, 11:450
88. Platt JL, Bach FH. Mechanisms of tissue injury in hyperacute xenograft rejection. In: Cooper DKC, et al. (eds): Xenotransplantation.Heidelberg, Springer-Verlag, 1991, p69
89. Cooper DKC, Good AH, Malcolm AJ et al. Identification of α-galactosyl and other carbohydrate epitopes that are bound by human anti-pig antibodies: relevance to discordant xenografting in humans. Transplant. Immunol. 1993, 1:198
90. Good AH, Cooper DKC, Malcolm AJ et al. Identification of carbohydrate structures that bind human antiporcine antibodies: implications for discordant xenografting in humans. Transplant. Proc. 1992, 24:559
91. Mozes M, Gewurz H, Gunnarsson A et al. Xenograft rejection by dog and man: isolated kidney perfusions with blood plasma. Transplant. Proc. 1971, 3:531
92. Cooper DKC. Depletion of natural antibodies in nonhuman primates–a step towards successful discordant xenografting in humans. Clin. Transplantation. 1992, 6:178
93. Platt JL, Fishel RJ, Matas AJ et al. Immunopathology of hyperacute xenograft rejection in a swine-to-primate model. Transplantation. 1991, 52:214
94. Linn BS, Jensen JA, Portal P et al. Renal xenograft prolongation by suppression of natural antibody. J. Surg. Res. 1968, 8:211
95. Zekorn T, Siebers U, Bretzel RG et al. Protection of islets of Langerhans from interleukin-1 toxicity by artificial membranes. Transplantation. 1990, 50:391
96. Lanza RP, Ecker D, Kuhtreiber WM et al. A simple method for transplanting discordant islets into rats using alginate gel spheres. Transplantation. 1995, 59:1486
97. Soon-Shiong P, Feldman E, Nelson R et al. Long-term reversal of diabetes by the injection of immunoprotected islets. Proc. Natl. Acad. Sci. USA. 1993, 90:5843
98. Soon-Shiong P, Heintz RE, Merideth N et al. Insulin independence in a type 1 diabetic patient after encapsulated islet transplantation. Lancet. 1994, 143:950
99. Calafiore R. Transplantation of microencapsulated pancreatic human islets for therapy of diabetes mellitus. ASAIO Journal 1992, 38:34
100. Lanza RP, Kuhtreiber WM, Ecker DM, Marsh JP, Chick WL. Successful bovine islet xenografts in rodents and dogs using injectable microreactors. Transplant. Proc. 1995, 27:3211

VII Pharmacologic Immunosuppression in Xenotransplantation

44 Pharmacologic Immunosuppressants in Xenotransplantation[1]

T.R. Brazelton, A. Cheung, and R.E. Morris

Introduction

Since the late 1980s a number of new immunosuppressive agents with novel mechanisms of action and distinct therapeutic efficacies have emerged [1–6]. Many of these offer the ability to prolong xenograft survival dramatically and have toxicity profiles compatible with their future use in clinical xenotransplantation [5, 7–10].

Xenografting is currently a very diverse field with a variety of different species and organ combinations, each with slightly different immunological mechanisms of rejection. However, several general observations can be made. For example, all xenografts can be roughly classified into one of four possible categories (Table 1). Species combinations have historically been functionally classified as concordant or discordant [11]. Concordant combinations typically occur among species that are more closely related such as hamster/rat combinations. In concordant combinations, the recipient lacks detectable natural antibodies against the donor and the recipient's alternative complement pathway is not activated by the donor graft [12]. In discordant combinations, preexisting natural antibodies and complement circulating in the recipient rapidly damage the donor graft immediately after xenografting [12, 13]. However, while the concordant-versus-discordant classification scheme is generally correct and will be used here, several recent studies of xenograft rejection indicate that each species combination produces an immune response that is dissimilar to somp extent from that produced by other species combinations [14].

Furthermore, different organ types demonstrate different susceptibilities to hyperacute and acute immune disruption. Liver and, to a lesser extent, lung grafts tend to be more resistant to antibody- and complement-mediated damage than do heart grafts (Table 2) [7, 14, 15]. However, this difference may be partially due to the different physiological endpoints used to identify graft loss. Xenografts using relatively resistant organs, for example livers, are termed "special," giving us the final two classes of xenografts: special concordant and special discordant. In addition, the special discordant category also includes a few distinct strain combinations in which, despite a relatively distant phylogenetic relationship between the species, xenoreactive antibodies and complement fail to damage the graft.

---

[1] T.R. Brazelton and A. Cheung contributed equally to this chapter.

Table 1. General classes of xenografts

Class	Comments
Concordant	Heart and kidney grafts between closely related species No xenoreactive natural antibodies or graft-induced complement activation Includes hamster/rat, mouse/rat, monkey/baboon, and chimp/human combinations
Special concordant	Liver and possibly lung grafts which display resistance to humorally mediated damage
Discordant	Heart and kidney grafts between less closely related species Natural antibody and complement activation lead to hyperacute rejection Includes guinea pig/rat, pig/baboon, and pig/rabbit combinations
Special discordant	Liver or lung grafts Heart and kidneys in rare strain combinations that are not related but in which hyperacute rejection is attenuated

Table 2. Typical xenograft survival times in untreated animals

Model	Survival times		
(donor/recipient)	Heart	Liver	Lung
Hamster/rat	2–4 days	6–8 days	5.4 days
Mouse/rat	4.5–7.5 days	–	–
Rat/mouse	2–4 days	–	–
Guinea pig/rat	8–21 min	2.5–16.7 h	53 min

Based on [14, 15, 40, 190].

To achieve long-term functioning xenografts, four major immunological barriers must be overcome: (1) hyperacute rejection, (2) delayed (or accelerated) vascular rejection, (3) acute cellular rejection, and (4) chronic rejection.

Hyperacute rejection, the first barrier, is mediated primarily by preexisting xenoreactive antibodies and the complement system, but phagocytic and natural killer cells also play a role [12]. Hyperacute rejection has been successfully overcome by a variety of techniques which prevent natural antibody- and complement-mediated injury (Fig. 1) [13, 16–19] (reviewed in [12]). Natural antibodies can be depleted by plasmapheresis, plasma exchange, organ perfusion, and immunoabsorption with affinity columns [12, 17–19]. Alternatively, natural antibody production can be inhibited by splenectomy, irradiation, lymphocyte-depleting antibodies, and immunosuppressive drugs [12, 16–22]. Complement-mediated injury can be prevented with cobra venom factor, soluble complement receptor type 1, heparin, complement regulatory proteins such as decay accelerating factor and homologous restriction factor, as well as several other types of complement inhibitors [12, 17, 19]. The creation of transgenic animal strains expressing complement-mediating proteins such as human decay-accelerating factor represents a recent approach to reduce complement-mediated injury [23,

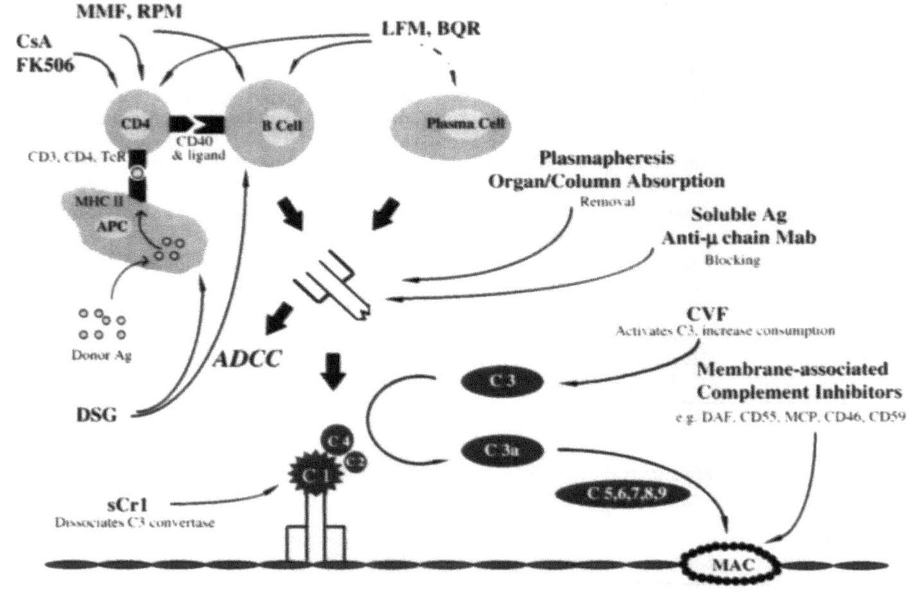

Fig. 1. Pathogenesis of humoral xenograft rejection. *CsA*, cyclosporin A; *MMF*, mycophenolate mofetil; *RPM*, rapamycin; *LFM*, leflunomide; *BQR*, brequinar sodium; *DSG*, 15-deoxyspergualin; *TcR*, T cell receptor; *APC*, antigen-presenting cell; *Ag*, antigen; *Mab*, monoclonal antibody; *CVF*, cobra venom factor; *sCr1*, soluble complement receptor 1; *DAF*, decay-accelerating factor; *MAC*, membrane attack complex; *C*, complement; *ADCC*, antibody-dependent cellular cytotoxicity

24]. And finally, the most commonly utilized method of avoiding hyperacute rejection has been the use of concordant xenograft combinations in which neither natural antibody nor complement is significantly active. In summary, due to advancements during the last decade, the hyperacute xenograft rejection barrier can be consistently overcome.

The second immunological barrier is *delayed (or accelerated) vascular rejection*, which typically occurs 1–5 days after xenografting and is mediated primarily by graft-induced xenoreactive antibodies [7, 17, 25–30]. This barrier has been breached by a variety of B cell-depleting treatments, such as splenectomy, irradiation, and anti-lymphocyte antibodies. Furthermore, short-term therapy with several immunosuppressive agents (reviewed below), notably deoxyspergualin, brequinar sodium, and leflunomide, are able to consistently bring xenografts beyond this barrier (Fig. 1).

Once a xenograft has avoided both hyperacute and delayed vascular rejection, the next challenge is to avoid the third barrier, *acute cellular rejection*, which is mediated primarily by the cellular arm of the immune system and is, in many ways, similar to the rejection seen in untreated allografts. The extensive experience gained with the use of immunosuppressive drugs to treat allograft rejection is applicable for the prevention of acute cellular rejection. Several of the immu-

Table 3. Summary of mechanisms of action, toxicity, and efficacy of immunosuppressive agents in preventing xenograft rejection

Agent	In vitro targets-effect	Efficacy in preventing xenograft rejection		Toxicity[a]
		Cellular	Humoral	
Cyclosporine	Calcineurin serine/threonine phosphatase - inhibits IL-2 transcription	+++	+/-	++
Tacrolimus	Calcineurin serine/threonine phosphatase - inhibits IL-2 transcription	+++	+/-	+
Sirolimus	? 70 kDa S6 and cyclin-dependent kinases - inhibits IL-2 transduction	+++	+	++
Deoxyspergualin	? Heat shock protein 70 and 90 - interferes with antigen processing/presentation	+	+++	+++
Mycophenolate mofetil	Inosine monophosphate dehydrogenase - inhibits purine biosynthesis	++	++	++
Brequinar	Dihydrooratate dehydrogenase - inhibits pyrimidine biosynthesis	++	+++	++
Leflunomide	? Dihydrooratate dehydrogenase - inhibits pyrimidine biosynthesis ? Tyrosine kinases inhibits IL-2 signal-transduction	++	+++	+/-

[a] The degree of toxicity relates to the toxic effects of the drug when used at a dosage that is typically successful in prolonging xenograft survival.
IL, interleukin.

nosuppressive agents, particularly cyclosporine, tacrolimus and sirolimus, effectively allow xenografts to surmount this barrier (Fig. 1).

The last barrier, *chronic rejection*, is being increasingly encountered in xenografting. Chronic rejection, which is the major barrier to long-term survival of allografts, is currently a subject of intense interest in the allograft transplantation community. Several new immunosuppressants, notably sirolimus, mycophenolate mofetil and leflunomide, are currently promising in their abilities to breach this final barrier.

The focus of this review is new immunosuppressants with efficacy and toxicity profiles consistent with their future use in clinical xenotransplantation (Tables 3, 4). We have chosen not to include cyclophosphamide or methotrexate in this review due to their narrow therapeutic indices. Azathioprine has not been included since it fails to prolong xenograft survival significantly [7, 31]. Cyclosporine (CsA) is primarily effective in xenografting when it is used in combination with other immunosuppressants, and it is mentioned where appropriate throughout this review.

Table 4. Summary of survival of hamster hearts xenografted into rats treated with various immunosuppressive regimens

Treatment	References	Median or mean survival ranges (days)	Individual means or medians (days)	Mortality and morbidity[a]
None	[7, 53, 54, 64, 83–88, 90, 106, 107, 158, 191, 192]	2–4	2, 3, 3, 3, 3, 3, 3, 3, 3, 3, 3, 3, 4, 4, 4, 4	None
CsA	[9, 10, 14, 38, 64, 86, 106, 107, 156, 158]	2–28	2, 3, 3, 4, 4, 5, 6, 7, 28	Significant
FK	[7, 38, 39, 45, 52, 53, 157]	3–5	3, 4, 4, 4, 5, 5, 5	Significant
DSG	[54, 64, 83–88, 90, 192]	4–14	4, 5, 5, 5, 7, 7, 9, 10, 13, 14	High
MMF	[7, 90]	9–12	9, 12	Significant
RPM	[9, 90, 130]	4–5	4, 5, 5	Minimal
BQR	[7, 9, 26, 146]	25 to >42	25, 27, 40, >42	Significant
LFM	[10, 30]	11–71	11, 71	Minimal
SPL	[45, 52–54, 84, 85, 87, 88, 90, 158]	5–6	5, 5, 5, 6, 6, 6, 6, 6, 6, 6	Minimal
CsA+SPL	[53, 86]	24–146	24, 146	Minimal
FK+CsA	[38]	5	5	Very high
FK+SPL	[41, 45, 52–54, 193]	33 to >100	33, 36, 37, 44, >70, >100	High
DSG+FK	[7, 54, 64]	14 to >70	14, 18, >70	Very high
DSG+MMF	[90]	7	7	NA
DSG+SPL	[53, 54, 84–86, 88, 90]	7–93	7, 10, 18, 18, 22, 23, 93	High
DSG+FK+SPL	[54]	17	17	Very high
DSG+MMF+SPL	[90]	27	27	Very high
MMF+CsA	[106, 107]	5–6	5, 6	Minimal
MMF+FK	[7]	>100	>100	Minimal
MMF+BQR	[106, 107]	10–11	10, 11	Moderate
MMF+SPL	[90]	7	7	NA
BQR+CsA	[106, 156, 158]	33 to >100	33, >49, >100	Moderate
BQR+FK	[7]	>100	>100	NA
BQR+SPL	[146]	15	15	High
BQR+CsA+SPL	[158]	>16	>16	Very high
BQR+MMF+CsA	[106, 107]	>20–40	>20, 40	Minimal
BQR+RPM+CsA	[9]	40	40	Minimal
LFM+CsA	[10, 30]	>90	>90, permanent	None

Studies using ineffective doses have not been included.
[a] Degree of toxicity seen in longer-surviving groups.
CsA, cyclosporine; FK, FK506, tacrolimus; DSG, deoxyspergualin, gusperimus (also includes deoxymethylspergualin); MMF, mycophenolate mofetil, mycophenolic acid; RPM, rapamycin, sirolimus; BQR, brequinar sodium; LFM, leflunomide; SPL, splenectomy; NA, data not available.

Tacrolimus (FK506)

History

Like most other immunosuppressive agents, tacrolimus is a microbial product. It was first isolated from *Streptomyces tsukubaensis* by Goto and Kino from Fujisawa Pharmaceuticals in 1984 [1]. In vitro, tacrolimus was found to be 50–100 times more potent than CsA in inhibiting mitogen stimulated T and B cell proliferation. It was found to effectively prolong skin, heart, liver, and kidney allograft survival in numerous small and large animal models. In addition, it is able to halt the development or reverse the effect of hereditary or induced autoimmune diseases in animals [31, 32]. Recently, tacrolimus has gained popularity among liver and kidney transplant physicians because of its superiority to CsA for the prevention and reversal of ongoing organ allograft rejection in several clinical trials.

Structure and Mechanisms of Action

Tacrolimus is a macrolactam with a molecular mass of 804 Da. Tacrolimus can be distinguished from other macrolactams, except rapamycin, by its hemiketal-masked, α,β-diketoamide in a 23-membered ring (Fig. 2). Since tacrolimus is hydrophobic it is formulated in alcohol and a surfactant for intravenous use. Orally, it is supplied in a hydroxypropylmethyl cellulose dispersion.

Tacrolimus is structurally unrelated to cyclosporine. However, tacrolimus's immunosuppressive action on lymphocytes is remarkably similar to CsA, i.e., inhibiting interleukin (IL)-2 gene transcription. At the cellular level tacrolimus first binds to a cytosolic protein, FK-binding protein (FKBP). Of the many FKBP isoforms, FKBP12 is believed to be the instrumental mediator of the immunosuppressive actions of tacrolimus. This tacrolimus–FKBP12 complex then binds to calcineurin and subsequently blocks IL-2 gene transcription [33–35]. T cell activation stimulates T cell receptor (TcR)-associated tyrosine kinase activity, leading to an influx of extracellular calcium and calcium mobilization intracellularly. The increase in intracellular calcium stimulates several calcium-dependent events including the activation of calmodulin/calcineurin's serine/threonine phosphatase which leads to dephosphorylation of transcription factors (NF-ATs). Dephosphorylated NF-ATs translocate into the nucleus and attach to the promoter region of cytokine genes, stimulating transcription and subsequent cytokine production. In addition to inhibiting IL-2 production, tacrolimus inhibits the production of IL-3, IL-4, IL-5, interferon (IFN)-γ, tumor necrosis factor (TNF)-α, and granulocyte-macrophage colony-stimulating factor (GM-CSF) [36, 37].

Tacrolimus in Xenografting

Tacrolimus is similar to CsA since, when both are used as single agents, they typically prolong xenograft survival ineffectively in all discordant and in stan-

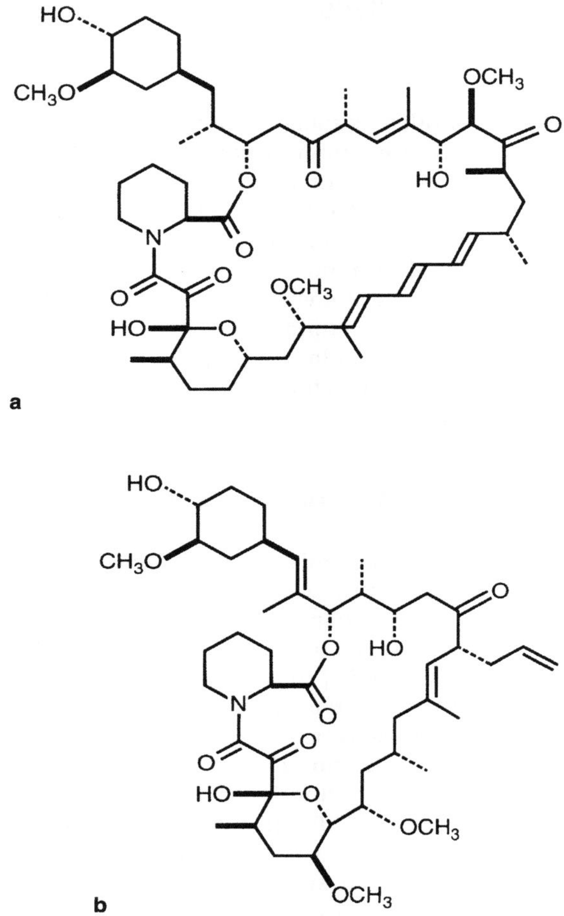

Fig. 2a,b. Molecular structures of **a** sirolimus and **b** tacrolimus

dard concordant combinations. However, both of these agents have had considerable success maintaining a variety of allografts. This discrepancy is explained by the observation that xenograft survival closely correlates with the suppression of T cell-independent anti-donor antibodies [7, 17, 25–30], while both tacrolimus and CsA act primarily against cellular immune responses and T cell-dependent humoral responses. Tacrolimus is able to inhibit rat popliteal lymph node swelling in response to hamster xenoantigen stimulation [38]. However, this is likely due to predominantly T cell inhibition, since hamster hearts xenografted into similarly treated rats do not survive longer than untreated controls [38]. Inhibition of the cellular response to a xenograft becomes important only if inhibition of the humoral response has been sufficient to allow the graft to survive long enough for cellular rejection to develop. Thus agents inhibiting the cellular response have proved most effective when used in combination with therapeutic regimens that inhibit antibody production.

In models of hamster and mouse cardiac xenografts into rats, neither tacrolimus nor CsA prolongs graft survival more than a day despite a variety of dosing regimens that have been attempted [7, 13, 38–44]. However, in special concordant situations, such as liver xenografts, which are somewhat resistant to humorally mediated rejection, tacrolimus alone is able to increase graft survival significantly [7, 39, 45]. In fact, as a monotherapy for hamster-to-rat liver xenografts, tacrolimus appears to be superior to brequinar, mycophenolate mofetil and cyclophosphamide [7]. Valdivia et al. [39] were consistently able to extend survival of hamster liver grafts in rats to over 100 days with tacrolimus alone. Furthermore, they found that a 2-week treatment of low-dose tacrolimus at the time of transplantation was able to extend mean graft survival to 47.2 days. Other groups xenografting hamster or mouse livers into rats have consistently extended mean graft survival times to over 30 days [40, 42, 45, 46]. However, Celli et al. [45] documented that most long-term recipients had severe jaundice and biliary proliferation but few signs of rejection when they died, and postulated that the liver damage was likely the result of the initial humoral attacks.

Interestingly, CsA has not been effective in these models of liver xenografting despite the similar actions of these two drugs [47, 48]. A possible explanation for this discrepancy is the observation that tacrolimus distributes preferentially to the liver relative to CsA [49]. Tacrolimus monotherapy has also successfully prolonged mouse skin graft survival in rats and fetal pig pancreatic graft survival in mice [50, 51]. Thus, while tacrolimus alone is able to control xenograft survival effectively in special situations such as concordant liver and nonvascularized xenografts, its ability to control xenograft rejection of other solid organs is limited [38].

However, when tacrolimus is combined with therapies that deplete antibodies or inhibit antibody production, xenograft survival improves dramatically. In fact, tacrolimus often displays a synergistic effect when used in such combinations [45, 52, 53]. This concept was first demonstrated by combining tacrolimus with splenectomy in a variety of animal models, the most popular of which is the hamster cardiac xenograft-to-rat model. In this model, splenectomy alone typically delays xenograft rejection until around day 5 or 6 [45, 52–54]. The addition of tacrolimus for the first 4 weeks post-transplant typically extends graft survival out to about 35 days [52, 54]. Furthermore, several groups have demonstrated that precisely timed splenectomies combined with tacrolimus treatment consistently results in indefinite cardiac xenograft survival (>100 days) [45, 53]. However, a significant increase in mortality was observed when tacrolimus was combined with splenectomy [52]. Once again, despite similar effects on allografts, this xenograft model found tacrolimus significantly superior to CsA, which failed to demonstrate a synergistic effect when used in combination with splenectomy [53]. In rhesus monkey recipients of baboon heart xenografts the efficacy of tacrolimus was potentiated by splenectomy [55].

However, while splenectomy serves as a useful experimental manipulation, other less invasive approaches are required if xenografting is to become a viable clinical option. The efficacy of both pretransplant plasmapheresis and plasma exchange has been demonstrated, but in both cases xenoreactive antibodies rapidly reappear in the recipient. In the last few years, several new immunosuppressive drugs with the ability to effectively inhibit antibody production have been tested in xenograft models. These new agents are most useful when used in combination with agents such as tacrolimus or CsA that inhibit the cellular immune response. These combination therapies are discussed below.

15-Deoxyspergualin

History

15-Deoxyspergualin (DSG), an analogue of the anti-neoplastic drug spergualin, was first isolated from a culture of *Bacillus laterosporus*. DSG was initially intended for use in cancer therapy [56]. However, in 1985 Umezawa et al. demonstrated that spergualin possessed immunosuppressive properties [2]. Subsequently, DSG was found to be more immunosuppressive than its parent compound [2, 57, 58]. Since then DSG has been shown to effectively prolong allo- and xenograft survival in numerous animal transplant models [57, 59–66].

Structure and Mechanisms of Action

DSG is a spermidine polyamine, has a molecular mass of 496 Da, and is highly soluble in aqueous solution. DSG is given intravenously in human subjects because of its poor oral bioavailability and short half-life of only 30 min. The major toxicities of DSG are adverse gastrointestinal effects and myelosuppression. DSG's toxicity correlates well with its peak concentration.

The mechanisms of action of DSG are not well defined. It is hypothesized that DSG acts directly on monocytes/macrophages and inhibits their ability to process and/or present antigen. Early studies indicated that DSG inhibited T and B cell proliferation in vitro. However, these in vitro studies were carried out in presence of polyamide oxidases (PAO), which metabolize DSG into toxic aldehydes [67, 68]. It is now known that DSG fails to inhibit lymphocyte proliferation in the absence of PAO, suggesting that DSG does not act directly on T cells [69]. DSG has consistently demonstrated its ability to inhibit immunoglobulin production in vivo [18, 20, 24, 70–72]. DSG is believed to affect both T cell-dependent and independent antibody production [73, 74]. Furthermore, in vitro studies have shown that DSG can inhibit antibody production independent of B cell proliferation [23]. In addition, once B cells become terminally differentiated into plasma cells, DSG fails to inhibit immunoglobulin secretion, suggesting that DSG affects B cells at an early stage of cell differentiation [11, 23]. However, the exact mechanisms of action of DSG on B cells remaine controversial.

Recent experiments have shown that while DSG pretreatment of tetanus- and diphtheria toxin-stimulated macrophages inhibits the macrophage's ability to stimulate T cell proliferation, DSG has no effect when added directly to a culture of T cells and prestimulated macrophages [75]. The role of DSG on IL-1 and IFN-γ synthesis, as well as on the expression of major histocompatibility (MHC) class II antigens from monocytes, remains controversial [76–79]. Another recent finding suggests that DSG may inhibit monocytes by binding to heat shock proteins

(Hsp) 70 and 90, which are believed to participate in antigen processing and presentation [80–82]. The exact role of this interaction is not entirely clear.

15-Deoxyspergualin in Xenografting

DSG monotherapy moderately prolongs xenograft survival in concordant strain combinations. Hamster-to-rat cardiac xenografts typically survive 5–12 days, compared to 3–4 days for untreated controls [54, 83–86]. The results tend to vary more among studies than for most other drugs. These variations are partially due to the different dosage schedules that have been used. Because toxicity is common when using DSG, many groups are still attempting to create better treatment schedules. Furthermore, instead of daily drug administration, the continuous infusion of a more stable derivative of DSG, deoxymethylspergualin, has led to slightly increased graft survival [87, 88]. The experience with the mouse-to-rat cardiac xenografts has been similar to the hamster-to-rat cardiac xenograft experience [70, 89]. However, Corry et al. [59] demonstrated that rat-to-mouse cardiac xenografts treated for 20 days postoperatively had a median survival time of >26 days compared to 5 days in the control group. Slightly prolonged survival of hamster-to-mouse islet cell xenografts has also been reported with DSG monotherapy [61, 62].

The addition of splenectomy has extended survival of DSG-treated grafts. However, a clear potentiated interaction, as is seen between tacrolimus and splenectomy, has not been consistently observed even though a few experiments suggest this possibility [53, 86]. This lack of potentiation may be due to the fact that neither DSG nor splenectomy strongly inhibits cell-mediated graft rejection. The combination of DSG and splenectomy typically results in hamster-to-rat cardiac xenograft survival for 18–22 days, while splenectomy alone extends graft survival to days 5 or 6 [45, 52–54, 84, 88].

However, disagreement exists regarding the efficacy of DSG and splenectomy for prolongation of hamster cardiac xenograft survival in rats. Two groups have found that mean graft survival is prolonged less than 11 days [85, 90]. In contrast, Thomas et al. [86] were able to maintain functioning grafts for an average of 94 days with only a 14-day DSG treatment when combined with splenectomy; furthermore, two out of the ten animals in this study were able to maintain their grafts indefinitely (>160 days) [86]. In accordance with current views on the central role of antibody in xenorejection, this study found an association between lower xenoreactive antibody titers in the early post-transplant period (days 0–40) and a lack of xenograft rejection. However, six of their animals that had graft survival of more than 100 days had xenoreactive antibody titers that were not significantly different from animals with rejecting grafts, indicating that the development of humoral accommodation had occurred [86]. Humoral accommodation, however, has proven to be difficult to achieve. Most investigators still find that the maintenance of low titers of xenoreactive antibodies is required for long-term graft survival [7, 25, 29, 91, 92]. However, increased morbidity and mortality have been observed when DSG is combined with splenectomy [85].

Furthermore, in one study, hamster-to-rat cardiac xenograft survival was extended to a mean of 26.3 days when DSG was combined with total lymphoid irradiation [63] despite the failure of total lymphoid irradiation alone to prolong graft survival. Animals receiving the combined treatment had significantly lower xenoreactive antibody titers at the time of rejection, and histopathology of rejected grafts indicated that rejection had been initiated predominantly by cellular-mediated immunity [63].

DSG has also been tested in a variety of discordant strain combinations. In guinea pig-to-rat cardiac xenografts DSG alone does not significantly affect graft survival [13, 93]. This finding is not surprising, since in this model the heart is hyperacutely rejected in 8–21 min [13, 14, 18] by mechanisms involving natural antibodies and complement. However, if complement is depleted by treatment with cobra venom factor prior to the transplant, DSG can extend graft survival to 5 days compared to 2 days for cobra venom factor alone [13, 19].

Interest has also been generated by DSG's ability to inhibit natural xenoreactive antibody production. DSG has been shown to decrease both natural antibodies in unstimulated animals and prevent an increase in xenophile antibodies in rats stimulated with human peripheral blood cells [18, 20, 93]. Similarly, DSG has been shown to inhibit the sensitization of rats receiving sequential mouse cardiac xenografts [70, 89]. Sensitized rats hyperacutely rejected a second mouse graft in less than 2 min. Only IgG deposition was found on the graft. Treatment with DSG from the time of the first cardiac xenograft resulted in mean survival times of 30–46 min for a subsequent xenograft. Furthermore, only weak IgM deposition was found on the rejected graft indicating that DSG had prevented both increased production of IgM as well as an immunoglobulin class switch to IgG. Furthermore, the administration of cobra venom factor to the DSG-treated recipients allowed the second grafts to survive a mean of 48 h [89].

DSG has also been used in combination with various other immunosuppressive agents. DSG is at least additive when combined with tacrolimus. The results of two studies indicate that hamster-to-rat cardiac xenografts can be maintained at a mean of 14 or 18 days [54,64] by DSG and tacrolimus compared to 3–5 days with either drug alone. However, Murase et al. [7] was able to extend four out of six hamster-to-rat cardiac xenografts to more than 70 days by using high-dose DSG for the first 3 days post-xenografting followed by 28 days of a moderate dose in combination with long-term tacrolimus treatment. It is notable that 3- to 4-week therapy with the induction dose of DSG plus tacrolimus resulted in 50% mortality from toxicity, while therapy with the moderate dose plus tacrolimus resulted in a mean graft survival of 5 days. This illustrates the quite narrow therapeutic window of DSG which makes its use difficult. Furthermore, the 70-day graft survival with DSG plus tacrolimus was close to that of tacrolimus plus mycophenolate mofetil, but the authors felt that the latter protocol was less toxic [7]. In another model of hamster-to-rat islet cell xenografts, DSG and tacrolimus extended graft survival to 31.4 days compared to 2.9, 13, and 7.8 days for no treatment, tacrolimus alone, or DSG alone, respectively [61].

DSG has also been used in combination therapy with mycophenolate mofetil. However, this combination failed to prolong hamster-to-rat cardiac xenograft survival [90]. Furthermore, this combination became extremely toxic when splenectomies were added to the regimen [90].

In summary, DSG has demonstrated moderate efficacy in maintaining xenografts as a monotherapy and high efficacy when used optimally in combination with tacrolimus or splenectomy. However, the use of DSG may be limited by its narrow therapeutic window, need for parenteral administration, and substantial toxicity associated with peak drug levels.

Mycophenolate Mofetil (RS-61443)

History

Mycophenolate mofetil (MMF) is metabolized to its active metabolite, mycophenolic acid (MPA), shortly after oral or intravenous administration. MMF has a mechanism of action distinct from all other immunosuppressive agents, except mizoribine. MMF was first isolated from cultures of *Penicillium* species by Gosio in 1896 [94]. Its immunosuppressive activity was briefly explored by Ohsugi et al. in 1972, in which MMF weakly suppressed skin allograft rejection in mice [95]. In the 1980s, researchers at Syntex began the development of MMF as an anti-rheumatoid drug. Its utility for use in transplantation had not been recognized until work was done at Stanford which demonstrated that MMF effectively prolonged rat and nonhuman heart allograft survival [3, 96]. In several clinical trails conducted in the United States, Canada, and Europe, MMF was found to reduce the incidence of biopsy-proven acute cadaveric renal allograft rejection and graft failure [97–99]. In 1995, MMF was approved for use in renal transplantation by the U.S. Food and Drug Administration.

Structure and Mechanisms of Action

MMF is a semi-synthetic small molecule that is relatively soluble in aqueous solution. Unlike CsA and tacrolimus, MMF does not inhibit cytokine production. Instead, it is a noncompetitive, reversible inhibitor of inosine monophosphate dehydrogenase (IMPDH), a key enzyme in the pathway for de novo purine synthesis (Fig. 3) [100–102]. Blockage of IMPDH by MPA can be reversed by the addition of exogenous guanosine nucleotides in vitro [103]. IMPDH catalyzes the conversion of inosine monophosphate to xanthine monophosphate, which then leads to the production of guanosine nucleotides. By blocking IMPDH, MMF produces changes in intracellular nucleotide levels which prevent cells from initiating DNA synthesis. Furthermore, the enzymes 5-phosphoribosyl-1-pyrophosphate (PRPP) synthetase and ribonucleotide reductase are allosterically regulated by guanosine nucleotides. By decreasing the pool of guanosine nucleotides, their catalytic activities are inhibited, leading to further reductions in DNA synthesis. MMF also interferes with the glycosylation of membrane proteins and the functions of adhesion molecules in vitro.

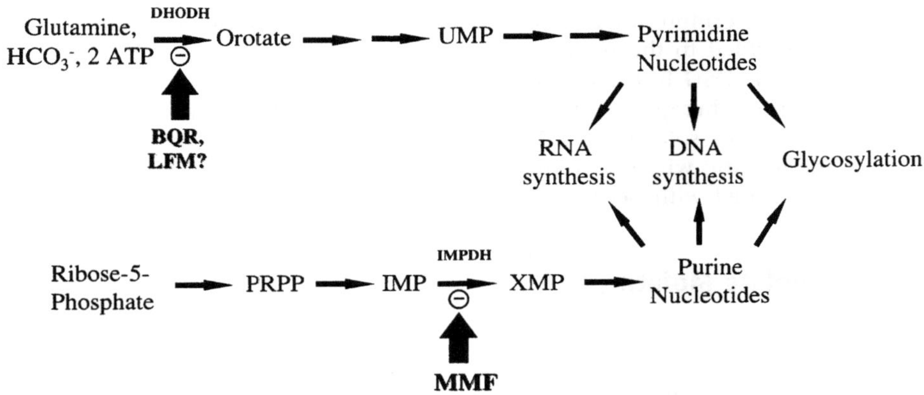

Fig. 3. De novo purine and pyrimidine nucleotide synthesis pathways. *BQR*, brequinar sodium; *LFM*, leflunomide; *DHODH*, dihydroorotate dehydrogenase; *UMP*, uridine monophosphate; *PRPP*, 5-phosphoribosyl-1-pyrophosphate; *IMP*, inosine monophosphate; *XMP*, xanthine monophosphate; *IMPDH*, inosine monophosphate dehydrogenase; *MMF*, mycophenolate mofetil.

The major toxicities of MMF are diarrhea and abdominal pain in humans, and myelotoxicity in rats. These side-effects can be minimized by reducing the dose or discontinuing the drug for short periods.

Mycophenolate Mofetil in Xenografting

High-dose MMF monotherapy is only able to prolong hamster-to-rat cardiac xenografts until approximately day 11 after transplant [7, 90]. Furthermore, a moderate dose of MMF appears to have no effect on hamster-to-rat liver xenograft survival [7]. Monotherapy also failed to prolong rat-to-mouse and hamster-to-mouse skin xenograft survival [104]. Five-day pretreatment with MMF in a fetal pig heart-to-rabbit model only slightly prolonged graft survival [105].

Despite its ineffectiveness as a monotherapy in various xenograft models, MMF has demonstrated considerable efficacy when used in combination with other immunosuppressants. MMF appears to be synergistic with tacrolimus in the hamster-to-rat model to prolong both heart and liver xenograft survival consistently and indefinitely (>100 days) [7]. MMF's performance in combination with tacrolimus was superior to azathioprine, DSG, mizoribine, and methotrexate, and it was comparable to brequinar sodium and cyclophosphamide [7]. In a cynomolgus monkey-to-baboon heterotopic cardiac xenograft model, treatment with CsA and methylprednisolone extended graft survival to 78 days [8]. The addition of MMF to the regimen allowed cardiac grafts to survive an average of 296 days, which was significantly longer than when azathioprine was added (mean, 94 days) [8].

In combination with splenectomy, MMF has the ability to steadily decrease the titers of natural xenoreactive antibodies [22]. In addition, when natural antibodies are depleted by plasma exchange in splenectomized rats, MMF prevents a subsequent rebound of natural antibodies [22]. Furthermore, MMF's efficacy in decreasing natural antibodies is potently increased when it is combined with brequinar [17]. MMF also demonstrates a potentiated interaction with CD4- and CD8-blocking antibodies when used to treat rat-to-mouse skin xenografts, extending graft survival to more than 120 days, despite the fact that when either MMF alone or both blocking antibodies together are used, graft survival is only 6 days [104]. Interestingly, this triple combination failed to prolong hamster-to-mouse skin xenografts more than 2 days longer than controls [104]. The reasons why the hamster skin xenograft failed are unclear. MMF may have at least an additive interaction with rapamycin, but fails to act synergistically with brequinar (discussed below).

However, despite MMF's ability to potentiate the efficacy of several immunosuppressive regimens, MMF plus CsA failed to prolong hamster-to-rat cardiac xenografts longer than a few days [106, 107]. It was noted, however, that the addition of MMF to CsA significantly reduced graft-induced xenoreactive antibody titers [106]. Furthermore, while brequinar plus CsA prolonged graft survival in this model to 33 days [106], the arteries of grafts surviving over 30 days showed remarkable medial and intimal smooth muscle cell proliferation. The addition of MMF to the CsA plus brequinar regimen extended graft survival to 40 days and, more importantly, dramatically reduced the incidence of vascular hyperplasia in these grafts [106]. However, significant toxicity was seen in this triple combination group.

Thus, MMF has demonstrated significant efficacy when used in combinations with other agents, particularly tacrolimus, in a variety of xenograft models. MMF's significant ability to inhibit chronic vascular changes and its moderate performance in preventing humoral responses combined with its moderate toxicity profile make it a good choice for many concordant combinations.

Sirolimus (Rapamycin)

History

Like tacrolimus, sirolimus is also a product of an actinomycete, *Streptomyces hygroscopicus*, which was isolated from soil samples of Easter Island. It was first isolated by Sehgal at Ayerest Pharmaceuticals in the mid-1970s as a result of a screen for new anti-fungal agents. Its toxic side-effects on lymphoid tissue prohibited its development into an anti-fungal agent. Its potential as an immunosuppressive agent was briefly examined in several animal autoimmune models. However, its potential as an immunosuppressant was not fully appreciated until the discovery of tacrolimus which bears structural similarity with sirolimus. In 1988, independent work at Stanford and Cambridge demonstrated the potential of sirolimus as a novel immunosuppressant for the control of allograft rejection [4, 108].

Structure and Mechanism of Action

Sirolimus bears remarkable structural similarity with tacrolimus (Fig. 2). It is a macrolactam consisting of an amide, a ketone, and a hemiketal. Its 31-membered ring contains a triene segment from C1-C6 which tacrolimus lacks. These subtle differences in structure may explain the entirely different mechanisms of action of the two compounds.

Like tacrolimus, sirolimus binds to cytosolic FKBPs. Interestingly, this sirolimus-FKBP complex does not inhibit calcineurin serine/threonine phosphatase activity [109]. Therefore, its effects on the immune system are not dependent on the inhibition of IL-2 transcription in the early cell cycle. Instead, sirolimus blocks the IL-2 receptor-coupled signal transduction pathway required for the progression of the cell cycle from G_1 to S phase. Support for this mechanism comes from experiments that demonstrated sirolimus's ability to arrest the growth of a murine IL-2-dependent T cell line and IL-3-dependent mast cells in the G_1 stage [110–112]. Even though the mechanism of this effect is not well understood, it may be related to the 70-kDa S6 kinases, which are key enzymes in the signal transduction pathway. Sirolimus was found to inhibit the phosphorylation of 70-kDa S6 kinases, which in turn interrupts protein synthesis [113–116]. The exact mode of interaction between sirolimus–FKBP complexes and 70-kDa S6 kinases is not completely understood. Recent reports by Morice et al. suggest that sirolimus-FKBP complex reduces the activity of cyclin A- and cyclin E-associated cyclin-dependent kinases, which are required for cytokine-activated cell progression from G_1 to S phase [117–119].

Sirolimus has proven to be effective in preventing and reversing acute allograft rejection in a number of small and large animal studies [108, 120–123]. Furthermore, it is very effective in preventing and reversing chronic rejection [124, 125]. This latter effect may be secondary to its anti-proliferative effect on vascular smooth muscle cells [124, 126, 127].

Unlike CsA and tacrolimus, sirolimus does not inhibit the function of calcineurin, leading one to suspect that it is less nephrotoxic. Indeed, this is supported by several studies in rodents [128, 129]. However, its safety in humans is not well established.

Sirolimus in Xenografting

Sirolimus alone has a limited effect on xenograft survival, prolonging hamster-to-rat cardiac xenografts only 1–2 days longer than untreated controls [9, 90, 130]. In addition, sirolimus minimally extends cardiac xenograft survival in a discordant pig-to-rabbit model [131]. While sirolimus fails to extend skin xenografts in rat-to-mouse models more than a few days, it displays a potent and effective ability to increase the survival of islet cell xenografts in both rat-to-mouse and hamster-to-mouse models [132–134]. Furthermore, sirolimus potently and effectively inhibits immunoglobulin production in vitro of all three major isotypes (IgG, IgM, IgA), suggesting sirolimus's usefulness for controlling antibody-mediated rejection [130, 135]. Blakely et al. [17] found that sirolimus's ability to reduce natural xenoreactive antibodies in rats was intermediate between brequinar sodium (BQR), which effectively inhibited natural antibodies, and MMF, which was less effective.

Ultimately, one of sirolimus's greatest strengths may prove to be its ability to both prevent and reverse intimal proliferation associated with chronic rejection [124, 125]. Recent work from our laboratory has demonstrated that rapamycin potently and effectively inhibits myofibroblast proliferation in a model of obliterative bronchiolitis in which a hamster trachea is heterotopically transplanted into the greater omentum of a recipient rat [136]. However, sirolimus's ability in this respect has not been tested in other xenograft models.

In combination therapies, sirolimus displays at least additive interactions with many immunosuppressants. Hamster-to-rat cardiac xenograft survival was significantly prolonged to 40 days by a combination of low-dose CsA, low-dose BQR, and sirolimus with no noticeable toxicity [9]. However, a moderate dose of BQR can also achieve 40-day graft survival in the same model with only mild toxicity [9]. A combination of sirolimus and MMF was able to extend cardiac xenograft survival in a discordant pig-to-rabbit model to a mean of 24.3 h versus means of 11.5 and 9.8 h for sirolimus and MMF monotherapies, respectively [131]. Sirolimus also interacts at least additively with anti-lymphocyte immunoglobulin to prolong skin xenografts [132, 133].

Brequinar Sodium

History

BQR is a novel immunosuppressant that is able to specifically inhibit de novo pyrimidine biosynthesis. Another novel anti-proliferative agent, leflunomide, may have a similar mode of action.

BQR was first intended to be developed as an anti-tumor agent by Du Pont-Merck [137–141]. Its use in cancer therapy was rather short-lived, and in 1988, Cramer et al. began to investigate BQR for potential use in transplantation. BQR was proven to be effective in inhibiting both T and B cell functions in vitro and in vivo [29, 142–150]. Furthermore, BQR's ability to inhibit antibody production may be valuable in presensitized hosts and xenotransplantation.

Structure and Mechanisms of Action

Rather than being a natural microbial metabolite, this 4-quinolinecarboxylic acid analog is produced completely by organic synthesis. BQR is water-soluble and has good oral bioavailability. It has a long half-life of 15 h due to its slow clearance, and no secondary active metabolite has been detected.

The primary action of BQR is the inhibition of dihydro orotate dehydrogenase (DHODH), which catalyzes the conversion of dihydro orotate to orotate [137, 139, 143, 144, 151, 152]. This inhibition is noncompetitive and reversible, and ultimately depletes the intracellular pool of pyrimidine nucleotides available for RNA and

DNA synthesis (Fig. 3). Activated lymphocytes appear to rely on both the salvage and de novo pathways to supply nucleotides for proliferation. By disarming one of the pathways, lymphocyte proliferation becomes retarded. Other modes of action of BQR have been postulated. BQR has been shown to block the progression of stimulated lymphocytes into S and G_2+M phase of the cell cycle [143]. Furthermore, BQR inhibits IL-2 receptor expression, but its role on IL-2 transcription remains a topic of discussion [143, 153, 154]. In addition, it has been demonstrated to inhibit IgM, IgG and IgE production potently and effectively *in vitro* and in vivo. These characteristics produced excellent results in extending graft survival in presensitized hosts and xenografts [26, 28, 29, 121, 147–150, 155, 156].

BQR's toxicity is primarily myelotoxic, causing leukopenia, thrombocytopenia and anemia. Gastrointestinal side effects, dermatitis and mucositis are also seen. BQR has a relatively narrow efficacy to toxicity ratio, which may limit its use in a clinical setting.

Brequinar in Xenografting

In the xenografting experience with BQR, has distinguished itself as a single agent to prevent xenograft rejection. Furthermore, demonstrates synergistic interactions with some other immunosuppressants, notably CsA and tacrolimus [7, 156].

In hamster-to-rat cardiac xenografts, BQR and leflunomide are the only monotherapies capable of significantly prolonging graft survival. However, the dosages of BQR required for monotherapy are associated with moderate toxicity. CsA, tacrolimus, DSG, MMF, and rapamycin all display significantly more limited capabilities as monotherapies [7, 9, 38, 41, 54, 65, 87, 88, 90, 106, 130, 157]. BQR monotherapy has been able to extend mean hamster-to-rat cardiac xenograft survival to more than 30 days consistently [7, 9, 26, 146]. Grafts surviving more than 100 days after BQR monotherapy are not uncommon.

However, several other groups using BQR monotherapy achieved mean survival times of less than 10 days [28, 92, 156, 158]. The efficacy of BQR is very dependent upon the dosing regimen, which may explain this discrepancy in survival times. Typically, survival with BQR treatment is increased if a loading dose is used for the first 4–7 days, if a higher dosage is used every other day instead of daily administration of a lower dosage, and if treatment is started a day prior to transplantation [9, 146, 156]. Toxicity with BQR can directly affect graft survival and varies greatly with different dosage regimens. Once again, this illustrates the relatively narrow therapeutic index of BQR [106].

Histopathology of hamster-to-rat cardiac xenografts effectively treated with BQR monotherapy found reduced myocyte necrosis, interstitial hemorrhage and vascular rejection, as well as weak IgM and IgG deposition [106]. In addition, these grafts demonstrated an increased mononuclear cell infiltrate compared to grafts treated with other immunosuppressants which rejected earlier [106]. These results suggest that BQR dramatically reduces the role of humoral rejection allowing a cell-mediated rejection process, not unlike that seen in rejected allografts, to occur. Furthermore, in BQR and CsA-treated cardiac xenografts which survived for more than 30 days, remarkable intimal and medial smooth muscle cell proliferation was noted, suggesting that BQR is unable to adequately control chronic vascular rejection [106]. Furthermore, in vitro, BQR does not have a significant ability to directly inhibit smooth muscle cell proliferation [102].

One of BQR's strengths lies in its ability to inhibit antibody production effectively. Several groups have demonstrated that BQR is able to markedly inhibit IgM and IgG production in xenografted animals. [7, 26, 28, 29, 92, 106, 146, 156, 158]. Cramer et al. found that the IgM levels in BQR-treated rats receiving hamster cardiac xenografts were about the same as the IgM levels in normal animals [146]. Furthermore, BQR potently inhibits IL-6-stimulated IgM production in vitro and this effect appears to be independent of B cell proliferation [28, 29].

When used in combination with other immunosuppressants, BQR can effectively prolong xenograft survival. BQR synergistically interacts with both tacrolimus and CsA, extending hamster-to-rat cardiac xenograft survival to more than 100 days [7, 92, 106, 156, 158]. Murase et al. were able to induce permanent survival in entire groups of hamster-to-rat cardiac xenografts using a combination of tacrolimus and BQR [7]. Their dosing regimen illustrates nicely the successful use of this combination treatment. Hamster-to-rat cardiac xenografts were treated with BQR starting on the day prior to xenografting and ending on day 30 post-transplant. Tacrolimus, in a progressively decreasing dose, is used for the duration of the graft. In this combination, BQR blocks humoral rejection while the anti-T cell agent (tacrolimus, or alternatively CsA) blocks cellular rejection. Once the antibody barrier is broken by day 30, BQR is no longer needed. Furthermore, Murase et al. [7] also found that when a liver xenograft was used in the hamster-to-rat model, the same combination of tacrolimus plus BQR (or alternatively MMF) produced indefinite survival (>100 days). However, if therapy with BQR or MMF was continued the full 30 days post-xenografting, graft survival was decreased. In the case of the liver xenografts, maximum survival was obtained by using BQR or MMF for only the first 13 days after xenografting. This may reflect the liver's higher resistance to antibody-mediated damage versus the effects of the toxicity of BQR or MMF.

BQR has an additive effect with MMF in the reduction of rat natural antibodies reactive with guinea pig xenoantigens [17]. The immunosuppressive efficacy of BQR is also potentiated by the addition of cytidine in xenograft animal models [28].

BQR has demonstrated an effective ability to prolong graft survival in a variety of xenograft models, both as a monotherapy and in combination with tacrolimus. Its greatest strength lies in its potent and effective ability to inhibit a variety of humoral responses. However, BQR's potentially high toxicity warrants close monitoring and may limit its application in clinical practice.

Leflunomide

History

Leflunomide (LFM) is one of the newest members of the small molecule immunosuppressant family. LFM is an isoxazole compound that was first developed by Hoechst in Germany for agricultural purposes. It was subsequently found to have anti-inflammatory properties and was developed to be used in autoimmune diseases [159–162]. It is very effective in both controlling and modifying autoimmune diseases in small animals. At present, its effectiveness in rheumatoid arthritis is being evaluated in advanced clinical trials in Europe and the United States.

LFM's potential in transplantation was first demonstrated in an experiment by Kuchle et al., in which LFM prolonged skin and kidney allograft survival in rats [6]. In our laboratory, we demonstrated that LFM alone or in combination with CsA effectively prevents and reverses ongoing allograft and xenograft rejection in several animal models [15, 124, 163, 164]. Studies by others have also shown LFM's effectiveness in extending allo- and xenograft survival in a variety of animal models [10,165–173]. Interestingly, LFM was found to be very effective in inhibiting B cell functions in vitro [174]. This property may have an important impact on xenotransplantation.

Structure and Mechanisms of Action

LFM is a synthetic isoxazole derivative, which is not water-soluble. It is readily absorbed after oral administration. LFM is metabolized by the intestinal mucosa to its active open-ring and water-soluble form, A771726, which is also the preparation used for in vitro experiments.

The mechanisms of action of LFM are not entirely understood and are being actively studied by us and other researchers. Earlier reports suggested that LFM inhibits the production of IL-2 and the expression of IL-2 receptors. However, these findings were not consistent [175–179]. Another possible site of action was believed to be at the IL-2 receptor-associated tyrosine kinases [174, 180, 181]. Recent work by our group and others has demonstrated that LFM neither inhibits the influx of calcium, a tyrosine kinase-dependent activity, nor IL-2 gene expression in Jurkat T cells. In addition, we have demonstrated that the addition of exogenous uridine reverses the anti-proliferative effects of LFM ex vivo [182]. The cumulative evidence suggests that LFM exerts its immunosuppressive properties in vitro by interfering with de novo pyrimidine nucleotide synthesis (Fig. 3) [183–187].

Thus far, the participants involved in human rheumatoid arthritis clinical trials have suffered few ill effects from taking leflunomide for an extended period of time. Several new analogues, the malononitriloamides, are being developed for use in transplantation and preliminary data show comparable pharmacological profiles to their parent compound. The application of the malononitriloamides in transplantation seems very promising.

Leflunomide in Xenografting

LFM also stands out in its efficacy when used as a monotherapy. In the few xenograft models in which it has been tested, it has rivaled BQR in its efficacy as a monotherapy while exhibiting minimal or no toxicity. Xiao et al. were able to achieve a mean survival of 76.5 days in a hamster-to-rat cardiac xenograft model [10, 173]. In addition, four other treatment groups with suboptimal doses of LFM alone had mean survival of more than 50 days [173]. However, when PVG instead of Lewis rats were used as recipients by Lin et al., a mean survival of only 11.4 days was achieved with LFM alone [30]. In both cases, minimal side effects were observed at effective doses and both graft-induced and circulating, xenoreactive IgM were reduced significantly [30, 173]. Furthermore, untreated hamster-to-rat cardiac xenografts were able to be rescued by LFM monotherapy 2 days after xenografting and survived a mean of 58 days [10]. In a hamster-to-rat lung xenograft model, LFM was able to extent xenograft survival to 15.8 days versus 5.4 days in untreated controls [15].

Several other experiments have indicated that LFM has the ability to effectively inhibit antibody production and reduce preexisting antibodies. Xenoreactive natural antibody levels in rats are potently inhibited by LFM [20, 188]. Furthermore, we have recently shown that LFM has the ability to prevent hyperacute rejection when administered only 1 day prior to heart allografting into presensitized rats with high levels of circulating anti-donor antibody [189].

Hamster-to-rat cardiac xenografts treated with LFM alone eventually succumbed to fibrosis and myocardial necrosis. However, the addition of CsA to LFM prevented this outcome [10]. In addition, initial therapy with LFM plus CsA followed by the subsequent discontinuation of LFM produced permanent xenograft survival [30]. Furthermore, the combination of LFM and CsA was able to extend hamster-to-rat lung xenografts to 30 days [15]. In rats with long-term hamster cardiac xenografts that had initially been treated with both LFM and CsA, and which were currently receiving maintenance therapy of CsA alone, the removal of CsA resulted in graft rejection in approximately 7 days [30].

In a subsequent experiment, a second hamster heart was xenografted into rat recipients carrying a long-term beating heart after induction therapy with LFM and CsA followed maintenance therapy with CsA alone [30]. These rats rejected the second hamster heart in 2–3 days without harming the initial xenograft and without producing detectable anti-hamster antibody [30].

In summary, the initial xenografting results indicate that LFM is extremely effective in prolonging xenograft survival with minimal toxicity. Furthermore, when used in combination, LFM and CsA have been able to provide complete control of xenoreactivity at undetectable drug toxicity [10].

Comment

Several novel immunosuppressants have emerged over the last decade with the potential to dramatically inhibit specific aspects of the xenograft rejection process. Furthermore, the current research on many of these drugs indicates that they have efficacy and toxicity profiles consistent with clinical use. The increasingly skilled use of combinations of these drugs in animal models, as well as the variety of new techniques able to overcome hyperacute rejection, currently offer novel opportunities to predictably and indefinitely prolong xenograft survival.

References

1. Kino T, Hatanaka H, Hashimoto M. A novel immunosuppressant isolated from a streptomyces. I. Fermentation, isolation, and physico-chemical and biological characteristics. J. Antibiotics 1987; 40: 1249
2. Umezawa H, Ishizuka M, Takeuchi T, et al. Suppression of tissue graft rejection by spergualin. J Antibiot (Tokyo) 1985; 38: 283
3. Morris RE, Hoyt G. Prolongation of rat heart allograft survival by RS-61443. Surg Forum 1989; 40: 337
4. Morris RE, Meiser BM. Identification of a new pharmacologic action of an old compound. Med Sci Res 1989; 17: 609
5. Cramer DV, Chapman FA, Makowka L. The use of brequinar sodium for transplantation. Ann N Y Acad Sci 1993; 696: 216
6. Kuchle CC, Thoenes GH, Langer KH. Prevention of kidney and skin graft rejection in rats by leflunomide, a new immunomodulating agent. Transplant Proc 1991; 23(1 pt 2): 1083
7. Murase N, Starzl TE, Demetris AJ, et al. Hamster-to-rat heart and liver xenotransplantation with FK506 plus antiproliferative drugs. Transplantation 1993; 55 (4): 701
8. McManus RP, O'Hair DP, Komorowski R, Scott JP. Immunosuppressant combinations in primate cardiac xenografts. A review. Ann N Y Acad Sci 1993; 696: 281
9. Wang M, Tu Y, Stepkowski SM, Kahan BD. Effect of cyclosporine alone or in combination with rapamycin and brequinar on survival of hamster heart xenograft in rats. Transplant Proc 1993; 25: 2876
10. Xiao F, Chong A, Foster P, et al. Effect of leflunomide in control of acute rejection in hamster-to-rat cardiac xenografts. Transplant Proc 1994; 26: 1263
11. Sterbenz KG, Tepper MA. Effect of 15-deoxyspergualin on antibody secretion by specific isotypes producing B-cell hybridomas and myelomas. Transplant Proc 1994; 26: 3218
12. Sterbenz KG, Tepper MA. Effects of 15-deoxyspergualin on the expression of surface immunoglobulin in 70Z/3.12 murine pre-B cell line. Ann N Y Acad Sci 1993; 685: 205
13. Hayashi S, Ito M, Yokoyama I, Takagi H. Evidence that combination therapy using cobra venom factor, splenectomy, and deoxyspergualin is effective in guinea pig to rat cardiac xenotransplantation. Transplantation 1994; 57: 777
14. Leventhal JR, Matas AJ. Xenotransplantation in rodents: a review and reclassification. Transplantation Reviews 1994; 8: 80

15. Yuh D, Morris R, Hoyt G, Guitierrez J, Robbins R. Leflunomide effectively prolongs pulmonary allo- and xenograft survival. The Journal of Heart and Lung Transplantation 1995; 14: 1136
16. Kawauchi M, Takeda M, Nakajima J, Matsumoto J, Furuse A. Cardiac xenotransplantation from pig to Japanese monkey with splenectomy, tacrolims, filtration plasmapheresis, and nafamstat mesilate. Transplant Proc 1994; 26: 1076
17. Blakely ML, Van der Werf WJ, Dalmasso AP, Bach FH. Anti-B cell agents: suppression of natural antibodies and prolongation of survival in discordant xenografts. Transplant Proc 1994; 26: 1374
18. Flores HC, Leventhal JR, Gruber SA, et al. Natural antibody production can be inhibited by 15-deoxyspergualin in a discordant xenograft model. Transplant Proc 1992; 24: 714
19. Hayashi S, Ito M, Yokoyama I, Uchida K, Takagi H. Effectiveness of combination therapy using cobra venom factor, splenectomy, and deoxyspergualin in guinea pig to rat cardiac xenografts. Transplant Proc 1993; 25 (1 Pt 1): 405
20. Ulrichs K, Wang H, Muller-Ruchholtz W. Down-regulation of xenophile antibodies by 15-deoxyspergualin in an experimental animal model. Transplant Proc 1994; 26: 994
21. Henretta J, Pittman K, McFadden T, Thomas J, Thomas F. Deoxyspergualin and rabbit antithymocyte globulin markedly prolong discordant pig pancreatic islet xenografts. Transplant Proc 1993; 25 (1 Pt 1): 412
22. Figueroa J, Fuad SA, Kunjummen BD, Platt JL, Bach FH. Suppression of synthesis of natural antibodies by mycophenolate mofetil (RS-61443). Its potential use in discordant xenografting. Transplantation 1993; 55: 1371
23. Morikawa K, Oseko F, Morikawa S. The suppressive effect of deoxyspergualin on the differentiation of human B lymphocytes maturing into immunoglobulin-producing cells. Transplantation 1992; 54: 526
24. Nemoto K, Ito J, Abe F, et al. Suppression of humoral immunity in dogs by 15-deoxyspergualin. J Antibiot (Tokyo) 1987; 40: 1065
25. Hasan RIR, Sriwatanawongsa V, Wallwork J, White DJG. Consistent prolonged "concordant" survival of hamster-to-rat cardiac xenografts by inhibition of anti-species antibodies with methotrexate. Transplant Proc 1993; 25 (1 Pt 1): 421
26. Cramer DV, Chapman FA, Jaffee BD, et al. The prolongation of concordant hamster-to-rat cardiac xenografts by brequinar sodium. Transplantation 1992; 54: 403
27. Monden M, Valdivia LA, Gotoh M, et al. A crucial effect of splenectomy on prolonging cardiac xenograft survival in combination with cyclosporine. Surgery 1989; 105: 535
28. Woo J, Valdivia LA, Pan F, et al. Cytidine potentiates the inhibitory effect of brequinar sodium on xeno-MLR, antibody production, and concordant hamster to rat cardiac xenograft survival. Ann N Y Acad Sci 1993; 696: 227
29. Tamura K, Woo J, Bakri MT, Thomson AW. Brequinar sodium inhibits interleukin-6-induced differentiation of a human B-cell line into IgM-secreting plasma cells. Immunology 1993; 79: 587
30. Lin Y, Sobis H, Vandeputte M, Waer M. Mechanism of leflunomide-induced prevention of xenoantibody formation and xenograft rejection in the hamster to rat heart transplantation model. Transplant Proc 1995; 27: 305
31. Lieberman I, Heil BV, Seow WK, Thong YH. Synergy between tetrandrine and FK506 in prevention of diabetes in BB rats. Life Sci 1993; 53: L453

32. Wakugami T, Islam MR, Higa S, Murakami K, Mimura G. Effect of FK506 on the development of diabetes in BB rats in comparison with that of cyclosporin. Tohoku J Exp Med 1993; 169: 21
33. Clipstone NA, Crabtree GR. Calcineurin is a key signalling enzyme in t lymphcyte activation and the target of the immunosuppressive drugs cyclosporin A and FK506. Ann NY Acad Sci 1993; 696: 20
34. Schreiber SL, Crabtree GL. The mechanism of action of cyclosporin A and FK506. Immunol Today 1992; 13: 136
35. Weiederrecht G, Lam E, Hung S. The mechanism of action of FK506 and cyclosporin A. Ann NY Acad Sci 1993; 696: 9
36. Minoda M, Ohno M, Tomioka Y, et al. Effects of gamma-interferon and FK506 on resting B cell proliferation of New Zealand black/white F1 mice. Microbiol Immunol 1992; 36: 885
37. Morikawa K, Oseko F, Morikawa S. The distinct effects of FK506 on the activation, proliferation, and differentiation of human B lymphocytes. Transplantation 1992; 54: 1025
38. Gudas VM, Carmichael PG, Morris RE. Comparison of the immunosuppressive and toxic effects of FK506 and cyclosporine in xenograft recipients. Transplant Proc 1989; 21 (1 Pt 1): 1072
39. Valdivia LA, Fung JJ, Demetris AJ, Starzl TE. Differential survival of hamster-to-rat liver and cardiac xenografts under FK 506 immunosuppression. Transplant Proc 1991; 23: 3269
40. Murase N, Demetris AJ, Tanabe M, et al. Effect of FK 506 and antiproliferative agents for heart and liver xenotransplantation from hamster to rat. Transplant Proc 1993; 25 (1 Pt 1): 425
41. Hayashi S, Ito M, Yasutomi M, et al. Evidence that donor pretreatment with FK506 has a synergistic effect on graft prolongation in hamster-to-rat heart xenotransplantation. J Heart Lung Transplant 1995; 14: 579
42. Pan F, Valdivia LA, Tsugita M, et al. FK 506 prolongs survival of liver but not heart mouse-to-rat vascularized xenografts. Transplant Proc 1994; 26: 1211
43. Hasan R, Van den Bogaerde JB, Wallwork J, White DJ. Evidence that long-term survival of concordant xenografts is achieved by inhibition of antispecies antibody production. Transplantation 1992; 54: 408
44. van den Bogaerde J, Aspinall R, Wang MW, et al. Induction of long-term survival of hamster heart xenografts in rats. Transplantation 1991; 52: 15
45. Celli S, Valdivia LA, Fung JJ, et al. Long-term survival of heart and liver xenografts with splenectomy and FK 506. Transplant Proc 1993; 25 (1 Pt 1): 647
46. Celli S, Valdivia LA, Kelly RH, et al. Mechanisms of protection from humoral rejection by a xenografted liver. Transplant Proc 1995; 27: 300
47. Valdivia LA, Monden M, Gotoh M, et al. Prolonged survival of hamster-to-rat liver xenografts using splenectomy and cyclosporine administration. Transplantation 1987; 44: 759
48. Monden M, Valdivia LA, Gotoh M, et al. Hamster-to-rat orthotopic liver xenografts. Transplantation 1987; 43: 745
49. Takada K, Usuda H, Oh-Hashi M. Distribution kinetics of FK-506, a novel immunosuppressant, after intravenous administration to rats in comparison with cyclosporin A. Biopharm Drug Dispos 1992; 13: 345

50. Akita K, Ogawa M, Mandel TE. Effect of FK506 and anti-CD4 therapy on fetal pig pancreas xenografts and host lymphoid cells in nod/Lt, CBA, and BALB/c mice. Cell Transplant 1994; 3: 61
51. Sakamoto K, Nakajima K, Ochiai T, Asano T, Isono K. Analysis of long-term acceptance of xenografts in rats induced by short-term administration of FK506. Transplant Proc 1989; 21 (1 Pt 1): 527
52. Nishimori H, Suzuki S, Kido K, et al. Combination therapy with FK 506 and splenectomy may induce tolerance in cardiac xenografts. Transplant Proc 1994; 26: 1064
53. Carobbi A, Araneda D, Quarantillo P, Thomas JM, Thomas FT. Synergism of splenectomy and immunosuppressive drugs in prolongation of cardiac xenograft survival. Transplant Proc 1992; 24: 527
54. Carobbi A, Araneda D, Patselas T, Thomas J, Mosca F, Thomas F. Effect of splenectomy in combination with FK 506 and 15-deoxyspergualin on cardiac xenograft survival. Transplant Proc 1991; 23 (1 Pt 1): 549
55. Kawauchi M, Gundry SR, de Begona JA, et al. Prolonged survival of orthotopically transplanted heart xenograft in infant baboons. J Thorac Cardiovasc Surg 1993; 106: 779
56. Umeda Y, Moriguchi M, Ikai K, et al. Synthesis and antitumor activity of spergualin analogues. III. Novel method for synthesis of optically active 15-deoxyspergualin and 15-deoxy-11-O-methylspergualin. J Antibiot (Tokyo) 1987; 40: 1316
57. Masuda T, Mizutani S, Iijima M, et al. Immunosuppressive activity of 15-deoxyspergualin and its effect on skin allografts in rats. J Antibiot (Tokyo) 1987; 40: 1612
58. Nemoto K, Abe F, Takita T, et al. Suppression of experimental allergic encephalomyelitis in guinea pigs by spergualin and 15-deoxyspergualin. J Antibiot (Tokyo) 1987; 40: 1193
59. Corry RJ, Cutkomp J, Oberholser JH, Kapelanski DP, Wakely E. Prolongation of allograft and xenograft survival with 15-deoxyspergualin. Transplant Proc 1989; 21 (1 Pt 1): 530
60. Gannedahl G, Karlsson-Parra A, Totterman TH, Tufveson G. 15-Deoxyspergualin and mouse to rat heart retransplantation. Transplant Proc 1992; 24: 710
61. Hisanaga M, Nakajima Y, Yabuuchi H, Nakano H. Successful combination therapy with FK 506 and 15-deoxyspergualin in pancreatic islet xenografting. Transplant Proc 1992; 24: 1043
62. Lu X, Borel JF. Prolongation of islet xenograft survival with combined treatment of 15-deoxyspergualin or cyclosporine and anti-CD4 monoclonal antibody. Transplant Proc 1995; 27: 298
63. Marchman W, Araneda D, DeMasi R, et al. Prolongation of xenograft survival after combination therapy with 15-deoxyspergualin and total-lymphoid irradiation in the hamster-to-rat cardiac xenograft model. Transplantation 1992; 53: 30
64. Nakajima K, Sakamoto K, Ochiai T, et al. Prolongation of cardiac xenograft survival in rats treated with 15-deoxyspergualin alone and in combination with FK506. Transplantation 1988; 45: 1146
65. Pruitt SK, Halperin EC, Bollinger RR. The effect of 15-deoxyspergualin on hamster-to-rat cardiac xenograft survival. Transplant Proc 1991; 23: 585
66. Sandberg JO, Korsgren O, Groth CG, Andersson A. 15-Deoxyspergualin prolongs pancreatic islet allo- and xenograft survival in mice. Pharmacol Toxicol 1993; 73: 24

67. Kunimoto S, Miura K, Iinuma H, Takeuchi T, Umezawa H. Cytotoxicity of spergualin and amine oxidase activity in medium. J Antibiot (Tokyo) 1985; 38: 899
68. Kunimoto S, Nosaka C, Xu CZ, Takeuchi T. Serum effect on cellular uptake of spermidine, spergualin, 15-deoxyspergualin, and their metabolites by L5178Y cells. J Antibiot (Tokyo) 1989; 42: 116
69. Tepper MA, Nadler S, Mazzucco C, Singh C, Kelley SL. 15-Deoxyspergualin, a novel immunosuppressive drug: studies of the mechanism of action. Ann N Y Acad Sci 1993; 685: 136
70. Gannedahl G, Karlsson-Parra A, Totterman TH, Tufveson G. 15-Deoxyspergualin inhibits antibody production in mouse to rat heart transplantation. Transplant Proc 1993; 25 (1 Pt 1): 778
71. Leventhal JR, Platt JL, Flores HC, et al. Inhibition of natural antibody synthesis by cyclophosphamide or 15-deoxyspergualin fails to prevent xenograft rejection in the guinea pig-to-rat model. Transplant Proc 1992; 24: 551
72. Makino M, Fujiwara M, Watanabe H, Aoyagi T, Umezawa H. Immunosuppressive activities of deoxyspergualin. II. The effect on the antibody responses. Immunopharmacology 1987; 14: 115
73. Nemoto K, Hayashi M, Abe F, et al. Immunosuppressive activities of 15-deoxyspergualin in animals. J Antibiot (Tokyo) 1987; 40: 561
74. Nishimura K, Tokunaga T. Mechanism of action of 15-deoxyspergualin. I. Suppressive effect on the induction of alloreactive secondary cytotoxic T lymphocytes in vivo and in vitro. Immunology 1989; 68: 66
75. Hoeger PH, Tepper MA, Faith A, et al. Immunosuppressant deoxyspergualin inhibits antigen processing in monocytes. J Immunol 1994; 153: 3908
76. Imamura M, Zhu X, Hashino S, et al. Effects of 15-deoxyspergualin on proliferative responses and cytokine gene expression in vitro. Immunobiology 1994; 192: 24
77. Morisaki F, Sakagami K, Orita K. Effect of 15-deoxyspergualin on class II antigen expression in hepati sinusoidal lining cells and on infiltration of mononuclear cells in s liver transplantation. Transplant Proc 1989; 21 (1 Pt 1): 1077
78. Nemoto K, Abe F, Nakamura T, et al. Blastogenic responses and the release of interleukins 1 and 2 by sple cells obtained from rat skin allograft recipients administered with 15-deoxyspergualin. J Antibiot (Tokyo) 1987; 40: 1062
79. Fandrich F, Waaga AM, Jacob S, et al. Impact of 15-deoxyspergualin on MHC class I and II antigen expression following small bowel transplantation in rats. Transplant Proc 1994; 26: 1592
80. Nadler SG, Cleaveland J, Tepper MA, Walsh C, Nadeau K. Studies on the interaction of the immunosuppressant 15-deoxyspergual with heat shock proteins. Ann N Y Acad Sci 1993; 696: 412
81. Nadler SG, Tepper MA, Schacter B, Mazzucco CE. Interaction of the immunosuppressant deoxyspergualin with a member of Hsp70 family of heat shock proteins. Science 1992; 258: 484
82. Nadeau K, Nadler SG, Saulnier M, Tepper MA, Walsh CT. Quantitation of the interaction of the immunosuppressant deoxyspergua and analogs with Hsc70 and Hsp90. Biochemistry 1994; 33: 2561
83. Walter P, Bernhard U, Seitz G, Dickneite G, Sedlacek HH. Xenogeneic heart transplantation with 15-deoxyspergualin. Prolongation of graft survival. Transplant Proc 1987; 19: 3993

84. Valdivia LA, Monden M, Gotoh M, et al. Prolonged cardiac xenograft survival by 15-deoxyspergualin combined with splenectomy. Transplant Proc 1989; 21 (1 Pt 1): 532
85. Suzuki S, Nishimori H, Hayashi R, Quinonez D, Amemiya H. Prolonged survival of cardiac allografts and xenografts in rat-to-rat and hamster-to-rat transplantation by treatment with deoxyspergualin. Transplant Proc 1992; 24: 1638
86. Thomas F, Araneda D, Quarantillo P. Long-term survival of disparate cardiac xenografts: induction of tolerance and humoral accommodation. Transplant Proc 1994; 26: 1220
87. Suzuki S, Nishimori H, Kido K, et al. Continuous administration of methyldeoxyspergualin prolongs xenograft survival in hamster-to-rat cardiac transplantation. Transplant Proc 1993; 25 (1 Pt 1): 430
88. Suzuki S, Nishimori H, Ohdan H, Niiya S, Amemiya H. Prolongation of cardiac xenograft survival in a hamster-to-rat combination by recipient treatment with deoxymethylspergualin. Transplantation 1993; 56: 1257
89. Gannedahl G, Karlsson-Parra A, Wallgren A, et al. Role of antibody synthesis and complement activation in concordant xenograft retransplantation. Transplantation 1994; 58: 337
90. Wang J, Morris RE. Effect of splenectomy and mono- or combination therapy with rapamycin, the morpholinoethyl ester of mycophenolic acid and deoxyspergualin on cardiac xenograft survival. Transplant Proc 1991; 23 (1 Pt 1): 699
91. Steinbruchel DA, Nielsen B, Salomon S, Kemp E. Sequential, morphological, and antidonor antibody analysis in a hamster-to-rat heart transplantation model. Transpl Int 1992; 5: 38
92. Cosenza CA, Tuso PJ, Chapman FA, et al. Prolonged xenograft survival following combination therapy with brequinar sodium and cyclosporine. Transplant Proc 1993; 25 (3 Suppl 2): 59
93. Leventhal JR, Flores HC, Gruber SA, et al. Evidence that 15-deoxyspergualin inhibits natural antibody production but fails to prevent hyperacute rejection in a discordant xenograft model. Transplantation 1992; 54: 26
94. Gosio B. Ricerche batteriologiche e chimiche sulle alterazoni del mais. Rivista d' Igiene e Sanita Pupblica Ann 1896: 825
95. Ohsugi Y, Hirose S, Fuji G. Immunosuppressive effect of mycophenolic acid. Prolongation of survival time of skin allografts. Transplant J 1972; 7: 257
96. Morris RE, Wang J. Immunosuppressive effects of the morphlinoethyl ester of mycophenolic acid (RS-61443) in rat and nonhuman primate recipients of heart allografts. Transplant Proc 1991; 2, supp 2: 19
97. Sollinger HW. Mycophenolate mofetil for the prevention of acute rejection in primary cadaveric renal allograft recipients. U.S. Renal Transplant Mycophenolate Mofetil Study Group. Transplantation 1995; 60: 225
98. Placebo-controlled study of mycophenolate mofetil combined with cyclosporin and corticosteroids for prevention of acute rejection. European Mycophenolate Mofetil Cooperative Study Group. Lancet 1995; 345: 1321
99. Halloran P. The tricontinental mycophenolate mofetil renal transplant study group. N Eng J Med (submitted) 1996
100. Franklin T, Cook JM. The inhibition of nucleic acid synthesis by mycophenolic acid. Biochem J 1969: 515

101. Allison AC, Kowalski WJ, Muller CD, Eugui EM. Mechanisms of action of mycophenolic acid. Ann N Y Acad Sci 1993; 696: 63
102. Allison AC, Eugui EM. Inhibitors of de novo purine and pyrimidine synthesis as immunosuppressive drugs. Transplant Proc 1993; 25 (3 Suppl 2): 8
103. Wu J. Mycophenolate mofetil: molecular mechanisms of action. perspect Drug Discovery Design 1994; 2: 185
104. Chen Z, Cobbold S, Waldmann H, Metcalfe S. Combined use of RS61443 with CD4 and CD8 MAbs to generate tolerance to skin xenografts from rat to mouse. Transplant Proc 1994; 26: 2433
105. Yatscoff RW, Wang S, Keenan R, Chackowsky P, Koshal A. Efficacy of rapamycin, RS-61443, and cyclophosphamide in the prolongation of survival of discordant pig-to-rabbit cardiac xenografts. Transplant Proc 1994; 26: 1271
106. Fujino Y, Kawamura T, Hullett DA, Sollinger HW. Evaluation of cyclosporine, mycophenolate mofetil, and Brequinar sodium combination therapy on hamster-to-rat cardiac xenotransplantation. Transplantation 1994; 57: 41
107. Hullett DA, Kawamura T, Fujino Y, Allison AM, Sollinger HW. Prolongation of allograft and xenograft survival with mycophenolate mofetil (RS-61443) and brequinar sodium (DUP-785). Transplant Proc 1993; 25 (1 Pt 1): 700
108. Calne RY, Collier DS. Rapamycin for immunosuppression in organ allografting. Lancet 1989; 2: 227
109. Dumont FJ, Staruch MJ, Kaprak SL. The immunosuppressive and toxic effects of FK506 are mechanistically related: pharmacology of a novel antagonist of FK506 and rapamycin. J Exp Med 1992; 3: 751
110. Terada N, Lucas JJ, Szepesi A. Rapamycin blocks cell cycle progression of activated T cells prior to events characteristic of the middle to late G1 phase of the cycle. J Cell Physio 1993; 1: 7
111. Albers MW, Brown EJ, Tanaka A, et al. An FKBP-rapamycin-sensitive, cyclin-dependent kinase activity that correlates with the FKBP-rapamycin-induced G1 arrest point in MG-63 cells. Ann N Y Acad Sci 1993; 696: 54
112. Hultsch T, Martin R, Hohman RJ. The effect of the immunophilin ligands rapamycin and FK506 on proliferation of mast cells and other hematopoietic cell lines. Mol Biol Cell 1992; 3: 981
113. Chung J, Kuo CJ, Crabtree GR. Rapamycin-FKBP specifically blocks growth dependent activation of and signalling by the 70 kd S6 protein kinases. Cell 1992; 69: 1227
114. Price DJ, Grove JR, Calvo V. Rapamycin-induced inhibition of the 70-kilodalton S6 protein kinases. Nature 1992; 358: 70
115. Terada N, Lucas JJ, Szepesi A. Rapamycin inhibits the phosphorylation of p70 S6 kinase in IL-2 mitogen-activated human T cells. Biochem Biophys Res Commun 1992; 3: 1315
116. Kuo CJ, Chung J, Fiorentino DF, et al. Rapamycin selectively inhibits interleukin-2 activation of p70 S6 kinase. Nature 1992; 358: 70
117. Morice WG, Wiederrecht G, Brunn GJ, Siekierka JJ, Abraham RT. Rapamycin inhibition of interleukin-2-dependent p33cdk2 and p34cdc2 kinase activation in T lymphocytes. J Biol Chem 1993; 268: 22737
118. Morice WG, Brunn GJ, Wiederrecht G, Siekierka JJ, Abraham RT. Rapamycin-induced inhibition of p34cdc2 kinase activation is associated with G1/S-phase growth arrest in T lymphocytes. J Biol Chem 1993; 268: 3734

119. Albers MW, Williams RT, Brown EJ, et al. FKBP-rapamycin inhibits a cyclin-dependent kinase activity and a cyclin D1-Cdk association in early G1 of an osteosarcoma cell line. J Biol Chem 1993; 268: 22825
120. Chen H, Wu J, Xu D, Luo H, Daloze PM. Reversal of ongoing heart, kidney, and pancreas allograft rejection and suppression of accelerated heart allograft rejection in the rat by rapamycin. Transplantation 1993; 56: 661
121. Cramer DV, Chapman FA, Makowka L. Prevention of vascularized allograft and xenograft rejection in rodents by brequinar sodium. Transplant Proc 1993; 25 (3 Suppl 2): 23
122. Granger DK, Cromwell JW, Chen SC, et al. Prolongation of renal allograft survival in a large animal model by oral rapamycin monotherapy. Transplantation 1995; 59: 183
123. Morris RE. Rapamycins: antifugal, antitumor, antiproliferative, and immunosuppressive macrolides. Transplant Review 1992; 6: 39
124. Morris RE, Huang X, Gregory CR, et al. Studies in experimental models of chronic rejection: use of rapamycin (sirolimus) and isoxazole derivatives (leflunomide and its analogue) for the suppression of graft vascular disease and obliterative bronchiolitis. Transplant Proc 1995; 27: 2068
125. Gregory CR, Huang X, Pratt RE, et al. Treatment with rapamycin and mycophenolic acid reduces arterial intimal thickening produced by mechanical injury and allows endothelial replacement. Transplantation 1995; 59: 655
126. Cao W, Mohacsi P, Shorthouse R, Pratt R, Morris RE. Effects of rapamycin on growth factor-stimulated vascular smooth muscle cell DNA synthesis. Inhibition of basic fibroblast growth factor and platelet-derived growth factor action and antagonism of rapamycin by FK506. Transplantation 1995; 59: 390
127. Morris RE, Cao W, Huang X, et al. Rapamycin (Sirolimus) inhibits vascular smooth muscle DNA synthesis in vitro and suppresses narrowing in arterial allografts and in balloon-injured carotid arteries: evidence that rapamycin antagonizes growth factor action on immune and nonimmune cells. Transplant Proc 1995; 27: 430
128. DiJoseph JF, Sharma RN, Chang JY. The effect of rapamycin on kidney function in the Sprague-Dawley rat. Transplantation 1992; 53: 507
129. Ryffel B, Weber E, Mihatsch MJ. Nephrotoxicity of immunosuppressants in rats: comparison of macrolides with cyclosporin. Exp Nephrol 1994; 2: 324
130. Chen H, Xu D, Wu J, Daloze P. Prolongation of hamster to rat xenograft survival by rapamycin. Transplant Proc 1992; 24: 715
131. Yatscoff RW, Wang S, Keenan R, et al. Efficacy of rapamycin, RS-61443 and cyclophosphamide in the prolongation of survival of discordant pig to rabbit cardiac xenografts. Can J Cardiol 1994; 10: 711
132. Bobbio SA, Porter JG, Monaco AP. Effect of rapamycin on islet and skin xenograft survival. Transplant Proc 1993; 25: 2745
133. Dono K, Wood ML, Ozato H, et al. Marked prolongation of rat skin xenografts induced by intrathymic injection of xenogeneic splenocytes and a short course of rapamycin in antilymphocyte serum-treated mice. Transplantation 1995; 59: 929
134. Lu X, Schuurman HJ, Borel JF. Effect of rapamycin on islet xenograft survival. Transplant Proc 1994; 26: 1128
135. Luo H, Chen H, Daloze P, et al. Inhibition of in vitro immunoglobulin production by rapamycin. Transplantation 1992; 53: 1071

136. Reichenspurner H, Soni V, Berry GJ, et al. Obliterative airway dsease after heterotopic tracheal xenotransplantation – pathogenesis and prevention using new immunosuppressive drugs. Transplantation (submitted) 1996
137. Lyons SD, Christopherson RI. Effects of brequinar and ciprofloxacin on de novo nucleotide biosynthesis in mouse L1210 leukemia. Biochem Int 1990; 22: 939
138. Pizzorno G, Wiegand RA, Lentz SK, Handschumacher RE. Brequinar potentiates 5-fluorouracil antitumor activity in a murine model colon 38 tumor by tissue-specific modulation of uridine nucleotide pools. Cancer Res 1992; 52: 1660
139. Peters GJ, Schwartsmann G, Nadal JC, et al. In vivo inhibition of the pyrimidine de novo enzyme dihydroorotic acid dehydrogenase by brequinar sodium (DUP-785; NSC 368390) in mice and patients. Cancer Res 1990; 50: 4644
140. Braakhuis BJ, van Dongen GA, Peters GJ, van Walsum M, Snow GB. Antitumor activity of brequinar sodium (Dup-785) against human head and neck squamous cell carcinoma xenografts. Cancer Lett 1990; 49: 133
141. Aungst BJ, Blake JA, Rogers NJ, Dusak BA. Effects of plasma protein binding displacement on the pharmacokinetics, tissue and tumor concentrations and efficacy of brequinar, a highly protein-bound antitumor agent. J Pharmacol Exp Ther 1990; 253: 230
142. Kahan BD, Tejpal N, Gibbons-Stubbers S, et al. The synergistic interactions in vitro and in vivo of brequinar sodium with cyclosporine or rapamycin alone and in triple combination. Transplantation 1993; 55: 894
143. Forrest TL, Ware RE, Howard T, Jaffee BD, Denning SM. Novel mechanisms of brequinar sodium immunosuppression on T cell activation. Transplantation 1994; 58: 920
144. Lakaschus G, Loffler M. Differential susceptibility of dihydroorotate dehydrogenase/oxidase to Brequinar Sodium (NSC 368 390) in vitro. Biochem Pharmacol 1992; 43: 1025
145. Eiras-Hreha G, Cramer DV, Cajulis E, et al. Correlation of the in vitro and in vivo immunosuppressive activity of brequinar sodium. Transplant Proc 1993; 25 (1 Pt 1): 708
146. Cramer DV, Chapman FA, Jaffee BD, et al. The effect of a new immunosuppressive drug, brequinar sodium, on concordant hamster-to-rat cardiac xenografts. Transplant Proc 1992; 24: 720
147. Nozaki S, Ito T, Kamiike W, et al. Effect of brequinar sodium on accelerated cardiac allograft rejection in presensitized recipients. Transplant Proc 1994; 26: 2333
148. Yasunaga C, Cramer DV, Cosenza CA, et al. Effect of brequinar sodium on in vivo antibody production. Transplant Proc 1993; 25 (3 Suppl 2): 40
149. Yasunaga C, Cramer DV, Chapman FA, et al. The prevention of accelerated cardiac allograft rejection in sensitized recipients after treatment with brequinar sodium. Transplantation 1993; 56: 898
150. Moudgil A, Toyoda M, Wang SJ, et al. Inhibition of in vitro immunoglobulin production by a novel immunosuppressive drug brequinar sodium. Transplant Sci 1994; 4: 116
151. Simon P, Townsend RM, Harris RR, Jones EA, Jaffee BD. Brequinar sodium: inhibition of dihydroorotic acid dehydrogenase, depletion of pyrimidine pools, and consequent inhibition of immune functions in vitro. Transplant Proc 1993; 25 (3 Suppl 2): 77
152. Chen SF, Perrella FW, Behrens DL, Papp LM. Inhibition of dihydroorotate dehydrogenase activity by brequinar sodium. Cancer Res 1992; 52: 3521

153. Lemster B, Woo J, Strednak J, et al. Cytokine gene expression in murine lymphocytes activated in the presence of FK 506, bredinin, mycophenolic acid, or brequinar sodium. Transplant Proc 1992; 24: 2845
154. Woo J, Lemster B, Tamura K, Starzl TE, Thomson AW. The antilymphocytic activity of brequinar sodium and its potentiation by cytidine. Effects on lymphocyte proliferation and cytokine production. Transplantation 1993; 56: 374
155. Yasunaga C, Cramer DV, Chapman FA, et al. Cardiac graft rejection in hypersensitized recipients: prevention of antibody response and graft rejection using brequinar sodium. Transplant Proc 1993; 25 (3 Suppl 2): 65
156. Cosenza CA, Cramer DV, Tuso PJ, et al. Combination therapy with Brequinar sodium and cyclosporine synergistically prolongs hamster-to-rat cardiac xenograft survival. J Heart Lung Transplant 1994; 13: 489
157. Hayashi S, Ito M, Yokoyama I, Uchida K, Takagi H. Synergistic effect of donor pretreatment using FK 506 in hamster-to-rat cardiac xenotransplantation. Transplant Proc 1994; 26: 1284
158. Schuurman HJ, Joergensen J, Kuipers H, et al. Vascular transplantation of Syrian hamster heart into Lewis rat: effect of brequinar, cyclosporine, cobra venom factor, and splenectomy. Transplant Proc 1994; 26: 1217
159. Bartlett RR, Schleyerbach R. Immunopharmacological profile of a novel isoxazol derivative, HWA 486, with potential antirheumatic activity–I. Disease modifying action on adjuvant arthritis of the rat. Int J Immunopharmacol 1985; 7: 7
160. Bartlett RR, Popovic S, Raiss RX. Development of autoimmunity in MRL/lpr mice and the effects of drugs on this murine disease. Scand J Rheumatol Suppl 1988; 75: 290
161. Popovic S, Bartlett RR. Disease modifying activity of HWA 486 on the development of SLE in MRL/1-mice. Agents Actions 1986; 19: 313
162. Thoenes GH, Sitter T, Langer KH, Bartlett RR, Schleyerbach R. Leflunomide (HWA 486) inhibits experimental autoimmune tubulointerstitial nephritis in rats. Int J Immunopharmacol 1989; 11: 921
163. Morris RE, Huang X, Cao W, Zheng B, Shorthouse RA. Leflunomide (HWA 486) and its analog suppress T- and B-cell proliferation in vitro, acute rejection, ongoing rejection, and antidonor antibody synthesis in mouse, rat, and cynomolgus monkey transplant recipients as well as arterial intimal thickening after balloon catheter injury. Transplant Proc 1995; 27: 445
164. Gregory C, Lirtzman RL, Morris RE. Combination leflunomide and cyclosporin immunosuppression prevents MLR mismatched allograft rejection in mongrel dogs. Transplant Proc; (in press)
165. D'Silva M, Candinas D, Achilleos O, et al. The immunomodulatory effect of leflunomide in rat cardiac allotransplantation. Transplantation 1995; 60: 430
166. Foster PF, Xiao F, Kociss K, et al. Leflunomide immunosuppression in rat small intestinal transplantation. Transplant Proc 1994; 26: 1599
167. He G, McAlister VC, Lee TD, et al. Oral leflunomide prevents small bowel allograft rejection in the rat. Transplant Proc 1994; 26: 1613
168. Lin Y, Sobis H, Vandeputte M, Waer M. Long-term xenograft survival and suppression of xenoantibody formation in the hamster-to-rat heart transplant model using a combination therapy of leflunomide and cyclosporine. Transplant Proc 1994; 26: 3202

169. McChesney LP, Xiao F, Sankary HN, et al. An evaluation of leflunomide in the canine renal transplantation model. Transplantation 1994; 57: 1717
170. Wennberg L, Wallgren AC, Sundberg B, et al. Immunosuppression with leflunomide and cyclosporine prevents pig-to-rat islet xenograft rejection. Transplant Proc 1995; 27: 3314
171. Williams JW, Xiao F, Foster PF, et al. Immunosuppressive effects of leflunomide in a cardiac allograft model. Transplant Proc 1993; 25 (1 Pt 1): 745
172. Williams JW, Xiao F, Foster P, et al. Leflunomide in experimental transplantation. Control of rejection and alloantibody production, reversal of acute rejection, and interaction with cyclosporine. Transplantation 1994; 57: 1223
173. Xiao F, Chong AS, Foster P, et al. Leflunomide controls rejection in hamster to rat cardiac xenografts. Transplantation 1994; 58: 828
174. Chong A, Xiao F, Xu X, Williams J. In vivo and in vitro immunosuppression with leflunomide. Recent development in transplantation medicine, New immunosuppressive drugs, edited by Przepiorka, D. Sollinger, E., Physicans and Scientists Publishing Co., Inc. 1994: p. 163
175. Chong AS, Gebel H, Finnegan A, et al. Leflunomide, a novel immunomodulatory agent: in vitro analyses of the mechanism of immunosuppression. Transplant Proc 1993; 25 (1 Pt 1): 747
176. Chong AS, Finnegan A, Jiang X, et al. Leflunomide, a novel immunosuppressive agent. The mechanism of inhibition of T cell proliferation. Transplantation 1993; 55: 1361
177. Cherwinski HM, McCarley D, Schatzman R, Devens B, Ransom JT. The immunosuppressant leflunomide inhibits lymphocyte progression through cell cycle by a novel mechanism. J Pharmacol Exp Ther 1995; 272: 460
178. Zielinski T, Muller HJ, Bartlett RR. Effects of leflunomide (HWA 486) on expression of lymphocyte activation markers. Agents Actions 1993; 38 Spec No: C80–2
179. Lang R, Wagner H, Heeg K. Differential effects of the immunosuppressive agents cyclosporine and leflunomide in vivo. Leflunomide blocks clonal T cell expansion yet allows production of lymphokines and manifestation of T cell-mediated shock. Transplantation 1995; 59: 382
180. Mattar T, Kochhar K, Bartlett R, Bremer EG, Finnegan A. Inhibition of the epidermal growth factor receptor tyrosine kinase activity by leflunomide. FEBS Lett 1993; 334: 161
181. Nikcevich D, Finnegan A, Chong A, Williams J, Bremer E. Inhibition of interleukin 2 (IL-2) stimulated tyrosine activity by leflunomide. Agents Action. In press
182. Silva HT, Cao W, Shorthouse R, Morris RE. Mechanism of action of leflunomide in vivo: In vivo uridine administration reverses LFM's inhibition of lymphocyte proliferation. Transplant Proc 1996; (in press)
183. Cherwinski HM, Cohn RG, Cheung P, et al. The immunosuppressant leflunomide inhibits lymphocyte proliferation by inhibiting pyrimidine biosynthesis. J Pharmacol Exp Ther 1995; 275: 1043
184. Greene S, Watanabe K, Braatz-Trulson J, Lou L. Inhibition of dihydroorotate dehydrogenase by the immunosuppressive agent leflunomide. Biochem Pharmacol 1995; 50: 861
185. Cherwinski HM, Byars N, Ballaron SJ, et al. Leflunomide interferes with pyrimidine nucleotide biosynthesis. Inflamm Res 1995; 44: 317

186. Zielinski T, Zeitter D, Muller S, Bartlett RR. Leflunomide, a reversible inhibitor of pyrimidine biosynthesis? Inflamm Res 1995; 44 Suppl 2: S207–8
187. Cao W, Kao P, Chao A, et al. Mechanism of antiproliferative action of leflunomide, A77 1726, the active metabolite of leflunomide, does not block T-cell receptor mediated signal transduction but its antiproliferative effects are antagonized by pyrimidine nucleotides. J Heart Lung Transplant 1995; 14 (6 part 1): 1016
188. Ulrichs K, Kaitschick J, Bartlett R, Muller-Ruchholtz W. Suppression of natural xenophile antibodies with the novel immunomodulating drug leflunomide. Transplant Proc 1992; 24: 718
189. Cheung A, Adams B, Brazelton TR, et al. Leflunomide abrogates hyperacute rejection in presensitized rats. Transplantation 1996; (in press)
190. Tsugita M, Valdivia LA, Demetris AJ, et al. Hepatocytes or liver nonparenchymal cells plus FK 506 prolong liver xenograft survival. Transplant Proc 1994; 26: 3371
191. DeMasi R, Araneda D, Gross U, et al. Improved xenograft survival with continuous infusion deoxyspergualin and RATG. J Invest Surg 1991; 4: 59
192. Valdivia LA, Wonden W, Gotoh M, et al. Suppressor cells induced by donor-specific transfusion and deoxyspergualin in cardiac xenografts from hamsters to rats. Transplant Proc 1991; 23 (1 Pt 1): 203
193. Yoshida Y, Kitamura S, Kawachi K, Taniguchi S, Kondo Y. Comparison of cardiac rejection in heart and heart-lung concordant xenotransplantation. J Heart Lung Transplant 1994; 13: 325

45 Use of Brequinar Sodium To Prevent Xenograft Rejection

D.V. Cramer

Introduction

The shortage of human donor organs has stimulated widespread interest in the use of xenografts for clinical transplantation. The use of non-human donors for human transplantation has been attempted in more than 30 cases with limited success. The early examples of xenotransplants usually failed within a few days, primarily because of technical complications or the onset of a vigorous host immune response to the foreign graft. Improvements in surgical techniques and the use of immunosuppressive drugs in one series of chimpanzee to human kidney xenotransplants was associated with extension of graft survival to a few weeks and, in one case, to 9 months [1]. These early studies demonstrated that the host response to the xenograft can be modified with vigorous immunosuppression and the grafts would function in a foreign physiological environment. There has been, however, little additional progress in prolonging the clinical survival of xenografts in the past 30 years. This is true despite marked improvements in surgical techniques and the development of immunosuppressive regimens that are highly effective for preventing allograft rejection.

The failure to provide for prolonged graft survival in more recent examples of xenotransplantation continues to be a lack of a clear understanding of the nature and severity of the host immune response to the graft and the development of effective therapeutic strategies to prevent graft rejection. Experimental and clinical studies of those drugs and immunosuppressive regimens that are effective for providing excellent allograft survival have demonstrated only modest effects on preventing the rejection of xenografts [2]. These studies have made it apparent that the initial recipient immune response to pig or baboon xenografts, the donor species most likely to be considered for human xenotransplantation, consist of anti-donor antibody produced in response to the new graft. This humoral anti-donor response is not adequately controlled by immunosuppressive regimens based upon the exclusive use of cyclosporine (CsA) or FK506. These immunosuppressive agents effectively prevent T cell-mediated immune responses but have little effect on antibody production. Accordingly, immunosuppressive regimens that have been shown to prolonged xenograft survival have often include aggressive means of immunosuppression, including irradiation, to allow for longer graft survival. Unfortunately, these aggressive regimens of treatment are considered by many to be unsafe for general use in xenotransplantation.

Despite the success seen with CsA on patient and graft survival following allotransplantation, there are frequent examples of adverse side effects in patients treated with these powerful drugs. Many recipients of allografts require immunosuppression schedules that can produce significant toxic side effects without preventing graft rejection. The aggressive nature of the host immune responses to xenografts is potentially less sensitive to the effect of these drugs and therefore more likely to induce serious side effects without effective prolongation of graft survival. These issues have created a recent interest in the development of more effective new immunosuppressive drugs for transplant recipients. Clearly, the emphasis of this new drug development is for allograft recipients although ultimately many of these new drugs may find provide an important role in the prevention of xenograft rejection.

Brequinar sodium (BQR) is one of a new group of immunosuppressive drugs that have been recently tested for their usefulness as adjuvant therapy for preventing allograft rejection [3, 4]. BQR acts as an antimetabolite, preventing nucleic acid synthesis and interfering with the proliferation of activated lymphocytes. The radiomimetic effect of BQR is distinct from the mechanisms of activity for CsA and FK506. The combination of two drugs with different immunosuppressive mechanisms provides the potential for synergistic interactions when the drugs are used in combination for preventing graft rejection. Experimentally BQR has been tested for its interaction with a number of immunosuppressive agents, including CsA and FK506, and many of these combinations exhibit significant improvements in immunosuppressive activity [5, 6]. BQR is particularly effective in preventing B cell function, a characteristic which might provide the potential of establishing effective immunosuppressive regimens for a broader spectrum of patients. There are many forms of transplant rejection, including the rejection of allografts in sensitized patients or xenografts, that depend to a greater extent on humoral responses and are therefore resistant to conventional immunosuppression. The following is a brief description of the experimental and clinical data available for BQR with a particular emphasis on that information that is most relevant for its future potential for use as an immunosuppressive agent for xenotransplantation.

Pharmacologic Characteristics

BQR was originally developed as an antineoplastic drug. It was tested extensively in cancer patients and a large body of pharmacokinetic and safety data has been accumulated for the drug [7, 8]. BQR specifically inhibits dihydroorotate dehydrogenase (DHO-DH), the fourth enzyme in the de novo pyrimidine biosynthetic pathway [9]. The inhibition of DHO-DH has important antiproliferative effect on dividing cells, particularly lymphocytes because of their dependence on the de novo pathway of pyrimidine biosynthesis. Like other antimetabolite drugs, the inhibition of DHO-DH is reversible and cessation of drug treatment is associated with a rapid return of enzyme function and recovery from the toxic side effects. The effect of BQR on DHO-DH inhibition can be measured directly by analysis of the intracellular lymphocyte pools of uridine, the distal metabolite of the drug.

The ability to measure the drug directly and its effect on the effector cells indirectly via uridine levels represent important pharmacologic features of the drug when compared to many of the newer agents.

The antiproliferative effect of BQR is seen with both T and B cells. A variety of in vitro and in vivo assays have demonstrated a selective effect of BQR on proliferating lymphocytes. The drug is water soluble and is readily and completely absorbed from the gastrointestinal tract. Peak levels of the drug are reached within 2–4 h following oral administration and the drug is excreted at a steady rate of approximately 22 ml/min [3]. While imprecise, there is a rough correlation between plasma levels of the drug and inhibition of in vitro measurements of lymphocyte proliferative activity. The correlation between the peak levels of the drug and the inhibition of lymphocyte function appear to be good for single doses but may be less informative when shorter intervals between doses are used. The relatively long half-life of BQR may have a residual effect on lymphocyte function. Treatment with small, repetitive doses of the drug to maintain steady plasma levels does not improve allograft survival. Instead, the more frequent treatment schedules are accompanied by an increase in the appearance of adverse side effects. The immunosuppressive activity of BQR may depend upon the peak levels of the drug and smaller, more frequent doses may increase the side effects without improving the therapeutic effectiveness.

In patients with stable organ allografts there is data to suggest a considerable variation in pharmacokinetics (PK) curves when dosing is based upon weight [3]. Patients with stable kidney or liver allografts receiving CsA and steroid therapy to prevent graft rejection were examined in phase I BQR trials. The kidney patients received BQR as single ascending intravenous doses of 0.5, 1.0, 2.0, or 3.0 mg/kg doses. After 1 week without treatment each group received multiple (15) doses of the drug orally on alternative days. Individual patients exhibited substantial variation in the area under the curve (AUC) drug concentration values, suggesting that a dosage schedule based upon weight is not an effective method to obtain consistent results. Accordingly, PK values were also examined in patients given a standard regiment of CsA and steroids plus 50, 100, or 200 mg/kg doses of BQR on alternative days starting within 48 h of transplantation. The BQR treatment levels were adjusted to provide for 24 h plasma levels of less than 2 μg/ml. A group of 32 patients was studied and there was evidence that the number of rejection episodes had been reduced significantly. Extension of these early results to other transplant centers, however, did not confirm these initial observations and the clinical trials involving the use of BQR for preventing allograft rejection have been suspended.

Immunosuppressive Activity

Allografts

One of the consistent features of the immunosuppressive activities of BQR has been the effectiveness of this compound in preventing antibody production. While disruption of humoral immune responses may play a reduced role in the prevention of first set acute allograft rejection, there are a number of important potential applications for this type of immunosuppressive compound in organ transplantation. These include the prevention of the rejection of vascularized organs in patients sensitized to donor histocompatibility antigens, transplantation across AB barriers, and suppression of the xenograft reaction. In each, an important component of the primary immune response of the host to the graft is anti-donor antibody production. The presence of preformed and/or antibody stimulated by placement of the donor graft has the potential to precipitate an accelerated rejection that is resistant to traditional immunosuppressive regimens.

BQR has been shown to be important components of strategies to prevent humoral forms of rejection because of it's ability to disrupt B cell proliferation and the subsequent production of antibody. The effect of BQR on antibody production was first demonstrated in mice where treatment with BQR was shown to be at least an order of magnitude more effective than CsA or azathioprine for preventing mouse antibody responses to immunization with sheep red blood cells (RBCs) or lipopolysaccharide [10]. These results led us to examine the effectiveness of BQR when tested in rodents to prevent the type of rejection expected to be seen in sensitized patients. Immunization of rats with allogeneic lymphocytes followed in 1 week with transplantation with a heart from the same donor strain is a well-described rodent model of accelerated rejection of heart and kidney grafts in presensitized patients [11]. In this model, the recipient animals developed circulating antidonor antibodies and the rejection of heart grafts is seen within 48 h, instead of rejection times of approximately 7 days in naive recipients. Treatment of graft recipients with BQR, either before or at the time of transplantation, effectively prolongs graft survival [12]. The prolongation of heart grafts in the sensitized recipients is closely associated with suppression of anti-donor antibody production. The most effective schedule of treatment begins prior to sensitization and extends 30 days post-transplantation. The ability of BQR to prevent the accelerated graft rejection is seen even when the start of the treatment is delayed until placement of the graft. The ability of the drug to prevent accelerated rejection in the face of preformed antibody suggests that similar treatment regimens could be developed for patients who have become sensitized to many potential donors or donor/recipient combinations that exhibit preformed antibody to AB blood group antigens.

Xenografts

One of the major potential applications of BQR in organ transplantation is use of this compound to prevent the rejection of xenografts. During the initial characterization of the immunosuppressive characteristics of BQR, we tested the ability of this drug to prevent the rejection of rodent heart xenografts [6, 13, 14]. BQR was as effective as any other immunosuppressive drug in prolonging xenograft survival when used as a single agent. Daily treatment with higher levels of the drug could delay heart xenograft rejection for a median of 26 days. While this studies demonstrated a significant prolongation of graft survival, therapy with BQR alone is not sufficient to allow for clinically useful xenograft survival.

The use of BQR in combination with CsA was then tested to provide for more effective immunosuppression. The use of these two drugs in combination led to the first demonstration that clinically acceptable immunosuppressive drugs could experimentally induce long-term xenograft (>100 days) survival [6, 15]. The ability of this immunosuppressive regimen to allow for long-term graft survival, like the rejection of allografts in sensitized recipients, was closely linked to the suppression of anti-donor antibody production. Therapeutic regimens that failed to adequately suppress antibody production or cessation of treatment resulted in a return of anti-donor antibodies and subsequent rejection of the grafts.

The ability of BQR and CsA to induce prolonged xenograft survival is not a unique feature of either drug or their use in combination. BQR behaves in a similar fashion when used combination with FK506 [5]. Other immunosuppressive drugs that interfere with B cell function when used in combination with FK506 have the capacity to induce prolonged xenograft survival. In each case, most important feature of the immunosuppressive regimen appears to be disruption in the ability of the host to make an effective anti-donor antibody response. In the hamster-to-rat combination the use of CsA or FK506 and BQR together allows for prolonged survival and the maintenance of good graft function. Liver xenografts function normally and can be shown to be actively producing hamster specific proteins [16]. The ability to prolong xenograft survival has also demonstrated that xenografts, like their allograft equivalents, may experience a low-grade, chronic rejection that manifests itself as a proliferative lesion in the graft vasculature. The immunopathologic features of transplant arteriosclerosis in xenografts is very similar to that seen in allografts, including a concentric intimal proliferation that constricts the vascular lumen [17]. One feature of the xenograft lesion that may differ from the allograft model is the demonstration of antibody directed at the donor vascular endothelium in the vascular lesions. The persistence of cellular infiltrates in the heart xenografts and the rapid appearance of transplant arteriosclerosis suggests that more effective schedules of treatment may be necessary to develop for application in larger species.

Comment

The development of new immunosuppressive drugs and treatment regimens may have an important impact on the implementation of xenotransplantation as a therapeutic strategy. Many new technologies are currently under development to reduce the intensity of the immune responses patients may mount against potential xenograft donors. These include the creation of transgenic lines of donor animals that express human complement regulatory proteins or have modifications in the expression of xenogeneic target antigens, pharmacologic or genetic strategies to disrupt the xenograft reaction, and the induction of immunological tolerance to donor tissues. It is unlikely, however, that any of these strategies, singly or in combination, will allow for successful xenotransplantation in the absence of some form of immunosuppression. Downregulation of the major target antigens and disruption of the immunological responses most responsible for the early rejection of xenografts are likely to allow for modest prolongation of graft survival. They are may also prove to be inadequate for long-term suppression of xenograft rejection, particularly for the reaction that may shift to other antigenic differences between donor and host. The evidence for chronic rejection, including cellular infiltrates in grafts and the occurrence of proliferative vascular lesions in long-term surviving xenografts suggest that xenografts, like allografts, many be subjected to host immune responses directed against multiple antigens.

The need to provide for effective immunosuppression for xenografts will requires additional efforts be directed at the characterization and preclinical testing of agents that may have the potential for use in a clinical setting. Because of differences in the nature of the host responses to allografts and xenografts, the present focus on the development of drugs for preventing allograft rejection is likely to have little application for xenografts. While the use of xenografts for permanent organ replacement in humans is a therapy that will not be in general use for many years, the current time schedules for new drug development in humans will require similar periods of time to bring drugs that are effective for preventing xenograft rejection to a stage of development that would allow for their use at the appropriate time. The intersection in the developmental processes for selected new immunosuppressive drugs, including BQR, and techniques allow for the use of xenogeneic donors is a unique opportunity for the implementation of a major new medical therapies.

References

1. Reemtsma K. Renal heterotransplantation from nonhuman primates to man. Ann.N.Y.Acad.Sci. 1969; 162: 412
2. Makowka L, Cramer DV. The pathogenesis of the xenograft reaction. In: Advances in Transplantation, Hackel B, AuBuchon J, eds. Bethesda, Amer Assoc Blood Banks, 1993; 93
3. Makowka L, Sher LS, Cramer DV. The development of Brequinar sodium as an immunosuppressive drug for transplantation. Immunological Reviews 1993; 136: 51
4. Makowka L, Cramer DV. Brequinar sodium: Mode of action and effects on graft rejection. In: Immunosuppressive Drugs: Developments in Anti-Rejection Therapy, Thomson AW, Starzl TE, eds. Kent, Edward Arnold, 1993; 177
5. Murase N, Starzl TE, Demetris AJ, et al. Hamster-to-rat heart and liver xenotransplantation with FK506 plus antiproliferative drugs. Transplantation 1993; 55: 701
6. Cosenza CA, Cramer DV, Tuso PJ, et al. Combination therapy with brequinar sodium and Cyclosporin A synergistically prolongs hamster-to-rat cardiac xenograft survival. J Heart Lung Transplant 1994; 13: 489
7. Schwartsmann G, Dodion P, Vermorken JB, et al. Phase I study with brequinar sodium (NSC 368390) in patients with solid malignancies. Cancer Chemother Pharmacol 1990; 25: 345
8. Arteaga CL, Brown TD, Kuhn JG, et al. Phase I clinical and pharmacokinetic trial of brequinar sodium (DUP 785; NSC 368390). Cancer Res 1989; 49: 4648
9. Chen S, Ruben R, Dexter D. Mechanism of action of the novel anticancer agent 6-fluoro-2-(2'-fluoro-1,1'-biphenyl-4-yl)-3-methyl-4-quinolinecarboxylic acid sodium salt (NSC 368390): Inhibition of de novo pyrimidine nucleotide biosynthesis. Cancer Res 1986; 46: 5014

10. Jaffee BD, Jones EA, Loveless SE, Chen SF. The unique immunosuppressive activity of brequinar sodium. Transplant Proc 1993; 25 (Suppl 2): 19
11. Hancock WW, DiStefano R, Braun P, et al. Cyclosporine and anti-interleukin 2 receptor monoclonal antibody therapy suppress accelerated rejection of rat cardiac allografts through different effector mechanisms. Transplantation 1990; 49: 416
12. Yasunaga C, Cramer DV, Chapman FA, et al. The prevention of accelerated cardiac allograft rejection in sensitized recipients after treatment with brequinar sodium. Transplantation 1993; 56: 898
13. Cramer DV, Chapman FA, Jaffee BD, et al. The effect of a new immunosuppressive drug, Brequinar sodium, on concordant hamster-to-rat cardiac xenografts. Transplant Proc 1992; 24: 720
14. Cramer DV, Chapman FA, Jaffee BD, et al. The prolongation of concordant hamster-to-rat cardiac xenografts by brequinar sodium. Transplantation 1992; 54: 403
15. Cosenza CA, Tuso PJ, Chapman FA, et al. Prolonged xenograft survival following combination therapy with brequinar sodium and cyclosporine. Transplant Proc 1993; 25(Suppl 2): 59
16. Valdivia LA, Lewis JH, Celli S, et al. Hamster coagulation and serum proteins in rat recipients of hamster xenografts. Transplantation 1993; 56: 489
17. Cramer DV, Wu GD, Makowka L. The immunopathologic characterization of transplant arteriosclerosis in cardiac xenografts. In: Abhandlungen der Rheinisch-Westfalischen Akademie der Wissenschaften, Anonymous Munster, 1994

46 Leflunomide and the Malononitriloamides in Xenotransplantation

R.R. Bartlett and E. Kemp

Introduction

Leflunomide is a novel drug that has shown efficacy in an array of animal models of autoimmune disease [1–9] and organ graft rejection [9–14]. This drug has demonstrated efficacy and good tolerability in clinical phase II trials in patients with rheumatoid arthritis [15]. Leflunomide is being developed for this indication and other autoimmune disorders. Recently, derivatives of leflunomide's primary metabolite, A77 1726 (Fig. 1), so-called malononitriloamides (MNAs), have been brought into development for potential use in organ transplantation (by Hoechst Marion Roussel). As far as is presently known, the activities of leflunomide and MNAs are identical, but the MNAs seem to have a shorter half-life. The long half-life of leflunomide in humans (about 14 days) could be a problem when applying this drug in combination with immunosuppressive agents.

Leflunomide exerts its effects primarily on B cells, reducing autoantibody [3–8], alloantibody [13], and xenoantibody [11, 14] formation. The mode of action of this drug is not fully understood, but there is strong evidence that it has inhibitory effects on de novo pyrimidine biosynthesis, specifically dehydroorotate-dehydrogenase (DHODH) [16–28], and inhibits certain tyrosine kinases responsible for signal transduction [19, 20]. Unlike cyclosporine (CsA), leflunomide inhibits CD28-induced T cell activation [21, 14, 26] and does not have inhibitory effects on cytokine production [9]. Further, the drug antagonizes the activity of several cytokines [2, 9].

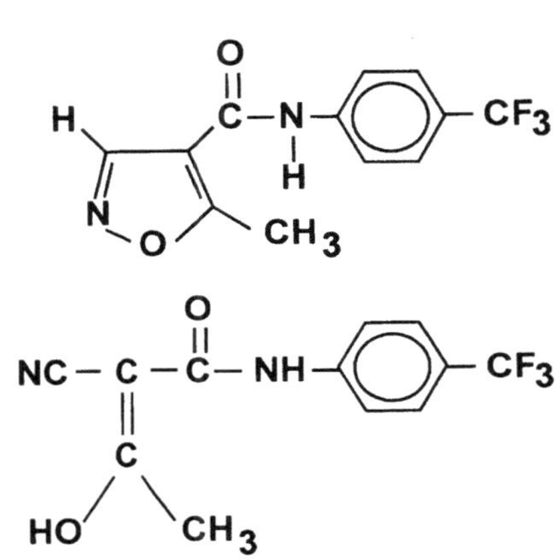

Fig. 1. Molecular structures of leflunomide (HWA 486, *top*) and its primary metabolite, A77 1726 (*bottom*)

Leflunomide in Allotransplantation

Acute Rejection

Leflunomide is a relatively new drug for use in experimental transplantation. The first indication that leflunomide has effects on reactions leading to transplantation rejection was observed in mice undergoing a chronic graft versus host disease (cGvHD) [22]. Due to these results it was reasoned by Küchle et al. [10] that this drug also must be efficient in preventing reactions leading to organ transplantation rejection. Using Lewis rats (RT 1) as host animals, kidneys from BN rats were transplanted. In the untreated rats, these allografts were rejected within 8 days, whereas treatment with leflunomide for 30 days prolonged the graft and thus the survival of all these animals for the duration of the experiment (>60 days). By following the plasma creatinine levels it was determined that the transplanted kidneys functioned normally, and histological studies revealed virtually no signs of rejection [10]. The results obtained from leflunomide therapy revieled that this drug was not only efficacious in suppressing kidney, but also skin rejection in rats.

Later, Schorlemmer et al. were able to provide data demonstrating leflunomide's ability to induce specific allograft tolerance in two skin graft models [12]. The authors also reported that this tolerance was adoptively transferable. This activity could not be observed using CsA.

We (E. Kemp et al., unpublished) have also observed long-term graft acceptance (tolerance?) in rats with heart allografts after short-term periods of treatment with a combination of leflunomide (5 mg/kg, p.o.) and CsA (12.5 mg/kg, i.m.). Using a treatment protocol in which the drug combination was applied daily for a period of 14 days (group 1), graft survival was considerably increased and in one animal the heart was still beating 348 days after being transplanted (Table 1). Much more consistent results were obtained when the animals (group 2) were administered the same drugs for short periods (14 days) at intervals (starting on post-transplant days 2, 50, 100, 200, 250, and 300). Five out of five grafts were still functioning more than 330 days after transplantation (Table 1).

Table 1. Results of heart allotransplantation in rats (Sprague-Dawley to Lewis) transplanted with a combination of leflunomide and cyclosporine

Group	Rats (*n*)	Treatment protocol	Survival (days)
1	5	Leflunomide 5 mg/kg p.o. daily for 14 days CsA 12.5 mg/kg i.m. three times weekly for 14 days.	52, 139, 155, 182, >348
2	5	As for group 1, but additional 14-day courses of leflunomide + CsA given at 50, 100, 200, 250, 300 days post-transplant	All >338. All sacrified with beating hearts.

Mean survival in untreated control experiments in this model was 9 days. Induction of an operationally tolerant state was seen in all animals in group 2.

In human organ allotransplantation it is necessary to use sufficient amounts of immunosuppressive agents to maintain organ function and prevent rejection. Over-immunosuppression is very often the outcome of such therapy, with its well-known complications. Induction of tolerance would be the best of all possibilities. Thus, if the data obtained in animals treated with leflunomide (with or without CsA) could be transferred to the human situation, this would be a medical breakthrough.

Chronic Rejection

Activities distinguishing leflunomide's actions from those of CsA are its efficacy in chronic allograft rejection. Swan et al. [23] used a rat model in which aortic allografts, transplanted across a major histocompatibility barrier, developed histological changes within the vascular wall mirroring those found in chronically rejected human allografts. This response lead to chronic intimal proliferation and subsequently to sclerosis. The authors reported that leflunomide significantly reduced the acute, adventitial inflammatory response in the transplanted aortic segment. Likewise, fibrointimal proliferation within the vascular wall, a characteristic of chronic rejection, was markedly diminished in these rats.

Recently, Xiao et al. [24] published data further supporting the efficacy of leflunomide on chronic rejection. They reported that when given at an oral dose of 10 mg/kg per day to Fisher-344 rats, grafted with hearts from Lewis rats, the smooth muscle cell and fibroblast proliferation in the intima was significantly inhibited by day 90 (therapy started on day 30). Using a non-inhibitory dose of leflunomide (5 mg/kg per day) in combination with 5 mg CsA/kg per day (which is ineffective as a monotherapy in this model at any dose), the efficacy was even better.

Leflunomide in Xenotransplantation

The first publication dealing with leflunomide's effect on xenotransplantation appeared in 1991 by Ulrichs et al.[11]. They reported that natural xenoantibodies against human leukocytes in rats could be greatly reduced by therapy with leflunomide, i.e., it lowered preformed xenoantibodies and prevented xenoantigen-induced xenoantibody production in rodents. Thus, it became apparent that leflunomide had other immunosuppressive characteristics than CsA, i.e., it could induce specific allograft tolerance and also be used in the prevention of xenograft rejection.

Concordant Models

In 1993, the Chicago-based group headed by Williams reported a marked influence of leflunomide on the survival of hamster hearts transplanted into rats [25]. Somewhat later, Waer's group, using the same concordant model, published similar results [26]. Both groups found that although monotherapy with leflunomide was effective, the combination with CsA led to more efficient suppression of xenoantibodies and long-term xenograft survival.

We have also studied the effects of leflunomide in the concordant hamster-to-rat heart xenograft model. In 1994, we published a comparative study of this drug with cyclophosphamide, CsA, rapamycin, and FK506 [27]. Leflunomide was superior to the other agents when used as single therapeutic agents. When four drugs were used in combination, almost normal morphology of the graft was found during the first weeks after transplantation, but over-immunosuppression was a problem. The best protection was observed when leflunomide was combined with CsA, with a mean graft survival of about 3 months. This combination was superior to all other combinations studied in our trial. In very recent experiments using this combination we have obtained even better results, indicating that rejection can be avoided as long as treatment is continued [28]. Moreover, splenectomy of leflunomide-treated xenograft recipients further prolonged graft acceptance. Additional treatment with donor cells from spleen, thymus, or bone marrow did not influence the survival time of the grafted hearts, and tolerance was not obtained in any of our studies [27].

Recently, Lin et al. [29] have provided evidence suggesting that early concordant heart xenograft rejection in rats is mainly provoked by T-independent xenoantibodies. Further, the B cells naturally secreting xenoantibodies are of CD5 phenotype, which produce IgM molecules. Their production could be greatly suppressed by leflunomide therapy, thus preventing xenograft rejection. In the same situation, CsA treatment had no effect on T cell-independent IgM antibody production and the xenograft was rejected. Even though the animals were treated with leflunomide, and little-to-no IgM xenoantibody was formed, after a few days a T cell-dependent class switch to IgG took place and the xenograft was rejected. In this case, the addition of CsA could prevent the class switch and the graft was not rejected. While CsA had no effect on the T-independent xenoantibody formation, it synergized with leflunomide to result in long-term xenograft survival and total absence of xenoantibody formation. This was most likely due to CsA's capacity to suppress late T-dependent antibody formation.

The complementary activities of CsA and leflunomide can explain their reported synergistic effects [13, 21, 26], i.e., CsA prevents the production of interleukin (IL)-2 and primarily prevents T cells from becoming activated, whereas leflunomide blocks T cell-independent B cell antibody formation and can inhibit active cells from proliferating.

Discordant Models

Not only concordant xenograft rejection has been suppressed by leflunomide, but also discordant rejection. Wright et al. demonstrated the monotherapeutic efficacy of this drug in a fish-to-mouse islet xenograft model [30]. More recently, the group headed by Groth reported that leflunomide, in combination with CsA, was effective in another discordant model [31]. These authors transplanted fetal porcine islet-like cell clusters under the kidney capsule of Lewis rats. Monotherapy with either CsA (15 mg/kg), leflunomide (20 mg/kg), or mycophenolate mofetil (40 mg/kg) had no or only marginal effects on the infiltration of mononuclear cells (primarily macrophages). This infiltration led to total destruction of the islets. In rats treated with leflunomide in combination with CsA, only a minimal cellular infiltration was observed and the majority of islet cells were morphologically intact. When mycophenolate mofetil was added to the other two drugs, even further improvement was recorded.

Tolerance induction in xenografts with leflunomide therapy seems to be much more difficult than tolerance induced in allograft models. We and both the Chicago and Leuven-based groups have attempted to induce xenotolerance by using leflunomide alone or in combination with CsA, but have been unsuccessful [25, 27, 32]. Long-term graft survival was observed as long as the drugs were administered. Even discontinuation of one drug, i.e. leflunomide, but continued therapy with CsA, prevented graft rejection. After discontinuation of both drugs, however, graft rejection took place [32].

Malononitriloamides

Studying the MNAs (X91 0279 and X92 0715) in transplantation, it has been reported that they are just as effective as leflunomide. We [33, 34] found their activities similar to that of leflunomide in both chronic and acute graft-versus-host disease. Further, Schorlemmer et al. [35] could demonstrate activity of the MNAs in a concordant skin xenograft model. For their experiments, skin grafts from NMRI-mice were transplanted onto the tails of Lewis rats. Monotherapy with MNAs (at oral doses of 5 or 10 mg/kg per day on days 0–9) resulted in mean graft survivals of 12 and 16 days, respectively (compared to 5 days in a vehicle-gavaged group). Furthermore, the combination of CsA (10 mg/kg per day on days 0–9) and MNAs (5 mg/kg per day on days 0–4) synergistically prolonged xenograft survival to about 19 days.

Lin et al. have also demonstrated the efficacy of X92 0715 in allo and xenograft models. The synergistic activity of this MNA with CsA was just as effective as that of leflunomide in both models. These drug combinations resulted in long-term survival of the transplanted allo- and xenografts (>30 days in both cases). Further, Morris et al. have reported the effects of leflunomide and the MNAs on the suppression of graft vascular disease and obliterative bronchiolitis in experimental models of chronic rejection [36].

These reports on MNAs' activity in acute and chronic allograft as well as xenograft rejection are encouraging and speak for their development in transplantation. As leflunomide and MNAs are rather unique for xenografting, one can look forward to a new class of drugs which, most likely, can be used with greater success than present therapies. Considering the advantage of the shorter half-lives of the MNAs, it is reasonable to expect an optimal combination therapy of these drugs together with other immunosuppressive agents (e.g., CsA) to prevent or reverse the rejection of xenografts in humans.

References

1. Bartlett, RR., Schleyerbach, R. Immunopharmacological profile of a novel Isoxazol derivative, HWA 486, with potential antirheumatic acvitity-1. Disease modifying action on adjuvant arthritis of the rat. Int J Immunopharmacol. 7:7,18,1985
2. Bartlett, RR., Anagnosotulos, H., Zielinski, T., Mattar, T., Schleyerbach, R. Effects of leflunomide on immune responses and models of Inflammation. Springer Sem.Immunopath. 14,381,1993
3. Glant,TT., Mikecz,K., Bartlett, RR., et al. Immunomodulation of proteoglycaninduces progressive polyarthritis by leflunomide. Immunopharmacol. 23,105, 1992
4. Ogawa, T., Inazu, M., Gotoh, K., Hayashi, S. Effects of leflunomide on glomerulonephritis induced by antibasement membrane antibody in rats. Agents Actions. 31,321,1990
5. Smith-Lang,L., Glaser, B., Weimer, LK., et al. Efficacy of novel immunomodulators leflunomide and rapamycin in autoimmune uveitis. FASEB J. 6,4,A1048, part 1, 1992
6. Thoenes, GH., Sitter, T., Langer, KH., Bartlett, RR., Schleyerbach, R. Leflunomide (HWA 486) inhibits experimental autoimmune tubulointerstitial nephritis in rats. Int J Immunopharmacol. 11,921,1989
7. Vidic-Dankovic, B., Kosec, D., Damjanovic, M., et al. Leflunomide prevents the development of experimentally induced myasthenia gravis. Int J Immunopharmacol. 17,273,1995
8. Bartlett, RR., Popovic, S., Raiss, RX. Development of autoimmunity in MRL/lpr mice and the effects of drugs on this murine disease. Scand J Rheumatol. 75,290,1988
9. Bartlett, RR., Zielinski, T., Campion, G., et al. Leflunomide: a novel immunomodulating drug. In: Non-Steroidal Anti-inflammatory Drugs II (eds. Lewis, AJ, Furst, D.) Marcel Dekker, Inc., New York. 349, 1994
10. Küchle, CCA, Thones, GH., Langer, KH., et al. Prevention of kidney and skin graft rejection in rats by leflunomide, a new immunomodulating agent. Transplant. Proc. 23,1083,1991
11. Ulrichs, K., Kaitschick, J., Bartlett, R., Müller-Ruchholtz, W. Suppression of natural xenophile antibodies with the novel immunosuppressive drug leflunomide. Transplant. Proc. 24,718,1992
12. Schorlemmer, HU., Seiler, FR., Bartlett, RR. Prolongation of allogenic transplanted skin grafts and induction of tolerance by leflunomide (HWA 486), a new immunosuppressive isoxazol derivative. Transplant. Proc. 25,763,1993
13. Williams, JW., Xiao, F., Foster, P., et al. S-F Leflunomide in experimental transplantation. Control of rejection and alloantibody production, reversal of acute rejection, and interaction with cyclosporine. Transplantation. 57,1223,1994
14. Lin, Y., Sobis, H., Vandeputte, M., Waer, M. Mechanism of leflunomide-induced prevention of xenoantibody formation and xenograft rejection in the hamster to rat heart transplantation model. Transplant. Proc. 27,305,1995
15. Mladenovic, V., Domljan, Z., Rozman, B., et al. Safety and efficacy of leflunomide in the treatment of patients with active rheumatoid arthritis. Arthritis Rheumatism. 38,1595,1995
16. Zielinski, T., Zeitter, D., Müllner, S., Bartlett, RR. Leflunomide, a reversible inhibitor of pyrimidine biosynthesis? Inflamm Res. 44, S207,1995

17. Cherwinski, HM., Byars, N., Ballaron, SJ., et al. Leflunomide interferes with pyrimidine nucleotide biosynthesis. Inflamm Res. 44,317,1995
18. Williamson, RA., Yea, CM., Robson, PA., et al. Dihydroorotate dehydrogenase is a high affinity binding protein for A77 1726 and mediator of a range of biological effects of the immunomodulating compound. J Biol Chem. 270,22467,1995
19. Mattar, T., Kochhar, K., Bartlett, RR., Bremer, EG., Finnegan, A. Inhibition of the epidermal growth factor receptor tyrosine kinase activity by leflunomide. FEBS 13234. 334,161,1993
20. Nikcevich, DA., Finnegan, A., Chong, ASF., Williams, JW., Bremer, EG. Inhibition of Interleukin 2 (IL-2)-stimulated tyrosine kinase activity by leflunomide. Agents Actions. 41,C279,1994
21. Chong, AS., Xiao, F., Xu, X., Williams, JW. In vivo and in vitro immunosuppression with leflunomide. In: Recent Developments in Transplantation Medicine. Vol. 1. New Immunosuppressive Drugs. eds. Sollinger, H., Przepiorke, D. Physicians & Scientists Publishing Co, Glenview, USA, 163,1994
22. Popovic, S., Bartlett, RR. The use of the murine chronic graft versus host (CGVH) disease, a model for systemic lupus erythematosis (SLE) for drug discovery. Agents Actions. 21,284,1987
23. Swan, SK., Carlos, GS., Guijarro, C., et al. Immunosuppressive effects of leflunomide in experimental chronic vascular rejection. Transplantation. 60,887,1995
24. Xiao, F., Chong, A., Shen, J., et al. Pharmacologically induced regression of chronic transplant rejection. Transplantation. 60,1065,1995
25. Xiao, F., Chong, AS., Foster, P., et al. Leflunomide controls rejection in hamster to rat cardiac xenografts. Transplant. Proc. 58,828,1994
26. Lin, Y., Sobis, H., Vandeputte, M., Waer, M. Long-term xenograft survival and suppression of xenoantibody formation in the hamster-to-rat heart transplant model using a combination therapy of leflunomide and cyclosporine. Transplant. Proc. 26,3202,1994
27. Kemp, E., Dieperink, H., Jensen, J., et al. Newer immunosuppressive drugs in concordant xenografting - Transplantation of hamster heart to rat. Xenotransplantation. 1,102, 1994
28. Kemp, E. Xenotransplantation. J Intern Med. 239,287,1996
29. Lin, Y., Waer, M. In vivo mechanisms of action of leflunomide (LF): selective inhibition of the capacity of B lymphocytes to make T-independent (TI) xenoantibody formation. Transplant. Proc. In press
30. Wright, JR., Kearns, H., McDonals, AS. Leflunomide and cyclosporin-A prolong fish-to-mouse islet xenograft survival in BALB/C mice. Transplant. Proc. 26,1310,1994
31. Wennberg, L., Wallgren, AC., Sundberg, B., et al. Immunosuppression with cyclosporin A in combination with leflunomide and mycophenolate mofetil prevents rejection of pig-islets transplanted into rats. Transplant. Proc. (in press)
32. Lin, Y., Sobis, H., Vandeputte, M., Waer, M. Induction therapy of leflunomide and cyclosporine allows for long-term xenograft survival under cyclosporine alone. Transplant. Proc. 26,3052,1994
33. Bartlett, RR, Brendel, S., Schorlemmer, H-U. Malononitriloamides, analogues of leflunomide's primary metabolite, prevent the development of murine systemic lupus erythematosis (SLE)-like diseases. Transplant. Proc. In press
34. Schorlemmer, H-U, Kurrle, R., Bartlett, RR. Effects of malononitriloamides on models of murine graft-versus-host (GVH) disease. Transplant. Proc. In press

35. Schorlemmer, H-U, Kurrle, R. Malononitriloamides (MNAs) control rejection of mouse-to-rat skin xenografts. Transplant. Proc. In press
36. Morris, RE, Huang, X., Cao, W., Zheng, B., Shorthouse, RA. Leflunomide (HWA 486) and its analog suppress T and B Cell proliferation in vitro, acute rejection, ongoing rejection, and antidonor antibody synthesis in mouse, rat, and cynomolgus monkey transplant recipients as well as arterial intimal thickening after balloon catheter injury. Transplant. Proc. 27,445,1995

VIII Genetic Engineering of the Xenograft Donor

47 Use of Transgenic Animals as Xenotransplant Donors

J.L. Platt and J.S. Logan

Introduction

One factor which has contributed to a recent surge in interest in xenotransplantation is the development of transgenic animals for use as xenotransplant donors. The development of these animals not only reflects a certain measure of technical advance, it also results from a rapid expansion of basic knowledge about the molecular hurdles to the xenotransplantation of organs from lower mammals into humans [1]. This chapter will review some of the ways in which genetic engineering can address the immunologic hurdles to xenotransplantation and in doing so further extend basic knowledge.

Use of Transgenic Animals To Modulate Expression of Antigens Recognized by Xenoreactive Antibodies

Hyperacute rejection of porcine organ by a primate is initiated by the binding to the graft of xenoreactive natural antibodies of the recipient leading to activation of the complement system. Most of the complement-fixing xenoreactive antibodies are of IgM isotype and are specific for Galα1–3Gal [2–4]. The synthesis of Galα1–3Gal is catalyzed by α1,3-galactosyltransferase which is expressed in functional form by lower animals such as pigs [5]. This enzyme adds galactose via an α-linkage to Galβ1–4GlcNAc-R to yield Galα1–3Galβ1–4GlcNAc-R. Humans, apes, and Old World monkeys do not have a functional α1,3-galactosyltransferase gene, but have two pseudogenes; these species make natural antibodies specific for Galα1–3Gal, whereas lower animals do not.

Some investigators have suggested that the α1,3-galactosyltransferase gene might eventually be disrupted by gene targeting [6]. However, gene targeting by homologous recombination in embryonic stem cells has not been possible in pigs due to the lack of an appropriate pluripotent embryonic stem cell. Sandrin and Hutchinson have suggested an alternative approach, the expression as the product of transgenes of other glycosyltransferases which would compete with α1,3-galactosyltransferase for synthesizing the terminus of oligosaccharide chains. For example, α1,2-fucosyltransferase (H transferase) utilizes Galβ1–4GlcNAc-R as does α1,3-galactosyltransferase; its expression in a cell might divert synthesis away from Galα1–3Galβ1–4GlcNAc to Fucα1,2Galβ1–4GlcNAc (H antigen). Studies in cultured cells and in transgenic mice suggest that this strategy is, in fact, effective – porcine and murine cells expressing human H transferase make substantially less Galα1–3Gal [7, 8]. We applied the same concept to the development of transgenic pigs, expressing H transferase under control of H-2Kb and chick β-actin promoters. Preliminary analysis of founder pigs demonstrates that a very significant decrease in expression of Galα1–3Gal has been achieved. The extent to which this approach actually decreases the binding of complement fixing xenoreactive antibodies to porcine cells and the implications for xenotransplantation remain to be tested; however, it seems not unlikely given the preliminary results that the method will be shown to decrease if not eliminate the humoral reactions initiated by natural antibodies.

Development of Transgenic Animals To Address the Susceptibility of a Transplant to Heterologous Complement

Activation of the complement system leads to deposition of C3 on the surfaces of foreign and autologous cells. The ability of complement to selectively mediate effector functions against foreign organisms and to spare host cells damage that might otherwise ensue depends on the functioning of complement regulatory proteins of which more than ten proteins have been described. For example, factor H, a 150-kDa plasma protein, inhibits the assembly of the alternative pathway C3 convertase on autologous cells, but fails to do so on many foreign cells, allowing the spontaneous hydrolysis of C3 and attachment to adjacent surfaces to bring about the assembly of alternative pathway C3 convertase on a foreign cell but inhibiting the assembly of this complex on autologous surfaces. So effective is the differential function of this protein that it may account for the explosive injury to a guinea pig organ transplanted into a rat while at the same time rat blood vessels remain inured to this process.

The activation of complement and complement-mediated injury to autologous cells is also inhibited by cell associated complement regulatory proteins. For example, decay-accelerating factor (DAF) is a 70-kDa phosphatidylinositol (PI)-linked cell membrane protein which forces the dissociation of C3 convertase complexes. Membrane cofactor protein, an integral component of cell membranes, serves as a cofactor for factor I mediated cleavage of C3b. CD59 (membrane inhibitor of reactive lysis) inhibits assembly of lytic complement complexes.

Most of the cell-associated complement regulatory proteins function more effectively against homologous complement than against heterologous complement. As a result, exposure of a cell to heterologous complement under a given set of conditions leads to far more damage and cell lysis than exposure to homologous complement under the same conditions. This type of specificity, called homologous restriction, discovered in the first decade of this century by Muir [9], is exploited in the design of cytotoxicity assays in which heterologous complement is used to achieve greater sensitivity than would be possible in an homologous system.

The idea of focusing on complement regulatory proteins as a potential hurdle to xenotransplantation was suggested by Miyagawa [10] and Dalmasso [11, 12]. The concept was that a xenograft would be more susceptible to complement-mediated injury than an allograft because the complement regulatory proteins expressed in the xenograft would fail to control activation of the recipient's complement system. One potential implication of this idea which the author suggested was that apart from the issue of xenoreactive antibodies and complement, which clearly are necessary for the hyperacute rejection of xenografts, perhaps the "incompatibility" of donor complement regulatory proteins might contribute an important, heretofore unrecognized step [13]. This later idea reflected the concept that in addition to rendering an organ more susceptible to complement-mediated injury, the complement regulatory proteins through their species specific functioning also contribute to immunorecognition.

Since hyperacute rejection occurs in homologous systems such as allografts in presensitized recipients, the availability of functioning regulatory proteins does not necessarily prevent its development. However, the failure of those proteins to function might, in the case of xenografts, convert a more benign lesion into the hyperacute rejection lesion. Until recently, the contribution of complement regulatory proteins to tissue homeostasis was poorly understood. While it was known that failure of the synthesis of DAF and CD59 on erythrocytes would lead to the clinical syndrome of paroxysmal nocturnal hemoglobinuria [14, 15], the role of complement regulatory molecules in protecting the nucleated cells comprising solid organs had yet to be shown. Recently, Matsuo took up this question in a rat model [16]. Administration of $F(ab')_2$ or Fab fragments of antibodies specific for rat homologue of DAF caused a rapid deposition of C3 on blood vessel walls, alteration in vascular tone and permeability and loss of leukocytes and platelets from the circulation. Further evidence for the importance of cell-associated complement regulatory proteins in protecting organs against complement mediated damage would emerge from studies in xenotransplantation.

Expression of Human Complement Regulatory Proteins in Heterologous Cells

The first experiments aimed at evaluating the potential importance of complement regulatory proteins in a xenogeneic model were carried out by Dalmasso [11]. DAF was isolated from human erythrocytes and, using a method adapted from Medof and coworkers [17], the protein was inserted through its PI anchor directly into the cell membrane of cultured porcine endothelial cells. Insertion of DAF into the endothelial cells caused dose-dependent inhibition of complement-mediated cytotoxicity and inhibition of iC3b-mediated neutrophil adhesion. Although isolation and insertion of DAF into endothelial cells might be carried out as an experimental procedure, it would probably be impractical as a clinical modality due to the large amounts of protein that would have to be isolated. In addition, the procedure would have to be carried out repeatedly because of the limited half-life of the extrinsically incorporated human protein. Thus it was suggested that the protein might be expressed as the product of a transgene [12].

As Dalmasso was carrying out his experiments, White and colleagues at Cambridge, U.K., began to test the ability of human DAF and membrane cofactor protein (MCP) to regulate the activation of human complement on heterologous cells [18]. Murine fibroblasts were transfected with human DAF or MCP. Cells expressing either protein were insensitive to lysis by human serum, whereas control transfectants were lysed as easily as nontransfected cells. Akami et al. [19] used a similar approach to study the protection that would be provided by introducing human CD59 into heterologous cells [20]. Expression of human CD59 by transfected murine cells effectively protected the cells from lysis by human serum [20]. Kennedy et al. used a retroviral vector to transfer human CD59cDNA to porcine endothelial cells [21]. The cells expressing CD59 exhibited resistance to lysis and to activation induced by the membrane attack complex. Other investigators transfected mouse cells with human DAF and MCP and demonstrated a protective effect against cell lysis by human complement [18, 22, 23]. The results of these studies in another system lent encouragement to the idea that human complement regulatory proteins might be used to control complement mediated injury in a xenogeneic organ. The next step would involve the introduction of human complement regulatory genes in mice.

Expression of Human Complement Regulatory Proteins in Transgenic Animals

Mice

To explore the concept of using human complement regulatory proteins to protect to protect a whole organ and to develop useful expression systems for such a purpose, various groups undertook the development of trangenic mice which would express these proteins. Using a modified version of the endogenous promoter of DAF to drive expression, Cary and White developed transgenic mice expressing human DAF in various tissues [24]. The lymphocytes of the transgenic mice were found to resist lysis by human complement. We developed transgenic mice expressing human DAF, CD59, and MCP using three modes of expression: (1) indirect expression using globin promoters, (2) direct expression using heterologous promoters, and (3) direct expression using modified homologous promoters [25–27]. Our experience is summarized below.

Kooyman used the human α-globin promoter, which yields erythroid-specific expression in pigs [28], to express human CD59 and DAF in transgenic mice [29]. As expected, the PI-linked proteins were expressed in murine erythrocytes. Surprisingly, the human proteins were also found on endothelial cells of murine heart, lung kidney and liver [25]. The mechanism mediating expression in parenchymal organs did not involve direct expression of the human proteins by murine cells as the murine tissues had no detectable RNA for these proteins. Rather, the PI-linked proteins were shown to transfer passively to endothelium [30]. The functional properties of the transferred protein were tested by McCurry [31]. When organs containing human DAF and CD59 expressed by the α-globin promoter were perfused with human plasma, the activation of complement at the level of C8/C9 was nearly completely inhibited; similar results were achieved when the organs were connected to baboons through an ex vivo circuit. The results provided the first evidence at the level at the whole organ that expression of human complement regulatory proteins might contribute to the control of complement. The observation that glycosylphosphatidylinositol (GPI)-linked proteins could transfer spontaneously from erythrocytes to endothelial cells also offers a novel approach which might be used to modify the composition of endothelial cell membranes.

Diamond used the control elements of the CD59 gene to drive expression of CD59 and other human proteins in transgenic animals [32]. The construct, a CD59 minigene, yielded widespread, but low-level constitutive expression of human genes in various parenchymal organs. Although the human genes were expressed at significantly lower levels than in human tissues, the organs from the transgenic mice exhibited significant ability to control activation of human and baboon complement [33].

Byrne used the chick β-actin promoter to control expression of CD59 and the H-2K promoter to control expression of DAF in transgenic mice [27]. Organs from the transgenic mice which expressed both of the human proteins exhibited resistance to the activation of human and baboon complement in ex vivo perfusion models [31].

These early experiments provided the first evidence that expression of human complement regulatory proteins in the blood vessels of lower animals might confer some protection against injury by human complement. How this approach might influence the biology of xenograft rejection remained to be analyzed. Recent experiments using pigs expressing this construct have shown that hyperacute rejection can be avoided with an overall outcome that is most encouraging.

Pigs

Testing whether the species specificity of complement regulatory proteins would actually contribute to the susceptibility of an organ to hyperacute rejection and whether this problem could be overcome by "genetic engineering" would require the development of transgenic pigs whose organs could be used for transplantation. The first successful effort to develop such animals was that of White and colleagues who developed transgenic pigs expressing human DAF under control of the DAF promoter [34]. Fodor et al. used the H-2K promoter to drive expression of CD59 in a transgenic pig [35]. In both systems, lymphocytes isolated from the transgenic pigs showed resistance to lysis by human complement.

Our own efforts allowed direct evaluation of a xenograft model. Using the erythroid-specific α-globin expression system, Kooyman and Martin developed transgenic pigs the erythrocytes of which expressed the human proteins at a level comparable to the level in human erythrocytes [25]. As in mice, the human proteins transferred spontaneously from the surface of erythrocytes to endothelium in various organs, although the level of expression of the human proteins in the tissues of the transgenic animals was considerably below the level observed in human organs. McCurry transplanted the hearts from three of these transgenic pigs into baboons [36]. In two cases the transplanted organs did not undergo hyperacute rejection but functioned for many hours. This result was achieved despite the only transient and low level expression of the proteins which could be achieved with this system. Also of import were the results of histologic studies which revealed that in all three cases the amount of tissue injury was markedly less than in xenografts of normal porcine hearts in unmodified baboons. Also of interest were the results of the immunopathology of these tissues which revealed the presence of the membrane attack complex in the grafts in which there was very significant protection against complement-mediated injury. This result is consistent with the concept that the kinetics of membrane attack complex formation rather than the total number of complexes formed determines the biological outcome [37, 38] and contrary to the simplistic idea that complement-mediated injury such that seen in hyperacute rejection is an obligatory outcome of membrane attack complex formation. The concept that it is the kinetics rather than absolute amount of membrane attack complex assembly that determines biological outcome probably also explains the observation that in ABO-incompatible allografts, hyperacute rejection usually does not occur, despite the deposition of significant amounts of membrane attack complex. Presumably, homologous complement regulatory proteins provide some, albeit incomplete, protection.

Transgenic pigs expressing CD59 alone under control of the CD59 minigene promoter expressed the human protein at a very low level (as few as 7000 molecules per cell) [33]. Nevertheless, the organs of these animals transplanted into baboons showed significant ability to control activation of baboon complement as deposits of the membrane attack complex were markedly decreased. Although some prolongation of graft function was observed the xenografts were still destroyed in a period of hours. These limited studies demonstrated that CD59 has a potent effect on the assembly of the membrane attack complex, but by itself this effect is probably insufficient to prevent some of the manifestations of complement-mediated injury particularly hyperacute rejection.

More recent studies using transgenic pigs expressing CD59 under control of the chick β-actin promoter and DAF under control of the H-2K promoter have yielded exciting initial results [39]. In all but one case studied so far, hyperacute rejection was not observed and the transgenic organs survived up to 3 days in otherwise unmodified recipients. The grafts from transgenic donors exhibited much less tissue injury than control grafts.

Comment

The results of our initial studies involving the transplantation of organs from pigs expressing human complement regulatory proteins suggested several conclusions which may be relevant to this field. First, the enduring survival of the xenografts despite the transient and low level of expression of human CD59 and DAF in these organs suggests that these proteins play a very important role in maintaining the integrity of a graft in the early post-transplant period. Given the importance of complement in mediating ischemia–reperfusion injury as well as hyperacute rejection, such a conclusion is not unexpected. However, the striking protection observed under these conditions suggests that the species specificity of the proteins is an important aspect of the susceptibility to hyperacute rejection and perhaps, as we conceive it [1], of immunorecognition. A second conclusion concerns our finding that the transgenic organ xenografts exhibited such protection even though significant amounts of complement, including C5b and the membrane attack complex, were deposited in the organ. This result is consistent with the idea that under conditions in which complement is activated in a graft, as for example in ABO-incompatible organ transplants, hyperacute rejection is not the invariable outcome and that intrinsic resistance to complement-mediated injury is indeed an important factor in avoiding hyperacute rejection. The third and in our view most important conclusion is that these results support a change in the approach to dealing with the hurdles to xenotransplantation. Clearly methods exist which allow therapy to be directed at the graft rather than at the recipient and to target with greater specificity the molecular basis of graft injury. Such a focus is ultimately bound to reduce at some of the complications of immunosuppression.

From the current vantage point we can anticipate further advances. We are now conducting studies using pigs expressing human complement regulatory proteins expressed permanently and at higher levels. The results which include much more effective and enduring interference with the complement cascade are correspondingly improved. Beyond this there will be animals whose organs resist other aspects of the rejection reaction.

Acknowledgments. Some of the work described in this paper was supported by grants from the National Institutes of Health (HL52297, HL50985 and Hl46810) and from Nextran, Princeton, N.J., USA.

References

1. Platt, J.L. Hyperacute Xenograft Rejection. R.G. Landes Company, Austin, 1995
2. Good, A.H., Cooper, D.K.C., Malcolm, A.J., et al. Identification of carbohydrate structures that bind human antiporcine antibodies: implications for discordant xenografting in humans. Transplant. Proc. 24, 559, 1992
3. Sandrin, M.S., Vaughan, H.A., Dabkowski, P.L.McKenzie, I.F.C. Anti-pig IgM antibodies in human serum react predominantly with Galα(1,3)Gal epitopes. Proc.Natl.Acad. Sci.USA 90, 11391, 1993
4. Collins, B.H., Parker, W.R.Platt, J.L. Characterization of porcine endothelial cell determinants recognized by human natural antibodies. Xenotransplantation 1, 36, 1994
5. Galili, U.Swanson, K. Gene sequences suggest inactivation of α-1,3-galactosyltransferase in catarrhines after the divergence of apes from monkeys. Proc.Natl.Acad.Sci.USA 88, 7401, 1991
6. Cooper, DKC., Good, AH., Koren, E., et al. Identification of α-galactosyl and other carbohydrate epitopes that are bound by human anti-pig antibodies: relevance to discordant xenografting in man. Transplant. Immunol. 1, 198, 1993
7. Sandrin, M.S., Fodor, W.L., Mouhtouris, E., et al. Enzymatic remodelling of the carbohydrate surface of a xenogeneic cell substantially reduces human antibody binding and complement-mediated cytolysis. Nature Med. 1, 1261, 1995

8. Sharma, A., Okabe, J.F., Birch, P., Platt, J.L.Logan, J.S. Expression of α1,2 fucosyltransferases in transgenic animals to reduce the number of Gal α1,3Gal epitopes. Proc. Natl.Acad.Sci.USA 93, 7190, 1996
9. Muir, R. On the relationships between the complements and immune-bodies of different animals. J.Path.Bact. 16, 523, 1911
10. Miyagawa, S., Hirose, H., Shirakura, R., et al. The mechanism of discordant xenograft rejection. Transplantation 46, 825, 1988
11. Dalmasso, A.P., Vercellotti, G.M., Platt, J.L.Bach, F.H. Inhibition of complement-mediated endothelial cell cytotoxicity by decay accelerating factor: Potential for prevention of xenograft hyperacute rejection. Transplantation 52, 530, 1991
12. Platt, J.L., Vercellotti, G.M., Dalmasso, A.P., et al. Transplantation of discordant xenografts: a review of progress. Immunol.Today 11, 450, 1990
13. Platt, J.L.Bach, F.H. The barrier to xenotransplantation. Transplantation 52, 937, 1991
14. Nicholson-Weller, A., March, J.P., Rosenfeld, S.I.Austen, F. Affected erythrocytes of patients with paroxysmal nocturnal hemoglobinuria are deficient in the complement regulatory protein, decay accelerating factor. Proc.Natl.Acad.Sci.USA 80, 5066, 1983
15. Pangburn, M.K., Schreiber, R.D.Muller-Eberhard, H.J. Deficiency of an erythrocyte membrane protein with complement regulatory activity in paroxysmal nocturnal hemoglobinuria. Proc.Natl.Acad.Sci.USA 80, 5430, 1983
16. Matsuo, S., Ichida, S., Takizawa, H., et al. In vivo effects of monoclonal antibodies that functionally inhibit complement regulatory proteins in rats. J.Exp.Med. 180, 1619, 1994
17. Medof, M.E., Kinoshita, T.Nussenzweig, V. Inhibition of complement activation on the surface of cells after incorporation of decay-accelerating factor (DAF) into their membranes. J.Exp.Med. 160, 1558, 1984
18. White, D.J.G., Oglesby, T., Liszewski, M.K., et al. Expression of human decay accelerating factor or membrane cofactor protein genes on mouse cells inhibits lysis by human complement. Transpl.Proc. 24, 474, 1992
19. Walsh, L.A., Tone, M.Waldmann, H. Transfection of human CD59 complementary DNA into rat cells confers resistance to human complement. Eur.J.Immunol. 21, 847, 1991
20. Akami, T., Sawada, R., Minato, N., et al. Cytoprotective effect of CD59 antigen on xenotransplantation immunity. Transplant Proc 24, 485, 1992
21. Kennedy, S.P., Rollins, S.A., Burton, W.V., et al. Protection of porcine aortic endothelial cells from complement-mediated cell lysis and activation by recombinant human CD59. Transplantation 57, 1494, 1994
22. Atkinson, J.P., Oglesby, T.J., White, D., Adams, E.A.Liszewski, M.K. Separation of self from non-self in the complement system: a role for membrane cofactor protein and decay accelerating factor. Clin.Exp.Immunol. 86 (Supp. 1), 27, 1991
23. Oglesby, T.J., Allen, C.J., Liszewski, M.K., White, D.J.G.Atkinson, J.P. Membrane cofactor protein (CD46) protects cells from complement-mediated attack by an intrinsic mechanism. J.Exp.Med. 175, 1547, 1992
24. Cary, N., Moody, J., Yannoutsos, N., Wallwork, J.White, D. Tissue expression of human decay accelerating factor, a regulator of complemenent activation expressed in mice: a potential approach to inhibition of hyperacute xenograft rejection. Transplant. Proc. 25, 400, 1993
25. Kooyman, D.L., Byrne, G.W., McClellan, S., et al. In vivo transfer of GPI-linked complement restriction factors from erythrocytes to the endothelium. Science 269, 89, 1995

26. Diamond, L.E., McCurry, K.R., Platt, J.L., et al. A human CD59 expressed in transgenic mousehearts inhibits activation of complement biologically functional complement regulatory protein in transgenic mice. Transplant Immunol 3, 305, 1995
27. Byrne, G.W., McCurry, K.R., Kagan, D., et al. Protection of xenogenic endothelium from human complement by expression of CD59 or DAF in transgenic mice. Transplantation 60, 1149, 1995
28. Logan, J.S.Martin, M.J. Transgenic swine as a recombinant production system for human hemoglobin. Methods Enzymol. 231, 435, 1994
29. Kooyman, D., Byrne, G.W., McClellan, S., et al. Erythroid-specific expression of human CD59 and transfer to vascular endothelial cells. Transplant. Proc. 26, 1241, 1994
30. Kagan, D.T., Platt, J.L., Logan, J.S.Byrne, G.W. Expression of complement regulatory factors using heterologous promoters in transgenic mice. Transplant. Proc. 26, 1242, 1994
31. McCurry, K.R., Kooyman, D.L., Diamond, L., et al. Transgenic expression of human complement regulatory proteins in mice results in diminished complement deposition during organ xenoperfusion. Transplantation 59, 1177, 1995
32. Diamond, L.E., Oldham, E.R., Platt, J.L., et al. Cell and tissue specific expression of a human CD59 minigene in transgenic mice. Transplant. Proc. 26, 1239, 1994
33. Diamond, L.E., McCurry, K.R., Oldham, E.R., et al. Characterization of transgenic pigs expressing functionally active human CD59 on cardiac endothelium. Transplantation 61, 1241, 1996
34. Rosengard, A.M., Cary, N.R.B., Langford, G.A., et al. Tissue expression of human complement inhibitor, decay-accelerating factor, in transgenic pigs. Transplantation 59, 1325, 1995
35. Fodor, W.L., Williams, B.L., Matis, L.A., et al. Expression of a functional human complement inhibitor in a transgenic pig as a model for the prevention of xenogeneic hyperacute organ rejection. Proc.Natl.Acad.Sci.USA 91, 11153, 1994
36. McCurry, K.R., Kooyman, D.L., Alvarado, C.G., et al. Human complement regulatory proteins protect swine-to-primate cadriac xenografts from humoral injury. Nature Med. 1, 423, 1995
37. Shin, M.L.Carney, D.F. Cytotoxic action and other metabolic consequences of terminal complement proteins. Prog.in Allergy 40, 44, 1988
38. Morgan, B.P. Complement membrane attack on nucleated cells: resistance, recovery and non-lethal effects. Biochem.J. 264, 1, 1989
39. Byrne, G.W., McCurry, K.R., Martin, M.J., et al. Expression of human CD59 and DAF in transgenic pigs: intrinsic regulation of complement activity. Submitted 1995

48 Engineering of Xenografts To Provide Organs for Human Transplantation

S.P. Squinto and W.L. Fodor

Clinical Need for Organs

Transplantation is clearly the treatment of choice for most patients suffering from end-stage organ failure. Significant progress in clinical allotransplantation has been achieved during the past decade. These pharmacological and surgical achievements have resulted in higher survival rates for the organ grafts as well as improved patient survival and quality of life. Additionally, organ transplantation provides significant cost-savings for the health care system in the treatment of patients with severe and debilitating diseases. For example, it has been projected that the broader use of kidney transplantation instead of dialysis could save the United States Federal Government $2 billion annually. The profound medical benefits as well as the potential cost-savings and public benefit of the advances made in allogeneic transplantation have been severely limited, however, by a persistent and serious problem - severe shortage of donor organs.

Many initiatives have been introduced to increase the donor organ supply, including publicity campaigns, distribution of donor cards, appointment of hospital-based transplant coordinators, implementation of procurement protocols and educational programs for hospital personnel. Although these factors have helped to increase donor availability, they have not been sufficient to significantly increase the donor supply. As a result, most patients who would benefit from organ transplantation do not even appear on a waiting list. The current need for organ transplantation is conservatively estimated to be at least 90 000 solid organ transplantations per year in the United States alone.

Genetically Engineered Xenografts – A Potential Solution to the Organ Shortage Problem

The serious shortage of human organs available for transplantation has created an intense search for alternative sources of suitable organs. Recent attention to the topic of animal-to-human transplantation has led to public awareness through newspaper articles, television exposure, and news-format magazines. Published public opinion surveys have revealed that individuals, when confronted with the potential loss of their own life, would generally accept a xenogeneic organ.

Therefore, we have developed a rational strategy to address the severe organ shortage problem which centers around the development of genetically engineered animals as organ donors. Among the species considered as potential donors of xenogeneic organs, the major interest has focused on the pig. This is due to several advantageous qualities, including large litter size, age of sexual maturity, disease resistance, domestication, and, most importantly, striking similarities between swine and human organ size and physiology [1]. Also, unlike primates, over 90 million pigs are already killed annually as a food source, making these animals an ethically acceptable alternative donor organ source.

Here we describe the development of transgenic pigs engineered to express human genes aimed at eliminating the human immune response to the foreign xenograft. Our research goals have been focused on achieving long-term survival of genetically engineered pig organs following transplantation in Old World primate model systems. If successful, the clinical transplantation of these engineered organs into humans can be anticipated.

Pig-to-Primate Transplantation

Immunological Barrier

The major barrier to xenogeneic transplantation is the phenomenon of hyperacute rejection (HAR). Studies of the immunological response to xenotransplanted tissue have shown that these transplants inexorably fail due to HAR [2, 3] (Chap. 2). The hyperacute response is triggered by the deposition of preformed recipient antibodies on the surface of the donor endothelium resulting in the subsequent activation of the classical pathway of the complement system [2]. Therefore, following transplantation of a vascularized xenogeneic donor pig organ into a primate recipient, the massive inflammatory response that ensues from natural antibody activation of the classical complement cascade leads to the activation and destruction of the vascular endothelial cells and ultimately of the donor organ within minutes to hours after revascularization.

Old World primates, including humans, have high levels of preexisting circulating "natural" antibodies that predominantly recognize carbohydrate determinants expressed on the surface of xenogeneic cells from discordant species [4] (Chap. 4). Evidence indicates that most, if not all, of these antibodies react with the carbohydrate epitope Galα1–3Gal (αGal), an epitope absent from Old World primates because of a lack of the functional α1,3-galactosyltransferase enzyme [5, 6]. The levels of these naturally circulating anti-αGal antibodies are approximately 1% of all the antibody in any given individual. The high titer of these antibodies is believed to arise from constant stimulation of the immune system to this epitope through naturally occurring infections, and from stimulation from the natural flora and fauna in the gastrointestinal tract. In studies of in vivo animal model systems aimed at assessing HAR, within 15 min of revascularization xenoreactive antibodies are deposited on the surface of the donor endothelium [2].

The result of antibody deposition is the subsequent activation of serum complement proteins. Activation of the complement cascade results in the deposition of complement at the site of antibody reactivity, i.e., the xenogeneic vascular endothelium. Following complement activation there is significant aggregation and adhesion of platelets to the damaged endothelium as well as formation of microthrombi and the migration of neutrophils and granulocytes into the interstitium [2]. Ultimately, endothelial cells are destroyed which results in tissue ischemia and necrosis of the donor organ. Additional detrimental effects of antibody deposition include the antibody-dependent cellular effects that arise from Fc receptor-bearing cells interacting with deposited antibodies, resulting in acute vasculitis and vessel occlusion. Therefore, any strategy aimed at the successful transplantation of xenografts into humans must aim to abrogate the binding of preformed human antibodies to the xenograft as well as provide for protection against activated human complement proteins.

Solution to the Immunological Challenge

The problem of natural antibody reactivity and subsequent complement activation that occurs during xenogeneic organ transplantation in the pig-to-primate model has prompted the development of several strategies aimed at preventing natural anti-αGal antibody reactivity and of inhibiting human complement. Most of these efforts to prevent HAR have focused on modifying the immune system of the host. For example, strategies for prolonging discordant xenograft survival have included depletion of the naturally occurring xenoreactive antibodies with plasma exchange, plasmapheresis, or donor organ absorption (Chaps. 25 and 26), and inhibition of complement with either cobra venom factor or soluble complement receptor type 1 [7, 8] (Chaps. 32 and 33). Other groups are proposing to treat patients with suprapharmacologic doses of antibody-binding carbohydrates potentially in combination with splenectomy [9] (Chap. 25). These approaches to block antibody-induced HAR have the following critical drawbacks and, therefore, make them clinically unattractive: (a) they only transiently reduce antibody titer, (b) they do not prevent rebound production of organ-binding antibodies, (c) they may result in globally decreased and compromised immune function, and (d) they could potentially result in increased susceptibility of the host to infection.

Rather than developing systemic immunosuppressive approaches to abrogating HAR, we and others have chosen to take advantage of an opportunity unique to xenotransplantation, that is the ability to genetically modify the donor organ. One such strategy employed by us and others has been to achieve high level expression of species-restricted human complement inhibitor proteins in vascularized pig organs via transgenic engineering [10–12]. We have demonstrated expression of the human complement inhibitor protein CD59 in several tissues of a transgenic pig, including the vascular endothelium, and showed that cells from this animal are resistant to human complement-mediated lysis in vitro [10]. Recently, we have conducted experiments that demonstrate the efficacy of high-level human CD59 vascular expression in the transgenic organ when the organ is perfused ex vivo with human blood [13] and transplanted either heterotopically (heart) or orthotopically (heart and lung) into Old World primates. Although prolonged survival was observed, incomplete protection resulted in the eventual rejection of the organ within hours to several days after transplantation. Non-transgenic control pig organs were typically hyperacutely rejected within 1–2 h after transplantation. As observed in these experiments and also with systemic complement depletion, organ failure appears to be related to an acute antibody-dependant vasculitis.

Another engineering strategy that has been proposed aims to eliminate the αGal epitope from the donor xenograft. However, unlike the successful expression of human complement inhibitor proteins in transgenic pigs, this strategy has been largely theoretical to-date. That is, the generation of αGal-negative pigs might be accomplished by disrupting the porcine α1,3-galactosyltransferase gene via homologous recombination. However, this approach requires the availability of porcine embryonic stem cells, which makes it currently impractical.

We chose to develop a strategy to downregulate the expression of the αGal epitope in porcine xenografts that would have a practical application toward the generation of αGal-deficient transgenic pigs. Our strategy takes advantage of an intracellular competition between the α1,3-galactosyltransferase (αGT) and the α1,2-fucosyltransferase (H transferase). We demonstrated that these enzymes can be co-expressed within a porcine cell and transgenically in mouse tissues and organs, and that the H transferase is dominant over the αGT [14] (Chap. 50). The result of this enzyme competition is a remodeling of carbohydrate structures on the cell surface of the xenograft such that the non-immunogenic H epitope (the product of the H transferase reaction) substitutes for the expression of the xenoreactive αGal epitope (the product of the αGT). The H transferase carbohydrate product, the H epitope, corresponds to the universal donor blood group O antigen. Therefore, our engineering strategy serves two purposes, elimination of the predominant xenoreactive epitope and concomitant replacement with a universally accepted antigen. Consequently, cells expressing the H epitope in place of the αGal epitope are no longer targets for human natural antibody binding and are significantly resistant to HAR.

In addition to developing a practical approach to downregulating the xenoreactive carbohydrate residues on the porcine graft, we have also developed a novel and robust approach to blocking human complement attack on the xenograft. Our data [10] and the results of others [11] have suggested that long-term xenograft survival will most likely require both the downregulation of the αGal residue as well as the expression of multiple human complement inhibitor proteins. The technical difficulties associated with engineering multiple complement inhibitors to be expressed on the vascular endothelium of a transgenic animal are substantial.

To overcome this problem, we have utilized genetic engineering approaches to develop a potent bifunctional novel complement inhibitor, termed DC, to block complement at two distinct points in the complement cascade. The DC molecule contains functional domains from decay-accelerating factor (DAF), a C3/C5 convertase inhibitor, and CD59, a terminal complement inhibitor [12]. In vitro experiments demonstrate that the DC molecule inhibits complement-mediated cell lysis when challenged with human serum, and that it retains both DAF and CD59 function. The development of the DC complement inhibitor, and the subsequent demonstration that it retains the activity of both the terminal complement inhibitor, CD59, and the human C3 convertase inhibitor, DAF (CD55), permits the development of a single transgenic animal which otherwise would require a double transgenic expressing two complement inhibitor genes in the appropriate tissues at sufficiently high levels. Recently, we have been successful in generating transgenic mice that express high levels of the DC inhibitor. The generation of DC transgenic pigs is in progress.

Achieving high-level cell surface expression of the DC bifunctional chimeric complement inhibitor and high-level expression of the H transferase enzyme in vascular endothelium of the pig organ will effectively eliminate both the antibody and complement components of the massive inflammatory response to the xenograft. The combination of the novel strategies discussed here provides a rational approach to the elimination of HAR and represents a critical first step toward making animal organ xenotransplantation a viable alternative to genetically matched human organ allotransplantation.

Comment

Elimination of HAR will establish inroads into understanding the cellular immune response towards the discordant tissue. Hypothetically, it is conceivable that immunosuppressive regimens that are routinely practiced with allotransplantation will also be effective drug therapies for xenotransplantation. Therefore, it is critical to develop a system that tests these possibilities in order to solve the ever-growing need for donor organs.

References

1. COZZI, E., WHITE, D.J.G. The generation of transgenic pigs as potential organ donors for pigs. Nature. Med. 1:964, 1995
2. PLATT, J.L., LINDMAN, B.J., CHEN, H., SPITALNIK, S., BACH, F. Endothelial antigens recognized by xenoreactive antibodies. Transplantation. 50:817, 1990
3. COMMERVILLE, C.A., D'APICE, A.J.F. Future directions in transplantation: xenotransplantation. Kidney Int. 44(suppl. 42):S112, 1993
4. ORIOL, R., YE, Y., KOREN, E., COOPER, D.K.C. Carbohydrate antigens of pig tissues reacting with human natural antibodies as potential targets for hyperacute rejection in pig-to-man xenotransplantation. Transplantation. 56:1433, 1993
5. LARSEN, R.D., RIVERRA-MARRERO, C.A., ERNST, L.K., CUMMINGS, R.D., LOWE, J.B. Frameshift and nonsense mutations in a human genomic sequence homologous to a murine UDP-Galβ Gal1,4-D-GlcNAcα1,3-galactosyltransferase cDNA. J. Biol. Chem. 265:7055, 1990
6. SANDRIN, M.S., VAUGHAN, H.A., McKENZIE, I.F.C. Identification of Galα(1–3)Gal as the major epitope for pig-to-human vascularized xenografts. Transplant. Rev. 8:134, 1994
7. LEVENTHAL, J.R., DALMASSO, A.P., CROMWELL, J.W., et al. Prolongation of cardiac xenograft survival by depletion of complement. Transplantation. 55:857, 1993
8. PRUITT, S.K., KIRK, A.D., BOLLINGER, R.R., et al. The effect of soluble complement receptor type 1 on hyperacute rejection of porcine xenografts. Transplantation. 57:363, 1994

9. COOPER, D.K.C., KOREN, E., ORIOL, R. Oligosaccharides and discordant xenotransplantation. Immunol. Rev. 141:31, 1994
10. FODOR, W.L., WILLIAMS, B.L., MATIS, L.A., et al. Expression of a functional human complement inhibitor in a transgenic pig as a model for the prevention of xenogeneic hyperacute organ rejection. Proc. Natl. Acad. Sci. USA. 91:11153, 1994
11. McCURRY, K.R., KOOYMAN, D.L., ALVARADO, C.G., et al. Human complement regulatory proteins protect swine-to-primate cardiac xenografts from humoral injury. Nature. Med. 1:423, 1995
12. FODOR, W.L., SQUINTO, S.P. Engineering of transgenic pigs for xenogeneic organ transplantation. Xeno. 3:23, 1995
13. KROSHUS, T.J., BOLMAN, R.M. III, DALMASSO, A.P., et al. Expression of human CD59 in transgenic pig organs enhances survival in an ex vivo xenogeneic perfusion model. Transplantation. In press
14. SANDRIN, M.S., FODOR, W.L., MOUHTOURIS, E., et al. Enzymatic remodelling of the carbohydrate surface of a xenogeneic cell substantially reduces human antibody binding and complement-mediated cytolysis. Nature. Med. 1:1261, 1995

49 Effect of Transgenic Expression of Human Decay-Accelerating Factor on the Inhibition of Hyperacute Rejection of Pig Organs

E. Cozzi, N. Yannoutsos, G.A. Langford, G. Pino-Chavez, J.Wallwork, and D.J.G. White

Introduction

Clinical xenotransplantation utilizing pig organs represents, in theory, a very attractive solution to the worldwide shortage of organs for human transplantation. The use of pigs as organ donors has several advantages over the choice of any other species [1]. The pig has a short gestation period, it produces large litters and its offspring grow very rapidly. Utilization of pigs would also eliminate the ethical and virological concerns associated with the use of organs from nonhuman primates [2]. However, hyperacute rejection (HAR), which occurs when transplanting between discordant xeno combinations, currently represents the major immunological barrier to the survival of pig organs into primates [3–5]. The binding of naturally occurring cytotoxic xenoreactive antibodies (XNA) mainly directed to the carbohydrate structure Galα1–3Galß1–4GlcNAc-R [6–8] on porcine endothelial cells and the activation of the recipient's complement cascade represent the sequence of immunological events which underlie HAR [5, 9, 10].

Recent advances in the field of biomolecular engineering have led to the opportunity to produce genetically modified animals expressing new characteristics which make their tissues biologically more compatible with humans and potentially suitable for clinical xenotransplantation [11]. The challenging hypothesis of constructing transgenic animals as a source of unlimited numbers of organs for transplanting into humans has represented the beginning of a new era for transplant immunology. In this regard, research in the field has essentially moved in two main directions. Some scientists have focused their efforts in attempts to alter the antigenic profile of pig cells, mainly by deleting or reducing the expression of the Galα1–3Galß1–4GlcNAc-R epitope, which is known to constitute the main immunological target of XNA [12–14].

Although encouraging results have been obtained by using this approach, the work is limited for two main reasons. Firstly, the genetic modification would only affect the naturally present xenoreactive immune response directed to the Galα1–3Galß1–4GlcNAc-R residue. Although this certainly represents the main immunogenic determinant expressed by pig cells, it is probably not the only one. Secondly, this approach does not take into account the detrimental effects to the xenograft resulting from activation of the alternative pathway of complement. Such activation has been shown to occur in the pig-to-human xenocombination [4, 15].

As a result of these considerations, other researchers, including ourselves, have attempted to overcome HAR using a totally different strategy which is based on the down-regulation of the recipient's complement cascade. This approach arose from a series of fundamental observations in animal models which clearly showed the pivotal role played by complement activation in the onset of HAR [5]. Indeed, the revascularization of the xenograft is generally accompanied by a reduction of the circulating complement factors in the blood [16, 17]. Similarly, a massive and early deposition in the xenograft of complement components is a consistent finding in HAR [16]. Xenograft rejection is delayed in animals congenitally deficient of some factors of the complement cascade [18, 19]. Moreover, xenograft survival is prolonged if complement activity is prevented by the use of cobra venom factor [20, 21], soluble complement receptor 1 [22], the utilization of anticomplement agents such as FUT-175 [23] or monoclonal antibodies directed to complement factors such as C5 or C8 [24, 25].

In humans, complement activation is finely downregulated by the existence of a series of species-specific proteins called regulators of complement activity (RCA) [26, 27]. Some of these proteins, such as decay-accelerating factor (DAF), membrane cofactor protein (MCP), and CD59 are membrane-bound and protect human cells from lysis deriving from complement activation on their surface. In patients with paroxysmal nocturnal hemoglobinuria (PNH), the deficiency of two of these molecules on the surface of human erythrocytes increases the sensitivity of these blood cells to autologous complement-mediated lysis. Considered together, these observations led us and others to hypothesize that expression of human RCA on pig cells could prevent their lysis as a result of human complement activation and thus potentially protect the xenograft from HAR [3, 28].

The validity of this approach was first investigated in vitro by expressing human RCA on porcine or murine cells. In one series of experiments, DAF was chemically isolated from human erythrocyte membranes and passively incorporated into porcine endothelial cells [3]. The functional activity of human DAF (HDAF) expressed by these cells was subsequently assessed by in vitro cytotoxicity assays using human serum as a source of complement. These studies demonstrated that expression of HDAF on pig endothelial cells could reduce the complement-mediated cytotoxicity by more than 80 %.

Experiments performed in our laboratories were aimed at expressing human RCA on nonhuman mammalian cells by genetic manipulation of the target cell [28]. Relying on the evidence that human chromosome 1 contains the sequences for several RCA, Wang et al. produced a mouse/human hybrid cell line expressing DAF. This cell line was obtained by fusion of a human B lymphoblastoid line with mouse myeloma cells and was found to have incorporated human chromosome 1. Expression of DAF on the surface of these cells was detected by fluorescence-activated cell sorter (FACS) analysis. Chromium release assays showed that these cells were protected from lysis by human complement. Specificity of the protection conferred to these lines by the expression of DAF was confirmed by blocking experiments using monoclonal antibodies. In a series of elegant in vitro studies, murine fibroblasts were transfected with DAF and MCP cDNA [29]. FACS analysis showed the expression of DAF and MCP on the surface of these cells. These proteins conferred protection against lysis from human complement in a specific fashion. These experiments demonstrated that, following appropriate genetic manipulation, it is possible to transfer the protective capacity of these species-restricted human molecules to the surface of nonhuman cells. All the above studies supported the hypothesis that expression of human RCA by transgenic pig organs could potentially protect them from the onset of HAR.

In contrast to those genetic manipulations aimed at reducing the expression of Galα1-3Galß1-4GlcNAc-R residues, the present approach should offer the advantage of conferring protection to the xenograft from humoral aggression regardless of the specificity of the XNA involved. In addition, the use of human RCA should also protect the organs from any damage resulting from the activation of the complement cascade via the alternative pathway. In the light of these promising data, we started a genetic manipulation program aimed at producing transgenic pig organs expressing large amounts of human RCA and thus resistant to the human complement activation-mediated attack and possibly to HAR.

Production of Transgenic Animals

The technology for the production of transgenic animals has now been available for more than 10 years. The microinjection of DNA directly into the pronucleus of a fertilized egg currently represents one of the most commonly used techniques to produce transgenic pigs and mice. In the production of these animals it is evident that the microinjected DNA construct is one of the key elements which determines the outcome of the genetic manipulation. In nature, the expression of a gene is dependent on its genomic integrity both in terms of intronic and exonic sequences and of its regulatory elements [30, 31]. These include locus control regions (LCR), promoters, enhancers, and intronic sequences. These regulatory regions are known to control the spatial and temporal expression of a gene and its expression in response to extracellular stimuli.

The central role of the LCR as a regulatory element has recently been illustrated in transgenic mice obtained by microinjection of constructs containing the LCR of the gene of interest. In contrast to the previous observations in transgenic models developed using minigene constructs, the level of expression of the transgene in these animals was independent of its site of integration into the recipient's genome but was related to the number of copies of the gene integrated [32]. In this context, transgenic mice were produced by microinjection of a construct in which the LCR region was inserted upstream of the human globin gene [33]. High levels of expression of the transgene were detected in erythroid cells. Expression of the globin gene was enhanced and all the animals which had incorporated intact copies of the transgene expressed human globin RNA.

In contrast, it was found that 30 %–70 % of transgenic mice produced using an alternative globin transgenic construct *not* containing the LCR did not express the transgene. While the LCR are generally considered to be located within 20–30 kb 5′ or 3′ of the gene, the promoters are directly upstream of the DNA sequence, usually within several hundred base pairs from the start of the coding sequence of the gene [30, 31, 34]. Conversely, enhancers can be located at a much greater distance than the promoter, either upstream or downstream of the gene.

It is therefore evident that the production of transgenic animals which express transgenic proteins with patterns similar to those observed in humans, theoretically requires the whole genomic sequence of the gene together with both these 3′ and 5′ sequences. It is estimated that the total exon-intron genomic length of each of the three major membrane-bound human RCAs is dispersed over a 45- to 50-kb area [35–37]. This ultimately implies that a transgene for any of these RCAs which contains both the entire gene and the appropriate regulatory elements should cover an area of approximately 80–90 kb (Fig. 1). Until recently, limitations of the techniques available have prevented the manipulation of genomic DNA sequences of this size. This was mainly due to the fact that the plasmid and cosmid vectors, which were the two main vehicles available to handle DNA elements, could not carry DNA sequences greater than 40–45 kb. These vectors were, therefore, clearly inadequate for the manipulation of the large stretches of DNA which we were interested in.

For this reason, most groups involved in the production of transgenic animals microinjected cDNA or minigene constructs which contained the cDNA sequences and some genomic DNA of interest. Experiments rapidly showed that the use of cDNA alone for the production of transgenic animals was generally not satisfactory [38]. It was found that a strong homologous or heterologous promoter and some intronic sequences are necessary for expression of the transgene since they increase both the level and the stability of its expression [39].

The production of transgenic animals using minigene constructs does have several advantages. These constructs are relatively quick to produce and, due to their small size, they are easy to manipulate. Moreover, following microinjection, minigenes readily incorporate into the host genome. As we will discuss later in this chapter, we have been able to use a minigene for HDAF to produce both transgenic mice and pigs which express significant levels of HDAF in all of their organs.

However, there are two major disadvantages associated with the production of animals utilizing these constructs. Firstly, as a result of the absence of the control elements which naturally regulate the levels of expression of the gene in humans, expression of the transgene is dependent on the site at which it integrates into the recipient's genome [34, 40]. Thus, if the minigene incorporates into an inactive chromosomal locus of the host's genome, it will never be expressed. Secondly, some minigene constructs do not code for all the mRNA splice variants that are coded for by the entire gene. It is well known, for instance, that several different protein isoforms of MCP naturally arise due to alternative splicing of MCP RNA [41, 42]. The two prevalent forms of MCP so far described have a molecular weight of 56 and 66 kOa, respectively. The advantage of expressing one isoform rather than the other has yet to be established. However, it is likely that most cDNA minigenes for this RCA will only code for one of the two isoforms of the protein.

One possible solution to this problem is represented by the use of new constructs such as P1 artificial chromosomes (PAC) and yeast artificial chromosomes (YAC), which can carry foreign DNA sequences with sizes ranging between 50 and more than 1000 kb [43, 44]. The genomic sequences incorporated into these constructs should contain all the transcription regulatory elements required for proper spatial and temporal expression and the appropriate splice donor and acceptor sites which are needed to generate the complete spectrum of alternatively spliced transcript.

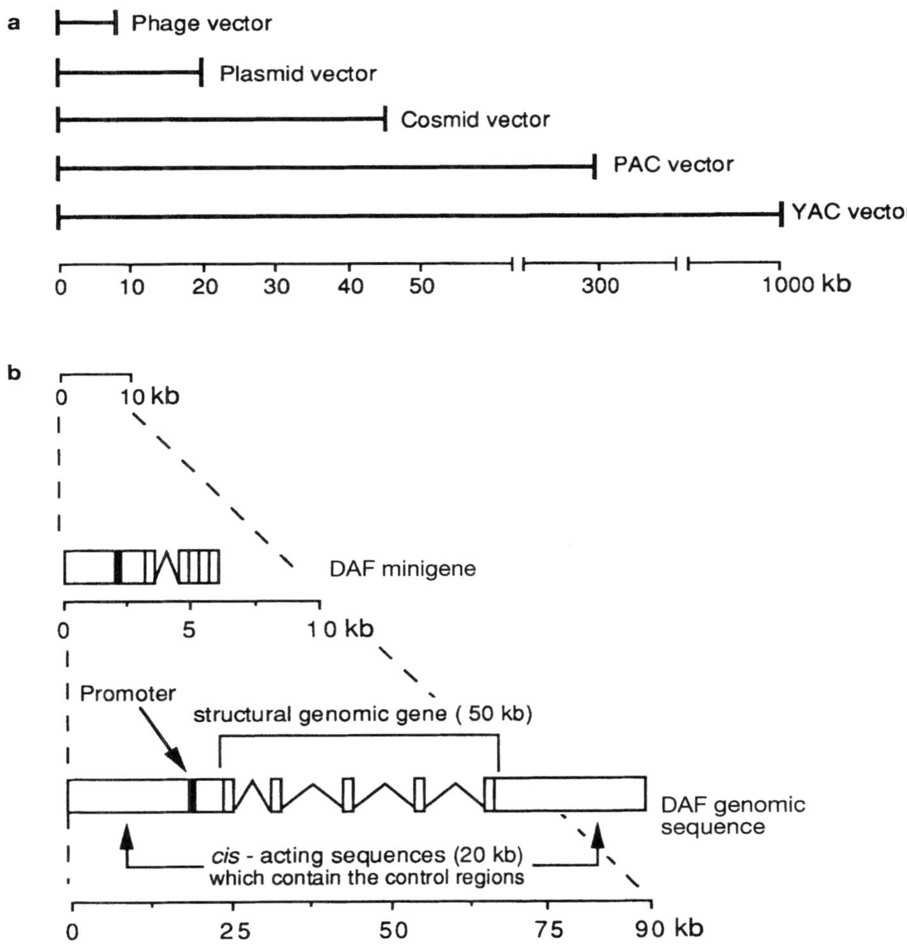

Fig. 1a,b. Preparation of DNA constructs for microinjection. **a** Most common expression vectors available for the transfer of genomic sequences. Represented is the maximum size of the DNA elements that each of these vectors can carry. *PAC*, P1 artificial chromosomes; *YAC*, yeast artificial chromosomes. **b** Human decay-accelerating factor (*DAF*) genomic sequence and human DAF minigene as used in the production of the transgenic pigs presented in this study. Note that the exon–intron genomic sequences are dispersed over a 45- to 50-kb area between the two *cis*-acting sequences which contain the control regions. To date, only plasmid and cosmid vectors able to carry DNA sequences of up to 45 kb have been available. For this reason, most constructs used so far contained cDNA sequences of the gene of interest and were missing most of the regulatory elements located at the 5′ or 3′ extremities of the gene

The first transgenic mice and pig lines carrying YACs for the MCP gene have been produced [45]. In addition, DAF YAC mice and pigs have also been obtained. Preliminary data have already shown that these animals contain the entire gene and that the gene is transcriptionally fully active. However, it must be pointed out that there are several difficulties surrounding the use of YAC constructs [45]. As a result of their large size, which can be 1000 kb or more, YAC DNA are more difficult to manipulate than minigenes. They are very susceptible to shearing during their preparation; thus methods are currently being developed in our laboratories to make the DNA more resistant to any damage. In addition, there are two further disadvantages associated with the use of YAC constructs:(1) some YAC libraries contain a high percentage of chimeric clones, which contain DNA from two or more different parts of the genome, and (2) some regions of the genome are unclonable or unstable and can be lost from the YAC. It is hoped that some of the problems associated with the utilization of YACs will be overcome with the recent introduction of the PAC technology [44]. Since PAC vectors are able to carry fragments of foreign DNA of up to 300 kb, it is expected that some PAC clones will be able to carry fragments of DNA as large as those containing the entire RCA gene and its 5′ and 3′ flanking regulatory sequences.

Production of Pigs Transgenic for Human Decay-Accelerating Factor

A 6.5-kb construct was prepared using approximately 4.3 kb of a HDAF genomic DNA sequence containing the 5′ untranslated region, the signal peptide, the first exon and intron of the gene. This fragment was linked to a cDNA fragment that coded for the remaining exons of the DAF gene and to 41 adenosines which constituted the mRNA poly-A tail. Pronuclear stage pig embryos were collected surgically from the oviducts of inseminated gilts superovulated with a regime of pregnant mare's serum gonadotrophin (PMSG) and human chorionic gonadotrophin (HCG). Using differential interference contrast optics (Nomarski microscopy), pronuclei were visualized within the stratified cytoplasm and the male pronucleus was injected with the DAF minigene construct. DNA was injected until the diameter of the ovum had increased by approximately 50% in size. Injected ova were transferred to both oviducts of recipient gilts, whose estrous cycles were either synchronous with or 24 h behind those of the donors.

Forty-nine gilts farrowed and 311 piglets were subsequently born. Forty-nine transgenic pigs were identified by dot blot analysis, using DNA isolated from ear biopsy samples. Slot-blot analysis of genomic DNA isolated from the liver, lung, kidney, spleen and heart of a founder transgenic pig killed during the course of the work indicated that the transgene was present in all of these tissues. Analysis of mRNA isolated from different tissues of transgenic animals showed that HDAF mRNA was present in all the organs (Fig. 2).

Expression of HDAF protein was subsequently investigated in the different tissues from 30 lines of transgenic pigs. The analysis was performed by double determinant radioimmunoassay using lysates from seven organs or tissues (heart, lung, liver, pancreas, kidney, small bowel, and muscle). Measurable levels

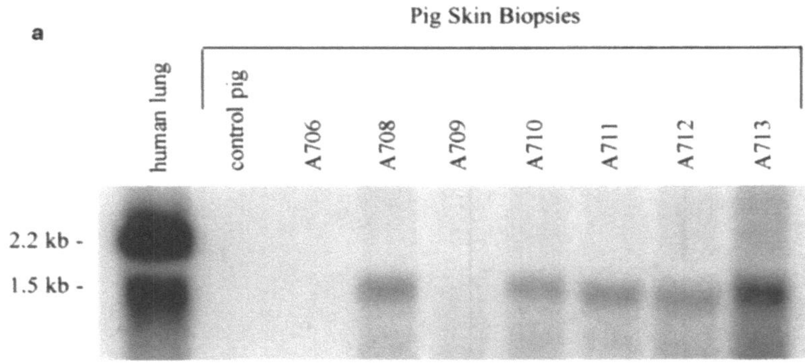

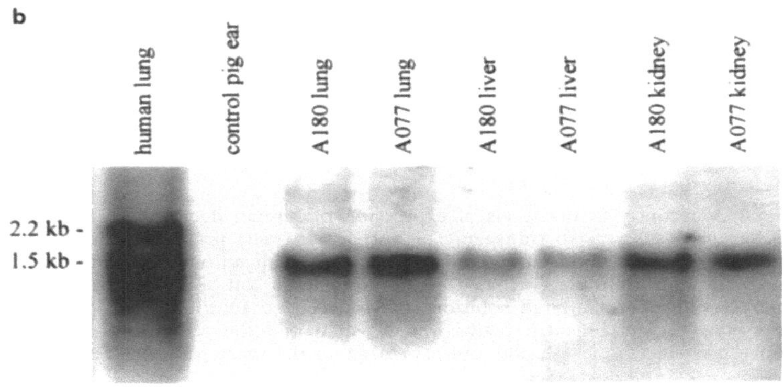

Fig. 2a,b. Northern blot analysis of human decay-accelerating factor (HDAF) mRNA extracted **a** from a human lung and from eight pig skin biopsies and **b** from a human lung, a control pig skin and three organs from transgenic pigs (A180 and A077). The positions of the naturally occurring transcripts produced in humans as a result of alternative splicing are shown in the first lane. These human transcripts consist of one mRNA species (1.6 kb), which includes an Alu sequence and produces a secreted form of HDAF protein and two mRNA species (1.5 and 2.2 kb) for the membrane-attached HDAF protein. The minigene construct microinjected into the pig zygotes contains the proximal major polyadenylation signal and lacks the Alu sequence, such that it only gives rise to the 1.5-kb transcript which codes for the phosphatidylinositol-linked membrane-anchored form of the HDAF protein

of HDAF were detected in 73% of the organs studied. However, the detailed analysis of these tissues showed that, within the same animal, there was considerable variability in the levels of expression of HDAF between the different organs (Fig. 3). In addition, for the same tissue, HDAF levels varied considerably from animal to animal (Fig. 4). Twenty-six organs from 12 different lines of pigs were found to express amounts of HDAF comparable with, or even greater than, those found in the same human tissue. FACS analysis performed on cultured endothelial cells from transgenic pigs showed that one line of pigs (A74) expressed levels of HDAF higher than that expressed by human umbilical

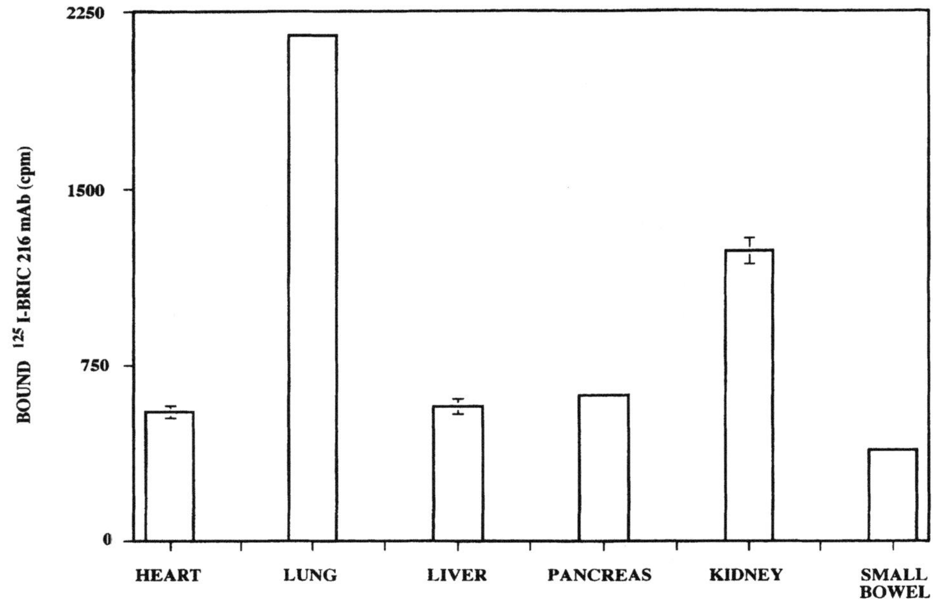

Fig. 3. Variability in the levels of expression of human decay-accelerating factor (HDAF) in the different tissues of J50 transgenic pigs. NP40 extracts prepared from heart, lung, liver, kidney, pancreas, small bowel, and striated muscle of each animal were incubated in triplicate on to 96-well microtiter plates coated with monoclonal antibody (mAb) IA10. After washing with 0.05% phosphate-buffered solution (PBS)-Tween 20 solution, ^{125}*I-BRIC* 216 mAb was added for 2 h at 4 °C. Subsequently, plates were washed and the remaining radioactivity was measured on a gamma counter. Results are expressed as the mean value of the measurements ±SEM

vein endothelial cells. The number of copies of the HDAF minigene incorporated was found to vary from two to 30 copies per line and, as already observed by others [46], the levels of expression of the transgenic protein did not correlate with the number of copies of the transgene incorporated into the porcine genome.

Protection from Complement

Protection conferred by HDAF expression on pig PBMC against human complement-mediated lysis was analysed using a chromium release assay. It is noteworthy that protection from lysis by human complement was observed in the PBMC of our transgenic pigs which expressed HDAF on the surface of these cells [47]. The protection against HAR conferred to pig organs by the expression of the transgene was investigated in ex vivo perfusion studies in which normal or HDAF transgenic pig hearts were perfused with fresh human blood in a working experimental model [48] (Fig. 5). Control pig hearts perfused with fresh human blood were shown to undergo a rapid decline in the cardiac output with the

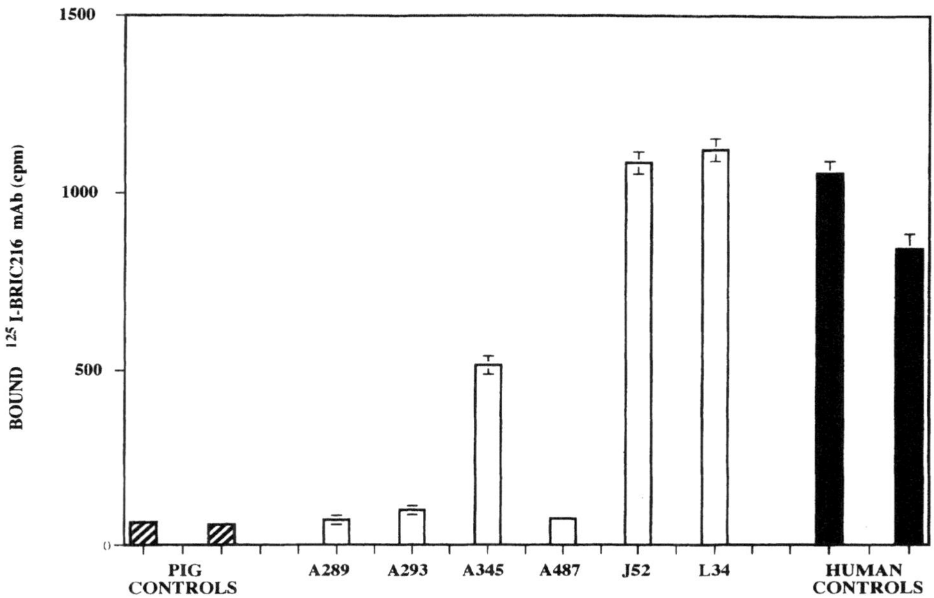

Fig. 4. Comparative analysis of the expression of human decay-accelerating factor (HDAF) in the hearts from two control pigs, six independently derived lines of transgenic pigs, and two human controls. The experiment was performed as described in the legend to Fig. 3. Results are expressed as the mean value of the measurements ±SEM

hearts ceasing to function within 69±18 min. Similarly, hearts from HDAF transgenic pigs which did not express the transgene ceased beating at 72±20 min. Significant variability in the cardiac output was found between transgenic organs taken from animals with different patterns of expression of HDAF. While transgenic pig hearts expressing HDAF only in the myocardium showed a moderate prolongation of the duration of the flow (97±48 min), an excellent protection of cardiac function was observed in animals with high expression of HDAF on endothelial cells (180±25 min).

The protective effect on damage deriving from the activation of the complement cascade conferred to the transgenic pig heart by the expression of HDAF was also confirmed by histological investigation. These studies demonstrated a massive destruction of all control pig hearts perfused with human blood. The histopathological picture was compatible with HAR of these organs with diffuse hemorrhage, edema, and vascular thrombosis. Widespread deposition of C3 in the graft was also observed at the time of cardiac failure. In contrast, a substantially normal cardiac structure was observed in the transgenic pig tissues expressing HDAF on endothelial cells perfused with human blood, and only minimal deposition of C3 was detected in these organs.

Taken together, these data confirmed the success of the genetic manipulation undertaken and allowed us to test in vivo in primates the starting hypothesis that

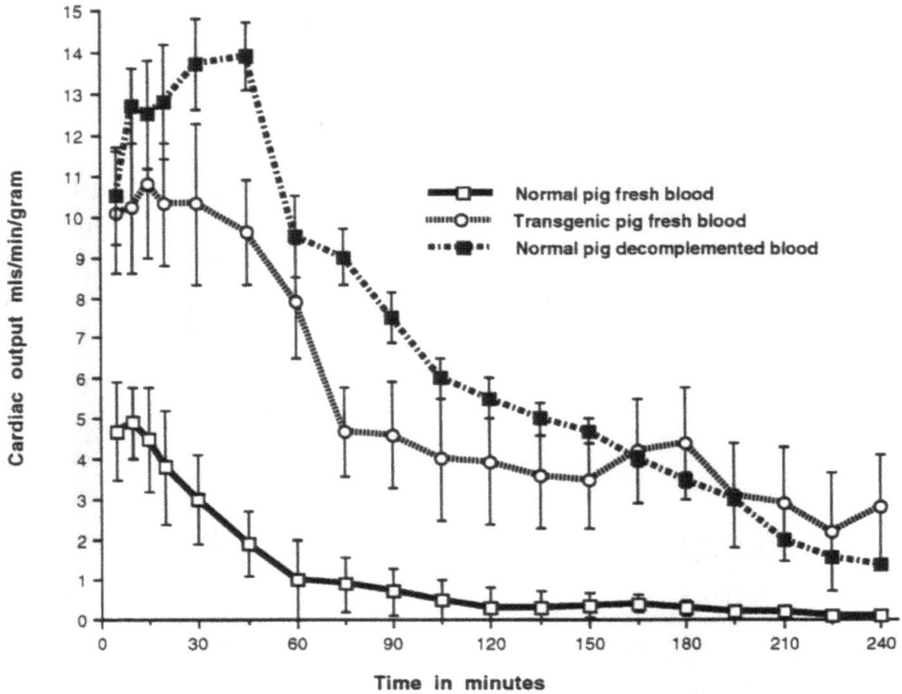

Fig. 5. Comparison of cardiac output of pig hearts perfused ex vivo with human blood. Normal pig hearts were perfused with fresh human blood or decomplemented human blood. Transgenic pig hearts were perfused with fresh human blood

pig organs transgenic for human RCA could be protected from complement activation and the subsequent HAR.

Organ Transplantation Studies

Hearts from new born heterozygote transgenic pigs or control animals were transplanted heterotopically into the abdomen of adult cynomolgus monkeys (*Macaca Fascicularis*). This species had been chosen in the light of our previous observations which had shown, in vitro, that complement from this species was down regulated by HDAF. Transplants were performed using a variant of the technique described by Ono [49]. In this technique the donor aorta is anastomosed to the recipient aorta and the donor pulmonary artery anastomosed to the inferior vena cava. The spleen was left in situ and care was taken to avoid any hemodilution from intravenous infusion of fluids at the time of surgery. Systemic heparinization of the recipient was also avoided as heparin can inhibit complement activity. Donor pigs were heparinized prior to excision of the heart.

Post-transplant, the abdominal heart was palpated 2-hourly for the first 24 h and then twice daily. Rejection of the heart was defined as the time at which a heart beat was no longer detectable by external palpation. Potential recipients were tested pre-transplant for the presence of antibodies directed against pig endothelium [50] or red blood cells [51]. Any monkey whose anti-pig antibody titer was not greater than that of a pool of four human sera was not used for this study. After transplantation, anti-pig RBC hemolytic antibodies were measured on alternate days (three times weekly). The experimental protocols for all the primate studies were approved by, and carried out under the supervision of, the Animal Inspectorate of the Home Office of England and Wales.

In the first series of experiments, eight transgenic hearts were transplanted heterotopically into non-immunosuppressed cynomolgus monkeys. Ten hearts from non-transgenic pigs were used as controls. None of the transgenic pig hearts was hyperacutely rejected and these organs had a median survival of 5.1 days (range, 97–126 h). In contrast, control hearts had a median survival of 1.6 days (range, 0.4–101 h). It is noteworthy that, of the ten control hearts, five were rejected in a mean of 2.6 ± 3 h, while the remaining five control hearts rejected in a mean of 86.4 ± 13.8 h. No recipient factor was found which could account for this bimodal distribution.

A possible explanation is in the genetic variability inherent in the use of outbred pigs. Staining of pig heart biopsies for the presence of Galα1–3Galß1–4GlcNAc-R residues with GS-I-B_4 lectin suggested that long-surviving control xenografts expressed less lectin binding residues than the organs which were hyperacutely rejected. The lesser immunogenicity of these organs could, therefore, explain this surprising finding. However, Platt and colleagues have recently pointed out a lack of correlation between GS-I-B_4 lectin and naturally present human anti-pig IgM antibodies in their binding profiles to Galα1–3Galß1–4GlcNAc-R epitopes [52]. The existence in some of these pigs of an increased expression of porcine "CD59-like" molecules, which are known to block human MAC formation [53], could represent another possibility. The classical histological patterns of HAR were demonstrated in all biopsies from the control hearts which failed within the first few hours subsequent to the transplant. In contrast, acute vascular rejection represented the usual picture in all the non-hyperacutely rejected grafts.

In another series of experiments, hearts from ten heterozygous transgenic pigs and five normal pigs were transplanted heterotopically into the abdomen of immunosuppressed cynomolgus monkeys. In these animals, triple immunosuppression with cyclosporin A cyclophosphamide and steroids was administered based on individual monitoring of clinical and immunological parameters. While cyclosporine was administered to achieve a trough level of 400 ng/ml, cyclophosphamide was administered at the dose needed to maintain the total white blood cell (WBC) count at a minimum of 2.0×10^9/l (Fig. 6). It must be pointed out that this minimum WBC count has recently been applied in the clinical immunosuppression of patients affected by autoimmune diseases such as systemic lupus erythematosus (SLE) [54], and that some authors have advanced as far as treating similar patients with pulse cyclophosphamide, considering a WBC count as low as 1.5×10^9/l as the minimum acceptable nadir for immunosup-

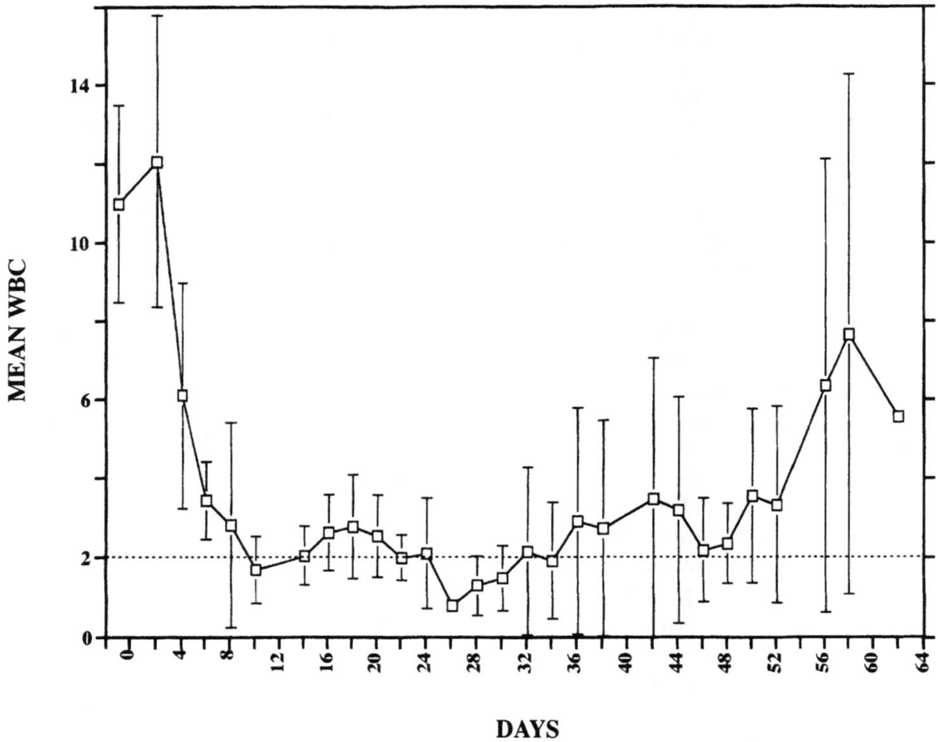

Fig. 6. Mean total number of circulating white blood cells (WBC) at different time points of the study in the ten immunosuppressed cynomolgus monkeys transplanted with transgenic pig hearts

pression [55]. Methylprednisolone was administered at 1 mg/kg on the day of transplant, reducing to 0.2 mg/kg by day 18.

Control pig hearts were rejected with a median survival of 55 min (range, 0.1–3 h), while transgenic hearts beat for a median of 40 days (6 to 62 days Fig. 7). Despite the presence of preformed anti-pig antibodies, HAR never occurred in monkeys transplanted with transgenic pig hearts while, in this study, all control pig hearts were hyperacutely rejected. Two of the ten transgenic pig hearts failed from rejection on days 6 and 62, respectively, showing significant deposition of C3 and C9. Both recipients had high titers of hemolytic anti-RBC antibodies at the time of rejection. One animal was killed on day 10 with an abscess on the apex of the transplanted heart. This was the only infection recorded in the study. One graft failed on day 54 for primary cardiomyopathy, and one graft failed on day 55 for unknown reasons. While this graft showed patchy histological evidence of immune attack, this was insufficient to account for graft failure. Histology showed that none of the other hearts was in any way affected by rejection. Five animals were euthanized in compliance with Home Office welfare gui-

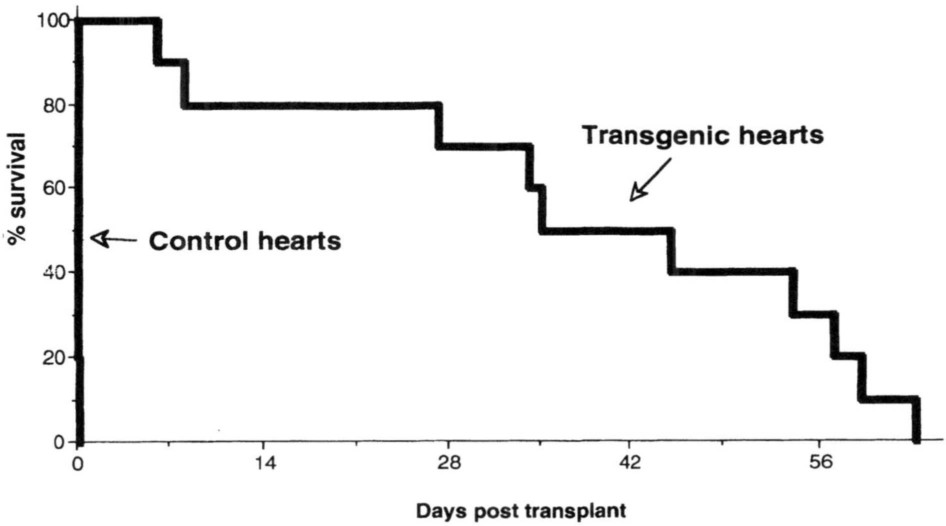

Fig. 7. Survival of pig hearts transplanted heterotopically into immunosuppressed cynomolgus monkeys. Hearts from decay-accelerating factor (DAF) transgenic pigs (n=10) had a median survival of 40 days, while those from normal pigs (controls, n=5) had a median survival of 55 min

dance, with their xenografted hearts still beating. In these five cases, the experiment was terminated because of gastrointestinal complications, possibly as a result of drug-related toxicity, adhesions or the abdominal position of the heart. In this respect, it may be of relevance that, in a clinical study, gastrointestinal complications were observed in 22 % of patients treated with cyclophosphamide [56]. In our study, repeated blood and stool cultures failed to reveal any infectious agent.

Postmortem histological examination of the gastrointestinal tract did not reveal any lesions compatible with bacterial or viral infection. All the control hearts which were rejected hyperacutely showed the classical histological lesions characteristic of HAR (Fig. 8A). However, histopathology of the transgenic hearts explanted at the time of euthanasia while still beating (Fig. 8B) showed normal cardiac architecture with no evidence of any cellular infiltrate or immune damage. While there were significant deposits of IgG and C4 on these hearts, staining for C3, C9, and P-selectin was negative.

Recently, we have initiated the transplantation of transgenic pig hearts into non human primates as life-supporting organs. In this context, it is worth mentioning that an orthotopically transplanted transgenic pig heart in a baboon treated with immunosuppression similar to that described above sustained life for 9 days, at which time the animal was euthanized with normal cardiac function. Finally, preliminary data obtained in nephrectomized cynomolgus monkeys, recipients of transgenic pig kidneys showed that these xenografts were able to sustain the life of these animals for up to 5 weeks.

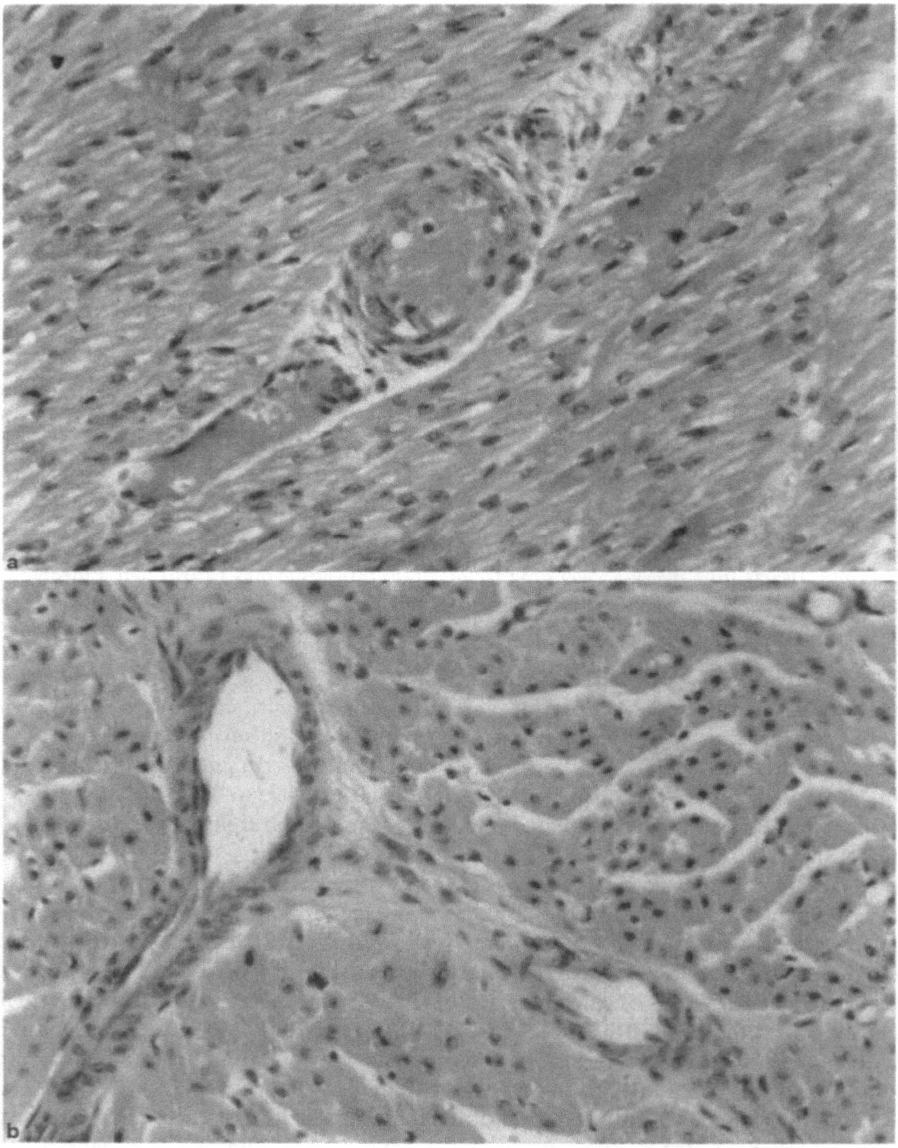

Fig. 8a,b. Light micrographs of pig hearts explanted from cynomolgus monkeys. **a** Hyperacute rejection of a control pig heart at cessation of heart beat (55 min following revascularization). Note the massive vascular thrombosis, the modest edema, the interstitial hemorrhage and the disparate infiltration of neutrophils. **b** Normal architecture of a transgenic pig heart explanted while still beating from a cynomolgus monkey euthanized on day 34. Note the integrity of the arteriolar endothelium, the absence of thrombosis, hemorrhage, or neutrophils and the conserved normal structure of the cardiac parenchyma

Comment

To the best of our knowledge, these data document the longest survival of pig-to-primate xenografts reported to date. The pig-to-primate model is undoubtedly a very challenging and difficult model. However, several conclusions can be made in the light of the results of our experience with transplanting pig organs into nonhuman primates. Firstly, expression of high levels of HDAF on the surface of transgenic pig organs is able to prevent the onset of HAR of pig xenografts transplanted into cynomolgus monkeys and baboons.

Secondly, the best previous survival of pig organs into primates recorded to date was by Alexandre et al. who achieved, in the premolecular engineering era, the remarkable survival of a pig kidney in a baboon for 22 days [57]. This was achieved utilizing a very complex experimental immunosuppressive approach which entailed splenectomy of the recipient, repeated preoperative plasmapheresis, rabbit anti human thymocyte serum, azathioprine, cyclosporine, soluble blood group substances A and B, and methylprednisolone. It is likely that this approach could never be applicable for clinical purposes. In contrast, with a simpler immunosuppressive approach developed in rodents [58], consisting of the utilization of three relatively common immunosuppressive drugs already utilized in clinical practice, we have managed to prolong to more than 8 weeks the survival of pig organs into primates.

We are aware of the fact that 50% of these animals experienced severe side-effects as a possible consequence of the long-term administration of cyclophosphamide. On the other hand, serious side-effects related to the utilization of cyclophosphamide have been reported in humans [54, 56, 59], and it is possible that the therapeutic index of this drug is further reduced in cynomolgus monkeys. However, we are confident that the utilization of one of the latest generation immunosuppressive molecules will probably mitigate these drug-related side-effects, allowing further improvement of the long-term survival of HDAF transgenic pig organs in primates.

Thirdly, while in both immunosuppressed and nonimmunosuppressed monkeys the rejection of a pig xenograft was always associated with a rise in the recipient's anti-pig RBC hemolytic antibodies, acute vascular rejection was not observed in the heart biopsies of some animals which had high titers of such hemolytic antibodies for several days prior to the time of their euthanasia. Clearly, the analysis of acute rejection of xenografts and its inhibition remains an exciting challenge for the future.

The data reported here suggest that transplantation into humans of organs from pigs transgenic for human RCA may represent a realistic therapeutic option in the not-too-distant future.

Acknowledgements. The authors would like to thank all of those involved in undertaking these studies; particularly Professor F. Grosveld, Mr J. Dunning, Mr V. Young, Mr P. Friend, Mr M. Tolan, Mr P. Waterworth, Mr P. Braidley, Dr C. Carrington, and Dr N. Cary. Finally, we wish to express our gratitude to Miss Helen Sykes for excellent secretarial assistance. This work was funded by Imutran.

References

1. Cooper DKC, Ye Y, Rolff LL, Zuhdi N. The pig as potential organ donor for man. In: Xenotransplantation, (First edition). Cooper DKC, et al. (eds). Heidelberg, Springer, 1991, p. 481
2. Allan JS. Xenotransplantation at a crossroads: Prevention versus progress. Nature Med 1996; 2: 18
3. Dalmasso AP, Vercellotti GM, Fischel RJ, et al. Mechanisms of complement activation in the hyperacute rejection of porcine organs transplanted into primate recipients. Am J Pathol 1992; 140(5): 1157
4. Zhao Z, Termignon JL, Cardoso J, et al. Hyperacute xenograft rejection in the swine-to-human donor-recipient combination. In vitro analysis of complement activation. Transplantation 1994; 57: 245
5. Platt JL, Bach FH. The barrier to xenotransplantation. Transplantation 1991; 52: 937
6. Good AH, Cooper DKC, Malcolm AJ, et al. Identification of carbohydrate structures which bind human anti-porcine antibodies: implications for discordant xenografting in man. Transplant Proc 1992; 24: 559
7. Sandrin MS, Vaughan HA, Dabkowski PL, McKenzie IFC. Anti-pig IgM antibodies in human serum react predominantly with Gal(α1–3)Gal epitopes. Proc Natl Acad Sci 1993; 90: 11391
8. Galili U. Interaction of the natural anti-Gal antibody with α-galactosyl epitopes: a major obstacle for xenotransplantation in humans. Immunol Today 1993; 14: 480
9. Bach FH, Blakely ML, Van Der Werf M, et al. Discordant xenografting: a working model of problems and issues. Xeno 1993; 1: 8
10. Auchincloss H Jr. Xenogeneic transplantation: a review. Transplantation 1988; 46: 1
11. Cozzi E, White DJG. The generation of transgenic pigs as potential organ donors for humans. Nature Med 1995; 1: 964
12. Oriol R, Ye Y, Koren E, Cooper DKC. Carbohydrate antigens of pig tissues reacting with human natural antibodies as potential targets for hyperacute vascular rejection in pig-to-man organ xenotransplantation. Transplantation 1993; 56: 1433
13. d'Apice AJF, Tange MJ, Chen C-G, et al. Gal(α1,3)Gal: elimination, suppression, masking or none of the above? Xeno 1995; 3: 113
14. Koike C, Hayashi S, Yokoyama I, et al. Converting α-Gal epitope of pig into H antigen. Transplant Proc 1996; 28: 553
15. Makowka L, Cramer DV, Hoffman A, et al. The use of a pig liver xenograft for temporary support of a patient with fulminant hepatic failure. Transplantation 1995; 59: 1654
16. Busch GJ, Martins ACP, Hollenberg NK, Wilson RE, Colman RW. A primate model of hyperacute renal allograft rejection. Am J Pathol 1975; 79: 31
17. Miyagawa S, Hirose H, Shirakura R, et al. The mechanism of discordant xenograft rejection. Transplantation 1988; 46: 825
18. Chartrand C, O'Regan S, Robitaille P, Pinto-Blonde M. Delayed rejection of cardiac xenografts in C6-deficient rabbits. Immunology 1979; 38: 245
19. Brauer RB, Baldwin WM, Daha MR, Pruitt SK, Sanfilippo F. Use of C6-deficient rats to evaluate the mechanism of hyperacute rejection of discordant xenografts. J Immunol 1993; 151: 7240
20. Leventhal JR, Dalmasso AP, Cromwell JW, et al. Prolongation of cardiac xenograft survival by depletion of complement. Transplantation 1993; 55: 857

21. Johnston PS, Lim SML, Wang MW, Wright L, White DJG. Hyperacute rejection of xenografts in the complete absence of antibody. Transplant Proc 1991; 23: 877
22. Pruitt SK, Kirk DA, Bollinger RR, et al. The effect of soluble complement receptor type 1 on hyperacute rejection of porcine xenografts. Transplantation 1994; 57: 363
23. Kobayashi T, Neethling FA, Koren E, et al. In vitro and in vivo investigation of anti-complement agents, FUT-175 and K76COOH, in the prevention of hyperacute rejection following discordant xenotransplantation in a nonhuman primate model. Transplant Proc 1996; 28: 604
24. Kroshus TJ, Rollins SA, Dalmasso AP, et al. Complement inhibition with an anti-C5 monoclonal antibody prevents acute cardiac tissue injury in an ex vivo model of pig-to-human xenotransplantation. Transplantation 1995; 60: 1194
25. Rollins SA, Matis LA, Springhorn JP, Setter E, Wolff DW. Monoclonal antibodies directed against human C5 and C8 block complement-mediated damage of xenogeneic cells and organs. Transplantation 1995; 60: 1282
26. Lachmann PJ. The control of homologous lysis. Immunol Today 1991; 12: 312
27. Morgan BP, Meri S. Membrane proteins that protect against complement lysis. In: Springer Seminars in Immunopathology.Heidelberg, Springer, 1994, p. 369
28. Wang M-W, Wright LJ, Sims MJ, White DJG. Presence of human chromosome 1 with expression of human decay- accelerating factor (DAF) prevents lysis of mouse/human hybrid cells by human complement. Scand J Immunol 1991; 34: 771
29. White DJG, Oglesby TJ, Tedja I, et al. Expression of human decay accelerating factor or membrane cofactor protein genes on mouse cells inhibits lysis by human complement. Transpl Int 1992; 5: 648
30. Lewin B. Organization of the eukaryotic genome. In: Genes V. Lewin B (ed). Oxford, Oxford University Press, 1994
31. Miller JFAP. Application of molecular genetics to transplantation immunology. Transplant Proc 1991; 23: 1717
32. Grosveld F, Blom van Assendelft G, Greaves DR, Kollias G. Position-independent, high-level expression of the human β-globin gene in transgenic mice. Cell 1987; 51: 975
33. Grosveld F, Antoniou M, Berry M, et al. Regulation of human globin gene switching. In: Cold Spring Harbor Symposia on Quantitative Biology, volume 58, 7. Cold Spring Harbor Laboratory Press, 1993
34. Pinkert CA. Transgenic pig models for xenotransplantation. Xeno 1994; 2: 10
35. Post TW, Arce MA, Liszewski MK, et al. Structure of the gene for human complement protein decay accelerating factor. J Immunol 1990; 144: 740
36. Liszewski MK, Post TW, Atkinson JP. Membrane cofactor protein (MCP or CD46): newest member of the regulators of complement activation gene cluster. Annu Rev Immunol 1991; 9: 431
37. Tone M, Walsh LA, Waldmann H. Gene structure of human CD59 and demonstration that discrete mRNAs are generated by alternative polyadenylation. J Mol Biol 1992; 227: 971
38. Vize PD, Michalska AE, Ashman R, et al. Introduction of a porcine growth hormone fusion gene into transgenic pigs promotes growth. J Cell Sci 1988; 90: 295
39. Brinster RL, Allen JM, Behringer RR, Gelinas RE, Palmiter RD. Introns increase transcriptional efficiency in transgenic mice. Proc Natl Acad Sci 1988; 85: 836
40. Pursel VG, Bolt DJ, Miller KF, et al. Expression and performance of transgenic pigs. J Reprod Fertil 1990; 40: 235

41. Post TW, Liszewski MK, Adams ME, et al. Membrane cofactor protein of the complement system: alternative splicing of serine/threonine/proline-rich exons and cytoplasmic tails produces multiple isoforms that correlate with protein phenotype. J Exp Med 1991; 174: 93
42. Russell SM, Sparrow RI, McKenzie IFC, Purcell DFJ. Tissue-specific and allelic expression of CD46 is controlled at the level of alternative splicing. Eur J Immunol 1992; 22: 1513
43. Burke DT, Olson MV. Preparation of clone libraries in yeast artificial chromosome vectors. Methods Enzymol 1991; 194: 251
44. Ioannou PA, Amemiya CT, Garnes J, et al. A new bacteriophage P1-derived vector for the propagation of large human DNA fragments. Nature Genetics 1994; 6: 84
45. Yannoutsos N, Ijzermans JNM, White D, Grosveld F. Using yeast artificial chromosomes to generate transgenic animals. Xeno 1995; 3: 107
46. Hammer RE, Pursel VG, Rexroad CE, et al. Production of transgenic rabbits, sheep and pigs by microinjection. Nature 1985; 315: 680
47. Cozzi E, Langford GA, Richards A, et al. Expression of human decay accelerating factor in transgenic pigs. Transplant Proc 1994; 26: 1402
48. White DJG, Langford GA, Cozzi E, Young VJ. Production of pigs transgenic for human DAF. A strategy for xenotransplantation. Xenotransplantation 1995; 2: 213.
49. Ono K, Lindsay L. Improved technique of heart transplantation in the rat. J Thorac Cardiovasc Surg 1969; 57: 225
50. Platt JL, Lindman BJ, Chen H, Spitalnik SL, Bach FH. Endothelial cell antigens recognized by xenoreactive human natural antibodies. Transplantation 1990; 50: 817
51. Van den Bogaerde JB, Aspinall R, Wang M-W, et al. Induction of long-term survival of hamster heart xenografts in rats. Transplantation 1991; 52: 15
52. Platt JL, Holzknecht ZE. Porcine platelet antigens recognized by human xenoreactive natural antibodies. Transplantation 1994; 57: 327
53. van den Berg CW, Morgan BP. Complement-inhibiting activities of human CD59 and analogues from rat, sheep and pig are not homologously restricted. J Immunol 1995; 152: 4095
54. Euler HH, Schroder OJ, Harten P, Zeuner RA, Gutschmidt HJ. Treatment-free remission in severe systemic lupus erythematosus following synchronization of plasmaphersis with subsequent pulse cyclophosphamide. Arthritis Rheumatism 1994; 12: 1784
55. Boumpas DT, Austin HA, Vaughn EM, et al. Controlled trial of pulse methylprednisolone versus two regimens of pulse cyclophosphamide in severe lupus nephritis. Lancet 1992; 340: 741
56. McCune WJ, Golbus J, Zeldes W, et al. Clinical and immunological effects of monthly administration of intravenous cyclophosphamide in severe systemic lupus erythematosus. N Engl J Med 1988; 318: 1423
57. Alexandre GPJ, Gianello P, Latinne D, et al. Plasmaphersis and splenectomy in experimental renal xenotransplantation. In: Xenograft 25. Hardy MA (ed). Amsterdam, Elsevier, 1989: p. 259
58. Hassan R, Van den Bogaerde JB, Wallwork J, White DJG. Evidence that long-term survival of concordant xenografts is achieved by inhibition of antispecies antibody production. Transplantation 1992; 54: 408
59. Hoffmann GS, Kerr GS, Leavitt RY, et al. Wegener's granulomatosis: an analysis of 158 patients. Ann Intern Med 1992; 116: 488

50 Overcoming the Anti-Galα(1–3)Gal Reaction To Avoid Hyperacute Rejection: Molecular Genetic Approaches

M.S. Sandrin, S. Cohney, N. Osman, and I.F.C. McKenzie

Introduction

As indicated previously, pig organs appear to be the most suitable to use for vascularized transplants for humans [1, 2]. The social need for this has been covered elsewhere in this volume, as has the major problem – hyperacute antibody mediated rejection (HAR). It has been known for many years that all humans have naturally occurring cytotoxic and hemagglutinating antibodies reacting with pig antigens [3], and it is clear that these antibodies would cause, within minutes, the rejection of vascularized pig tissues such as heart, liver, kidney, pancreas, or lung after transplantation to humans. Examples of HAR in pig to human transplantation, particularly for kidney and liver, are described elsewhere in this volume. The interacting components in HAR are: (a) antigen, (b) IgG and IgM antibodies, and (c) complement (C). There is little doubt that if there were neither antigen (the subject of this chapter), nor antibody or C [4, 5], then HAR would not occur, the graft would survive for days (at least) and other mechanisms of rejection would then come into play. The modes of removal of antibodies and/or C are described elsewhere; here we will discuss modifying the antigens to prevent HAR; we do not discuss antigens involved in the later phases of rejection which could involve both antibody and cellular mechanisms as the primary components.

One would think that, as there are so many obvious differences between humans and pigs, there would be many xenoantigenic differences (i.e., antigens important in the human immune response to pigs). This prediction is wrong, as it appears that the major, if not the only, antigen of importance when pig tissue is transplanted to humans is the carbohydrate epitope Galα(1,3)Gal [6–8] (also described in Chaps. 4 and 25). The importance of this epitope was clearly shown by the following:

1. The identification of large amounts of natural antibodies to Galα(1,3)Gal, an observation made originally by Landsteiner, but more recently by Galili [9–11] and others [6–8, 12, 13]; it is now clear that both IgG and IgM antibodies are present to Galα(1,3)Gal [6–13]; IgA antibodies have also been described [14].
2. The demonstration that, in vitro and in vivo, the presence of Galα(1,3)Gal inhibits HAR [15–19]; this is strong evidence that Galα(1,3)Gal is the major target in HAR.
3. Studies showing Galα(1,3)Gal expressed in monkey COS cells, (produced by transfection of the α1,3-galactosyltransferase cDNA [12, 20]) gave differential reactions with human serum compared with nontransfected COS cells and that Galα(1,3)Gal^{+} COS cells could absorb all the antibodies, from human serum, capable of reacting with pig cells [21].

4. Removal of anti-Galα(1,3)Gal antibodies by plasmapheresis absorption to Galα(1,3)Gal columns delays graft rejection in monkeys [16] (Third International Congress for Xenotransplantation poster 1995).

Thus, if the Galα(1,3)Gal epitope could be removed by either masking, blocking or prevention of synthesis, then HAR would not occur. In practical terms, how difficult a problem is this? Several points need to be made:

1. Galα(1,3)Gal epitopes are found on many cell surface molecules in the pig [22, 23]. Pigs (and indeed in all species except human, Old World monkeys, and some other species including bacteria) express Galα(1,3)Gal. In species with a functional α1,3-galactosyltransferase, Galα(1,3)Gal is a normal component of glycosylation of many glycoproteins and glycolipids.
2. As there are so many molecules expressing Galα(1,3)Gal [22], it is not practical to deal with these individually; a strategy is required that will stop Galα(1,3)-Gal being expressed on all molecules. To do this, the sugar itself can be targeted, the transferase that transfers galactose to the appropriate substrate, or the processing pathway (Table 1, Fig. 1). These approaches are possible because all molecules are galactosylated by a single α1,3-galactosyltransferase encoded by a single gene (Fig. 1). As will become apparent, it is possible to target the α1,3-galactosyltransferase and its gene.

Methods To Avert Hyperacute Rejection by Altering the Genes of Donor Animals

As shown in Fig. 1, there are a number of sites to attack Galα(1,3)Gal expression – from the gene encoding the transferase to the final product, the sugar; most of these involve genetic engineering techniques, particularly introducing "transgenes" to express a foreign gene with its own or a different promoter. The opposite approach is to stop expression entirely by inactivating the gene through the

Table 1. Summary of approaches to reduce Galα(1,3)Gal in pigs

Site of action	Method	Galα(1,3)Gal expression	*N*-acetyl-lactosamine expression	Feasibility
Gene				
α1,3-Galactosyltransferase gene	Gene knockout	None	↑↑↑	No
RNA				
Antisense RNA[a]	Transgenesis	↓	↑↑	Yes
Antisense oligonucleotides	Infusion	↓	↑↑	Yes
Protein				
Inhibitor of α1,3-Galactosyltransferase	Infusion	↓↓	↑↑↑	No[b]
Carbohydrate				
α1,2-Fucosyltransferase	Transgenesis	↓↓↓	None	Yes
α-Galactosidase	Transgenesis	↓↓	↑↑	Yes

↑, Increase in expression; ↓, decrease in expression.
[a] Theoretical possibility, as little efficacy in vitro.
[b] No specific inhibitor of α1,3-galactosyltransferase currently known.

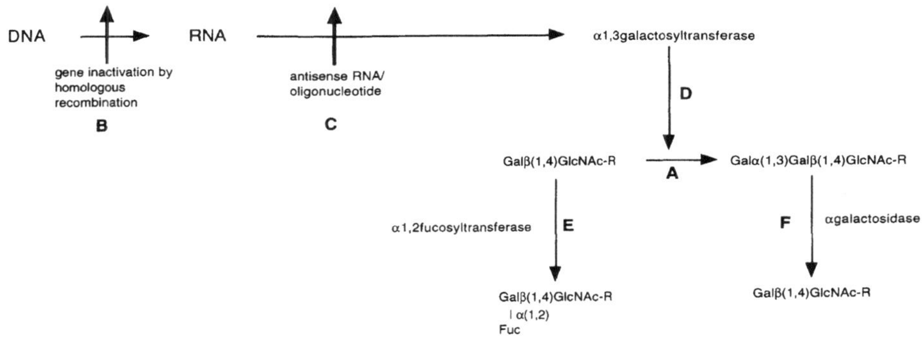

Fig. 1. Biosynthetic pathway for synthesis of Galα(1,3)Gal. Pathway begins with *N*-acetyl lactosamine (Galβ(1,4)GlcNAc). The α1,3-galactosyltransferase enzyme adds galactose to generate Galα(1,3)Gal (*A*). Both gene inactivation by homologous recombination (*B*) and transgenic approaches to inhibit/breakdown RNA (*C*) would prevent production of α1,3-galactosyltransferase and eliminate Galα(1,3)Gal. Potentially specific α1,3-galactosyltransferase inhibitors could act upon the enzyme (*D*). Also shown is an alternative transgenic approach to utilize the substrate of α1,3-galactosyltransferase by α1,2-fucosyltransferase (*E*). Galα(1,3)Gal could be eliminated by α-galactosidase (*F*)

process of homologous recombination, the "gene knockout" (GKO) technique. As these methods are central to this chapter they will be briefly described. We will not discuss the use of direct inhibitors of the α1,3-galactosyltransferase enzyme itself (Table 1, Fig. 1).

Transgenesis

Transgenesis is the integration of a foreign gene (transgene) into the germline of an animal such that the gene is expressed, and is transmitted to the offspring. To date, the transgenic technology has been applied to both plants and animals: mice, rats, rabbits, pigs, sheep, cows, goats, chickens, and fish. The method for producing transgenic animals is similar for all species, and the production of transgenic mice is described here (for more detail, see [24–28]); it is the same procedure for pigs.

The commonest approach for producing transgenic mice is by the microinjection of cloned DNA into the pronucleus of a fertilized mouse egg (Fig. 2). Immature female mice are superovulated with hormones (to produce more eggs) by the sequential administration of follicle stimulating hormone/luteinizing hormone and human chorionic gonadotrophin, and are then mated with fertile male mice. Twenty-four hours later, the females are operated upon, and fertilized eggs are flushed from the oviducts into tissue culture medium and are assessed for their suitability for injection by microscopy. A microneedle loaded with a suspension of the transgene plasmid DNA is injected into the male pronucleus of a single-celled fertilized mouse embryo. Surviving embryos are incubated for 8–18 h until division to the two-cell stage has occurred, and then surgically

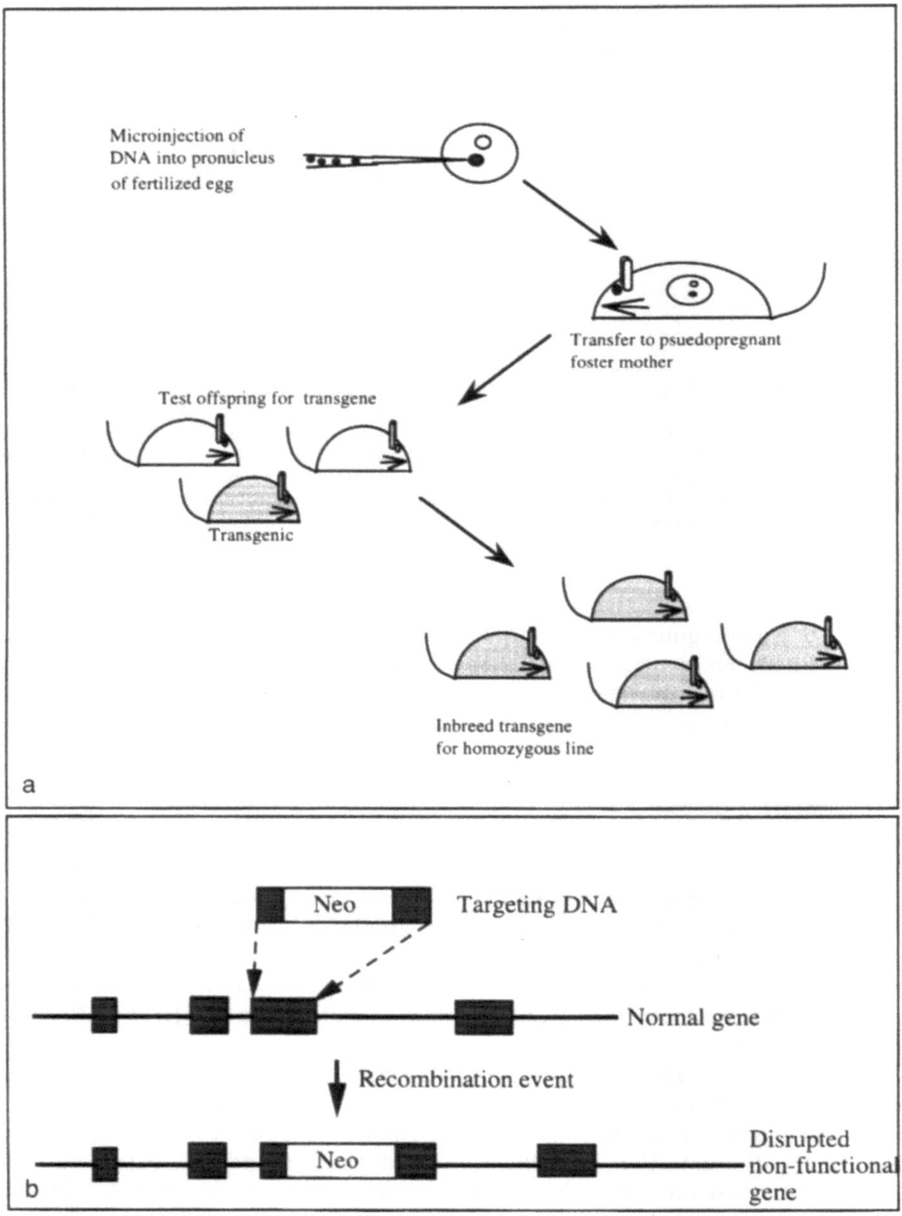

Fig. 2. **a** Method of transgenesis. **b** Gene knockout and homologous recombination

transferred to the oviducts of pseudopregnant foster mothers (produced by mating female mice with vasectomized male mice). Transgenic mice are born 19 days later and are evaluated for transgene incorporation (see below). An efficiency of 0.5%–3.7% is reported in mice [29], e.g., in one series 3342 eggs were isolated and microinjected, 874 fetuses developed, and 502 had DNA integration [29]. An important factor in transgenic efficiency is the strain of mouse used, the production of transgenic mice being more efficient with F_1 or F_2 zygotes than with zygotes of inbred strains.

DNA integration into the genome is random and insertion at a single site with multiple head-to-tail copies of the transgene is usual. One to several hundred copies of the transgene may integrate, but copy number is not always proportional to transgene expression. Insertion of the transgene in multiple sites of the genome is less common, and integration may be delayed for several cleavage divisions after microinjection, resulting in the transgene being present in only a fraction of the cells. The host genome may have deletions, duplications, rearrangements, or translocations at the transgene insertion site, with the possible consequence of disruption of an essential gene. Insertion of the transgene adjacent to gene regulatory sequences can result in unexpected patterns of transgene expression.

After obtaining DNA from the tail of mice at any time after birth, identification of transgenic mice can be made several ways: by polymerase chain reaction (PCR) analysis of crude DNA preparations, dot blotting of genomic DNA, or Southern blotting of genomic DNA digested with restriction enzymes. The latter method is the most stringent test of transgene integration. Histological or other studies of protein expression can be made on transgenic mouse tissues to assess transgene expression, or northern blot analysis to assay for mRNA. Subsequent breeding of transgenic founder mice determines whether the transgene can be transmitted to the next generation.

Several types of DNA constructs can be used in the generation of transgenic animals and to some extent the type of construct dictates the questions that can be addressed using transgenic animals models. Constructs consisting of complete genomic clones, containing all exons, introns and related 5′ and 3′ sequences contain all the information required to synthesize the gene product in the appropriate cells and tissues, and accordingly the expression of the transgene produce can be assessed. Minigene constructs comprised of cDNA sequences linked to 5′ regulatory sequences can also be used, however the inclusion of some intron sequence is a requirement for high level gene expression. Alternatively, the gene coding region for a protein of interest can be linked to the promoter sequences from another gene, i.e., a heterologous promoter, to provide different tissue and cell specific expression relative to wild type, and thereby help reveal the normal function of the gene as well as showing the consequences of ectopic expression of the transgene (e.g., using an H2 class I promoter). Given the simplicity of the procedure from a practical viewpoint, it is not surprising that many different transgenic animals have been produced. Transgenic pigs have been produced using scaled up (and more expensive) facilities than described above. As indicated in this volume, pigs transgenic for the human complement components CD46 (membrane cofactor protein, MCP), CD55 (decay-accelerating factorDAF), and CD59 have been described and used in functional studies. The transgenic approaches which could be used to avoid Galα(1,3)Gal expression are described below.

Gene Inactivation by Homologous Recombination

As discussed above, the transgenic approach requires the injection of a gene (or cDNA) into an egg; the gene is incorporated randomly and functions under its "own" promoter (i.e., the promoter in the DNA construct). For homologous recombination [30–32], the additional requirements are: (a) the gene to be targeted depends on the recombinant gene "finding" its target, an event which occurs with a frequency of 1×10^{6}–10^{7}; in this case, the transgene cannot be inserted randomly, but has to be in the correct site; (b) extensive in vitro screening has to be done to find the one (in 10^{6-7}) recombinant; (c) the cell containing the recombinant DNA has to be maintained and then introduced into a blastocyst. This is done by the use of embryonic stem (ES) cells derived from the mouse strain 129/SvSn, which, in culture, can differentiate into teratocarcinoma cells. These cells are maintained in the non-differentiated stare by various media, cells (fibroblast feeders), and agents such as leukemia inhibitory factor (LIF). On injection, some of the ES cells are incorporated into the developing blastocyst; the resultant offspring are chimeras containing the ES DNA (and hopefully the recombinant gene) and blastocyst DNA.

The procedure is complex and laborious with the following steps:

1. Production of a nonfunctional gene as similar as possible to the gene to be targeted. The gene can be rendered nonfunctional by different means – excising a segment, altering the reading frame but usually, by the insertion of the neomycin (neo)gene (Fig. 2), which also functions as a selectable marker to the gene, which allows growth, in selective media, of cells which have the neo gene present, irrespective of where the gene is integrated.
2. Maintenance of ES cells in a nondifferentiated state.
3. Introduction of gene–neo construct into ES cells, usually by electroporation. It will be noted that the gene-neo construct can integrate anywhere (random integration), but may also recombine with the gene to be targeted (homologous recombination). The frequency of recombination is increased with the greater similarity of the two gene sequences; thus if 129/SvSn ES cells are used, it is preferable to use DNA of 129/SvSn origin.
4. Selection in G418-containing media for gene incorporation. G418 acts by blocking protein synthesis by interfering with ribosomal function; the expression of the neo gene (bacterial aminoglycoside phosphotransferase) in transfected cells results in the detoxification of G418 [33].
5. Testing of G418-resistant cells for recombinants of the normal gene with the gene-neo construct (PCR or Southern analysis). This can be tedious – with hundreds of reactions to be performed. With PCR, primers are used which use the new gene-neo (e.g., sequences in neo) and sequences adjacent to the site of integration so that a band will be amplified only if homologous recombination has occurred.

6. Microinjection of selected ES cells into blastocysts for transgenesis.
7. Examination of offspring – coat color chimera (if ES and blastocysts have different coat color genes) or by DNA testing.
8. Breeding of chimeras to show germline transmission, and then inbreeding of mice which have the new homologous recombination gene in place of the normal gene.

Using this method, many genes of immunological interest have been targeted:

- β2M (class I MHC)
- 1A (class I major histocompatibility complex, MHC)
- CD3, 4, 5, 8
- Ly1
- Fc receptor
- CD18 (lymphocyte function-associated antigen-1, LFA-1; intercellular adhesion molecule 1, ICAM-1)
- Perforin
- Granzyme B
- Cytokines interleukin (IL)-2, -4, -5, -6, -7R, -10, -12, γ-interferon (IFN), tumor necrosis factor (TNF)
- Galα(1,3)Gal transferase

At present the technology is only available in mice – most "knockouts" being done in 129/SvSn ES cells leading, usually, to chimeras on a mixed genetic background, requiring many generations of backcrossing. C57BL/6 ES cells can also be used, and if injected into C57BL/6 blastocysts, the offspring will have C57BL/6 background genes. Intercrossing two founder mice will produce progeny homozygous -/- for the gene of interest, and be coisogenic with C57BL/6. This technology cannot currently be performed in pigs so that only transgenes can be used in studies of xenotransplantation.

There are several other problems with the homologous recombination technique that deserve mention. Firstly, some genes are crucial for either development or maintenance of life and the knockout is lethal. For example, deletion of the *N*-acetyl glucosaminyltransferase I (found in both N- and O-linked sugars of mammals) is lethal in utero [34]. Secondly, some genes considered to be crucial for life (or at least for an immune response), when nonfunctional do not appear to be accompanied by any particular phenotype. For example, IL-2 is considered a key cytokine in T cell-dependent immune responses. In the IL-$2^{-/-}$ mice there is severe ulcerative colitis [35], but the mice are otherwise normal [36]. Presumably, in such mice, compensatory mechanisms develop in utero so that the effect of the missing gene is minimized.

There are now several methods under development to induce gene dysfunction in adults and these have appeal, for if the genes could be turned on or off at will, then their effects can be fine-tuned, much like adjusting the dose of immunosuppressive agents. Such systems include the cre/lox system where the cre gene can lead to recombination in lox containing transgenes, and irreversibly splice out the gene of interest – the homologous recombination method being used to target the gene of interest using lox containing constructs [37–39]. The system is such that if the recombination inducing gene lox is under an externally inducible promoter (e.g., metallothionein which responds to heavy metals in the drinking water, or under tetracycline responsive genes) [39], then the mere addition of these materials to the food intake can turn on the gene. It remains to be seen how these procedures can apply to xenografts.

Gene Homologous Recombination Approaches to Xenotransplantation

α1,3-Galactosyltransferase Enzyme

As described above, and elsewhere in this volume, the majority of natural human anti-pig antibodies recognize Galα(1,3)Gal [6–8]. Approaches to overcome HAR produced by anti-Galα(1,3)Gal antibodies requires an understanding of the enzyme which produces the carbohydrate epitope. Galα(1,3)Gal is used to terminate the nonreducing end of *N*-glycans, *O*-glycans, and glycolipids on many different molecules, and is used by cells, as an alternative to sialic acid, to provide an uncharged terminal carbohydrate residue. The Galα(1,3)Gal residues are synthesized by α1,3-galactosyltransferase, which catalyses the addition of a terminal α-linked galactose to *N*-acetyl lactosamine (Fig. 1). The substrate specificity of the α1,3-galactosyltransferase has been examined in vitro, and is any unbranched galactose in a β-linkage with either *N*-acetyl glucosamine or *N*-acetyl galactosamine [40]. Approaches to inhibit the action of this enzyme can focus on the gene or on the expression of the mRNA (Table 1, Fig. 1).

Molecular Cloning of α1,3-Galactosyltransferase cDNA

cDNA clones encoding α1,3-galactosyltransferase have now been isolated from the mouse [41, 42], ox [43], pig [20, 44], and New World monkeys [45], all containing open reading frames which encode a predicted protein with a domain structure common to all glycosyltransferases thus far cloned [46]. α1,3-galactosyltransferase is a typical type II integral membrane protein (amino terminal orientated towards the cytoplasm) comprising a short cytoplasmic tail (six amino acids), a transmembrane region (16 amino acids), a stalk region, and a carboxyl-terminal catalytic domain (that resides within the lumen of the Golgi).

Using a series of truncated cDNA clones, Galili et al. [45] were able to demonstrate that the active site (catalytic domain) of α1,3-galactosyltransferase commences 67 amino acids from the putative transmembrane domain, residing in the 277 amino acid carboxyl terminal domain. Comparison of the amino acid sequences of pig, mouse, ox, and marmoset shows that the highest sequence identity between all the cloned α1,3-galactosyltransferases is in the carboxyl portion which contains the catalytic domain, with an overall identity of 78 %.

Related to α1,3-galactosyltransferase is B blood group transferase, which also catalyses the addition of terminal α1,3-linked galactose [47]. However, in contrast to α1,3-galactosyltransferase, which uses *N*-acetyl lactosamine as the acceptor substrate, the B blood group α1,3-galactosyltransferase can only use fucosylated *N*-acetyl lactosamine as a substrate (H substance) [47]. The distinguishing feature of these two transferases (which have 65 % amino acid identity) is that even though both can transfer a terminal α1,3-linked galactose, neither can utilize the other's substrate, an observation used as an alternative approach to functional inactivation of the α1,3-galactosyltransferase enzyme (see below).

Structure of the α1,3-Galactosyltransferase Gene

The murine α1,3-galactosyltransferase gene (the best characterized) is a single gene composed of nine exons spanning approximately 35 kb of chromosome 2 [42]. There is evidence that the enzyme has at least 4 alternatively spliced isoforms in the mouse [42], and comparison of the published sequences [20, 44] suggests that there are at least two splice variants in the pig. Genomic sequences homologous to murine α1,3-galactosyltransferase gene have been reported in humans, defining two nonlinked pseudogenes [48, 49]; one located on chromosome 9q33–34 and the other on chromosome 2q14–15 [50]. It is interesting to note that the pseudogene on chromosome 9 is linked to the A and B blood group transferases, suggesting an evolutionary relationship between all of these transferase genes [8, 48].

In the mouse, the first three exons of the α1,3-galactosyltransferase gene encode the 5′ untranslated sequence of mRNA, with the next six exons encoding the protein [42]. The catalytic domain of the α1,3-galactosyltransferase is encoded within the last exon (exon 9) [42], which makes this the ideal exon to target for gene knockout strategies (see below).

Expression of Galα(1,3)Gal

It is clear from several studies that endothelial cells of almost all vessels in the pig, including capillaries, arterioles and venules express Galα(1,3)Gal [51, 52]. As this would be the first site of interaction in vascularized transplantation, vigorous rejection would be assured because of the dense distribution of Galα(1,3)-Gal. The parenchyma in some tissues were also positive -particularly the liver and kidney which contained large amounts [51]. In the kidney this was differentially distributed and found strongest in the proximal convoluted tubules, lesser amounts elsewhere; in the liver there was uniform distribution of the parenchyma and in the hepatic ducts. Heart muscle was nonreactive; in the lung, the lining of alveoli and bronchioles was strongly staining, as were the vessels. The one glandular tissue that was different was the pancreas, where adult pancreas, apart from the vessels and ducts, was virtually nonreactive – the exocrine and endocrine tissue (islets) did not stain at all [51].

There are major differences in the expression of Galα(1,3)Gal in mice and pigs. While pig tissues fixed in formalin or examined fresh expression copious amounts of the epitope, mouse tissues fixed in formalin give very poor reactivity compared with fresh tissue (I.F.C. McKenzie et al., unpublished). Finally, there are major species differences in that mouse kidney and liver are virtually nonreactive, whereas in the pig they are strongly reactive. Similar results have been described using fluorescein isothiocyanate (FITC)-labeled IB4 lectin [53], and in mRNA expression (by northern blot analysis) [54]; however, using reverse transcriptase (RT)-PCR, signals have been detected in most tissue [42]. The relevance of the mouse work is in the homologous recombination experiments to produce Galα(1,3)Gal⁻ mice. However, while the murine model will be of some use, one should be cautious in extrapolating experimental results from mouse to pig.

α1,3-Galactosyltransferase$^{-/-}$ Mice Produced by Homologous Recombination

Mice deficient in α1,3-galactosyltransferase (gal$^{-/-}$ mice) after gene inactivation by homologous recombination have been reported from two centers [55, 56], both targeting exon 9 (the exon encoding the catalytic domain) for disruption. Several important observations arose from the studies of these mice:

1. In contrast to the inactivation of some glycosyltransferases [34], inactivation of the α1,3-galactosyltransferase gene is not lethal. This result was predicted [6, 8], as the gene had been inactivated by naturally occurring mutations in humans and Old World monkeys, without deleterious effects [48, 49, 57].
2. Inactivation of the α1,3-galactosyltransferase gene leads to the lack of expression of Galα(1,3)Gal in all tissues examined, not an unexpected finding as there is only one α1,3-galactosyltransferase gene in the mouse [42].
3. The gal$^{-/-}$ mice produce natural anti-Galα(1,3)Gal antibodies [55]. Whether these are induced by bacterial infection, or without antigenic stimulus is not clear, but it is apparent that the occurrence of these antibodies in these gal$^{-/-}$ mice parallels the observations in humans and Old World monkeys.
4. Although gal$^{-/-}$ mice do not bind purified human anti-Galα(1,3)Gal antibodies [55, 56], when examined with whole human serum, some antibody binding was still observed [56]. This reaction is probably due to the binding of natural human anti-*N*-acetyl lactosamine antibodies, which are present in substantial amounts in all humans tested [58], but are not observed in normal mice as *N*-acetyl lactosamine is not a terminal carbohydrate.

Clearly, gene inactivation of the α1,3-galactosyltransferase alone is not the ultimate solution to generate animals suitable to be transplant donors, particularly as the technique is currently not available in pigs (Table 1). However, these studies are important as they indicate what carbohydrates will be expressed by pig organs if the technique ever becomes available.

Transgenic Approaches to Xenotransplantation

As homologous recombination is not available in pigs, transgenic approaches which could be used to produce pigs expressing reduced amounts of Galα(1,3)Gal are necessary and will be discussed.

Antisense RNA

RNA–RNA interactions have been shown to be important in several processes. The discovery in 1978 [59] that an oligonucleotide, complementary to the coding strand of Rous sarcoma virus, could inhibit the replication of the virus led to the use of antisense oligonucleotides as potential antiviral therapeutic agents (an

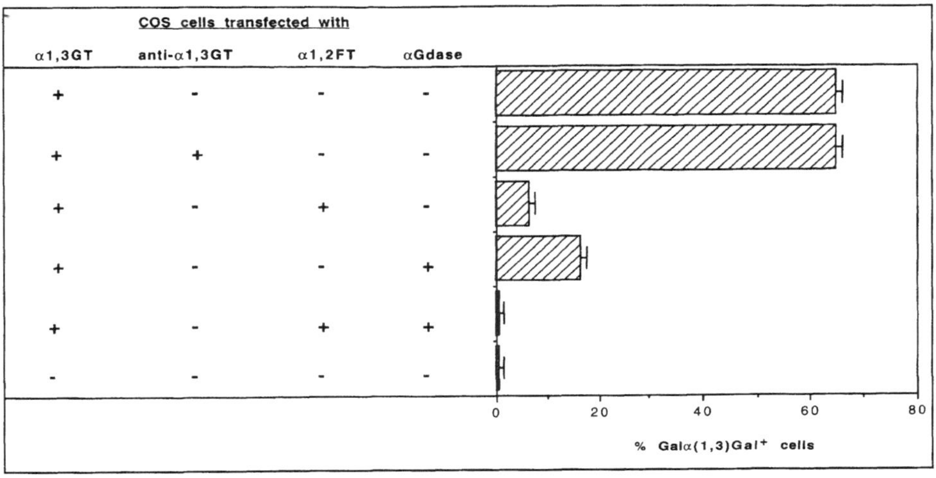

Fig. 3. Expression of Galα(1,3)Gal on COS cells after transfection. The cDNA clones used were: *α 1,3GT*, α1,3-galactosyltransferase; *anti-α1,3GT*, antisense α1,3-galactosyltransferase; *α1,2FT*, α1,2-fucosyltransferase; *αGdase*, α-galactosidase A

antisense RNA is defined as an RNA molecule which interferes with the activity of another RNA). Antisense RNA constructs have been used to inhibit gene function in both plants [60] and animals [61].

Of relevance to the α1,3-galactosyltransferase gene would be to use an antisense cDNA to α1,3-galactosyltransferase mRNA which, when used as a transgene, would be produced in the cell and bind irreversibly with RNA and block its transcription (Table 1, Fig. 1), a phenomenon not as yet described. In our hands, antisense RNA, produced by transfecting COS cells with cDNA for the noncoding strand of α1,3-galactosyltransferase, inhibits Galα(1,3)Gal expression in vitro (Fig. 3; M.S. Sandrin and I.F.C. McKenzie, unpublished). Alternatively, extraneous antisense oligonucleotides (administered intravenously) could be used. In vitro, such oligonucleotides have been reported to decrease the level of cell surface Galα(1,3)Gal by 40 % in pig endothelial cells [62, 63], but this is not a major or useful decrease. Whether such approaches will be of use in the production of transgenic pigs remains to be seen as the level of decreased expression of Galα(1,3)Gal will lead to an increased expression of *N*-acetyl lactosamine, to which humans have antibodies (Table 1; also see above).

Transgene Expression of α1,2-Fucosyltransferase

Another method for reducing expression of the Galα(1,3)Gal epitope is by the competitive removal of its precursor with another glycosyltransferase. As described above, both α1,3-galactosyltransferase and the α1,2-fucosyltransferase (H transferase) utilize *N*-acetyl lactosamine as their acceptor substrate (Fig. 1).

While the former generates (the antibody reactive) Galα(1,3)Gal epitope, the α1,2-fucosyltransferase is responsible for the production of a fucosylated structure (H substance/H antigen) – well known as the O blood group antigen. Furthermore, the α1,3-galactosyltransferase enzyme is unable to utilize *N*-acetyl lactosamine once it has been fucosylated [40], leading to the concept that the over-expression of H transferase may lead to a reduction in the formation of the terminal Galα(1,3)Gal epitopes [6, 8].

Thus studies from our laboratory have shown, both in vitro and in vivo, that not only was there competition between these two transferases, but that when both transferases are present there is preferential expression of H substance leading to a marked decrease in Galα(1,3)Gal expression [64–66]. The major findings were:

1. When cDNA clones encoding both porcine α1,3-galactosyltransferase and human α1,2-fucosyltransferase were transfected simultaneously into COS cells or pig kidney cells, the cell surface expression of Galα(1,3)Gal was reduced by more than 90 % (Fig. 3) while the level of H substance was unaffected [64, 65]. The preferential expression of the product of the α1,2-fucosyltransferase over that of the α1,3-galactosyltransferase seems to be related primarily to the topographical organization of these transferases within the Golgi complex of the cell [67].
2. There was a significant decrease in the susceptibility of the pig kidney cell lines to lysis by human serum [64].
3. Transgenic mice expressing human α1,2-fucosyltransferase were produced using the cDNA encoding this transferase under the control of the H-2K^b promoter, and expression of H antigen demonstrated on erythrocytes, peripheral blood lymphocytes, splenocytes, and thymocytes, which contrasted with its absence from cells of normal mice and nontransgenic littermates [64, 66]. More importantly, the surface expression of Galα(1,3)Gal was reduced by approximately 90 %. In addition, immunohistological studies showed high levels of expression of H substance on liver, spleen, kidney, and heart, with a concomitant reduction in levels of Galα(1,3)Gal [66]. Importantly, Galα(1,3)-Gal staining on endothelium was reduced, though still detectable [66].

It is not clear whether the remaining amount of Galα(1,3)Gal epitope present in an H transgenic animal would be sufficient to react with human antibody to trigger hyperacute rejection. However, the transgenic strategy should also succeed in the pig, and allow evaluation of porcine to primate organ transplants.

Removing Galα(1,3)Gal with α-Galactosidase

Another approach to eradicating HAR would be to reduce the amount of Galα(1,3)Gal using α-galactosidase (Table 1, Fig. 1), an enzyme which cleaves terminal α-linked galactosyl residues from the adjacent carbohydrate. Treatment of erythrocytes, lymphocytes and endothelial cells with α-galactosidase (of coffee bean or bacterial origin) removes Galα(1,3)Gal from these cells and negates their reaction with human serum both in vitro and in vivo [52, 68–70]. We have demonstrated the efficacy of using α-galactosidase cDNA in vitro [71], as a prelude for use in a transgenic approach to the removal of Galα(1,3)Gal, and have shown the following:

1. Human α-galactosidase A enzyme [72] in vitro is as effective as the bacterial or plant enzymes used in other studies for the cleavage of Galα(1,3)Gal from the cell surface [71].
2. Coexpression of human α-galactosidase and pig α1,3-galactosyltransferase cDNA clones in COS cells resulted in a 75% reduction in Galα(1,3)Gal expression (Fig. 3) [71].
3. The susceptibility to lysis by human serum of COS cells coexpressing human α-galactosidase and pig α1,3-galactosyltransferase cDNA clones was markedly reduced (71).

These findings suggest that α-galactosidase enzyme expressed within the appropriate subcellular fraction can cleave the terminal galactose from Galα(1,3)-Gal. In addition, the simultaneous expression of α-galactosidase and α1,2-fucosyltransferase (Fig. 3) should eliminate the expression of Galα(1,3)Gal. This approach has the potential to be used in the production of transgenic pigs, a viable alternative to α1,3-galactosyltransferase gene inactivation by homologous recombination.

Comment

To totally reduce Galα(1,3)Gal to levels which do not react in deleterious ways with antibodies it will be necessary to use a number of strategies shown in Table 1 in combination, e.g., a method for removal of Galα(1,3)Gal, such as the gene knockout (should it become technically feasible) or α-galactosidase transgene (both of which may unmask other immunogenic epitopes), together with the H transgene, which would result in the conversion of any free *N*-acetyl lactosamine groups to H substance (the universal donor antigen). Alternatively, the H transferase may be used with the human complement regulators (as described in Chap. 49, this volume) in a composite transgenic animal.

However, whether these sophisticated transgenic approaches will be required is not all that clear. Firstly, antibodies can be removed by plasmapheresis, or absorption, leading to prolonged survival of pig organ transplants in monkeys, as shown years ago in Belgium, with survival up to 24 days [73], and more recently in the Sachs' tolerance studies [74]. However, heavy immunosuppression was required to prevent the reemergence of antibodies in both studies. Whether a combination of plasmapheresis/absorption and immunosuppression (which can be done very effectively now) is better than sophisticated transgenic approaches (not proven or not yet available) remains to be seen. Secondly, while animals with no expression of Galα(1,3)Gal, or of other antigens to which there are antibodies, will have organs resistant to anti-Galα(1,3)Gal or other antibodies, care will have to be taken that they do not produce organisms (such as retroviruses) that also lack Galα(1,3)Gal and will therefore not be eradicated by the natural immune reactivity of anti-Galα(1,3)Gal antibodies. A theoretical possibility only? Perhaps so, but it should be noted that a recent study demonstrated the inability of human serum to neutralize murine retroviruses which had been passaged through α1,2-fucosyltransferase-expressing mouse cells, in contrast to those grown in normal mouse cells, which are readily neutralized by anti-Galα(1,3)Gal antibodies, suggesting the role of these antibodies as a barrier to the horizontal transmission of retroviruses [75].

It is clear that either simple mechanical procedures or sophisticated transgenic/GKO techniques should soon provide pigs which are suitable as donors for organ transplantation, as overcoming HAR is now an achievable goal. We await the description of the residual problems in organ transplants which may then be revealed. "Where lurks aging, and yet noble facts? As thence, here can I ponder and build better cases" (Anon).

References

1. YE, Y., NIEKRASZ, M., KOSANKE, S., et al. The pig as a potential organ donor for man. A study of potentially transferable disease from donor pig to recipient man. Transplantation. 57, 694, 1994
2. SACHS, D.H. The pig as a potential xenograft donor. Vet. Immunol. Immunopathol. 43, 185, 1994
3. McKENZIE, I.F.C., STOCKER, J., TING, A., MORRIS, P.J. Human lymphocytotoxic and hemagglutinating activity against sheep and pig cells. Lancet. 2, 386, 1968
4. COZZI, E., WHITE, D.J.G. The generation of transgenic pigs as potential organ donors for humans. Nature Med. 1, 964, 1995
5. RYAN, U.S. Complement inhibitory therapeutics and xenotransplantation. Nature Med. 1, 967, 1995
6. SANDRIN, M.S., McKENZIE, I.F.C. Galα(1,3)Gal, the major xenoantigens recognized in pigs by human natural antibodies. Immunol. Rev. 141, 169, 1994
7. COOPER, D.K.C., KOREN, E., ORIOL, R. Oligosaccharides and discordant xenotransplantation. Immunol. Rev. 141, 31, 1994
8. SANDRIN, M.S., VAUGHAN, H.A., McKENZIE, I.F.C. Identification of Galα(1,3)Gal as the major epitope for pig-to-human vascularized xenografts. Transplant. Rev. 8, 134, 1994
9. GALILI, U., RACHMILEWITZ, E.A., PELEG, A., FLECHNER, I. A unique natural human IgG antibody with anti-α-galactosyl specificity. J. Exp. Med. 160, 1519, 1984
10. GALILI, U., MACHER, B.E., BUEHLER, J., SHOHET, S.B. Human natural anti-α-galactosyl IgG II. the specific recognition of α(1,3)-linked galactose residues. J. Exp. Med. 162, 573, 1985
11. GALILI, U. Evolution and pathophysiology of the human natural anti-α-galactosyl IgG (anti-Gal) antibody. Springer Semin. Immunopathol. 15, 155, 1993
12. SANDRIN, M.S., VAUGHAN, H.A., DABKOWSKI, P.L., McKENZIE, I.F.C. Anti-pig IgM antibodies in human serum reacts predominantly with Galα(1,3)Gal epitopes. Proc. Natl. Acad. Sci. USA. 90, 11391, 1993
13. COOPER, D.K.C., GOOD, A.H., KOREN, E., et al. Identification of alpha-galactosyl and other carbohydrate epitopes that are bound by human anti-pig antibodies: relevance to discordant xenografting in man. Transpl. Immunol. 1, 198, 1993
14. KOREN, E., NEETHLING, F.A., RICHARDS, S., et al. Binding and specificity of major immunoglobulin classes of preformed human anti-pig heart antibodies. Transplant. Int. 6, 351, 1993

15. VAUGHAN, H.A., LOVELEND, B.E., SANDRIN, M.S. Galα(1,3)Gal is the major xenoepitope expressed on pig endothelial cells recognized by naturally occurring cytotoxic human antibodies. Transplantation. 58, 879, 1994
16. NEETHLING, F.A., KOREN, E., YE, Y., et al. Protection of pig kidney (PK15) cells from the cytotoxic effect of anti-pig antibodies by α-galactosyl oligosaccharides. Transplantation. 57, 959, 1994
17. NEETHLING, F.A., KOREN, E., ORIOL, R., et al. Immunoadsorption of natural antibodies from human serum by affinity chromatography using specific carbohydrates protects pig cells from cytotoxic destruction. Transplant. Proc. 26, 1378, 1994
18. RIEBEN, R., von ALLMEN, E., KORCHAGINA, E.Y., et al. Detection, immunoabsorption, and inhibition of cytotoxic activity of anti-αGal antibodies using newly developed substances with synthetic Galα1-3Gal disaccharide epitopes. Xenotransplantation. 2, 98, 1995
19. GOOD, A.H., COOPER, D.K.C., MALCOLM, A.J., et al. Identification of carbohydrate structures that bind human antiporcine antibodies: implications for discordant xenografting in humans. Transplant. Proc. 24, 559, 1992
20. SANDRIN, M.S., DABKOWSKI, P.L., HENNING, M.M., MOUHTOURIS, E., McKENZIE, I.F.C. Characterization of cDNA clones for porcine α1,3galactosyltransferase: the enzyme generating the Galα(1,3)Gal epitope. Xenotransplantation. 1, 81, 1994
21. McKENZIE, I.F.C., VAUGHAN, H.A., SANDRIN, M.S. How important are anti-Galα(1-3)Gal antibodies in pig to human xenotransplants? Xeno. 2, 107, 1994
22. VAUGHAN, H.A., McKENZIE, I.F.C., SANDRIN, M.S. Biochemical studies of pig xenoantigens detected by naturally occurring human antibodies and the galactoseα(1-3)galactose reactive lectin. Transplantation. 59, 102, 1995
23. PLATT, J.L., LINDMAN, B.J., CHEN, H., SPITALNIK, S.L., BACH, F.H. Endothelial cell antigens recognized by xenoreactive human natural antibodies. Transplantation. 50, 817, 1990
24. PALMITER, R.D., BRINSTER, R.L. Germ-line transformation of mice. Ann. Rev. Genet. 20, 465, 1986
25. JAENISCH, R. Transgenic animals. Science. 240, 1468, 1988
26. SIGMUND, C.D. Major approaches for generating and analyzing transgenic mice. Hypertension. 22, 599, 1993
27. MULLINS, J.J., MULLINS, L.J. Transgenesis in non-murine species. Hypertension. 22, 599, 1993
28. FIRST, N.L., HASELTINE, F.P. Transgenic Animals. Reed Publishing, Inc., 1991
29. BRINSTER, R.L., CHEN, H.Y., TRUMBAUER, M.E., YAGLE, M.K., PALMITER, R.D. Factors affecting the efficiency of introducing foreign DNA into mice by microinjecting eggs. Proc. Natl. Acad. Sci. USA. 82, 4438, 1985
30. CAPECCHI, M.R. Altering the genome by homologous recombination. Science. 244, 1288, 1989
31. MANSOUR, S.L. Gene targeting in murine embryonic stem cells: introduction of specific alterations into the mammalian genome. Genet. Anal. 7, 219, 1990
32. ROBERTSON, E.J. Using embryonic stem cells to introduce mutations into the mouse germ line. Biol. Reprod. 44, 238, 1991
33. SOUTHERN, P.J., BERG, P. Transformation of mammalian cells to antibiotic resistance with a bacterial gene under control of the SV40 early region promoter. J. Mol. Appl. Gen. 1, 327, 1982

34. IOFFE, E., STANLEY, P. Mice lacking N-acetylglucosaminyltransferase I activity die at mid-gestation, revealing an essential role for complex or hybrid N-linked carbohydrates. Proc. Natl. Acad. Sci. USA. 91, 728, 1994
35. SADLACK, B., MERZ, H., SCHORLE, H., et al. Ulcerative colitis-like disease in mice with a disrupted interleukin-2 gene. Cell. 75, 253, 1993
36. KUNDIG, T.M., SCHORLE, H., BACHMANN, M.F., et al. Immune responses in interleukin-2-deficient mice. Science. 262, 1059, 1993
37. FUKUSHIGE, S., SAUER, B. Genomic targeting with a positive-selection lox integration vector allows highly reproducible gene expression in mammalian cells. Proc. Natl. Acad. Sci. USA. 89, 7905, 1992
38. KUHN, R., SCHWENK, F., AGUET, M., RAJEWSKY, K. Inducible gene targeting in mice. Science. 269, 1427, 1995
39. SHOCKETT, P., DIFILIPPANTONIO, M., HELLMAN, N., SCHATZ, D.G. Modified tetracycline-regulated system provides autoregulatory, inducible gene expression in cultured cells and transgenic mice. Proc. Natl. Acad. Sci. USA. 92, 6552, 1995
40. BLANKEN, W.M., VAN den EIJNDEN, D.H. Biosynthesis of terminal Galα1–3Galβ1–4GlcNAc oligosaccharide sequences on glycoconjugates. Purification and acceptor specificity of a UDP-Gal:N-acetyllactosaminide α1–3-galactosyltransferase from calf thymus. J. Biol. Chem. 260, 12927, 1985
41. LARSEN, R.D., RAJAN, V.P., RUFF, M., et al. Isolation of a cDNA encoding a murine UDPgalactose:β-D-galactosyl-1,4-N-acetyl-glucosamide-α1,3-galactosyltransferase: expression cloning by gene transfer. Proc. Natl. Acad. Sci. USA. 86, 8227, 1989
42. JOZIASSE, D.H., SHAPER, N.L., KIM, D., VAN den EIJNDEN, D.H., SHAPER, J.H. Murine α1,3galactosyltransferase: a single gene locus specifies four isoforms of the enzyme by alternative spicing. J. Biol. Chem. 267, 5534, 1992
43. JOZIASSE, D.H., SHAPER, J.H., VAN den EIJNDEN, D.H., VAN den TUNEN, A.J., SHAPER, N.L. Bovine α1,3galactosyltransferase: isolation and characterization of a cDNA clone. Identification of homologous sequences in human genomic DNA. J. Biol. Chem. 264, 142990, 1989
44. STRAHAN, K.M., GU, F., PREECE, A.F., et al. cDNA sequence and chromosome localization of pig alpha 1,3 galactosyltransferase. Immunogenetics. 41, 101, 1995
45. HENION, T.R., MACHER, B.A., ANARAKI, F., GALILI, U. Defining the minimal size of catalytically active primate α1,3galactosyltransferase: structure-function studies on the recombinant truncated enzyme. Glycobiology. 4, 193, 1994
46. JOZIASSE, D.H. Mammalian glycosyltransferase: genomic organization and protein structure. Glycobiology. 2, 271, 1992
47. YAMAMOTO, F., CLAUSEN, H., WHITE, T., MARKEN, J., HAKAMORI, S. Molecular genetic basis of the histo-blood group ABO system. Nature. 345, 229, 1990
48. JOZIASSE, D.H., SHAPER, J.H., JABS, E.W., SHAPER, N.L. Characterization of an α1,3-galactosyltransferase homologue on human chromosome 12 that is organized as a processed pseudogene. J. Biol. Chem. 266, 6991, 1991
49. LARSEN, R.D. RIVERRA-MARRERO, C.A., ERNST, L.K., CUMMINGS, R.D., LOWE, J.B. Frameshift and nonsense mutations in a human genomic sequence homologous to a murine UDP-Gal:β-D-Gal1,4-D-GlcNAcα1,3-galactosyltransferase cDNA. J. Biol. Chem. 265, 7055, 1990

50. SHAPER, N.L., LIN, S.P., JOZIASSE, D.H., KIM, D.Y., YANG-FENG, T.L. Assignment of two human alpha-1,3-galactosyltransferase gene sequences (GGTA1 and GGTA1P) to chromosomes 9q33-q34 and 12q14-q15. Genomics. 12, 613, 1992
51. McKENZIE, I.F., XING, P.X., VAUGHAN, H.A., PRENZOSKA, J., DABKOWSKI, P.L., SANDRIN, M.S. Distribution of the major xenoantigen (gal(α1–3)gal) for pig to human xenografts. Transpl Immunol 2, 81, 1994
52. ORIOL, R., YE, Y., KOREN, E., COOPER, D.K.C. Carbohydrate antigens of pig tissues reacting with human natural antibodies as potential targets for hyperacute vascular rejection in pig-to-man organ xenotransplantation. Transplantation. 56, 1433, 1993
53. PETERS, B.P., GOLDSTEIN, R. The use of Bandeiraea simplicifolia B4-isolectin as a histochemical reagent for the detection of α-D-galactopyranosyl groups. Exp. Cell. Res. 120, 321, 1979
54. IKEMATSU, S., KANAME, T., OZAWA, M., et al. Transgenic mouse lines with ectopic expression of α-1,3-galactosyltransferase: production and characteristics. Glycobiology. 3, 575, 1993
55. THALL, A.D., MALY, P., LOWER, J.B. Oocyte Galα1,3Gal epitopes implicated in sperm adhesion to the zona pellucida glycoprotein ZP3 are not required for fertilization in the mouse. J. Biol. Chem. 270, 21437, 1995
56. TEARLE, R.G., TANGE, M.J., ZANNETTINO, Z.L., et al. The α1,3-galactosyltransferase knockout mouse: implications for xenotransplantation. Transplantation. 61, 13, 1996
57. GALILI, U., SWANSON, K. Gene sequences suggest inactivation of a 1,3-galactosyltransferase in catarrhines after divergence of apes from monkeys. Proc. Natl. Acad. Sci. USA. 88, 7401, 1991
58. SANDRIN, M.S., PATTON, K., MOUHTOURIS, E., McKENZIE, I.F.C. Natural human anti-N-acetyl lactosamine antibodies react with xenogeneic cells after removal of Galα(1,3)Gal. Transplantation. Submitted 1995
59. ZAMECNIK, P.C., STEVENSON, M.L. Inhibition of Rous sarcoma virus replication and cell transformation by a specific oligodeoxynucleotide. Proc. Natl. Acad. Sci. USA. 75, 280, 1978
60. DAY, A.G., BEJARANO, E.R., BUCK, K.W.K., BURRELL, M., LICHTENSTEIN, C.P. Expression of an antisense viral gene in transgenic tobacco confers resistance to the DNA virus tomato golden mosaic virus. Proc. Natl. Acad. Sci. USA. 88, 6721, 1991
61. HAN, L., YUN, J.S., WAGNER, T. Inhibition of Moloney murine leukemia virus-induced leukemia in transgenic mice expressing antisense RNA complementary to the retroviral packaging sequences. Proc. Natl. Acad. Sci. USA. 88, 4313, 1991
62. STRAHAN, K.M., GU, F., ANDERSSON, L., GUSTAFSSON, K. Pig α1,3galactosyltransferase: sequence of a full-length cDNA clone, chromosomal localization of the corresponding gene, and inhibition of expression in cultured pig endothelial cells. Transplant. Proc. 27, 245, 1995
63. STRAHAN, K.M., PREECE, A.F., XU, Y., GUSTAFSSON, K. Antisense inhibition of pig α1,3galactosyltransferase leads to a reduction in expression of the major target for human natural antibodies on pig vascular endothelial cells. Xenotransplantation. 2, 143, 1995
64. SANDRIN, M.S., FODOR, W.L., MOUHTOURIS, E., et al. Enzymatic remodeling of the carbohydrate surface of a xenogenic cell substantially reduces human antibody binding and complement-mediated cytolysis. Nature Med. 1, 1261, 1995

65. SANDRIN, M.S., FODOR, W.L., COHNEY, S., et al. Reduction of the major porcine xenoantigen Galα(1,3)Gal by expression of α(1,2)fucosyltransferase. Xenotransplantation. 3, 134, 1995
66. COHNEY, S., PATTON, K., PRENZOSKA, J., et al. Reduction of Galα(1,3)Gal in vivo by transgenic expression of α1,2fucosyltransferase. Transplantation. In press, 1996
67. OSMAN, N., MOUHTOURIS, E., McKENZIE, I.F.C., SANDRIN, M.S. Switching amino-terminal cytoplasmic domains of α1,2fucosyltransferase and α1,3galactosyltransferase alters the expression of H substance and Galα(1,3)Gal. J. Biol. Chem. In press, 1996
68. CAIRNS, T. HAMMELMANN, D., GRAY, K., WELSH, K., LARSON, G. Enzymatic removal from various tissues of galactose α1,3-galactose target antigens of human anti-species antibodies. Transplant. Proc. 26, 1279, 1994
69. HOLZKNECHT, Z.E., PLATT, J.L. Identification of porcine endothelial cell membrane antigens recognized by human xenoreactive natural antibodies. J. Immunol. 154, 4565, 1995
70. SATAKE, M., KAWAGISHI, N., RYDBERG, L., et al. Limited specificity of xenoantibodies in diabetic patients transplanted with fetal porcine islet cell clusters. Main antibody reactivity against a-linked galactose-containing epitopes. Xenotransplantation. 1, 89, 1994
71. OSMAN, N., IOANNOU, Y.A., DESNICK, R.J., McKENZIE, I.F.C., SANDRIN, M.S. Reduction in the cell surface expression of Galα(1,3)Gal with α-galactosidase A cDNA. Transplantation. In press, 1995
72. IOANNOU, Y.A., BISHOP, D.F., DESNICK, R.J. Over-expression of human α-galactosidase A results in its intracellular aggregation, crystallization in lysosomes, and selective secretion. J. Cell. Biol. 119, 1137, 1992
73. GIANELLO, P.R., LATINNE, D., ALEXANDRE, G.P.J. Pig-to-baboon renal xenografts. Xeno. 3, 26, 1995
74. SACHS, D.H. Pig-to-primate xenotransplantation: tolerance through mixed chimerism. Xeno. 3, 52, 1995
75. ROTHER, R.P., FODOR, W.L., SPRINGHORN, J.P., et al. A novel mechanism of retrovirus inactivation in human serum mediated by anti-α-galactosyl natural antibody. J. Exp. Med. 182, 1345, 1995

51 Galα1–3Gal Xenoepitope: Donor-Targeted Genetic Strategies

M.J. Tange, M.J. Pearse, and A.J.F. d'Apice

Introduction

Anti-αGal antibody has been identified as the dominant xenoantigen in pig-to-human transplantation [1, 2]. It binds to terminal Galα1–3Galβ1–4GlcNAc-R [3]. This structure is not present in humans as the enzyme which creates it, α1,3-galactosyltransferase (αGT) has undergone frameshift and nonsense mutations [4]. The epitope is, however, widely distributed in the animal kingdom up to and including New World monkeys [5]. Humans develop anti-Gal antibodies as they are continually exposed to the α-galactosyl epitope on gut bacteria [6]. Although Galili first described anti-αGal as an IgG antibody occurring at a frequency of up to 1% of total IgG, it also has IgM and IgA components [7].

Anti-αGal has been variably estimated to account for 70%–90% of the total human anti-pig xenoantibody [7], and its functional capacity has been demonstrated both in vitro in cell cytotoxicity assays [8] and in ex vivo models in baboons [9]. The following is an overview of our research on the αGal xenoantigen, which initially focused on defining its relevance as a porcine xenoantigen and subsequently on various methods of genetically eliminating it.

Histological Studies

A tissue survey of porcine organs using affinity-purified anti-αGal antibody and anti-αGal-depleted serum revealed strong staining with anti-αGal antibody on the endothelium of all organs, in a perinuclear pattern in the heart and in small bile ductules in the liver. The strongest staining was seen in the proximal convoluted tubule of the kidney (Fig. 1a). However, there was almost no staining seen with serum which had been depleted of anti-αGal by affinity chromatography (Fig. 1b). These observations were confirmed by the demonstration that the reactivity of either purified anti-αGal antibodies or of whole human serum could be blocked by α-galactosyl sugars, such as melibiose, but not by irrelevant sugars, such as lactose. These studies demonstrated that the αGal epitope was the dominant porcine xenoantigen recognized by human xenoantibodies. A variety of other approaches, predominantly by Cooper's and Sandrin's groups [2, 8, 10, 11], have been published and unequivocally demonstrate the dominant position of the αGal epitope in this clinically relevant xenocombination.

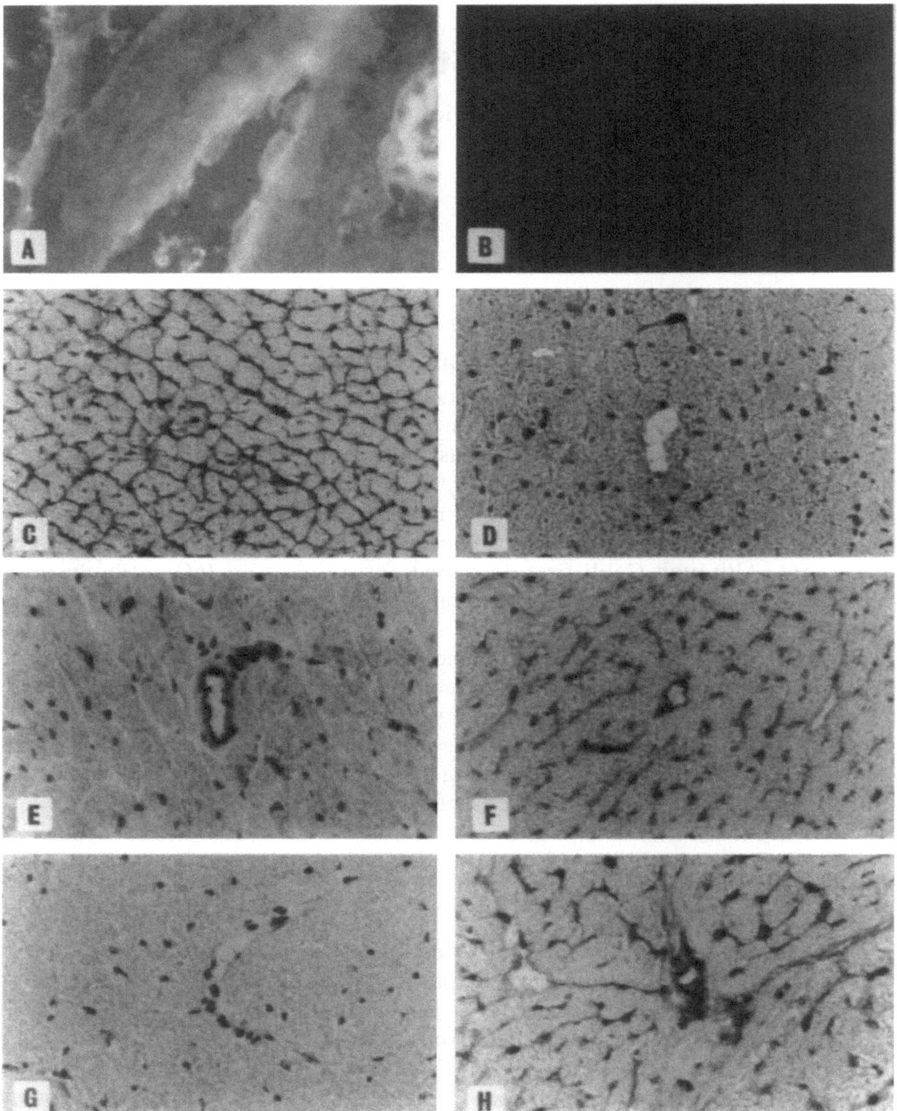

Functional Studies

To determine whether these xenoantibodies had functional capability which could mediate hyperacute rejection, ^{51}Cr release lysis assays were performed on porcine aortic endothelial cells (PAEC), using either whole human serum, anti-αGal depleted serum or purified anti-αGal antibody, together with pig spleen cell absorbed rabbit serum as the source of complement. Figure 2 demonstrates

◀ **Fig. 1. a** Indirect immunofluorescence staining of 2-μm pig renal cortex sections with anti-αGal antibody (200 μg/ml) and fluorescein isothiocyanate (FITC)-conjugated sheep anti-human IgG $F(ab)^2$ fragment. Section shows strong staining of endothelium of small artery and brush border of adjacent proximal convoluted tubules. Original magnification, ×500. **b** Indirect immunofluorescence staining of 2-μm pig renal cortex sections with anti-αGal-depleted serum (200 μg/ml) and FITC-conjugated sheep anti-human IgG $F(ab)^2$ fragment. Section shows no staining of any structure in the renal cortex. Original magnification, ×500. Immunoperoxidase staining of 4-μ m sections of **c** H transferase transgenic and **d** wild-type mouse hearts with FITC-conjugated *Ulex europaeus* 1 lectin (3 μg/ml; Sigma, St. Louis, MO, USA) and horseradish peroxidase-conjugated anti-FITC (1:300). 3,3′-Diaminobenzidine tetrachloride was used as the chromogen and Harris' hematoxylin as the counterstain. There is strong staining of the endothelium of small and large vessels in **c** the transgenic heart which is absent in **d** the nontransgenic heart. Original magnification, ×600. Immunoperoxidase staining of 4-μm sections of **e** H transferase transgenic and **f** wild-type mouse hearts with FITC-conjugated IB_4 lectin (1.25 μg/ml; Sigma, St. Louis, MO, USA) and horseradish peroxidase-conjugated anti-FITC (1:300). There is no staining on the endothelium of capillaries and small vessels. However, **e** there is staining of the endothelium of arterioles in wild-type hearts, while **f** there is IB_4 lectin staining of the endothelium of all vessels in transgenic hearts. Original magnification, ×600. Immunoperoxidase staining of 4-μm sections of **g** αGal knockout and **h** wild-type mouse heart with FITC-conjugated IB_4 lectin (20 μg/ml) and horseradish peroxidase-conjugated anti-FITC (1:300). There is no staining of the endothelium of any vessel in **e**, in contrast to **h**, where the endothelium of all vessels is positive. Original magnification, ×600

dose-dependent lysis of PAEC by human serum which is due to anti-αGal. The cytotoxicity of anti-αGal antibody is due to the IgM component since disruption of the IgM with 10 m*M* dithiothreitol abolished lysis. Finally, using an ex vivo model in which a mouse heart is perfused with human plasma in a Langendorff apparatus [12], we have demonstrated a substantial prolongation of survival when hearts are perfused with human plasma depleted of anti-αGal antibodies (32.5±6.7 min) compared to normal plasma (13.3±4.6 min; $p<0.01$) [13]. Taken together, these relatively simple studies strongly implicate anti-αGal as the key xenoantibody in hyperacute rejection of pig xenografts by humans and therefore a major barrier to clinical xenotransplantation.

Strategies To Inhibit Gal Expression

Inhibition of this xenoantibody-xenoantigen interaction clearly has the potential to prevent hyperacute rejection. There are a number of different approaches to achieve this goal which can be divided broadly into those which target the xenoantibody and those attacking the xenoantigen. We have taken the view that antibody depletion, antigen blockade and other therapies directed at the recipient depend on a temporary and possibly incomplete effect being sufficient and have the potential to further compromise recipients, who must in any case face substantial immunosuppression to prevent cell-mediated rejection. We have therefore focused on strategies directed at the xenograft donor, which are permanent and do not place the recipient at any greater risk. Strategies directed at recipient xenoantibodies are discussed in other chapters.

Broadly, the xenograft donor-directed strategies that we have investigated involve genetic manipulation so that the αGal epitope is either not expressed at all or is expressed at a very low level. We have examined two approaches.

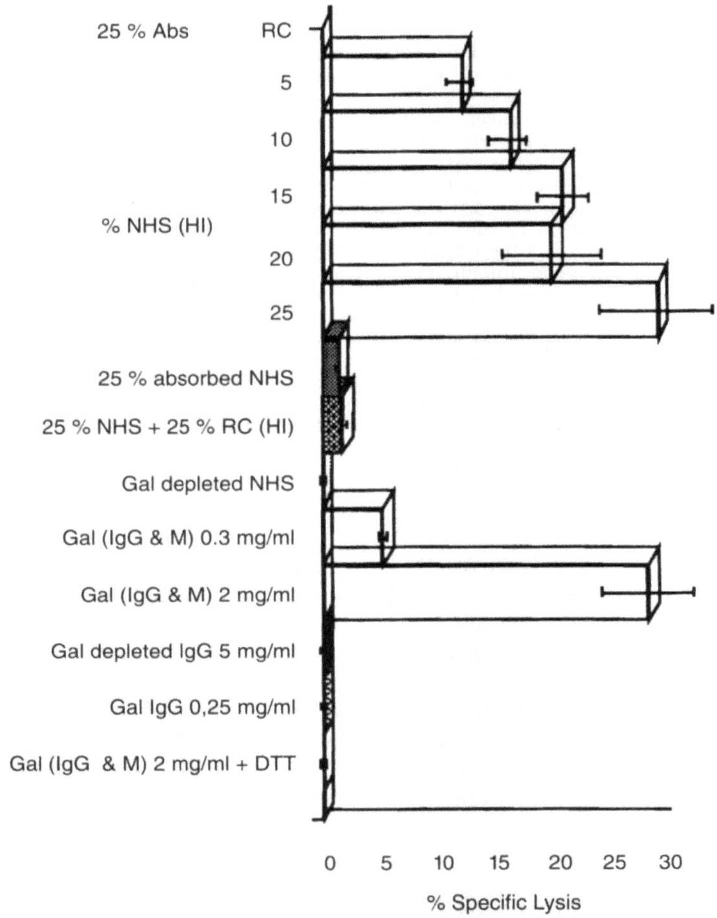

Fig. 2. ^{51}Cr release assay of lysis of pig aortic endothelial cells by human xenoantibodies in the presence of pig spleen cell-absorbed rabbit complement. Results are expressed as mean ± SD. *DTT*, dithiothreitol; *Abs*, antibodies

The first is gene inactivation (knockout) in which the αGT enzyme which creates the αGal epitope is disrupted by homologous recombination. The second is suppression of the αGal epitope by transgenic expression of the human H transferase gene. Other approaches which we have not attempted and will not discuss here are suppression of production or destruction of αGT by antisense RNA [14] and ribozymes [15], respectively.

H Transferase Transgenics

Sandrin's group initially proposed this novel method of suppressing production of the Gal epitope [16, 17]. In human endothelial cells, where αGT is absent, H transferase (α1,2-fucosyltransferase) fucosylates the Galβ1-4GlcNAc-R (*N*-acetyllactobiose) substrate and produces H substance. This enzyme is not present in pig endothelium, although another homologous α1,2-fucosyltransferase, Se transferase, is present in exocrine tissue. Sandrin demonstrated that transfection of a pig cell with human H transferase resulted in expression of H substance and suppression of the Gal epitope, presumably by completion for the common *N*-acetyllactobiose substrate. The advantage of this approach is that the H transferase gene can be introduced into pigs by existing transgenic technology and does not require embryonic stem cell technology. We have recently tested this hypothesis both by transfection and transgenesis in mice [18].

Murine NSO myeloma cells which express high levels of the αGal epitope were transfected with human H transferase. There was strong expression of H substance and an 80%–90% reduction in αGal epitope expression. Transgenic mice were made in which the H transferase gene was under control of the ubiquitously expressing murine H2-K^b promoter. Figure 3 shows strong expression

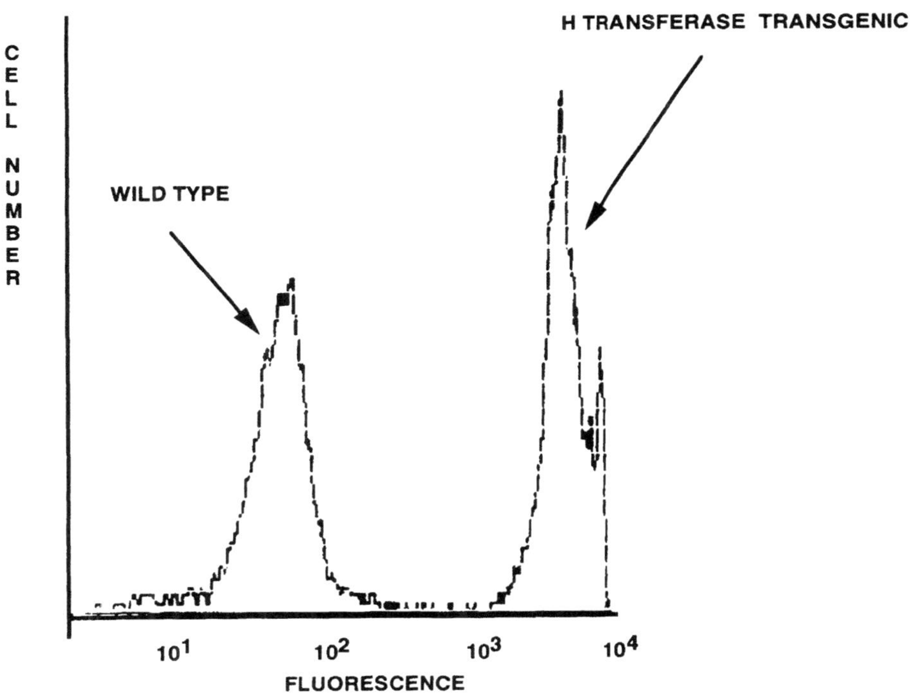

Fig. 3. Expression of H substance on peripheral blood leukocytes (PBL) of an H transferase transgenic mouse compared to a wild-type control. Fluorescein isothiocyanate (FITC)-*Ulex europaeus* lectin and flow cytometry

Fig. 4. Expression of αGal epitope on peripheral blood leukocytes (PBL) of an H transferase transgenic mouse compared to a wild-type control. Fluorescein isothiocyanate (FITC)-IB_4 lectin and flow cytometry

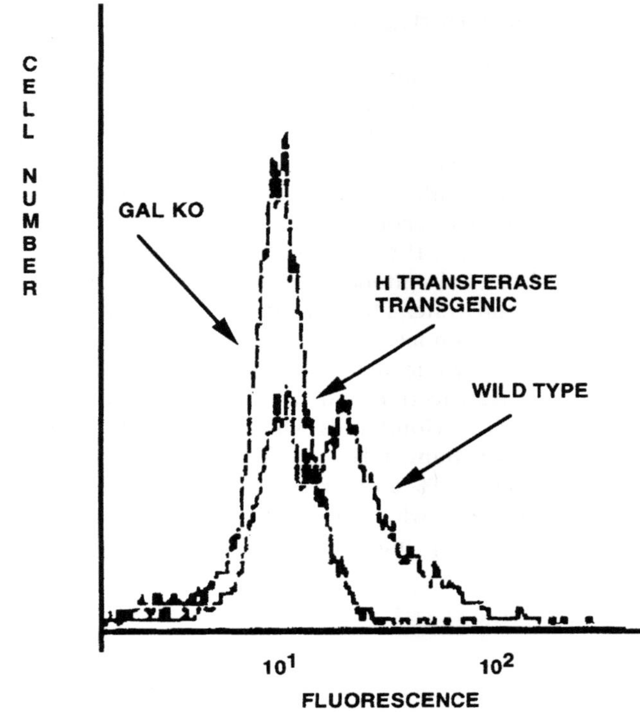

of H substance on peripheral blood leukocytes (PBL), with suppression of αGal epitope expression (Fig. 4). However, despite strong expression of H substance on the endothelium of all blood vessels (Fig. 1c,d), a diminution in the level of αGal expression as detected by IB_4 lectin only occurred in capillaries and not in larger vessels (Fig. 1e,f). There appeared to be an inverse relationship between the amount of αGal normally expressed on the endothelium and the ability of transgenically expressed H transferase to suppress it. It is not clear whether the failure to suppress the αGal epitope on larger vessels simply represents a difference in substrate supply or whether endothelium from different types of blood vessels express glycosyltransferases at different sites in the Golgi apparatus.

Another unexpected finding was an increase in binding of human IgM to the splenocytes of the H transferase transgenic mice compared to controls. This was accompanied by an increase in complement activation as measured by C3c binding. These findings strongly suggest that the genetic manipulation has created or exposed a new xenoantigen. So far this theoretically elegant approach has posed more problems than solutions and it needs further assessment to determine its utility.

αGal Knockout Mice

We have recently reported the generation of mice in which the αGT gene has been inactivated by homologous recombination [19]. These αGal knockout (KO) mice are viable and fertile and the only phenotypic abnormality observed to date is the universal development of cortical cataracts by 6 weeks of age. The finding that the αGal knockout mice are fertile argues strongly against αGal being critical for fertilization as has recently been suggested [20]. Histological surveys have not revealed any other abnormalities. Importantly, αGT mRNA was not detected by reverse transcriptase PCR and the αGal epitope was not detectable by IB_4 lectin on all cells (Fig. 5) and organs examined (e.g., Fig. 1g,h). Thus, as hoped, the αGal epitope has been completely depleted by inactivation of the αGT gene and is not regenerated by another unsuspected redundant glycosyltransferase.

The αGal knockout mice were then used to examine human serum for other non-αGal xenoantibodies. At very high serum concentrations (50%), binding of human IgM was markedly higher on αGal knockout compared to normal splenocytes. At serum concentrations below 20% NHS, spleen cells from αGal knockout mice showed an approximate 60% reduction in both IgM and IgG binding compared to normal mouse splenocytes with a typical prozone

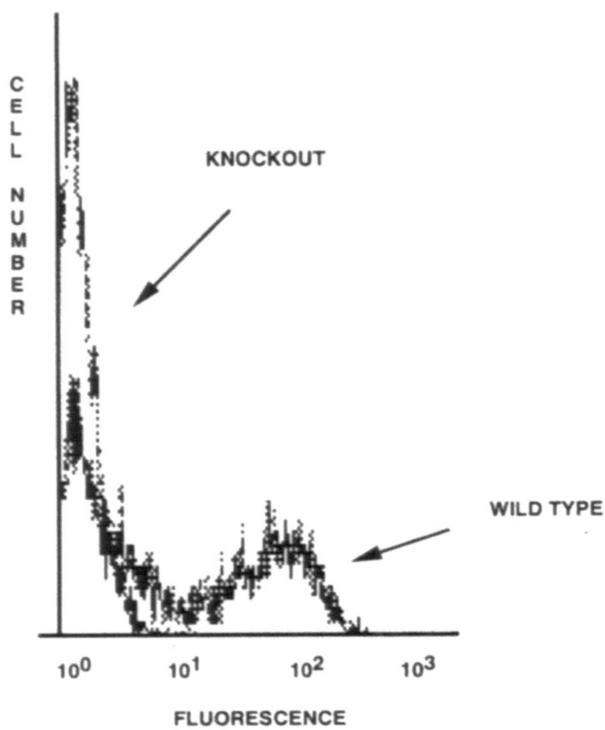

Fig. 5. Absence of expression of αGal epitope on peripheral blood leukocytes (PBL) of a Gal knockout mouse compared to a wild-type control. Fluorescein isothiocyanate (FITC)-IB_4 lectin and flow cytometry

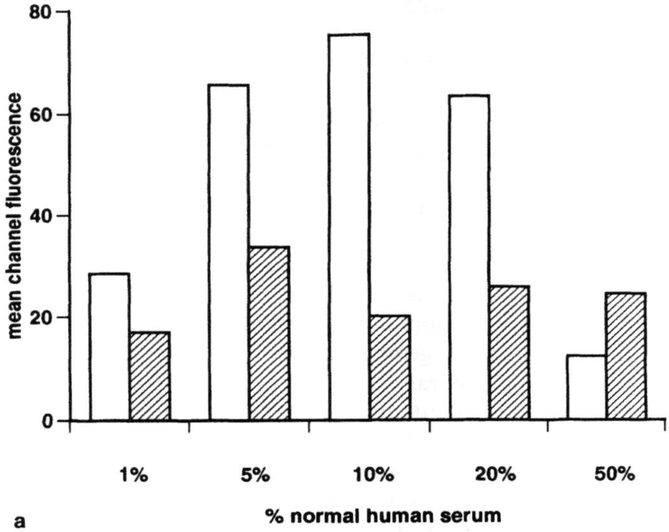

a

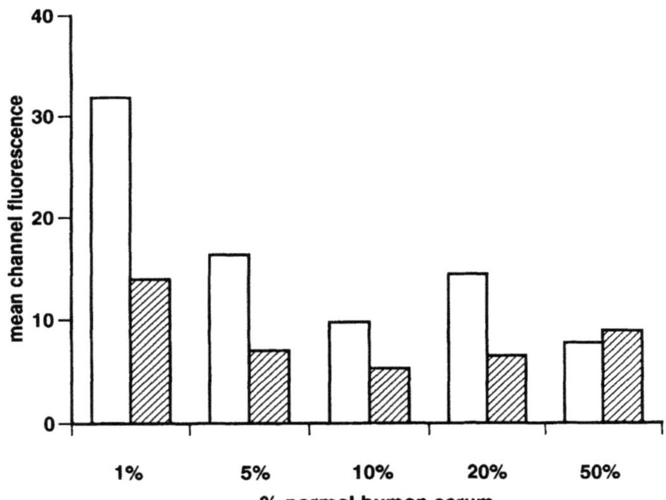

b

Fig. 6a,b. Flow cytometry binding assays of **a** human serum IgM and **b** IgG with splenocytes of αGT knockout (*hatched bars*) and wild-type mice (*open bars*)

(Fig. 6). As with the H transferase transgenic mice, deletion of the αGal epitope by gene inactivation is not completely effective in reducing xenoantigenicity.

These results suggest that two different types of "new" xenoantigens have been created or exposed. Firstly, there is the new xenoantigen reactive with very low titer IgM xenoantibodies. Secondly, there is the xenoantigen(s) detected by non-αGal IgG and IgM xenoantibodies at high titer. There is a strong suggestion that this represents either a new xenoantigen or one which has been exposed in increased amounts, as the reduction in high titer xenoreactivity of human sera with cells from αGal knockout mice (by approximately 60 %) is substantially less than would be predicted from earlier in vitro studies in which it was shown that depleting human serum of anti-αGal xenoantibodies almost completely abolished xenoreactivity (Figs. 1, 2).

When histological sections of organs from αGT knockout mice are reacted with 10 % human serum there is little apparent difference in the intensity of staining for bound human IgG or IgM.

Functional Studies

The decrease in IgM binding to αGal KO splenocytes at serum concentrations below 20 % is paralleled by a decrease in complement activation. C3 binding to KO mouse splenocytes is reduced by 30 %–50 % compared to wild-type splenocytes, depending on the serum concentration (Fig. 7).

Protection was also demonstrated using the ex vivo Langendorff model in which hearts were perfused with increasing concentrations of normal human plasma up to a total concentration of 13 %. αGal knockout heart survival was significantly prolonged compared to wild type mice (26.7±9.3 min vs. 8.3±1.3 min; $p<0.001$). There was an accompanying decrease in IgM and C3 binding in αGal knockout hearts compared to wild-type hearts. However, there was little decrease in the IgG binding between the two groups.

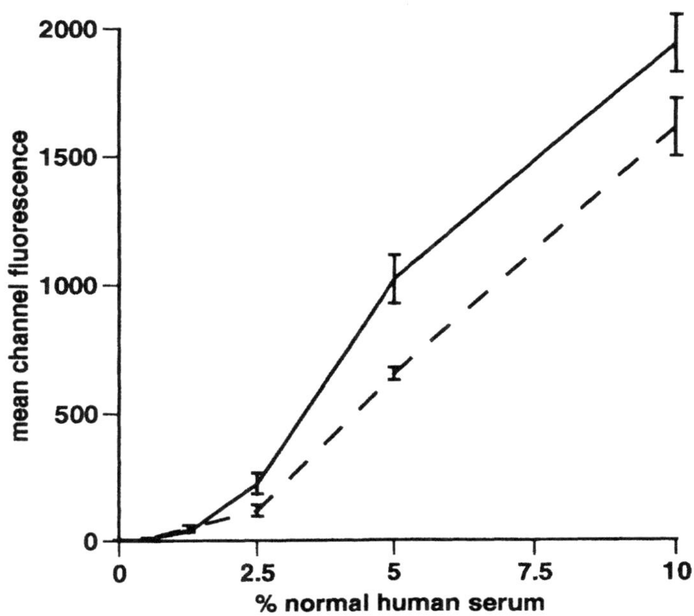

Fig. 7. Flow cytometry binding assay of C3 deposition (mean channel fluorescence) on splenocytes of wild-type (*solid line*) and αGal knockout (*broken line*) mice after reaction with human serum. Results are mean ±SEM of four experiments

Specificities of Non-αGal Xenoantibodies

Both genetic manipulations have had an effect on the αGal epitope - complete abolition in αGal knockout mice, and partial (and apparently tissue-dependent) reduction in H transferase transgenics. However, in both, the effect on "total xenoantigenicity," as determined by reactivity with pooled human serum or plasma, has been less than would be predicted from studies of the reactivity of anti-αGal-depleted human serum with pig cells and tissues. What are the possible explanations?

Firstly, it must be said that the expectations of massive reduction in total xenoantigenicity are derived from studies of the dominance of the αGal xenoantigen in the human–pig combination, and here we are dealing with human anti-mouse xenoantigenicity. It is clear that αGal is much more strongly expressed in pigs than mice [21] and therefore the proportion of xenoantibodies which react with non-αGal xenoantigens is much greater in the mouse than the pig. Studies are in progress to determine the contribution of anti-mouse$^{(+)}$/pig$^{(-)}$ xenoantibodies to this phenomenon. Secondly, if these genetic manipulations have generated "new" xenoantigens or uncovered or increased the expression of preexisting otherwise minor xenoantigens, the fundamental differences in the genetic manipulations would predict quite different consequences in this regard. Broadly, the H transferase transgenic approach might allow the generation of an entirely "new" xenoantigen, because a new non-native structure is being generated, while the αGal knockout approach would be more likely to favor increased expression of previously minor xenoantigens or exposure of preexisting but cryptic xenoantigens. So far, the nature of these non-αGal xenoantigens is unknown but provides for interesting speculation.

A wild card candidate for a "new" xenoantigen which might be generated in H transferase transgenics in human blood group A. Some pigs certainly have A transferase, but its expression is limited to tissues of endodermal origin such as exocrine tissue where its substrate, H substance, is generated by Se transferase (an α1,2-fucosyltransferase) [1]. However, they do not express blood group A on blood and endothelial cells because, unlike humans, they do not have the mesodermal α1,2-fucosyltransferase known as H transferase. If pigs (or mice) express A transferase in endothelium or blood cells and do not generate a product because its substrate is not generated (due to lack of H transferase), provision of the latter by transgenesis would create blood group A - a "new" xenoantigen!

Candidates for over-expression or uncovering of previously lowly expressed or cryptic antigens in αGal KO mice are the T, Tn, I/i, p^k, and Forsmann antigens. The structures of these are shown in Table 1. Humans are known to have naturally occurring antibodies to T (Thomsen-Friedenreich) antigen [22], Tn antigen [23], I/i (the core structures of the ABO antigen system which are fucosylated by H transferase to generate H substance) [24], the P group substances (including p^k antigen [24]), and in some individuals Forssman glycolipid [2,26]. A change in the xenoantigen composition may be accompanied by a change in the characteristics of the relevant xenoantibodies. For example, we have noticed that when αGal knockout mouse splenocytes are incubated with human serum at 37 °C,

Table 1. Candidate xenoantigens in αGal knockout mice

Antigen	Structure
Tn antigen (± sialic acid)	GalNAc-R 6 ± | 2NeuAc
Thomsen-Friedenreich (T) antigen	Galβ1-3GalNAc-R
I antigen	Galβ1-4GlcNAcβ1-3Galβ1-4GlcNAc-R β1 | 3Galβ1-4Glc-1Cer
i antigen	Galβ1-4GlcNAcβ1-3Galβ1-4GlcNAc-R 6 β1 / | Galβ1-4GlcNAcβ1 3Galβ1-4Glc-1Cer
P^{k} antigen	Galα1-4Galβ1-4Glcβ1-1Cer
Forssman antigen	GalNAcα1-3GalNAcβ1-3Galα1-4Galβ1-4Glcβ1-1Cer

there is little residual IgM binding compared to that seen at 4 °C, suggesting that they are anti-I antibodies which can behave as a cold agglutinin [24].

Comment

In pig-to-human xenotransplantation the dominant xenoantigen recognized by naturally occurring human xenoantibodies is the αGal epitope. This has been demonstrated in vitro by immunohistochemistry and flow cytometry using anti-αGal-depleted serum and inhibition by specific sugars. Anti-αGal antibody depletion in in vitro experiments protects pig endothelial cells from lysis by human serum, and in an ex vivo heart perfusion model it prolongs heart survival.

Both the αGT knockout and H transferase transgenesis approaches are effective in reducing αGal epitope expression. The former is clearly superior as its effects are complete and uniform. Unfortunately, gene knockout is at present not achievable in the pig because pig embryonic stem cells, which are critical for this technology, are not yet available. Despite the success of both approaches in abolishing or reducing expression of the αGal epitope, the effect on total xenoantigenicity is substantially less than expected from the in vitro studies using anti-αGal-depleted sera. both genetic manipulations appear to have been confounded to different degrees by the appearance of "compensatory" xenoantigenicity, the basis of which is still uncertain. "Candidate" xenoantibody-antigen combinations include cold reactive IgM, Thompson-Friedenreich antibody, anti-Tn, anti-p^{k}, and anti-I antibodies.

References

1. ORIOL, R., YE, Y., KOREN, E., COOPER, D.K.C. (1993) Carbohydrate antigens of pig tissues reacting with human natural antibodies as potential targets for hyperacute vascular rejection in pig-to-man organ xenotransplantation. Transplantation.56:1433
2. COOPER, D.K.C., GOOD, A.H., KOREN, E., et al. (1993) Identification of alpha galactosyl and other carbohydrate epitopes that are bound by human anti-pig antibodies: relevance to discordant xenografting in man. Transplant. Immunol.1:198
3. GALILI, U., RACHMILEWITZ, E.A., PELEG, A., FLECHNER, I. (1984) A unique natural human IgG antibody with an anti-alpha galactosyl specificity. J. Exp. Med.160:1519
4. LARSEN, R.D. RIVERA-MARRERO, C.A., ERNST, L.K., CUMMINGS, R.D., LOWE, J.B. (1990) Frameshift and nonsense mutations in a human genomic sequence homologous to a murine UDP-G D-Gal(1,4)-D-GlcNAc alpha(1,3)-galactosyltransferase cDNA. J. Biol. Chem.265:7055
5. GALILI, U., SHOHET, S.B., KOBRIN, E., STULTS, C.L.M., MACHER, B.A. (1988) Man, apes and Old World monkeys differ from other mammals in the expression of alpha galactosyl epitopes on nucleated cells. J. Biol. Chem.263:17755
6. GALILI, U., MANDRELL, R.E., HAMADEH, R.M., SHOHET, S.B., GRIFFITH, J.Mc.L. (1988) Interaction between the human natural anti-alpha galactosyl IgG (anti-Gal) and bacteria of the human flora. Infect. Immun.57:1730
7. SANDRIN, M.S., VAUGHAN, H.A., DABKOWSKI, P.L., McKENZIE, I.F.C. (1993) Anti-pig IgM antibodies in human serum react predominantly with Gal(α1–3)Gal epitopes. Proc. Natl. Acad. Sci. USA.90:11391
8. NEETHLING, F.A., KOREN, E., YE, Y., et al. (1994) Protection of pig kidney (PK15) cells from the cytotoxic effect of anti-pig antibodies by alpha-galactosyl oligosaccharides. Transplantation.57:959
9. YE, Y., NEETHLING, F.A., NIEKRASZ, M., et al. (1994) Evidence that intravenously administered alpha galactosyl carbohydrates reduce baboon serum cytotoxicity to pig kidney cells (PK15) and transplanted pig hearts. Transplantation.58:330
10. VAUGHAN, H.A., LOVELAND, B.E., SANDRIN, M.S. (1994) Gal alpha(1,3)Gal is the major xenoepitope expressed on pig endothelial cells recognized by naturally occurring cytotoxic human antibodies. Transplantation.58:879
11. SAMUELSSON, B.E., RYDBERG, L., BREIMER, M.E., et al. (1994) Natural antibodies and human xenotransplantation. Immunol. Rev.141:151
12. ROMANELLA, R., AMINIAN, A., ADAM, W.R., PEARSE, M.J., d'APICE, A.J.F. Evidence for involvement of the alternate pathway of complement in an ex vivo model of hyperacute xenograft rejection. Submitted for publication
13. TANGE, M.J., AMINIAN, A., ROMANELLA, R., ADAM, W.R., PEARSE, M.J., d'APICE, A.J.F. Demonstration of the functional importance of the Gal epitope in an ex vivo model of xenotransplantation. Xenotransplantation. In press
14. STRAHAN, K.M., PREECE, A.F., XU, Y., GUSTAFSSON, K. (1994) Antisense inhibition of pig α1,3 galactosyltransferase leads to a reduction in expression of the major target for human natural antibodies on pig vascular endothelial cells. Xenotransplantation.2:143
15. HAYASHI, S., NAGASAKA, T., NAMII, Y., et al. (1995) Effect of antisense ribozyme to pig α1,3 galactosyltransferase gene on the expression of Galα1,3Gal epitope. Third International Congress for Xenotransplantation. (Abstract), p. 78

16. SANDRIN, M.S., MOUHTOURIS, E., OSMAN, N., et al. (1995) Elimination of the major porcine xenoantigen, Gal alpha 1,3Gal by expression of alpha 1,2 fucosyltransferase. Glycoconjugate. J.12:468
17. SANDRIN, M.S., FODOR, W.L., MOUHTOURIS, E., et al. (1995) Enzymatic remodelling of the carbohydrate surface of a xenogeneic cell substantially reduces human antibody binding and complement-mediated cytolysis. Nature. Med. 1:1261
18. CHEN, C.G., FISICARO, A., SHINKEL, T.A., et al. (1996) Expression of H transferase reduction in Gal α1,3Gal epitope expression in transgenic mice expressing human H-transferase. Xenotransplantation. 3:69
19. TEARLE, R.G., TANGE, M., ZANETTINO, Z., et al. (1996) Analysis of the α1,3 galactosyltransferase knock-out mouse. Transplantation. 61:13
20. BLEIL, J.D., WASSARMAN, P.M. (1988) Galactose at the nonreducing terminus of O-linked oligosaccharides of mouse egg zona pellucida glycoprotein ZP3 is essential for the glycoprotein's sperm receptor activity. Proc. Natl. Acad. Sci. USA. 85:6788
21. McKENZIE, I.F.C., KOULMANDA, M., MANDEL, T., XING, P.X., SANDRIN, M. (1995) Comparative studies of the major xenoantigen Galα(1,3)Gal in pigs and mice. Transplant. Proc. 27:247
22. LEVENE, C., LEVENE, N.A., BUSKILA, D., MANNY, N. (1988) Red cell poly agglutination. Transfusion Med. Rev.2:176
23. BOORMAN, K.E., DODD, B.E., LINCOLN, P.L. Blood Group Serology.Fifth Edition. Churchill Livingstone, Edinburgh, 1977, p. 228
24. BRAY, J., LEMIEUX, R.U., McPHERSON, T.A. (1981) Use of a synthetic hapten in the demonstration of the Thomsen-Friedenreich (T) antigen on neuraminidase-treated human red blood cells and lymphocytes. J. Immunol.125:1966
25. RYDBERG, L., BREIMER, M.E., CEDERGREEN, B., et al. (1992) Serological and immunochemical characterization of PP_1P^k (anti-Tj^a) antibodies in blood group little p individuals. Blood group A type 4 recognition due to internal binding. Mol. Immunol.29:1273
26. YOUNG, W.W. Jr., HAKOMORI, S., LEVENE, P. (1979) Characterization of anti-Forssman antibodies in human serum: their specificity and possible changes in patients with cancer. J. Immunol.123:92

IX Aspects of Xenotransplantation in Humans

52 Evolution: Its Complexity and Impact on Xenotransplantation

C. Hammer

Introduction

The goal of xenotransplantation is to resolve the shortage of donor organs. Success would lead to a major revolution in transplantation. The current enthusiasm, however, has to be viewed in the light of the results actually achieved during the past 33 years of effort. All clinical attempts since 1963 have ended in lethal rejection (due to insufficient immunosuppression) or in deadly infection (due to overimmunosuppression). Survival and, in particular, function time of discordant xenografts have been insignificantly prolonged to date.

More than 250 reports about new immunosuppressive drugs and schedules of administration in xenotransplantation have been published in the last 5 years alone. Most have been related to experience in small rodent models. Progress made in small laboratory animals, however, shows only inconsistent correlation with controlled in vivo studies in large mammals or with clinical efforts. Even the reports in large animal studies and humans have to be regarded with caution, because either the organs were not transplanted orthotopically or their function was suboptimal, necessitating support by artificial measures until the lethal end.

The reasons for this disappointingly slow progress can be directed to the bewildering complexity of hyperacute xenogeneic rejection, which is related in great part to the presence of evolutionary hurdles. This chapter will attempt to review our limited knowledge in the field of comparative physiology, biochemistry, and anatomy, but can at best describe discrepancies in these interspecies interactions only in mosaic form.

Evolution has set severe obstacles to xenotransplantation. Even in closely related species combinations, significant differences in metabolism and interaction of mediators exist which can profoundly disturb physiological, biochemical, and even immunological interactions between graft and recipient [2]. In models in which widely divergent species are used, major adverse reactions are observed within a very short period after reperfusion with xenogeneic blood [3]. Furthermore, cell-mediated reactions have not yet been sufficiently investigated in vivo because none of these organs has achieved a long enough survival time. Therefore, the mechanisms involved in late xenogeneic rejection of discordant primary and secondary vascularized organs can only be assumed and/or composed as hypotheses [4].

Evolution

Numerous components of evolution influence the progress of xenotransplantation. Genetics, physiology, and anatomy all separately relate to evolution and (in regard to xenotransplantation) have to be understood as an integrated whole, with an increasing complexity developed over evolutionary time. Evolution's own dilemma is the continuing conflict of retaining the advantages that have been achieved but at the expense of what might be achieved. Total constancy of living material would eliminate any future change, while unlimited variation would jeopardize what has been attained already. The phylogeny of mankind depends on improvements and adaptations arising from accidental and spontaneous mutations.

The rate of evolution per unit of absolute time is, however, unpredictable and peculiar to each species. It depends on the environmental niche chosen. Only very approximate estimations can be made of the time required to effect a morphological change. The rates of evolution of the external appearance of man and animals are rather similar, although the rates of genetic and immunologic modifications are different [5].

Molecular evolution can proceed with a remarkable regularity.

It has been found that the amino acid sequences of albumin change to a similar degree over a given period of time in different groups of animals, such as primates and dogs [6]. The more recent the common ancestor that the two species share, then the greater the structural resemblance between the albumins. This difference can even be expressed as "index of dissimilarity" or "immunological distance." It has also been called the "immunological clock" [5] (Table 1). This

Table 1. Index of dissimilarity (ID) and rates of albumin evolution in primates and canines

Species	ID
Primates	
Man	1.00
Gorilla	1.09
Chimpanzee	1.14
Orangutan	1.22
Baboon	2.23
Chapuchin monkey	5.00
Tupaia	11.00
Cattle	32.00
Pig	>35.00
Canine	
Dog	1.00
Coyote	1.06
Wolf	1.16
Jackal	1.18
Fox	1.20

process of molecular evolution is discontinuous. In other words, the minimum change is the substantiation of one amino acid after the other. Serum albumin is involved in the transport of steroid hormones, cholesterol, bilirubin, etc., and is responsible for the maintenance of blood osmolarity, and yet, despite all of these useful functions, is fully dispensable [7]. Individuals totally lacking serum albumin have been described in several species (humans, dogs, and rats) without impairment of any essential capacity to support life.

Selection of a Suitable Donor Species

Nature did not anticipate that humans would one day wish to develop xenotransplantation, particularly when this involves a widely divergent relationship. Natural selection over 3 billion years has achieved 2–5 million animal species on earth today. But from approximately 4100 mammal species, one quarter are small rodents and are not suitable for the purpose of clinical xenotransplantation. Only very few species, mainly those domesticated by man, would be suitable as organ donors on the basis of their anatomical characteristics (Fig. 1).

The classification of the phylogenetic relationship between a donor animal species and man, and the impact of this relationship on the functioning of organs and cells in a different environment, are possibly the most fundamental problems in xenotransplantation. Xenograft survival time seems to be inversely proportional to the evolutionary time divergency (or phylogenetic distance) between the two species [8]. Transplants between individuals of one zoological family or between zoologically closely related creatures are rejected acutely, usually in

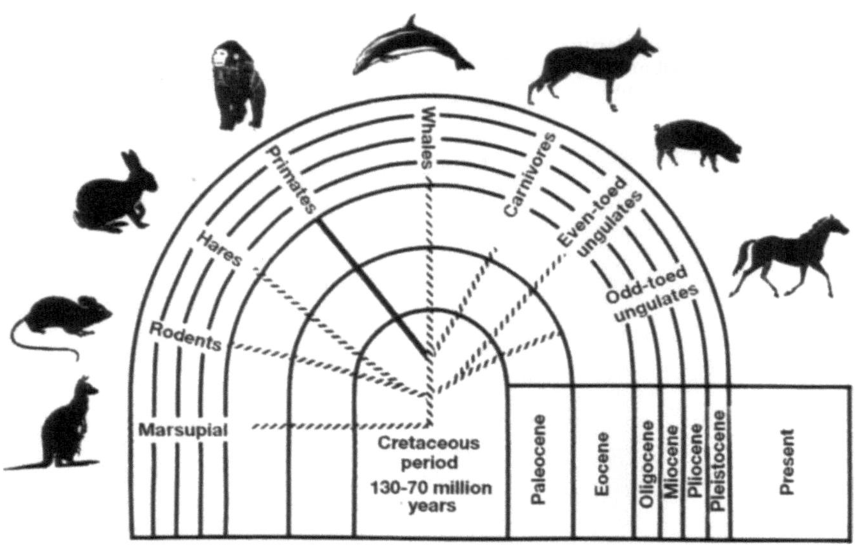

Fig. 1. Evolutionary relationship between species suitable for xenotransplantation in man

a cellular fashion. Transplants between members of two families within one moderately related zoological order are rejected in a mixed humoral/accelerated cellular fashion, while transplants between two widely divergent zoological orders are destroyed hyperacutely by purely humoral mechanisms (or possibly even nonimmunological mechanisms) [9].

Within this general pattern, however, lie many inconsistencies. For example, hearts transplanted from rat to mouse survive for 7.5 days but vice versa for only 3.5 days. Rabbit hearts function in rats for 3 days, while rabbits reject rat hearts hyperacutely [10]. Wolf kidneys survive in mongrel dogs for 20 days without immunosuppression, while wolves reject dog kidneys in 12 days [11]. Guinea pig organs are rejected by Old World rodents (such as rats and mice) hyperacutely, a paradox which must be related to the ancient separation of the American continent from Eurasia and the different chromosomal evolutionary processes in these rodents [5]. Hearts from New World monkeys transplanted into Old World primate species are also rejected hyperacutely [12].

The rates of morphological, biochemical, and physiological change are relatively rapidly (in evolutionary terms) simply under the pressure of the environment, for example during domestication, or as seen in the contrast in the presence of αGal1-3Gal epitopes between Old and New World primates after continental shifting. In the absence of such pressures, however, features may remain unchanged for millions of years [6]. Most domestic animals differ completely in their phenotype from their wild ancestors (e.g., domestic dog and wolf, pig and wild boar), while their genetic background has changed little. This indicates that domestic breeding or "farming" of appropriate donors would allow us to modify organ size in a relatively short time without, for example, altering the phenotype of the major histocompatibility complex [13].

Anatomical Differences

The *size* of potential donor species is an important aspect of xenotransplantation. Domestication has shown that nature would allow appropriately sized donors to be produced in a relatively short time, but their genetic skeleton would not change so rapidly. The original shape, structure, and texture, as well as the basic mechanical and functional characteristics, would still exist [14]. Anatomical differences may impede successful surgical techniques. Organs incompatible for size are prone to be either compressed in the new recipient (in the case of large organs) or unphysiologically enlarged by edema or hemorrhage (in the case of small organs) as is known from the experience with liver transplantation [15]. In addition, most parenchymal organs depend on rhythmic heartbeat or muscle tone to produce undulating tissue pressure [16].

The human upright *posture* is exceptional in the animal kingdom, and could influence the suitability and successful transplantation of organs from animals of horizontal bearing. Only humans, primates, and kangaroos have adapted to a permanently upright position. As a result, their anatomical characteristics are quite different from other mammals of comparable size to man. A comparison of heart valves (originating from the upright kangaroo and the horizontal

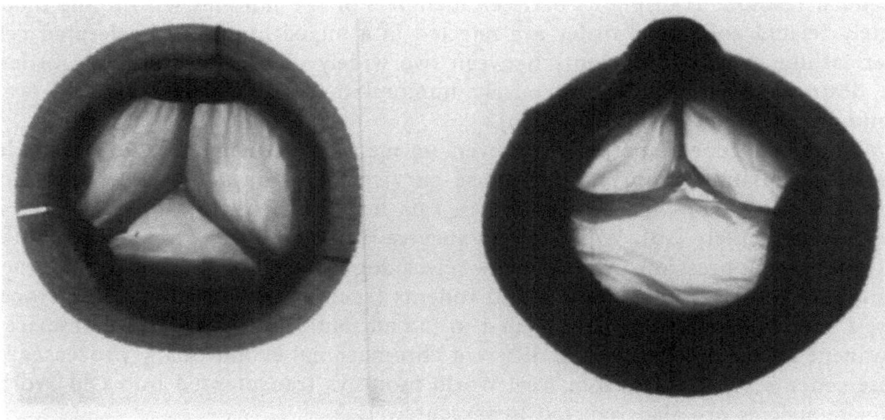

Fig. 2. Heart valves (aortic) from pig (*left*) and kangaroo (*right*). Note the 17% reduction in the orifice of the pig valve due to the presence of muscle tissue

pig) transplanted into sheep demonstrated that the effective orifice of a kangaroo aortic valve is 17% larger than that of a pig valve of the same diameter. Thus the stroke volume is higher and the resulting transvalvar pressure gradient is lower, which reduces the demand on the host heart muscle [17] (Fig. 2).

Posture also influences blood circulation. In the human lung, for example, blood flow varies in three distinguishable zones. For example, the lower third of the lung has both a larger change in volume during inhalation and exhalation and a smaller resting volume than the apex. The different pressures measured in each zone are related to upright posture and affect the capillaries variously. The pressure of the blood vessels is more pulsatile in upright than in horizontal lungs. Together with species-specific differences in resistance at the blood-gas barrier, different hemoglobins, and varying blood viscosity, gas transport could be disturbed if the lungs or heart from a horizontal animal are transplanted into an upright recipient [18].

The transplantation of baboon livers to humans has also resulted in unsatisfactory technical outcomes [2]. Transplanting rodent hearts into guinea pigs heterotopically has proved to be technically difficult, possibly because of the extremely low blood pressure found in the guinea pig. Many other examples of difficulties will probably be discovered.

Physiological/Biochemical Differences

If we disregard the immunological problems, or assume that immunological tolerance in xenotransplantation can one day be achieved, we still do not know whether the physiological mechanisms of the organ and its new host will be compatible. Very few data exist which would allow the accurate assessment of the physiological function of xenografts in man. The short survival times experienced in most xenotransplation models to date have not enabled predictions to be made about metabolic compatibility between species. The function of multicellular organs and organisms depends on the ability of cells to communicate with each other, which requires a controlled basic metabolism which is universal in all mammals. Therefore, most metabolic activities, such as pH, osmolarity, organ blood flow, and cardiac output per unit, may have little impact on the results of xenotransplantation [14].

These basic metabolic characteristics will remain similar in different mammalian species, however, only through the controlled growth and organization of communication through cell-to-cell contact. The secreted messenger molecules must be compatible with the receptor of the target. This humoral "concert" involves myriad signal molecules, with most being species-specific proteins. Because of their potent action, the activated molecules (once they have fulfilled their function) have to be destroyed, again by a species-specific inhibitor. Some signals, such as neurotransmitters, cooperate only with the adjacent cell, while others, such as hormones and cytokines, circulate in the bloodstream. Due to their individual receptors, parenchymal cells respond differently from, for example, lymphoid cells to the same signal [20]. Examples of such signals are neurointestinal hormones and interleukins. Responses to these may change not only from parenchymal to lymphoid cells but from species to species.

For the transport of many of these molecules, and because of their variable solubility, binding and transport molecules are needed, which are also species-specific and have to be secreted by a "compatible" liver. Due to the extremely fast evolutionary rate of these phylogenetically "modern" molecules, large differences exist between species. [21]. Such variations and lack of suitable transport molecules could nullify the action of hormones in a xenogeneic environment.

Selected examples of physiological and biochemical variations between species include blood viscosity, blood groups, liver metabolism, enzymes, and hormones.

Blood Viscosity

Blood viscosity varies from 5.9 mPa/s in pigs to 4.7 mPa/s in humans and dogs to 3.4 mPa/s in rabbits. Viscosity depends on the various blood components, including total protein and the size and number of red (RBCs) and white blood cells (WBCs). The numbers of RBCs and WBCs vary significantly between species. It has also been demonstrated in perfusion experiments that the size of the foreign RBC can be critical and can interfere mechanically with the microcirculation. Hematocrit comprises 30 % of blood volume in pigs and 40 % in man. Due to the increased viscosity of human blood, a reduced hemoperfusion of pig organs has to be expected. This would be especially critical for coronary blood flow [22].

Blood Groups

The blood groups of most domestic animals have been studied [23] and more closely resemble the rhesus system than the ABO system of humans and primates. However, human anti-ABO antibodies seem to play no role in the rejection of pig organs.

Liver Metabolism

Livers of different animal species exhibit differences of metabolism. For example, the highest concentrations of serum cholesterol are typically found in humans, (at 200 mg/100 ml). Cholesterol levels are extremely low in pigs (45 mg/100ml), while in dogs, horses and cattle (at approximately 90 mg/100 ml) and sheep (at 64 mg/100 ml), concentrations are in the middle range. Blood sugar levels are similar in man and pig (at 80–100 mg/100 ml) but lower in sheep and cattle (at 30–60 mg/100 ml). Lipase levels differ between man and rat and man and pig by 46 % and 28 %, respectively. Apolipoprotein concentration in man differs by 40 % from that in the pig and rat. Albumin levels differ significantly even between humans and primates [24].

Enzymes

All highly developed animals possess innumerable proteolytic enzymes which interact in a species-specific fashion. A mammalian liver, whether transplanted or not, is able to produce about 2500 enzymes, which are released mostly as precursor molecules or proenzymes, to be activated by other active enzymes, hormones or peptides. Their tissue specificity is highly expressed and they are well known as isoenzymes. Because of this specificity, isoenzymes may not function adequately in a transplanted organ. Organs from different species show varying combinations of enzymes. Fetal tissue can contain enzymes and isoenzymes which barely function even in adults of the same species. In addition, isoenzymes differ in substrate specifity and inhibitory behaviour [25].

Enzymes need careful control. Most have stereospecific characteristics and qualities. If they do not build a coherent system in which to function (in which they are interdependent), the total effect of their activities can be chaos. Extracellular enzymes are highly discriminative. Each enzyme catalyses only one type of reaction and is active for only one of the numerous substances in the body [25] (Fig. 3).

To what extent these mechanisms might upset the metabolism of the xenograft recipient is unknown. However, studies on the renin-angiotensin system show that such enzyme cascades can be incompatible between species, even within the rodent family. The effect of foreign enzymes on the circulation and metabolism of an animal cannot be predicted [26].

Extensive cross-reactions among enzymes have been observed in 12 species, including primates and pig. The many analogous enzymes with similar substrate

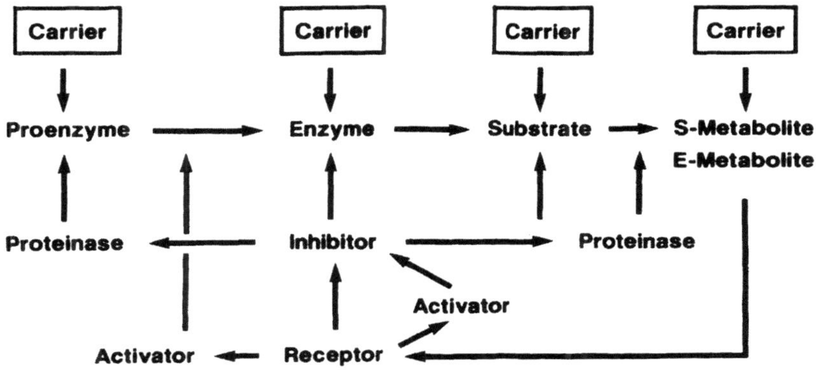

Fig. 3. Species-specific interactions during enzyme activation and inhibition

specifity show considerable variation between different animal species in regard to their electrophoretic mobility. A range of immunological cross-reactions occurs in closely related species, especially primates, and even greater degrees of antigenic diversity are found between widely divergent species. In the case of alkaline phosphatase, immunological cross-reactions occur even between members of one zoological family [27].

Proteolytic enzymes have many physiological functions (starting with general protein digestion), ranging from activation of complement and blood coagulation, and extending to the release of hormones and pharmacologically active peptides and their precursor molecules. Underlying all functions, however, are specific and multivarious control mechanisms. If uncontrolled, such enzymes can destroy the protein components of the cells and tissue, as is reflected in the hyperacute rejection that occurs between widely divergent species [28].

During phylogeny and ontogeny, changes in amino acid sequence, three dimensional structure, and even enzymatic reaction, indicate the existence of distinct families of these proteins.

In addition, changes in molecular structure bring about variation in species-specific inhibitors. Proteases are believed to have arisen in the earliest phase of biological evolution. In the course of evolutionary development, they have adapted from having a purely digestive function to become complex physiological regulators. Their heterogeneity (despite enzymatic specificities), their ontogeny and tissue differentiation are of wide biological influence. Their tissue specificity is highly expressed and well known (as isoenzymes). Most of the different organs and tissues in adult vertebrates show a characteristic distribution and activity of enzymes. This individuality not only differs in organs but also changes during ontogeny. Fetal tissue can contain isoenzymes that barely function in adults of the same species [29]. The embryonic form of *lactate dehydrogenase* (LDH) in cattle, for example, develops in a unidirectional way into the adult form, whereas in rabbits and pigs embryonic LDH remains well represented at all stages of ontogeny.

Another example is provided by ovine embryos, which are less well oxygenated than rabbit or cavian (guinea pig) embryos. This is reflected in the embryonic isoenzyme status and the A- and B-type contributions of the subunit of LDH, which indicate an indirect effect of oxygen on the biosynthesis of LDH [30].

Carboxylesterases exhibit the most extensive multiplicity of all of the esterases in vertebrate tissue, and show considerable species variation with respect to the electrophoretic properties of the isoenzymes, their tissue distribution, degree of multiplicity and, therefore, immunogenicity. Carboxylesterase type 5, for example, exists in two forms in pig, sheep, horse, ox and possum (with molecular weights of 80 000 and 160 000) but only as one isoenzyme (with a molecular weight of 80 000) in the guinea pig and rat [31, 27].

Catalase may be the most extensively investigated enzyme. It exists as five major isoenzymes in such species as horse, rat and rabbit, whereas most other mammalian species display only a single form of catalase. Its distribution in the cell and subcellular organelles in various species varies as markedly as its activity. Catalase exists at a low level in the early stages of postneonatal development, but increases during sexual maturation and reaches a maximum in the adult male.

Such multiplicity and heterogeneity, overlapping with substrate specificity, is probably common to most enzymes in the form of primary or secondary modifications of protein structure and therefore of immunogenicity. Only forms which are not involved in such differences are likely to function in an undisturbed manner in a foreign host.

Variations in physiological function reflect the degree of divergency of the species and also the pressure of "selection" in particular biological environments and, furthermore, specific developmental events in vertebrate animals. It should be emphasized that the activators and inhibitors of enzymes probably show similar species differences. Their functions, however, have not been explored and are poorly understood.

Hormones

The spectrum of *steroid hormones* seems to be biologically similar in all mammals, but these molecules occur in different concentrations [32]. A few species need specific steroid hormones. For example, horses require species-specific steroid metabolites, such as equilin or equilinin. However, the synthesis (and probably the metabolism) of steroid hormones is almost the same in all vertebrates. Hormone-binding proteins, however, are not present in all species. Where they exist, they seem to be specific transport molecules [33].

The situation is totally different for *peptide hormones*. Members of this group can vary from tripeptides to polypeptides of 100 amino acids and more. Their fast action is regulated by similarly fast inhibitors. In most cases, both peptide hormones and their inhibitors are species-specific (Fig. 4). The peptide molecule released and activated from the prehormone by a releasing factor must exist in a stable form and fit its receptor, this latter requirement being necessary for specific cellular functions and membrane expression. Add to this the specialisation

Fig. 4. Species-specific factors involved in the control of hormone release

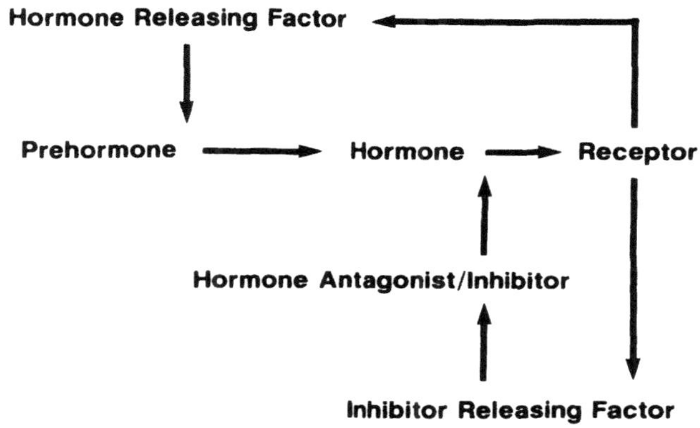

of the target cell, the complex chains of intermediate molecules and enzymes which have to be integrated to effect a satisfactory result, and one can appreciate how even one disparate factor can disrupt such a sequence [34].

Growth hormones differ between primates in their amino acid sequence by only 2 %, between man and whale by 34 %, between man and pig by 19 %. Powerful evidence of this incompatibility is provided by the fact that the growth factors of one species will not function on an organ of another. It must be remembered that antigenic determinants of growth factors may comprise only a few amino acids, and that the sequence may not include that part of the molecule responsible for biological activity. Nevertheless, it is antigenic even in closely related species.

The measurement of locally produced xenogeneic hormones circulating in blood is unlikely to be rewarding. It could reflect nothing but a trivial spillover from the xenogeneic site of action. It poses the question as to whether hormones released from a xenograft are physiologically meaningful. We do not know whether a single hormone can act at different sites within a xenogeneic organism or whether it has different local functions, some possibly unphysiological or even pathological.

The function of growth hormone is not only to control body and organ growth, but also to influence the metabolism of protein, carbohydrates and fat. Experiments show that transgenic mice carrying bovine or porcine growth hormone gene constructs develop into giant mice [35]. The gene products are not recognized as foreign due to neonatal tolerance, and no immunological reaction occurs. However, there is no downregulation by physiological inhibitors, thus leading to the overproduction of a functional molecule which is associated with marked nephropathy (obsolescence of numerous glomeruli, massive dilatation of the renal tubules) and liver hypertrophy. Fifty percent of the animals die from malignancies. However, bovine growth hormone does not function in humans. This raises the question of whether transplanted xenogeneic fetal or adult animal organs would grow satisfactorily or, conversely, become giant organs under the influence of human growth hormone [36].

To function, most hormones require a releasing factor which is species-specific, as is the subsequent releasing inhibitor. Releasing factors produced by foreign cells induce reduced receptor binding and hormone liberation. Releasing factors are similar between some species, but different between others. The corticotrophin releasing factor, for example, is identical in man and rat, but differs by 25% between man and sheep. Encephalins from man and pig also differ by 25%. Growth hormones in man are identical with 98% of those in primates, 81% in pigs, and 61% in rats.

Purified thyroglobulins (TG) from man cross-react to various degrees with those of other mammalian species and also those of reptiles, but to a lesser extent with avian types. Sheep and pig TGs (both ungulates) are more closely related than others. In order to inactivate rabbit anti-sheep TG-antibodies in vitro, a 200-fold concentration of reptilian TG is needed as compared with sheep TG. Rabbit TG, in contrast, is less effective than python TG. To inactivate rabbit anti-pig TG-antibodies, however, all the TGs are equally effective. This apparent inconsistency indicates the complexity of the correlation between phylogeny and the molecular evolutionary history of proteins [37, 38].

Immunological Differences

Immunological differences are clearly another obstacle to successful xenotransplantation. The heterogeneity, different avidity and affinity, and variable specificity of preformed natural antibodies, for example, depend on the antigenic relationship of donor and recipient. The interaction of preformed natural antibodies from one species with the complement from another can cause dysfunction or extreme opsonisation of transplanted tissues.

Preformed Natural Antibodies

Preformed natural antibodies (PNAb) trigger the activation of endothelial cells (EC) [39–41]. Recent work has described carbohydrate epitopes on EC as the target of PNAb [42–45]. Calculations have, shown, however, that only approximately 1% of immunoglobulin molecules bind to these carbohydrate epitopes [46, 47]. Most xenogeneic antibody types, such as hemagglutinins, cytotoxins, etc., are eliminated through absorption by red blood cells or whole organs, but EC absorb only a small number of PNAb [48].

Reduction of PNAb by plasmapheresis, isovolemic hemodilution, or immunoadsorption delays the typical hyperacute rejection (HAR) [49–52]. Newborn unsuckled piglets, not yet possessing PNAb, are able to reject dog kidneys hyperacutely [53]. PNAb bind to EC and other structures, such as xenogeneic corneas, myocytes and hepatocytes and lyse the targets. Again, some exceptions exist. In vitro, only 50% of EC are killed while the rest are activated to produce large amounts of typical mediators [54].

PNAb are involved in the triggering of HAR, though their primary target is on the vascular endothelial cell. Their possible impact on parenchymal cells, however, has not been well investigated and is poorly understood. In spontaneously beating cardiomyocytes from neonatal rats, PNAb (in the sera of man, pig and other species) induce a stereotypic pattern of altered contractility with a temporary halt in beating for a few minutes. An experimental series performed with human serum proved that the break in contractions could be prevented by the prior absorption of PNAb but not by complement inactivation. The cessation of beating could be overcome by a big increase in the extracellular Ca^{2+} concentration, but not by extracellular electrical stimulation. After spontaneously resuming contractility, the cells of the syncytial monolayer then beat asynchronously for at least 12 h. The main electrophysiological effect of PNAb is an enhanced excitation threshold, so that temporary intracellular electrical stimulation is no longer sufficient to elicit action potentials [55].

In contrast to PNAb, antibodies specifically induced against fractions of fetal rat cardiomyocytes stop the contractions of beating cardiomyocytes within less than 30 min and lead to cell lysis.

Thus PNAb reduce the electrical excitability of beating cardiomyocytes by binding to the cell surface membrane. This lowering of the excitation threshold results from a general reduction of excitability of the myocytes rather than from the inhibition of a specific ionic conductance. PNAb and antibodies induced specifically against fetal rat cardiomyocytes have totally different actions on parenchymal cells, i.e., beating cardiomyocytes. While PNAb, which are primarily IgM, inhibit the contractility of beating cardiomyocytes, antibodies induced specifically against fetal rat cardiomyocytes, which are IgG, are cytotoxic. The effects of these different antibodies will have an important impact on xenogeneic cardiac grafts between widely divergent species [56].

Complement

The complement cascade is currently one of the most intensively studied mechanisms involved in hyperacute rejection. This system of proteinases is activated by the classical, or more commonly the alternative, pathway in a complex loop, with many triggering factors and multiplying proteins, such as factor B or properdin. The activity of the system is controlled by species-specific factors and inhibitors [57]. Cobra venom factor activates the alternative pathway and depletes the levels of C3 and factor B, with loss of function of both the classical and alternative pathways. (The early part of the classical pathway is, however, not affected by CVF [58]).

Complement regulatory proteins (CRP), such as decay-accelerating factor (DAF), membrane cofactor protein (MCP), and protectin, have species-specific functions. They protect against complement-mediated injuries, but only in the same or closely related species. In the case of widely divergent xenografted organs, these protective mechanisms are absent, and complement is able to induce hyperacute rejection.

The approach of transferring human genes for these CRP into donor species, and breeding transgenic animals expressing human DAF, MCP, or both, on their EC, has prolonged survival time of the xenografted organ by decreasing complement activation. However, all other systems, such as those involving adhesion molecules, interleukins and antibody binding, remain unchanged. Transgenic animals expressing CRP on the surface of cells (mainly endothelial cells) are described as being viable and functional, maybe because in addition they continue to carry their own species-specific molecules. Knock-out mice deficient in adhesion molecules, in contrast, are prone to be infertile.

Interleukins

Differences in interleukins between species are also expected to cause problems. These proteins vary considerably, even between animal species of the same order. Although bioassays can detect interleukins, they often cannot be recognized by enzyme-linked immunosorbent assay (ELISA). With regard to function and antigenicity, interleukins are usually incompatible beyond the taxonomic level of the order (for example, between humans and dog, sheep or pig) [59].

Adhesion Molecules

Leukocytes are equipped with receptors for adherence to vascular endothelium. The receptors are responsible for the homing and recirculation of leukocytes to different (lymphoid) organs [60]. New molecules of this category (not always with clearly defined functions) are detected at intervals. Human integrins are one protein family that have a relatively broad distribution. Their function is not specific and they show a striking diversity [61]. Studies of other species have revealed multiple related but distinct adhesion molecules, some of which have no homologue in the human species.

Since their interactions are likely to have an important influence on cell integration and the microcirculation in the postcapillary venules, they are probably responsible for triggering parts of the blood clotting system. It has to be assumed that they also produce microcirculatory disturbances with systemic hemodynamic effects, and therefore need to be intensively investigated [62, 63].

Cytokines

Cytokines are extremely potent factors produced by a number of cells, such as EC, leukocytes and fibroblasts, whose multiple functions are not limited to the immunological system. In contrast to immunoglobulins, they are not antigen specific. They act either in an autocrine or paracrine fashion, and are in most cases species specific. Interleukin (IL)-1, as an example of this type of protein, is known to participate in a variety of immune and inflammatory reactions, and also has many functions outside the immune system. In some species, such as mouse,rabbit and pig, IL-1 is represented by an α and β form, with a homology of 60 % and 70 %, respectively, between the species [59]. These two distinct polypeptide chains are species specific and are different, for example, between man and mouse by 38 % and 77 % of the amino acid sequence in each chain. Despite this difference, their function remains the same. Such conservation of bioactivity is also documented for TNF-α and β [64].

Many reports suggest that a variety of IL-1-responding target cells possess specific IL-1 receptors in quantities ranging from 100 to 5000 receptors per cell. Therefore, different IL-1 concentrations initiate different biological responses. The homology between man and mouse IL-1 indicates that cytokines existed before human/mouse speciation and that there was (and is) a strong selective pressure for continuance of different functional genes with similar bioactivity. There exist, however, monoclonal antibodies that are able to identify the different molecules, a process which would occur after xenogeneic immunization following xenografting. Precursors of IL-1 are not biologically active but are antigenic, a similar situation to insulin and preproinsulin.

Pig thyrocytes carry receptors for IL-1β. Human recombinant IL-1β is able to bind to these porcine receptors with a capacity of 822 molecules per cell, while the capacity of human IL-1β to bind to receptors on human thyrocytes is 2000–6000 molecules per cell. The function of the pig thyrocytes is not markedly changed by human IL-1β. In contrast, human IL6 cannot act on pig cells [64].

Eicosanoids

Eicosanoids, derived from various precursor fatty acids, play a key role in regulating hemostasis, and are not species-specific. Their interaction with the endothelium has a significant impact on blood coagulation [65]. Modulation of their synthesis capacity and downregulation, as well as the regulation of receptors, are important mechanisms in vasoconstriction during hyperacute rejection. Eicosanoids available locally have a short but strong biological activity and have to be inactivated quickly. Their role is comparable in all mammals, although metabolism, localization in tissues, and interaction with other mediators might differ.

Blood Coagulation

Most of the biochemical mechanisms mentioned above contribute to blood clotting, which is the final event of hyperacute rejection. Blood clotting is one of the most primitive requirements for the survival of mammals. It is responsible for the preservation of vascular integrity, i.e., hemostasis. The activation of the extrinsic and intrinsic coagulation protease cascades is mediated by cells expressing tissue factors (TF) [66]. There is a high-affinity receptor for factor VIIa and, as a consequence, also for factors IX and X. Human, murine, and rabbit TF molecules show only small degrees of conservation. Also, their tissue distribution varies, with the highest levels of functional TF being in the brain and the heart. Despite significant conservation, differences exists between rabbit and man (71 %) and between man and mouse (58 %). The mouse is much less efficient at forming catalytic binary complexes with human factor VII than is man.

An intensive study of the coagulation system is important for xenogeneic transplantation. In several species it has been demonstrated that most coagulation factors, and the balance between specific factors and inhibitors, are not the same as in humans. Surprisingly, the hemostatic system in the pig is very similar to those of both adult and fetal humans. In contrast, in species such as the rabbit and dog, the coagulation system is immature at birth and has many important differences from that of man [67]. The coagulation systems in closely related species (such as hamster and rat or within primates), however, seem to be similar. Clotting occurs after xenogeneic transplantation of a hamster liver into a rat, indicating that the clotting proteins of both animals interact [68, 69].

Kallikrein

Plasma and tissue kallikrein can be involved in blood clotting and in the complement system. Kallikrein varies greatly among mammals and has changed rapidly during mammalian evolution. However, some of the primary determinants of this serine protease are conserved between species, including man and pig. The action of tissue kallikrein depends on its organ localisation. Its function and its species-specific action at multiple sites of regulation are not clearly understood. In xenotransplantation, deregulation would have many side effects, because such chemically controlled systems are characterized by a great diversity of signals, a shorter or larger reaction time, and less precise connections than those provided by species-specific molecules [70].

Fibrinopeptides

Fibrinopeptides are proteolytically removed by thrombin from fibrinogen, forming the insoluble fibrin gel at the end of hyperacute rejection. There exist clear differences in the amino acid sequences involved in this process even between rather closely related species. Since the cleavage is limited to special amino acid combinations, this procedure is species specific, as indicated by the rapid interaction that occurs only between fibrinopeptides and homologous thrombin [71].

Superoxide Dismutase

In most experiments in which xenogeneic blood has been used, blood clotting has had to be prevented by the use of heparin. Heparin leads, however, to a prompt increase in extracellular superoxide dismutase (EC-SOD). Endothelial cell surfaces are the likely source of the released enzyme, which has the function of protecting against superoxide radicals in the extracellular space. Superoxide radicals are major molecules produced during hyperacute rejection and reperfusion. This complicated process varies much between species. Even the pathogenic importance of extracellularly formed superoxide radicals may differ considerably between species.

With the wide diversity of EC-SOD in the vascular systems of mammals (with regard to the total amount, division into fractions, and distribution as soluble or endothelium-fixed forms), it is not surprising that EC-SOD from pig, cat, rabbit, guinea pig and mouse have been found to be heterogeneous with regard to heparin affinity. Very large interspecies differences in EC-SOD activity have been documented. The reason for this heterogeneity is unknown [72].

Circulating Xenogeneic Proteins

Even if enzyme and hormone incompatibilities could be overcome, the problem of circulating foreign antigens released from the xenograft would remain. Various experiments show that within a short time, even under immunosuppression, antibodies are produced (a) against the foreign γ-globulins, (b) in the form of hemagglutinins and hemolysins against erythrocytes, or (c) in the form of cytotoxic antibodies against white blood cells, especially lymphocytes. Antibodies will also probably be produced against species-specific hormones and enzymes. Suppression of such reactions has not been attempted.

Class I and II antigens vary considerably between different species, even between closely related primates. After xenotransplantation, these antigens are shed into the circulation. If the soluble forms of these molecules or receptors play a part in xenogeneic rejection, further investigation will be required.

Comment

Today, possibly on the eve of successful clinical xenotransplantation, at the beginning of the xenogeneic era, only simple and, in most cases, single, observations in the fields of comparative physiology, biochemistry, and even anatomy, have been made. In addition, only few data are informative enough to hint at the effects that differences between donor and recipient will have on the patient, especially their influence on survival time.

In the pig-to-primate model, little convincing organ function has been achieved. The hope that transgenic manipulation of one or several factors can lead to success remains to be proved. Today's approaches are not convincing. Even if multiple factors can be knocked out, transferred or modified, the remaining myriad donor-specific characteristics, with all their consequences and products, will remain. As much as the application of xenografts is desirable, the problems seem many and perhaps insoluble. Intensive research in this field may lead to surprising, and as yet unforseen, solutions which might overcome the fail-safe and redundant mechanisms which nature has developed to protect the individual from "non-self." The perfection of these potential solutions will be a major undertaking. We have set ourselves a difficult task – we have to outwit evolution.

References

1. Sheil A.G.R., 1993. Human xenotransplantation. Transplant. Soc. Bull. 1, 8
2. Starzl T., 1993. Liver allo- and xenotransplantation. Transplant. Proc. 25, 15
3. Hammer C., Suckfüll M., Saumweber D., 1992. Evolutionary and immunological aspects of xenotransplantation. Transplant. Proc. 24, 2397
4. Auchincloss H., 1993. Are we ready to try clinical xenotransplantation? Xeno. 1, 2
5. Kimura M., 1976. Molecular evolutionary clock and neutral theory. J. Mol. Evol. 26, 24
6. Sarich VM., Wilson AC., 1967. Rates of albumin evolution in primates. Proc. Natl. Acad. Sci. USA. 58, 142
7. Blauer G., Lavie E., Silfen J., 1977. Relative affinities of bilirubin for serum albumins from different species. Biochem. Biophys. Acta. 492, 64
8. Chaline J., Houssin D., 1994. Organ xenografting between rodents:an evolutionary perspective. Transplant. Int. 7, 216
9. Hammer C., 1989. Evolutionary considerations in xenotransplantation. In Hardy (ed), Xenograft 25. Elsevier, Amsterdam, p. 115
10. Sugimoto K., Shelby J., Corry RJ., 1985. The effect of cyclosporine on cardiac xenograft survival. Transplantation. 39, 218
11. Hammer C., Chaussy C., Weber H., et al., 1981. Exceptionally long survival time in xenogeneic organ transplantion. Transplant. Proc. 13, 881
12. Collins BH., Cotterell AH., McCurry KR. et al., 1995. Hyperacute rejection of cardiac xenografts performed beween primate species. (Abstract) 21st Annual Meeting, Am. Soc. Transpl. Surg. p. 117
13. Herre W., Röhrs M., (eds), 1973. Haustiere Zoologisch Gesehen. Gustav Fischer Verlag, Stuttgart
14. Kirkman RL., 1989. Of swine and man: organ physiology in different species. In: Hardy M (ed). Xenograft 25. Elsevier, Amsterdam, p. 125
15. Starzl TE., Tzakis A., Fung JJ. et al., 1994. Prospects of clinical xenotransplantation. Transplant. Proc. 26, 1082
16. Abouna GM., Cook JS., Fisher JM., Still WJ., Costa G., Hume DM, 1972. Treatment of acute heptic coma by ex vivo baboon and human liver perfusions. Surgery. 71, 537
17. Weinhold C., Weingartner J., Hammer C. et al, 1986. In vivo investigation of kangaroo aortic valve xenoprostheses: An experimental animal model. In: Bodnar E, Yacoub M (eds) Biologic and bioprosthetic valves. Yorke Med, New York, p. 669
18. West JB. (ed), 1985. Respiratory Physiology. 3rd Ed. Williams and Wilkins, Baltimore
19. Braidley PC., Dunning J., Wallwork J., et al., 1994. Phylogenetic disparity does not always equate with hyperacute rejection in transplantation. Transplant. Proc. 26, 1230
20. Hemler ME., 1988. Adhesive protein receptors on hematopoetic cells. Immunol. Today. 9, 109
21. Tanabe O., Akira S., Kamiya T. et al., 1988. Genomic structure of the murine IL 6 gene. J. Immunol. 141, 3875
22. Schilling A., Land W., Pielsticker K., 1975. Experimental xenografting in widely divergent species; interaction of humoral factors in hyperacute xenograft rejection in the rat-dog system. Res. Exp. Med. 156, 79

23. Otte K., Andersen N., Jorgensen KA. et al., 1990. Xenoperfusion of pig kidney with human AB or O whole blood. Transplant. Proc. 22, 1091
24. Triulzi DJ., Jochum EA., Marino IR., Starzl TE., 1995. Heteroagglutinins and their significance in baboon hepatic xenotransplantation. Transplantation. 60, 127
25. Monod J., 1971. Le Hazard et la Necessite. Editions du Seuil, Paris
26. Barrington EJW., 1986. The phylogeny of the endocrine system. Experientia. 42, 775
27. Holmes RS., Masters CJ., 1969. A comparative study of the multiplicity of mammalian esterases. Biochem. Biophys. Acta. 151, 147
28. Walsh KA., 1975. Proteases and biological control. In: E. Reich, D. Rifkin, E. Shaw Eds. Cold Spring Harbor, New York, p 1
29. Markert CK., Shaklee JB., White GS., 1975. Evolution of a gene. Multiple genes for LDH isoenzymes - a model of the evolution of gene structure, function and regulation. Science. 189, 102
30. Wilson AC., Kaplan NO., Levine L., et al., 1964. Evolution of lactic dehydrogenase. Fed. Proc. 23, 1258
31. Masters CJ., Holmes RS., 1979. Peroxisomes. Trends Biochem. Sci. 4, 233
32. Santa-Coloma TA., Muschietti JP., Carreau EH., 1986. Sex steroid binding from Bufo arenarum: Further characterization. Comp. Biochem. Physiol. 85A, 401
33. Baumann G., 1990. Growth hormone binding proteins and various forms of growth hormone: implications for measurements. Acta. Paediatr. Scand. 370, 72
34. De Vos AM., Ultsch M., Kossiakoff AA., 1992. Human growth hormone and extracellular domain of its receptor. Science. 255, 306
35. Wanke R., Hermanns W., Folger S. et al., 1991. Accelerated growth and visceral lesions in transgenic mice expressing foreign genes of the growth hormone family: A review. Ped. Nephrol. 5, 513
36. Brem G., Wanke R., Wolf E., et al., 1989. Multiple consequences of human growth hormone expression in transgenic mice. Mol. Biol. Med. 6, 531
37. Torresani J., Gorbman A., Lachiver F. et al., 1973. Immunological cross-reactivity between thyreoglobulins of mammals and reptiles. Gen. Comp. Endocrin. 21, 530
38. Wilson AC., Sarich VM., Maxson LR., 1974. The importance of gene rearrangement in evolution: Evidence from studies on rates of chromosomal, protein, and anatomical evolution. Proc. Nat. Acad. Sci. USA. 71, 3028
39. Platt JL., Lindman BJ., Chen H. et al., 1990. Endothelial cell antigens recognized by xenoreactive human natural antibodies. Transplantation. 50, 817
40. Platt JL., Fischel RJ., Matas AJ. et al., 1991. Immunopathology of hyperacute xenograft rejection in a swine-to-primate model. Transplantation. 52, 214
41. Geller RL., Bach FH., Turman MA. et al., 1993. Evidence that polyreactive antibodies are deposited in rejected discordant xenografts. Transplantation. 55, 168
42. Cooper DKC., Ye Y., Niekrasz M. et al., 1993. Specific intravenous carbohydrate therapy. Transplantation. 56, 769
43. Laus R., Ulrichs K., Müller-Ruchholtz G., 1988. Carbohydrate-specific human heterophile antibodies in normal human sera that react with xenogeneic cells. Int Arch Allergy Appl Immunol, 85, 201–207
44. Holgersson J., Cairns TDH., Karlsson EC. et al., 1992. Carbohydrate specificity of human immunoglobulin-M antibodies with pig lymphocytic activity. Transplant. Proc. 24, 605

45. Good AH., Cooper DKC., Malcolm AJ. et al., 1992. Identification of carbohydrate structures that bind human antiporcine antibodies: Implications for discordant xenografting in humans. Transplant. Proc. 24, 559
46. Galili U., Shohet SB., Korbin E. et al., 1988. Man,apes and Old World monkeys differ from other mammals in the expression of αGal epitopes on nucleated cells. J. Biol. Chem. 263, 17755
47. Galili U., 1993. Interaction of the natural anti-Gal antibody with α-galactosyl epitopes: a major obstacle for xenotransplantation in humans. Immunol. Today. 14, 480
48. Hammer C., Höbel G., Csapo C., 1992. Fixation of mammalian natural antibodies to porcine endothelial cells. Transplant. Proc. 24, 588
49. Fischel RJ., Matas AJ., Platt JL. et al., 1992. Cardiac xenografting in the pig-to-rhesus monkey model: Manipulation of anti-endothelial antibody prolongs survival. J. Heart Lung Transplant. 11, 965
50. Tuso PJ., Cramer DV., Yasunaga C. et al., 1993. Removal of natural human xenoantibodies to pig vascular endothelium by perfusion of blood through pig kidneys and livers. Transplantation. 55, 1375
51. Messmer K., Hammer C., Land W. et al., 1971. Modification of hyperacute kidney rejection. Transplant. Proc. 3, 542
52. Alexandre GPJ., Gianello P., Latinne D. et al., 1985. Plasmapheresis and splenectomy in experimental xenotransplantation. In Hardy M (ed). Xenograft 25. Elsevier, Amsterdam, p. 259
53. Johnston PS., Lim S., Wang M. et al., 1991. Hyperacute rejection of xenografts in the complete absence of antibody. Transplant. Proc. 23, 877
54. Oriol R., Barthold F., Bergemer AM. et al., 1994. Monomorphic and polymorphic carbohydrate antigens on pig tissues: implications for organ xenotransplantation in the pig to man model. Transplant. Int. 7, 405
55. Müller U., Klein D., Zander M. et al., 1994. Preformed natural antibodies: their impact on beating fetal rat cardiomyocytes. Transplant. Proc. 26, 1000
56. Müller-Werdan U., Klein D., Zander M. et al., 1994. Beating neonatal rat cardimyocytes as a model to study the role of xenoreactive natural antibodies in xenotransplantation. Transplantation. 58, 1403
57. Farries TC., Atkinson JP., 1991. Evolution of the complement system. Immunol. Today. 12, 295
58. White D., 1992. The role of complement in xenograft rejection. UNOS Update 1992. 8, 6
59. Hammer C., Dommer S., Allmeling A., 1996. Cross species interaction of xenogeneic interleukins. Transplant. Proc. 28, 868.
60. Pardi R., Inverardi L., Bender JR., 1992. Regulatory mechanisms in leukocyte adhesion: flexible receptors for sophisticated travelers. Immunol. Today. 13, 224
61. Vestweber M., 1992. Selectins: cell surface lectins which mediate the binding of leukocytes to endothelial cells. Cell Biol. 3, 211
62. v. Andrian U., Hansell P., Chambers JD. et al., 1992. L-Selectins function is required for β2-integrin-mediated neutrophil adhesion at the physiological shear rates in vivo. Am. J. Physiol. 263, H1034
63. Marzi I., Takei Y., Rücker M. et al., 1994. Endothelin-1 is involved in hepatic sinusoidal vasoconstriction after ischemia and reperfusion. Transplant. Int. (Suppl), 7, 503

64. Beutler B., Cerami A., 1987. Physiological properties and evolutionary conservation of cachectin. Lymphokines. 14, 209
65. Foegh ML., Alijani MR., Helfrich GB. et al., 1984. Eicosanoids and organ transplantation. Ann. Clin. Res. 16, 318
66. Andrews BS., Rehemtulla A., Fowler BJ. et al., 1991. Conservation of tissue factor primary sequence among three mammalian species. Gene. 98, 265
67. Massicotte P., Mitchel L., Andrew M., 1986. A comparative study of coagulation systems in new born animals. Ped. Res. 20, 961
68. Dodds JW., 1982. The pig model for biochemical research. Fed. Proc. 41, 247
69. Valdivia LA., Lewis JH., Celli S. et al., 1993. Hamster coagulation and serum proteins in rat recipients of hamster xenografts. Transplantation. 56, 489
70. MacDonald RJ., Margolius HS., Erdös EG., 1988. Molecular biology of tissue kallikrein. Biochem. J. 253, 313
71. Doolittle RF., Blombäck B., 1964. Amino acid sequence investigations of fibrinopeptides from various mammals: evolutionary implications. Nature. 202, 147
72. Karlsson K., Marklund L., 1988. Extracellular superoxide dismutase in the vascular system of mammals. Biochem. J. 253, 223

53 Xenotransplantation and Infectious Diseases

L.E. Chapman and J.A. Fishman

Introduction

The use of tissues of nonhuman origin in humans expands the spectrum of infectious diseases confronted in allotransplantation to include diseases derived from other animal species. Concerns have been raised about the potential for the introduction of zoonotic diseases into the transplant recipient and into the general human population. This concern is based, in part, on experience with the human immunodeficiency virus (HIV)/acquired immunodeficiency syndrome (AIDS) pandemic and on heightened interest in novel or "emerging" infectious diseases. Questions of public health risk include evaluation of the potential for the introduction or development of previously unknown human pathogens into the general population via xenotransplantation [1–6].

The major "source" animals under consideration for use in organ procurement for xenotransplantation are non-human primates and swine. While this discussion will include specific reference to these species, it is possible to frame general criteria and approaches which are relevant to all potential "donor" species.

The terms "xenosis" and "xenozoonosis" have been proposed to describe these unique xenogeneic infections: xenograft-derived infections with infectious agents of animals that are not recognized to cause human infection under natural conditions [1, 7]. Particular concerns have been expressed regarding the inadvertent spread of novel pathogens from the individual xenograft recipient into the human population [6, 7]. The development of a scientific basis for substantiating and quantifying any infectious risks associated with xenotransplantation is possible during the process of addressing the immunologic road blocks to successful clinical xenotransplantation.

Infection in Allotransplantation as a Model for Xenogeneic Infection: Likely Pathogens

Risk of Opportunistic Infection

Successful allotransplantation requires a balance between the immune suppression needed to maintain graft function and the risks of opportunistic infections and cancer posed by that level of suppression. The risk of opportunistic infection in the transplant recipient is a function of the infectious burden and the "net state of immune suppression." The infectious burden includes such factors as the native *virulence* of a potential pathogen(s), the *quantity* of the organism(s), and the *route* of exposure. The net state of immune suppression is a function of all factors - pharmacologic, immunomodulatory viral infections, metabolic factors, or underlying anatomic defects - which contribute to the host's susceptibility to infection. Until strategies for the induction of tolerance (specific immunologic unresponsiveness) to xenogeneic organs are perfected, immune suppression will continue to be needed to maintain graft function. Interspecies transplantation will likely require a level of exogenous immune suppression greater than that currently used for allotransplantation. As a direct result, the risk of opportunistic infections and cancers classically associated with allotransplantation may be enhanced following xenotransplantation.

The risk of opportunistic infection in xenotransplantation may also be increased due to the introduction of organisms normally *not* associated with human disease (xenosis) directly into the human host [1]. The basis for this increased risk may include: (a) organisms not routinely culturable or identifiable in clinical laboratories, (b) the absence of serologic or other microbiologic tests for these organisms, (c) the development of novel clinical syndromes due to the involvement of novel pathogens and the impact of alterations in host responses, (d) the potential for changes in the organism (at the molecular level) and/or in the biologic behavior of the organism due to mutational "adaptation" or recombinational events within the human hosts, (e) the lack of need for vector-based transmission of common zoonotic pathogens, and (f) the absence of preexisting immunity in most humans to many animal-derived pathogens [2].

A meaningful measurement of the likelihood that specific organisms derived from a source species will contribute to human disease in the xenotransplant setting is an uncertain process at best. However, some predictions can be based on four criteria for the organisms likely to cause disease in humans: (1) organisms known to cause human infection under natural conditions (the zoonoses, such as *Toxoplasma gondii*), (2) organisms thought likely to cause infection based on similarity to organisms causing infection in clinical allotransplantation, (3) organisms of broad host range or thought likely to be able to "adapt" to the human host, and (4) organisms known to be capable of establishing replicative infection in human cell lines in vitro.

Early Infection

The organisms associated with opportunistic infection following allotransplantation can be divided into categories based on the time elapsed from surgery and the level of immune suppression needed to maintain graft function [8, 9]. In the first month following allotransplantation, bacterial, fungal, and parasitic infections, both nosocomial and graft-derived, predominate. Many of these organisms are common to most species (*Staphylococcus aureus*, streptococci, *Klebsiella* species, *Escherichia coli*) while others are species specific. These common pathogens do not pose a *unique* health risk to either the individual or the community. However, diseases due to novel microbial species which are not routinely cultured by clinical laboratories, or due to common organisms in the setting of altered host responses, may go unrecognized and diagnosis may be delayed - a critical event in immunocompromised patients. Infection will complicate and further amplify any technical difficulties related to surgery, e.g., hematomas, lymphoceles, indwelling catheters, or pulmonary atelectasis.

Late Infection

In the period from 1–6 months post-allotransplant, particularly during steroid or antilymphocyte treatments for acute graft rejection, the customary infections in the immediate postoperative period are replaced by common parasitic and fungal pathogens (*Pneumocystis carinii*, *Toxoplasma gondii*, *Cryptococcus neoformans*) and less common bacterial agents (mycobacteria, *Nocardia*, *Listeria*, *Legionella* sp.). In addition, latent viral infections released from host immune control following immune suppression may have a great impact. Most of these viruses have immunomodulatory effects and have analogs in nonhuman species [10, 11]. These viruses (cytomegalovirus, CMV; hepatitis B and C; herpes simplex virus, HSV; Epstein-Barr virus, EBV) may cause systemic clinical syndromes (e.g., the "mono" syndrome). In addition, they are globally immunosuppressive and may contribute to the development of other life-threatening opportunistic infections (e.g., *Pneumocystis* pneumonia, *Toxoplasma* encephalitis) and to the development of graft injury and rejection. Analogous animal-derived viruses, if present in the xenograft, may be expected to be activated by immune suppression, ischemic injury, and/or graft rejection. Whether these non-human viruses can infect the recipient host tissue, can cause disease in the recipient, and/or will be transmitted from the xenograft recipient to other humans, in addition to infecting the tissues of the xenograft, must be defined on a virus-specific basis. Such factors as the nature and presence of the viral receptors in the human host, or the requirement of the virus for specific host-derived, cellular factors for nucleic acid transcription or replication, may determine the infectivity and virulence of viruses spread between species.

Each species that has been studied has similar persistent cell-associated viruses, often carried in a latent state by a high proportion of individuals within that species. These include, most prominently for this discussion, the herpesviruses and retroviruses, but also may include hepatitis viruses, adenoviruses, Pseudorabies and rabies viruses, reovirus, papovavirus, and others. Whether and to what extent most non-human viruses pose a risk for human infection and disease is largely undefined. Human infections have been documented with simian immunodeficiency virus (SIV) and Cercopithecine herpesvirus 1 (B virus) [12–13], and infectivity for human cells (and, possibly, humans working with nonhuman primates) has been demonstrated with primate foamy virus [14]. Infection of human neuronal cells in vitro with porcine pseudorabies has been detected [15]. Interspecies transmission of a number of viruses has also been identified in other model systems [12, 16–22].

Alterations in Viral Pathogenesis

Under immune suppression, in addition to clinical reactivation of latent virus infections, prolonged carriage and shedding of viruses normally associated with self-limiting acute infections may occur. For example, prolonged infection with, and shedding of, influenza virus has been documented in immunocompromised hosts, with the accumulation of viral mutants over time [23, 24]. The accumulation of viral mutants is accelerated in influenza virus, which has a propensity for rapid evolution surpassed only by HIV. However, such an accumulation of viral mutants will occur whenever immunosuppression allows persistent viral replication. As a result, the viral population shed late in the course of any persistent viral infection may have different biologic characteristics from the progenitor viral variant that originated the infection.

Temporal modulation of viral virulence in association with the evolution of viral variants has not been well studied in the setting of immune compromise. However, viruses shed late in the course of an infection, or following passage through a host or tissue, have often been observed to have *attenuated* pathogenicity compared with wild type. If this attenuation of pathogenicity over time is a consistent phenomenon, the risk of disease resulting from human-to-human transmission of xenoses may *decrease* over the duration of sentinel human infections, even if transmissibility persists.

While virulence may decrease over time and passage, the potential for other viral alterations, with clinical and epidemiologic implications, may accrue. RNA virus polymerases and reverse transcriptases lack the editing precision of DNA virus polymerases; as a result, mutations accumulate more rapidly in RNA viruses (such as influenza or retroviruses) than in DNA viruses [25, 26]. These mutations may be detrimental to viral survival or may encode altered viral behavior. In large populations of viruses, mutants may emerge based on new biologic characteristics which are advantageous to viral persistence, or due to selective pressure such as pre-existing immunity or antiviral antibiotic exposure.

Viral antigens or tissue specificity may be altered by recombination (i.e., gene reassortment) between human and animal strains during passage in other species. Viruses resulting from antigenic recombinations may have a selective advantage in circumventing preexisting host immunity to species-familiar antigens. For example, the influenza A strain responsible for the 1917–18 human pandemic ("Spanish flu") was antigenically homologous to strains usually infecting swine; the variant of influenza A associated with a 1980 harbor seal die-off contained antigens usually present on avian influenza strains [27].

Antiviral therapy has been documented to result in shedding of drug-resistant viral variants of HSV-2. When antiviral pressure is removed, the shed virus may revert to the antiviral-sensitive wild type, or the antiviral resistance may persist. Thus, in the setting of persistent viral shedding in the immunocompromised host, antiviral therapy may result in the development of viral variants with clinical and epidemiologic implications for other infected humans [24, 28].

Endogenous retroviruses are presumed to represent exogenous viruses that became permanently integrated into the host germ line of most, if not all, mammalian species during the course of evolution. These are then transmitted vertically. They are thought to be benign in the host species, but may be xenotropic (able to infect other species). Sequencing of baboon endogenous virus, a xenotropic endogenous retrovirus present in all baboon cells, suggests that it is the chimeric result of recombination events that occurred during viral evolution [29–31]. Such observations raise questions regarding the potential for recombination or complementation of xenograft-derived endogenous retroviruses with viruses present in human tissues.

The extent to which selective pressures favoring mutant or recombinant strains may occur in human hosts following transplantation is unknown. For this reason, xenotropic or defective viruses in the donor species cannot a priori be excluded as pathogenic risks for the human recipient. Many conditions associated with retroviral activation (e.g., immune suppression, graft-versus-host disease, graft rejection, viral coinfection, cytotoxic therapy) are present in the transplant recipient [32–35]. The course of accidentally transmitted HIV-1 infection has been accelerated in allotransplant recipients, and other xenogeneic retroviruses may also exhibit decreased latency in the transplant setting [36, 37]. Conversely, the manifestations of retroviral infection may be clinically inapparent, including altered gene regulation, oncogenesis, or recombination with other viruses. The activation of latent viruses and the development of clinical manifestations, if any, may be delayed for a decade or more.

The oncogenic potential of viruses is recognized in the allotransplantation recipient beyond 6 months after transplantation. The roles of the immunomodulatory human viruses in the pathogenesis of cancer, particularly EBV and lymphoma, are well established. The oncogenic potential of animal-derived viruses introduced into immunosuppressed humans remains undefined. Because many of the retroviruses, particularly the oncoviruses, have long latency periods (one or more decades) the impact in humans of such viruses derived from animals is unknown and unmeasurable.

Novel Infectious Considerations in Xenotransplantation

In contrast with the natural spread of zoonotic infection between species, the transmission of xenoses with viable tissues may be uniquely efficient. The xenograft itself may serve as a "culture plate" from which such organisms can spread in the human host, avoiding the need for a vector to achieve disease transmission [1]. The migration of cells from the graft to other sites in the host (chimerism) may carry cell-associated infection throughout the host even in the absence of true viremia or propagation of virus along nerve routes (as occurs with disseminated herpesvirus infections). The history of human exposure to unsterilized biologic products (SV40 in vaccine, viral contamination of fetal calf serum) without recognized ill-effects is somewhat reassuring [38–44]. However, these may not be the most appropriate models by which to measure the infectious risks associated with xenotransplantation, where transplanted tissue may serve as a continuing nidus of infection, and where direct cell-to-cell interactions and the development of microvasculature bridging between the host and the xenograft may increase the efficiency of host infection.

Human xenograft recipients are unlikely to have preexisting immunity to most animal-derived microbes, rendering them more susceptible to infection both with zoonoses and xenoses, and increasing the probability that more severe disease will follow infection. This susceptibility is further enhanced by the impaired ability to mount protective responses after transplantation due to immune suppression.

Latent viral infections, including a variety of exogenous and endogenous retroviruses and herpesviruses, have been identified in each of the animal species proposed as sources of xenografts. Up to 30 strains of retroviruses have been described in primates. The ability of most of these to infect and propagate in human tissues has been incompletely explored. However, the ubiquitous nature and genetic homologies of the primate retroviruses (SIV; simian T lymphotropic virus, STLV; endogenous viruses), and the ability of these pathogens to infect other species, suggests a potential risk for human infection. Retroviral infections of swine have been less throughly explored, and to date only type C retroviruses have been recognized in swine [45–48]. One porcine retrovirus isolated from a transformed cell line has been associated with the induction of B and T cell lymphomas in wild boars [49]. Additional retroviruses from normal swine have been described recently (Fishman, unpublished data, R. Weiss unpublished data). The short life expectancy of the average domestic pig minimizes the opportunity to observe clinical manifestations, such as cancers, immunodeficiency states, or neurologic degeneration, that might result from infections with such retroviruses, prions or other agents characterized by long periods of clinical latency. These and other known and unknown infectious agents present in xenografts, but not recognized as human pathogens under natural conditions, pose an unknown risk to humans under the conditions of xenotransplantation.

The commercial production of animals, notably swine, which have been genetically engineered to lessen graft rejection raises questions of whether the genetic manipulations intended to minimize the rejection of xenografts may also influence the expression of latent infections or the presence of receptors for novel pathogens or alter the immunologic defenses against infections with xenogeneic pathogens [50]. Inserted or deleted transgenes may encode receptors for infectious agents [50, 51]. Natural antibodies that provide a major transplantation barrier to the use of vascularized organs from swine in humans may also be a part of an intrinsic defense mechanism against exogenous retroviral (and bacterial) infections [52–57]. Techniques which remove these antibodies may alter the risk of retroviral activation or other xenogeneic infections [58].

In the xenotransplant setting, the diagnosis and management of familiar zoonoses may be complicated by immunologic manipulations that alter the clinical presentation of illness, the reliability of antibody testing, and the response to therapy. It is likely that the absence of appropriate diagnostic reagents will be a major impediment to clinical evaluation of the xenograft recipient.

Approaches to the Development of Source Animals with Decreased Risk of Human Infections

Clinical experience with recognized zoonotic pathogens exists, and diagnostic assays are available for their identification. Therefore, infections with these pathogens should be relatively preventable, and their occurrence should be identifiable. The use of closed and isolated herds, screened for likely pathogens will minimize the chance of graft-derived infections with known pathogens. Infections may be more efficiently excluded from prospectively evaluated donor herds than from individual animals that are wild caught or raised in open herds allowing unregulated contact with other species. The development of closed, microbiologically well-characterized herds of source animals that are free of a list of selected organisms, or are "designated pathogen free" (DPF), will minimize the risks of transmission of both classic zoonoses and of new xenogeneic infections through xenotransplantation [2]. Such closed herds can undergo microbiologic screening using individual immunocompetent and/or immunosuppressed sentinel animals as representatives of the herd. It is important to recognize that the concept of DPF herds is narrowly focused, and the resultant protection incurred is relative. The significant gain in terms of disease prevention is made through the use of a healthy, microbiologically defined herd as opposed to a microbe free or "gnotobiotic" herd. A completely gnotobiotic herd is "organism free," but tends to be less robust and more susceptible to disease than herds of animals with normal microbiologic colonization, and is probably unnecessary. Further, a closed herd which is free of designated known pathogens, will remain undefined in terms of most latent or unrecognized pathogens with potential for infection in the human host.

Many potential pathogens are identifiable by routine microbiological methods, and animals carrying such pathogens can be excluded as potential donors. Reagents (both serologic and nucleic acid-based) for viral agents of swine and primates are available primarily on a research basis, but are potentially adaptable for clinical use. The ability to develop diagnostic tests for clinical use and for use in screening potential source animals is central to defining the margin of safety that can be established for xenotransplantation.

A variety of criteria can be used to develop microbiologic exclusion criteria to guide the development of source animal herds. Some of these have been discussed previously, e.g., the exclusion of animals carrying organisms of broad host range or similar to those causing infection in allograft recipients [1, 2]. The exclusion criteria will vary depending on the species, the tissues, and the specific use for which the xenograft is intended. Such a species- and application-specific list of designated pathogens provides a basis for microbiologic screening of breeding colony herds, individual donor-animals, and/or xenograft tissues. The manner in which the level of safety created by the exclusion criteria and lists of organisms is achieved need not be uniform as long as the transplanted tissues do not pose a known microbiologic hazard to the recipient. The risks of introducing antibiotic-resistant organisms can also be reduced by appropriate herd maintenance policies limiting the use of antimicrobial agents.

The presence of acute infections in individual animals used to provide xenografts can be monitored by: (a) herd surveillance indicating the presence or absence of infection in the herd from which the individual source animal is selected, (b) clinical examination and treatment of individual source animals, and (c) the use of appropriate individual animal quarantine periods accompanied by screening for the presence of clinically latent infections of concern. Microbiologic isolation will need to be maintained during transportation of source animals to minimize the extent to which the protection insured by the closed breeding colony is compromised. Additional quarantine and screening may be necessary upon arrival at the clinical facility. Aseptic tissue procurement is important.

All xenografts do not need identical handling or screening. For example, cellular transplants might be screened *after* isolation from the donor. Specific organs might merit unique considerations, e.g., for Mycoplasma species in lung xenografts or Coxsackie viruses in heart xenografts.

Advantages of Xenotransplantation

In addition to unlimited supply, xenogeneic organs may offer other advantages over allografting in specific settings. Animal-derived organs will exhibit species-specific resistance to infection by many common pathogens of human origin. For example, neither human hepatitis B or HIV-1 appear to infect baboons in vivo [59, 60]. The ability of various CMV and herpes viruses to infect across species lines may be restricted [1, 61]. This species specificity may reflect the absence of receptors or cellular machinery necessary for viral replication in a novel host, and may be exploited to advantage in certain clinical situations. Resistance to CMV, EBV, HIV, and the hepatitis viruses would provide a unique therapeutic advantage to xenotransplantation over traditional allotransplantation. As a result, reconstitution of the immune system of HIV-1-infected humans via transplantation of baboon bone marrow and the transplantation of a baboon liver into an HIV-1-infected human with hepatic failure due to fulminant hepatitis B have been attempted [62, 63].

Public Health Issues in Xenograft Transplantation

Xenotransplant-associated infections restricted to the recipient would constitute an additional factor influencing the risks and benefits of transplantation only to the individual. Zoonotic viruses that are not notably pathogenic in their host species have been agents of epidemic human disease. In these outbreaks, the first generation of human-to-human transmission has been from the patient to the medical staff or the patient's family, with subsequent generations of transmission extending into the greater community. It is this undefined potential for epidemic human disease which raises public health concerns in association with xenotransplantation [7].

Life-long post-transplantation clinical surveillance of the initial xenotransplant recipients will be needed to monitor for events suggestive of xenogeneic infection. The xenograft recipients must be willing to participate in such an enduring experiment. In addition, when xenogeneic agents of unknown pathogenicity for humans (e.g., baboon endogenous virus, primate foamy virus) are known or suspected to be present in the transplanted tissue, an active post-transplantation laboratory surveillance program directed toward the detection of sentinel human infections with these agents will be needed.

The pathogens responsible for the majority of common infectious episodes among the general population are never identified. Recipients of xenografts will remain at risk for routine community-acquired infections, complicating the assessment of potential xenoses. When the source of a significant illness remains obscure despite standard diagnostic testing, consideration of further diagnostic testing, infection control precautions, and additional investigations will be needed to determine whether xenogeneic infection can be identified. Post-transplantation testing of archived biologic specimens (tissues, leukocytes, and sera) from the source animal and the xenograft recipient may be indicated in response to a clinical episode possibly representing a xenogeneic infection. Such testing should be conducted in the context of a broader epidemiologic investigation in collaboration with appropriate public health authorities. Disease evaluations may require diagnostic tests based on nucleic acid detection or cell culture methodologies and other nonstandard techniques. These investigations may require consultation with persons experienced in the laboratory identification of unknown infectious agents, including the appropriate management of associated biosafety hazards.

Healthcare workers and laboratory personnel who handle the animal tissues prior to transplantation will also be at risk of infection, albeit more limited. This risk will be definable and equivalent to that of commercial meat preparers, animal care, veterinary, or abattoir workers routinely exposed to the source animal species. The risk to immunologically normal healthcare workers who provide direct or indirect care to xenogeneic tissue recipients post-transplantation is undefined but likely to be significantly less than for the immunocompromised host. Strict adherence to standard ("universal") precautions will reduce the risk of transmission of xenogeneic infections as well as that of other blood-borne pathogens in the hospital setting. The need for additional infection control or isolation precautions (e.g., airborne, droplet, contact) in specific instances must be continuously assessed by the xenotransplant team, especially by infectious disease specialists and hospital epidemiologists.

The introduction of xenogeneic retro- and herpesviruses into human hosts via xenotransplantation is a particular public health concern due to the uncertainty regarding their pathogenic potential and the long period of clinical latency typical of these infections. These characteristics may allow for prolonged periods of silent human-to-human transmission prior to recognition of infection. The importance of such transmission is unknown. Standardized diagnostic testing is not available for most of these animal viruses, which reduces the likelihood that human infections with them will be readily identified.

Few data exist on the presence or absence of prion-associated disease in potential donor animal species. Like retroviruses, prion encephalopathies have protracted clinical latency. No diagnostic tests are available. Transmission has been documented both between species and through transplanted tissue [64]. However, the epidemic potential of prion transmission is less than that of competent retroviruses.

Surveillance of populations of xenogeneic tissue recipients for clustering of adverse health outcomes and monitoring of individual recipients for unexplained illnesses are important public health tools available to address unknown infectious risks. To be adequate, surveillance would need to detect xenogeneic infections in recipients before these infections spread into the general population. Detection of untoward events would allow the suspension of the specific associated procedure (e.g., transplant operation), or the use of a particular donor species (e.g. pig) or donor tissue (e.g., kidney) pending the development of adequate methods for prevention and control, thereby reducing the risk of further infections. Existing collaborations between transplant surgeons, transplant physicians, and immunologists must be augmented to include the expertise of infectious disease physicians, veterinarians, epidemiologists, and microbiologists to address these concerns. Systematic record maintenance linking records of the recipients, the source animals, the herd surveillance, and the occupational health program is needed to provide the database for epidemiologic investigations.

Risk Assessment/Research Needs

Research intended to define and quantify infectious risks must be developed for each source species and application. Such studies can proceed in conjunction with the development of specific clinical applications for the use of xenogeneic tissue in humans. Inherent to the concept of assessing the infectious risk of xenotransplantation is the recognition and consideration of the characteristics of the infectious agents present, and of both the donor and the recipient species.

Studies should attempt to define the microbial flora of specific donor species, to characterize the potential for identified agents to infect human hosts, and to assess the likelihood that such infections will result in human disease and in the human-to-human transmission of infection. Diagnostic tools adequate to monitor post-transplantation infections in humans must be developed. Diagnostic tests that are molecular or antigen based rather than serologic are required for the immunocompromised host.

Preclinical animal models using primates as recipients may be optimal for studies aimed at developing an understanding of cross-species transmission risks and the detection of emerging agents, endogenous viral recombinants, and complemented escape mutants. Progress in the development of clinical applications of xenotransplantation can be achieved with enhanced safety as the knowledge base related to the definition and quantification of microbiologic risks is developed.

References

1. Fishman JA: Miniature swine as organ donors for man: Strategies for prevention of xenotransplant-associated infections. Xenotransplantation 1:47, 1994
2. Fishman JA: Preventing infections in xenotransplantation: xenosis from miniature swine. Xeno 3:72, 1995
3. Michaels MG, Simmons RL: Xenotransplant-associated zoonoses: strategies for prevention. Transplantation 57:1, 1994
4. Ye Y, Niekrasz M, Welsh R, et al: A practical study of zoonoses that could complicate pig-to-man organ transplantation. Transplant Proc 26:1312, 1994

5. Ye Y, Niekrasz M, Kosanke S, et al: The pig as a potential organ donor for man. A study of potentially transferable disease from donor pig to recipient man. Transplantation 57:694, 1994
6. Allan JS: Xenotransplantation at a crossroads: prevention versus progress. Nature Med 2:18, 1996
7. Chapman LE, Folks TM, Salomon DR, et al: Xenotransplantation and xenogeneic infection. New Engl J Med 333:1498, 1995
8. Fishman JA, Rubin R: Opportunistic infections. In Bahn A, Colvin R (eds): Diagnostic Immunopathology. Plenum, New York, p. 283, 1995
9. Rubin RH, Tolkoff-Rubin NE: Antimicrobial strategies in the care of organ transplant recipients. Antimicrob Agents Chemother 37:619, 1993
10. Allan JS: Xenograft transplantation and the infectious disease conundrum. ILAR J 37:37, 1995
11. Kalter SS: The nonhuman primate as potential organ donor for man: virological considerations. In Cooper DKC, et al. Xenotransplantation. Heidelberg, Springer, 1991, p 457
12. Khabbaz RF, Heneine W, George JR, Parekh B, Rowe T, et al: Infection of a laboratory worker with simian immunodeficiency virus. New Eng J Med 330:172, 1994
13. Holmes GP, Chapman LE, Steward JA, et al: The B virus working group: guidelines for the prevention and treatment of B-virus in exposed persons. Clin Infect Dis 20:421, 1995
14. Neumann-Haefelin D, Fleps U, Renne R, Schweizer M: Foamy viruses. Intervirology 35:196, 1993
15. Subramanian G, Fuller AO: Method of transfecting human cells utilizing recombinant vector of a pseudorabies virus. U.S. Patent 8/506,556:1995
16. Weiss RA, Wong AL: Phenotypic mixing between avian and mammalian RNA tumor viruses: 1. Envelope pseudotypes of Rous sarcoma virus. Virology 76:826, 1977
17. Levy JA: Murine xenotropic typc C viruses. III. Phenotypic mixing with avian leukosis and sarcoma viruses. Virology 77:811, 1977
18. Lusso P, Di Marzo Veronese F, Ensoli B, et al: Expanded HIV-1 cellular tropism by phenotypic mixing with murine endogenous retroviruses. Science 247:848, 1990
19. Spector DH, Wade E, Wright DA, et al: Human immunodeficiency virus pseudotypes with expanded cellular and species tropism. J Virol 64:2298, 1990
20. Levin JL, Hilliard JK, Lipper SL, Butler TM, Goodwin WJ: A naturally occurring epizootic of simian agent 8 in the baboon. Lab Animal Sci 38:394, 1988
21. McClure MO, Sattentau QJ, Beverley PC, et al: HIV infection of primate lymphocytes and conservation of the CD4 receptor. Nature 330:487, 1987
22. Barnett SW, Murthy KK, Herndier BG, Levy JA: An AIDS-like condition induced in baboons by HIV-2. Science 266:642, 1994
23. Rocha E, Cox NJ, Black RA, et al: Antigenic and genetic variation in influenza A (H1N1) virus isolates recovered from a persistently infected immunodeficient child. J Virol 65:2340, 1991
24. Klimov AI, Rocha E, Hayden FG, et al: Prolonged shedding of amantadine-resistant influenza A viruses by immunodeficient patients: detection by polymerase chain reaction-restriction analysis. J Infect Dis 172:1352, 1995
25. Domingo E, Holland JJ: High error rates, population equilibrium and evolution of RNA replication systems. In Domingo E, Holland JJ, Ahlquist P (eds): RNA Genetics. Vol 3, Boca Raton, CRC Press, 1988, p 3

26. Steinhauer DA, Holland JJ: Rapid evolution of RNA viruses. Annu Rev Microbiol 41:409, 1987
27. Shortridge KF: Pandemic influenza: a zoonosis? Semin Respir Infect 17:11, 1992
28. Kost RG, Hill EL, Tigges M, Strauss SE: Brief report: recurrent acyclovir-resistant genital herpes in an immunocompetent patient. N Engl J Med 329:1777, 1993
29. Huang L, Silberman J, Rothschild H, Cohen JC: Replication of baboon endogenous retroviruses in human cells. J Biol Chem 264:8811, 1989
30. Cohen JC, Murphey-Corb M: Targeted integration of baboon endogenous virus in the BEV1 locus on human chromosome 6. Nature 301:129, 1983
31. Kato S, Matsuo K, Nishimua N, Takahashi N, Takano T: The entire nucleotide sequence of baboon endogenous virus DNA: a chimeric genome structure of murine type C and simian type D retroviruses. Jpn J Genet 62:127, 1987
32. Hirsch MS, Ellis DA, Black PA, Monaco AP, Wood ML: Leukemia virus activation during homograft rejection. Science 180:500, 1973
33 Hirsch MS, Phillips SM, Solnik C, et al: Activation of leukemia viruses by graft-versus-host and mixed lymphocyte reactions in vitro. Proc Natl Acad Sci 69:1069, 1972
34. Hirsch MS: Immunologic activation of endogenous oncogenic viruses. Ann NY Acad Sci 276:529, 1976
35. Olding LB, Jensen FC, Oldstone MB: Pathogenesis of cytomegalovirus infection. I. Activation of virus from bone-derived lymphocytes by in vitro allogeneic reaction. J Exp Med 141:561, 1975
36. Schwarz A, Offermann G, Keller F, et al: The effect of cyclosporine on the progression of human immunodeficiency virus type 1 infection transmitted by transplantation – data on four cases and review of the literature. Transplantation 55:95, 1993
37. Bowden RA, Coombs RW, Nikora BH, et al: Progression of human immunodefiency virus type-1 infection after allogeneic marrow transplantation. Am J Med 88:5–49N, 1990
38. Levings RL, Wessman SJ: Bovine viral diarrhea virus contamination of nutrient serum, cell culures and viral vaccines. Developments in Biological Standardization 75:177, 1991
39. Shah K, Nathanson N: Human exposure to SV40: review and comment. Am J Epidemiol 103:1, 1976
40. Geissler E, Staneczek W: SV40 and human brain tumors. Arch Gschwulstforsch 58:129, 1988
41. Farwell JR, Dohrmann GJ, Marrett LD, Meigs JW: Effect of SV40 virus-contaminated polio vaccine on the incidence and type of CNS neoplasms in children: a population-based study. Trans Amer Neurolog Assoc 104:261, 1979
42. Mortimore EA, Jr., Lepow ML, Gold E, et al: Long-term follow-up of persons inadvertently inoculated with SV40 as neonates. N Engl J Med 305:1517, 1981
43. Rosa FW, Sever JL, Madden DL: Absence of antibody response to simian virus 40 after inoculation with killed-poliovirus vaccine of mothers of offspring with neurologic tumors. N Engl J Med 318:1469, 1988
44. Melnick JL, Butel JS: Neurologic tumors in offspring after inoculation of mothers with killed-poliovirus vaccine. N Engl J Med 319:1226, 1988
45. Todaro GJ, Benveniste RE, Lieber MM, Sherr CJ: Characteristics of a Type C virus released from the porcine cell line PK(15). Virology 58:65, 1974
46. Bouilant AMP, Grieg AS, Lieber MM, Todaro GJ: Type-C virus production by a continuous line of pig oviduct cells (PFT). J Gen Virol 27:173, 1975

47. Lieber MM, Sherr CH, Benveniste RE, Todaro CJ: Biologic and immunologic properties of porcine type C virus. Virology 66:616, 1975
48. Suzuka I, Sekiguchi K, Kodama M: Some characteristics of a porcine retrovirus from a cell line derived from swine malignant lymphomas. FEBS 183:124, 1985
49. Kaeffer B, Bottreau E, Thanh LP, Olivier M, Salmon H: Histocompatible miiature boar model: selection of transformed cell lines of B and T lineages producing retrovirus. Int J Cancer 46:481, 1990
50. McCurry KR, Kooyman DL, Alvarado CG, et al: Human complement regulatory proteins protect swine-to-primate cardiac xenografts from humoral injury. Nature Med 1:423, 1995
51. Rosengard AM, Cary NRB, Langford GA, et al: Tissue expression of human coplement inhibitor, decay-accelerating factor, in transgenic pigs. A potential approach for preventing xenograft rejection. Transplantation 59:1325, 1995
52. Rother RP, Fodor WL, Springhorn JP, et al: A novel mechanism of retrovirus inactivation in human serum mediated by anti-a-galactosyl natural antibody. J Exp Med 182:1345, 1995
53. Welsh RM, Jensen FC, Cooper NR, Oldstone MBA: Inactivation and lysis of oncornaviruses by human serum. Virology 74:432, 1976
54. Welsh RM, Cooper NR, Jensen FC, Oldstone MBA: Human serum lyses RNA tumour viruses. Nature 257:612, 1975
55. Galili U, Clark MR, Shohet SB, Buehler J, Macher BA: Evolutionary relationship beteen the natural anti-Gal antibody and the GalaGal epitope in primates. Proc Natl Acad Sci , USA 84:1369, 1987
56. Snyder HW, Jr., Fleissner E: Specificity of human antibodies to oncovirus glycoproteins: recognition of antigen by natural antibodies directed against carbohydrate structures. Proc Natl Acad Sci USA 77:1622, 1980
57. Barbacid M, Bolognesi D, Aaronson SA: Humans have antibodies capable of recognizing oncoviral glycoproteins: demonstration that these antibodies are formed in response to cellular modification of glycoproteins rather than as consequence of exposure to virus. Proc Natl Acad Sci USA 77:1617, 1980
58. Sandrin MS, Fodor WL, Mouhtouris E, et al: Enzymatic remodelling of the carbohydrate surface of a xenogenic cell substantially reduces human antibody binding and complement-mediated cytolysis. Nature Med 1:1261, 1995
59. Michaels MG, Lanford R, Demetris AJ, et al: Lack of susceptibility of baboons to infection with hepatitis B virus. Transplantation 61:350, 1996
60. Morrow WJW, Homsy J, Eichberg JW, et. al. Long term observation of baboons, rhesus monkeys, and chimpanzees incoulated with HIV and given periodic immunosuppressive treatment. AIDS Res and Hum Retroviruses 5:233, 1989
61. Subramanian G, LeBlanc R, Wardley R, Fuller AO: Defective entry of herpes simplex types 1 and 2 into porcine cells and lack of infection in infant pigs indicates species tropism. J General Virol 76:2375, 1995
62. Lehrman S: AIDS patient given baboon bone marrow [news]. Nature 378:756, 1995
63. Lanford RE, Michaels MG, Chavez D, et al: Persistence of extrahepatic hepatitis B virus DNA in the absence of detectable heaptic replication in patients with baboon liver transplants. J Med Virol 46:207, 1995
64. Prusiner SB: The prion diseases. Sci Am 272:48, 1995

54 Nucleic Acid-Based Discovery Techniques for Potential Xenozoonotic Pathogens[1]

D.H. Persing

Introduction

In recent years, a veritable phalanx of emerging infectious agents has made national and international headlines as they acquire new mechanisms of drug resistance, are discovered in previously nonendemic geographic locations, or are identified as important variables in the equation of a new disease association [1–8]. In some cases, the science and practice of medicine is affected profoundly, as in the management of patients with infection with hepatitis C virus [9–11] or *Helicobacter pylori* [12–15]. In addition, specific interactions with pathogens may lead to an increased likelihood of development of neoplasia, as in chronic infection with human hepatitis viruses B and C [16, 17], human papillomaviruses [18, 19], and *Helicobacter pylori* [12, 20, 21]. The recent discovery of several previously unrecognized pathogens illustrates the fact that humans do not travel through life alone; the development of a better understanding of the interactions of human "flora" with their hosts , along with an understanding of other host and environmental determinants of pathogenicity, represents an increasingly important intersection of infectious disease research with the human genome project.

The recognition of the prevalence of previously undetected pathogens has had an impact on other fields as well. One of the greatest potential obstacles to the implementation of xenotransplantation has revolved around the infectious risk associated with transplantation of animal organs to humans, especially in the case of closely related donor-recipient species [22–25]. Pathogens such as foamy virus [26–28], simian Epstein-Barr virus [29], simian cytomegalovirus [23], simian T-cell lymphotropic virus [30–33], a novel reovirus [35], and a new species of babesia that is closely related to a known human pathogen have been proposed as potential xenozoonotic agents that could be transmitted in a baboon-to-human xenotransplant. Since these pathogens are now known entities, screening tests based on polymerase chain reaction (PCR) or other sensitive nucleic acid-based assays can be developed for the purpose of donor selection and implementation of selective breeding practices.

A potentially less tractable problem arises from our insecurity related to yet unknown pathogens, especially retroviruses. From phylogenetic studies of simian retroviruses, much has been discovered in recent years about the zoonotic origin of human T cell lymphotropic viruses (HTLV-1 and -2) and human immunodefi-

[1] Some material in this chapter was presented at the conference *Xenograft Transplantation: Science, Ethics,and Public Policy*, organized by the Institute of Medicine, National Academy of Sciences, June 1995.

ciency viruses (HIV-1 and -2) from higher primates [31, 36–39]. This, in turn, has engendered considerable concern that the real-life equivalent of an "andromeda strain" could, in a worst-case scenario, manage to: (a) cross species boundaries during xenotransplantation, (b) replicate within the immunocompromised host, and then (c) mutate rapidly to adapt to non-immunocompromised human hosts. Indeed, it is difficult to argue that such a scenario could not occur, because of the preponderance of evidence that it has already occurred in the past.

Fortunately, increasingly powerful tools necessary to discover previously unknown pathogens are now becoming available. DNA sequencing, in part facilitated by direct amplification of pathogens and host-specific genes from tissues, has provided an unprecedented glimpse of the genetic diversity of many pathogens, and in some cases their evolution in real time into "quasispecies" during the course of infection. Pathogen discovery techniques, such as broad range PCR and representational difference analysis (RDA), are allowing us to discover new pathogens and to begin to assess their effects on pathways of inflammation. Animal models, based on the severe combined immunodeficiency (SCID) mouse, may allow us to recover and to study some of these newly discovered pathogens within transplanted human tissues [40–48]. This convergence of new technologies and classical experimental approaches is likely to lead to many new discoveries.

Pathogen Discovery Techniques

In recent years, methods have been used to identify new pathogens and to characterize previously recognized uncultured infectious agents. Despite the large number of known infectious microorganisms, there is considerable evidence for the existence of far greater numbers of extant species, many of which do not grow in culture. A classic study of thermal vent bacteria demonstrated that of the organisms present within a thermophilic environment that could be detected by PCR, only about 5% could be recovered in culture [49]. With the possibility that currently uncharacterized organisms may play a role in the development of important human diseases, it becomes important to support efforts aimed at the identification and characterization of potential infectious components. It is anticipated that the use of these techniques in the next few years will contribute to a tremendous expansion of knowledge regarding the etiologic basis of many human diseases.

Nucleic acid-based pathogen discovery techniques used to date fall into two general categories: consensus PCR (also known as broad-range PCR) and RDA. Consensus PCR techniques exploit the presence of conserved nucleic acid sequences within infectious microorganisms and have been applied to identification of viral, parasitic and bacterial pathogens (for recent reviews, see [6, 50–52]). The RDA technique recovers pathogen-specific sequences by exploiting the kinetics of logarithmic amplification of pathogen nucleic acids within a reaction in which host genomic DNA sequences are amplified in a much slower, linear fashion [53–55]. These methods will be described in greater detail in the following sections.

Broad-Range Polymerase Chain Reaction

An important development in the field of nucleic acid-based genotypic pathogen discovery revolves around the use of conserved DNA target sequences within phylogenetically informative loci, such as the large (23S) and small (16S) subunit ribosomal RNA (rDNA) genes of bacteria [6, 51, 52, 56–60]. These genes encode important structural RNA molecules whose variation is subject to severe constraints. Analysis of the 16S and, to a lesser extent, the 23S genes has led to the identification of genus and species-specific regions that can be used in studies of bacteria classification and taxonomy [61]. Moreover, conserved regions of these genes facilitate amplification from a wide range of organisms; highly variable regions (signature sequences) within the amplicon permit phylogenetic analysis and in many cases, species-level identification. As with all PCR applications, the level of specificity is dictated by the design of the two oligonucleotide primers that anneal to complementary sequences flanking the target and then catalyze target replication. Depending upon the choice of primer sequences, amplification-based bacterial identification methods can operate at nearly any level of specificity – strain, species, genus, or all members of a domain. Some regions within the rRNA operon are so highly conserved as to be found in all free-living life forms.

Discovered or Characterized Using Ribosomal RNA Gene Targets

By using the consensus PCR approach, several novel, fastidious or uncultivated bacterial pathogens have been identified directly from infected human tissue or blood. *Mycobacterium genavense* , which has been implicated in disseminated mycobacterial infections in immunocompromised patients was identified in acid-fast stain positive tissues from acquired immunodeficiency syndrome (AIDS) patients [62–67]. Several additional members of the Mycobacterium genus have now been identified by using similar approaches [68–70]. *Bartonella henselae,* an important member of the Rickettsia family, was originally identified by direct amplification of single-stranded (ss)-rDNA sequences from tissues of AIDS patients affected by bacillary angiomatosis and peliosis hepatis [71–75]. Subsequent clinical and epidemiological studies, facilitated by the direct detection capabilities of PCR, have implicated this organism as the agent of common cat scratch disease [73, 76–80]. *Tropheryma whippelii* is an organism related to actinomycetes that is found in diseased tissues from patients with Whipple's disease, a chronic multisystem inflammatory disorder involving the central nervous system (CNS), musculoskeletal system, and duodenum [8, 82]. To date, this organism has eluded all attempts at in vitro cultivation; however, PCR-based tests can be used to diagnosis this disease accurately and to monitor the course of therapy in patients with the disease [82, 83]. A rickettsia-like agent implicated in human granulocytic ehrlichiosis was recently identified by ss-rDNA amplification of a blood specimen from a patient with visible inclusions (morulae) in circulating granulocytes [84, 85]. Other novel rickettsial organisms have now been identified by using similar consensus PCR approaches.

rDNA-based consensus PCR can also be used to identify eukaryotic pathogens, albeit with somewhat more difficulty, since the conditions used to amplify eukaryotic pathogen sequences from infected tissues often result in coamplification of host DNA. Broad-range PCR was used recently to identify from human blood specimens a novel tick-transmitted piroplasm that is related to organisms of the genus *Babesia* [86, 87]. Phylogenetic analysis of the piroplasm-specific region showed the organism to be a newly recognized member of the of the genus *Babesia*, and to be secondarily related to piroplasms of the genus *Theileria*, which cause a leukemia-like disease in African cattle. The phylogenetic analysis of sequences derived from this organism correlated with antigenic cross-reactivity studies (see below). Consensus PCR was also used recently to derive signature nucleotide sequences from the large subunit rDNA for a large number of pure cultures of pathogenic fungi; this information could be used to develop genus- and species-specific probes for direct detection, culture confirmation, and for pathogen discovery [88]. Similar broad-range PCR studies of *Entamoeba* [89–92], *Cryptosporidium* [93, 94], and *Toxoplasma* [95–98] have now been described.

Other Broad-Range Polymerase Chain Reaction Targets

All nonviral human pathogens contain a variety of routine maintenance or "housekeeping" genes, such as those encoding heat-shock proteins or DNA and RNA polymerases. These sequences, if sufficiently conserved, can also serve as detection targets for broad-range PCR studies. The bacterial gene *rpoB* , which encodes the β-subunit of RNA polymerase, has been recovered from a wide variety of mycobacterial and non-mycobacterial organisms [99–103]. This sequence displays many strain-specific polymorphisms that may be useful for phylogenetic analysis [101]. Similar approaches have been applied to the study of mycobacteria heat-shock proteins [104–107] and to the citrate synthetase gene of rickettsia-like organisms [99, 108, 109]. Analysis of these loci may offer certain advantages, especially when closely related organisms display few differences by phylogenetic analysis of ss-rDNA.

Viral pathogens can also be detected by broad-range PCR approaches. Although rDNA and housekeeping genes are not available for detection of new viruses, highly conserved sequence motifs that are present in many virus families allow detection of novel viral infectious agents or new sequence variants within a virus family. Highly conserved regions within conserved regions of overlapping reading frames of hepatitis B virus (HBV) have allowed for detection of novel HBV variants [110]. Consensus PCR has been the primary means of discovery of new strains of human papillomaviruses (HPV) which have been implicated in the development of cervical cancer; PCR amplification protocols directed against conserved regions of the L1 region of the HPV genome facilitated the discovery of many novel HPV variants [19, 111–114]. Conserved regions of the 5′ untranslated and NS5 regions of hepatitis C virus have allowed classification of HCV into multiple subtypes and facilitated the discovery of many novel subtypes [11, 115, 116]; classification of HCV may be important for predicting disease outcomes and likelihood of response to therapy [17, 79, 117–120]. Novel HIV variants have been identified by using similar consensus PCR approaches to amplification of conserved portions of the gene encoding the envelope glycoprotein gp120 [121, 122]. Discovery of new alpha herpesviruses [123], flaviviruses such dengue and tick-borne encephalitis virus [124, 125], and hantaviruses [126] may be facilitated greatly by the use of consensus PCR.

Representational Difference Analysis

In 1984, subtractive hybridization was first used to identify unique DNA sequences on the human Y chromosome by hybridization of excess female DNA to restriction-digested fragments of male DNA used [127]. Since then, subtractive hybridization has been used in many other settings for identification of large mutations in genetic disorders and for studying differences in gene expression. The theoretical basis of subtractive hybridization can best be described as the molecular equivalent of a digital background subtraction technique, in which excess "driver" DNA is used to subtract common sequences from a nucleic acid mixture containing a unique sequence from, for instance, a pathogen (the "tester"). Such an approach could be used to identify pathogen-specific sequences in diseased tissue. However, for the purposes of pathogen discovery, conventional subtractive hybridization techniques are usually not sensitive enough to recover small numbers of microbial genomes in a background of host nucleic acid sequences.

Substantial enrichment for the unique DNA or RNA sequences can be accomplished by so-called "kinetic enrichment" in a process that has been termed representational difference analysis (RDA) [53–55, 128]. RDA is performed by generating "representations" of genetic material from diseased and normal tissues via PCR amplification of restriction fragments. The amplified restriction fragment mixture from the diseased tissue is ligated to a priming sequence and then annealed with an excess of DNA fragments derived from tissues not involved in the disease process. It is preferable that the control tissues come from the same individual so that random genetic variability between individuals does not contribute to background. While sequences unique to the diseased tissue will rapidly re-anneal to themselves (a reaction that is facilitated in part by the short size of the restriction fragments), sequences common to both diseased and non-diseased tissues will hybridize to each other. Since the normal tissue lacks primer binding sites, the result of self-annealing between clones from background DNA of diseased and non-diseased tissues will lead to duplexes with only one primer binding sequence. On the other hand, unique sequences within the diseased tissue will re-anneal to themselves to form duplexes with primer binding sequences at both ends. PCR amplification of this molecular mixture results in linear amplification of background DNA hybridization products, but logarithmic amplification of unique sequences occurs since only these sequences contain both primer binding sites. The process is repeated with different primer adapter sequences to enrich for sequences that are found only in the diseased tissue [129–132].

Detection of a Novel Herpesvirus Associated with Kaposi's Sarcoma

RDA was used to identify a novel member of the herpes virus family in AIDS-associated Kaposi's sarcoma (KS) tissues [53, 133–136]. Building on the suspicion that AIDS-associated KS may have an infectious etiology independent of HIV infection, Chang et al [53] performed RDA on KS and normal tissue to identify for KS-associated RDA products after *BamHI* digestion. Two of the clones hybridized specifically with KS tissues. One of the clones was 50 % identical by amino acid homology to a capsid protein of herpes virus Samurai, a gammaherpes virus associated with fulminant lymphoma in monkeys. Overall, 74 %–78 % of the AIDS KS specimens hybridized to the two probes, compared to 4 % of controls. Nearly all the tissues were positive by PCR. Subsequent studies have validated this original finding and have shown HHV-8 to be present in KS lesions from non-AIDS patients as well [134].

Identification of a Novel Flavivirus Associated with Hepatitis

The first transmissible agent associated with hepatitis that was successfully propagated in primates was originally obtained from the serum of a 34-year-old surgeon after the development of acute hepatitis. RDA was recently used to identify unique viral sequences within infectious plasma from an infected tamarin [55, 137]. After conversion of RNA extracted from plasma into cDNA by random primed reversed transcription, three rounds of RDA were used to amplify flavivirus-specific sequences selectively; virus-specific sequences could be observed after a single round of amplification, presumably because of the low background content within plasma. Sequence analysis of the clones showed some similarity to hepatitis C virus [55, 137). Recent molecular and seroepidemiologic studies have suggested that risk factors for acquisition of infection with the virus or its relatives may be similar to that of hepatitis C virus; coinfection with this virus, which is now termed hepatitis G virus, may occur in a significant number of patients with hepatitis C virus. Further studies will be required to determine the extent to which infection with this virus is associated with acute and chronic hepatitis or other disease.

Phylogenetic Analysis and Antigenic Relatedness: A New Paradigm

Once new sequence information pertaining to a novel pathogen has been obtained, phylogenetic analysis can be performed to assess the relationships between the new organism and those already characterized by similar means [138–150]. Each of the phylogenetic analysis programs has certain advantages and disadvantages, depending on the type of data being analyzed [151–153]. Thus it is reasonable to use multiple analytic methods during the initial analysis of a newly derived sequence. Several excellent and up-to-date reviews are available on this subject [61, 150, 152].

By phylogenetic analysis, similarities and differences between organisms can be inferred. These genetic similarities have, on a few occasions, been extrapolated to identify antigenic relationships as well, which can be exploited for further study of infected individuals.

Ehrlichia chaffeensis, a cause of human monocytic ehrlichiosis, is genetically closely related to *Ehrlichia canis*, and the two organisms are antigenically cross-reactive [154–157]. The agent of human granulocytic ehrlichiosis, ribosomal sequences of which were recovered directly from human clinical specimens, is more closely related to *Ehrlichia equi* and *Ehrlichia phagocytophila*. These latter two organisms are antigenically distinct from *Ehrlichia canis/chaffeensis*, as demonstrated in recent serological cross-comparisons [158]. However, *Ehrlichia equi* antigen can be used as a substrate for detection of antibody to the human granulocytic agent for confirmation of molecular analyses and for determination of past exposure to this newly discovered class of organism [84, 85, 158, 159]. Thus, in the case of *Ehrlichia* spp., phylogenetic analysis based on DNA sequencing of small subunit ribosomal genes directly from clinical specimens can be used to identify the appropriate antigen substrate to be used for immunologic follow-up, as well as for seroepidemiologic studies.

Another example of the correlation of phylogenetic analysis with immunologic cross-reactivity was described recently for a new member of the piroplasm family [86, 87, 160]. In this case, phylogenetic analysis of small subunit ribosomal DNA sequences directly from clinical specimens predicted that a new member of the piroplasm family was genetically related to a strain that had been recovered previously from a patient in Washington State (strain WA1) [160]. Antibody cross-reactivity studies showed that sera from patients infected with the newly identified organism crossreacted with the WA1 strain. In contrast, serologic testing with *Babesia microti* antigen was negative in these patients, consistent with the substantial phylogenetic distance between WA1 and *B. microti* [86].

Collectively, this approach of the use of phylogenetic information to predict antigenic relatedness represents a new paradigm that can be used to develop tests for detection of humoral and cellular immune responses to new pathogens. As more uncultured pathogens are discovered, it becomes increasingly important to demonstrate host responses during an infectious process associated with the presence of organism-specific nucleic acid sequences. Representational difference analysis as described above, may take things a step further – this method may be capable of recovering pathogen-specific nucleic acid sequences encoding immunodominant antigens directly from tissues. Alternatively, genes expressed selectively in tissues can be isolated. Presumably, by the use of inferred antigenic relationships (via phylogenetic analysis of broad-range PCR products) or by direct recovery of antigen genes from tissues, a battery of immunodiagnostic tests could be developed for a pathogen that has yet to be recovered in culture.

Comment

In reductionist terms, some infectious diseases can now be viewed as "horizontally acquired genetic disorders," in which nucleic acid sequences from a pathogen comingle with those of the host to produce, in some cases, inflammation and disease and, in others, no symptoms whatsoever. The use of pathogen discovery techniques will undoubtedly contribute greatly to our understanding of the huma flora, especially those organisms whose presence has been heretofore unrecognized. Likewise, the use of these techniques to better characterize xenotransplant donor animals may lead to a greater understanding of the diversity of microbial flora that are potentially zoonotic, how they can best be recognized, and ultimately perhaps eliminated from the donor pool.

Endemic human viruses and other pathogens have been known for many years. It is interesting to note that some human viruses, such as the Old and New World human retroviruses [38], human papillomaviruses [18, 19], and hepatitis C viruses [161, 162] show features of "zoonotic" diseases; for these viruses, major differences exist between viral strains found within different socially - and geographically - separated human populations. Potentially, a viral variant that is well adapted to a local human populatation could exhibit greater or lesser virulence in hosts with different immunogenetic profiles. In light of this, it is important to consider the perspective that, although human-to-human transmission of many types of infectious agents has been well documented after transplantation of human organs, no mutation or activation of a more virulent strain of a human retrovirus has been documented to date. Nonetheless, the use of nucleic acid-based pathogen discovery techniques, as described here, may go far toward the characterization of the uncultured flora of xenotransplant donor animals.

It is no coincidence that many of the applications of the described pathogen discovery methods have been for the identification of zoonotic pathogens, since the organisms involved are typically difficult or impossible to cultivate in vitro. The use of the above described methods (as well as others that will certainly be developed in the future) for zoonotic pathogen discovery in the area of xenotransplantation is a natural extension of the paradigm. Perhaps, as a first project, potential donor species with one or more known infectious agents (e.g., STLV-1 or foamy virus or both) should be examined to define the sensitivity and specificity of the approaches being used and to gain experience with the methods. Once the sensitivity of the methods is established, the pathogen discovery process could begin with appropriate combinations of cases and controls. By the systematic application of the nucleic acid-based pathogen discovery techniques, it may indeed become possible to expand significantly our understanding of the range of microbial agents residing in animal donors, with the ultimate goal of avoiding or interrupting their potential transmission during xenotransplantation.

References

1. BEARDSLEY, T. Paradise lost? Microbes mount a comeback as drug resistance spreads (news). Sci. Amer.267, 18, 1992
2. BURKE, J.P., LEVY, S.B. Summary report on worldwide antibiotic resistance: international task forces on antibiotic use. Rev. Infect. Dis.7, 560, 1985
3. MURRAY, B.E. Can antibiotic resistance be controlled? N. Engl. J. Med.330, 1229, 1994
4. NEU, H.C., DUMA, R.J., JONES, R.N., et al. Antibiotic resistance. Epidemiology and therapeutics (comment). Diag. Microbiol. Infect. Dis.15, 53S, 1992

5. OFFICE OF TECHNOLOGY ASSESSMENT, U.S. Congress Impacts of antibiotic resistant bacteria. Government Printing Office, Washington, DC, 1995
6. RELMAN, D.A. The identification of uncultured microbial pathogens (Review). J. Infect. Dis.168, 1, 1993
7. RICHMAN, D.D. Drug resistance in viruses (Review). Trends Microbiol.2, 401, 1994
8. WALKER, D.H., DUMLER, J.S. Emerging and reemerging rickettsial diseases (editorial comment). N. Engl. J. Med.331, 1651, 1994
9. De MITRI, M.S., POUSSIN, K., BACCARINI, P., et al. HCV-associated liver cancer without cirrhosis. Lancet.345, 413, 1995
10. GROSS, J.B. Jr., PERSING, D.H. Hepatitis C: advances in diagnosis (Review). Mayo Clinic Proc.70, 296, 1995
11. SIMMONDS, P. Variability of hepatitis C virus genome (Review). Curr. Studies Hematol. Blood Trans. 61, 12, 1994
12. BOLIN, T.D., HUNT, R.H., KORMAN, M.G., et al. Helicobacter pylori and gastric neoplasia: evolving concepts (Review). med. J. Australia.163, 253, 1995
13. De KOSTER, E., BUSET, M., FERNANDES, E., DELTENRE, M. Helicobacter pylori: the link with gastric cancer (Review). Eur. J. Cancer Prevent.3, 247, 1994
14. FENNERTY, M.B. Helicobacter pylori (Review). Arch. Intern. Med.154, 721, 1994
15. THIJS, J.C., KUIPERS, E.J., VAN SWET, A.A., PENA, A.S., de GRAFF, J. Treatment of helicobacter pylori infections (Review). QJM88, 369, 1995
16. HAYDON, G.H., JARVIS, L.M., SIMMONDS, P., HAYES, P.C. Association between chronic hepatitis C infection and hepatocellular carcinoma (Letter). Lancet.345, 928, 1995
17. ZEIN, N.N., POTERUCHA, J.J., GROSS, J.J., WIESNER, R.H., PERSING, D.H. Increased risk of hepatocellular carcinoma in patients infected with hepatitis C genotype b. Submitted for publication
18. BERNARD, H.U., CHAN, S.Y., MANOS, M.M., et al. Identification and assessment of known and novel human papillomaviruses by polymerase chain reaction amplification, restriction fragment length polymorphisms, nucleotide sequence, and phylogenetic algorithms. J. Infect. Dis.170, 1077, 1994
19. MANOS, M.M., WALDMAN, J., ZHANG, T.Y., et al. Epidemiology and partial nucleotide sequence of four novel genital human papillomaviruses. J. Infect. Dis.170, 1096, 1994
20. BAYERDORFFER, E., NEUBAUER, A., RUDOLPH, B., et al. Regression of primary gastric lymphoma of mucosa-associated lymphoid tissue type after cure of helicobacter pylori infection. MALT Lymphoma Study Group. Lancet.345, 1591, 1995
21. BOOT, H., de JONG, D., VAN HEERDE, P., TAAL, B. Role of helicobacter pylori eradication in high-grade MALT lymphoma (Letter). Lancet.346, 448, 1995
22. DELL, R.B., KORNFELD, D.S. Guidelines for xenotransplantation (Letter). Science.268, 349, 1995
23. MICHAELS, M.G., McMICHAEL, J.P., BRASKY, K., et al. Screening donors for xenotransplantation. The potential for xenozoonoses. Transplantation.57, 1482, 1994
24. STARZL, T.E., FUNG, J., TZAKIS, A., et al. Baboon-to-human liver transplantation. Lancet.341, 65, 1993
25. YE, Y., NIEKRASZ, M., KOSANKE, S., et al. The pig as a potential organ donor for man. A study of potentially transferable disease from donor pig to recipient man. Transplantation.57, 694, 1994

26. AGUZZI, A. The foamy virus family: molecular biology, epidemiology and neuropathology (Review). Biochem. Biophys. Acta.1155, 1, 1993
27. AGUZZI, A., BOTHE, K., WAGNER, E.F., RETHWILM, A., HORAK, I. Human foamy virus: an underestimated neuropathogen? (Review). Brain Pathol.2, 61, 1992
28. BIENIASZ, P.D., RETHWILM, A., POTMAN, R., et al. A comparative study of higher primate foamy viruses, including a new virus from a gorilla. Virology.207, 217, 1995
29. EBERLE, R., BLACK, D.H., LIPPER, S., HILLIARD, J.K. Herpesvirus papio 2, an SA8-like alpha-herpesvirus of baboons. Arch. Virol.140, 529, 1995
30. FRANCHINI, G. Molecular mechanisms of human T-cell leukemia/lymphotropic virus type I infection (Review). Blood.86, 3619, 1995
31. FRANCHINI, G., REITZ, M. Jr. Phylogenesis and genetic complexity of the nonhuman primate Retroviridae (Review). Aids Res. Human Retrovirus.10, 1047, 1994
32. MONE, J., WHITEHEAD, E., LELAND, M., HUBBARD, G., ALLAN, J.S. Simian T-cell leukemia virus type I infection in captive baboons. Aids. Res. Human Retrovirus.8, 1653, 1992
33. SCHATZL, M., YAKOVIEVA, L., LAPIN, B., et al. Detection and characterization of T-cell leukemia virus-like proviral sequences in PBL and tissues of baboons by PCR. Leukemia.6, 158S, 1992
34. DUNCAN, R., MURPHY, F.A., MIRKOVIC, R.R. Characterization of a novel syncytium-inducing baboon reovirus. Virology.212, 752, 1995
35. HARRISON, C., KOLBERT, C.P., MAGERA, J., et al. Identification of an endemic piroplasm of domestic baboons, 1996
36. KORALNIK, I.J., BOERL, E., SAXINGER, W.C., et al. Phylogenetic associations of human and simian T-cell leukemia/lymphotropic virus type I strains: evidence for interspecies transmission. J. Virol.68, 2693, 1994
37. LIU, H.F., VANDAMME, A.M., VAN BRUSSEL, M., DESMYTER, J., GOUBAU, P. New retroviruses in human and simian T-lymphotropic viruses (Letter). Lancet.344, 265, 1994
38. MIURA, T., FUKUNAGA, T., IGARASHI, T., et al. Phylogenetic subtypes of human T-lymphotropic virus type I and their relations to the anthropological background. Proc. Natl. Acad. Sci. USA.91, 1124, 1994
39. YANAGIHARA, R., SALTOU, N., NERURKAR, R., et al. Molecular phylogeny and dissemination of human T-cell lymphotropic virus type I viewed within the context of primate evolution and human migration. Cell. Moll. Biol.41, S145, 1995
40. BONYHADI, M.L., SU, L., AUTEN, J., McCUNE, J.M., KANESHIMA, H. Development of a human thymic organ culture model for the study of HIV pathogenesis. Aids Res. Human Retrovirus.11, 1073, 1995
41. BRANDSMA, J.L., BROWNSTEIN, D.G., XIAO, W., LONGLEY, B.J. Papilloma formation in human foreskin xenografts after inoculation of human papillomavirus type 16 DNA. J. Virol.69, 2716, 1995
42. BUTCHER, G.A., COUCHMAN, A.F., VAN PELT, J.F., FLECK, S.L., SINDEN, R.E. The SCID mouse as a laboratory model for development of the exoerythrocytic stages of human and rodent malaria. Exp. Parasitol.77, 257, 1993
43. KRESINA, T.F., WISNEWSKI, A., LOVE-HOMAN, L., RAMIREZ, B., NEIL, G.A. Induction of hepatic pathology in SCID-Hu mice engrafted with peripheral blood lymphocytes of patients with Schistosomiasis japonica. J. Infect. dis.170, 733, 1994
44. MOSIER, D.E., PICCHIO, G.R., KIRVEN, M.B., et al. EBV-induced human B cell lymphomas in hu-PBL-SCID mice (Review). Aids. Res. Human Retrovirus. 8, 735, 1992

45. REVILLA, Y., PENA, L., MAMPASO, F., VINUELA, E., MARTINEZ-ALONSO, C. Swine-reconstituted SCID mice as a model for African swine fever virus infection. J. Gen. Virol.75, 1983, 1994
46. TSUJI, M., ISHIHARA, C., ARAI, S., HIRATAI, R., AZUMA, I. Establishment of a SCID mouse model having circulating human red blood cells and a possible growth of Plasmodium falciparum in the mouse. Vaccine.13, 1389, 1995
47. TSUJI, M., TERADA, Y., ARAL, S., IKADA, H., ISHIHARA, C. Use of the Bo-RBC-SCID mouse model for isolation of a Babesia parasite from grazing calves in Japan. Parasitol.81, 512, 1995
48. WILLIAMS, A., McBRIDE, B.W., HALL, G., FITZGEORGE, R.B., FARRAR, G.H. Experimental Legionnaire's disease in SCID-beige mice reconstituted with human leukocytes. J. Med. Microbiol.42, 433, 1995
49. WAGNER, M., AMANN, R., LEMMER, H., SCHLELFER, K.H. Probing activated sludge with oligonucleotides specific for proteobacteria: inadequacy of culture-dependent methods for describing microbial community structure. Appl. Environ. Microbiol.59, 1520, 1993
50. ROWLEY, A.H., WOLINSKY, S.M., RELMAN, D.A., et al. Search for highly conserved viral and bacterial nucleic acid sequences corresponding to an etiologic agent of Kawasaki disease. Pedia. Res.36, 567, 1994
51. SCHMIDT, T.M., RELMAN, D.A. Phylogenetic identification of uncultured pathogens using ribosomal RNA sequences (Review). Methods. Enzymol.235, 205, 1994
52. WILSON, K.H. Detection of culture-resistant bacterial pathogens by amplification and sequencing of ribosomal DNA (Review). Clin. Infect. Dis.18, 958, 1994
53. CHANG, Y., CESARMAN, E., PESSIN, M.S., et al. Identification of herpesvirus-like DNA sequences in AIDS-associated Kaposi's sarcoma. Science.266, 1865, 1994
54. LISITSYN, N.A., LISITSINA, N.M., DALBAGNI, G., et al. Comparative genomic analysis of tumors: detection of DNA losses and amplification. Proc. Natl. Acad. Sci. USA.92, 151, 1995
55. SIMONS, J.N., PILOT-MATIAS, T.J., LEARY, T.P., et al. Identification of two Flavivirus-like genomes in the GB hepatitis agent. Proc. Natl. Acad. Sci. USA.92, 3401, 1995
56. FREDRICKS, D.N., RELMAN, D.A. Sequence-based identification of microbial pathogens: a reconsideration of Koch's postulates. Clin. Microbiol. Rev.9, 1996
57. KIRSCHNER, P., SPRINGER, B., VOGEL, U., et al. Genotypic identification of mycobacterial by nucleic acid sequence determination: report of a 2-year experience in a clinical laboratory. J. Clin. Microbiol.31, 2882, 1993
58. MEIER, A., PERSING, D.H., FINKEN, M., BOTTGER, E.C. Elimination of contaminating DNA within polymerase chain reaction reagents: implications for a general approach to detection of uncultured pathogens. J. Clin. Microbiol.31, 646, 1993
59. RELMAN, D.A., FALKOW, S. Identification of uncultured microorganisms: expanding the spectrum of characterized microbial pathogens (Review). Infect. Agents Dis.1, 245, 1992
60. SOINI, H., BOTTGER, E.C., VILJANEN, M.K. Identification of mycobacteria by PCR-based sequence determination of the 32-kilodalton protein gene. J. Clin. Microbiol.32, 2944, 1994
61. PERSING, D.H., HERWALDT, B.L., GLASER, C., et al. Infection with a Babesia-like organism in northern California. N. Engl. J. Med.332, 298, 1995

62. BOTTGER, E.C. Mycobacterium genavense: an emerging pathogen (Review). Eur. J. Clin. Microbiol. Infect. Dis.13, 932, 1994
63. BOTTGER, E.C., HIRSCHEL, B., COYLE, M.B. Mycobacterium genavense sp. nov. Int. J. System. Bacteriol.43, 841, 1993
64. COYLE, M.B., CARLSON, L.C., WALLIS, C.K., et al. Laboratory aspects of "mycobacterium genavense", a proposed species isolated from AIDS patients. J. Clin. Microbiol.30, 3206, 1992
65. EMIER, S., BOTTGER, E.C., BROERS, B., et al. Growth-deficient mycobacteria in patients with AIDS: diagnosis by analysis of DNA amplified from blood or tissue. Clin. Infect. Dis.20, 772, 1995
66. HOOP, R.K., BOTTGER, E.C., OSSENT, P., SALFINGER, M. Mycobacteriosis due to mycobacterium genavense in six pet birds. J. Clin. Microbiol.31, 990, 1993
67. MASCHEK, H., GEORGII, A., SCHMIDT, R.E., KIRSCHNER, P., BOTTGER, E.C. Mycobacterium genavense. Autopsy findings in three patients. Amer. J. Clin. Pathol.101, 95, 1994
68. HAAS, W.H., KIRSCHNER, P., ZIESING, S., BREMER, H.J., BOTTGER, E.C. Cervical lymphadenitis in a child caused by a previously unknown mycobacterium. J. Infect. Dis.167, 237, 1993
69. KIRSHNER, P., TESKE, A., SCHRODER, K.H., et al. Mycobacterium confluents sp. nov. Internat. J. System. Bacteriol.42, 257, 1992
70. MEIER, A., KIRSCHNER, P., SCHRODER, K.H., et al. Mycobacterium intermedium sp. nov. Internat. J. System. Bacteriol.43, 204, 1993
71. RELMAN, D.A. Bacillary angiomatosis and Rochalimaea species (Review). Curr. Clin. Topics in Infect. Dis.14, 205, 1994
72. RELMAN, D.A., FALKOW, S., LEBOTT, P.E., et al. The organism causing bacillary angiomatosis, peliosis hepatis, and fever and bacteremia in immunocompromised patients (Letter). N. Engl. J. Med.324, 1514, 1991
73. RELMAN, D.A., SCHMIDT, T.M., MACDERMOTT, R.P., FALKOW, S. Identification of the uncultured bacillus of Whipple's disease. N. Engl. J. Med.327, 293, 1992
74. TAPPERO, J.W., KOEHLER, J.E. Rochalimaea infections (Letter). Ann. Int. Med.119, 535, 1993
75. TAPPERO, J.W., KOEHLER, J.E., BERGER, T.G., et al. Bacillary angiomatosis and bacillary splenitis in immunocompetent adults. Ann. Int. Med.118, 363, 1993
76. ADAL, K.A., COCKERELL, C.J., PETRI, W. Jr. Cat scratch disease, bacillary angiomatosis and other infections due to Rochalimaea (Review). N. Engl. J. Med.330, 1509, 1994
77. ANDERSON, B., KELLY, C., THRELKEL, H., EDWARDS, K. Detection of Rochalimaea henselae in cat scratch disease skin test antigens. J. Infect. Dis.168, 1034, 1993
78. ANDERSON, B., SIMS, K., REGNERY, R., et al. Detection of Rochalimaea henselae DNA in specimens from cat scratch disease patients by PCR. J. Clin. Microbiol.32, 942, 1994
79. KOEHLER, J.E., GLASER, C.A., TAPPERO, J.W. Rochalimaea henselae infection. A new zoonosis with the domestic cat as reservoir. JAMA.271, 531, 1994
80. RAOULT, D., TISSOT DUPONT, H., ENEA-MUTILLOD, M. Positive predictive value of Rochalimaea henselae antibodies in the diagnosis of cat scratch disease (Letter). Clin. Infect. Dis.19, 355, 1994
81. RELMAN, D.A., SCHMIDT, T.M., MACDERMOTT, R.P., FALKOW, S. Identification of the uncultured bacillus of Whipple's disease. N. Engl. J. Med.327, 293, 1992

82. RICKMAN, L.S., FREEMAN, W.R., GREEN, W.R., et al. Brief report: uveitis caused by Tropheryma whippelii (Whipple's bacillus). N. Engl. J. Med.332, 363, 1995
83. RAMZAN, N.N., LOFTUS, E.J., BURGHART, L., et al. Molecular diagnosis and monitoring of Whipple's disease. In press
84. BAKKEN, J.S., DUMIER, J.S., CHEN, S.M., et al. Human granulocyte ehrlichiosis in the upper Midwest United States. A new species emerging? JAMA.272, 212, 1994
85. CHEN, S.M., DUMLER, J.S., BAKKEN, J.S., WALKER, D.H. Identification of a granulocytotropic Ehrlichia species as the etiologic agent of human disease. J. Clin. Microbiol.32, 589, 1994
86. PERSING, D.H., HERWALDT, B.L., GLASER, C., et al. Infection with a Babesia-like organism in northern California. N. Engl. J. Med.332, 298, 1995
87. THOMFORD, J.W., CONRAD, P.A., TELFORD, S.E., et al. Cultivation and phylogenetic characterization of a newly recognized human pathogenic protozoan. J. Infect. Dis.169, 1050, 1994
88. SANDHU, G.S., KLINE, B.C., STOCKMAN, L., ROBERTS, G.D. Molecular probes for diagnosis of fungal infections. J. Clin. Microbiol.33, 2913, 1995
89. CLARK, C.G., DIAMOND, L.S. Ribosomal RNA genes of ‚pathogenic' and ‚nonpathogenic' Entamoeba histolytica are distinct. Mol. Biochem. Parasitol.49, 297, 1991
90. CRUZ-REYES, J.A., SPICE, W.M., REHMAN, T., GISBORNE, E., ACKERS, J.P. Ribosomal DNA sequences in the differentiation of pathogenic and nonpathogenic isolates of Entamoeba histolytica. Parasitology.104, 239, 1992
91. MEZA, I. Entamoeba histolytica: phylogenetic considerations. A review. Arch. Med. Res.23, 1, 1992
92. QUE, X., REED, S.L. Nucleotide sequence of a small subunit ribosomal RNA (16S-like rRNA) gene from Entamoeba histolytica: differentiation of pathogenic from nonpathogenic isolates. Nucleic Acid Res.19, 5438, 1991
93. BARTA, J.R., JENKINS, M.C., DANFORTH, H.D. Evolutionary relationships of avian Eimeria species among other Apicomplexa protozoa: monophyly of the Apicomplexa is supported. Molecular Biol. Evolut. 8, 345, 1991
94. TENTER, A.M., BAVERSTOCK, P.R., JOHNSON, A.M. Phylogenetic relationships of Sarcocystis species from sheep, goats, cattle, and mice based on ribosomal RNA sequences. Int. J. Parasitol.22, 503, 1992
95. ELLIS, J., LUTON, K., BAVERSTOCK, P.R., et al. The phylogeny of Neurospora caninum (published erratum appears in Mol Biochem Parasitol, 67, 341, 1994). Mol. Biochem. Parasitol.64, 303, 1994
96. ELLIS, T.J., LUTON, K., BAVERSTOCK, P.R., et al. Phylogenetic relationships between Toxoplasma and Sarcocystis deduced from a comparison of 18S rDNA sequences. Parasitology.110, 521, 1995
97. MARSH, A.E., BARR, B.C., SVERLOW, K., et al. Sequence analysis and comparison of ribosomal DNA from bovine Neurospora to similar coccidial parasites. J. Parasitol.81, 530, 1995
98. TENTER, A.M., LUTON, K., JOHNSON, A.M. Species-specific identification of Sarcocystis and Toxoplasma by PCR amplification of small subunit ribosomal RNA gene fragments. Appl. Parasitol.35, 173, 1994
99. DEMKIN, V.V., RYDKINA, E.B., LIKHODED, L.Y., et al. Genotypic characterization of rickettsiae by DNA probes generated from Rickettsia prowazekii DNA. Acta. Virol.38, 65, 1994

100. GUERRERO, C., STOCKMAN, L., MARSHESI, F., et al. Evaluation of the rpoB gene in rifampicin-susceptible and -resistant Mycobacterium avium and Mycobacterium intracellulare (Letter). J. Antimicrob. Chemotherap.33, 661, 1994
101. HUNT, J.M., ROBERTS, G.D., STOCKMAN, L., FELMLEE, T.A., PERSING, D.H. Detection of a genetic locus encoding resistance to rifampin in mycobacterial cultures and in clinical specimens. Diag. Microbiol. Infect. Dis.18, 219, 1994
102. KAPUR, V., LI, L.L., LORDANESCU, S., et al. Characterization by automated DNA sequencing of mutations in the gene (rpoB) encoding the RNA polymerase beta subunit in rifampin-resistant Mycobacterium tuberculosis strains from New York City and Texas. J. Clin. Microbiol.32, 1095, 1994
103. MILLER, L.P., CRAWFORD, J.T., SHINNICK, T.M. The rpoB gene of Mycobacterium tuberculosis. Antimicrob. Agents Chemotherap.38, 805, 1994
104. BOORSTEIN, W.R., ZIEGELHOFFER, T., CRAIG, E.A. Molecular evolution of the HSP70 multigene family. J. Mol. Evolut.38, 1, 1994
105. GUPTA, R.S., GOLDING, G.B. Evolution of HSP70 gene and its implications regarding relationships between Archaeobacteria, eubacteria, and eukaryotes. J. Mol. Evolut.37, 573, 1993
106. HUGHES, A.L. Contrasting evolutionary rates in the duplicate chaperonin genes of Mycobacterium tuberculosis and M. leprae. Mol. Biol. Evolut.10, 1343, 1993
107. RENSING, S.A., MAIER, U.G. Phylogenetic analysis of the stress-70 protein family. J. Mol. Evolut.39, 80, 1994
108. JIN, S., SONENSHEIN, A.L. Identification of two distinct Bacillus subtilis citrate synthase genes. J. Bacteriol.176, 4669, 1994
109. REGNERY, R.L., SPRUILL, C.L., PLIKAYTIS, B.D. Genotypic identification of rickettsiae and estimation of intraspecies sequence divergence for portions of two rickettsial genes. J. Bacteriol.173, 1576, 1991
110. CHIRARA, M.M., CHETSANGA, C.J. Variant of hepatitis B virus isolated in Zimbabwe. J. Med. Virol. 42, 73, 1994
111. MEHAL, W.Z., LO, Y.M., HERRINGTON, C.S., et al. Role of human papillomavirus in determining the HLA associated risk of cervical carcinogenesis. J. Clin. Pathol. 47, 1077, 1994
112. PEYTON, C.L., WHEELER, C.M. Identification of five novel human papillomavirus sequences in the New Mexico triethnic population. J. Infect. Dis. 170, 1089, 1994
113. RADY, P.L., ARANY, I., HUGHES, T.K., TYRING, S.K. Type-specific primer-mediated direct sequencing of consensus primer-generated PCR amplicons of human papilloma viruses: a new approach for the simultaneous detection of multiple viral type infections. J. Virol. Methods.53, 245, 1995
114. ZHENG, P.S., LI, S.R., IWASAKA, T., et al. Simultaneous detection by consensus multiplex PR of high-and low-risk and other types of human papilloma virus in clinical samples. Gynecol. Oncol. 58, 179, 1995
115. SIMMONDS, P., ALBERTI, A., ALTER, H.J., et al. A proposed system for the nomenclature of hepatitis C viral genotypes (Letter). Hepatology.19, 1321, 1994
116. SIMMONDS, P., HOLMES, E.C., CHA, T.A., et al. Classification of hepatitis C virus into six major genotypes and a series of subtypes by phylogenetic analysis of the NS-5 region. J. Gen. Virol.74, 2391, 1993

117. FERAY, C., GIGOU, M., SAMUEL, D., et al. Influence of the genotypes of hepatitis C virus on the severity of recurrent liver disease after liver transplantation. Gastroent.108, 1088, 1995
118. LAURENT-PUIG, P., DUSSAIX, E., ALTMAN, C., et al. Host and viral characteristics affecting the response to interferon therapy in chronic hepatitis C. Eur. J. Gastroent. Hepatol.7, 335, 1995
119. POZZATO, G., MORETTI, M., CROCE, L.S., et al. Interferon therapy in chronic hepatitis C virus: evidence of different outcome with respect to different viral strains. J. Med. Virol.45, 445, 1995
120. QU, D., HANTZ, O., GOUY, M., et al. Heterogeneity of hepatitis C virus genotypes in France. J. Gen. Virol.75, 1063, 1994
121. BRUCE, C., CLEGG, C., FEATHERSTONE, A., et al. Presence of multiple genetic subtypes of human immunodeficiency virus type 1 proviruses in Uganda. AIDS Res. Human Retrovir.10, 1543, 1994
122. GURTLER, L.G., HAUSER, P.H., EBERLE, J., et al. A new subtype of human immunodeficiency virus type 1 (MVP-5180) from Cameroon. J. Virol.68, 1581, 1994
123. AONO, T., MURAKAMI, S., YANAGIHARA, N., YAMANISHI, K. Detection of human alpha-herpesvirus DNA using consensus primers and specific probes. Acta. Oto. Laryngologica Suppl.514, 132, 1994
124. CHOW, V.T., SEAH, C.L., CHAN, Y.C. Use of NS3 consensus primers for the polymerase chain reaction amplification and sequencing of dengue viruses and other Flaviviruses. Arch. Virol.133, 157, 1993
125. FULOP, L., BARRETT, A.D., PHILLPOTTS, R., et al. Rapid identification of flaviviruses based on conserved NS5 gene sequences. J. Virol. Methods.44, 179, 1993
126. ARTHUR, R.R., LOFTS, R.S., GOMEZ, J., et al. Grouping of hantaviruses by small (S) genome segment polymerase chain reaction and amplification of viral RNA from wild-caught rats (published erratum appears in Am J Trop Med Hyg, 48, 5, 1993). Am. J. Trop. Med. Hygiene.47, 210, 1992
127. LAMAR, E.E., PALMER, E. Y-encoded, species-specific DNA in mice: evidence that the Y chromosome exists in two polymorphic forms in inbred strains. Cell.37, 171, 1984
128. LISITSYN, N., LISITSYN, N., WIGLER, M. Cloning the differences between two complex genomes. Science.259, 946, 1993
129. BROWN, P.O. Genome scanning methods (Review). Curr. Opinion Genet. Develop.4, 366, 1994
130. CHALLONER, P.B., SMITH, K.T., PARKER, J.D., et al. Plaque-associated expression of human herpesvirus 6 in multiple sclerosis. Proc. Natl. Acad. Sci. USA.92, 7440, 1995
131. HUBANK, M., SCHATZ, D.G. Identifying differences in mRNA expression by representational difference analysis of cDNA. Nucleic Acids Res.22, 5640, 1994
132. TSUCHLYA, H., TSUCHLYA, Y., KOBAYASHI, Y., KLKUCHI, Y., HINO, O. Isolation of genes differentially expressed between the Yoshida sarcoma and long-survival Yoshida sarcoma variants: origin of Yoshida sarcoma revisited. Jap. J. Cancer Res.85, 1099, 1994
133. CESARMAN, E., CHANG, Y., MOORE, P.S., SAID, J.W., KNOWLES, D.M. Kaposi's sarcoma-associated herpesvirus-like DNA sequences in AIDS-related body-cavity-based lymphomas. N. Engl. J. Med.332, 1186, 1995

134. MOORE, P.S., CHANG, Y. Detection of herpesvirus-like DNA sequences in Kaposi's sarcoma in patients with and without HIV infection. N. Engl. J. Med.332, 1181, 1995
135. SCHALLING, M., EKMAN, M., KAAYA, E.E., LINDE, A., BIBERFELD, P. A role for a new herpesvirus (kshv) in different forms of Kaposi's sarcoma. Nature. Med.1, 707, 1995
136. WHITBY, D., HOWARD, M.R., TENANTFLOWERS, M., et al. Detection of Kaposi's sarcoma associated herpesvirus in peripheral blood of HIV-infected individuals and progression to Kaposi's sarcoma. Lancet. 346, 799, 1995
137. MUERHOFF, A.S., LEARY, T.P., SIMONS, J.N., et al. Genomic organization of GB viruses A and B: two new members of the Flaviviridae associated with GB agent hepatitis. J. Virol.69, 5621, 1995
138. CAVALL-STORZA, L.L., EDWARDS, W.F. Phylogenetic analysis: models and estimation procedures. Evolution.32, 550, 1987
139. FARRIS, J.S. HENNIG86.Port Jefferson Station, NY, 1988
140. FELSENSTEIN, J. PHYLIP (Phylogeny Inference Package), 3,4 ed. University of Washington, Seattle, WA, 1988b
141. FELSENSTEIN, J. Phylogenies from molecular sequences: inference and reliability. Ann. Rev. Genetics. 22, 521, 1988a
142. FELSENSTEIN, J. Phylogenies from restriction sites: a maximum-likelihood approach. Evolution.46, 159, 1992
143. FITCH, W.M., MARGOLIASH, E. Construction of phylogenetic trees. Science.155, 279, 1967
144. FITCH, W.M., YE, J. Weighted parsimony. Does it work? In: Phylogenetic Analysis of DNA Sequences. M.M. Mlyamoto and J. Cracraft (eds). Oxford University Press, Oxford, 1992
145. JIN, L., NEL, M. Limitations of the evolutionary parsimony method of phylogenetic analysis. Mol. Biol. Evol.7, 82, 1990
146. SAITOU, N. A theoretical study of the underestimation of branch lengths by the maximum parsimony principle. Syst. Zool.38, 1, 1989
147. SAITOU, N., NEI, M. The neighbor-joining method: a new method for reconstructing phylogenetic trees. Mol. Biol. Evol.4, 406, 1987
148. SNEATH, P.H.A., SOKAL, R.R. Numerical Taxonomy: the Principles and Practice of Numerical Classification.W.H. Freeman, San Francisco, CA, 1973
149. SWOFFORD, D.L. Phylogenetic Analysis Using Parsimony (PAUP).3.0s ed, Champaign, 1991
150. SWOFFORD, D.L., OLSEN, G.J. Phylogeny reconstruction. In: Molecular Systematics.D.M. Hills and G. Moritz (eds). Sinauer Associates, Sunderland, MA, 1990
151. HILLIS, D.M., BULL, J.J., WHITE, M.D., BADGETT, M.R., MOLINEUX, I.J. Experimental phylogenetics: generation of a known phylogeny. Science.255, 589, 1992
152. HILLIS, D.M., HUELSENBECK, J.P., CUNNINGHAM, C.W. Application and accuracy of molecular phylogenies (Review). Science.264, 671, 1994
153. HILLIS, D.M., HUELSENBECK, J.P., SWOFFORD, D.L. Hobgoblin of phylogenetics? (Letter). Nature. 369, 363, 1994
154. ANDERSON, B.E., DAWSON, J.E., JONES, D.C., WILSON, K.H. Ehrlichia chaffeensis, a new species associated with human ehrlichiosis. J. Clin. Microbiol.29, 2838, 1991
155. DUMLER, J.S., BAKKEN, J.S. Ehrlichia diseases of humans: emerging tick-borne infections (Review). Clin. Infect. Dis.20, 1102, 1995

156. FISHBEIN, D.B., DAWSON, D.E., ROBINSON, L.E. Human ehrlichiosis in the United States, 1985 to 1990. Ann. Int. Med.120, 736, 1994
157. STANDAERT, S.M., DAWSON, J.E., SCHAFFNER, W., et al. Ehrlichiosis in a golf-oriented retirement community. N. Engl. J. Med.333, 420, 1995
158. DUMLER, J.S., ASANOVICH, K.M., BAKKEN, J.S., et al. Serologic cross-reactions among Ehrlichia equi, Ehrlichia phagocytophila, and human granulocytic Ehrlichia. J. Clin. Microbiol.33, 1098, 1995
159. PANCHOLI, P., KOLBERT, C.P., MITCHELL, P.D., et al. Ixodes dammini as a potential vector of human granulocytic ehrlichiosis. J. Infect. Dis.172, 1007, 1995
160. QUICK, R.E., HERWALDT, B.L., THOMFORD, J.W., et al. Babesiosis in Washington State: a new species of Babesia? Ann. Int. Med.119, 284, 1993
161. KAO, J.H., CHEN, P.J., LAI, M.Y., WANG, T.H., CHEN, D.S. Quasispecies of hepatitis C virus and genetic drift of the hypervariable region in chronic type C hepatitis. J. Infect. Dis.172, 261, 1995
162. SIMMONDS, P., SMITH, D.B., McOMISH, F., et al. Identification of genotypes of hepatitis C virus by sequence comparisons in the core, E1 and NS-5 regions. J. Gen. Virol.75, 1053, 1994

55 Comments on Ethics in Human Xenotransplantation

C. Hammer

Introduction

In 1993, two baboon liver xenotransplantations carried out in Pittsburgh, which resulted in the death of the patients, provoked the protest of 3000 U.S. medical doctors, who called for an end to the transplantation of such xenografts. The leader of these 3000 members of the "Committee of Doctors for Responsible Medicine" said that such an operation had no chance of succeeding. The protesters claimed that performing experimental surgery on someone who may have felt that he had little choice was inappropriate and unethical. They said that even when organs are taken from closely related animal species, too much immunosuppression is required to prevent rejection; the heavy immunosuppression leaves the body unable to fight off severe infections, which leads to death. The Committee of Doctors for Responsible Medicine said that the time for the use of animal organs has not yet come [1].

In the same year, Professor A.G.R. Sheil, Chairman of the Ethics Committee of the International Transplantation Society, published guidelines on the use of xenografts in humans. Xenografts, including those from nonhuman primates, would be considered acceptable in controlled cicumstances. Among other recommendations, the committee recommended that (a) the feasibility of human xenotransplantation should have been demonstrated before clinical trials by success in an appropriate nonrodent animal xenograft model and that (b) the clinical procedures should be carried out by groups with fully coordinated preclinical and clinical programs, with local institutional and/or State or National Ethics Review Board approval, and with informed recipient consent. The Ethics Committee discouraged isolated attempts at xenografting in humans, emphasizing that uncontrolled application with failure would result in a powerful negative impact on the field of transplantation in general.

What Are "Ethics"?

"Ethics" refer to principles of justice and are attempts to establish standards with reference to the individual character and its development in accordance with generally accepted human behavior. Ethics are a yardstick for daily life, without being a positive rule, and ask the question: "What would a rational human being do?" Ethics aim to guide us toward what is right and what is common sense. Situations and emotional factors, as well as ethical fundamentals, change constantly. New realities of life (for example, the results of new biomedical research, new technical advances, and other intellectual and emotional attitudes) modify what is rational. Principles that were once important in life suddenly become unimportant, and hitherto unimportant problems become central overnight.

Ethics in Relation to Human Xenotransplantation

The shortage of organs for transplantation has precipitated a rather theoretical field of research - xenotransplantation - into the spotlight of clinical hope. The use of animal organs would open up a totally new dimension in the treatment of terminally ill patients. Some see xenotransplantation as a victory for medical research in its fight against lethal diseases, others simply as an extension of the current organ transplant practices. But the prospect also triggers sharp and negative reactions in many minds, with some seeing xenotransplantation as a form of hybridism, carrying with it terrible dangers.

With regard to xenotransplantation, we have to consider: (a) the rights of animals, (b) the rights of critically ill patients with end-stage organ failure (who are in a different situation from young and healthy critics of xenografting, including some doctors), (c) the rights of the surgeon and others in the medical team, (d) national ethics, (e) religious ethics, and (f) international and global ethics.

Ethics Must Catch up with Technology

The doctors' protest over the baboon liver transplants highlights the fact that, while we have made rapid progress in developing xenograft surgery techniques, decisions on the ethics of the procedure have lagged well behind. Medicine is simply moving faster than its regulators. No domestic or international law exists that deals expressly with xenotransplantation. No one can be certain that the lawfulness of this practice will never be called into doubt. But scientists and doctors are not waiting for governments or the courts to decide whether xenotransplantation is legal. Futuristic surgery is being carried out now, before the immunological and other biological processes are fully understood. It is still not certain whether xenotransplantation will one day be able to prolong life for periods similar to those achieved with allografts. The dream of an endless supply of animal organs has not yet become a scientific reality.

If medical professionals are to avoid opposition, both from their colleagues and the outside community, to what critics may perceive as misuse of patients, then some self-imposed controls, based on ethics, must be exercised.

Xenotransplantation Ethics Versus Allotransplantation Ethics

The ethics of xenotransplantation are more complex than those of allogeneic organ transplantation. Is it justifiable to kill animals so that their organs can be transplanted into humans? Is it ethical to create a chimera, and how will the recipient and his or her relatives, friends, and colleagues react?

If an abundant supply of animal organs were available in the future, this would create a far more equitable situation than that which exists at present, where the worldwide shortage of human organs means that some patients will remain on dialysis or die.

The prospect of an unlimited supply of animal organs could, however, prompt patients or relatives to ask for (and the doctor to offer) a xenograft which may be unwarranted and/or unethical. For example, an animal organ could be sought for a fetus, a newborn baby, a drug addict, a mentally deficient patient, or an extremely aged man or woman. In all cases but the latter, how could these potential candidates be fully informed of the benefits and risks and decide whether they wish to accept an animal organ? Is a transplant for them ethical [2]? In the cases of the alcoholic, the drug addict, or the elderly, is their community prepared to pay the considerable costs of surgery and after-care, and sacrifice the life of an animal, for an individual whose illness may be self-inflicted or who is likely to die within a short time anyway?

Animal Rights

Today, we treat diabetic patients throughout their lives with porcine insulin. We also routinely transplant pig heart valves into patients. Recently, pig pancreatic islets have been transplanted into humans. Is it not also moral, then, to transplant a complete pig heart? In some centers, we currently transplant organs from anencephalic or cortically dead newborn infants. If we are able to do this, it would be nonsensical to refuse to use animal organs.

Although xenotransplantation creates an apparent imbalance favoring humans over animals, the removal of organs from animals is lawful. It is reasonable to save the life of a human at the expense of an animal life. Even the most fervent protector of animals would probably not dispute the legitimacy of xenotransplantation to benefit humans. A prerequisite for using animals, however, is that they must be treated with full regard to the prevention of suffering, pain, distress, or long-lasting harm [3–5].

The Ethics Committee of the Transplantation Society recommended that (a) the care and humane treatment of animals must always be of the highest standards, (b) all animal studies in transplantation must be approved by an institutional and/or State or National Review Board, (c) endangered species should not be used, (d) animals bred for the purpose of transplantation should be the preferred source, and (e) research designed to diminish the need for the use of animals in experimentation should be encouraged.

Gene Transfer

Any interference with genetic heritage that could be transmissible to subsequent generations must be prohibited [6]. A taboo must remain on (a) the transfer or implantation of human embryos into the uterus of another species, (b) the introduction of foreign genes into human sperm, (c) xenogeneic brain transplantation, and (d) the creation of human hybrids.

Patient and Community Ethics

For some members of the community, xenotransplantation is unethical [7]. Some may complain that not only is it experimental, but it is cruel to both animals and patients. If we could successfully transplant animal organs into humans, would the surviving recipient still be a human? The patient must have the freedom to accept or reject the idea of becoming a chimera. A minority of individuals would find this inhumane or regard it as a degrading form of therapy.

However, the expectation of a high quality of life and longevity has become so dominant in our culture that most patients would accept (a) an organ from a transgenic pig, (b) the transfusion of xenogeneic bone marrow, and (c) the state of mixed chimerism [8].

Coping with Chimerism

In deciding whether to go ahead with any operative procedure, the surgeon has to take into account what is right for the individual patient – in this case, how he or she will cope with chimerism. How will recipients react if they are constantly reminded, perhaps by themselves or by colleagues or relatives, that they have a pig heart in their chest or that they see the world through the cornea of a monkey? A recipient may more readily accept other xenografted organs, such as the kidney or liver. A total of 30%–50% of transplanted patients go back to work. The recipient of an animal organ could be subjected to constant teasing and annoyance by colleagues.

Personal relationships can be jeopardized even after allotransplantation. Will marital breakdown rates be even higher among those receiving a xenograft? Can the partner live with a chimera, love somebody who has a pig heart? Transplantation of the heart may have a special meaning. For the layman, this organ is still the place of sentiment and conscience, of good and bad, of love, courage, and bravery, and the organ on which life depends. It is the nucleus of an individual. It is not only the most important organ, it is a symbol. The lay person may have serious reservations. A father may wonder "Will my son still respect me if I have a porcine heart?" A mother offered a pig heart may doubt that she will be able to continue to love her children "with all her heart."

Ethics and the Transplant Surgeon

The transplant surgeon has to take into consideration the potential reaction – of the patient, the patient's relatives, and his or her own colleagues – to chimerism. What level of support will he receive from others in the medical team? Will a nurse be willing to care for a patient with a porcine liver? Will the surgeon's formerly loyal colleagues support his or her future career?

As progress is made in medicine, the demands on doctors increase. The transplant surgeon could be begged by a dying patient to transplant an animal organ. The surgeon may have to act immediately and could be rushed into hasty, ill-advised action. Responsibility to the patient has to be weighed against medical feasibility. As scientists, surgeons have to develop new techniques but, if attempting an experiment, they have to inform the patient about all the potential problems, side effects, and danger to life. They have to ask themselves what value the treatment has for each particular patient.

Surgeons have to consider the dignity of their patients. Even when the Ethics Committee has given its approval, the surgeon has to calculate the risk of harming the patient's physical or physiological integrity. Perhaps for most physicians the test of whether their behavior is ethical is whether they can personally justify their actions.

A novel procedure could be in the best interests of a critically ill patient and ethically justified in the eyes of both patient and surgeon, but may be seen by some as amoral. In contrast, an amoral procedure may be applauded in some quarters because it contributes toward knowledge. Widely differing views of the same procedure may be the result of differences in race, religion, or nationality.

There have been examples of doctors (in the field of transplantation and elsewhere) being corrupted by money, by the hope of a better career, by the temptation of power. Those who offend ethical norms and who carelessly misuse the lives of their patients, are amoral [2]. Only those surgical procedures and medical therapies that have treatment and cure as their objective should be acceptable.

Financing Xenografts

Questions may arise over financial aspects of xenotransplantation. For example, might the poor be relegated to receiving animal organs (which may be less expensive, but will probably function for fewer years than allografts), while the rich receive the perfectly matched allograft?

Scientific Ethics

Xenotransplantation should attempt to save lives, but should be realistic, and the benefits should be calculable. However, the scientist has a responsibility to provide new information, not only for today, but also for tomorrow. It would be unethical to avoid this responsibility. The scientist must have the right to investigate, to create new therapies. To do this, he or she must have the freedom to propose and develop ideas.

In Germany, there is an increasing objection to current biological research, particularly with regard to the manipulation of life. This is probably reflected in the dramatic decrease in organ donation. According to public opinion, there is too much technical medicine. Large sections of the population believe that health engineering is bordering on the inhumane [9]. Fear of the abuse of scientific and technical advances in medicine has led to heightened sensitivity. The public is asking: "Are there morals governing science?"

Anxiety, and even resentment, with regard to xenotransplantation can be better understood if we list the techniques that may possibly be involved in the successful transplantation of a widely divergent xenograft: (a) extracorporeal immunoadsorption, (b) complement inhibition with cobra venom factor, (c) the use of organs from genetically engineered animals, (d) heavy immunosuppression, possibly involving total lymphoid irradiation, followed by xenogeneic bone marrow transplantation, (e) chimerism, and (f) transplantation in the fetus to achieve neonatal xenotolerance [7]. Some form of bioethical control is certainly necessary.

In Germany, modern medicine seems to suffer not from a deficiency, but rather from an excess of success and power. Ethics are in danger of being neglected or ignored because of the spectacular discoveries being made by scientists.

National Ethics

As we have learned from the fields of organ donation and organ sharing between nations, some countries will have difficulty in establishing xenotransplantation. The selection of species to supply organs might not only depend on the national income, but also on the feasibility, for climatic or religious reasons, of breeding the appropriate animals.

Presently, no national or international law exists to govern the use of animal organs for xenotransplantation. The Council of Europe, for example, simply states that research on human beings must keep the risk to a minimum. For animals, it declares that when any animal is used or is intended for use in any experimental or other scientific procedure that may cause pain, suffering, distress, or lasting harm, the risk has to be kept to a minimum.

International/Cultural Ethics

In different cultures we find different attitudes towards life, a different respect for death, and a different view of transplantation. Western culture is based on science, and its scientific community will undoubtedly continue its work, constantly looking for favorable cost-benefit ratios or valid alternatives in medicine. Xenotransplantation could be one such alternative to the shortage of human organs.

The future of xenotransplantation is probably not a question of technology, but of motivation and morals. What is moral and ethical for one society and culture may not be so for another. We have to respond as citizens within a pluralistic world, where cultural value systems in developing countries have to be considered. All human beings should have equal rights to live by their own cultural standards [6].

Ethics in medicine is not a recent invention. The need for ethical guidelines exists as soon as a group of people begin living together. The first written record on ethics originates from a Hindu physician in 1500 B.C. The oath of Hippocrates is still largely valid for doctors after almost 3500 years and has spread all around the globe.

The Nuremberg Code (1945), the Universal Bill of Human Rights (1948), and the Declaration of Helsinki (1967) are accepted worldwide and protect the individual as a research subject. Global ethics have to protect the dignity of man, but with the heterogeneity of cultures and the freedom of choice provided by democracy, there is no uniform approach.

Religious Ethics

From the Christian point of view, no fundamental opposition exists to the voluntary donation of an organ. Objections evolve from the possibility of misusing donors or patients.

For the theologist or religious individual who believes in God, however, xenotransplantation might be unacceptable. In the Christian religion, all human beings and their bodies have their dignity. They have to go before God as a God-like person, as they were born – perhaps not with an animal organ.

A halachic view on baboon liver transplantation was published by Rabbi Moshe David Tendler from New York [9]. The Talmud commands that species constancy must be respected and does not allow hybridizing of the species. However, no biblical law takes precedence over the obligation to save a life. This halachic view indicates that animal organs, even of porcine origin, could be transplanted in emergencies to save sick human beings.

The Christian church has not published such a clear ruling. Nor have Moslems reported any statement about the use of animal organs or transplants [11]. Moslem jurists, however, have sanctioned many modern methods of medicine, even blood transfusion, though blood is considered "dirty." Islam believes diseases to be natural phenomena. The Prophet declares that there is a cure for every illness, though we may not know it at the time. He encourages mankind to search for the cure. New treatments should be searched for and, if early attempts prove successful, generally applied.

Comment

The purpose of ethics is to guide us towards behaving in a manner acceptable to the rest of our community. This community includes our patients, our colleagues, the community (nation) in which we live and work, and perhaps religious and international communities. Scientific and medical ethics might allow what some may consider an "amoral" procedure on a fetus or on a chronically ill patient if it is likely to provide new and rich knowledge and might save or improve the quality of life of the patient. The procedure itself must not be harmful or unethical, and the patient must not be misled or given false hope about the outcome.

Ethics would allow us to offend the dignity of man, e.g., by xenotransplantation, because the wish to live is often greater than the desire to retain dignity, yet xenotransplantation should not be used to overcome death if such a treatment is inhumane. Ethics in medicine, including xenotransplantation, must be based above all on the patient's needs, whether the patient is rich or poor.

With regard to xenotransplantation, technically we have already traveled to the ends of the earth, but in terms of the development of our ethics, we are still in the Stone Age [12].

References

1. News. Deutsches Ärzteblatt, 90, 558, 1993
2. A. Gellorn. Medical ethics, so what's the story. In Vitro 13, 588–594, 1977
3. P. Singer. Xenotransplantation and speciesism. Transplant. Proc. 24, 728–732, 1992
4. P. Singer. Practical Ethics. Cambridge University Press, Cambridge, 1979
5. J. Goodall. Ethical concerns in the use of animals as donors. In: Xenograft 25, M. Hardy (ed), Elsevier, New York, p. 335, 1991
6. S. Elias, G.J.Annas. Perspectives on fetal surgery. Am. J. Obstet Gynecol. 145, 807, 1982
7. W. Cartwright. The ethics of xenografting in man. In: Organ Replacement Therapy: Ethics, Justice, Commerce. W. Land, J.B. Dosseter (eds), Springer, Berlin, p. 519, 1991
8. J.S. Najarijan. Overview of in vivo xenotransplantation studies. Prospect for the future. Transplant. Proc. 24, 733–738, 1992
9. D.J. Rothman. Xenograft, the social and ethical dimensions. In: Xenograft 25, M. Hardy (Ed), Elsevier, New York, p. 321, 1991
10. M.D. Tendler. A halachic view on recent baboon liver transplantation. UNOS Update. 8, 31, 1991
11. M.A. Abar. Islamic view an organ transplantation. In: Organ Transplantation, G.M. Abouna, M.A. Kumar, A.G. White (eds), Klüwer, Dordrecht, 1990
12. K.H.Tscheliessnigg. Ethik in der Medizin. Osterr Transplant. 1, 17, 1995

X Clinical Experience

56 Clinical Xenotransplantation – A Brief Review of the World Experience

S. Taniguchi and D.K.C. Cooper

Introduction

The ability to use animal organs, such as from the pig, for the purpose of transplantation in humans would clearly overcome the major shortage of human organs that greatly restricts transplantation programs worldwide. Recent experimental advances have raised the possibility of renewed attempts at organ xenotransplantation in humans within the near future. In this chapter, prior clinical experience, dating back to 1906, is briefly reviewed. Experience with extracorporeal xeno-liver perfusion is reviewed elsewhere in this volume by Abouna (Chap. 57). The limited experience with extracorporeal xeno-kidney perfusion [1–3] will not be discussed, but all of the world's early experience with extracorporeal xeno-organ perfusion has been reviewed by Dubernard et al. [4], who provide an excellent source of reference.

Clinical Concordant Organ Xenotransplantation

Several attempts have been made to provide humans with organs from closely-related species (Tables 1–3). Those that took place during the early part of the century have mostly been reviewed previously [4, 5]. The classical early studies by Reemtsma (Fig. 1) et al. [6], who used chimpanzees as donors of kidneys (Table 1), and of Starzl (Fig. 2) et al. [7], who used baboons as donors, demonstrated that the greater the phylogenetic disparity between donor and recipient, then the more aggressive was the rejection response. Chimpanzee donor kidneys were in general rejected more slowly and by a cellular mechanism, whereas baboon donor kidneys were rejected more aggressively. Reemtsma et al. demonstrated that acute cellular rejection of a chimpanzee kidney could be reversed by a course of increased steroid therapy. Survival of the patients ranged from 11 days to 2 months, with one patient surviving almost 9 months. The majority of deaths were related to rejection or infection. Baboon kidneys, in general, were rejected more aggressively, with patient survival ranging from 19 to 60 days.

The first heart transplant performed in man by Hardy (Fig. 3) et al. in 1964 [8] (Table 2) utilized a chimpanzee as the donor, but the heart proved too small to support the patient's circulation. Further attempts using closely related donor species were made by Marion [9] and Barnard (Fig. 4) et al. [10] without significant success. It should be remembered that these attempts, as well as those of Reemtsma and Starzl, were carried out in the precyclosporine era and therefore

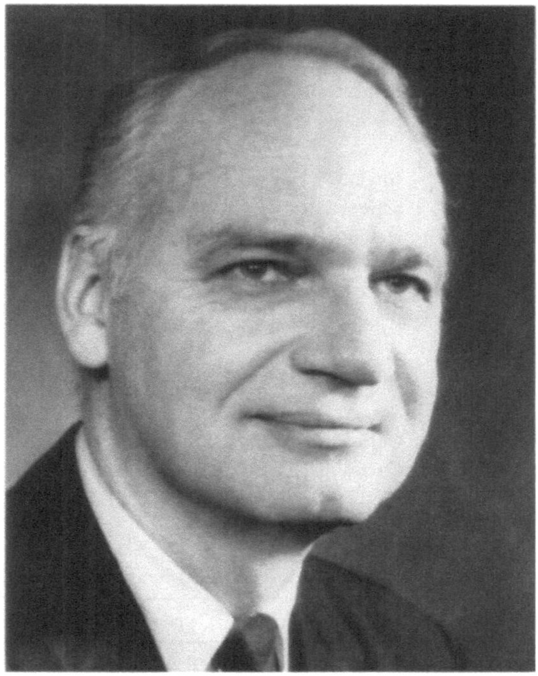

Fig. 1. Keith Reemtsma headed the group at Tulane University in New Orleans, which was the first to explore xenotransplantation in a scientific manner. Their clinical work, carried out between 1963 and 1965, on kidney transplantation using chimpanzees as donors stimulated many other experimental and clinical studies during the subsequent decade

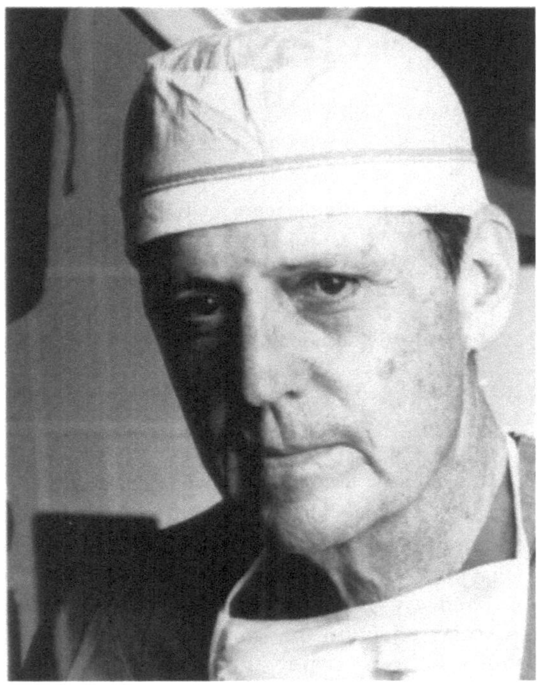

Fig. 2. Thomas Starzl, one of the major surgical pioneers of organ transplantation, led the teams that carried out the first attempts at clinical liver xenografting using chimpanzees as donors

Table 1. World experience in clinical renal xenotransplantation

Year	Surgeon	Donor	*n*	Patient survival	Reference
1905	Princeteau	Rabbit (slices)	1	16 days	[26]
1906	Jaboulay	Pig	1	<3 days	[27]
		Goat	1	<3 days	
1910	Unger	Monkey	1	<2 days	[28]
1913	Schonstadt	Monkey	1	?	[29]
1923	Neuhof	Sheep	1	<9 days	[30]
1964	Reemtsma	Chimpanzee	12	≤9 months	[6]
		Monkey	1	10 days	
1964	Hitchcock	Baboon	1	5 days	[31]
1964	Starzl	Baboon	6	<60 days	[7]
1964	Hume	Chimpanzee	1	1 day	[32]
1964	Traeger	Chimpanzee	3	<49 days	[33]
1965	Goldsmith	Chimpanzee	2	4 months	[34]
1966	Cortesini	Chimpanzee	1	31 days	[35]

Modified from [36].

Table 2. World experience in clinical heart xenotransplantation

Year	Surgeon	Donor	Type	Patient survival	Reference
1964	Hardy	Chimpanzee	OHT	Functioned 2 h (heart too small)	[8]
1968	Cooley	Sheep	OHT	Immediate cessation of function (vascular rejection?)	[37]
1968	Ross	Pig	HHT	Cessation of function within 4 min (vascular rejection?)	[38, 39]
1968	Ross	Pig	Perfused with human blood but not transplanted	Immediate cessation of function (vascular rejection?)	
1969	Marion	Chimpanzee	OHT?	Rapid failure (4 h) (raised pulmonary vascular resistance?)	[9]
1977	Barnard	Baboon	HHT	Functioned 5 h (heart too small)	[10]
1977	Barnard	Chimpanzee	HHT	Functioned 4 days (probable vascular rejection)	[10]
1984	Bailey	Baboon	OHT	Functioned 20 days (vascular rejection)	[11]
1992	Religa	Pig	OHT	Functioned 24 h (cause of failure uncertain)	[20]

Modified from [36].
OHT, orthotopic heart transplantation; HHT, heterotopic heart transplantation.

the immunosuppression utilized was relatively primitive. In 1984, however, Bailey (Fig. 5) et al. [11] performed a baboon heart transplant in a newborn infant and utilized cyclosporine therapy. The heart functioned for 20 days but failed from vascular rejection that may have been related, at least in part, to ABO incompatibility between donor and recipient.

Table 3. World experience in clinical liver xenotransplantation

Year	Surgeon	Donor	Type	Patient survival (days)	Reference
1966	Starzl	Chimpanzee	HLT	<1	[12]
1969	Starzl	Chimpanzee	OLT	9	[13]
		Chimpanzee	OLT	<2	[14]
1969	Bertoye	Baboon	HLT	<1	[40]
1970	Leger	Baboon	HLT	3	[41]
1970	Marion	Baboon	HLT	<1	[9, 42]
1971	Poyet	Baboon	HLT	<1	[43]
1971	Motin	Baboon	HLT	3	[44]
1974	Starzl	Chimpanzee	OLT	14	[15]
1992	Starzl	Baboon	OLT	70	[17–19]
1993	Starzl	Baboon	OLT	26	[18, 19]
1993	Makowka	Pig	HLT	<2	[21, 22]

OLT, orthotopic liver transplantation; HLT, heterotopic (auxiliary) liver transplantation.

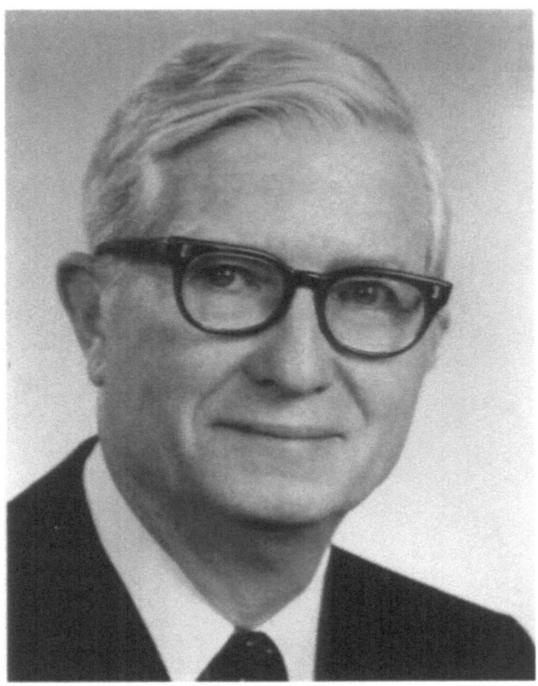

Fig. 3. James Hardy, who, in 1964, led the surgical team that performed the world's first heart transplant, using a chimpanzee as donor. In the previous year, Hardy and his group had carried out the world's first single lung allotransplant

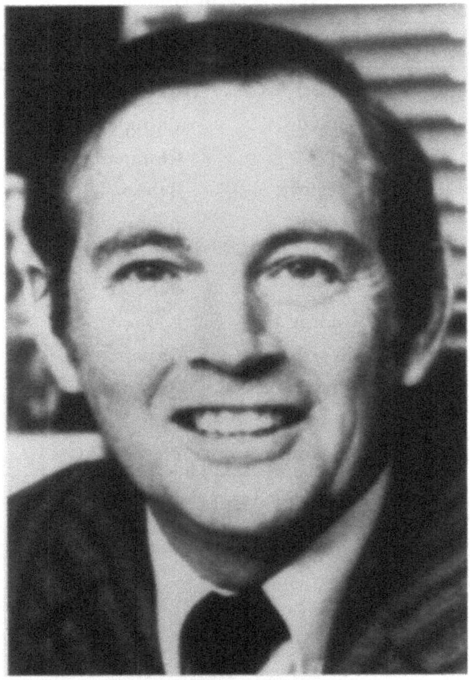

Fig. 4. Christiaan Barnard, who, in 1977, made two attempts to support failing human hearts with primate hearts placed in the heterotopic position

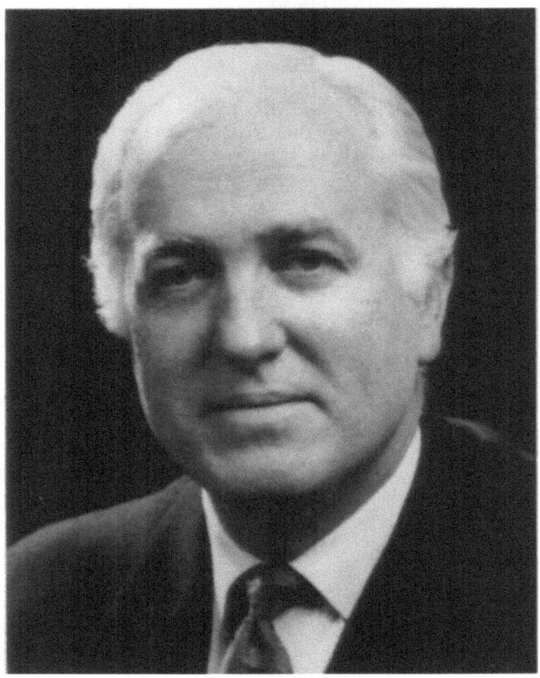

Fig. 5. Leonard Bailey performed heart transplantation using a baboon as donor in Baby Fae in 1984

Starzl and his colleagues [12–16] were again pioneers in the field of clinical orthotopic and heterotopic liver xenotransplantation, performing four chimpanzee liver transplants in humans between 1966 and 1974, with the grafts functioning from 1–14 days (Table 3). In two of these cases, only minimal pathologic lesions were seen in the xenografted liver. Other early attempts involved heterotopic placement of baboon livers (Table 3) and have been reviewed briefly by Dubernard et al. [4].

In 1992 and 1993, Starzl's group utilized the baboon as donor in two orthotopic liver transplants with patient survival for 70 days and 26 days, respectively [17–19] (Chap. 58). The first of these two cases can be considered a relative success in that there was little pathologic evidence of rejection in the liver at any stage, but this was achieved probably at the expense of overimmunosuppression, the patient dying of overwhelming sepsis. The second case was less successful as the patient did not regain consciousness or renal function during the postoperative period, but again there was little histopathologic evidence of rejection in the transplanted liver.

Clinical Discordant Organ Xenotransplantation

The early attempts at clinical xenotransplantation using a widely-disparate animal species as a donor for humans were all doomed to early failure [4] (Tables 1–3).

The most recent attempt at clinical cardiac xenotransplantation (Table 2) was reported in 1992 by a Polish group and involved the transplantation of a pig heart [20]. The patient suffered from Marfan's syndrome and severe aortic valve insufficiency. His condition was exceedingly poor, and it was decided to proceed with xenografting as no allograft was available. Prior to the transplant he received an experimental regimen of homogenized embryonal fetal calf thymus therapy in addition to cyclosporine and azathioprine. Initially, extracorporeal immunoadsorption was carried out by perfusing the patient's blood through a pig heart to eliminate antibodies against donor-species' antigens. The heart from a second pig, that had also been treated with fetal calf thymus, was then orthotopically transplanted into the patient. He died from a low cardiac output syndrome just under 24 h after transplantation. Histopathologic examination was reported not to show any features of rejection of the transplanted heart.

Fulminant hepatic failure is considered to be a condition in which xenotransplantation may play a bridging role. A suitable hepatic allograft may not become available during the short period of time in which the patient rapidly deteriorates and dies. Under such conditions, Makowka and his colleagues [21, 22] (Table 3) inserted an auxiliary pig liver to support a patient with fulminant hepatic failure until an allograft became available, at which time it was planned to perform orthotopic transplantation and remove the auxiliary pig liver. Following ex vivo perfusion of pig organs with the patient's blood to eliminate anti-pig antibodies, a pig liver was heterotopically transplanted. The liver was hyperacutely rejected within 30 h and the patient died before an allograft became available.

There have been no recent attempts at discordant kidney xenotransplantation.

Comment

There would appear to be a growing acceptance of xenotransplantation amongst the public. A "Partnership for Organ Donation Survey" in the United States in 1993 confirmed that, whereas 79 % of those questioned said they would accept an organ allograft, 51 % said they would accept an organ transplant from an animal if a suitable human organ was not available [23].

Clearly, attempts at xenotransplantation can best be justified if (a) the patient will die rapidly without organ transplantation or (b) failure of the xenografted organ will not result in death of the patient. In cases of rapidly increasing cardiac failure or fulminant hepatic failure, xenotransplantation could therefore be considered, particularly as a bridge to allotransplantation. In patients with diabetes mellitus or chronic renal failure in whom allotransplantation is precluded, perhaps by a high degree of allosensitization, then once again xenografting may be justified as failure of the graft will not necessarily lead to death of the patient.

This latter approach has been pursued by the Stockholm group who have performed pig islet cell transplants in patients with diabetes mellitus [24, 25] (Chap. 59). As the pig is a source of insulin that successfully controls hyperglycemia in human subjects, this is a logical step forward. This clinical trial, however, has to date not been successful in providing long-term insulin production by pig islet cells, but is a sensible approach for future clinical studies.

The problems inherent in clinical xenotransplantation remain considerable but, if they can be overcome, the rewards will be enormous.

References

1. LAVENDER, A.R., FORLAND, M., RAMS, J.J., et al. Laboratory and clinical studies in perfusion of the isolated kidney. In: Organ Perfusion and Preservation J.C. Norman (ed), Appleton Cnetury Crofts, New York, 1968, p. 330
2. PICHLMAIER, R. Sources de rein. Ass. Franc. Urol. Masson Ed, Paris, 1969, p. 167
3. MONAKHENKO, F.P. Symposium on extracorporeal organs. Leningrad. 1970. (Quoted by Dubernard et al. [4])
4. DUBERNARD, J.M., BONNEAU, M., LATOUR, M. Heterografts in primates. Villeurbanne, Fondation Merieux, 1974, p. 43
5. REEMTSMA, K. Xenotransplantation – a brief history of clinical experiences: 1900–1965. In: Xenotransplantation, 1st edn. Cooper, D.K.C. et al (eds), Springer, Heidelberg, 1991, p. 9
6. REEMTSMA, K., McCRACKEN, B.H., SCHLEGEL, J.U., et al. Renal heterotransplantation in man. Ann. Surg. 160, 384, 1964
7. STARZL, T.E., MARCHIORO, T.L., PETERS, G.N., et al. Renal heterotransplantation from baboon to man: experience with 6 cases. Transplantation. 2, 752, 1964
8. HARDY, J.D., KURRUS, F.E., CHAVEZ, C.M., et al. Heart transplantation in man: developmental studies and report of a case. J. Am. Med. Ass. 188, 1132, 1964
9. MARION, P. In: Les transplantations cardiaques et les transplantations hepatiques. Lyon Med. 222, 585, 1969

10. BARNARD, C.N., WOLPOWITZ, A., LOSMAN, J.G. Heterotopic cardiac transplantation with a xenograft for assistance of the left heart in cardiogenic shock after cardiopulmonary bypass. S. Afr. Med. J. 52, 1035, 1977
11. BAILEY, L.L., NEHLSEN-CANNARELLA, S.L., CONCEPCION, W., JOLLEY, W.B. Baboon-to-human cardiac xenotransplantation in a neonate. J. Amer. Med. Assoc. 254, 3321, 1985
12. STARZL, T.E., MARCHIORO, T.L., FARTS, T.D., McCARDLE, M.J., IWASAKI, Y. Avenues of future research in homotransplantation of the liver. Amer. J. Surg. 112, 391, 1966
13. STARZL, T.E. Orthotopic heterotransplantation. In Experience in Hepatic Transplantation. Saunders, Philadelphia, 1969, p. 408
14. GILES, G.R., BOEHMIG, H.J., AMEMIYA, H., et al. Clinical heterotransplantation of the liver. Transplant. Proc. 2, 506, 1970
15. STARZL, T.E., ISHIKAWA, M., PUTNAM, C.W., et al. Progress in and deterents to orthotopic liver transplantation, with special reference to survival, resistance to hyperacute rejection, and biliary duct reconstruction. Transplant. Proc. 6, 129, 1974
16. CRAMER, D.V., SHER, L., MAKOWKA, L. Liver xenotransplantation: clinical experience and future considerations. In (Cooper, D.K.C, et al. eds.) Xenotransplantation. Springer, Heidelberg, 1991, p. 559
17. STARZL, T.E., FUNG, J.J., TZAKIS, A., et al. Baboon-to-human liver transplantation. Lancet. 341, 65, 1993
18. STARZL, T.E., TZAKIS, A., FUNG, J.J., et al. Human liver transplantation. Xeno. 1, 4, 1993
19. STARZL, T.E., TZAKIS, A., FUNG, J.J., et al. Prospects of clinical xenotransplantation. Transplant. Proc. 26, 1082, 1994
20. CZAPLICKI, J., BLONSKA, B., RELIGA, Z. The lack of hyperacute xenogeneic heart transplant rejection in a human. J. Heart Lung Transplant. 11, 393, 1992
21. MAKOWKA, L., WU, G.D., HOFFMAN, A., et al. Immunohistopathologic lesions associated with the rejection of a pig-to-human liver xenograft. Transplant. Proc. 26, 1074, 1994
22. MAKOWKA, L., CRAMER, D.V., HOFFMAN, A., et al. The use of a pig liver xenograft for temporary support of a patient with fulminant hepatic failure. Transplantation. 59, 1654, 1995
23. THE GALLUP ORGANIZATION, INC., The American public's attitudes toward organ donation and transplantation. Conducted for the Partnership for Organ Donation, Boston, MA, 1993
24. GROTH, C.G., ANDERSSON, A., KORSGREN, O., et al. Transplantation of porcine fetal islet-like cell clusters into eight diabetic patients. Transplant. Proc. 25, 970, 1993
25. SATAKE, M., KAWAGISHI, N., RYDBERG, L, et al. Limited specificity of xenoantibodies in diabetic patients transplanted with fetal porcine islet cell clusters. Main antibody reactivity against α-linked galactose-containing epitopes. Xenotransplantation. 1, 89, 1994
26. PRINCETEAU, M. Greffe renale. J. Med. Bordeaux. 26, 549, 1905
27. JABOULAY, M. Greffe de rein au pli du coude par suture de l'artere et de la veine. Lyon Med. 39, 575, 1906
28. UNGER, I. Transplantation des vaisseaux et des organes. B. Fur. Chir. 46, 1367, 1908
29. MOREL, L., PAPIN, E. Les applications physiologiques et chirurgicales des transplantations renales. Biol. Med. 10, 397, 1913. (Quoted by Dubernard et al. (4))

30. NEUHOF, H. The transplantation of tissues. Appleton, New York, 1923
31. HITCHCOCK, C.R., KISER, J.C., TELANDER, R.L., et al. Baboon renal grafts. JAMA. 189, 934, 1964
32. HUME, D.M. Discussion of Reemtsma paper. Ann. Surg. 160, 384, 1964
33. TRAEGER, J., FRIES, D., PERRIN, J. Heterotransplantation chex l'homme. Premiers resultats. Proc. Eur. Dial. Transplant. Assoc. 2, 214, 1965
34. MILLARD, C., SHUMWAY, N.E., STARZL, T.E., et al. Xenografts: review of the literature and current status. JAMA. 254, 3353, 1985
35. CORTESINI, R., CASCIANI, C., CUCCHIARA, G. Heterotransplantation in primates: current state of affairs. In (Balner, H. ed.) Infection and Immunosuppression in Subhuman Primates. Murksgaard, Copenhagen, pp. 239, 1969
36. COOPER, D.K.C., YE, Y. Experience with clinical heart xenotransplantation: In (Cooper, D.K.C., et al. eds) Xenotransplantation. Springer, Heidelberg, 1991, p. 541
37. COOLEY, D.A., HALLMAN, G.L., BLOODWELL, R.D., et al. Human heart transplantation: experience with 12 cases. Am. J. Cardiol. 22, 804, 1968
38. ROSS, D.N. In: (Shapiro, H., ed), Experience With Human Heart Transplantation. Butterworths, Durban, 1969, p. 227
39. COOPER, D.K.C. The first heart transplants in the United Kingdom, 1968–1980 – the role of Guy's graduate's. Part 2. Guy's Hospital Gazette. 109, 114, 1995
40. BERTOYE, A. Essais de traitement de certaines insuffisances hepatiques graves par greffe hepatique heterologue. Lyon. Med. 222, 345, 1969
41. LEGER, L., CHAPUIS, J.P., LENRIOT, J.P. Greffe heterotopique d'un foie de babouin sur une malade atteinte d'hepatite fulminante. Chirurgie. 96, 249, 1970
42. MARION, P., BERTOYE, A., MIKAELOFF, Ph., et al. Traitement du coma hepatique par transplantation auxiliaire heterologue du foie. Chirurgie. 96, 152, 1970
43. POUYET, M., BERARD, Ph. Deux cas de transplantation heterologues du foie de babouin au cours d'hepatites aigues malignes. Lyon. Chir. 67, 287, 1971
44. MOTIN, J. (Quoted by Dubernard et al. [4])

57 Extracorporeal Xenogeneic Liver Perfusion for the Treatment of Hepatic Failure

G.M. Abouna

Introduction

It is estimated that in the United States some 27 000 patients die annually from liver disease, many as a result of chronic hepatic failure while others as a consequence of acute fulminant hepatic failure (FHF). Of the latter, some 2000 patients die from acute viral hepatitis, which is potentially reversible. In addition, some 20 % of patients who are on the liver transplant waiting list die every year from complications of liver failure while awaiting a suitable hepatic allograft [1–4].

FHF is usually a terminal event of severe liver dysfunction with resultant encephalopathy, accumulation of toxic metabolites, failure of synthesis of vital substances (including essential amino acids and clotting factors), failure in neurotransmission, renal failure, increased intracranial pressure, cerebral edema and death [5–7].

In the early 1960s and 1970s, several extracorporeal techniques were tried for the treatment of patients with FHF, including hemodialysis, exchange transfusion, cross-circulation with a human or primate partner, hemofiltration through charcoal or resin columns, and extracorporeal xenogeneic liver perfusion [8–21]. It soon became clear that, of all these techniques, extracorporeal xenogeneic liver perfusion was the most effective in reversing deep hepatic encephalopathy. The extracorporeal liver performed all of the functions of a normal liver, thus giving the patient's failing liver sufficient time to regenerate and resume normal function. Unfortunately, with the subsequent rapid development and improved success of liver transplantation in the 1980s, many patients with FHF were treated by emergency hepatic transplantation, and the procedure of extracorporeal liver perfusion was abandoned [22–25]. While this did improve the survival rate of patients with FHF, treatment by liver transplantation is clearly complicated, expensive, and deprives other, possibly more suitable, patients from receiving a liver graft. Also, liver transplantation may not always be indicated since some patients with FHF might recover spontaneously if they could be supported for a short time by an extracorporeal hepatic "device" until their own liver regenerated (thus avoiding the need for hepatectomy, liver transplantation, and life-long immunosuppression). Today a realization has once again emerged of resuming extracorporeal hepatic support procedures as the most logical and cost-effective method of supporting the ever-increasing number of patients with FHF and those awaiting liver transplantation [26–28].

Three techniques of liver support are now being evaluated:

1. The revival of extracorporeal xenogeneic and allogeneic hepatic perfusion techniques [29–31].
2. Bioartificial liver devices in which xenogeneic hepatocytes (obtained by digestion of a whole liver followed by culture, storage, and preparation) are either entrapped within gel capsules or are suspended on a microcarrier matrix and then placed in a cartridge around hollow fiber tubes which are perfused with the patient's plasma (after its separation by plasmapheresis) [32–37]. These devices, which contain some 50–150 g liver tissue, have been used as a bridge to liver transplantation, but complete recovery from grade IV hepatic coma has not been clearly demonstrated [38–40]. From our own experience and the observations of other investigators, we believe it is unlikely that the bioartificial liver device (which contains less than 10 % of normal liver tissue and which is prepared in a complicated process of liver digestion, preservation, culture, and encapsulation) can replace or substitute for the patient's own diseased liver (as is possible with a fresh whole extracorporeal xenogeneic liver when used in a well-designed liver perfusion circuit) in the patient with FHF [27–31, 42, 43].
3. Hepatocyte transplantation using encapsulated xenogeneic or allogeneic hepatocytes [41]. This may prove useful for patients with early liver failure from congenital and hereditary liver disease, but is unlikely to benefit patients with FHF.

Technique of Clinical Extracorporeal Xenogeneic Liver Support for Fulminant Hepatic Failure

As a result of several years of experimental studies in the late 1960s [10–12], and following clinical applications in the early 1970s [13–21], we were able to define the conditions necessary for optimum function of an isolated perfused xenogeneic liver. Such a liver can carry out most of the major detoxifying and synthetic functions of a normal liver for many hours without any deleterious effect on the patient providing that certain important conditions prevail. These include: (a) gentle donor hepatectomy, (b) well-preserved xenogeneic graft, using cold oxygenated electrolyte solution containing high potassium, low sodium, and added Dextran and insulin as the perfusate, (c) the perfusion circuit must contain inflow and outflow pumps and heat exchanger, (d) the liver is perfused with the patient's whole blood at 38 °C, with regional heparinization through both hepatic artery and portal vein, maintaining physiologic inflow pressures and outflow hepatic venous pressure at a flow rate of 0.6–1 ml per min. In these studies, it was documented that hepatic artery perfusion is essential for good hepatocyte function (Fig. 1).

Using the above guidelines, 33 clinical xenogeneic and allogeneic liver perfusions were carried out for treatment of 21 episodes of grade IV hepatic coma in ten patients with FHF (from acute viral and toxic hepatitis), as a bridge to liver transplantation in patients with decompensated chronic active hepatitis, and for patient support following ischemic necrosis after a failed liver transplant. During

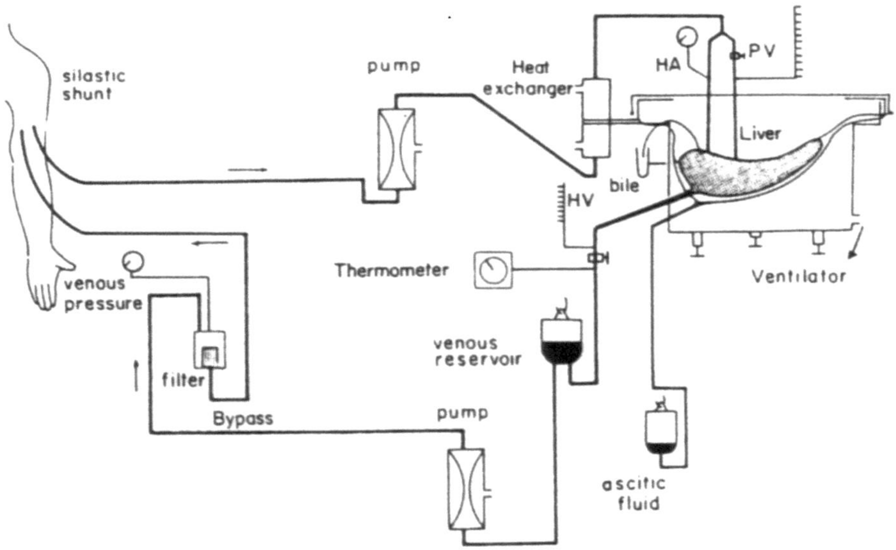

Fig. 1. Optimum circuitry for clinical xenogeneic liver perfusion. Note perfusion through hepatic artery and vein, and inflow and outflow pneumatic pumps, which maintain physiologic pressures in the hepatic artery (*HA*) and in the portal (*PV*) and hepatic veins (*HV*)

this experience, several important parameters were analyzed, including the rate of clinical recovery in relation to the length of perfusion, the type of donor animal species used, the number of perfusions required for each episode of coma, the incidence and type of xenograft rejection, the immunologic changes in the recipients, and possible methods of removing xenogeneic pre-formed antibodies prior to perfusion.

Extracorporeal xenogeneic liver perfusion (using livers from different species including pig, calf, baboon, and human) consistently and repeatedly reversed deep encephalopathy when all other measures had failed [16–18]. One patient was brought out of grade IV coma on seven separate occasions over a period of 11 weeks while awaiting a liver transplant [13]. Of the 21 episodes of coma treated by these techniques, complete recovery of consciousness was seen in 13 (62%), and improvement in the level of consciousness in another four (19%) (Table 1).

When the results were analysed with regard to the liver species used, it was found that with a porcine liver successful perfusion could be maintained for 5–12 h with full recovery in three of ten episodes of coma (30%), and improvement in consciousness in another four (40%). Using baboon livers, successful perfusion could be maintained for up to 24 h, with full recovery of consciousness in every patient. With human livers, successful perfusion could be continued for up to 51 h, with full recovery of consciousness after each single perfusion. Following pig liver perfusions, recovery of consciousness could be maintained for 1–2 weeks before the patient relapsed into coma, while in the four patients who were treated with baboon perfusions all recovered full consciousness, survived

Table 1. Results of extracorporeal xenogeneic and allogeneic hepatic perfusion used in 21 episodes of grade IV hepatic coma in ten patients

Liver donor species	Episodes of coma treated	Duration of perfusion (h)	Episodes of coma completely reversed		Episodes of coma improved	
			(*n*)	(%)	(*n*)	(%)
Pig	10	5–12	3	30	4	40
Baboon	7	13–24	7	100[a]	–	–
Human	2	35–51	2	100	–	–
Calf	1	6	1	100	–	–
Monkey	1	3	0	0	0	0
Total	21	3–51	13	62	4	19

[a] Baboon liver perfusion was 100 % successful in a total of four patients, two of whom were long-term survivors.

for at least one month, and two left the hospital with normal liver function and are long-term survivors [14, 18, 19]. While recovery of consciousness required the use of one to four consecutive porcine liver perfusions, only one baboon liver perfusion was sufficient to bring the patient out of deep hepatic coma, remain awake, and talk and take oral fluids while still on the baboon liver circuit.

Immunological studies showed that, in the case of porcine xenogeneic liver perfusion, preformed xenoantibody in the patients was quickly adsorbed by the liver, with a secondary rise after repeated perfusions. However, no lymphocytotoxic antibody to human lymphocytes was detected after several porcine and baboon perfusions, indicating that cross-sensitization to human alloantibody does not occur and thus subsequent liver allotransplantation could be carried out safely. Pathological studies of these livers showed that many porcine livers maintained normal histology for up to 9 h of perfusion. However, immunofluorescence studies did show deposition of IgG and complement. In the case of baboon livers, even after 24 h of perfusion there was no hepatic cell damage, but some lymphocyte infiltration developed around the portal tracts, indicating mild cellular rejection. Xenogeneic liver perfusions were more successful when the patient was pretreated with an exchange transfusion, which most probably reduced the titer of preformed xenogeneic antibody in the recipient.

Current Status of Liver Perfusion for Treatment of Fulminant Hepatic Failure

The advent of successful liver transplantation resulted in a temporary cessation of extracorporeal liver perfusion therapy. However, the high incidence of death from liver failure in patients awaiting orthotopic hepatic allotransplantation has stimulated several centers to revive the technique of ex vivo hepatic perfusion as a bridge to liver transplantation, using the pig liver or an ABO-incompatible human liver, with some success [29–31]. Those centers using the perfusion criteria which we developed in the early 1970s have achieved the greatest success, whereas those that have taken "short-cuts", such as using portal perfusion only and inadequate maintenance of physiologic inflow and outflow pressures, have had much less success [31].

Future of Extracorporeal Xenogeneic Liver Perfusion

From our own experience, and that of several other investigators who have since used the technique, there is no doubt that extracorporeal perfusion through a whole normal xenogeneic liver is the preferred therapy for the support of patients with FHF (with the potential for spontaneous recovery of their own liver) or who develop acute-on-chronic liver decompensation while on a liver transplant waiting list. We believe that the use of extracorporeal xenogeneic liver perfusion in patients with FHF, besides being simpler and more cost-effective than liver transplantation, will help identify those patients who may have permanent cortical brain damage and are thus not suitable for transplantation. Our observations also indicate that extracorporeal baboon liver perfusion is always successful in reversing coma, and is thus the ideal therapy for patients with FHF or as a bridge to liver transplantation. Unfortunately the use of the baboon will most likely face strong disapproval from members of the public, thus making the pig or the calf the only sources of "extracorporeal" livers.

The porcine liver has definite limitations due to the presence of heterologous preformed xenoantibodies in the recipient which, together with complement, may cause accelerated xenograft rejection. It is possible, however, that the effect of these preformed antibodies can be greatly diminished by several methods which are now under investigation:

1. Performing an exchange blood transfusion using homologous blood with a low anti-porcine antibody titer
2. Adsorption of the preformed antibody by first perfusing the kidneys of the pig with the patient's blood until they are rejected, and then connecting the patient to the extracorporeal pig liver
3. Inactivating the naturally occurring antibody using synthetic sugars to block the α-galactose, the target epitope for the antibody/antigen reaction [44, 45)
4. Depletion of both complement and xenoantibody, as described by Bach [46]
5. Pretreatment of the liver graft with the Fab_2 fragment of the naturally occurring porcine antibody in order to mask the porcine xenoantigens [47]
6. Using transgenic pigs with a human DNA construct [42, 48]

It is, of course, very important that the donor animals used for extracorporeal perfusion are bred in special farms and are tested for the presence of infectious organisms [49].

Comment

Extracorporeal xenogeneic whole liver perfusion is the most physiologic (and thus most likely to be successful) treatment of FHF, and should be more widely used in the future, especially when methods of preformed antibody depletion become available. The need for revitalising the technique of extracorporeal xenogeneic perfusion is particularly important at the present time, not only because of the large number of young patients who die every year from potentially reversible acute viral and toxic hepatitis, but also because of the large number of potential liver transplant recipients who die from liver failure while on the waiting list (due to the ever-widening gap between organ demand and organ supply). For these reasons and for the fact that, once the extracorporeal liver perfusion circuitry is constructed, the actual procedure is simple and relatively inexpensive, we strongly believe that the time has come for this form of liver support technology to be reintroduced and used widely in institutions with an interest in the treatment of hepatic failure and hepatic transplantation.

It is very unlikely that the currently available bioartificial liver containing isolated xenogeneic hepatocytes will be able to provide the necessary complete hepatic support that is required and which can be obtained by xenogeneic whole liver perfusion. We are in full agreement with the many investigators who believe that the bioartificial liver devices containing 50–150 g semiviable encapsulated porcine hepatocytes (instead of 1500 g normal adult liver) can never substitute for the myriad of complicated and essential functions of a normal liver, particularly when these artificial devices are devoid of important accessory cells, such as bile ducts, Kupffer cells, and endothelial cells, which are known to contribute to the overall function of a normal liver [27, 29, 36, 42]. Clearly, a final and definitive conclusion to this matter should be possible through a well-designed and controlled trial comparing the bioartificial liver cartridge with whole liver perfusion, and involving either an experimental animal model of acute, but potentially reversible, liver failure (as described previously [20]) or actual patients with FHF in a multicenter project.

Finally, as the great liver physiologist Claude Bernard (1813–1878) rightly said: "When the human liver fails, only another normal liver can take its place." And as my former associate, Giovanni Costa, more recently put it: "The good Lord gave man 1500 g of hepatocytes. It is very unlikely that man will do as well with only 50 g. We also must remember that while a bridge to liver transplantation is good, a bridge to a regenerating liver is much better" [43].

References

1. National Center for Health Statistics. Monthly Vital Stat. Report. 1991; 39:1
2. Lee W M. Acute liver failure. N. Engl. J. Med. 1993; 329:1862
3. Hoofnagle JH, Carithers RL, Shapiro C, Asher N. Fulminant hepatic failure: summary of a Workshop. Hepatology. 1995; 21:240
4. Sherlock S. Fulminant hepatic failure. Adv. Int. Med. 1993; 38:245
5. Aggarwal S, Kremer D, Yonas H, et al. Cerebral hemodynamic and metabolic changes in fulminant hepatic failure: a retrospective study. Hepatology. 1994; 19:80
6. O'Grady J G, Schalm S, Williams R. Acute liver failure: redefining the syndromes. Lanet. 1993; 342:273
7. Mousseau D D, Buttworth R F. Current theories on the pathogenecis of hepatic encephalopathy. Proc. Soc. Exp. Biol. Med. 1994; 206:329

8. Marks M I, Mauer S M, Goldman H. Exchange transfusion in the treatment of hepatic coma. J. Pediatr. 1969; 75:418
9. Eiseman B, Liem D S, Ruffucci F. Heterologous liver perfusion in treatment of hepatic failure. Ann. Surg. 1965; 162:329
10. Abouna G M. Extracorporeal liver perfusion using a new perfusion chamber. preliminary communication. Lancet. 1968; 2:1211
11. Abouna G M. Pig liver perfusion with human blood. Brit. J. Surg. 1968; 55:761
12. Abouna G M. Improved techniques of exchange transfusion for hepatic coma. Surg. Gynecol. Obstet. 1972; 134:658
13. Abouna G M, Ashcroft T, Hull C, et al. The assessment of function of the isolated perfused porcine liver. Brit. J. Surg. 1969; 56:289
14. Abouna G M, Serrou B, Boehmig H G, et al. Long-term hepatic support by intermittent multi-species liver perfusions. Lancet. 1970; 2:391
15. Abouna G M, Fisher L McA, Still W J, Hume D M. Acute hepatic coma successfully treated by extracorporeal baboon liver perfusions. Brit. Med. J. 1972; 1:23
16. Hume D M, Mendez G, Gayle W E, et al. Current methods for support of patients in hepatic failure. Transplant. Proc. 1971; 111:1525
17. Abouna G M, Amemiya H, Andres G, et al. Immunological studies in patients receiving repeated allogenic and xenogenic liver hemoperfusions. Transplantation. 1974; 185:395
18. Abouna G M, Fisher L McA, Porter K A, Andres G. Experience in the treatment of hepatic failure by intermittent liver hemoperfusions. Surg. Gynecol. Obstet. 1973; 137:741
19. Abouna G M, Cook J S, Fisher L M A, et al. Treatment of acute hepatic coma by ex-vivo baboon and human liver perfusions. Surgery. 1972; 71:537
20. Abouna G M, Barabas A Z, Alexander F, et al. Animal models of hepatic failure for evaluation of artificial liver support techniques. In: Artificial Organs Kenedi, RH, et al. (eds), Macmillan, UK, 1977, p. 351
21. Abouna G M, Barabas A Z, Boyd N, et al. Resin and charcoal haemoperfusion in the treatment of hepatic coma. In: Artificial Organs. Kenedi, RH, et al. (eds), Macmillan, UK, 1977, p. 363
22. Castells A, Salmeron J M, Navasa M, et al. Liver transplantation in acute liver failure: analysis of applicability. Gastroenterology. 1993; 105:532
23. Detre K, Belle S, Beringer K, Daily O P. Liver transplantation for fulminant hepatic failure in the United States: October 1987 through December 1991. Clin. Transplantation. 1994; 8:274
24. Williams R, Wendon J. Indications for orthotopic liver transplantation in fulminant liver failure. Hepatology. 1994; Suppl 58:108
25. Pauwels A, Mostefa-Kara N, Florent C, Levy V G. Emergency liver transplantation for acute liver failure: evaluation of London and Clichy criteria. Hepatology. 1993; 17:124
26. Pappas S C. Fulminant hepatic failure and the need for artificial liver support. Mayo Clinic Proc. 1988; 63:613
27. Cattral M S, Levy G A. Artificial liver support – pipe dream or reality? N. Engl. J. Med. 1994; 331:268
28. Davies E, Hodgson H J F. Artificial livers – what's keeping them? Gut. 1995; 36:168
29. Burdick J F, Fair T H. Xenoperfusion, the pig as a bridge. Xeno. 1994; 2:3

30. Fox I J, Langnas A N, Ozaki C F, et al. Successful application of extracorporeal liver perfusion for the treatment of fulminant hepatic failure: a technology whose time has come. Am. J. Gastroenterol. 1993; 88:1876
31. Chari R S, Collins B H, Magee J C, et al. Brief report: treatment of hepatic failure with ex vivo pig liver perfusion followed by liver transplantation. N. Engl. J. Med. 1994; 331:234
32. Arnaout W S, Moscioni A D, Barbour R L, Demetriou A A, Development of bioartificial liver: bilirubin conjugation in Gunn rats. J. Surg. Res. 1990; 48:379
33. Chang T M S. Hybrid artificial cells: microencapsulation of living cells. ASAIO J. 1992; 38:128
34. Matthew H W T, Basu S, Peterson W D, Salley S O, Klein M D. Performance of plasma-perfused, microencapsulated hepatocytes: prospects for extracorporeal liver support. J. Paed. Surg. 1993; 28:1423
35. Rozga J, Holzman M D, Ro M-S, et al. Development of a hybrid bioartificial liver. Ann. Surg. 1993; 217:502
36. Tompkins R G, Yarmush M L. Prospects for an artificial liver. Transplant. Rev. 1993; 7:191
37. Rozga J, Williams F, Ro M-S, et al. Development of a bioartificial liver: properties and function of a hollow-fiber module inoculated with liver cells. Hepatology. 1993; 17:258
38. Neuzil D F, Rozga J, Moscioni A D, et al. Use of a novel bioartificial liver in a patient with acute liver insufficiency. Surgery. 1993; 113:340
39. Rozga J, Podesta L, Lepage E, et al. A bioartificial liver to treat severe acute liver failure. Ann. Surg. 1994; 219:538
40. Nyberg S L, Peshwa M V, Payne W D, Hu W-S, Cerra F B. Evolution of the bioartificial liver: the need for randomized clinical trials. Am. J. Surg. 1993; 166:512
41. Mito M, Kusano M, Sawa M. Hepatocyte transplantation for hepatic failure, Transplant. Rev. 1993; 7:35
42. White D J G. Xenografting – present and future. Xeno. 1994; 2:1
43. Costa G (Modena, Italy) 1996 – Personal communication
44. Cooper D K C, Good A H, Koren E, et al. Identification of α-galactosyl and other carbohydrate epitopes that are bound by human anti pig antibody. Transpl. Immunol. 1993; 1:198
45. Cooper D K C. Depletion of natural antibody in non-human primates – a step towards successful discordant xenotransplantation in humans. Clin. Transplantation. 1992; 6:178
46. Hancock W W, Bach F. The immunobiology of discordant xenograft rejection. Xeno. 1994; 2:68
47. Faustman D, Coe C. Prevention of xenograft rejection by masking donor antigen HLA class 1 using Fab2. Science. 1991; 252:1700
48. Fodor W L, Squinto SP. Engineering of transgenic pigs for xenogeneic organ transplantation. Xeno. 1995; 3:23
49. Smith D M. Endogenous retroviruses in xenografts. N. Engl. J. Med. 1993; 328:142

58 Baboon Liver Xenotransplantation in Humans: Clinical Experience and Principles Learned

I.R. Marino, H.R. Doyle, B. Nour, and T.E. Starzl

Introduction

The significant advances achieved in the field of liver transplantation have led to an increased demand for organs, and created a wide gap between organ availability and supply [1, 2]. As of 3 January 1996, there were 44 025 patients on the United Network for Organ Sharing (UNOS) waiting list (the agency that coordinates organ allocation in the United States), up from 13 115 on 31 December 1987, an increase of 335%. Of these, 5715 awaited liver transplantation, up from 449 in 1987 (12-fold increase). The supply of organ donors, on the other hand, underwent a marginal increase between 1988 and 1990 (from 4085 to 4514), and has remained relatively stable (4531 in 1991, 4521 in 1992, 4849 in 1993, and 4891 in 1994) thereafter. A wider availability of organs for transplantation would allow an expansion [3, 4] rather than a contraction of the indications for transplantation, and at the same time a relaxation of the patient selection criteria [5–7]. All these facts clearly justify the renewed interest in xenotransplantation observed in the last decade [8, 9].

The first three attempts at whole organ xenotransplantation were made in France and Germany between January and April 1906, using a pig, a goat, and a macaque as kidney donors [10, 11]. None of these kidneys functioned because of almost immediate vascular thrombosis, and the human recipients died in less than 3 days. In a further attempt in 1923 by Neuhof [12], a lamb was used as a kidney donor, and the patient died 9 days later. On 16 February 1963, Hitchcock transplanted the kidney of a baboon into a 65-year-old woman. The organ functioned for 4 days before its artery clotted [13]. A few months later, on 8 October 1963, Reemtsma of Tulane University used a rhesus monkey as kidney donor for a human recipient, who survived 12 days. Reemtsma tried again with a series of six consecutive chimpanzee kidney grafts [14], one of which functioned for 270 days.

In December 1963 and January 1964, six patients received baboon kidneys at the University of Colorado in Denver [15]. Each of these kidneys functioned immediately and sustained a dialysis-free life for 10–60 days. The patients were treated with high doses of azathioprine and prednisone; four of them died of sepsis, while rejection was mainly responsible for the other two deaths. However, the pathology of the rejection was not qualitatively different from that observed in allografts [16].

In fact, although the pathology of the rejection process was not well understood during the early era of xenotransplantation, the descriptions of the rejected xenografted kidneys, from both baboons and chimpanzees, are consistent with the pathophysiology of xenograft rejection as we describe it today. Lymphocytotoxic antibodies as a cause for antibody-mediated rejection of allografts were actually not recognized until 1965 [17]. In the Denver baboon-to-human kidney xenotransplant series mentioned above, heterospecific antibodies could be detected bound to the kidney xenografts [15, 16]. Summarizing that experience, Dr. Kendrick Porter concluded:

> In the resulting [heterograft] rejection process, cellular infiltration and peritubular capillary destruction are prominent early pathologic features, but by nine days the vasculonecrotic element is marked. There is circumstantial evidence to suggest that, whereas the peritubular capillary damage is mediated by cell-bound antibody, the fibrinoid necrotic vascular lesions are caused by circulating antibody.

Porter also noted that the rejected xenografts showed variability in the histology, from total infarction, cellular infiltrates, interstitial edema and tubular necrosis, to only intimal hypertrophy. The antibody component of rejection has been the central issue of xenotransplantation since that time.

A pig kidney and a pig heart, transplanted in the 1960s by Kuss [18] and Ross [19], respectively, were hyperacutely rejected in a matter of minutes, demonstrating that the pig was not, and will not be, an easy donor for a human recipient.

In 1968, the guidelines for defining brain death were published in the *Journal of the American Medical Association* [20]. Almost overnight, the availability of brain-dead, heart-beating cadaver donors eliminated the need to continue the quest for nonhuman donor organs. Widespread access to dialysis and United States government financing of the end-stage renal disease program allowed patients with kidney failure to live and wait for kidney transplantation, whereas previously kidney transplantation was the only alternative to death. Interest in xenotransplantation of kidneys gave way to pretransplant management with dialysis, and more timely transplantation with optimally functioning human kidney allografts. However, in the following two decades, the success achieved with allotransplantation triggered a new organ shortage crisis, highlighted by the increasing number of patients dying while waiting for a human organ. This is particularly disturbing in certain candidate populations, such as neonates and small children, where donor scarcity is even more severe. Such was the rationale for the only attempt at human xenotransplantation in the cyclosporine era, when the shortage of neonatal hearts induced Bailey and coworkers [21] to use a baboon heart in a 2.2-kg neonate recipient in 1984. In spite of the cyclosporine, steroid, azathioprine, and antithymocyte globulin treatment, immunopathological events similar to the ones observed by Porter [16] 20 years before brought the baboon heart to irreversible failure within 3 weeks. No further attempts were made for almost a decade, until three human liver xenotransplantations, using two baboons and one pig, were performed in 1992 and 1993 [22–24]. The description of the two baboon-to-human liver xenotransplantations, and the principles learned with this experience, are the subject of this chapter.

Work in the Laboratory and the Consensus Process

In 1969, Sir Peter Medawar [25] stated:

> A new solution is therefore called for: the use of heterografts – that is to say, of grafts transplanted from lower animals into man. Of the use of heterografts I can say only this: that in the laboratory we are achieving greater success with grafts *between* species today than we achieved with grafts *within* 15 years ago. We shall solve the problem by using heterografts one day if we try hard enough, and maybe in less than 15 years.

However, the laboratory work performed at different institutions in the following 15–20 years did not bring results that could encourage further clinical trials.

In May 1992, a study performed in Pittsburgh by Murase et al. [26], using a hamster-to-rat xenotransplant model, was discussed at the meeting of the American Society of Transplant Surgeons in Chicago. Murase's work clearly showed that indefinite survival under tacrolimus (formerly FK506) was routinely achievable if it was combined, for the first two post-transplant weeks, with either of two "antiproliferative" drugs: mycophenolate mofetil (an inhibitor of purine synthesis) or brequinar sodium (an inhibitor of pyrimidine synthesis). The use of cyclophosphamide, an alkylating agent with considerable B cell specificity [27, 28], allowed similar consistent chronic survival after either heart or liver xenotransplantation. Particularly significant was the fact that a single large dose of cyclophosphamide, given 10 days before the xenotransplant, allowed success in almost 100% of the animals with only daily administration of tacrolimus. This work, together with the previous experience with cyclophosphamide [29, 30] as an effective drug in clinical transplantation, justified its use in a clinical xenograft trial.

Pittsburgh Clinical Trial

Planning

Starting from this premise, in November 1991 the Pittsburgh Transplantation Institute notified the National Institute of Diabetes and Digestive and Kidney Diseases of the National Institutes of Health (J. Hoofnagle and P. Gordon), the Food and Drug Administration (R. Lieberman and G. Burke), and the Secretary of the Department of Health and Human Services (L. Sullivan) of the intention to proceed with the clinical liver xenotransplant project. Eight months were then needed to present the scientific documentation to the appropriate government agencies in the United States, the Institutional Review Board and the Ethics Committee of the University of Pittsburgh Medical Center, and members of the United States Congress with special interest in health care problems [31]. Also, in March 1992, a committee formed by six eminent European and American surgeons, coordinated by Keith Reemtsma of Columbia University, was brought together to hear the opinions of other experts before sanctioning the first clinical baboon liver xenotransplant.

After making several modifications to the initial protocol, on the basis of suggestions made by the various experts consulted, the first xenotransplant was performed on 28 June 1992, and the second on 10 January 1993. During the long interval between the first and the second, and despite authorization to perform four consecutive liver xenotransplants [32], it was chosen to bring together the same group of experts previously consulted, this time at the New York Academy of Medicine, so that they could analyze the results obtained in the first xenotransplant. On this occasion, the Pittsburgh Transplantation Institute was advised to continue the clinical trial.

The protocol for this human trial (approved by the Institutional Review Board of the University of Pittsburgh Medical Center [32] allowed baboon-to-human liver transplantation for the treatment of end-stage cirrhosis related to chronic active hepatitis B virus. In many areas of the world, infection with hepatitis B virus is endemic. Over 250 million people are affected by this disease worldwide [33], and it is also the most common cause of advanced liver disease and hepatocellular carcinoma. Recurrence of infection after liver transplantation is high in this patient population, especially in the subset with positive viral replication markers (e.g., hepatitis B "e" antigen and/or hepatitis B DNA positivity) [34, 35]. In many institutions this disease is considered a contraindication for liver allotransplantation. Because the baboon liver is thought to be resistant to the development of chronic active hepatitis B [22], the principal benefit to the patients enrolled in this trial was the possibility that the xenotransplanted liver would not be reinfected by the viral disease. The transplant was therefore planned as a permanent replacement for the failing human liver.

Choice of Donor Species

Nonhuman primates, by sharing many physiologic and genetic characteristics with humans, seemed to qualify as donors for this attempt. Primates are comprised of two suborders, *Prosimii* and *Anthropoidea*. Prosimian primates resemble squirrels or rats more than true monkeys. The *Anthropoidea* suborder can be further subdivided into families: New World monkeys, Old World monkeys, lesser apes, great apes, and man. From an investigational standpoint, the most frequently used species are the Old World monkeys. This family includes rhesus monkeys (*Macaca mulata*), cynomologus monkeys (*Macaca fascicularis*), and baboons (*Papio cynocephalus*, *Papio sphinx*, *Papio gelada*, and *Papio hamadryas*) [36]. Great apes include the chimpanzee (*Pan troglodytes*) and gorilla (*Gorilla gorilla*), but are not used in great numbers for research because of their endangered classification, although their genome and their size approximate those of humans more than lesser apes.

The liver anatomy in all primates is similar, with a right and left lateral lobe placed dorsally and a single large ventral central lobe. The liver of the Macaca and Papio is notable for lobation, with four identifiable lobes. In the higher order of primates, the central lobe fuses with the right and left lateral lobes. The quadrate lobe is much narrower in non-human primates than in man, and the caudate lobe may fully encircle the inferior vena cava. The ligamentous attachments are similar to those described in man. The portal venous system is essentially identical in the higher order of primates. The hepatic venous drainage is similar to man, with small short hepatic venous tributaries draining the right and central lobes, with two large hepatic venous branches, one right and one left. In all primates, the gallbladder lies closely attached to the right or central lobe. The gallbladder arterial supply is usually from a branch of the right hepatic artery. The common bile duct empties into the duodenum.

The chimpanzee is most likely the best donor in biological terms, due to the very small genetic differences between this species and humans. However, their endangered status prevents their widespread use for scientific purposes. In the United States, only 25–50 chimpanzees may be used annually in biomedical research, including those used in acquired immunodeficiency syndrome (AIDS) research [37], and it is estimated that only 70 chimpanzees would be available worldwide as organ donors each year [38]. Therefore, it was decided that the donor in the Pittsburgh clinical trial would be the baboon, *Papio cynocephalus*.

Donor Baboon Selection Criteria

The baboons used as donors came from the Southwest Foundation for Research and Education, San Antonio, Texas, the same institution that supplied the baboons used in the previous kidney xenotransplant trial [15]. All the baboons used during donor selection were born in the United States [36].

Baboons have group A, B, and AB antigens weakly expressed in all cells, with group O baboons being extremely rare [39–41]. However, ABO incompatibility did not affect the results of previous clinical xenotransplant trial [15, 42]. An ABO match is desirable in a baboon-to-human xenotransplant, but its absence does not constitute an absolute contraindication. Both of our human recipients in this trial, blood group A and B, respectively, received livers from compatible histo-blood group donors.

In addition to histo-blood group, donor selection criteria included a lymphocytotoxic crossmatch, as well as a complete biochemical, viral and bacteriological evaluation of the animals [22]. In particular, infectious disease screening was performed at the Virus Reference Laboratory of the Southwest Foundation for Research and Education, San Antonio, Texas. All potential donors were screened for retroviruses (simian T lymphocytic virus, STLV; human T lymphocytic virus, HTLV; simian immunodeficiency virus, SIV; SRV-1; SRV-2; SRV-5; human immunodeficiency virus-1, HIV-1; HIV-2; foamy virus), herpesviruses (SA-8; herpes simplex virus, HSV; B virus; rCMV, cytomegalovirus; human CMV, hCMV; Epstein-Barr virus, EBV; varicella-zoster virus, VZV), and hepatitis A (HAV), B (HBV), and C (HCV) viruses. In addition, the baboons were examined to exclude tuberculosis and toxoplasmosis, and routine cultures of blood and feces were performed [43].

Baboons are physically smaller than humans. The maximum weight of an adult male baboon is about 30–35 kg. However, a liver from a smaller donor can rapidly grow to accommodate the size of a larger recipient [44]. A number of suitable donors were selected and quarantined before the xenotransplant.

Case Reports

Donor Procedure

The donor operation was performed using the traditional technique described by our group [45, 46]. The operations on the donor and the recipient were performed simultaneously, in two different operating rooms. Cold ischemia times were 80 min in the first case and 231 min in the second. University of Wisconsin solution was used to preserve the organs, as is done in our routine clinical practice.

Recipient Selection

The first patient was a 35-year-old white male, who had undergone a splenectomy in 1989 following a motor vehicle accident. The patient was found to be HIV positive, but his CD4 lymphocyte count was normal, as were in vitro mitogen responses. The second patient was a 62-year-old white male with no previous abdominal surgery. Both patients had end-stage liver disease secondary to chronic active hepatitis B. In both patients, the principal complications of the liver disease were poorly controlled edema, fatigue, ascites, encephalopathy, and gastrointestinal bleeding.

Operative Technique

The liver xenotransplants were performed using a modification of the standard method [47], described 33 years ago [48], and employing a venovenous bypass [49]. The difference in diameter between the vessels of donor and recipient, and the small size of the donor's liver (600 cm^3 and 450 cm^3 in the first and second cases, respectively) made it necessary to use the piggy-back method [50]. In both cases the right suprahepatic vein of the recipient was closed with a running suture, while the left and middle suprahepatic veins were used to perform the suprahepatic vena cava anastomosis. In the first patient, given the considerable size discrepancy between the recipient and donor portal veins, the latter was anastomosed end-to-end onto the recipient's left portal branch, and the right branch was closed with a running suture. In the second case, a smaller discrepancy made it possible to perform a normal end-to-end portal anastomosis.

The donor's celiac axis was anastomosed end-to-end onto the recipient's common hepatic artery in the first case, and end-to-side onto the supraceliac recipient aorta (using a donor carotid artery interposition graft) in the second. In both cases, the liver reperfused uniformly and produced bile on the operating table. The biliary anastomosis was done using a choledochojejunostomy on a Roux loop. In the second case, a small (3.5F) diameter catheter was placed into the biliary anastomosis and brought out through the abdominal wall (Fig. 1), in order to gain direct access to the bile duct to study its anatomy and take bile samples during the postoperative period.

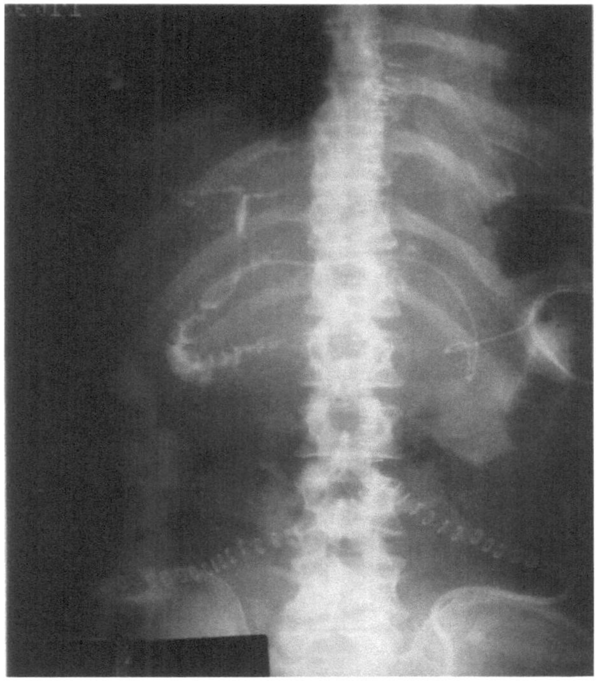

Fig. 1. Second liver xenograft (baboon-to-human) recipient. Cholangiogram performed on postoperative day 18 by injection through a percutaneous biliary catheter. This catheter was placed during the xenotransplant operation (10 January 1993) across the choledochojejunostomy and allowed study of the biliary anatomy as well as daily collection of bile samples after the xenotransplantation. (From [96])

Immunosuppressive Therapy

The immunosuppressive protocol comprised four drugs: cyclophosphamide, tacrolimus, methylprednisolone, and prostaglandin E_1. Cyclophosphamide was begun 2 days prior to the transplant, and administered for a total of 56 days in the first case and 10 days in the second, at a dosage varying between 0.07 and 10.6 mg/kg per day. Tacrolimus, steroids, and prostaglandin were started on the day of the transplant, using the same protocol we follow in clinical liver allotransplantation. Detailed descriptions of the immunosuppressive drug dosing and blood levels obtained are shown in Figs 2 and 3.

Postoperative Course

The first patient was extubated 17 h after the operation, he was placed on an oral diet on the fifth post-transplant day, and lived for 70 days. He spent most of this time in a regular hospital ward and had an almost normal plasma bilirubin level for the majority of the 70 days that he survived. The second patient, who was much older, never regained consciousness, remained icteric, and survived for only 26 days. Figures 2 and 3 illustrate their postoperative courses. The alkaline phosphatase was always very high in the first patient [51] (Fig. 2), while in the second patient it was not as conspicuously high, although it was always above normal limits.

The first patient underwent five liver biopsies, while the second had seven. Only the biopsy obtained from the first patient on the 12th postoperative day

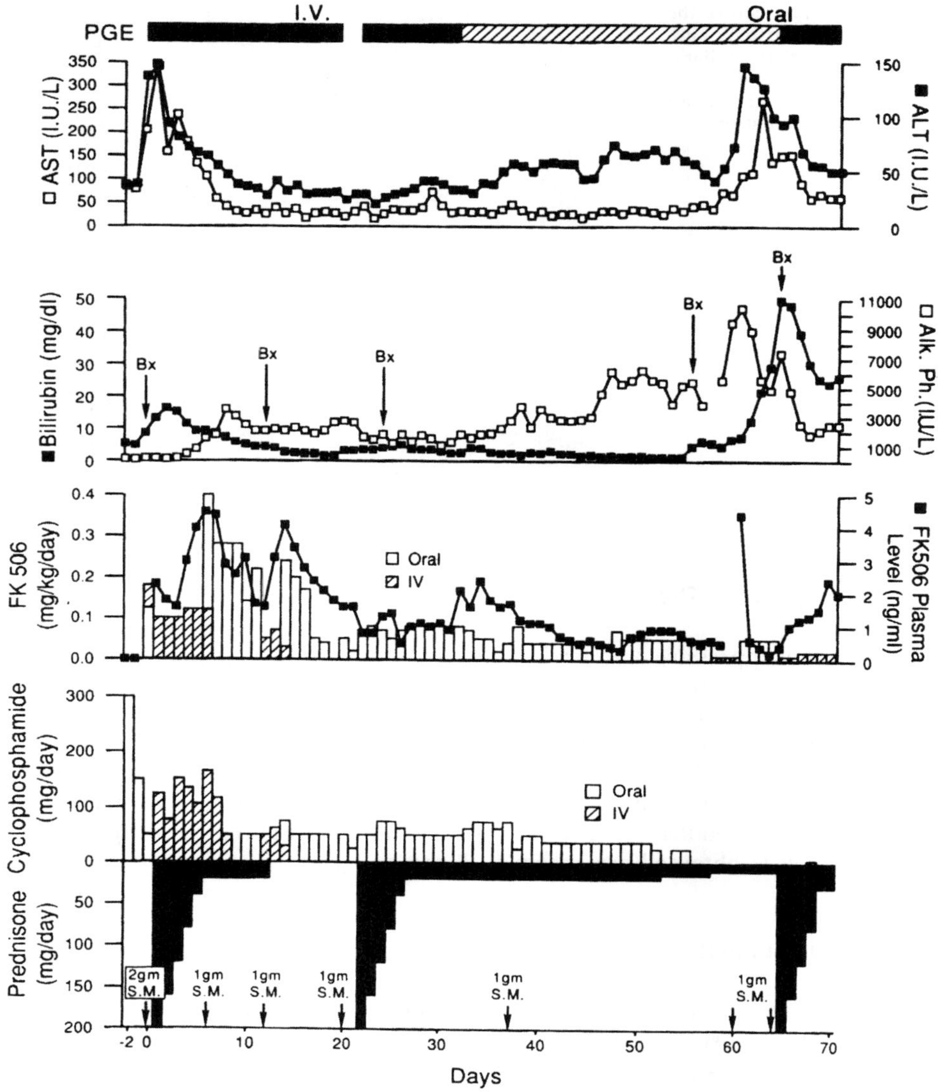

Fig. 2. Clinical course of the first liver xenograft (baboon-to-human) recipient (28 June 1992). *S.M.*, Solumedrol (methylprednisolone); *PGE*, prostaglandin E_1; *Bx*, biopsy; *AST*, aspartate aminotransferase; *ALT*, alanine aminotransferase; *Alk. Ph.*, alkaline phosphatase; *FK506*, tacrolimus. (From [22])

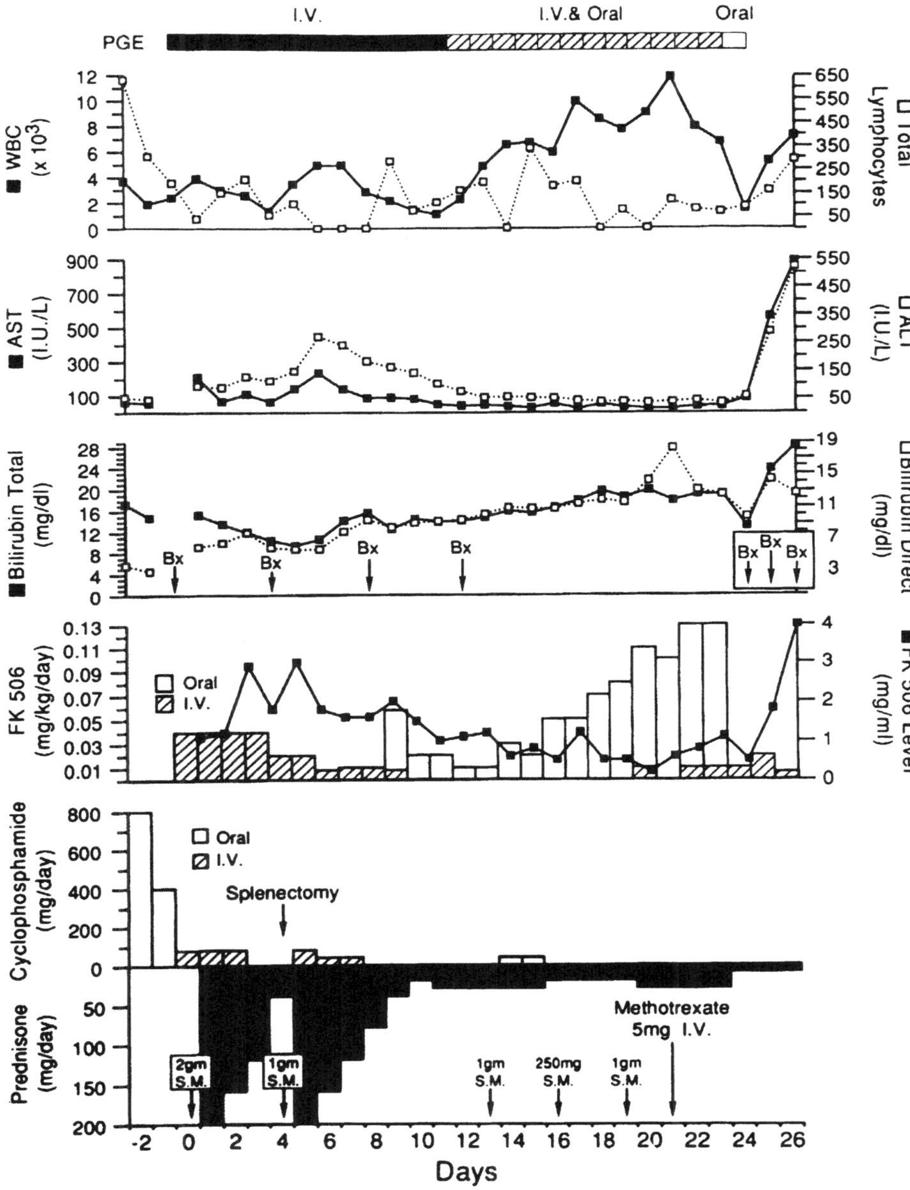

Fig. 3. Clinical course of the second liver xenograft (baboon-to-human) recipient (10 January 1993). *S.M.*, Solumedrol (methylprednisolone); *PGE*, prostaglandin E_1; *Bx*, biopsy; *AST*, aspartate aminotransferase; *ALT*, alanine aminotransferase; *WBC*, white blood cells; *FK506*, tacrolimus. (From [52])

showed signs of mild focal cellular rejection, while no evidence of acute cellular rejection (according to the criteria routinely used in liver allotransplantation), was detected in any of the other biopsies from either patient [22, 23, 31, 52]. However, direct immunofluorescence demonstrated the presence of endothelial deposits of immunoglobulins (IgG>IgA>IgM) and complement (particularly Clq) in both cases [53]. No evidence of HBV reinfection was detectable by immunoperoxidase staining in the liver tissue at any time. Since the period of follow-up was short, no definitive conclusions can be reached regarding the possibility of long-term resistance of the baboon liver to hepatitis B recurrence. However, the most sensitive assay using polymerase chain reaction (PCR) could not detect hepatitis B DNA in the transplanted livers [54].

Macroscopically, considerable hepatic regeneration was noted in both cases, with a significant increase in the volume of the baboon organs. Computed tomography (CT) was used to calculate the volume of the transplanted livers [55]. Both livers showed an extremely rapid growth, as normally occurs when a human liver is transplanted into a recipient with a larger abdomen than the donor [44]. Figures 4 and 5 show the CT performed on the two recipients on the 26th and 14th postoperative days, respectively. The first patient's liver grew from an initial volume of 600 cm^3 to 1555 cm^3 in 26 days. The second patient's liver grew from an initial volume of 450 cm^3 to 1741 cm3 in 14 days. An angiogram performed on postoperative day 59 in the first patient showed that the vasculature of the transplanted xenograft had scaled up appropriately, i.e., the architectural relationships were preserved as the liver increased in volume.

Papio cynocephalus normally produces elevated levels of factor VII and low levels of factors IX and XI, as compared to humans. Coagulation profiles were measured in both recipients preoperatively and several times postoperatively. Our results [56] showed that the baboon's coagulation pattern was acquired by

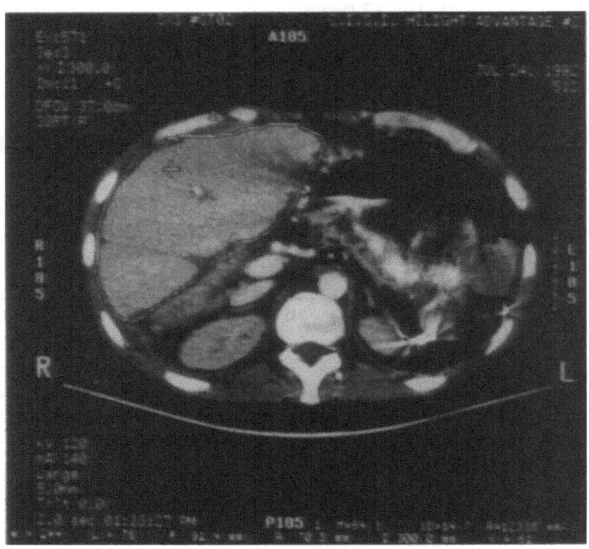

Fig. 4. First liver xenograft (baboon-to-human) recipient. Abdominal computed tomography (CT) on postoperative day 26. The liver volume has increased to 1555 cm^3, from an initial value of 600 cm^3. (From [96])

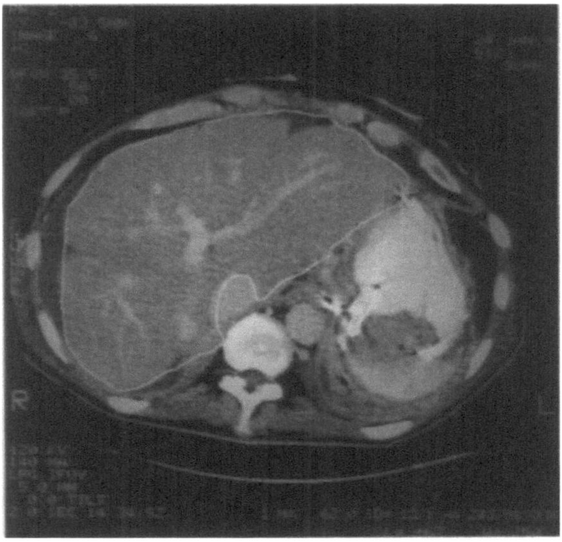

Fig. 5. Second liver xenograft (baboon-to-human) recipient. Abdominal computed tomography (CT) on postoperative day 14. The liver volume has increased to 1741 cm^3, from an initial value of 450 cm^3. (From [96])

the patients after liver xenografting, but this did not affect their clotting ability. No adverse effects of the presence of baboon proteins, such as immune-mediated kidney injury, could be detected at any time.

In both patients there was evidence of an adequately functioning liver mass, such as: (a) normalization of coagulation with normal prothrombin time, (b) correction of hyperammonemia, (c) normal arterial ketone body ratio (a reflection of hepatic energy stores) [57], and (d) clearance of serum lactate. However, both patients suffered from hypoalbuminemia and needed to receive frequent albumin infusion. The baboon liver did impact on the protein profile of both patients. Liver-specific proteins could be shown to be of baboon origin by serum protein electrophoresis (Fig. 6). Total complement levels were depleted for 1–2 weeks after liver xenotransplantation, similar to that reported in liver allotransplantation across a positive lymphocytotoxic crossmatch [9, 22, 23, 52, 53, 58].

The first patient went into renal failure on postoperative day 21, while the second patient became anuric immediately after surgery. Both patients suffered a number of infectious complications. Many of the organisms involved were typical of the agents seen after allotransplantation, e.g., *Staphylococcus*, *Candida*, CMV, *Enterococcus*, and *Aspergillus*. In the first patient, both the recipient and donor were CMV positive. Attempts to determine the origin of the subsequent CMV infection to either human or baboon origin failed because of inability to culture the CMV from clinical samples in sufficient quantity to subtype. However, the susceptibility of both baboon and human CMV to ganciclovir makes the origin of this virus of lesser practical importance.

The causes of death in both patients were multifactorial. In the first, a rise in both the alkaline phosphatase and total bilirubin prompted a percutaneous transhepatic cholangiogram on the 61st post-transplant day. Within 1 h after the pro-

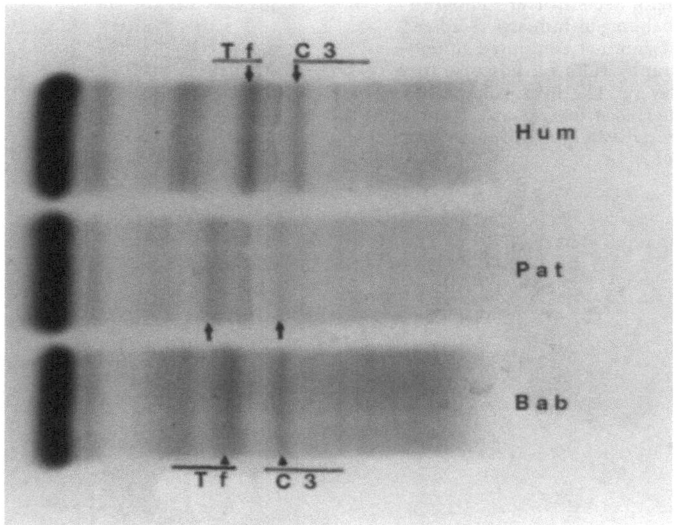

Fig. 6. First liver xenograft (baboon-to-human) recipient. Protein electrophoresis of normal human (*Hum*), baboon donor (*Bab*), and patient serum (*Pat*). *C3*, complement; *Tf*, transferrin. (From [22])

cedure, the patient became hypotensive, febrile, and coagulopathic. He was intubated, stabilized, and his clinical condition improved significantly. A positive culture for *Aspergillus flavus* was noted, and amphotericin treatment was started. On the last day of his life (post-transplant day 70), the patient was hemodynamically stable and was being weaned from the ventilator. Early in the afternoon he suddenly deteriorated neurologically, and a CT scan of the head revealed a massive subarachnoid bleed. The autopsy showed, as cause of death, a subarachnoid hemorrhage due to angioinvasive aspergillosis. In this patient, two foci of aspergillosis were found in the lungs, with focal dissemination to the kidneys and brain. The intrahepatic bile ducts were slightly dilated, and numerous bile infarcts were detected. Although the patient was in renal failure, the kidneys were intact and there was no evidence of immune complex deposition.

The second patient died on the 26th post-transplant day from complications from peritonitis. It is likely that the high doses of corticosteroids used to control early immunologic damage were responsible for poor tissue healing, leading to a leak from the enteric anastomosis.

There were some differences in the immunologic circumstances between the two cases. As mentioned before, the first patient had a splenectomy in 1989 following a motorcycle accident, whereas the second patient still had his spleen, which was subsequently removed 4 days after the xenotransplant.

The first patient was also HIV positive. Our center traditionally does not refuse transplantation to HIV-positive patients [59], but analysis of the immunological parameters obviously differs in the case of an allotransplant. Although this first xenotransplant patient was considered immunocompetent at the time of the transplant and had no change in this state during his postoperative course [22], it is difficult to judge whether his condition provided a natural immunosuppression, and whether or not this represented an advantage.

After completing the vascular anastomoses the second patient was given an infusion of bone marrow cells from the donor baboon (3×10^8/kg body weight). This was aimed at increasing the natural tolerogenicity induced by the liver transplant [60]. It is believed the liver has certain advantages in immunological terms on account of the large number of dendritic cells it possesses. These cells abandon the transplanted organ and participate in a two-way cell traffic, which gives rise to microchimerism [61, 62]. The autopsy on the first patient confirmed this expectation, since baboon DNA was found (using PCR amplification of baboon-specific DNA) in the patient's heart, kidneys, lungs, and lymph nodes. All blood samples taken from the second patient during the postoperative course showed the presence of xenogeneic baboon DNA.

Analysis of the Two Cases and Strategies For Future Clinical Xenotransplantation

The most disquieting fact in our baboon-to-human liver transplant experience was the disparity between the paucity of the histopathologic findings of rejection (which was very encouraging), and the discouraging functional deficiencies of these xenotransplants, which suggested incomplete control of xenograft rejection. The pathology of the transplanted baboon livers was compared to that of six baboon kidney xenografts transplanted in Denver in 1963 [15, 16]. These kidneys, as we mentioned before, functioned for 10–60 days. The key pathological finding was an occlusive endothelialitis of the graft vessels, presumably antibody mediated. The pathology of those kidneys removed in 1964 [16] showed distal ischemia, caused by the vascular injury, that appeared to be responsible for the patchy gangrene of the xenografts. In the two recent liver xenotransplants, polymorphonuclear leukocytes were seen in the sinusoids immediately after reperfusion, and biliary sludging was detected at the autopsy. Both the sludging and the appearance of polymorphonuclear leukocytes were compatible with a diagnosis of an aborted hyperacute (humoral) rejection. Complement studies were also consistent with this possibility, showing that total complement was depleted for most of the critical first 2 weeks. While the complement system was restored, irreversible damage to the graft may have been already done [9, 22, 23, 53]. Although these baboon liver xenografts looked macroscopically normal, closer inspection showed a very fine microsteatosis, which was particularly obvious in the second patient. This may represent a sub-lethal immunological injury that precluded long-term success in both cases.

We suspect that these livers were acutely damaged by an incomplete version of a form of rejection that was described in 1964 in ABO-incompatible kidneys [63, 64], and seen later in kidney allografts transplanted across a positive lymphocytotoxic crossmatch [17]. These were the first descriptions of hyperacute kidney rejection by preformed antigraft antibodies. A few years later, hyperacute rejection was defined in a more sophisticated way as a complement activation syndrome, analogous to the Shwartzman and local Arthus reactions [65, 66]. It was pointed out that, although hyperacute allograft rejection was usually associated with antigraft antibodies, this was not an absolute requirement - a heretical statement at that time. However, the distinction between hyperacute rejection *with* and *without* preformed antibodies is merely the difference between the classical pathway of complement activation, in which the first steps are antibody dependent, and the alternative pathway, which does not require an antibody trigger or the participation of complement components C1, C2, and C4. These hyperacute rejection syndromes, *with* or *without* preformed antigraft antibodies, are not fundamentally different from those seen after xenotransplantation of organs between genetically diverse species [9].

Many methods of manipulating the xenograft recipient have been tried and retried since the 1960s, without any definite success. These methods include antibody suppression [67], antibody depletion [68–79], inhibition of the complement cascade [80–85], and inhibition of the inflammatory response [86, 87]. Alteration of the xenograft before its implantation, mainly by blocking antibody binding sites with recipient $F(ab')_2$ immunoglobulin fragments [76, 88, 89], has also been unsuccessful.

The introduction of the concept of systemic chimerism has heightened interest in designing strategies aimed to alter the cell composition of the graft. The creation of a transgenic pig, to be utilized as a source of organs for clinical xenotransplants, has already been started in a few laboratories [90, 91]. The scientists working on this project have embarked on a program to produce pigs transgenic for human regulators of complement activation (e.g., decay-accelerating factor, DAF; CD59; membrane cofactor protein, MCP). This is achieved by microinjection of human genomic DNA fragments into the pronuclei of fertilized porcine oocytes [92–94]. However, only one of the components of the xenotransplant barrier could be overcome by this strategy (namely, the complement cascade); therefore it is difficult to hope that a complete control of rejection will be achieved by this method alone.

One other extremely fascinating possibility is the production of chimeric organs. Human-to-baboon bone marrow transplantation has already been performed at the Pittsburgh Transplantation Institute laboratories, after conditioning with nonlethal irradiation [95]. In this experiment, two baboons preconditioned with 7.4 Gy total lymphoid irradiation were given unaltered human bone marrow cells at the dose of 6×10^8 cells/kg body weight, without any subsequent treatment. Donor DNA was found widely distributed in the tissues of both animals when killed 18 months later. It is also interesting to note that graft-versus-host disease (GvHD) did not occur in either animal. As recently stated elsewhere [9], "it remains to be seen if incomplete or even full chimerism will change the image of baboon organs enough to make them viewed as allografts by humans."

Acknowledgements. We wish to acknowledge the immeasurable debt of gratitude to our two patients for their heroism and their families for their admirable strength. This work was aided by research grants from the Veterans Administration and Project Grant No. DK29961 from the National Institutes of Health, Bethesda, Maryland.

References

1. UNOS update, 1994; 10(11):58
2. Marino IR, Doyle HR, Kang Y, Kormos RL, Starzl TE. Multiple organ procurement. In: Ayres CM, Grenvik A, Holbrook PR, Shoemaker WC, eds. Textbook of Critical Care. 3rd ed. (Section XIV Transplantation), Chapter 178, Philadelphia: WB Saunders Company, 1995:1610
3. Land W, Hammer C, Brynger H, eds. Indication for organ transplantation. Transplant. Proc.1986; 18(suppl 3):1
4. Marino IR, Doyle HR, Rakela J, Fung JJ, Starzl TE. Liver transplantation: indications and results. In: Hess W, Cirenei A, Rohner A, Akovbiantz A, eds. Diseases of the Biliary Tract and Pancreas.Padua: Piccin Publishing. In press
5. Merriken KJ, Overcast TD. Patient selection for heart transplantation. When is a discriminatory choice discrimination? J. Health Polit. Policy Law.1985; 10:7
6. Starzl TE, Todo S, Gordon R, et al. Liver transplantation in older patients. (Letter) N. Engl. J. Med.1987; 316:484
7. Doyle HR, Morelli F, McMichael J, et al. Hepatic retransplantation – an analysis of risk factors associated with outcome. Transplantation. 1996; 61:1499
8. Auchincloss H. The scientific study of xenografting: 1964–1988. In: Cooper DKC, Kemp E, Reemtsma K, White DJG, eds. Xenotransplantation.Heidelberg, Springer, 1991, p. 23
9. Starzl TE, Valdivia L, Murase N, et al. The biological basis of and strategies for clinical xenotransplantation. Immunol. Rev.1994; 141:212
10. Jaboulay M. Greffe de reins au pli du coude par soudures arterielles et veineuses. Lyon Med.196; 107:575
11. Unger E. Nierentransplantationen. Klin. Wochenschr.1910; 47:573
12. Neuhof H. The Transplantation of Tissues.New York: Appleton, 1923, p. 260
13. Hitchcock CR, Kiser JC, Telander RL, Seljeskog EL. Baboon renal grafts. JAMA. 1964; 189:158
14. Reemtsma K, McCracken BH, Schlegel JU, et al. Renal heterotransplantation in man. Ann. Surg.1964; 160:384
15. Starzl TE, Marchioro TL, Peters GN, et al. Renal heterotransplantation from baboon to man. Experience with 6 cases. Transplantation.1964; 2:752
16. Porter KA. Pathological changes in transplanted kidneys. In: Starzl TE, ed. Experiences in Renal Transplantation.Philadelphia: WB Saunders, 1964, p. 346
17. Terasaki PI, Marchioro TL, Starzl TE. Serotyping of human lymphocyte antigens: preliminary trials on long-term kidney homograft survivors. In: Russell PS, Winn HJ, Amos DB, eds. Histocompatibility Testing 1965.Washington, DC: National Academy of Science, 1965, p. 83
18. Kuss' case is reported in: Starzl TE. Editorial. Animal to human transplantation. In: Organ Transplantation and Tissue Grafting.Herve P, Vuitton DA, Rifle G, eds. Inserm Publishers, John Libbey, Paris-London, 1992
19. Ross DN. In: Experience With Human Heart Transplantation.Shapiro H, ed. Durban: Butterworths, 1969, p. 228
20. Ad Hoc Committee of the Harvard Medical School. A definition of irreversible coma. Report of the Ad Hoc Committee of the Harvard Medical School to examine the definition of brain death. JAMA.1968; 205:337

21. Bailey LL, Nehlsen-Canarella SL, Concepcion W, Jolley WB. Baboon-to-human cardiac xenotransplantation in a neonate. JAMA.1985; 254:3321
22. Starzl TE, Fung J, Tzakis A, et al. Baboon to human liver transplantation. Lancet. 1993; 341:65
23. Starzl TE, Tzakis AG, Fung JJ, et al. Prospects of clinical xenotransplantation. Transplant. Proc.1994; 26:1082
24. Makowka L, Cramer DV, Hoffman A, et al. The use of a pig liver xenograft for temporary support of a patient with fulminant hepatic failure. Transplantation.1995; 59:1654
25. Reemtsma K. Heterotransplantation. Transplant. Proc.1969; 1:251
26. Murase N, Starzl TE, Demetris AJ, et al. Hamster to rat heart and liver xenotransplantation with FK506 plus anti-proliferative drugs. Transplantation.1993; 55:701
27. Marino IR, Doyle HR. Conventional immunosuppressive drugs. In: Thomson AW, Starzl TE, eds. Immunosuppressive Drugs: Advances in Anti-Rejection Therapy.London: Edward Arnold Publishers, 1994, p. 1
28. Putnam CW, Halgrimson CG, Groth CG, et al. Immunosuppression with cyclophosphamide in the dog. Clin. Exp. Immunol.1975; 22:323
29. Starzl TE, Putnam CW, Halgrimson CG, et al. Cyclophosphamide and whole organ transplantation in human beings. Surg. Gynecol. Obstet.1971; 133:981
30. Starzl TE, Groth CG, Putnam CW, et al. Cyclophosphamide for clinical renal and hepatic transplantation. Transplant. Proc.1973; 5:511
31. Starzl TE. The future of xenotransplantation. Editorial for the Surgical Residents issue. Ann. Surg.1992; 3:10
32. Starzl TE, Todo S, Tzakis AG, et al. Orthotopic baboon to human heterotransplantation. Institutional Review Board Protocol #920301. University of Pittsburgh, 1992
33. Fung JJ, Eghtesad B, Todo S, et al. Hepatitis B virus (HBV) reinfection following liver transplantation: theory and practice. Clin. Transplant.1995; 9:262
34. Todo S, Demetris AJ, Van Thiel DH, Fung JJ, Starzl TE. Orthotopic liver transplantation for patients with hepatitis B virus (HBV) related liver disease. Hepatology.1991; 13:619
35. Samuel D, and the Investigators of the European Concerted Action on Viral Hepatitis Study. Liver transplantation in European patients with the hepatitis B surface antigen. N. Engl. J. Med.1993; 329:1842
36. Kalter SS. The baboon. Microbiology, clinical, chemistry, and some hematological aspects. In: Goldsmith EI, Moor-Jankowski J, eds. Primates in Medicine. Vol. 8.Basel: Karger, 1973
37. Starzl TE. Baboon renal and chimpanzee liver heterotransplantation. In: Hardy MA, ed. Xenograft 25.Amsterdam, New York, Oxford: Elsevier, 1989, p. 17
38. Auchincloss H, Jr. Xenogenic transplantation. Transplantation.1988; 46:1
39. Socha WW, Moor-Jankowski J, Ruffie J. Blood group of primates: present status, theoretical implications and practical applications. J. Med. Primatol.1984; 13:11
40. Triulzi DJ, Jochum EE, Marino IR, Starzl TE. Compatibility testing in baboon xenotransplantation. Transfusion.1993; 33(s):43S
41. Triulzi DJ, Jochum EE. Red cell compatibility testing in baboon xenotransplantation. Transfusion.1995; 35:756
42. Kirkpatrick CH, Wilson WEC. Immunologic studies of baboon-to-man renal heterotransplantation. In: Starzl TE, ed. Experience in Renal Transplantation. Philadelphia: WB Saunders, 1964, p. 284

43. Michaels MG, Simmons RL. Xenotransplant-associated zoonoses: strategies for prevention. Transplantation.1994; 57:1
44. Van Thiel DH, Gavaler JS, Kam I, et al. Rapid growth of an intact human liver transplanted into a recipient larger than the donor. Gastroenterology.1987; 93:1414
45. Starzl TE, Miller C, Broznick B, Makowka L. An improved technique for multiple organ harvesting. Surg. Gynecol. Obstet.1987; 165:343
46. Marino IR, Doyle HR, Fung JJ. Liver. In: Higgins RSD, Sanchez JA, Lorber MI, Baldwin JC, eds. The Multiorgan Donor.Blackwell Science, Cambridge, Massachusetts. In press
47. Marino IR, Doyle HR, Starzl TE. Liver transplantation: surgical technique. In: Diseases of the Biliary Tract and Pancreas.Hess W, Cirenei A, Rohner A, Akovbiantz A, eds. Piccin Publishing, Padua. In press
48. Starzl TE, Marchioro TL, Von Kaulla KN, et al. Homotransplantation of the liver in humans. Surg. Gynecol. Obstet.1963; 117:659
49. Shaw BW Jr, Martin DJ, Marquez JM, et al. Venous bypass in clinical liver transplantation. Ann. Surg.1984; 200:524
50. Tzakis A, Todo S, Starzl TE. Piggyback orthotopic liver transplantation with preservation of the inferior vena cava. Ann. Surg.1989; 210:649
51. Mercer DW, Tang M, Marino IR, et al. Changes in biliary (high-molecular-mass) and liver isoforms of alkaline phosphatase after baboon-to-human liver transplantation. Clin. Chem.1994; 40:1335
52. Starzl TE, Tzakis A, Fung JJ, et al. Human liver xenotransplantation. Xeno.1993; 1:4
53. Triulzi DJ, Jochum EE, Marino IR, Starzl TE. Heteroagglutinins and their significance in baboon hepatic xenotransplantation. Transplantation.1995; 60:127
54. Lanford RE, Michaels MG, Chavez D, et al. Persistence of extrahepatic hepatitis B virus DNA in the absence of detectable hepatic replication in patients with baboon liver transplants. J. Med. Virol.1995; 46:207
55. Van Thiel DH, Hagler NG, Schade RR, et al. In vivo hepatic volume determination using sonography and computed tomography: validation and a comparison of the two techniques. Gastroenterology.1985; 88:1812
56. Bontempo FA, Lewis JH, Marino IR, et al. Coagulation factor pattern in baboon-to-human liver transplant: acquisition of baboon pattern by recipient. The American Society of Hematology, 34th Annual Meeting. Blood.1992; 80(suppl 1):309
57. Asonuma K, Takaya S, Selby R, et al. The clinical significance of the arterial ketone body ratio as an early indicator of graft viability in human liver transplantation. Transplantation.1991; 51:164
58. Manez R, Kobayashi M, Takaya S, et al. Humoral rejection associated with antidonor lymphocytotoxic antibodies following liver transplantation. Transplant. Proc.1993; 25:888
59. Tzakis AG, Cooper MH, Dummer JS, et al. Transplantation in HIV+ patients. Transplantation.1990; 49:354
60. Fontes P, Rao A, Demetris AJ, et al. Augmentation with bone marrow of donor leukocyte migration for kidney, liver, heart, and pancreas islet transplantation. Lancet. 1994; 344:151
61. Starzl TE, Demetris AJ, Murase N, et al. Cell migration, chimerism and graft acceptance. Lancet.1992; 339:1579
62. Starzl TE, Murase N, Demetris AJ, et al. Drug development and testing in relation to cell migration and chimerism. Transplant. Proc.1993; 25:469

63. Starzl TE, Marchioro TL, Holmes JH, et al. Renal homografts in patients with major donor-recipient blood group incompatibilities. Surgery.1964; 55:195
64. Starzl TE. Patterns of permissible donor-recipient tissue transfer in relation to ABO blood groups. in: Starzl TE, ed. Experience in Renal Transplantation.Philadelphia: WB Saunders, 1964, p. 37
65. Starzl TE, Lerner RA, Dixon FJ, et al. Schwartzman reaction after human renal transplantation. N. Engl. J. Med.1968; 278:642
66. Starzl TE, Boehmig HJ, Amemiya H, et al. Clotting changes including disseminated intravascular coagulation, during rapid renal-homograft rejection. N. Engl. J. Med.1970; 283:383
67. Starzl TE. Role of excision of lymphoid masses in attenuating the rejection process. In: Starzl TE, ed. Experience in Renal Transplantation.Philadelphia: WB Saunders, 1964, p. 126
68. Merkel FK, Bier M, Beavers DC, et al. Modification of xenograft response by selective plasmapheresis. Transplant. Proc.1971; 3:534
69. Bier M, Beavers DC, Merriman WG, et al. Selective plasmapheresis in dogs for delay of heterograft response. Trans. Am. Soc. Artif. Intern. Organs.1970; 16:325
70. Alexandre GPJ, Latinne D, Gianello P, Squifflet JP. Preformed cytotoxic antibodies and ABO-incompatible grafts. Clin. Transplantation.1991; 5:583
71. Bygren P, Freiburghaus C, Lindholm T., et al. Goodpasture's syndrome treated with staphylococcal protein A immunoadsorption. (Letter) Lancet.1985; 2:1295
72. Fischel RJ, Bolman RM, Platt JL, et al. Removal of IgM anti-endothelial antibodies results in prolonged cardiac xenograft survival. Transplant. Proc.1990; 22:1077
73. Giles GR, Boehmig JH, Lilly J, et al. Mechanism and modification of rejection of heterografts between divergent species. Transplant. Proc.1970; 2:522
74. Cooper DKC, Human PA, Lexer G, et al. Effects of cyclosporine and antibody adsorption on pig cardiac xenograft survival in the baboon. J. Heart Transplant.1988; 7:238
75. Tuso PJ, Cramer DV, Yasunaga C, et al. Removal of natural human xenoantibodies to pig vascular endothelium by perfusion of blood through pig kidneys and livers. Transplantation.1993; 55:1375
76. Corman JL, Kashiwagi N, Porter KA, et al. Unsuccessful attempts to control hyperacute rejection of human renal homografts with F $(ab)_2$ and citrate organ pretreatment. Transplantation.1973; 16:60
77. Starzl TE, Weil, R III, Koep LJ, et al. Thoracic duct fistula and renal transplantation. Ann. surg.1979; 190:474
78. Starzl TE, Koep LJ, Weil R III, Halgrimson CG, Franks JJ. Thoracic duct drainage in organ transplantation: will it permit better immunosuppression? Transplant. Proc.1979; 1:276
79. Soares M, Lu X, Havaux X, et al. In vivo IgM depletion by anti-m monoclonal antibody therapy: the role of IgM in hyperacute vascular rejection of discordant xenografts. Transplantation.1994; 57:1003
80. Kux M, Boehmig HJ, Amemiya H, et al. Modification of hyperacute canine renal homograft and pig-to-dog heterograft rejection by the intra-arterial infusion of citrate. Surgery.1971; 70:103
81. Belitsky P, Popovtzer M, Corman J, Launois B, Porter KA. Modification of hyperacute xenograft rejection by intra-arterial infusion of disodium ethylenediaminetetraacetate. Transplantation.1973; 15:248

82. Leventhal JR, Dalmasso AP, Cromwell JW, et al. Prolongation of cardiac xenograft survival by depletion of complement. Transplantation.1993; 55:857
83. Pruitt SK, Kirk AD, Bollinger RR, et al. The effect of soluble complement receptor type I on hyperacute rejection of porcine xenografts. Transplantation.1994; 57:363
84. Xia W, Fearon DT, Kirkman RL. Effect of repetitive doses of soluble human complement receptor type I on survival of discordant cardiac xenografts. Transplant. Proc.1993; 25:410
85. Miyagawa S, Shirakura R, Matsumiya G, et al. Prolonging discordant xenograft survival with anticomplement reagents K76COOH and FUT175. Transplantation.1993; 55:709
86. Mundy AR. Prolongation of cat to dog renal xenograft survival with prostacyclin. Transplantation.1980; 30:226
87. Makowka L, Miller C, ChapChap P, et al. Prolongation of pig-to-dog renal xenograft survival by modification of the inflammatory mediator response. Ann. Surg.1987; 206:482
88. Shaipanich T, Vanwijck RR, Kim JP, et al. Enhancement of rat renal allografts with $F(ab)_2$ fragment of donor specific antikidney serum. Surgery.1971; 70:113
89. Gambiez L, Salame E, Chereau C, et al. The role of natural IgM in the hyperacute rejection of discordant heart xenografts. Transplantation.1992; 54:577
90. Pierson RN III, Dunning JJ, Konig WK, et al. Mechanisms governing the pace and character of pig heart-lung rejection by human blood. Transplant. Proc.1994; 26:2337
91. White DJG. Xenografting: present and future. Xeno.1994; 2:1
92. Langford GA, Yannoutsos N, Cozzi E, et al. Production of pigs transgenic for human decay accelerating factor. Transplant. Proc.1994; 26:1400
93. White DJG, Langford GA, Cozzi E, Young VJ. Protective effects of human DAF in transgenic pigs. Xeno.1995; 3:48
94. Cozzi E, White DJG. The generation of transgenic pigs as potential organ donors for humans. Nature. Med.1995; 1:964
95. Fontes P, Rao AS, Ricordi C, et al. Human-to-baboon bone marrow transplantation after conditioning with nonlethal irradiation. Transplant. Proc.1994; 26:3367
96. Marino IR, Tzakis AG, Fung JJ, et al. Hepatic xenotransplantation: clinical experience. In: Liver Transplantation, Procedures and Management.D'Amico DF, Bassi N, Tedeschi U, Cillo U, eds. Masson, Milan, 1994, p. 221

59 Clinical Islet Xenotransplantation – Transplantation of Porcine Islets into Diabetic Patients

C.G. Groth, O. Korsgren, A. Tibell, F. Reinholt, L. Wennberg, M. Satake, E. Moller, L. Rydberg, B. Samuelsson, A. Andersson, and C. Hellerström

Introduction

A logical method to cure insulin-dependent diabetes would be to transplant insulin-producing islets to the patient. For 20 years, considerable efforts have been invested into making such transplantations feasible. If this procedure is to be widely used, the supply of human islet tissue will not be sufficient. Animal tissue would then have to be relied upon. There are good reasons to believe that islets from animals can perform their physiological function in humans. Also, at this stage, islet transplantation is clearly the safest means of performing clinical trials in xenotransplantation.

The transplanted islets are initially not vascularized, but subsequently become vascularized by vessels originating from the host. Thus the hyperacute rejection seen with a vascularized xenograft should not occur. Indeed, in vitro data from our laboratory indicate that although human natural anti-pig antibodies bind to fetal pig islet cells, they do not cause cell death [1].

With regard to islet xenotransplantation, the pig offers advantages as the donor animal: (a) porcine and human insulin are structurally similar, (b) pigs and humans have a similar glucose metabolism and a similar regulation of insulin release, and (c) porcine insulin has been used successfully over many years for the treatment of diabetes mellitus in humans.

Porcine and bovine fetal pancreatic tissues have been transplanted into several diabetic patients in east European countries. There is, however, only limited scientific documentation concerning these cases, and they will not be discussed further here. A series of well-documented clinical xenoislet transplantations has recently been performed in Stockholm/Uppsala in Sweden. This chapter will summarize the clinical, metabolic and immunological events in the ten patients included in this series.

Preclinical Studies

Initial studies demonstrated that when the fetal pig pancreas was first digested with collagenase and then placed in tissue culture, a large number of islet-like cell clusters (ICCs) were formed. When such ICCs were transplanted into alloxan-diabetic nude mice, the majority of the fetal cells differentiated into β cells, and the animals became normoglycemic after 4–8 weeks [2, 3].

Before pig ICCs could be transplanted to patients, the risk of transferring pathogens from animal to human had to be considered. To address this problem, a microbiological screening program was developed in a population of Swedish landrace pigs. These studies indicated that the transmission of identifiable infectious agents could be avoided if a stringent control program was used [4].

If the porcine material was to be given by an intraportal injection, there was also the possibility of disturbing liver function and the coagulation system of the recipient. This question was explored in a pig-to-dog model, and no adverse effects were found [5].

On the basis of these findings, a clinical trial with transplantation of porcine ICCs to ten diabetic patients was initiated in 1990 [6] with the approval of the Human Ethics Committee of the Karolinska Institute in Stockholm.

Clinical Studies

Xenograft, Patients, and Transplant Procedure

Fetal porcine pancreatic tissue was obtained from pig fetuses (Swedish landrace) at a gestational age of 66–81 days (full term is approximately 120 days). The uterus was removed under sterile conditions. The average yield of ICCs from one fetus was about 10 000. For a single transplantation, pancreases from 39–100 fetuses (4–8 litters) were used.

All ten human recipients had long-standing insulin-dependent (type 1) diabetes mellitus (IDMM) and had developed end-stage diabetic nephropathy. There were nine women and one man aged 30–47 years (mean, 40 years). The duration of IDMM was 21–40 years (mean, 30 years). The first eight patients had undergone cadaveric or living-related renal transplantation between 2–17 years earlier and were receiving conventional immunosuppression with cyclosporine, prednisolone, and azathioprine. These eight patients were given the ICCs through a catheter placed (a) in the portal vein by percutaneous transhepatic puncture (six patients) or (b) in a mesenteric vein exposed by a small midline laparotomy (two patients).

In two patients, the ICCs were placed under the capsule of a simultaneously transplanted living-related kidney allograft. Again, immunosuppression was with the same triple drug therapy. All ten patients were given adjunctive immunosuppressive treatment at the time of the xenoislet transplantation, with either rabbit antithrombocyte globulin (ATG) or 15-deoxyspergualin.

In the first six patients, the number of ICCs transplanted intraportally varied between 330 000 and 520 000. In the last two patients, the numbers of ICCs were increased to 800 000 and 1 000 020, respectively. Signs of transient portal congestion occurred in the last patient. The numbers of ICCs placed under the kidney capsule were 200 000 and 410 000, respectively. Intravenous insulin was given for 2 weeks to optimize metabolic control after transplantation.

Clinical Course After the Xenoislet Transplantation

In seven of the eight patients given an intraportal injection of the xenogeneic ICCs, clinical vital signs, portal pressure, or electrocardiogram were all unaffected. Clotting parameters and liver function tests remained undisturbed. The patient who received the largest volume of ICCs (6.1 ml tissue) had a transient increase in portal pressure and some abdominal discomfort. Kidney graft function remained stable. As a consequence of the increased steroid doses given after transplantation, blood glucose levels rose and insulin doses had to be increased in all recipients. When the dose of the immunosuppressive drugs had been tapered to maintenance levels, insulin requirements were similar to those before xenotransplantation.

Graft function was assessed by analyses of porcine C peptide in serum and urine. Porcine C peptide in serum was not detected in any of the patients and the insulin requirements were not affected by the xenotransplant. However, small amounts of porcine C peptide were excreted into the urine of four of the eight patients who had received their ICCs intraportally. The duration and magnitude of the C peptide excretions are shown in Fig. 1.

Neither of the two patients who had received the ICCs under the renal capsule showed any C peptide excretion. In one renal biopsy obtained on day 21, clusters of morphologically intact epithelial cells were identified. These cells stained positively for insulin, glucagon, and chromogranin. A moderate infiltrate consisting mainly of mononuclear cells and eosinophilic granulocytes was seen adjacent to the xenogeneic cells (Fig. 2).

Today (March 1996), 3–5 years after islet xenotransplantation, all ten patients are well with functioning renal grafts.

Development of Xenoantibodies

In all ten patients, irrespective of the immunosuppressive drugs given and whether C peptide excretion occurred, specific xenoantibodies were formed [7] (Fig. 3). Increases in the lymphocytotoxic antibody titers began after 10–14 days, with a peak reactivity occurring after 30–50 days. High titers of antibody-dependant cellular cytotoxicity (ADCC) against porcine lymphoblasts developed in all patients, and the titers remained elevated for at least 100 days. There was no increase in the titers of alloantibodies, as evidenced by a panel-reactive lymphocytotoxic antibody test. In all patients, an increase in titers of isohemagglutinins was recorded. especially against blood group B antigens.

In vitro absorption studies showed that xenoreactivity present in healthy individuals could not be blocked by absorption with human red blood cells (RBCs) [7]. However, in the transplanted patients, xenoreactivities against pig antigens were partly inhibited by absorption with human RBCs, particularly of the blood group B. These data indicate that the increase in isohemagglutinins resulted from cross-reactivity with xenogeneic antigens. Using an enzyme-linked immunosorbent assay (ELISA) assay, increased antibody titers were also present against purified pig major histocompatibility complex (MHC) class I antigens.

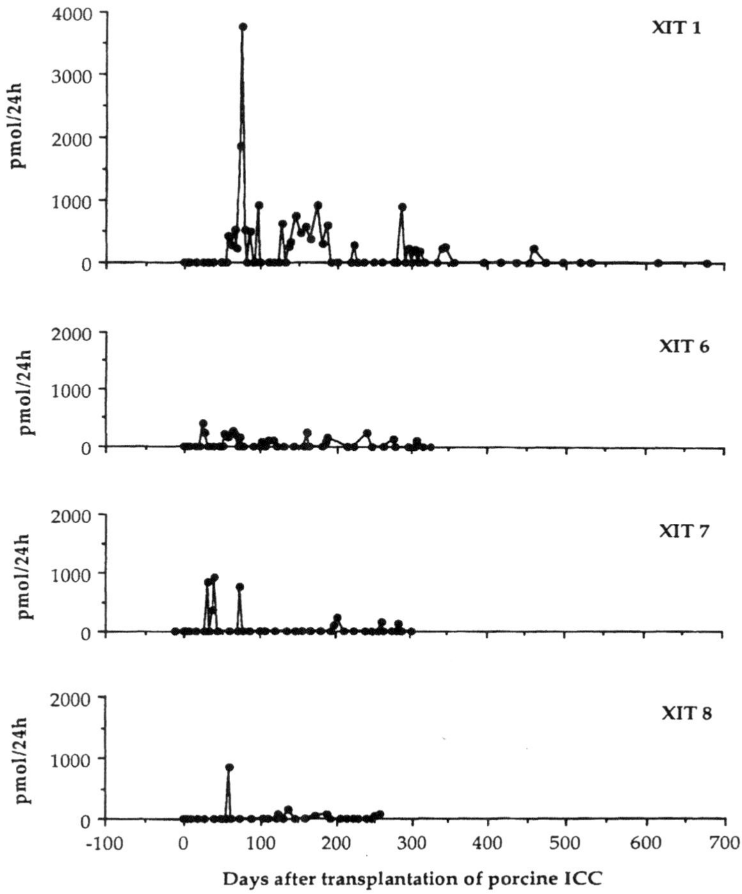

Fig. 1. Urinary excretion of porcine C peptide in four patients transplanted with fetal porcine islet-like cell clusters (*ICC*) intraportally. (Healthy individuals excrete up to 43 000 pmol C peptide per 24 h)

Titer increases were also detected against pig thyroglobulin, but not against actin, myoglobin, or haptenated bovine serum albumin (BSA) [8]. Antibody titers against tetanus toxoid were unaffected. The reactivity against porcine RBCs could be completely blocked by absorption with pig thyroglobulin. Since pig thyroglobulin contains the Galα1–3Gal antigen, the reactivity against RBCs was most probably mainly due to antibodies against this oligosaccharide epitope. These conclusions were substantiated by the finding that the antigenic determinant of the pig thyroglobulin was completely destroyed by treatment with α-galactosidase, but not with β-galactosidase. Further studies showed that immune reactivity against pig RBCs, platelets, islet cells, endothelial cells, and pig MHC class I molecules caused by xenoimmunization was almost completely blocked

Fig. 2. a Insulin- and **b** glucagon-positive cells in a biopsy specimen from a kidney allograft with fetal porcine islet-like cell clusters placed under the capsule. ×450

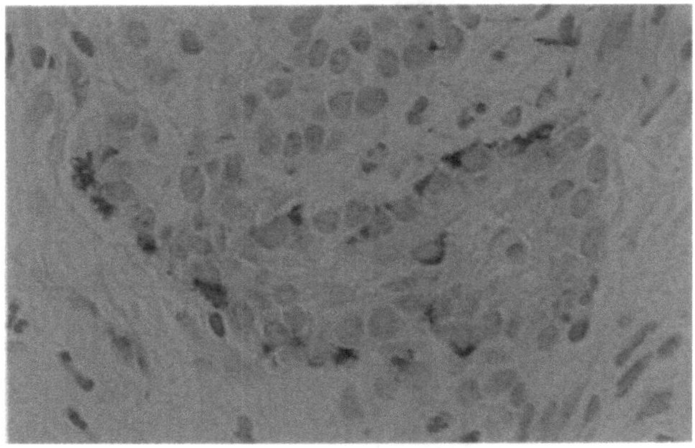

a

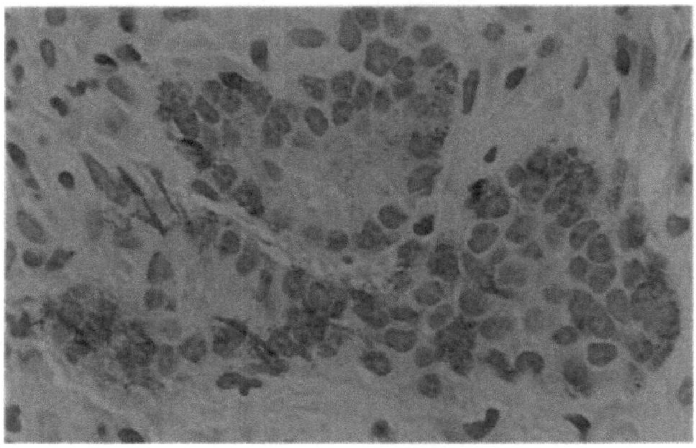

b

either by absorption of antibodies on a Sepharose column with beads coated with Galα1–3Gal or by pretreatment of the antigen with α-galactosidase [8] (Fig. 4).

Western blot experiments revealed that both the natural and xenoimmune antibodies reacted with a large number of different glycoproteins [8]. There was no difference in heterogeneity of the response when comparisons were made between pre- and post-transplantation sera, nor was there any difference in patterns caused by IgM or IgG antibodies. Absorption studies revealed that the Galα1–3Gal epitope was present in a large number of different glycoproteins, a conclusion verified by staining with the eluate from a thyroglobulin-immunoabsorbent column. No direct evidence was found of reactivity against any porcine proteins nor of specific immunization against porcine MHC peptides [8].

When glycosphingolipid antigens were prepared from various pig organs and separated on thin layer plates, both IgM and IgG antibodies in the pretransplant sera bound to several glycolipid fractions from the tri-, tetra-, and pentasaccharide regions, but also to compounds with longer carbohydrate chains [9]. In the post-transplant serum samples, stronger binding, compared to the pretransplant samples, was noted for both Ig classes. Strong binding was seen in the pentasac-

Fig. 3a,b. Kinetics of IgM (*white circles*) and IgG (*black circles*) antibody production after transplantation of porcine islet-like cell clusters in a patient. **a** Peripheral blood leukocyte (PBL) membrane components and **b** purified pig major histocompatibility complex (MHC) class I molecules served as the target antigens. *OD*, optical density

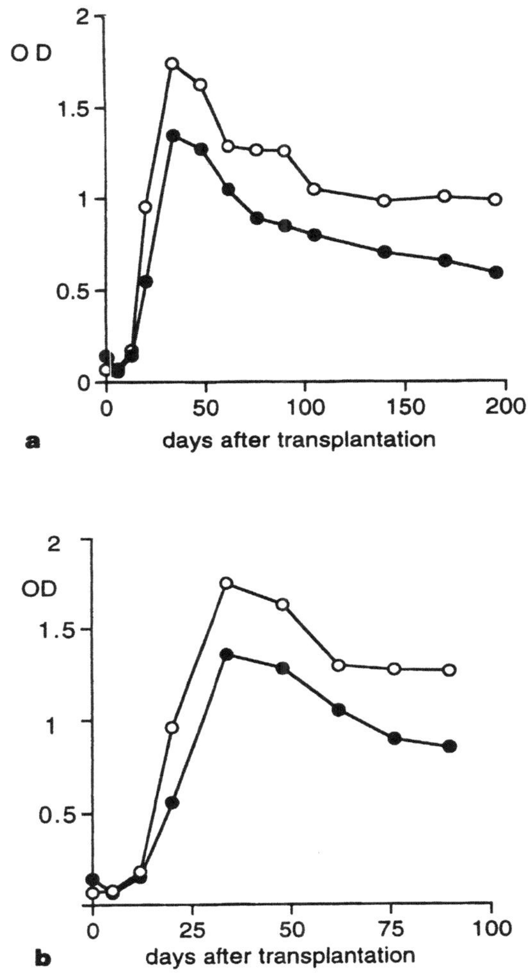

charide region known to contain the ("linear B") Galα1–3Galβ1–4GlcNAcβ1–3Galβ1–4Glcβ1–1Cer. There was no convincing evidence of the recognition of new specificities. Adsorption of patient serum to a Synsorb column with Galα1–3Gal specificity did not grossly change the binding pattern of the IgG antibodies in the effluate. However, the eluate from the column showed strong binding to the "linear B" compound but also to glycolipids with longer carbohydrate chains prepared from porcine aorta and presumably carrying the same terminal epitope, Galα1–3Gal [9].

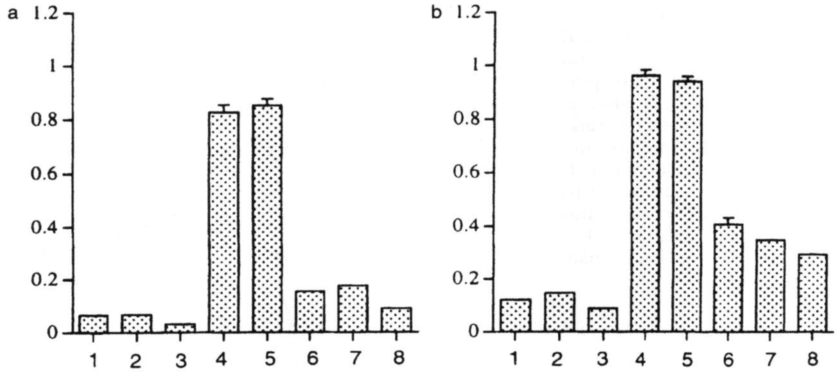

Fig. 4a,b. Xenoreactivity (IgG + IgM) measured by enzyme-linked immunosorbent assay (ELISA) and expressed as optical density (OD) in sera from a patient transplanted with porcine islet-like cell clusters. **a** Islet cells or **b** endothelial cells served as targets (see text). *Columns 1–3* represent pretransplant sera: *1*, unmodified antigen; *2*, α-galactosidase-treated antigen; *3*, Galα1,3Gal-absorbed serum, unmodified antigen. *Columns 4–8* represent post-transplant sera: *4*, unmodified antigen; *5*, β-galactosidase-treated antigen; *6*, α-galactosidase-treated antigen; *7*, Galα1,3Gal-absorbed serum, unmodified antigen; *8*, Galα1,3Gal-absorbed serum, α-galactosidase-treated antigen

Comment

Our evidence suggests that some transplanted pig ICCs remained viable for several months. Thus porcine C peptide was excreted in the urine of four of the recipients. The fact that several weeks passed before C peptide was excreted is compatible with the findings in our experimental studies [2, 3]. This delay presumably represents the time required for fetal precursor cells to mature and differentiate into insulin-producing cells.

The identification of viable insulin- and glucagon-containing cells under the kidney capsule in one of the biopsy specimens provides further evidence that the transplanted porcine cells could survive in humans. Somewhat surprisingly, there was only a moderate inflammatory reaction around the pig cells.

All patients developed a prolonged xenoantibody response against pig antigens. The antibody response was directed mainly against carbohydrate antigens on the pig cells, and seemed to detect a limited number of epitopes, with Galα1–3Gal being the major target. However, other structures may also be targets for xenoreactive antibodies. The immunization caused by the porcine cells did not initiate antibody production against new carbohydrate epitopes, but rather an increased production by the existing antibody-forming clones [10].

Our experience indicates that fetal pig islet-like cell clusters can be safely transplanted into diabetic patients, intraportally or under the kidney capsule. Following such transplantation, the porcine cells can survive for weeks or months. In human alloislet transplantation, the intraportal route has been favored by most investigators. Portal congestion, however, may occur, as happened in our patient given the largest amount of tissue. In rodents, the subcapsular renal site has been found to be effective. This site has the advantage of allowing for graft monitoring by percutaneous graft biopsies.

Thus further trials with pig-to-human islet transplantation seem justifiable. To achieve clinical benefit, however, a greater and more lasting insulin production is needed. Several measures might improve the clinical results. These include the depletion (or blocking) of the xenogeneic antibody before transplantation, and the use of other new, potent immunosuppressive drugs. Recent studies in our laboratory have shown that combination therapy with cyclosporine and 15-deoxyspergualin, mycophenolate mofetil, rapamycin or leflunomide can prevent xenoislet rejection in a pig-to-rat model [11, 12]. Other alternatives include in vitro immune modulation of the xenograft, or its immune isolation by the use of encapsulation. The use of islets from transgenic pigs expressing a human complement inhibitor might offer an advantage, and adult pig islets might provide earlier and better function. However, the problem of obtaining a sufficient number of islets of good quality from the adult pig pancreas remains to be solved.

References

1. SATAKE, M., KUMAGAI-BRAESCH, M., KORSGREN, O., ANDERSSON, A., MOLLER, E. Characterization of humoral antiporcine xenoreactivity. Clin. Transplant. 7:281, 1993
2. KORSGREN, O., SANDLER, S., SCHNELL-LANDSTROM, A., JANSSON, L., ANDERSSON, A. Large-scale production of fetal porcine pancreatic islet-like cell clusters. Transplantation. 45:509, 1988
3. KORSGREN, O, JANSSON, L., EIZIRIK, D., ANDERSSON, A. Functional and morphological differentiation of fetal porcine islet-like cell clusters after transplantation into nude mice. Diabetologia. 34:379, 1991
4. BJOERSDORFF, A., KORSGREN, O, ANDERSSON, A., et al. Microbiological screening as preparatory step for clinical xenografting of porcine fetal islet-like cell clusters. Transplant. Proc. 24:647, 1992
5. TOLLEMAR, J., GROTH, C.G., KORSGREN, O., et al. Injection of xenogeneic endocrine pancreatic tissue into the portal vein -effects on coagulation, liver function and hepatic hemodynamics. A study in the pig to rat model. Transplantation. 53:139, 1992
6. GROTH, C.G., KORSGREN, O., TIBELL, A., et al. Transplantation of porcine fetal pancreas to diabetic patients. Lancet. 344:1402, 1994
7. SATAKE, M., KAAGASHI, N., RYDBERG, L., et al. Limited specificity of xenoantibodies in diabetic patients transplanted with fetal porcine islet cell clusters. Main antibody reactivity against α-linked galactose-containing epitopes. Xenotransplantation. 1:89, 1994
8. SATAKE, M., KUMAGAI-BRAESCH, M., KAWAGISHI, N., et al. Kinetics and character of xenoantibody formation in diabetic patients transplanted with fetal porcine islet cell clusters. Xenotransplantation. 1:24, 1994
9. RYDBERG, L., CAIRNS, T.D.H., GROTH, C.G., et al. Specificities of human IgM and IgG anticarbohydrate xenoantibodies found in the sera of diabetic patients grafted with fetal pig islets. Xenotransplantation. 1:69, 1994
10. GALILI, U., TIBELL, A., SAMUELSSON, B., RYDBERG, L., GROTH, C.G. Increased anti-gal activity in diabetic patients transplanted with fetal porcine islet cell clusters. Transplantation. 59:1549, 1995

11. WENNBERG, L., WALLGREN, A.C., SUNDBERG, B., et al. Efficacy of immunosuppressive drugs in islet xenotransplantation: a study in the pig-to-rat model. Xenotransplantation. 2:222, 1995
12. WENNBERG, L., WALLGREN, A.C., RAFAEL, E., et al. Immunosuppression with leflunomide and cyclosporine prevents pig-to-rat islet xenograft rejection. Transplant. Proc. 27:3314, 1995

60 Conceptual Scientific Development of the Xenotransplantation Project in Goteborg

M.E. Breimer, L. Rydberg, S. Björck, C.T. Svalander, M. Aurell, and B.E Samuelsson

Introduction

The knowledge of blood group A_2 erythrocytes having a "weak" A antigen expression, together with the work of Ceppelini [1, 2] describing successful A_2 to O skin transplantations, were the incitements to start a clinical trial with A_2 to O human kidney transplantations [3]. The trial was successful, but at first impossible to publish in internationally well-renowned scientific journals, as reviewers were afraid of dismantling the well-known and safe selection rules of Landsteiner [4].

In 1987, two international conferences (Philadelphia, USA and Göteborg, Sweden) took place on the subject of ABO-incompatible organ transplantations. These two conferences showed beyond doubt that the blood group ABO barrier could be surpassed either by carefully selecting donor (subgroup A2) and recipient (low titers of anti-A antibodies) or by extensive immunosuppression. In editing the proceedings of the two meetings, two of us (B.E. Samuelsson, M.E. Breimer) had several stimulating discussions with Felix Rappaport, editor in chief of *Transplantation Proceedings*, discussions that were decisive for us. This was the first time we realized the conceptual similarity between ABO-incompatible human allo- and xenotransplantations, as formulated in the foreword to the proceedings of the two conferences [5]:

> "We do, however, strongly believe that with these basic, experimental and clinical studies on ABO-incompatible transplants, and the ability to delete or neutralize preformed antibodies, we have a unique opportunity to study basic biologic and immunologic phenomena in man, which ultimately will open up new vistas in the field of allo- as well as xenotransplantation"

Our studies concerning the A2 to O kidney transplants had at that time already revealed structurally new blood group ABH antigens in human kidney [6, 7], and later we also showed an individual specific distribution of these antigens in single human kidneys [8–10]. We also elucidated the humoral immune response against the incompatible A antigens, showing the fine specificity of immune antibodies [8, 9, 11, 12]. The incompatible glycosyltransferase was in these cases also shown to be immunogenic [13]. The phenomenon of accomodation in ABO-incompatible organ transplantation turned out to be a reality, since expression of A antigens in the presence of circulating antibodies was shown in some of these patients [10].

On pursuing our core line of scientific work, aiming towards an understanding of the expression of glycosphingolipid-based carbohydrate antigens in different cells, organs, and species, pig intestinal mucosa was used as a rich source for glycosyltransferases in biosynthetic experiments [14, 15]. After some time we became aware of trials in England (later published in [16, 17]), where a pig kidney was extracorporeally coupled to a human recipient after removal of plasma anti-pig xenoantibodies. The similarity between ABO-incompatible organ transplantation and xenotransplantation was the background for a turn in our research direction into the xenotransplantation field. The description of the carbohydrate antigen expression in pig kidney was the first example of this change [18].

In 1989, Ken Welsh, David Taube, and Per Gjörstrup visited our laboratory with a specific request of collaboration to define the carbohydrate antigen in pigs against which human natural anti-pig antibodies were directed. Their precise definition of the problem was based on experiences from the Dulwich "ex vivo" experiments [16, 17], in which pig kidneys had been extracorporeally connected to a volunteer dialysis patient. A collaboration was initiated and the hypothesis of sulphatides being one target xenoantigen was the first result of this collaboration [19]. The collaboration has continued [20–22].

In the summer of 1989, Holgersson in our laboratory started agglutination studies of pig red blood cells with human serum. This was initiated by the papers of Galili et al. about the Galα1–3Gal epitope expression in New World monkeys and lower vertebrate animals, but not in Old World monkeys and higher primates, and the reciprocal appearance of anti-gal antibodies along the evolutionary tree [22–26]. His results indicated that human serum contained IgM antibodies which could be absorbed on Galα1– solid phase columns and that the antibodies eluted from the column had the capacity to agglutinate pig red blood cells. Although enthusiastic at first, we were discouraged by the discovery of the glycoproteins gp115–130, which were described as the target antigens for human anti-pig antibodies [27], although a terminal galactose seemed to play a role. Furthermore, our basic biochemical education misled us to believe our red cell agglutination data to be unreliable and "soft." In spite of our awareness of Galα1– being a potential xenoepitope and the obvious presence of biochemical data, our first structural paper on glycolipids in pig kidney [18] did not contain this information. At the time of publication this was realized, but we were not permitted to add an erratum [28]. The structure of the Galα1– pentaglycosylceramide was described later both in pig kidney [21, 29] and in pig aorta [21, 22]. The excellent early data produced by Cooper et al., Oriol et al., and McKenzie et al. [30–34] strengthened our view and convinced us that carbohydrate antigens in general and the Galα1–3Gal epitope in particular were important mediators in the hyperacute rejection phenomenon.

An important contribution to our conceptual understanding of the problem of xenotransplantation was the experiments performed by Alexandre et al. showing that pig kidneys could be transplanted to monkeys [35] using the same immunosuppressive protocol as for major ABO-incompatible human allotransplantation [36].

In 1991, a collaboration was established with the transplant unit at Huddinge Hospital, Stockholm, on fetal islet-like cell transplantations to diabetic patients, with the aim to define the carbohydrate specificity of antibodies being produced after infusion of cells. The main findings in those studies are presented in Chap. 59 (this volume); they confirmed the Galα1–3Gal antigen to be of major importance in pig-to-man xenotransplantation [37].

A Human Trial

Planning

Reconsidering the Dulwich experiments (see above) [16, 17], it became obvious to us that these had to be repeated. These were two single experiments using one recipient and one donor animal. Were the conceptually very important findings of a singular or general nature? A problem in the interpretation was the extensive immunosuppression used, which would undoubtedly mask a multitude of biological events not necessarily all forseeable. We also stated that basic human experiments without interference of drugs must be performed. After almost a year of intellectual "build up," we decided to start preparing for such human experiments in 1993. Ken Welsh, David Taube, Richard Binns, and Tom Cairns generously shared their experience with us, and Ken Welsh later took part in our first trial as an observer.

Several groups were created, encompassing nephrologists, transplant surgeons, serologists, immunologists, pathologists, anesthesiologists, and others. A patient-oriented group was responsible for patient selection, information, preparation, ethical issues, etc. A pig kidney perfusion group was created with the object to study kidney physiology, perfusion characteristics, reaction with autologous blood and with human blood manipulated in several different ways. This group also took the responsibility for the experimental setup in the final human experiments and for questions about microbiology and virology. Another group established techniques for monitoring of anti-pig antibodies. At this time Gunnar Tufvesson was head of the transplant clinic and was an active member of the planning group. Experiments were set up by this group to study the removal of antibodies by plasmapheresis and immunoadsorption [38]. The effect of antibody blocking with soluble saccharides was also studied [39].

After an additional 1.5 years of preparation, we were ready to start. The ethical committee of the Medical Faculty gave us permission to perform two initial experiments. These experiments were performed in 1995 and are described briefly below and in detail elsewhere (xenotransplantation 1996 accepted).

Establishment of an In Vitro Pig Kidney Perfusion Model

The initial work was to develop an in vitro pig kidney perfusion model for xenotransplantation studies. We found it important to characterize kidney function both by physiological and histological techniques [39]. This work also trained us in all the practical details necessary for the human experiments.

Another important issue was the risk of transferring any infectious disease to the volunteer patients. Furthermore, this issue is of great importance concerning immunosuppressed organ recipients in the future. After reviewing the literature, we decided to use pigs which had been bred under a defined microbiological environment and were known to be free from a number of known bacterial, viral, and parasitic pathogens. A test operation under routine surgical conditions was performed, and the pig kidney tissue was delivered to the Department of

Microbiology for investigation. The pig had received two doses of antibiotic before the operation. The kidney tissue was investigated using all the techniques available, including inoculation into cultures of human and monkey cell lines and culture for extremely slow-growing bacterial and virus species. All these studies were negative.

Patient Selection Criteria and Pretreatment

The selection of dialysis patients was based on several important points. Except for their kidney disease, the patients had to have no other potentially serious disease and be in good condition for the experiment. He or she should be on hemodialysis using a well-functioning arteriovenous (AV) fistula and should be known to tolerate dialysis without problem. Another very important criterion was that the patient should have an intact intellectual capacity, be mentally strong and independent, and have the capability to refuse to participate in the trial. The patients were pretreated by daily plasmapheresis on days −2, −1, and 0 to remove the preformed anti-pig xenoantibodies. Some clinical data are listed in Table 1.

Extracorporeal (Ex Vivo) Perfusion of Pig Kidneys

The pig kidney was connected to the patient's AV fistula by two dialysis pumps, similar to the system used in ordinary dialysis. The perfusion pressure was controlled by the speed of the pump. Permeable membrane ports were located before and after the kidney for blood sampling. The patient was supervised by continous electrocardiographic, blood pressure, and pulse oximetry recording. A pulmonary artery catheter was used for central hemodynamic monitoring. No drugs, except for i.v. heparin, were given before or during the experiment.

Table 1. Selected clinical data of the two patients who participated in the pig kidney perfusion trial

Characteristic	Patient 1	Patient 2
Age (years)	44	47
Sex	M	M
Disease	CGN	CGN
Previous allografts (*n*)	1	0
Anti-pig lympocytotoxic titer at start of perfusion	2	1
Anti-pig red blood cell titer at start of perfusion	4	1
Kidney perfusion time (min)	65	15

CGN, chronic glomerulonephritis.

Patient 1. After an initial high blood flow for 5 min, the pump speed had to be reduced to keep a perfusion pressure of 100 mmHg. When a minimum pump flow of 30 ml/min was reached after 25 min, the perfusion pressure continously increased and the perfusion was terminated after 65 min at a pressure of 200 mmHg. Clear urine was produced by the pig kidney until the perfusion pressure rose above 100 mmHg, which resulted in hematuria. The patient revealed no subjective discomfort, and no changes in objective clinical monitoring parameters were observed. ^{51}Cr clearance studies revealed the kidney to be nonfunctioning at the end of the experiment. A slight fall in platelet count was seen, while the hemoglobin and leukocyte counts were not affected. Light microscopy examination of the kidney revealed a picture of a delayed hyperacute rejection.

A few weeks after perfusion, the humoral immune response of patient 1 showed a strongly increased reactivity against pig cells. Immunochemical analysis of pre- (before apheresis treatment) and postperfusion serum samples is shown in Fig. 1. Strong increases of binding to the pig kidney and to rabbit small intestine are seen in the postperfusion serum sample. Rabbit tissues are known to express large amounts of Galα1–3Gal determinants.

Patient 2. The blood flow was initially about 170 ml/min at a perfusion pressure of 100 mmHg, and increased thereafter during the first few minutes and remained stable at 200 ml/min. Clear urine, which became increasingly yellow, was produced. At 14 min the patient did not feel well, developed chest and abdominal pain, and vomited and the blood pressure started to decline. The perfusion was terminated. Transient electrocardiographic signs of myocardial ischemia appeared. The patient was transferred to the intensive care unit and recovered quickly. No laboratory or electrocardiographic signs of myocardial tissue damage were found, and his physical and mental status is now identical to that prior to the experiment. ^{51}Cr clearance studies revealed an increase in clearance value to about 12 ml/min at the end of the experiment. A considerable consumption of platelets was noted as measured in blood samples taken before and after perfusion of the pig kidney. Light microscopy examination showed very minor structural changes compared to the contralateral reference kidney of the same donor pig.

Comment

The results of the first two ex vivo perfusions indicated:

1. The importance of removing anti-pig antibodies to a sufficiently low level
2. The possibility of other carbohydrate antigens, besides Galα1–3Gal, being important for the acute/chronic rejection (data to be published)
3. The phenomenon of platelet trapping/destruction as a non-antibody-mediated xenoreaction between pig endothelial cells and human platelets

To explore these issues, experiments at basic cell biological and biochemical levels are needed. We are pursuing the issue of platelet interaction with pig endothelial cells. We are also investigating additional target antigens in pigs and other animals.

A perfusion medium which does not contain any biologically active compounds (based on a buffer solution, colloids and oxygen transporter) for

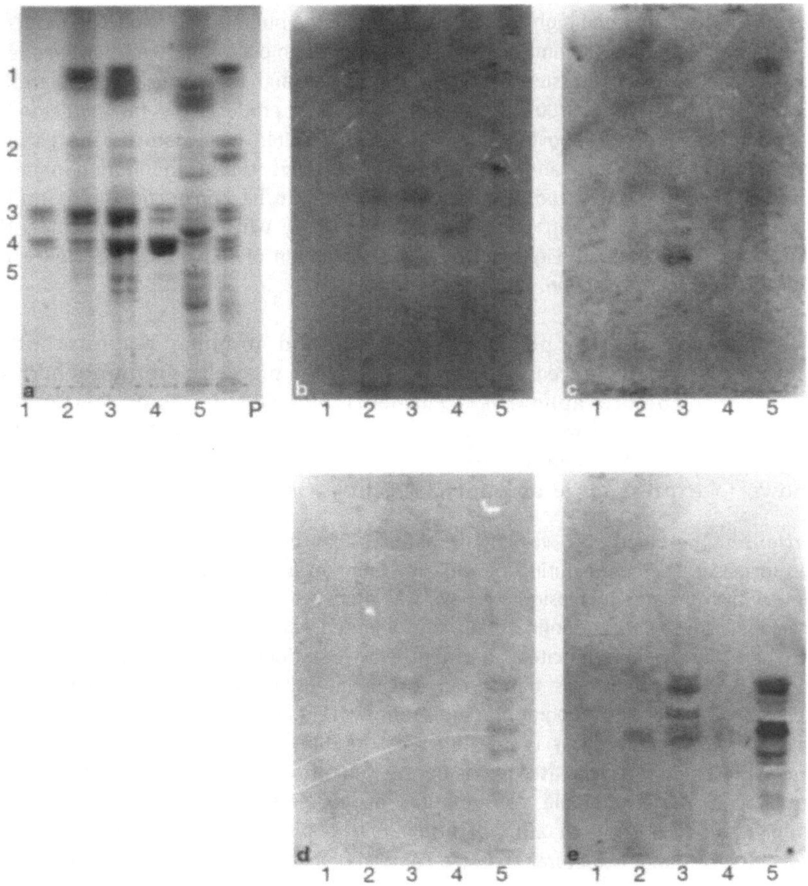

Fig. 1. a Thin-layer plate with a chemical (anisaldehyde) staining. *Lane P*, total neutral glycolipids from human A1 Le(a-b+) plasma. The figures to the *left* indicate the approximate number of sugars in each band. Binding of **b,c** IgM antibodies and **d,e** IgG antibodies. Chromatogram binding assays obtained **b,d** before apheresis and **c,e** 5 weeks after the perfusion experiment, showing binding of serum to glycolipid antigens from different pig organs and rabbit small intestine. The amount of each glycolipid applied was 20 µg. Serum samples were used in a 1:20 dilution. *Lane 1*, total neutral glycolipids from pig aorta; *lane 2*, total neutral glycolipids from pig serum; *lane 3*, total neutral glycolipids from pig kidney; *lane 4*, total neutral glycolipids from pig erythrocytes; *lane 5*, total neutral glycolipids from rabbit small intestine

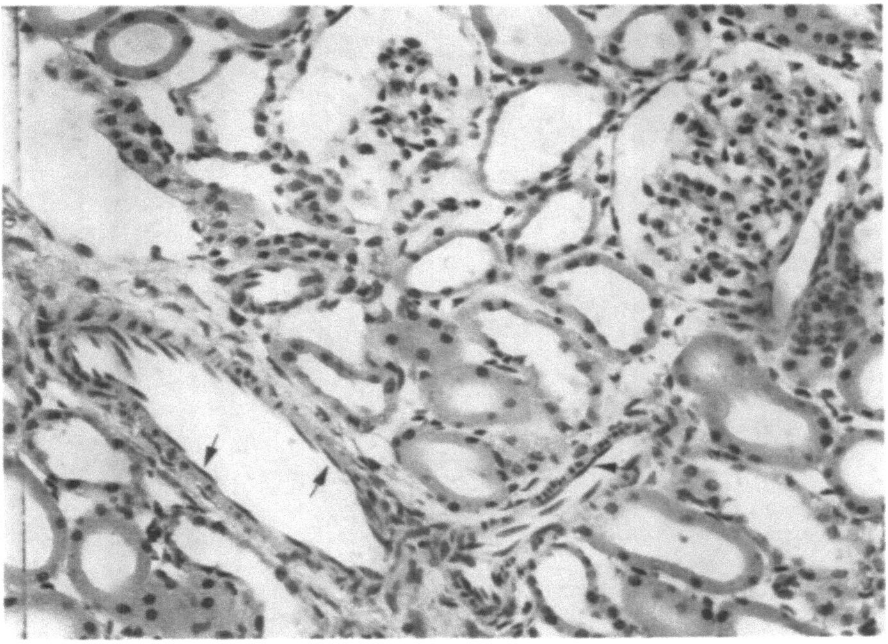

Fig. 2. Light micrograph of a pig kidney perfused for 55 min at 37 °C with a perfusion medium consisting of Tyrodes solution, bovine serum albumin, orosomucoid, urea, and human erythrocytes. The kidney was flushed with Euro-Collins solution after the perfusion. Very little structural damage to the tissue is seen. The nuclei of the endothelial cells are present in the intima of both the interlobular artery and the arteriole (*arrows*), indicating that the cells are intact. The glomeruli, peritubular capillaries, and the tubular epithelium are also well preserved. H&E; original magnification, ×350

short-term kidney perfusion is under development (Figs. 2, 3). Various reagents, such as mono-/polyclonal antibodies, platelets, and leukocytes (and combinations of these), could be added to this medium, and their interaction with the vascular endothelium studied. Additional extracorporeal ex vivo human perfusion experiments with pig kidneys are planned with the purpose to elucidate (a) the effect of solid-phase adsorption with synthetic carbohydrates, (b) the effects of different types of drugs on the immune response, and (c) the stability of platelets. An obvious continuation of the human trials would be to use pig strains transgenic with respect to human complement inhibitory proteins [40].

Acknowledgement. Financial support was provided by the Swedish Medical Research Council (project No. 6521 and 11612), the IngaBritt and Arne Lundberg Foundation for Medical Research, and the L.-E. Gelin Memorial Foundation.

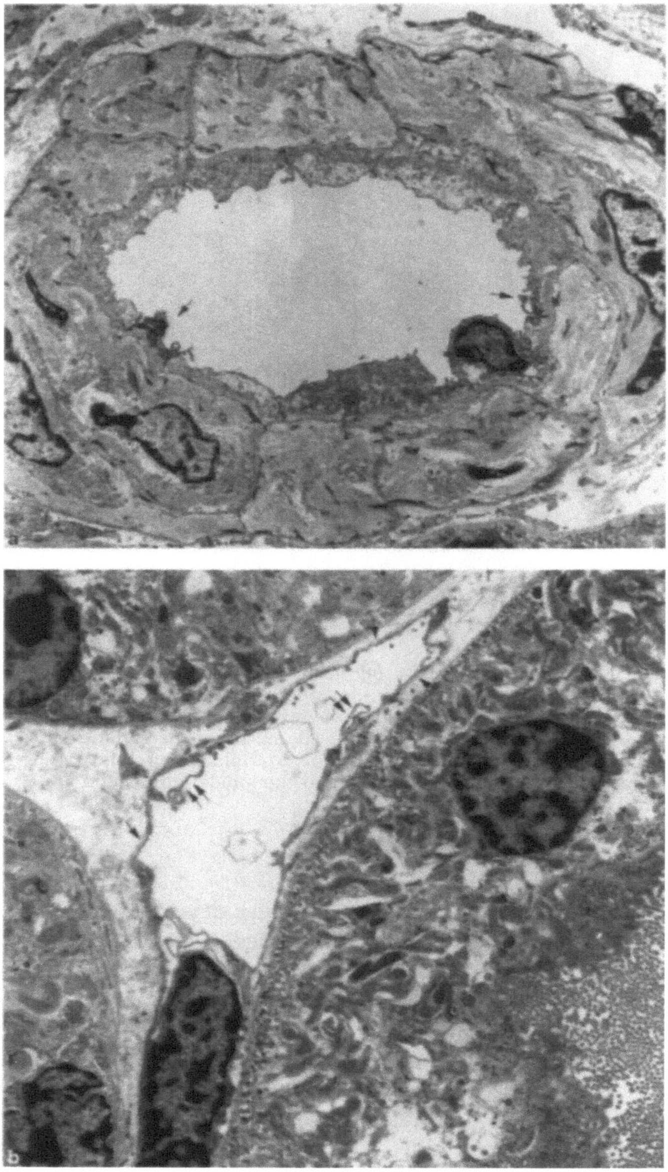

Fig. 3a,b. Electron micrograph of the same kidney as described in Fig. 2. **a** A small arteriole showing intact endothelium but with damage to individual endothelial cells (*arrows*). Several of the remaining endothelial cells show vacuoles, indicating cell damage. ×4450. **b** Peritubular capillary with an endothelial cell nucleus (*lower*). An intact cell basement membrane extends around the capillary (*single arrows*). Signs of activation/damage with projections of the endothelial cell membrane are seen in some areas (*double arrows*). Note the intact brush border of the proximal tubule epithelium at the *lower right*. OsO_4 fixative, contrasted with uranyl and lead. Original magnification, ×5750

References

1. Visetti, M., Leigheb, G., Scudeller, G., Ceppellini, R. (1967) Importanza dei sottogruppi A1-A2e delle reazioni crociate A-B per la sporavvivenza di alloinnesti di cute. Minerva Dermatologica. 42, 563
2. Ceppellini, R., Bigliani, S., Curtoni, E.S., Leigheb, G. (1969) Experimental allotransplantation in man: II. The role of A1, A2 and B antigens; III. Enhancement by circulation antibody. Transplant. Proc. 1, 390
3. Brynger, H., Rydberg, L., Samuelsson, B.E., Sandberg, L. (1984) Experience with 14 renal transplants with kidneys from blood group A (subgroup A2) to O recipients. Transplant. Proc. 16, 1175
4. Landsteiner, K. (1945) The Specificity of Serological Reactions, Harvard University Press, Cambridge, p. 1
5. Bannet, A.D., McAlack, R.F., Brynger, H., Breimer, M.E., Samuelsson, B.E. (1987) Foreword Transplant. Proc. 19, 4397
6. Jovall, P.Å., Breimer, M.E. (1985) Structural characterization of a blood group A heptaglycosylceramide with globo-series structure. The major glycolipid based blood group A antigen of human kidney. FEBS Lett. 179, 165
7. Holgersson, J., Jovall, P.-Å., Samuelsson, B.E., Breimer, M.E. (1991) Blood group type glycosphingolipids of human kidneys. Glyconconj. J. 8, 424
8. Rydberg, L., Breimer, M.E., Samuelsson, B.E., Brynger, H. (1987) Blood group ABO-incompatible (A2-O) kidney transplantation in humans: a clinical, serological and biochemical approach. Transplant. Proc. 19, 4528
9. Breimer, M.E., Brynger, H., Le Pendu, J., et al. (1987) Blood group ABO incompatible kidney transplantation. Biochemical and immunochemical studies of blood group A glycolipid antigens in human kidney and characterization of the antibody response (antigen specificity and antibody class) in O recipients receiving A2 grafts. Transplant. Proc. 19, 226
10. Ulfvin, A., Bäcker, A.E., Clausen, H., et al. (1993) Expression of glycolipid blood group antigens in single human kidneys. Change in antigen expression of rejected ABO incompatible kidney grafts. Kid. Int. 44, 1289
11. Rydberg, L., Breimer, M.E., Holgersson, J., et al. (1992) Characterization of the anti-A antibody response following an ABO incompatible (A2 to O) kidney transplantation. Mol. Immunol. 29, 547
12. Rydberg, L., Breimer, M.E., Brynger, H., Samuelsson, B.E. (1990) ABO incompatible kidney transplantation (A2 to O): qualitative and semiquantative studies on the humoral immune response against different blood group A antigens. Transplantation. 49, 954
13. Rydberg, L., Samuelsson, B.E. (1991) Presence of glycosyltransferase inhibitors in the sera of patients with long-term surviving ABO incompatible (A2 to O) kidney grafter. Transfusion Med. 1, 177
14. Samuelsson, B.E. (1987) Glycosyltransferase assay – solid-phase biosynthesis on high performance thin-layer plates of blood group glycosphingolipids III. Methods Enzymol. 138, 567
15. Samuelsson, B.E. (1984) Solid-phase biosynthesis on high performance thin-layer plates of blood group glycosphingolipids II. FEBS Lett. 167, 47

16. Welsh, K.I., Taube, D.H., Thick, M., et al. Human antibodies to pig determinants and their association with hyperacute rejection of xenografts. In: Xenotransplantation. (eds. Cooper, D.K.C., Kemp, E., Reemtsma, K., White, D.J.G.) Springer, Berlin, 1991, p. 501
17. Cairns, T.D., Taube, D.H., Stevens, N., Binns, R., Welsh, K.I. (1991) Xenografts - future prospects for clinical transplantation. Immunol. Lett. 29, 167
18. Holgersson, J., Jovall, P.-Å., Samuelsson, B.E., Breimer, M.E. (1990) Structural characterization of non-acid glycosphingolipids in kidneys of single blood group O and A pigs. J. Biochem. (Tokyo). 108, 766
19. Holgersson, J., Cairns, T.D.H., Karlsson, E.C., et al. (1992) Carbohydrate specificity of human IgM antibodies with pig lymphocytotoxic activity. Transplant. Proc. 24, 605
20. Cairns, T., Karlsson, E., Holgersson, J., et al. (1994) Confirmation of a major target epitope of human natural IgG and IgM anti-pig antibodies: terminal galactose alpha1,3-galactose. Transplant. Proc. 26, 1384
21. Samuelsson, B.E., Rydberg, L., Breimer, M.E., et al. (1994) Natural antibodies and human xenotransplantation. Immunol. Rev. 141, 151
22. Karlsson, E., Cairns, T., Holgersson, J., Welsh, K., Samuelsson, B.E. (1993) Pig to human xenotransplantation. Confirmation of the major target epitope of preformed human natural IgG and IgM anti-pig-terminal galactoseα1–3galactose. Glyconconj. J. 10, 297
23. Galili, U., Macher, B.A., Buehler, J., Shohet, S.B. (1985) Human natural anti-alpha-galactosyl IgG. II. The specific recognition of alpha(1–3)-linked galactose residues. J. Exp. Med. 162, 573
24. Galili, U., Basbaum, C.B., Shohet, S.B., Buehler, J., Macher, B.A. (1987) Identification of erythrocyte Galα1–3Gal glycosphingolipids with a mouse monoclonal antibody, Gal-13. J. Biol. Chem. 262, 4683
25. Galili, U., Buehler, J., Shohet, S.B., Macher, B.A. (1987) The human natural anti-Gal IgG. III. The subtelty of immune tolerance in man as demonstrated by crossreactivity between natural anti-Gal and anti-B antibodies. J. Exp. Med. 165, 693
26. Galili, U., Shohet, S.B., Kobrin, E., Stults, C.L., Macher, B.A. (1988) Man, apes and Old World monkeys differ from other mammals in the expression of alpha-galactosyl epitopes on nucleated cells. J. Biol. Chem. 263, 17755
27. Platt, J.L., Lindman, B.J., Chen, H., Spitalnik, S.L., Bach, F.H. (1990) Endothelial cell antigens recognized by xenoreactive human natural antibodies. Transplantation. 50, 817
28. Holgersson, J. Blood group ABH and related glycosphingolipid antigens. (1991) Ph.D. Thesis. University of Göteborg, Sweden
29. Jalali-Araghi, K., Macher, B.A. (1994) Characterization of porcine kidney neutral glycosphingolipids: identification of a carbohydrate antigen recognized by human natural antibodies. Glycoconj. J. 11, 266
30. Good, A.H., Cooper, D.K.C., Malcolm, A.J., et al. (1992) Identification of carbohydrate structures which bind human anti-porcine antibodies: implications for discordant grafting in man. Transplant. Proc. 24, 559
31. Sandrin, M.S., Vaughan, H.A., Dabowski, P.L., McKenzie, I.F.C. (1993) Anti-pig IgM antibodies in human serum react predominantly with Galα1–3Gal epitopes. Proc. Natl. Acad. Sci. USA. 90, 11391
32. Koren, E., Kujundzic, M., Koscec, M., et al. (1994) Cytotoxic effects of human preformed anti-Gal IgG and complement on cultured pig cells. Transplant. Proc. 26, 1336

33. Cooper, D.K.C., Good, A.H., Ye, Y., et al. (1993) Specific intravenous carbohydrate therapy - a new approach to the inhibition of antibody-mediated rejection following ABO-incompatible allografting and discordant xenografting. Transplant. Proc. 25, 377
34. Oriol, R., Ye, Y., Koren, E., Cooper, D.K.C. (1993) Carbohydrate antigens of pig tissues reacting with human natural antibodies as potential targets for hyperacute vascular rejection in pig-to-man organ transplantation. Transplantation. 56, 1433
35. Alexandre, G.P.J., Gianello, P., Latinne, D., et al. (1989) Plasmapheresis and splenectomy in experimental renal xenotransplantation. In: Xenograft 25. (M.A. Hardy, ed.), Elsevier, Amsterdam, p. 259
36. Alexandre, G.P.J., Squifflet, J.P., De Bruyère, M., et al. (1987) Present experiences in a series of 26 ABO-incompatible living donor renal allografts. Transplant. Proc. 19, 4538
37. Rydberg, L., Cairns,T.D.H., Groth, C.-G., et al. (1994) Specificities of human IgM and IgG anti-carbohydrate antibodies in diabetic patients grafted with pig fetal islets. Xenotransplantation. 1, 69
38. Rydberg, L., Hallberg, E., Björck, S., Magnusson, S., Samuelsson, B.E., Breimer, M.E. (1995) Studies on the removal of anti-pig antibodies in the human by plasmapheresis/immunoadsorption. Xenotransplantation. 2, 253
39. Breimer, M.E., Svalander, C.T., Haraldsson, B., Björck, S. (1996) Physiological characterization of a pig kidney in vitro perfusion model and studies of the effects of ANP (atrial natriuretic peptide) on the kidney function. Scand. J. Urol. Nephrol. 30, 213
40. Rosengard, A.M., Cary, N.R.B., Langford, G.A., et al. (1995) Tissue expression of human complement inhibitor, decay-accelerating factor, in transgenic pigs. Transplantation. 59, 1325

Subject Index

D

E

MIX
Papier aus verantwortungsvollen Quellen
Paper from responsible sources
FSC® C105338

If you have any concerns about our products,
you can contact us on
ProductSafety@springernature.com

In case Publisher is established outside the EU,
the EU authorized representative is:
Springer Nature Customer Service Center GmbH
Europaplatz 3, 69115 Heidelberg, Germany

Printed by Libri Plureos GmbH
in Hamburg, Germany